NUTRITION AND HEALTH

Adrianne Bendich, Ph.D., FACN, FASN,
Connie W. Bales, Ph.D., R.D., SERIES EDITORS

The Nutrition and Health series has an overriding mission in providing health professionals with texts that are considered essential since each is edited by the leading researchers in their respective fields. Each volume includes: (1) a synthesis of the state of the science, (2) timely, in-depth reviews, (3) extensive, up-to-date fully annotated reference lists, (4) a detailed index, (5) relevant tables and figures, (6) identification of paradigm shifts and consequences, (7) virtually no overlap of information between chapters, but targeted, inter-chapter referrals, (8) suggestions of areas for future research and (9) balanced, data driven answers to patient/health professionals questions which are based upon the totality of evidence rather than the findings of a single study.

Nutrition and Health is a major resource of relevant, clinically based nutrition volumes for the professional that serve as a reliable source of data-driven reviews and practice guidelines.

More information about this series at http://www.springer.com/series/7659

Saskia de Pee · Douglas Taren · Martin W. Bloem
Editors

Nutrition and Health in a Developing World

Third Edition

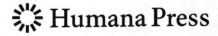 Humana Press

Editors
Saskia de Pee
Nutrition Division
World Food Programme
Rome
Italy

and

Friedman School of Nutrition Science and Policy
Tufts University
Boston, MA
USA

Douglas Taren
Mel and Enid Zuckerman College of Public Health
University of Arizona
Tucson, AZ
USA

Martin W. Bloem
Nutrition Division
World Food Programme
Rome
Italy

and

Department of International Health, Bloomberg
    School of Public Health
Johns Hopkins University
Baltimore, MD
USA

and

Friedman School of Nutrition Science and Policy
Tufts University
Boston, MA
USA

Nutrition and Health
ISBN 978-3-319-82898-5   ISBN 978-3-319-43739-2   (eBook)
DOI 10.1007/978-3-319-43739-2

Printed on acid-free paper

This Humana Press imprint is published by Springer Nature
The registered company is Springer International Publishing AG
The registered company address is: Gewerbestrasse 11, 6330 Cham, Switzerland

To our parents, who pursued a better life for the next generation: Leendert de Pee and Rijnie de Pee-Klaver, who encouraged their children to pursue a higher education than they had been able to enjoy and take great interest in the learnings of their children and grandchildren; Sid and Elizabeth Taren who expounded the value of helping others and propelled their children to be first generation children to attend college and obtain advanced degrees, and Jacqueline Bloem and the late Alexander Bloem, Dutch Indonesians and survivors of the Sumatra railway "work camp," the Kramat camp, and the sinking of the Yunyo Maru *by the British submarine* HMS Tradewind *off the west coast of Sumatra.*

Foreword

The challenges we face as a global community demand sophisticated responses against a backdrop of unrivalled complexity. The sheer scale and speed of change—cultural, political, social and technological—means we must constantly reassess old certainties in the light of new developments.

That is the environment against which we must achieve the Sustainable Development Goals, adopted by the United Nations in September 2015 as a call to action to end poverty, protect the planet and ensure food security and good nutrition for all.

Our collective efforts to achieve the Agenda 2030 goals—including number two, achieving Zero Hunger—require responses that take account of the trends currently reshaping society and shrinking the world, such as climate change, migration, urbanization and rising economic inequality.

Globalization has dispelled the illusion that these challenges are separate and geographically confined. Instead, we have come to learn that they are interconnected and common to us all. These interdependent relationships have profound implications: never before have health and nutrition professionals been called upon to respond to issues of such complexity and find new solutions to them.

For the third edition, the book has been retitled *Nutrition and Health in a Developing World*, to reflect this rapidly changing landscape and to acknowledge that it is not just low- and middle-income countries that must face these challenges. Twenty new chapters have been included, while some topics from the second edition have been contributed by new authors and other chapters have been updated. Chapters such as Developing Capacity in Nutrition and Ending AIDS by 2030: Partnerships and Linkages with SDG 2 analyze the implications of the complex shifts for specialists working in the field.

The drive to eradicate hunger and achieve food security for all illustrates this phenomenon. Consider why 3 million children under the age of five still die each year from causes attributable to malnutrition. Poverty, of course, but a variety of other factors also contribute to food insecurity, ranging from conflict and political instability, to lack of educational opportunity and gender discrimination. All of these issues represent hugely complex structural challenges which require a multidisciplinary response, underpinned by a clear understanding of their causalities and the interplay between them.

An effective and coordinated response also requires professionals to combine scientific knowledge with relevant social, cultural, and ethical insights to ensure that activities are tailored appropriately. It is not enough to have a strong grasp of the latest nutritional research findings, it must come with a solid understanding of the context in which they are applied. Local circumstances are just as important as global trends.

In relation to food assistance programs, for example, it means providing foods that contain the right nutrients, but which are also a familiar part of the everyday diet of the people we serve. I remember meeting a Syrian baker in the Zaatari refugee camp in Jordan, who complained to me because the bread we were handing out was made to a Jordanian rather than a Syrian recipe. The next day we changed the recipe to one that he provided. This broader cultural and social awareness can make a critical difference to the success or failure of an initiative.

The third edition of this book will make a valuable contribution towards ensuring that the next generation of specialists are equipped with the practical and theoretical tools necessary to deliver effective nutrition and public health policies and programs. This integrated forward looking focus is credit to the combination of practical and academic experience of the editors, which includes for Saskia de Pee and Martin W. Bloem already more than 10 years of working with the World Food Programme while also continuing to be involved in research and academic training and for Douglas Taren more than 25 years in academic research and undergraduate and graduate education programs in public health and medicine.

Well-trained young professionals, grounded in a multidisciplinary approach, are vital if we are to achieve the 17 SDGs by 2030—and realize the vision of the United Nations of a world free from hunger and poverty for all.

Rome, Italy   Ertharin Cousin

Preface

In September 2015, the General Assembly of the United Nations adopted the Sustainable Development Goals (SDGs). This was the first time that the UN had developed a set of Global Goals and not a series of goals only for low- and middle-income countries (LMICs) in contrast with the Millennium Development Goals (MDGs). The first two editions of this textbook, published in 2001 and 2008, were produced against the background of the MDGs and this was reflected in the title: *Nutrition and Health in Developing Countries*. In the 1990s, most development concepts and ideas were still based on a philosophy that problems in certain parts of the world were independent of the rest of the world. Despite the title, Semba and Bloem already embraced the complexity of the world of public health and nutrition, but the SDGs urged us to expand the scope of this third edition to the world as it is developing today, and include various new chapters and not include a revised version of some of the chapters of the second edition.

Climate change, pollution, hunger, food systems, Ebola and Zika viruses, etc., have taught us that the world is interconnected and interdependent. The security problems in the world, e.g., Syria and South Sudan, do not only lead to destroyed cities, infrastructure, high number of deaths, food insecurity etc., but also to increased migration of millions of people to Europe and other countries. What does this mean for public health specialists?

Students in the field of public health, nutrition, development practice, and related fields can no longer be trained and educated only in domestic or local problems whether they live in the US, Europe, Africa, Latin America, or Asia. For example, the influx of many immigrants have changed the morbidity 'landscape' in US and Europe, e.g. tuberculosis. The Zika virus epidemic shows that frequent travel of migrants from their home countries in Latin America contributes to the spread of the virus and complicates the management of the epidemic. The Ebola crisis of 2014/15 in West Africa led to global travel restrictions, which were impossible to control and maintain.

The evolving complexity and interconnectedness of our world requires a different approach of public health. In this edition we have therefore included a variety of topics which are related with public health but are often on their own the center of multiple other related areas, such as urbanization, supermarkets and food value chains. We realize that we can never be complete and fully comprehensive but are hoping that *Nutrition and Health in a Developing World* can help the next generation of public health and nutrition specialists to be trained in such a way that they will be able to contribute sound and in-depth knowledge of specific areas in health and nutrition while approaching problems in a multidisciplinary way through collaborating with other fields.

While the focus of public health is on populations, public health practitioners need to understand the etiology, treatment and political and social implications of health and nutrition problems in several domains, e.g., individual, household and community level, as well as at a systems level. Scientific progress, economic growth as well as various communication platforms in each domain influence what could be appropriate strategies for addressing the problem. For example, treatment availability and accessibility has enormous consequences for how individuals and communities are responding to public health threats. In the case of the Ebola epidemic in West Africa in 2014/15, for which no treatment or vaccine was available, including a medical anthropologist on the team for containing the outbreak turned out to be essential. The infected and affected populations had started to distrust the health facilities since the disease also spread from there. Good understanding of the communities through anthropological assessments eventually enabled gaining control of the epidemic. Another example is perception of overweight and obesity by different populations in the world. In the past two decades, obesity has become a problem of lower socioeconomic strata in high-income countries but is still a problem of the middle-class in low-income countries. Perceptions are, however, changing and having a healthy lifestyle and not being overweight increasingly becomes the goal among more affluent populations in low- and middle-income countries. Historical perspective is also an important tool of the public health practitioner.

The major drivers of public health and nutrition problems in the next 15 years are (i) the implications of climate change, (ii) increase of inequity in the world, (iii) political instability between and within states, (iv) migration, (v) urbanization, and (vi) challenges to achieving sustainable food systems. We will observe both an increase of non-communicable diseases and infectious diseases and in the field of nutrition, undernutrition will remain a problem while the obesity epidemic will continue, increasing the double burden of malnutrition in many low- and middle-income countries. We have never seen such a complexity of health and nutritional problems in the world, and we have to propose, pilot, and find new solutions.

Nutrition and Health in a Developing World, Third Edition, starts with a historical overview of nutrition by Richard Semba. We have recognized that many students in public health and international nutrition are overwhelmed by the magnitude of the problems of undernutrition, infectious diseases, and poor infrastructure in LMICs. It is, however, not enough appreciated that the prevalence and etiology of nutritional deficiencies, including stunting, as well as of infectious diseases, including tuberculosis, in the early 20th Century in Europe and the US were very similar.

We can still learn many lessons from the past but too often we are reinventing the wheel. An interesting example of Semba's chapter is how the ideas on the role of amino acids/proteins in malnutrition have changed in the past 50 years. In the late 1960s and early 1970s, there was a lot of interest in protein deficiency as one of the key determinants of undernutrition. Based on this interest, researchers from the Americas designed one of the most important studies in the nutrition field: The Institute of Nutrition of Central America and Panama's (INCAP) 1969–1977 nutritional supplementation trial. Four rural villages from eastern Guatemala were randomly selected to receive either a high-protein supplement (Atole) or an alternative supplement devoid of protein (Fresco) [1]. During the implementation of this study, the Lancet published an editorial in 1974, entitled "The protein fiasco" [2] which argued that when energy intake would be adequate, so would protein intake, and as a result, the UN stopped focusing on proteins and changed the focus to calories, which meant staple food in agricultural terms. The nutritionists changed their attention to micronutrients, particularly vitamin A, iron, iodine and zinc, including ourselves. The impact of the Guatemala trial was, however, quite impressive and has been extensively published. The long-term impact of "Atole", as assessed among adults who had participated in the study during their early childhood, was not only a better nutritional and health status but it also had positive economic implications [3], and many of the recommendations made by the 2008 and 2013 Lancet nutrition series were based on the long-term results observed from the INCAP supplementation trial. This did not yet lead, however, to a renewed interest in proteins. In 2016, Semba and co-workers published a number of papers on the associations between stunting and lower levels of circulating amino acids, which is most probably the beginning of a renewed focus and interest on the role of amino acids, and protein quality, in malnutrition.

The second part—Contextualizing international nutrition—considering benefit-cost, evidence-base and capacity, consist of three chapters: Economics of Nutritional Interventions by Sue Horton;

Nutrition Evidence in Context by Saskia De Pee and Rebecca Grais; and Developing Capacity in Nutrition by Jessica Fanzo and Matt Graziose.

Since 2014, the International Food Policy Research Institute (IFPRI) has published the Global Nutrition Report (GNR), a new annual publication that started as a result of the Nutrition for Growth meeting in London in 2012. The GNR has shown that malnutrition in all its forms is a public health problem in almost all countries of the world. The 2015 GNR showed that the field has made progress but there is still a great need for more funding if the world intends to reach the nutrition goal of SDG2. Horton in her chapter argues that analysis of the economic costs of undernutrition can be used to advocate for more resources for nutrition investments, and to prioritize cost-effective programming.

Over the past two decades, more and more attention is given to evidence-based programs. While evidence-based programming is important, De Pee and Grais explain that for interventions that aim to change dietary intake using foods the evidence-based medical paradigm has several limitations. Their chapter is exemplary for the philosophy of *Nutrition and Health in a Developing World*. They argue that the choice of interventions should be guided by situation analysis of the most likely causes of the specific nutrition problems among different subgroups of the population, and a good understanding of what can be delivered and accepted by the target population. They recommend that researchers should use various designs to collect evidence on implementation and impact, with particular emphasis on characterizing and assessing the role of context, both for choice of interventions and for assessing their contribution to addressing malnutrition.

Since the increase of interest in nutrition in the world, various global nutrition experts were concerned about the lack of capacity and availability of trained professionals in nutrition at all levels. In 2014, we organized a workshop to discuss this topic in the context of the changing world in preparation for the SDGs. The chapter by Fanzo and Graziose reflects many of the discussions we had at this workshop. Capacity development will remain a critical feature of nutrition and development agendas in the coming decades and *Nutrition and Health in a Developing World* is an important contribution to achieving this goal.

The third part—Malnutrition, nutrients and (breast)milk explained—consists of 12 chapters: Malnutrition spectrum by Douglas Taren and Saskia de Pee; Child Growth and Development by Mercedes De Onis; Overweight and Obesity by Colleen Doak and Barry Popkin; Nutrient Needs and Approaches to meeting them by Saskia de Pee; Vitamin A by Amanda C Palmer, Ian Darnton-Hill and Keith P West, Jr; Iron by Melissa Young and Usha Ramakrishnan; Zinc by Sonja K. Hess; Iodine by Michael Zimmermann; Vitamin D by John M. Pettifor and Kebashni Thandrayen; Essential Fatty Acids by Ettie Granot and Richard Deckelbaum; Role of Milk in Nutrition by Benedikte Grenov, Henrik Friis, Christian Mølgaard and Kim F Michaelsen; The role of Breastfeeding in a developing world by Douglas Taren and Chessa Lutter.

As previously mentioned, the second Sustainable Development Goal includes nutrition and it is recognized that nutrition should be tackled through many different platforms. The Scaling up Nutrition (SUN) Movement, Committee of Food Security (CFS) and the International Congress of Nutrition (ICN2) are specific platforms of nutrition but there are other platforms, which are critical for sustainable progress in nutrition, e.g., on climate change, every woman every child, HIV AIDS, etc. To understand the importance of the strategies, which focus on the underlying and basic causes of malnutrition, analysis of the direct causes of the various forms of malnutrition is critical. This part of twelve chapters deals with the different forms of malnutrition and discusses specific nutrients and their deficiencies, i.e., one of the two direct causes of malnutrition.

Taren and de Pee describe the spectrum of malnutrition, ranging from undernutrition to overweight and obesity and at the level of individual nutrients from deficiencies to toxicity, and describe indicators of different aspects of nutritional status and their use at individual as well as population level. De Onis discusses child growth and reviews many concepts including indicators, growth standards, the magnitude and geographical distribution of suboptimal growth, its short- and long-term consequences, and interventions aimed at promoting healthy growth and development. In 2012, the World

Health Assembly (WHA) adopted global nutrition targets to measure progress at the country level, using many growth indicators, i.e., stunting, wasting, and overweight in children under age 5; low birth weight; and in addition anemia in women of reproductive age; and exclusive breastfeeding.

Doak and Popkin describe recent trends in obesity. An important observation is that there is a shift in low- and middle-income countries from the urban elite to the middle and lower classes. Particularly interesting is that they show that obesity trends are similar in urban and rural areas, and that more research is needed to understand these various trends in overweight and obesity. Simple conclusions that dietary patterns are changing to a more Western type diet are not anymore enough. Global trends are critical but context analysis is as critical. Most probably, the underlying causes of the obesity epidemic in the Middle East are not the same as in the US, for example. Doak and Popkin conclude therefore that the policies and programs that contribute to and may alter these patterns may be best understood by examining the situation in different settings around the world.

In the 1970s, nutritionists developed a causal framework of malnutrition, which has been extensively used and advocated by UNICEF and is well known as 'the UNICEF framework'. The Lancet series on Nutrition in 2013 adjusted it to a more comprehensive framework and many authors in *Nutrition and Health in a Developing World* have used this framework as the basis for their chapters. The framework uses a three-level causality model: immediate causes, underlying causes, and basic causes. Dietary intake and morbidity are considered as direct, or immediate, causes in this framework. De Pee in her chapter focuses on nutrient intake recommendations and how they can be achieved. The chapters by Palmer, Darnton-Hill and West, Young and Ramakrishnan, Hess, Zimmermann, Pettifor and Thandrayen, and Granot and Deckelbaum each focus on specific nutrients.

As mentioned above, the UNICEF framework of nutrition has been shown to be a useful tool in nutrition programming and analysis but it is critical to understand that interventions at the level of the basic and underlying causes eventually have to lead to an adequate intake of nutrients and a morbidity level that does not interfere with the uptake and utilization of the nutrients. Adequate intake of nutrients is, therefore, a prerequisite in the prevention of malnutrition in all its forms. De Pee's chapter is, therefore, not only very important for every student in the field of public health and nutrition but a critical read for everyone who works in the field of nutrition education. Behavior change and education programs in nutrition can only be successful if they eventually lead to consumption of a diet that provides the right types and amounts of nutrients. Dietary reference intakes have been established for normal, healthy people of different age, sex, physiological state and physical activity groups. People who suffer from malnutrition or frequent or chronic infections have higher nutrient needs, and for some of these groups specific intake recommendations have been proposed. De Pee concludes that meeting nutrient intake recommendations requires consumption of a diverse diet, which for many target groups also needs to include some fortified commodities.

While work on vitamins started early in the twentieth century, it was in the 1970s that the significance of micronutrients deficiencies and their consequences was really recognized. Vitamin A, iron, zinc, iodine, and vitamin D were considered the most important vitamins and minerals. Alfred Sommer, an ophthalmologist trained in epidemiology, was one of the pioneers in the field of vitamin A deficiency. He carried out several vitamin A surveys in Haiti, El Salvador, and Indonesia as the technical advisor to the American Foundation for Overseas Blind (now Helen Keller International). Sommer's findings that even mild vitamin A deficiency leads to an increased risk of childhood mortality and that a high dose of vitamin A could prevent mortality by on average 23% changed the field of micronutrient deficiencies. West's chapter is an excellent overview of the history of vitamin A deficiency and discusses the many strategies that can and are being used to combat this problem.

The excellent Chapters by Young and Ramakrishnan, Hess, Zimmermann, and Pettifor and Thandrayen elucidate that the fight against micronutrient deficiencies is far from over. Although the scientific knowledge in this field is far greater than 50 years ago, micronutrient deficiencies remain public health problems and achieving an adequate intake, whether from the diet and/or supplements, i.e., through food or health systems, remains an important bottleneck.

Essential fatty acids play an important role in diverse biologic processes and metabolic pathways that are relevant to both health and disease. Granot and Deckelbaum provide an excellent overview and recommendations about the role of essential fatty acids during pregnancy, infancy and childhood, including in undernourished populations.

Since the development of ready to use therapeutic foods (RUTFs) for treating severe acute malnutrition, nutritionists have renewed their interest in the role of milk and its different components in the treatment and prevention of undernutrition. While the chapter by Kiess (in part VI) discusses the use of different ready-to-use foods in the context of the humanitarian crises, Grenov and colleagues particularly discuss the role of human and animal milks. Taren and Lutter discuss in their chapter the many benefits but also the programmatic obstacles of achieving good rates of appropriate breast-feeding practices.

The fourth part—Tuberculosis, HIV and the role of nutrition—has four chapters: Tuberculosis by Eyal Oren and Joann McDermid; HIV—medical perspective by Louise C. Ivers and Daniel Dure; HIV and Nutrition by Anupama Paranandi and Christine Wanke; Tuberculosis and Nutrition by Anupama Paranandi and Christine Wanke. Infectious diseases are increasingly a public health concern and in the second edition, we had covered diarrheal diseases, respiratory diseases, measles, malaria, HIV, and tuberculosis. For this edition, we have chosen to include only HIV and Tuberculosis because we believe that these two diseases are good examples of the philosophy of *Nutrition and Health in a Developing World*. These chapters, together with the chapters by Semba, and by Mehra, De Pee and Bloem (in Part VI) cover both HIV and TB from different perspectives, which can also be applied to other common diseases. We believe that many lessons learned from these chapters are applicable to other infectious diseases, e.g., Ebola, Zika, etc.

The fifth part—Nutrition and health in different phases of the lifecycle—has six chapters: Reproductive health by Satvika Chalasani and Nuriye Ortayli; Maternal nutrition and birth outcomes by Usha Ramakrishnan, Melissa Young, and Reynaldo Martorell; Small for Gestational Age: Scale and consequences for mortality, morbidity and development by Ines Gonzalez-Casanova, Usha Ramakrishnan, and Reynaldo Martorell; Developmental disabilities by Burris Duncan, Jennifer Andrews, Heidi Pottinger and F. John Meaney; Adolescent health and nutrition by Jee Rah, Satvika Chalasani, Vanessa M. Oddo and Vani Sethi; Nutrition in the Elderly from Low- and Middle-income Countries by Odilia Bermudez and Noel Solomons.

The development and pathology of nutrition and health problems are different in the various phases of the life cycle. The size of the human body increases rapidly during the first 1000 days, starting at conception, which is the best window for prevention of stunting. However, Ramakrishnan and colleagues show in their chapters that SGA is a key determinant of stunting that is associated with maternal nutritional status and needs to be tackled starting even before conception. Teenage pregnancies are very common in countries with a high prevalence of stunting and nutrition and health programs need to focus on this difficult to reach adolescent population. The chapter by Duncan et al. on developmental disabilities illustrates a new appreciation of how epigenetics, culture, and nutrition are interconnected to prevent and manage the health of a population that has been underrepresented on a global scale until the UN ratified The Convention on the Rights of Persons with Disabilities. Rah et al. discuss the period of adolescence, both from a biological and a social perspective and its implications for programming that aims to improve nutrition of adolescents for themselves as well as for the next generation. While many interventions during pregnancy aim to improve birth outcomes, Chalasani and Ortayli describe the impact of nutrition on the woman's own health. The nutritional status of the elderly has not received much attention but since life expectancy is increasing in all countries in the world, it is good to give more attention to this phase of the life cycle. Bermudez and Solomons have given an update on our current knowledge on this age group and the gaps.

The sixth part—Tackling health and nutrition issues in an integrated way in the era of the SDGs—consists of four chapters: Evaluation of nutrition sensitive interventions by Deanna Olney, Jef Leroy and Marie T. Ruel; Integrated approaches to health and nutrition: Role of communities by Olivia

Lange, Divya Mehra, Saskia de Pee and Martin W. Bloem; Nutrition in humanitarian crises by Lynnda Kiess, Natalie Aldern, Saskia de Pee and Martin W. Bloem; and Ending AIDS by 2030: Partnerships and Linkages with SDG2 by Divya Mehra, Saskia de Pee and Martin W. Bloem.

The SDGs show that many problems are interdependent and this is particularly valid for health and nutrition problems. Olney and colleagues describe the importance of nutrition-sensitive interventions and emphasize that good designs of evaluations of these programs are critical for understanding their contribution to improving nutrition and being cost-effective. The health field has since Alma Ata recognized the importance of communities, and in the 80s and 90s, many community-based programs were developed with the purpose to have lower cost, effective programs. As mentioned previously, an understanding of community dynamics was critical in the 2014/15 Ebola outbreak. Mehra and colleagues in both chapters have examined the many aspects of communities and how public health specialists have to understand not only the supply but also the demand side to ensure effective delivery and uptake of services. Communities are dynamic, not only the geographically defined communities but also the virtual communities. Emergencies are a good example of the need for a deep understanding of these affected communities and Kiess and colleagues explain the many determinants and solutions for malnutrition in humanitarian settings.

The seventh part—Trends in urbanization and development, impacts on the food value chain and consumers, and private sector roles—consists of five chapters: Urbanization patterns and strategies for ensuring adequate nutrition by Sunniva K. Bloem and Saskia de Pee; Urbanization, Food Security and Nutrition by Marie T. Ruel, James Garrett, Sivan Yosef and Meghan Olivier; The Impact of Supermarkets on nutrition and nutritional knowledge: a food policy perspective by Peter Timmer; Value chain focus on food and nutrition security by Jessica Fanzo, Shauna Downs, Quinn Marshall, Saskia de Pee and Martin W. Bloem; Role of foundations and initiatives by the private sector for improving health and nutrition by Kalpana Beesabathuni, Kesso Gabrielle van Zutphen and Klaus Kraemer.

The Sustainable Development Goals have recognized that more and more people are moving from rural areas to cities. This has led to SDG 11: Make cities inclusive, safe, resilient, and sustainable. While currently half of humanity already lives in urban areas, by 2030, almost 60% of the world's population will live in cities. This speed and scale of urbanization has been unprecedented. Originally, in high-income countries, cities developed close to and were linked to rural areas with high levels of agricultural produce. In many LMICs, however, many cities have grown independently and largely disconnected from rural areas and agricultural produce, with many already facing the double burden of malnutrition. The role of the private sector in health and nutrition is different in the rural areas as compared to urban areas, and disparities vary widely within cities. Health care in cities is often privatized and the role of the food industry is much larger as most people participate in the market economy. The chapters by Bloem and De Pee, Ruel and colleagues, Timmer, and Fanzo and colleagues, examine various components of urbanization. The rise of supermarkets as part of a modern value chain has raised many concerns but is a development that the global community has to deal with. Recently, a couple of countries have developed new nutrition policies and included dialogue with the private sector as a key strategy. Beesabathuni and colleagues argue that the private sector and foundations should and can play a critical role in the prevention and control of malnutrition and describe interesting examples.

Two of us have worked for an extensive time for the United Nations and one of us has spent a quarter of a century in academic research developing undergraduate and graduate education programs in public health and medicine and we feel that human rights should be the basis for every public health strategy. One of the components of a human rights approach is research. Doherty and Chopra have presented the history of ethics particularly in research in the last chapter of the book. Human rights should be at the basis of every health strategy.

We wish to thank our Series Editor, Adrianne Bendich, and the colleagues of Springer, Connie Walsh and Samantha Lonuzzi, for their encouragement, interest, and hard work to complete this volume. Adrianne's dedication, keen interest and deep knowledge of nutrition and health as well as her trust in the editors are very encouraging and inspiring. Additionally, we extend our gratitude and thanks to all the chapter authors for their extensive, thoughtful and analytical reviews and for their dedication to supporting the next generations who will continue to work to improve the lives of people throughout this developing world.

As editors, we hope that *Nutrition and Health in a Developing World* will instill curiosity, a desire to develop in-depth expertise, and appreciation for the need to approach public health and nutrition problems from multidimensional angles and with a multi-sectoral team. With that, public health professionals and others working to improve the world's development should be confident and well equipped to design comprehensive and effective policies, programs, and research across various sectors to reach the Sustainable Development Goals by the year 2030.

Rome, Italy   Saskia de Pee, Ph.D.
Tucson, USA   Douglas Taren, Ph.D.
Rome, Italy   Martin W. Bloem, M.D., Ph.D.

References

1. Martorell R, Rivera fJ. History, design, and objectives of the INCAP follow-up study on the effects of nutrition supplementation in child growth and development. Food Nutr Bull. 1992;14(3):254–7.
2. McLaren DS. The great protein fiasco. Lancet. 1974 Jul 13;2(7872):93–96.
3. Hoddinott J, Maluccio JA, Behrman JR, Flores R, Martorell R. Effect of a nutrition intervention during early childhood on economic productivity in Guatemalan adults. Lancet 2008;371-411-6.

Series Editor Preface

The great success of the Nutrition and Health Series is the result of the consistent overriding mission of providing health professionals with texts that are essential because each includes: (1) a synthesis of the state of the science, (2) timely, in-depth reviews by the leading researchers and clinicians in their respective fields, (3) extensive, up-to-date fully annotated reference lists, (4) a detailed index, (5) relevant tables and figures, (6) identification of paradigm shifts and the consequences, (7) virtually no overlap of information between chapters, but targeted, inter-chapter referrals, (8) suggestions of areas for future research and (9) balanced, data-driven answers to patient as well as health professionals questions which are based upon the totality of evidence rather than the findings of any single study.

The series volumes are not the outcome of a symposium. Rather, the editors have the potential to examine a chosen area with a broad perspective, both in subject matter as well as in the choice of chapter authors. The international perspective, especially with regard to public health initiatives, is emphasized where appropriate. The editors, whose trainings are both research and practice oriented, have the opportunity to develop a primary objective for their book; define the scope and focus, and then invite the leading authorities from around the world to be part of their initiative. The authors are encouraged to provide an overview of the field, discuss their own research and relate the research findings to potential human health consequences. Because each book is developed *de novo*, the chapters are coordinated so that the resulting volume imparts greater knowledge than the sum of the information contained in the individual chapters.

"Nutrition and Health in a Developing World, Third Edition" edited by Dr. Saskia de Pee, Ph.D., Dr. Douglas Taren, Ph.D. and Dr. Martin W. Bloem, M.D., Ph.D. is a welcome addition to the Nutrition and Health Series and fully exemplifies the series' goals. This unique volume is a very timely update of the second edition that was published in 2008. Over the past nine years, there has been a significant increase in public health understanding of the huge role of digital communication. Enhanced communication capabilities permit populations from different economic states to share in the new benefits, as well as threats, in this digital age. As examples, climate change, pollution, hunger, contaminated food systems, and Ebola and Zika virus infections have shown that the world is interconnected and interdependent. War-like aggressions in certain parts of the world not only led to destroyed cities and infrastructure, high number of deaths of adults as well as children and severe food insecurity, but also to increased migration of millions of people to Europe and other countries. Moreover, in 2015, the global Sustainable Development Goals were adopted and resulted in a shifting of the focus by UN member nations from disease specific interventions and poverty in low- and middle-income communities to addressing issues of sustainability, human rights, social inclusion and justice and ensuring "no one is left behind". Thus, with these global critical issues in mind, the editors have decided to not only update the relevant chapters from the second edition, but also to add new, timely chapters as well as adapt the volume title to better reflects today's interconnected and developing world and the current thinking of public health professionals.

The internationally recognized public health nutrition researchers who serve as the editors of this volume have identified key areas that will gain in importance due to current critical issues including the implications of climate change, increase of inequity in the world, political instability between and within states, numerous mass migrations of nutritionally at-risk populations, urbanization, outbreaks of new infectious diseases, continued health issues related to obesity among those that were mal-nourished as children, and challenges to achieving sustainable food systems. Moreover, the editors have chosen the most respected and knowledgeable authors for the volume's 36 insightful chapters. Thus, this volume addresses these critical issues with objective, data-driven chapters that reflect the goals of public health nutrition today and for the future. The chapters contain both Learning Objectives as well as Discussion Points as it is the intention of the editors that this volume serves as an important resource for educators and students.

The editors of this comprehensive volume are uniquely qualified to develop this 3rd Edition with its broader perspective. The editors have worked together and are well respected by their peers; each has been involved in international nutrition research, collectively, for more than a century and have each contributed greatly to enhancing the nutritional status and overall health of literally millions of children and adults in populations at-risk for nutritional and economic deficiencies. All three editors have extensive lists of peer-reviewed publications including original clinical research studies. Dr. Saskia de Pee serves as Senior Technical Advisor, Nutrition and HIV/AIDS for the United Nations World Food Programme (WFP) that focuses on improving the nutritional quality of food assistance provided by the WFP. Her responsibilities includes representing the WFP in global technical/scientific and policy-related meetings that ensure that policy and programming are in-line with the latest scientific evidence; coordinating technical aspects of nutrition-focused public–private partnerships; designing programs with new commodities with specific Country Offices, including evaluation of implemen-tation and outcomes; developing new public private partnership opportunities in nutrition and preparing technical communications for WFP colleagues. Dr. de Pee is Adjunct Associate Professor at the Friedman School of Nutrition Science and Policy, Tufts University, Boston, MA. Prior to joining the WFP, she was a consultant to the Global Alliance for Improved Nutrition (GAIN) and served on their Independent Review Panel for Infant and Young Child Nutrition Program proposals as well as evaluating the China Soy Sauce Fortification Project. She was also Scientific Advisor for Helen Keller International in the Asia Pacific and New York offices. Dr. Douglas L. Taren, Ph.D. currently serves as Associate Dean for Academic Affairs in the Mel and Enid Zuckerman College of Public Health, Professor of Public Health and Director of the Western Region Public Health Training Center at the University of Arizona, Tucson, AZ. Dr. Taren, during his 25+ year career, has been conducting nutritional research in low- and middle-income countries. He has been a member of NIH study and numerous grant review committees. His research includes work with the CDC on breastfeeding by HIV positive mothers and a related study in a breastfeeding counseling program to decrease perinatal HIV transmission in Kisumu, Western Kenya. Dr. Taren has served as the Director of graduate and postgraduate level training programs that include distance learning programs. Additionally, he has led a program that integrated and evaluated nutrition education into a medical curriculum and directed several training programs including the distance learning program on maternal and child health as part of a certificate program. Dr. Martin W. Bloem is the Global Coordinator of WFP in UNAIDS which is responsible for leading the UN's AIDS efforts to bring together, in the AIDS response, the efforts and resources of ten UN system organizations. He also serves as Senior Nutrition Advisor of the United Nations World Food Programme in Rome, Italy. He is Adjunct Associate Professor at the Friedman School of Nutrition Science and Policy at Tufts University, Boston, MA and at Johns Hopkins Bloomberg School of Public Health, Baltimore. Dr. Bloem previously served as Senior Vice President, Chief Medical Officer and Regional Director for Asia Pacific in Singapore for Helen Keller International. Dr. Bloem co-edited, with Dr. Richard Semba, the first and second editions of Nutrition and Health in Developing Countries and therefore Dr. Bloem has served as an esteemed editor for the Nutrition and Health Series for the past 15 years.

This comprehensive volume contains 36 chapters that are organized in eight parts: History of Nutrition; Contextualizing International Nutrition- Considering Benefit-Cost, Evidence Base and Capacity; Malnutrition, Nutrients and (Breast) Milk Explained; Tuberculosis, HIV and the Role of Nutrition; Nutrition and Health in Different Phases of the Lifecycle; Tackling Health and Nutrition Issues in an Integrated Way in the Era of Sustainable Development Goals; Trends in Urbanization and Development, Impacts on Food Value Chains and Consumers, and Private Sector Roles; and Ethics-Critical to Making Progress in Public Health.

Part I History of Nutrition

The first part in this volume contains a comprehensive review by Dr. Richard Semba, who co-edited the first two editions of this volume. We are reminded that within the last two centuries, there has been a general improvement in the health of people worldwide that can be attributed largely to changes in nutrition including food safety and availability, clean water and personal as well as population-based improvements in basic hygiene and public health including vaccination programs and dietary guidelines, as well as increased numbers of graduate and postgraduate students in the various fields of nutrition. At the beginning of the nineteenth century, the burden of morbidity and mortality from infectious diseases such as malaria, cholera, measles, tuberculosis, and diarrheal disease, and nutritional deficiency diseases such as scurvy, pellagra, rickets, goiter and vitamin A deficiency were relatively high in Europe, North America, and much of the rest of world. By the end of the twentieth century, these diseases were largely eradicated from industrialized countries. Unfortunately, many of these diseases and their associated morbidity and mortality continue to be major problems in low- and middle-income countries. The chapter, which includes over 200 relevant references and many helpful figures, reviews the development of understanding of the role of food, diet and essential nutrients in the practice of preventive medicine during the past 200 years in Europe and the US and describes the major scientists and physicians who initiated the development of public sewers, sterilization of surgical utensils and food preparation methods to avoid contamination and spoilage. The initiation of the fields of microbiology and immunology and the discovery of the vitamins and other essential nutrients and their roles in reducing infant mortality and links to chronic diseases are also discussed.

Part II Contextualizing International Nutrition—Considering Benefit-Cost, Evidence-Base and Capacity

Part II contains three chapters that concentrate on challenges to achieving optimal nutritional status for the world's population and sustaining that level of nutritional adequacy. Chapter 2 examines the importance of developing an economic model that quantifies the economic benefits of nutrition interventions. Economic analysis can assist nations in deciding how best to allocate investments to improve nutrition among competing programs, and how to use public funding most effectively. Methods, including cost-effectiveness analysis and cost-benefit analysis, are reviewed and outcomes, including increased cognition and educational achievement versus death and hospitalizations averted, are examined in depth. The next chapter, co-authored by one of the book's editors, discusses the methodologies needed to choose nutritional interventions, implementation strategies and assessment tools for a preventive approach among large numbers of at-risk individuals. The important role of evidence-based medicine and the development of systematic reviews of data based upon the hierarchy of study types is stressed and its implications (plusses and minuses) for nutrition interventions are examined. Chapter 4 continues to examine the critical issues that currently face the global nutrition community with emphasis on the 2015 Sustainable Development Goals, and examines the future needs for training a professional workforce to deal with these multi-sectoral dimensions of public health nutrition. Factors reviewed include climate change; population growth; extreme poverty; energy-intensive dietary patterns; water scarcity; land and natural resource degradation; rising prices of food, fuel and fertilizer; and political instability. These factors are predicted to contribute to a shift in the global burden of disease, both in type and locus, and an increase in food insecurity in many parts of the world. There is an examination of the bidirectional relationship between climate variability and agriculture, which affects health and nutritional status, commonly called the diet–environment–health trilemma, and how effectively dealing with this requires professionals that understand, and to some extent speak the language of, the different disciplines.

Part III Malnutrition, Nutrients and (Breast)Milk Explained

Part III includes twelve chapters that examine the continuing risk of childhood malnutrition and its consequences on growth and development even in the face of obesity. There are six chapters that review key individual essential nutrients followed by two chapters related to breast and other sources of milk during infancy and childhood. Chapter 5, written by two of the volume's editors, comprehensively reviews the most widely acceptable and used assessment tools for nutritional status, to measure different aspects of the spectrum of malnutrition. Information about the use and interpretation of indicators of food security, dietary intake, anthropometry, and biomarkers to assess nutritional status at the global, national, household and individual level are compared. There are also discussions of new areas of research regarding nutritional assessment such as metabolomics and gut microbiota that can help understand and identify links between nutritional status, dietary patterns, and other factors. The indicators have significant variation across the world and can help to determine global and national prevalence of different forms of malnutrition. These indicators are used to track progress towards improving nutrition and to assess the impact of nutrition interventions, whether they are part of research studies or public health programs. Accurate use of nutritional indicators is dependent upon accounting for the population's rate of response as well as individual factors including the participant's age, sex and non-nutritional factors. The chapter includes nine valuable tables and figures. Chapter 6 follows with a broad overview of the consequences of child growth retardation and how it affects the individual throughout their lifespan. The chapter reviews indicators and growth standards for assessing impaired fetal and child growth; describes the magnitude and geographical distribution of growth retardation in developing countries; outlines the main health and social consequences of impaired growth in terms of morbidity, mortality, child physical and mental development and adult-life consequences; and reviews interventions aimed at promoting healthy growth and development. There is an in-depth discussion of the three most commonly used indicators to assess childhood growth status: weight-for-height, height-for-age, and weight-for-age and the standards for these measurements as well as other key standards are included in the 10 informative figures and tables.

The seventh chapter examines the prevalence of adult obesity around the world using the WHO standard grading definitions. Currently, the greatest prevalence of overweight and above occurs in the Middle East and North Africa, Latin America and the Caribbean and in Central Asia. In contrast, countries in South Asia and sub-Saharan Africa have the lowest prevalence of overweight and obesity. The chapter contains detailed information concerning populations affected and certain health consequences that appear in extensive tables and figures. Chapter 8, written by a co-editor, examines the nutrient needs and approaches to meeting required nutrient intakes established by FAO/WHO, the Institute of Medicine (IOM) in the US and other regulatory bodies. The IOM uses terms including estimated average requirement (EAR) and upper intake levels (UL) that are explained in detailed. In terms of risk, the EAR and UL are very different. The EAR is the midpoint of required intake. At this level of intake, the risk of inadequacy is 50% and the negative consequences of inadequate macro or micronutrient intakes are well established. The risk of an intake close the UL, however, is negligible because it includes an uncertainty factor lower than the intake at and above which adverse effects may be expected. Moreover, if there was an absence of adequate safety data, a high uncertainty factor was applied for those micronutrients. The terms nutrient density and energy density are defined and examples of adequately nutritious foods for different population groups are included.

The next six chapters review the consequences of deficiencies in vitamin A, iron, zinc, iodine, vitamin D, and essential fatty acids and also provide mechanisms for the prevention of deficiencies. Chapter 9 reminds us that vitamin A deficiency still affects an estimated 190 million preschool-aged children and 10 million pregnant women in low-income countries. Prevalent cases of vitamin A deficiency blindness (xerophthalmia) in young children is believed to be about 5 million and remains the leading cause of preventable pediatric blindness in the developing world. Vitamin A deficiency remains an underlying cause of at least 157,000 early childhood deaths annually due to diarrhea, measles, malaria and other infections. This comprehensive chapter, that includes over 400 references and 24 key tables and figures, describes the chemical structure of vitamin A and its precursors, provides an historical review of the discovery and identification of the vitamin, dietary sources, absorption, metabolism and functions, followed by discussions of the epidemiology of vitamin A deficiency and its role in morbidity and mortality. The chapter concludes with insights on its diagnosis, treatment, and approaches for prevention through dietary improvement, supplementation, fortification, and biofortification. Iron is reviewed in Chap. 10 and includes eight comprehensive tables and figures that help to illustrate iron's biological functions, metabolism and regulation, assessment methods, prevalence of deficiency, key risk factors/etiology, functional consequences, along with evidence-based strategies for the prevention and control of iron deficiency and anemia. The likely causes of childhood anemia, new delivery systems for iron including biofortification, delayed cord clamping at birth and analysis of safety issues are included in this comprehensive chapter. Zinc is another essential mineral and Chap. 11 provides the rationale for reducing the risk of zinc deficiency especially for infants, young children and pregnant women. The reason for the attention to zinc status in recent years is the increased understanding that zinc is involved in hundreds of metabolic processes and acts as a catalyst, regulatory ion, and/or structural element of proteins. Over 300 metalloenzymes require zinc as a catalyst, and about 2500 genetic transcription factors require zinc for their structural integrity. The chapter, with 135 references, outlines the major causes of zinc deficiency and includes details concerning assessment tools, strategies for preemptive prevention as well as treatments for marginal as well as frank zinc deficiency.

Chapter 12 reviews the essentiality of iodine and reminds us that iodine is an essential component of thyroid hormones. Iodine deficiency has multiple adverse effects due to inadequate thyroid hormone production. Iodine deficiency during pregnancy and infancy impairs growth and neurodevelopment (especially higher brain functions) and increases the risk of infant mortality. Deficiency during childhood reduces growth, cognitive and motor functions. Mild-to-moderate iodine deficiency in adults results in goiter and an increase in thyroid hyperplasia. Overall, iodine deficiency produces widespread adverse effects in individuals, including decreased learning, apathy, and reduced work productivity. The major sources of iodine are salt extracted from sea water and sea life. If the majority of a population does not have access to iodine-containing foods, most of the population will be iodine deficient and population-wide interventions are needed. Assessment of iodine status is reviewed and implementation of iodized salt strategies is discussed. Chapter 13 describes the current global prevalence of nutritional rickets and the related effects of vitamin D and calcium deficiencies.

Nutritional rickets remains a major cause of infant and young child morbidity and mortality in several low- and middle-income countries across the world. A major environmental factor is that vitamin D production in the exposed skin is significantly less at high latitudes in the temperate zones. Another factor in the Middle East and in some population groups in other countries is the religious custom of covering the body that results in reduced sun exposure, which is particularly detrimental to infants and young children, adolescents and pregnant women. Low dietary calcium intakes and relative vitamin D deficiency exacerbates and promotes the development of rickets. Currently, effective prevention programs are not in place in most low-income countries. The chapter includes 165 relevant references and six important figures that provide strong support for more effective programs to reduce the two essential micronutrient deficiencies of vitamin D and calcium. Chapter 14 focuses on basic research and clinical/epidemiological studies relating to essential polyunsaturated fatty acids, with an emphasis on areas of importance to low- and middle-income countries, specifically those pertaining to mother and child health. Assessment of dietary requirements of essential fatty acids during the life time, and assuring adequate intakes especially during pregnancy, lactation and early childhood in vulnerable middle- and low-income populations, are included. The chapter reviews the roles of the elongated omega-3 fatty acids, eicosapentanoic acid (EPA) and docosahexaenoic acid (DHA), in the development of the brain, heart and immune system; the major sources of these fatty acids and the mechanisms to provide these essential nutrients to at-risk populations.

The final two chapters in Part III discuss the importance of breast milk and animal milk especially for infants and young children in low- to middle-level economies. The nutritional and immunological composition of breast milk is presented in detail as is the compositions of milks from cow, buffalo, sheep and goat that are often used in rural settings and increasingly included as ingredients in special nutritious foods for older infants and young children. The WHO recommendations are included: exclusive breastfeeding for 6 months and continued breastfeeding until the age of 2 years or beyond. Studies and recommendations from WHO and several national bodies are included. These find consistent reductions in child mortality and morbidity in those infants provided with breastfeeding and it has been estimated that 800,000 children die every year due to suboptimal breastfeeding practices. Chapter 16, co-authored by the volume's co-editor, containing more than 150 references, provides strong support for breastfeeding based upon an objective review of the literature. The WHO and national, community and local recommendations and implementation strategies for helping lactating women understand the many benefits of their efforts for their baby as well as themselves are reviewed. The importance of breastfeeding as a major component of the Sustainable Developmental Goals to be reached by 2030 is highlighted.

Part IV Tuberculosis, HIV and the Role of Nutrition

The four chapters in Part IV provide in-depth examination of tuberculosis and HIV with two chapters on each of these serious, chronic diseases; the first two chapters provide the medical perspective of the disease and then each disease is discussed with regard to the nutritional consequences and potential for treatment enhancement. Chapter 17 summarizes the history and major symptoms and effects of infection with tuberculosis, and outlines key barriers to further reduction of the global burden. There is a discussion of the epidemiology and major risk factors associated with *Mycobacterium tuberculosis* transmission, establishment of infection, and progression to active clinical disease, pathogenesis, diagnosis and treatment; over 160 relevant references and insightful figures are included. Current tuberculosis control strategies, including vaccination, are reviewed. Drug-resistant tuberculosis and tuberculosis within vulnerable populations including HIV co-infection, young children, diabetics, and those affected by poverty and/or special socioeconomic circumstances are also addressed in this comprehensive chapter. With regard to Human

Immunodeficiency Viral infection (HIV), Chap. 18 includes a brief history of the HIV/AIDS epidemic and access to care; HIV virology, transmission and pathogenesis; clinical history of HIV infection; global epidemiology; comprehensive HIV care and the HIV care continuum; prevention of HIV; overlapping epidemics, and special issues in women and children. Currently, individuals living with HIV infection can have a life expectancy that is similar to those without HIV infection if they have access to early, high quality care and treatment. The serious inequities that continue to exist globally that cause certain groups to remain particularly vulnerable to infection are examined.

Chapter 19 reviews the well-documented importance of nutrition in all aspects of tuberculosis infection. Malnutrition, involving both macro- and micronutrient deficiencies increases the risk of contracting the disease as well as the risk of developing active disease. Undernutrition results in worsened tuberculosis-related outcomes, including cachexia and death. Negative social and economic factors, such as food insecurity, help promote malnutrition and tuberculosis infection, which adds to the vicious cycle. Children and pregnant or lactating women are more vulnerable to the dual effects of tuberculosis and malnutrition. The effects of malnutrition are further compounded in those co-infected with HIV and tuberculosis, with an even higher risk of morbidity and mortality compared to those with either disease alone. Both medical treatment and adequate nutritional intake to achieve and maintain normal body mass index (BMI) and nutritional status, as recommended by the WHO, are required for prevention and successful treatment. The chapter reviews the efforts required to expand treatment and nutritional care to all infected people to ensure that tuberculosis is controlled and no longer a health threat to the global community. As with the patient with tuberculosis, those who are undernourished have a greater risk of becoming infected with HIV than the adequately nourished individual. However, unlike tuberculosis which can be cured, current therapies cannot cure HIV. Treatment must be lifelong and the treatment of HIV is complicated by nutritional issues. The HIV infected individual experiences lifelong nutritional issues related to the chronic viral infection and the treatment. The chapter includes an in-depth discussion of the chronic use of antiretroviral therapy that is required to maintain life, and may overcome the causes of weight loss, reduction in key essential nutrients and the risk of cachexia. Also included are discussions of co-infection with tuberculosis, maternal to child transmission of HIV and WHO guidelines to address these issues.

Part V Nutrition and Health in Different Phases of the Lifecycle

The six chapters in the fifth part examine the importance of nutrition for men and women of childbearing potential to help assure a healthy pregnancy, birth outcome and successful lactation. Malnutrition, be it undernutrition or obesity, significantly increases the risks for adverse pregnancy outcomes including, but not limited to, infant prematurity, small for gestational age, congenital malformations and other developmental disabilities that are also addressed in chapters in this part. Nutrition has become a well-accepted key to a healthy pregnancy and the importance of the pre-pregnancy window has especially been recognized since the findings of the benefits of peri-conceptional folic acid intake, for example from fortified flours, for the prevention of neural tube birth defects. The nutritional needs of the woman who is an adolescent when she becomes pregnant are reviewed as are numerous specific foods and dietary ingredients including harmful ones, such as alcohol. Adolescence growth spurts and the additional nutritional needs as well as those of seniors who may be at risk for food insecurity are also reviewed in separate chapters. Chapter 21 reviews the relationship between nutritional status and reproductive well-being during the phases of the reproductive cycle starting from the onset of puberty in both sexes, to the menstrual cycle and pregnancy. The chapter also examines the role of nutrition in the prevention and treatment of sexually transmitted infections and reproductive organ cancers in both sexes. The interplay of genetics, hormone production, and nutritional status of the mother during pregnancy as well as the adolescent are reviewed in detail. Evidence from clinical interventions involving supplementation and the importance of essential vitamins and minerals are also reviewed.

The next two chapters describe adverse effects on neonatal growth associated with maternal undernutrition and provide thoughtful recommendations to lower these risks. Chapter 22 concentrates on the myriad of nutritional factors that have been linked to healthy pregnancy outcomes for both the mother as well as the infant and places the science into the context of developing and implementing public policies in low- and middle-income countries. The need to identify better ways to overcome barriers to program implementation with improved methods for targeting and measuring program effectiveness for maternal nutrition before and during pregnancy is stressed. The authors provide key nutrition research areas and strongly recommend that nutrition and health programs that focus on improving birth outcomes should strengthen linkages with other sectors such as agriculture, water and sanitation, family planning, education, and social protection. Chapter 23 describes the major causes of neonates being born small for gestational age (SGA). SGA is defined as a birth weight for gestational age below the 10th percentile of the reference and is used as an indicator of inadequate intrauterine growth. It is estimated that over 27% of live births are SGA in developing countries, with important short- and long-term repercussions for health and development. The chapter describes the challenges to assess SGA, its main consequences, epidemiology and nutritional determinants especially in low- and middle-income countries. Methods to assess gestational age are described; factors that increase risk including preeclampsia, maternal diabetes (gestational or preexisting), anemia and/or other nutritional deficiencies, toxins, such as tobacco, alcohol and environmental toxins, fetal and placental factors are all reviewed. Along with numerous increased risks of adverse health effects following birth, being born SGA is also associated with an increased risk of childhood stunting and wasting, which in turn has been associated with increased morbidity and mortality. The chapter includes over 100 relevant references and 8 helpful tables and figures.

The next three chapters examine the consequences of undernutrition (and obesity where relevant) on the health of vulnerable populations including those with developmental disabilities, adolescents, especially females, and seniors. Chapter 24, with 130 references and 7 comprehensive tables and figures, provides a sensitive, in-depth analysis of the consequences to individuals who are considered to have developmental disabilities in low- or middle-economic environments where resources are limited. The authors cite the US definition of developmental disability: a severe, chronic disability that can be mental or physical or a combination of the two; that manifests itself prior to age 22; is likely to be permanent; and results in a substantial limitation in three or more of the specific areas (self-care, receptive and expressive language, learning, mobility, self-direction, capacity for independent living, and economic self-sufficiency); and that requires a combination of interdisciplinary services for an extended period of time that may be lifelong. In addition to genetic and genomic causes, the effects of malnutrition are discussed as well as the interactions between genetic and environmental causes, as illustrated by mutations in folate-related genes and lack of use of prenatal multivitamins that has been associated with increased risk of autism in the case of mothers with a specific genotype or genome. The nutrient deficiencies often found in children with these disabilities are reviewed as are the support systems that may be available for severely disabled children in their communities. Chapter 25 reviews the current needs for enhancing the nutritional status of adolescents with emphasis on females in low- and middle-income countries. The current evidence suggests that the prevalence of undernutrition, overweight, and micronutrient deficiencies are considerable among adolescents. Rapid growth and development during puberty increases physiological demands for energy and micronutrients, which is often coupled with suboptimal food and nutrient intake. The inability to meet nutrition requirements due to physiological changes are further complicated in females by child marriage and adolescent pregnancy. In low-income countries, many adolescents enter pregnancy with poor nutritional status and have a limited intake of nutrients during pregnancy and lactation. As discussed in the above chapters, both pregnant and lactating adolescents and their infants are likely to have suboptimal growth and nutritional status. The chapter stresses the need to improve adolescent nutrition with a range of effective, large-scale, complementary nutrition-specific and -sensitive interventions. Older adults represent another population group at-risk for nutritional inadequacies and Chap. 26 reviews the physiological changes associated with the ways that the older body handles nutrients as there is a decline in the functioning of the digestive system that impacts the utilization of critical, specific nutrients. Many of the affected organs are involved in the metabolism of food including the stomach and small intestine, liver, heart, kidneys, skin, immune system, and oral cavity. Older adults often experience a decline in gastric hydrochloric acid secretion that can result in a decline in the bioavailability of vitamin B12. Older adults may be at a compromised status for vitamin D, and consequently, for calcium absorption. Changes in body composition (decreased lean muscle mass and increased fat mass) result in decreased basal metabolic rates, energy needs, and capacity for physical activity. Depending upon the economic status of the individual and access to medical care in low- and middle-income countries, there may also be increased use of prescription and non-prescription medications, chronic drug therapy, and decreased capacity of the liver to metabolize drugs. The chapter stresses the risks of undernutrition during aging and provides tables that describe the WHO recommendations for intakes for seniors.

Part VI Tackling Health and Nutrition Issues in an Integrated Way in the Era of the Sustainable Developmental Goals

The four chapters in this part examine the major questions that are currently driving global efforts to reduce the risk of malnutrition for populations that may be acutely or chronically at risk. Chapter 27 provides options for determining the effectiveness of nutrition programs in low- and middle-income countries. Although most affected nations agree that there is a need to invest in nutrition-sensitive programs to address the underlying causes of undernutrition, the evidence of what works, how these work and the economic cost of the programs is not well documented. There is a detailed discussion of the many complexities of evaluating nutrition-sensitive programs, impact and process evaluations, and cost evaluations. The chapter puts forth a plan for building a strong body of evidence from rigorous, theory-based comprehensive evaluations of different nutrition-sensitive program models that bring together interventions from sectors including health, education, agriculture, social protection, women's empowerment, water and sanitation, and other relevant programs. There are study designs included that have the potential to build a strong body of evidence on what works to improve nutrition, how it works and at what cost. The next three chapters are co-authored by two of the co-editors. Chapter 28 concentrates on the role of communities in enhancing nutrition programs. The chapter discusses the role of geographically bounded communities in providing health resources. The changing global dynamics with respect to population demographics, health trends, urbanization, global health policy, technology, and analyses are reviewed. The concept of virtual communities is discussed within the health context. The authors propose an integrated supply and demand-oriented framework for the future role of communities in advancing health and nutrition outcomes. The importance of the community health worker is stressed using "Child Health Days" as an example, where multiple maternal and child health interventions were provided during a few days per year. This program is representative of an effective setting for providing routine services such as vaccinations, high-dose vitamin A capsule distribution, growth monitoring and nutrition education. These programs, administered by the community health workers have been documented to result in significant reductions in childhood under-5 mortality. Other major programs include those dealing with severe infections including HIV/AIDS and tuberculosis and acute childhood malnutrition. The chapter includes a detailed comparison between the earlier Millennium Development Goals and the 2015 Sustainable Development Goals and how the change in goals will impact communities and their role in supporting health and nutrition of its members.

Chapter 29 provides a compelling and up-to-date examination of the scope and effects of humanitarian crises. We learn that in 2016, the United Nations Office for the Coordination of Humanitarian Affairs reported that the global humanitarian appeal provided life-saving humanitarian assistance to over 87 million people across 37 countries, most of which remain in conflict. These figures do not include the expected humanitarian needs associated with the El Niño weather pattern in 2016 that affected Southern and East Africa, Southeast Asia and Central America. Those anticipated needs represent a massive increase from 2007, when 26 million people required assistance. In addition to more frequent crises affecting larger numbers of people, a greater share of crises are complex and protracted and the people affected require prolonged support and assistance. Forced displacement due to conflict and natural disaster is also increasing, and totaled 60 million people by the end of 2014. Climate change alone is expected to impact crop yields, water supply, greatly intensifying droughts, floods and heat waves and also impact the frequency and severity of existing diseases and the introduction of new health threats such as Zika virus mentioned above. The chapter reviews the prioritization of nutritious food resources, first to infants and toddlers during the first 1000 days of life, and describes the importance of reviewing the situation of nutrition, health and food systems that existed prior to the crisis as part of planning and preparing for a response to a crisis as well as in anticipation of potential crises.

Chapter 30 concludes this part with the examination of the potential to reach the third sustainable development goal of good health and well-being. The goal includes the commitment to end the HIV, malaria, and TB epidemics and address non-communicable diseases by 2030. The UNAIDS Fast-Track approach aims to achieve ambitious targets by 2020, including fewer than 500,000 people newly infected with HIV, fewer than 500,000 people dying from AIDS-related illnesses, and eliminating HIV-related discrimination. The chapter includes a description of the matrix framework that can help to bring about the United Nations Secretary General's Zero Hunger Challenge aimed at achieving the vision of a Zero Hunger world by uniting around clear, measureable zero-based targets that would reject inequities and aims to eliminate childhood stunting; ensure that food is accessible to all; and that food systems are sustainable.

Part VII Trends in Urbanization and Development, Impacts on Food Value Chains and Consumers, and Private Sector Roles

Part VII contains five chapters that examine the current world status and the future nutritional needs of low- and medium-income countries around the globe. Chapter 31 co-authored by one of the volume's editors, examines the capacity of urban development patterns to help policy makers prepare for and achieve better urban nutrition, especially for the urban poor, by analyzing city size, urban infrastructures, trade, and rural–urban linkages. This chapter is especially important as we learn that by 2050, 6.3 billion people, or two thirds of the world's population, will be living in cities. Today more than half of the world's people live in urban areas and 90% of the urban growth between now and 2050 will take place in Africa and Asia. The double burden of undernutrition and obesity is greater in cities and the topics of food waste, food security and food safety, water and sanitation are reviewed. The consequences of city size are examined in depth. Chapter 32 continues with a deep examination of the effects of urbanization on nutrition as well as access to sufficient nutritious food. The chapter reviews the status of poverty, food security and malnutrition in urban compared to rural areas; provides an overview of the unique challenges and opportunities for urban dwellers to generate income and achieve food security and nutrition; and discusses the implications for urban programs, policies and research. The chapter reaffirms the findings of a rapid rise in overweight and obesity in urban areas, while undernutrition and micronutrient deficiencies persist and highlights critical gaps in knowledge and understanding of the distinctive factors and conditions that shape poverty, food security, and nutrition in cities. The increased diversity of foods and higher incomes in urban areas results in diets that are less affected by seasonality than rural ones. The availability of a wide range of foods and the shift away from traditional diets also meets consumer desires for greater food choices especially in large urban areas, even among the poor. Conversely, physical activity levels are documented to be lower in urban versus rural areas. This comprehensive chapter, with 140 important references, expands upon the cultural changes in women's roles in the urban compared to rural areas and how these affect the nutritional status of the woman and her family.

The importance of the emergence of supermarkets in low- and middle-income countries is addressed in Chap. 33 that provides an analytical and policy perspective on supermarkets and their modern supply chains, and the subsequent impact on food security and nutritional well-being. On the positive side, supermarkets and modern supply chains offer significantly enhanced food safety, the opportunity to fortify basic food staples and food for specific target groups with essential vitamins and minerals, and the potential to stabilize food prices, thus contributing to food security. On the negative side, supermarkets offer many choices of foods that may contribute to the obesity epidemic and non-communicable chronic diseases such as diabetes and cardiovascular disease. The chapter includes an in-depth analysis of the economic effects as well as government and non-governmental agency policy development in light of the increased globalization of food availability in the face of local farmer and poor community members' nutritious food access. Chapter 34 concentrates on the need to add nutritional value to the food value chains in order to get the full benefit of the value chain system for consumers. Food value chains that include the nutrition component have a role to play in terms of identifying innovative ways to improve the availability, affordability and acceptability of nutritious foods both in the context of undernutrition and over-eating. The chapter reviews the potential for developing policies that support actions along the food value chain that can contribute to healthier consumption patterns; the role of the private sector in producing, processing, packaging, and distributing food is key. The chapter authors, that include two volume editors, discuss the potential benefits of applying a business perspective to nutrition to identify opportunities for integrating nutrition into the value chain with the goal of increasing the availability, affordability and acceptability of nutritious foods for the population. For readers who are not familiar with production methodologies that include adding value at each step, this chapter is a key primer.

The last chapter in this part, Chap. 35, provides a unique perspective on the importance of private sector involvement in enhancing the Sustainable Development Goals of 2015. The chapter covers both corporate foundations and major corporate initiatives by Fortune 500 companies that play a key role in improving nutrition and health in low- and middle-income countries. The areas covered include the provision of goods and services, financial and in-kind contributions, the advance of advocacy tools, driving innovation and novel approaches, and the proliferation of public–private partnerships. Foundations such as the Rockefeller Foundation and Ford Foundation are reviewed as these were early leaders in the field of health. Recently, the largest private global health foundation, the Bill & Melinda Gates Foundation, has made significant investments in nutritional health. Extensive review of programs and investments are provided and the benefits are outlined. In order for corporate foundations' role to be further strengthened and improved in the public health arena in the future, the chapter authors include an analysis of procedures that should be considered: conflicts of interest must be mitigated and addressed; transparency and accountability are encouraged across all sectors to acknowledge the interests of all stakeholder groups, including civilians, government, donor organizations and the private sector; trust and accountability should be strengthened by adopting reporting mechanisms where the social impact of investment is measured; independent audits should regularly measure the scope and management of conflicts of interest with private foundations; the authors recommend the institution of a transparent public health code of ethics that would provide guidance to mitigate conflicts of interest.

Part VIII Ethics—Critical to Making Progress in Public Health

The final chapter in this excellent, comprehensive volume examines the importance of ethics especially in public health research. Chapter 36 reviews the historical development of ethical codes of conduct for clinical research and their implications for today's clinical investigators. During the Nuremberg War Crime Trials following World War II, the Nuremberg code was drafted as a set of standards for judging physicians and scientists who had conducted biomedical experiments on concentration camp prisoners. The central feature of the Nuremberg Code was the protection of the integrity of the person participating in research. The Nuremberg code was endorsed by the World Medical Association which published the Declaration of Helsinki in 1964. This ethical standard is particularly relevant as there has been a significant increase in the number of international collaborative health research studies involving high-income country sponsors and scientists at low- and middle-income country institutions and subjects. The inherent inequality of the relationship between these two groups has drawn attention to the ethics of research sponsored (or conducted) by groups in high-income countries but carried out in low- and middle-income country institutions. Practical considerations, including the development of Institutional Review Boards, Informed Consent, standards of care and confidentiality are reviewed and case studies are provided. This sensitive chapter is of great value for any investigator who plans to embark on a clinical trial.

Conclusions

The above description of the volume's 36 chapters attests to the depth of information provided by the 59 well-recognized and respected chapter authors. Each chapter includes complete definitions of terms with the abbreviations fully defined and consistent use of terms between chapters. Key features of this comprehensive volume include over 200 detailed tables, boxed explanations and informative figures, an extensive, detailed index and more than 3300 up-to-date references that provide the reader with excellent sources of worthwhile information that will be of great value to the public health researcher, health provider, government food and nutrition policy leader as well as graduate and medical students.

In conclusion, "Nutrition and Health in a Developing World, Third Edition" edited by Dr. Saskia de Pee, Ph.D., Dr. Douglas Taren, Ph.D. and Dr. Martin W. Bloem, M.D., Ph.D. provides health professionals in many areas of research and practice with the most up-to-date, well-referenced volume on the importance of nutrition as a key component of health especially in populations living in low- and middle-income countries. The chapters review the role of diet, food, essential and nonessential nutrients, water and other components of the diet in maintaining the overall health of the populations that are examined with regard to public health nutrition. There is an overriding goal of evaluating the multiple adverse effects of malnutrition, from undernutrition to obesity throughout the lifecycle, so that targeted progress can be made in improving the health of those at greatest risk of nutritional deficits. Areas emphasized include nutritional impacts on maternal and infant health, adolescent health, and the health of older individuals as well as those with physical and mental disabilities in the context of limited national resources. The importance of optimal dietary intakes in those suffering from tuberculosis or HIV/AIDS or both are discussed along with chapters that address the increased rates of non-communicable diseases, especially cardiovascular disease, diabetes and obesity. The advent of the 2015 Sustainable Development Goals has resulted in the inclusion of updated chapters that examine the role of communities as more people move to urban centers and purchase their food in supermarkets; nutrition-based food value chains, and ethical guidelines in the changing world economics. Unique chapters review the implications of applying an evidence-based medicine approach to nutrition, and the essentiality of nutrient-rich foods for humanitarian crises and for fostering elimination of certain infectious diseases. The volume serves the reader as the benchmark in this complex area of interrelationships between nutrients, foods, social issues, ethnic factors, public policies, physical activity, pregnancy, older adults, adolescents, children, controversies within the nutrition research community, private foundations that impact nutrition programs, and the critical area of food safety. The editors, Dr. Saskia de Pee, Ph.D., Dr. Douglas Taren, Ph.D. and Dr. Martin W. Bloem, M.D., Ph.D. and the excellent chapter authors are applauded for their efforts to develop the most authoritative and unique resource on the importance of nutrition in today's interconnected and developing world and this excellent text is a very welcome addition to the Nutrition and Health Series.

Adrianne Bendich, Ph.D., FACN, FASN
Editor

About the Series Editors

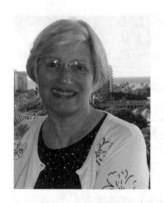

Dr. Adrianne Bendich, Ph.D., FASN, FACN has served as the "Nutrition and Health" Series Editor for 20 years and has provided leadership and guidance to more than 200 editors that have developed the 70+ well respected and highly recommended volumes in the Series.

In addition to "Nutrition and Health in a Developing World, Third Edition" edited by Dr. Saskia de Pee, Ph.D., Dr. Douglas Taren, Ph.D. and Dr. Martin W. Bloem, M.D., Ph.D., major new editions published from 2012–2017 include:

1. "Nitrite and Nitrate in Human Health and Disease, Second Edition" edited by Nathan S. Bryan, Ph.D. and Joseph Loscalzo, M.D., Ph.D., 2017
2. "Nutrition in Lifestyle Medicine" edited by James M. Rippe, M.D., 2016
3. "L-Arginine in Clinical Nutrition" edited by Vinood B. Patel, Victor R. Preedy, Rajkumar Rajendram, 2016
4. "Mediterranean Diet: Impact on Health and Disease" edited by Donato F. Romagnolo, Ph.D. and Ornella Selmin, Ph.D., 2016
5. "Nutrition Support for the Critically Ill" edited by David S. Seres, M.D., and Charles W. Van Way, III, MD, 2016
6. "Nutrition in Cystic Fibrosis: A Guide for Clinicians", edited by Elizabeth H. Yen, M.D. and Amanda R. Leonard, MPH, RD, CDE, 2016
7. "Preventive Nutrition: The Comprehensive Guide For Health Professionals, Fifth Edition", edited by Adrianne Bendich, Ph.D. and Richard J. Deckelbaum, M.D., 2016
8. "Glutamine in Clinical Nutrition", edited by Rajkumar Rajendram, Victor R. Preedy and Vinood B. Patel, 2015
9. "Nutrition and Bone Health, Second Edition", edited by Michael F. Holick and Jeri W. Nieves, 2015
10. "Branched Chain Amino Acids in Clinical Nutrition, Volume 2", edited by Rajkumar Rajendram, Victor R. Preedy and Vinood B. Patel, 2015
11. "Branched Chain Amino Acids in Clinical Nutrition, Volume 1", edited by Rajkumar Rajendram, Victor R. Preedy and Vinood B. Patel, 2015
12. "Fructose, High Fructose Corn Syrup, Sucrose and Health", edited by James M. Rippe, 2014
13. "Handbook of Clinical Nutrition and Aging, Third Edition", edited by Connie Watkins Bales, Julie L. Locher and Edward Saltzman, 2014

14. "Nutrition and Pediatric Pulmonary Disease", edited by Dr. Youngran Chung and Dr. Robert Dumont, 2014
15. "Integrative Weight Management" edited by Dr. Gerald E. Mullin, Dr. Lawrence J. Cheskin and Dr. Laura E. Matarese, 2014
16. "Nutrition in Kidney Disease, Second Edition" edited by Dr. Laura D. Byham-Gray, Dr. Jerrilynn D. Burrowes and Dr. Glenn M. Chertow, 2014
17. "Handbook of Food Fortification and Health, volume I" edited by Dr. Victor R. Preedy, Dr. Rajaventhan Srirajaskanthan, Dr. Vinood B. Patel, 2013
18. "Handbook of Food Fortification and Health, volume II" edited by Dr. Victor R. Preedy, Dr. Rajaventhan Srirajaskanthan, Dr. Vinood B. Patel, 2013
19. "Diet Quality: An Evidence-Based Approach", volume I edited by Dr. Victor R. Preedy, Dr. Lan-Ahn Hunter and Dr. Vinood B. Patel, 2013
20. "Diet Quality: An Evidence-Based Approach", volume II edited by Dr. Victor R. Preedy, Dr. Lan-Ahn Hunter and Dr. Vinood B. Patel, 2013
21. "The Handbook of Clinical Nutrition and Stroke", edited by Mandy L. Corrigan, MPH, RD Arlene A. Escuro, MS, RD, and Donald F. Kirby, MD, FACP, FACN, FACG, 2013
22. "Nutrition in Infancy, volume I" edited by Dr. Ronald Ross Watson, Dr. George Grimble, Dr. Victor Preedy and Dr. Sherma Zibadi, 2013
23. "Nutrition in Infancy, volume II" edited by Dr. Ronald Ross Watson, Dr. George Grimble, Dr. Victor Preedy and Dr. Sherma Zibadi, 2013
24. "Carotenoids and Human Health", edited by Dr. Sherry A. Tanumihardjo, 2013
25. "Bioactive Dietary Factors and Plant Extracts in Dermatology", edited by Dr. Ronald Ross Watson and Dr. Sherma Zibadi, 2013
26. "Omega 6/3 Fatty Acids", edited by Dr. Fabien De Meester, Dr. Ronald Ross Watson and Dr. Sherma Zibadi, 2013
27. "Nutrition in Pediatric Pulmonary Disease", edited by Dr. Robert Dumont and Dr. Youngran Chung, 2013
28. "Magnesium and Health", edited by Dr. Ronald Ross Watson and Dr. Victor R. Preedy, 2012.
29. "Alcohol, Nutrition and Health Consequences", edited by Dr. Ronald Ross Watson, Dr. Victor R. Preedy, and Dr. Sherma Zibadi, 2012
30. "Nutritional Health, Strategies for Disease Prevention, Third Edition", edited by Norman J. Temple, Ted Wilson, and David R. Jacobs, Jr., 2012
31. "Chocolate in Health and Nutrition", edited by Dr. Ronald Ross Watson, Dr. Victor R. Preedy, and Dr. Sherma Zibadi, 2012
32. "Iron Physiology and Pathophysiology in Humans", edited by Dr. Gregory J. Anderson and Dr. Gordon D. McLaren, 2012

Earlier books included "Vitamin D, Second Edition" edited by Dr. Michael Holick; "Dietary Components and Immune Function" edited by Dr. Ronald Ross Watson, Dr. Sherma Zibadi and Dr. Victor R. Preedy; "Bioactive Compounds and Cancer" edited by Dr. John A. Milner and Dr. Donato F. Romagnolo; "Modern Dietary Fat Intakes in Disease Promotion" edited by Dr. Fabien De Meester, Dr. Sherma Zibadi, and Dr. Ronald Ross Watson; "Iron Deficiency and Overload" edited by Dr. Shlomo Yehuda and Dr. David Mostofsky; "Nutrition Guide for Physicians" edited by Dr. Edward Wilson, Dr. George A. Bray, Dr. Norman Temple and Dr. Mary Struble; "Nutrition and Metabolism" edited by Dr. Christos Mantzoros and "Fluid and Electrolytes in Pediatrics" edited by Leonard Feld and Dr. Frederick Kaskel. Recent volumes include: "Handbook of Drug-Nutrient Interactions" edited by Dr. Joseph Boullata and Dr. Vincent Armenti; "Probiotics in Pediatric Medicine" edited by Dr. Sonia Michail and Dr. Philip Sherman; "Handbook of Nutrition and Pregnancy" edited by Dr. Carol Lammi-Keefe, Dr. Sarah Couch and Dr. Elliot Philipson; "Nutrition and Rheumatic Disease" edited by Dr. Laura Coleman; "Nutrition and Kidney Disease" edited by

Dr. Laura Byham-Grey, Dr. Jerrilynn Burrowes and Dr. Glenn Chertow; "Nutrition and Health in Developing Countries" edited by Dr. Richard Semba and Dr. Martin W. Bloem; "Calcium in Human Health" edited by Dr. Robert Heaney and Dr. Connie Weaver and "Nutrition and Bone Health" edited by Dr. Michael Holick and Dr. Bess Dawson-Hughes.

Dr. Bendich is President of Consultants in Consumer Healthcare LLC, and is the editor of ten books including "Preventive Nutrition: The Comprehensive Guide for Health Professionals, Fifth Edition" co-edited with Dr. Richard Deckelbaum (www.springer.com/series/7659). Dr. Bendich serves on the Editorial Boards of the Journal of Nutrition in Gerontology and Geriatrics, and Antioxidants, and has served as Associate Editor for "Nutrition" the International Journal; served on the Editorial Board of the Journal of Women's Health and Gender-based Medicine, and served on the Board of Directors of the American College of Nutrition.

Dr. Bendich was Director of Medical Affairs at GlaxoSmithKline (GSK) Consumer Healthcare and provided medical leadership for many well-known brands including TUMS and Os-Cal. Dr. Bendich had primary responsibility for GSK's support for the Women's Health Initiative (WHI) intervention study. Prior to joining GSK, Dr. Bendich was at Roche Vitamins Inc. and was involved with the groundbreaking clinical studies showing that folic acid-containing multivitamins significantly reduced major classes of birth defects. Dr. Bendich has co-authored over 100 major clinical research studies in the area of preventive nutrition. She is recognized as a leading authority on antioxidants, nutrition and immunity and pregnancy outcomes, vitamin safety and the cost-effectiveness of vitamin/mineral supplementation.

Dr. Bendich received the Roche Research Award, is a *Tribute to Women and Industry* Awardee and was a recipient of the Burroughs Wellcome Visiting Professorship in Basic Medical Sciences. Dr. Bendich was given the Council for Responsible Nutrition (CRN) Apple Award in recognition of her many contributions to the scientific understanding of dietary supplements. In 2012, she was recognized for her contributions to the field of clinical nutrition by the American Society for Nutrition and was elected a Fellow of ASN. Dr. Bendich is Adjunct Professor at Rutgers University. She is listed in Who's Who in American Women.

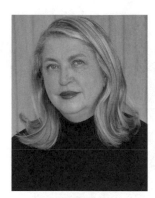

Connie W. Bales, Ph.D., R.D., is Professor of Medicine in the Division of Geriatrics, Department of Medicine, at the Duke School of Medicine and Senior Fellow in the Center for the Study of Aging and Human Development at Duke University Medical Center. She is also Associate Director for Education/Evaluation of the Geriatrics Research, Education, and Clinical Center at the Durham VA Medical Center. Dr. Bales is a well-recognized expert in the field of nutrition, chronic disease, function, and aging. Over the past two decades her laboratory at Duke has explored many different aspects of diet and activity as determinants of health during the latter half of the adult life course. Her current research focuses primarily on the impact of protein-enhanced meals on muscle quality, function, and other health indicators during obesity reduction in older adults with functional limitations. Dr. Bales has served on NIH and USDA grant review panels and is a member of the American Society for Nutrition's Medical Nutrition Council. Dr. Bales has edited three editions of the *Handbook of Clinical Nutrition in Aging* and is Editor-in-Chief of the *Journal of Nutrition in Gerontology and Geriatrics.*

About the Editors

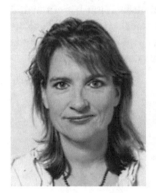

Dr. Saskia de Pee, Ph.D. has worked in public health nutrition for more than 20 years, focusing on science as well as practical applications, policies and strategies. Her areas of expertise include complementary feeding, micronutrients, fortification, food and nutrient security, nutrition in the context of social protection, HIV/AIDS and tuberculosis, and 'evidence for nutrition'. She works for the Nutrition Division of the United Nations World Food Programme (WFP), is Adjunct Associate Professor at the Friedman School of Nutrition Science and Policy, Tufts University, Boston and co-editor of the third edition of Nutrition and Health in a Developing World (in press). Prior to joining WFP in 2007 she worked for Helen Keller International in the Asia Pacific region for 10 years. She has co-authored more than 150 scientific publications and holds a Ph.D. in Nutrition from Wageningen University, the Netherlands.

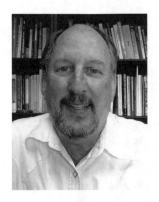

Dr. Douglas Taren, Ph.D. has 30 years of experience conducting research and developing educational programs in low- and middle-income countries. He has directed several graduate and post-graduate level training programs in colleges of medicine and public health. He has worked extensively on local food systems, the prevention of HIV transmission, infant growth, and maternal and child health. He has led studies using a variety of nutritional assessment methods and survey techniques as part of clinical and epidemiological studies. He has served as a resource person for the World Health Organization Nutrition Guidance Expert Advisory Group Monitoring and Evaluation Subgroup, and the United States (US) Centers for Disease Control and Prevention. He has evaluated food aid programs for the United Nations World Food Programme and the US Agency for International Development. His research and teaching have included field work in Latin America, Africa and South Asia. Dr. Taren received his BS (microbiology) and MS (nutritional sciences) from the University of Arizona and his Ph.D. (international nutrition) from Cornell University. He is the Associate Dean for Academic Affairs and Professor of Public Health at the University of Arizona Mel and Enid Zuckerman College of Public Health and the Director of the Western Region Public Health Training

Center that includes the six US Associated Pacific Islands. He resides in Tucson, Arizona, a UNESCO City of Gastronomy.

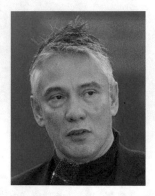

Dr. Martin W. Bloem, M.D., Ph.D. is the Senior Nutrition Advisor and Global Coordinator HIV/AIDS at the United Nations World Food Programme, in Rome, Italy. He holds a medical degree from the University of Utrecht and a doctorate from the University of Maastricht and has joint faculty appointments at both Johns Hopkins University and Tufts University. Martin has more than two decades of experience in nutrition research and policy. He was the Senior Vice President Chief Medical Officer of Helen Keller International prior to his appointment at the World Food Programme. Martin has devoted his career to improving the effectiveness of public health and nutrition programs through applied research. He has participated in task forces convened by many organizations, including Columbia University, international non-governmental organizations, the Scaling Up Nutrition Movement, the United Nations Children's Fund (UNICEF), the United States Agency for International Development (USAID), and the World Health Organization (WHO).

Contents

Part I   History of Nutrition

1   **Nutrition and Development: A Historical Perspective**   3
    Richard D. Semba

**Part II   Contextualizing International Nutrition—Considering Benefit-Cost,
            Evidence-Base and Capacity**

2   **Economics of Nutritional Interventions**   33
    Susan Horton

3   **Nutrition Evidence in Context**   47
    Saskia de Pee and Rebecca F. Grais

4   **Developing Capacity in Nutrition**   67
    Jessica C. Fanzo and Matthew M. Graziose

Part III   Malnutrition, Nutrients and (Breast)Milk Explained

5   **The Spectrum of Malnutrition**   91
    Douglas Taren and Saskia de Pee

6   **Child Growth and Development**   119
    Mercedes de Onis

7   **Overweight and Obesity**   143
    Colleen M. Doak and Barry M. Popkin

8   **Nutrient Needs and Approaches to Meeting Them**   159
    Saskia de Pee

9   **Vitamin A Deficiency**   181
    Amanda C. Palmer, Ian Darnton-Hill and Keith P. West, Jr.

10 **Iron**   235
    Melissa Fox Young and Usha Ramakrishnan

11 **Zinc Deficiency**   265
    Sonja Y. Hess

12 **Iodine**   287
    Michael B. Zimmermann

13 **Nutritional Rickets and Vitamin D Deficiency** 297
    John M. Pettifor and Kebashni Thandrayen

14 **Essential Fatty Acids** 321
    Esther Granot and Richard J. Deckelbaum

15 **The Role of Human and Other Milks in Preventing and Treating
    Undernutrition** 337
    Benedikte Grenov, Henrik Friis, Christian Mølgaard and Kim Fleischer Michaelsen

16 **The Role of Breastfeeding Protection, Promotion and Support
    in a Developing World** 361
    Douglas Taren and Chessa K. Lutter

Part IV   Tuberculosis, HIV and the Role of Nutrition

17 **Tuberculosis** 385
    Eyal Oren and Joann M. McDermid

18 **HIV—Medical Perspective** 413
    Louise C. Ivers and Daniel Duré

19 **Tuberculosis Infection and Nutrition** 437
    Anupama Paranandi and Christine Wanke

20 **HIV and HIV/TB Co-infection in Relation to Nutrition** 449
    Anupama Paranandi and Christine Wanke

Part V   Nutrition and Health in Different Phases of the Lifecycle

21 **Reproductive Health and Nutrition** 469
    Satvika Chalasani and Nuriye Ortayli

22 **Maternal Nutrition and Birth Outcomes** 487
    Usha Ramakrishnan, Melissa Fox Young and Reynaldo Martorell

23 **Small for Gestational Age: Scale and Consequences for Mortality,
    Morbidity, and Development** 503
    Ines Gonzalez-Casanova, Usha Ramakrishnan and Reynaldo Martorell

24 **Developmental Disabilities** 523
    Burris R. Duncan, Jennifer G. Andrews, Heidi L. Pottinger and F. John Meaney

25 **Adolescent Health and Nutrition** 559
    Jee Hyun Rah, Satvika Chalasani, Vanessa M. Oddo and Vani Sethi

26 **Nutrition in the Elderly from Low- and Middle-Income Countries** 579
    Noel W. Solomons and Odilia I. Bermudez

**Part VI   Tackling Health and Nutrition Issues in an Integrated Way
            in the Era of the SDGs**

27 **Evaluation of Nutrition-sensitive Programs** 603
    Deanna K. Olney, Jef L. Leroy and Marie T. Ruel

28 **Integrated Approaches to Health and Nutrition: Role of Communities** 625
    Olivia Lange, Divya Mehra, Saskia de Pee and Martin W. Bloem

29 Nutrition in Humanitarian Crises 647
Lynnda Kiess, Natalie Aldern, Saskia de Pee and Martin W. Bloem

30 Ending AIDS by 2030: Partnerships and Linkages with SDG 2 665
Divya Mehra, Saskia de Pee and Martin W. Bloem

**Part VII   Trends in Urbanization and Development, Impacts on Food Value
                Chains and Consumers, and Private Sector Roles**

**31 How Urbanization Patterns Can Guide Strategies for Achieving Adequate
      Nutrition** 685
Sunniva Bloem and Saskia de Pee

32 Urbanization, Food Security and Nutrition 705
Marie T. Ruel, James Garrett, Sivan Yosef and Meghan Olivier

**33 The Impact of Supermarkets on Nutrition and Nutritional Knowledge:
      A Food Policy Perspective** 737
C. Peter Timmer

34 Value Chain Focus on Food and Nutrition Security 753
Jessica C. Fanzo, Shauna Downs, Quinn E. Marshall, Saskia de Pee
and Martin W. Bloem

**35 Role of Foundations and Initiatives by the Private Sector for Improving
      Health and Nutrition** 771
Kalpana Beesabathuni, Kesso Gabrielle van Zutphen and Klaus Kraemer

Part VIII   Ethics—Critical to Making Progress in Public Health

36 Ethics in Public Health Research 793
Tanya Doherty and Mickey Chopra

Index 809

Contributors

Natalie Aldern Nutrition Division, World Food Programme, Rome, Italy

Jennifer G. Andrews Department of Pediatrics, University of Arizona, Tucson, AZ, USA

Kalpana Beesabathuni Gurgaon, Haryana, India

Odilia I. Bermudez Public Health and Community Medicine, Tufts University, Boston, MA, USA

Martin W. Bloem Nutrition Division, World Food Programme, Rome, Italy; Department of International Health, Bloomberg School of Public Health, Johns Hopkins University, Baltimore, MD, USA; Friedman School of Nutrition Science and Policy, Tufts University, Boston, MA, USA

Sunniva Bloem The Global Alliance for Improved Nutrition (GAIN), Utrecht, The Netherlands

Satvika Chalasani Technical Division, United Nations Population Fund, New York, NY, USA; Sexual and Reproductive Health Branch, Technical Division, United Nations Population Fund, New York, NY, USA

Mickey Chopra World Bank, Washington, DC, USA

Ian Darnton-Hill Institute of Obesity, Nutrition & Exercise, University of Sydney, Sydney, NSW, Australia

Mercedes de Onis Department of Nutrition, World Health Organization, Geneva, Switzerland

Saskia de Pee Nutrition Division, World Food Programme, Rome, Italy; Friedman School of Nutrition Science and Policy, Tufts University, Boston, MA, USA

Richard J. Deckelbaum Institute of Human Nutrition, Departments of Pediatrics and Epidemiology, Columbia University Medical Center, New York, USA

Colleen M. Doak Department of Health Sciences, VU University, Amsterdam, The Netherlands

Tanya Doherty Health Systems Research Unit, South African Medical Research Council, Parow, Cape Town, South Africa

Shauna Downs Berman Institute of Bioethics, Johns Hopkins University, Baltimore, MD, USA

Burris R. Duncan Health Promotion Sciences, Mel & Enid Zuckerman College of Public Health, University of Arizona Health Sciences Center, Tucson, AZ, USA

Daniel Duré Medical Education and Infectious Disease, Mirebalais Teaching Hospital (HUM), Mirebalais, Plateau Central, Haiti

Jessica C. Fanzo Berman Institute of Bioethics and School of Advanced International Studies, Johns Hopkins University, Washington, DC, USA

Henrik Friis Department of Nutrition, Exercise and Sports, Science, University of Copenhagen, Frederiksberg, Copenhagen, Denmark

James Garrett Bioversity International, Maccarese, Italy

Ines Gonzalez-Casanova Department of Global Health, Emory University, Atlanta, GA, USA

Rebecca F. Grais Epicentre (Medecins sans Frontieres), Paris, France

Esther Granot Department of Pediatrics, Kaplan Medical Center, Rehovot, Hebrew University— Hadassah Medical School, Jerusalem, Israel

Matthew M. Graziose Health and Behavior Studies, Teachers College Columbia University, New York, NY, USA

Benedikte Grenov Department of Nutrition, Exercise and Sports, Science, University of Copenhagen, Frederiksberg, Copenhagen, Denmark

Sonja Y. Hess Nutrition Department, University of California Davis, Davis, CA, USA

Susan Horton Balsillie School of International Affairs, University of Waterloo, Waterloo, ON, Canada

Louise C. Ivers Department of Global Health and Social Medicine, Harvard Medical School, Brigham and Women's Hospital, Boston, MA, USA

F. John Meaney Department of Pediatrics, University of Arizona, Tucson, AZ, USA

Lynnda Kiess Nutrition Division, World Food Programme, Rome, Italy

Klaus Kraemer Basel, Switzerland

Olivia Lange Nutrition Division, World Food Programme, Rome, Italy

Jef L. Leroy Poverty, Health and Nutrition Division, International Food Policy Research Institute (IFPRI), Washington, DC, USA

Chessa K. Lutter Food and Nutrition, Non-Communicable Diseases and Mental Health, Pan American Health Organization, Washington, DC, USA

Quinn E. Marshall Nutrition Division, World Food Programme, Rome, Italy

Reynaldo Martorell Hubert Department of Global Health, Rollins School of Public Health, Emory University, Atlanta, GA, USA; Nutrition & Health Sciences Program, Graduate Division of Biological & Biomedical Sciences, Emory University, Atlanta, GA, USA

Joann M. McDermid Department of Medicine, Division of Infectious Diseases and International Health, School of Medicine, University of Virginia, Charlottesville, VA, USA

Divya Mehra Nutrition Division, World Food Programme, Rome, Italy

Kim Fleischer Michaelsen Department of Nutrition, Exercise and Sports, Science, University of Copenhagen, Frederiksberg, Copenhagen, Denmark

Christian Mølgaard Department of Nutrition, Exercise and Sports, Science, University of Copenhagen, Frederiksberg, Copenhagen, Denmark

Vanessa M. Oddo International Health, Johns Hopkins Bloomberg School of Public Health, Baltimore, MD, USA

Meghan Olivier Poverty, Health and Nutrition Division, International Food Policy Research Institute, Washington, DC, USA

Deanna K. Olney Poverty, Health and Nutrition Division, International Food Policy Research Institute (IFPRI), Washington, DC, USA

Eyal Oren Department of Epidemiology and Biostatistics, Mel & Enid Zuckerman College of Public Health, University of Arizona, Tucson, AZ, USA

Nuriye Ortayli Technical Division, United Nations Population Fund, New York, NY, USA

Amanda C. Palmer Department of International Health, Johns Hopkins University, Baltimore, MD, USA

Anupama Paranandi Department of Medicine, Saint Mary's Hospital, Waterbury, CT, USA

John M. Pettifor MRC/Wits Developmental Pathways for Health Research Unit, Department of Paediatrics, Faculty of Health Sciences, University of the Witwatersrand, Johannesburg, South Africa

Barry M. Popkin Department of Nutrition, University of North Carolina at Chapel Hill, Chapel Hill, NC, USA

Heidi L. Pottinger Health Promotion Sciences, Mel & Enid Zuckerman College of Public Health, Tucson, AZ, USA

Jee Hyun Rah Child Development and Nutrition, UNICEF India Country Office, New Delhi, India

Usha Ramakrishnan Hubert Department of Global Health, Rollins School of Public Health, Emory University, Atlanta, GA, USA; Nutrition & Health Sciences Program, Graduate Division of Biological & Biomedical Sciences, Emory University, Atlanta, GA, USA

Marie T. Ruel Poverty, Health and Nutrition Division, International Food Policy Research Institute (IFPRI), Washington, DC, USA

Richard D. Semba Johns Hopkins University School of Medicine, Baltimore, MD, USA

Vani Sethi Child Development and Nutrition, UNICEF India Country Office, New Delhi, India

Noel W. Solomons Center for Studies of Sensory Impairment, Aging and Metabolism (CeSSIAM), Guatemala City, Guatemala

Douglas Taren Mel and Enid Zuckerman College of Public Health, University of Arizona, Tucson, AZ, USA

Kebashni Thandrayen Department of Paediatrics, Chris Hani Baragwanath Academic Hospital, Faculty of Health Sciences, University of the Witwatersrand, Johannesburg, Gauteng, South Africa

C. Peter Timmer Economics, Harvard University, Kenwood, CA, USA

Kesso Gabrielle van Zutphen Geneva, Switzerland

Christine Wanke Medicine/Infectious Diseases, Tufts Medical Center, Boston, MA, USA

Keith P. West Jr. Department of International Health, Johns Hopkins University, Baltimore, MD, USA

Sivan Yosef International Food Policy Research Institute, Washington, DC, USA

Melissa Fox Young Hubert Department of Global Health, Rollins School of Public Health, Emory University, Atlanta, GA, USA; Nutrition & Health Sciences Program, Graduate Division of Biological & Biomedical Sciences, Emory University, Atlanta, GA, USA

Michael B. Zimmermann Department of Health Sciences and Technology, ETH Zurich, Zurich, Switzerland

Part I
History of Nutrition

Chapter 1
Nutrition and Development: A Historical Perspective

Richard D. Semba

Keywords Diet · Hygiene · Infectious diseases · Nutritional deficiencies · Public health

Learning Objectives

- The idea of progress in public health has its roots in the French Enlightenment. French scientists conducted early work on preventive medicine and public health and demonstrated the relationship of social disparities with mortality in Paris.
- Infectious diseases such as malaria, yellow fever, tuberculosis, and cholera, and nutritional deficiencies such as rickets, pellagra, goiter/cretinism, and nutritional blindness, were major diseases in Europe, Great Britain, and the United States during the nineteenth century.
- In nutrition, the first half of the twentieth century was focused on the characterization of the vitamins, followed by two decades of emphasis on protein malnutrition. Under the assumption that children received enough protein and only needed more energy, much protein work was abandoned. The last four decades have focused mostly on micronutrient malnutrition.

Introduction

In the last two centuries, there has been a general improvement in the health of people worldwide that has been attributed largely to changes in nutrition, hygiene, and public health. At the beginning of the nineteenth century, the burden of morbidity and mortality from infectious diseases such as malaria, cholera, measles, tuberculosis, and diarrheal disease, and nutritional deficiency diseases such as pellagra, rickets, and vitamin A deficiency, were relatively high in Europe, North America, and much of the rest of world. By the end of the twentieth century, these diseases were largely eradicated from industrialized countries, but many of these diseases and their associated morbidity and mortality continue to be major problems in developing countries today. Mortality rates from infectious diseases have generally been declining in industrialized countries over the last 200 years, and improved nutrition and resistance to disease as well as better hygiene and sanitation have been cited as the main factors for a reduction in infectious disease mortality rather than technological advances in medicine [1–4].

R.D. Semba (✉)
Johns Hopkins University School of Medicine, 400 N. Broadway, M015, Baltimore, MD 21287, USA
e-mail: rdsemba@jhmi.edu

© Springer Science+Business Media New York 2017
S. de Pee et al. (eds.), *Nutrition and Health in a Developing World*,
Nutrition and Health, DOI 10.1007/978-3-319-43739-2_1

The purpose of this chapter is to provide a brief historical overview of major ideas and events that have shaped public health over the last two centuries, with an emphasis on developments related to nutrition and infectious disease. As a concise review, this chapter is limited to selected highlights from the last 200 years, and for a more detailed overview, the reader is referred to general texts on the history of public health [5–7], medicine [8], infectious disease [9, 10], and geographical medicine [11], as well as to more specialized sources dealing with protein and energy [12], scurvy [13], pellagra [14], food [15–17], and hunger [18]. Most of this review will focus on developments in Great Britain, the United States, and France, as these countries have drawn the most attention of historians of public health and nutrition.

The Idea of Progress in Public Health

The idea of progress in public health largely rose during the Enlightenment in France among the *philosophes* such as Denis Diderot (1713–1784) and Jean le Rond d'Alembert (1717–1783). Earlier antecedents were found in the methods of the French rationalist philosopher and mathematician René Descartes (1596–1650) [19]. Diderot and d'Alembert edited the monumental *Encyclopédie, ou Dictionnaire raisonné des sciences, des arts et des métiers*, which was published between 1751 and 1772. The *Encyclopédie*, a major work of the Enlightenment, was meant to benefit future generations with a compendium of human knowledge [20], and it included some issues relating to health, such as the duration of life, the health of infants, and growth of population.

One of the greatest *Encyclopedists* was Marie Jean Antoine Nicolas Caritat, Marquis de Condorcet (1743–1794), a French statesman, philosopher, and mathematician who wrote the *Esquisse d'un tableau historique des progrès de l'esprit humain* (*Sketch for a History of the Progress of the Human Mind*) [21]. A critic of Robespierre and the Jacobins, Condorcet had been accused of treason and was sentenced *in absentia* to the guillotine. During a period of hiding in Paris in 1792, Condorcet wrote the remarkable *Esquisse* in which he argued for the infinite perfectability of man. Condorcet predicted that there would be equality between men and women, the abolition of war, the end of colonialism and the slave trade, more equal distribution of wealth, and the eradication of disease through progress in medical science [21]:

> No one can doubt that, as preventive medicine improves and food and housing become healthier, as a way of life is established that develops our physical powers by exercise without ruining them by excess, as the two most virulent causes of deterioration, misery and excessive wealth, are eliminated, the average length of human life will be increased and a better health and a stronger physical constitution will be ensured. The improvement of medical practice, which will become more efficacious with the progress of reason and of the social order, will mean the end of infectious and hereditary diseases and illnesses brought on by climate, food, or working conditions. It is reasonable to hope that all other diseases may likewise disappear as their distant causes are discovered [22].

Condorcet's work was published posthumously in 1795 and became a seminal work in the idea of progress in Western thought [19, 23].

The assumption that "the happiness of the human species is the most desirable object for human science to promote" was expressed by William Godwin (1756–1836) in *An Enquiry Concerning Political Justice, and Its Influence on General Virtue and Happiness* [24]. Godwin noted the vast inequality in property and the role of political institutions in favoring these conditions, and he envisioned a future where intellectual and moral improvement and reform of government would reduce inequality, war, and injustice. According to Godwin, the perfectability of man was intrinsic to the human species, and political and intellectual state of man was presumed to be in a course of progressive improvement.

Instead of indefinite progress, Thomas Robert Malthus (1766–1834), a British economist, predicted overpopulation, misery, famine, and war, and his views first appeared in an anonymous book, *An Essay on the Principle of Population, as It Affects the Future Improvement of Society, with Remarks on the Speculations of Mr. Godwin, M. Condorcet, and Other Writers*, which was published in 1798 [25]. Malthus believed that the population was growing greater than the ability of the earth to provide subsistence. Preventive checks upon population included moral restraint, such as the postponement of marriage and avoidance of extramarital relationships. Later, Malthus was to concede that more personal and social action could prevent much of the grim scenario that he had predicted, and the debate about Malthus is frequently revived [26].

A central idea of social medicine—an outgrowth of Enlightenment thought—was that government could use medical knowledge to improve the health of the people. A comprehensive social medicine approach was described by Johann Peter Frank (1745–1821), a German physician, in *System einer vollständigen medicinischen Polizey* (*A System of Complete Medical Police*) [27]. Frank's recommendations for sanitary, social, and economic reforms were broad, and based on the idea that medical police, a benevolent form of despotism, could provide for the health and protection of the people from cradle to grave. Frank was Director General of Public Health of Austrian Lombardy and Professor of Clinical Medicine at the University of Padua, and his social concerns are clearly stated in his graduation address *De populorum miseria: morborum genitrice* (*The People's Misery: Mother of Diseases*) in 1790:

> Starvation and sickness are pictured on the face of the entire laboring class. You recognize it at first sight. And whoever has seen it will certainly not call any one of these people a free man. The word has become meaningless. Before sunrise, after having eaten a little and always the same unfermented bread that appeases his hunger only half- way, the farmer gets ready for hard work. With emaciated body under the hot rays of the sun he plows a soil that is not his and cultivates a vine that for him alone has no reward. His arms fall down, his dry tongue sticks to the palate, hunger is consuming him. The poor man can look forward to only a few grains of rice and a few beans soaked in water. And to this he can add only very sparingly the condiment with which nature has provided mankind in such a liberal way...

> Scarcity of food, however, and a quality of food that has no nutritional value make the citizens physically unfit for any sustained effort and predispose them for catching any matter of diseases. The weaker the organism and the more exhausted from troubles the human machine is, the sooner miasmas and contagions penetrate it like a dry sponge. Hence famine—sterility of the fields increased under an unfortunate constellation—is immediately followed by epidemics in the provinces [28].

Among the myriad recommendations made by Frank in the *System* were that wells and springs used by the public should be examined regularly, and that rivers and ponds be kept clean and protected against sewage, industrial discharges, and refuse. The medical police were to be responsible for ensuring that an abundant and pure food supply was available, and observations were to be made whether certain kinds of foods eaten by different classes might predispose to serious ills or greater mortality. Frank also emphasized the importance of breastfeeding of infants. Although Frank's work on "medical police" was considered somewhat outmoded by the time it was completely published, it was influential in setting a standard for broad approaches to public health [29].

The underlying theme of this book—nutrition and health in a developing world—implies the prevailing model for development, where knowledge is cumulative and progress in nutrition and health generally proceeds in a linear fashion where the world is destined for improved nutrition, better health, more equity, and greater justice. Such precepts are implicit in the mission of large organizations such as the United Nations Children's Fund, the World Health Organization, the United States Agency for International Development, the Overseas Development Agency, the World Bank, and the Food and Agricultural Organization.

The Rise of Statistics and Probability

The importance of keeping statistical records of health problems, including births, deaths, and other statistics relating to population, was emphasized by William Petty (1623–1687), an economist and physician, and John Graunt (1620–1674), a merchant, in England [30, 31]. In this early work on vital statistics, Graunt used detailed parish records to show the major causes of death, that mortality rates were higher in urban than rural areas, that more boys are born than girls, and that death rates varied by season [32]. Early attempts to enumerate all births and deaths and determine total population were undertaken in Sweden in the middle of the eighteenth century, and other efforts were made in France and Holland [33]. The use of "political arithmetic," or "the art of reasoning by figures upon things relating to government" [34], continued into the nineteenth century.

By 1836 the registration of births, marriages, and deaths had been made compulsory in England, and William Farr (1807–1883), a physician and compiler of abstracts in the Registrar General's office, became an advocate for social reform using statistics. Farr used life tables, an innovation introduced by the English astronomer Edmund Halley (1656–1742) [35], to show the relative health of districts, and infant mortality rates were used as a primary indicator of health [36]. Better statistics would help improve health and assist in the efforts of preventive medicine, and Farr assigned a greater role in public health to physicians [37]:

> It has been shown that external agents have as great an influence on the frequency of sickness as on its fatality; the obvious corollary is, that man has as much power to prevent as to cure disease. That prevention is better than cure, is a proverb; that it is as easy, the facts we had advanced establish. Yet medical men, the guardians of public health, never have their attention called to the prevention of sickness; it forms no part of their education. To promote health is apparently contrary to their interests: the public do not seek the shield of medical art against disease, nor call the surgeon, till the arrows of death already rankle in the veins. This may be corrected by modifying the present system of medical education, and the manner of remunerating medical men.

> Public health may be promoted by placing the medical institutions of the country on a liberal scientific basis; by medical societies co-operating to collect statistical observations; and by medical writers renouncing the notion that a science can be founded upon the limited experience of an individual. Practical medicine cannot be taught in books; the science of medicine cannot be acquired in the sick room.

Vital statistics were also examined by Adolphe Quetelet (1796–1874), a Belgian astronomer and mathematician, who showed that the distribution of observations around a mean could be expressed as the distribution of probabilities on a probability curve. In *Sur l'homme et le développement de ses facultés, essai d'une physique sociale* (*On Man and the Development of his Faculties: An Essay on Social Physics*), Quetelet investigated different aspects of "social physics," such as birth and death, height and weight, and health and disease. In this work he elaborated the important concept that the average man, or *l'homme moyen*, could be expressed mathematically [38]. Statistics became the means to study the condition of the population, especially the working classes, and early Victorian Britain saw the formation of the Statistical Society of Manchester in 1833 and the Statistical Society of London in 1834 [39].

Modern mathematical statistics arose largely from biometry in the late nineteenth century [40]. Francis Galton (1822–1911), an English scientist and explorer of Africa, originated the concepts of regression and correlation, tools which were being developed to study heredity [41]. Karl Pearson (1857–1936), a statistician at University College, London, continued to study the concepts of variation, correlation, and probability, and he introduced the term "standard deviation" in 1893 and defined the correlation coefficient mathematically in 1896 [42]. Other important developments in statistics were the chi-square test in 1900, and the t-test and its distribution was defined by W.S. Gosset (Student) in 1908 [43]. Analysis of variance derives from a paper by Ronald A. Fisher (1890–1962), a British geneticist and statistician, in 1918. An important development in statistical methods was the integration of statistics with experimental design in *The Design of Experiments* by Fisher, in which the idea of randomization was promoted in experimental design [44]. The idea of alternative hypotheses and two types of error was developed in the late 1920s [45] and was important in the determination of sample size and power calculations for experimental studies. The concepts of randomization, sample size and power, and placebo controls helped to refine the controlled clinical trial as the basis for scientific evaluation of new therapies [46].

Early Foundations of Preventive Medicine

The modern movement in preventive medicine and public health largely began in France in the first half of the nineteenth century, largely inspired by the Enlightenment approach to health and disease [47, 48]. Louis René Villermé (1782–1863) used a numerical approach to show that there was a large gap in health between the rich and poor. Villermé was a former French army surgeon who was familiar with the psychological and social consequences of famine during the war [49]. Shortly after leaving the military, Villermé showed in a large demographic study of Paris, *Recherches statistiques sur la ville de Paris* (*Statistical Researches in the City of Paris*), that mortality rates were highest in the poorest *arrondissements*, or districts, and lowest in the wealthy *arrondissements* [50]. Thus, the differences between the rich and poor clearly extended far beyond financial position into matters of life and death. Louis François Benoiston de Châteauneuf (1776–1862), a physician and contemporary of Villermé, showed that there were large differences in diet in Paris [51], and the differences in diet became incorporated into sociomedical investigations of mortality [52]. According to Villermé [53], famine was followed by epidemics, and the poor were always hit the hardest by hunger and epidemics. He argued that a high state of civilization reduces epidemics and called for reforms so that people would be protected against the high price of food, which, for the poor, meant the same as famine. Some of Villermé's and Benoiston's work appeared in France's first journal of public health, *Annales d'hygiène publique et de médecine légale*, founded in 1829. In 1840, the appalling health conditions of textile workers were reported by Villermé [54], leading to a law the following year limiting child labor in France.

In the kingdom of Naples, an important early survey was conducted in 1811 by the government of Joachim Murat (1767–1815) that addressed the relationship between nutrition and disease [55, 56]. In 1765, one year after a terrible famine killed thousands in the kingdom of Naples, Antonio Genovesi (1713–1769), a local leader of the Enlightenment, expressed the proto-Malthusian idea that an equilibrium exists between the population of the state and the availability of resources [57]. An attempt was made to address such a relationship in a survey, which showed that there was widespread nutritional deprivation in the kingdom, especially in rural areas. In one area, famine was so common it was said that "*tanto li contadini che li artieri pria degli occhi, aprono la bocca* (*upon awakening peasants and workers alike open their mouths before they open their eyes*)." This survey was an early analysis of the mutual relationships among environmental, social variables, nutrition, and public health, and nutritional deprivation was identified as a main factor predisposing to disease [56].

The Sanitary Idea

During the early industrialization of England, Jeremy Bentham (1748–1832), a writer on jurisprudence and utilitarian ethics, expressed the belief that laws should be socially useful and that actions should support "the happiness of the greatest number" [58]. Edwin Chadwick (1800–1890), a follower of Bentham, became Secretary of the Royal Commission to investigate the Elizabethan Poor Laws, legislation from the early seventeenth century in which relief for the indigent was to be provided by the local parish, and employment of the poor was provided by workhouses. As the population grew, the problems of urban overcrowding and deterioration of food, sanitation, and housing became a major crisis by the nineteenth century. In 1842, Chadwick published *Report on the Sanitary Condition of the Labouring Population of Great Britain* which described the unsanitary living conditions among the poor [59]. As in Villermé's report, higher mortality was shown among the poorer classes than among the wealthy classes. The report recommended that the highest priority be given to practical measures such as drainage, removal of refuse, and improvement in the water supply, and it was emphasized that much disease among the poor could be prevented by public health measures. As Chadwick put it, "...*all* smell is disease" [60]. Legislation followed in the wake of the report, including the British Public Health Act (1848), which established a general board of health, and legislation aimed at food adulteration, regulation of slaughterhouses and other trades, water supplies, and sewers.

The sanitary movement in the United States largely echoed the efforts in France and England. In 1850 a major plan for public health, *Report of the Sanitary Commission of Massachusetts*, was presented to the government of Massachusetts State by Lemuel Shattuck (1793–1859), a teacher, bookseller, and genealogist [61]. The report reviewed the sanitary movement abroad and in the United States, disease in the state of Massachusetts, and made recommendations for promotion of public health through creation of state and local boards of health, conduct of a regular census, better collection of vital statistics, improved sanitation, water, and housing, and other measures. The main basis for the report was that "...measures for prevention will effect infinitely more, than remedies for the cure of disease." Although Shattuck was unable to have many of the recommendations enacted into law immediately, the report was a harbinger for a comprehensive public health policy in the United States.

The first census in the United States by the federal government took place in 1790, and a nationwide census was decreed in the constitution to occur every 10 years [62]. In Great Britain the first nationwide census was undertaken in 1801, and periodic national censuses gained authority in France after 1840 [52]. National registration systems and their vital statistics were used to bring attention to problems in public health in Europe, Great Britain, and the United States, and a greater need for accurate statistics was noted after the arrival of the worldwide cholera pandemics in the mid-nineteenth century [63].

Contagion Versus Miasma

By the nineteenth century, epidemics of plague were gone from Europe, but other epidemic diseases such as scarlet fever, typhoid, typhus, and measles continued in outbreaks. Malaria was present in both Europe and the United States, and yellow fever was present in the south of the United States. Great pandemics of cholera swept large parts of the world in dates approximating 1817–1823, 1826–1837, 1846–1863, 1865–1875 [64], and later. The theory that epidemic disease was caused by miasmas rising from decaying organic matter was a dominant belief in the middle of the nineteenth century and a strong impetus behind the reforms of the sanitarians [6, 9]. Another major theory of epidemic disease was the contagionist theory in which an animate organism caused disease and was spread by person-to-person contact [65, 66]. Further credence to the contagionist theory was provided by epidemiological studies of measles, cholera, diphtheria, and typhoid fever.

A measles epidemic affected the Faroe Islands in 1846, and a medical commission was sent by the Danish government to investigate. The commission included two Danish physicians who had just finished medical school, 26-year-old Peter Ludwig Panum (1820–1885) and 25-year-old August Henrik Manicus (1821–1850). In what is considered a classic study in epidemiology [9], Panum described the incubation period of measles and noted that transmission of measles was through person-to-person contact [67]. He noted that measles attacked individuals of all ages, but those with a history of a previous attack of measles from a previous epidemic in 1781 were immune. Manicus observed that mortality was highest in a village that had the greatest poverty and poor diet, and he noted that diarrheal disease was mild among well-to-do islanders but was severe and persistent in the poorer villages [68]. Both Panum and Manicus concluded that measles was contagious and not miasmatic in origin.

Other studies that further may have changed perceptions about the contagiousness of disease were an investigation of cholera in London by John Snow (1813–1858), an English physician and anesthetist [69], and investigations of cholera by William Budd (1811–1880), a physician in Bristol. Budd thought that cholera was caused by a specific living organism that was found in the human intestinal tract and was spread through contaminated drinking water [70]. During the cholera epidemic of 1854 in London, Snow demonstrated that the number of deaths from cholera was related to the amount of pollution from the Thames River among the different private companies supplying drinking water. Nearly, all the victims had used water from the Broad Street pump in Soho. Snow concluded that cholera was carried in water contaminated by excreta of cholera patients, and that cholera was transmitted by ingestion of contaminated water and food and not through miasmata. Snow persuaded the local authorities to remove the handle from the Broad Street pump—presumably averting further deaths—but the epidemic was already in decline.

The contamination of the Thames by sewage and industrial waste was acknowledged by a London Commission in 1828 and became the subject of satire (Fig. 1.1). The Metropolis Water Act of 1852 required London water companies to draw their water supplies from cleaner nontidal reaches of the Thames and to filter all water supplies for domestic use [71], and the cholera outbreak of 1854 occurred before all companies could comply with the 1852 act. The findings of Snow and Budd regarding the contagious nature of cholera did not lead to a sudden revolution in water science as has been generally believed [72, 73], but these studies gave additional weight to the contagion theory. In the ensuing years, many international experts continued to hang on to the idea that miasmas were the cause of cholera [74]. Other detailed investigations that reinforced the contagion theory of epidemic disease were those of diphtheria by Pierre Fidèle Bretonneau (1778–1862), a physician in Tours, France [75], and of typhoid fever by William Budd [76].

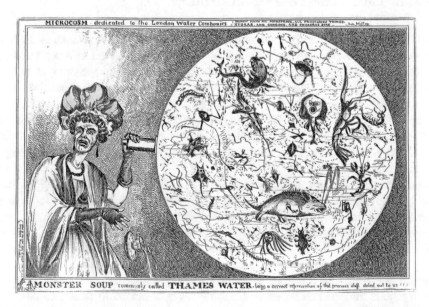

Fig. 1.1 A Monster soup commonly called Thames Water, by William Heath (1795–1840), circa 1828. Gift of Mrs. William Horstmann to Philadelphia Museum of Art, Object Number 1955-103-4, public domain

Advances in Microbiology

Further foundations for microbiological investigations were laid by Jacob Henle (1809–1885), a pathologist in Zurich, who thought that conclusive proof for an organism being responsible for a disease required three conditions: constant presence of the parasite, isolation from foreign admixtures, and reproduction of the disease with the isolated parasite [77]. These postulates were further developed by his student, Robert Koch (1843–1910) [78]. Louis Pasteur (1822–1895), a French chemist and microbiologist, further elaborated the germ theory of disease through broad studies that included the fermentation of beer and wine and diseases of silkworms. The last quarter of the nineteenth century was characterized by a rapid period of microbiological investigations, during which descriptions were made of the organisms responsible for anthrax [79], malaria [80], tuberculosis [81], and cholera [82]. Other organisms including streptococcus, staphylococcus, *Escherichia coli*, leprosy, diphtheria, and *Yersinia* were described, and investigation was facilitated by the development of new staining techniques and culture media [5, 65].

Strategies to control infectious diseases by the turn of the century included reporting of cases, isolation of affected individuals, and disinfection of the premises. Compulsory notification of infectious diseases was enacted in London, Berlin, and Paris within the last quarter of the nineteenth century [83]. The ways in which diseases could be transmitted through contaminated water, ice, milk, and uncooked food were outlined by William Sedgwick (1855–1921), a biologist [84]. In 1887, the first systematic monitoring of the public water supply in the United States was conducted by Sedgwick for the Massachusetts Board of Health, and his techniques for measurement and filtration of bacteria in the water supply became a standard for the country. In his influential treatise, *The Sources of Modes of Infection* [85], Charles V. Chapin (1856–1941), the Superintendent of Health in Providence, Rhode Island, emphasized the role of the carrier and further clarified the idea that diseases could be transmitted through lack of hygiene, by direct and indirect contact, by fomites, through the air, in food and drink, and by insects.

Nutritional Science in the Nineteenth Century

Modern nutritional science has early roots in experimental physiology in France at the beginning of the nineteenth century, when ideas surrounding nutrition were subjected to examination by animal experimentation [86]. François Magendie (1783–1855), professor of anatomy at the Collège de France, attempted to differentiate between various kinds of food and made a clear distinction between nitrogenous and non-nitrogenous foods [87]. In an early experiment that hinted at the existence of vitamin A, Magendie found that dogs fed only sugar and distilled water developed corneal ulcers and died [88]. The importance of nitrogenous foods was further recognized by Gerrit Jan Mulder (1802–1880), a Dutch physiological chemist, who coined the term "protein" to describe nitrogenous substances in plants and animal foods [89].

The German chemist, Justus von Liebig (1803–1873) considered food to be divided into "plastic" foods (plant and animal proteins), and "respiratory" foods (carbohydrates and fat). Liebig's main doctrine was that protein was used to build up the organism or repair tissues, whereas carbohydrates and fats served as fuels to facilitate the respiratory process [90]. The definition of food was further refined by Carl von Voit (1831–1908), a physiologist in Munich: "The foodstuffs are those substances which bring about the deposition of a substance essential to the composition of the body, or diminish and avert the loss thereof" [91]. A former pupil of Voit's, Wilbur Olin Atwater (1844–1907) conducted investigations into the caloric value of food using a bomb calorimeter and derived food and nutrient composition for an "average diet," and the energy-yielding functions of food were emphasized [92]. By the end of the nineteenth century, the prevailing notion was that food consisted of proteins, carbohydrates, fats, salts, and water.

Improved nutrition was considered to strengthen resistance to disease, and Germain Sée (1818–1896), a French physician, made dietary recommendations for individuals with specific diseases [93]. The influence of Liebig and Voit could be seen in some approaches; sufficient nourishment was thought to prevent "tissue waste" during a fever. Milk was given paramount importance as a dietary component [94]. Modern knowledge of nutrition was used to recommend diets for institutions such as schools, hospitals, prisons, and asylums. Special diets high in milk, whey, and egg yolk were recommended for certain diseases [95]. In the early twentieth century, influential textbooks in nutrition put heavy emphasis on the caloric value of food for human health [96, 97].

Infant Mortality and Social Reform

In the late eighteenth century, infant mortality became the target of social reform in France, England, and the United States [98, 99]. A major cause of infant mortality was diarrheal disease, which often occurred in epidemic proportions during the summer in cities of England, Europe, and the United States. Using data from Paris (Fig. 1.2) and Finsbury, a poor area of Bedfordshire where he worked as medical officer of health, George Newman (1870–1948) argued that breastfed infants suffered less from summer diarrhea than infants who were fed artificial formula or cow's milk [100]. The high infant mortality rate was considered to be mainly a problem of motherhood, and he emphasized proper training of mothers and promotion of breastfeeding. Newman argued that the infant mortality rate was gauge of health of a community, not the general death rate, and he considered it a sign of social degeneration that Great Britain should have a falling overall death rate but little change in the infant mortality rate over the preceding 50 years. Arthur Newsholme (1857–1943), Newman, and others [101] implicated fecal contamination of food and milk in the epidemics of summer diarrhea [102].

Similar concerns over infant mortality were voiced in Europe and the United States and led to the formation of national and international organizations devoted to the study and prevention of infant mortality, including the Ligue Française contre Mortalité Infantile (1902), the German Union for the Protection of Infants (1908), and the American Association for the Study and Prevention of Infant Mortality (1910). Among the measures sought by these groups were the education of mothers, the promotion of breastfeeding, improved prenatal care, and widespread gathering and compilation of vital statistics [98, 99]. Testing of the milk supply in large cities had revealed high bacterial counts in milk, and reform was aimed at providing a more pure milk supply through pasteurization [98].

The Emergence of the Vitamins

The late nineteenth and early twentieth century was marked by the emergence of the vitamin theory and the characterization of the vitamins. Although descriptions of scurvy, beriberi, night blindness and keratomalacia, and rickets—manifestations of vitamin C, thiamin, vitamin A, and vitamin D deficiencies, respectively—and their empirical treatments are known in the older medical literature, it was not until the last quarter of the nineteenth century that major progress commenced in the characterization of vitamins and vitamin deficiency diseases.

In the nineteenth century, beriberi was widespread in eastern and southeast Asia, and it was especially a problem for sailors on long voyages. In 1882, a Japanese naval vessel, *Riujo*, sailed from

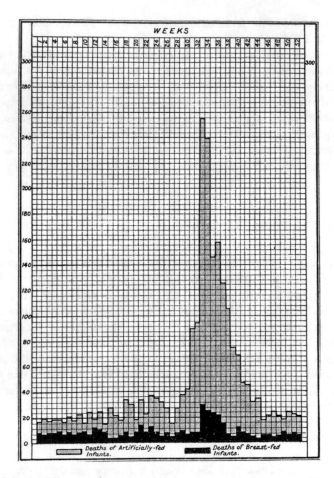

Fig. 1.2 Epidemics of diarrheal disease in Paris described by Newman in 1906. Adapted from [100]

Japan to Honolulu via New Zealand and Chile, and after 272 days of navigation, 60% of the ship's 276 crew members developed beriberi and 25 died [103]. A Japanese naval surgeon, Kanehiro Takaki (1849–1920) (Fig. 1.3), conducted epidemiological investigations of beriberi on different warships and examined clothing, living quarters, weather records, and rank. Takaki concluded that beriberi was related to the quality of food, particularly an insufficient intake of nitrogenous foods. In 1884, he persuaded the Japanese government to provide additional meat and dry milk on a training ship, *Tsukuba*, which sailed the same route of the ill-fated *Riujo*. When the *Tsukuba* arrived in Japan 287 days later, there were a handful of cases of beriberi and no deaths. After Takaki's dietary reforms were introduced, the cases of beriberi plummeted sharply in the Japanese navy [104, 105].

In 1886, Christiaan Eijkman (1858–1930), a Dutch army physician, was sent to the Dutch East Indies to investigate beriberi, which was generally thought at that time to be due to an unidentified bacterial infection. Eijkman demonstrated that chickens raised on polished rice alone developed a paralytic disorder similar to human beriberi and that this disorder could be corrected by a diet of unpolished rice. The bran portion of rice contained a substance which could prevent beriberi, and Eijkman originally thought that the polished rice contained a toxin that was neutralized by a substance in the bran portion [106]. His colleague, Gerrit Grijns (1865–1944), believed that the diseases affecting chickens and human beriberi were both due to an absence in the diet of a factor present in the rice polishings [107].

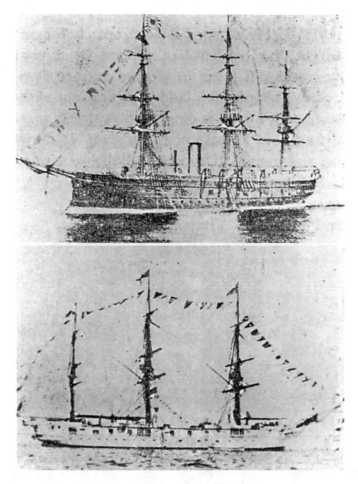

Fig. 1.3 Vessels involved in Navy research on beriberi by Kanehiro Takaki in the late nineteenth century

From the time of the early experiments of Magendie, the contributions of several investigators over many decades helped to characterize vitamin A [108, 109]. Nicholai Ivanovich Lunin (1853–1937) (Fig. 1.4), working in the laboratory of Gustav von Bunge (1844–1920) at the University of Dorpat, determined that mice cannot survive on purified diet of fats, carbohydrates, proteins, and salts alone; however, he noted that mice could survive when milk was added. Lunin concluded "other substances indispensable for nutrition must be present in milk besides casein, fat, lactose, and salts" [110]. Lunin's conclusion was disseminated widely in von Bunge's *Lehrbuch der physiologischen und pathologischen Chemie* [111]. Another student performed experiments with simplified diets in mice and found that there was an unknown substance in egg yolk that was essential for life [112]. At the University of Utrecht, Cornelius Pekelharing (1848–1922) conducted experiments that showed that mice are able to survive on diets in which small quantities of milk are added [113], and Wilhelm Stepp (1882–1964) showed that if the milk supplied to mice was extracted with alcohol ether (thus removing the fat-soluble substance later known as vitamin A), the mice could not survive [114].

The most explicit statement of the theory regarding the existence of vitamins came in 1906, when Frederick Gowland Hopkins (1861–1947), a biochemist at Cambridge University, who—on the basis of his own unpublished experiments and other observations—expressed the belief that there were "unsuspected dietetic factors" besides proteins, carbohydrates, fats, and minerals that were vital for

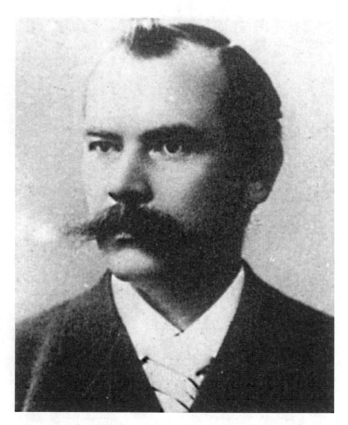

Fig. 1.4 Nicholai Ivanovich Lunin (1853–1937)

health [115]. In 1911, Casimir Funk (1884–1967) thought he had isolated the dietary factor involved in beriberi and coined the name "vitamine" for it [116]. Further exposition of the vitamin theory came in 1912, when Funk presented the idea that beriberi, scurvy, and pellagra were all nutritional deficiency diseases [117]. Later in 1929, Eijkman and Hopkins jointly received the Nobel Prize for their early pioneering scientific research on vitamins [118].

In the United States, Thomas Osborne (1859–1929) and Lafayette Mendel (1872–1935), working at Yale University, showed that a fat-soluble substance in butterfat was needed to support the growth of rats [119, 120]. After a period of illness, Hopkins published work he undertook in 1906–1907, which showed that mice could not survive on a purified diet without milk. Hopkins postulated the existence of what he called "accessory factors" in foods that were necessary for life [121]. In studies with eggs and butter, Elmer McCollum (1879–1967), a biochemist at the University of Wisconsin, noted that their data "supports the belief that there are certain accessory articles in certain food-stuffs which are essential for normal growth for extended periods" [122]. The "accessory factor" was later named "fat-soluble A" by McCollum, but it actually contained both vitamins A and D, leading to initial belief that "fat-soluble A" was responsible for rickets [123, 124]. In 1922, it was shown that cod liver oil contained both vitamin A, an anti-xerophthalmic factor, and vitamin D, an anti-rachitic factor [125]. Soon the term "fat-soluble A" was combined with Funk's designation to become "vitamine A" and later "vitamin A." The molecular structure of vitamin A was deduced in 1931 [126, 127], and vitamin A was eventually crystallized in 1937 [128].

Further Research on Nutritional Deficiency Diseases

Pellagra, a syndrome characterized by dermatitis, diarrhea, dementia, and death, was described in Europe as early as the eighteenth century, and it was often ascribed to spoilt maize [129]. With the rise of the germ theory of disease, it was thought that pellagra might also be attributable to an infection [130]. In the early part of the twentieth century, pellagra was increasingly recognized in the United States, especially in the South [131], and by 1916, it was second among the causes of death in South Carolina. Outbreaks of pellagra seemed to occur more commonly in asylums, jails, and poorhouses [132]. The Pellagra Commission of the State of Illinois conducted investigations in 1911 and concluded that pellagra was attributable to an infection [133], and another investigation in South Carolina implicated poor sanitation [134]. In 1914, Joseph Goldberger (1874–1929), a physician in the U.S. Public Health Service [135], conducted investigations of pellagra in South Carolina and showed that pellagra could be prevented by supplying milk, butter, and lean meat in the diet [136]. Careful study showed that household ownership of a cow was protective against pellagra. Further investigations among prison volunteers revealed that pellagra could be produced by a restricted, mainly cereal diet [137]. In later animal studies, niacin was implicated as the deficient dietary factor involved in the etiology of pellagra [129].

The Rise and Fall of Protein Malnutrition

After World War II, the main focus in nutrition shifted away from vitamins toward dietary protein [12]. The syndrome of kwashiorkor—edema, wasting, diarrhea, and peeling of the skin—was described by Cicely Williams (1893–1992), an English physician, among children in the Gold Coast of West Africa [138]. High mortality was noted among these children, and those affected appeared to be mostly one to four years old, weaned early, and fed entirely on white corn gruel. Williams noted that children recovered when given milk and cod liver oil; thus she suspected kwashiorkor was caused by an amino acid or protein deficiency. Subsequent surveys in Africa and Latin America showed that kwashiorkor was relatively common [139]. Protein malnutrition was the main theme of child nutrition conferences held by United Nations agencies from the 1950s through the mid-1970s. The United Nations Protein Advisory Group was established in 1955 [140]. International efforts began to focus upon closing the "protein gap" or addressing the "protein crisis" through high protein sources such as fish, soybean, and peanuts [141]. In a 1974 editorial in *The Lancet* titled "The Great Protein Fiasco," Donald S. McLaren made a withering attack on the UN Protein Advisory Group and declared that the "protein gap" was a fallacy [142]. The following year, John Waterlow, who led much of the effort to study protein malnutrition, admitted that children needed more energy, not protein [143]. As a consequence, the effort to address dietary protein was largely abandoned under the assumption that children received adequate dietary protein [139]. The UN Protein Advisory Group was quietly disbanded, and the protein conferences disappeared [139, 140]. The pendulum swung in the direction of micronutrient malnutrition, which became the dominant paradigm for nutrition in developing countries for four decades [139].

Nutritional Immunology

Nutritional immunology, the study of the relationship between nutrition and immunity, was a discipline that arose largely during the early twentieth century. Although it had been observed over the centuries that famine would reduce an individual's resistance to epidemic diseases, more specific clues were provided with the advent of animal experimentation using controlled diets. The recognition of specific vitamins and developments in immunology made it possible to study the effects of single or multiple vitamin deficiencies upon immune function. By the end of the nineteenth century, humoral antitoxic antibodies in the serum of immunized animals had been described, and this led to the development of serological tests involved in the diagnosis of infectious disease and measurement of immunological protection [144]. Experimental infections were soon conducted in animals on controlled diets, and serological tests allowed assessment of the effect of dietary deprivation on immunity to infection. By the mid-1930s, animal studies suggested that deficiencies of some of the vitamins reduced resistance to infection [145–147].

Vitamin A and Reduction of Child Mortality

Two Danish physicians, the pediatrician Carl Bloch (1872–1952) and the ophthalmologist Olaf Blegvad (1888–1961), dealt with a large number of children with clinical vitamin A deficiency in Denmark in the period 1910–1920. They noted that children with vitamin A deficiency had greatly increased mortality and that mortality among them could be reduced by providing the children with vitamin A-rich foods such as cod liver oil, whole milk, cream, and butter [148–151].

In the late 1920s, vitamin A was recognized to have an effect on immunity to infection, and vitamin A became known as the "anti-infective" vitamin [152]. Largely through the influence of Edward Mellanby (1884–1955), a professor of physiology at Sheffield University (Fig. 1.5), vitamin A underwent a period of intense clinical investigation. Between 1920 and 1940, at least 30 trials were conducted to determine whether vitamin A could reduce the morbidity and mortality from infectious diseases, including respiratory disease, measles, puerperal sepsis, and tuberculosis [153]. These trials were conducted prior to the time when many of the innovations known to the modern controlled clinical trial, such as randomization, sample size and power calculations, and placebo controls were widely known.

By the 1930s, it was firmly established that vitamin A supplementation could reduce morbidity and mortality in young children. In 1932, Joseph Ellison (b. 1898), a physician in London, showed that vitamin supplementation reduced the mortality of vitamin A-deficient children with measles [154]. During the 1931–1932 measles epidemic in London, Ellison assigned 600 children with measles at the Grove Fever Hospital to one of two groups of 300 each. One group received vitamin A and the other group did not receive vitamin A. Overall mortality rates in the vitamin A and control groups were 3.7 and 8.7%, respectively, representing a 58% reduction in mortality with vitamin A treatment. Ellison's study, published in the *British Medical Journal* in 1932, was the first trial to show that vitamin A supplementation reduces mortality in young children with vitamin A deficiency [155].

Vitamin A became a mainstream preventive measure: cod liver oil was part of the morning routine for millions of children—a practice promoted by physicians and popularized by the pharmaceutical industry [155]. The production and importation of cod liver oil in the U.S. totaled 4,909,622 lb in 1929 [156]. In the early 1930s in England, the annual consumption of cod liver oil was 500,000 gallons per year [157]. Much of the world's supply of cod liver oil, and hence, vitamins A and D, came from the commercial fisheries of New England, Norway, and Newfoundland. As noted in the *British Medical Journal*, "cod-liver oil was in use in almost every working-class household, and local authorities spent considerable sums in purchasing bulk supplies for hospitals and sanitoriums" [158]. In England, a proposal to tax cod liver oil in the Ottawa Agreements Bill in the House of Commons in 1932 raised protests, as there was concern that child mortality would increase if the price of cod liver oil increased and it became less accessible to poor people. As reported in both *The Lancet* and the *British Medical Journal*, one legislator who supported an amendment to exempt cod liver oil from the proposed taxation noted that many a child in the north of England "owed its life to being able to

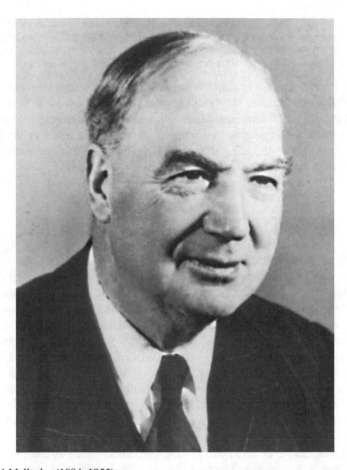

Fig. 1.5 Dr. Edward Mellanby (1884–1955)

obtain cod-liver oil" [157, 159]. Two British physicians also supported the amendment in letters published in *The Lancet* [157]. One expert from the Lister Institute of Preventive Medicine noted "It is evident that any steps which may raise the price and lower the consumption of cod-liver oil, especially in the winter, would have deleterious effect upon the health of the population, involving particularly the well-being of the children of the poorer classes" [157]. The concerns of physicians and legislators alike that children receive sufficient vitamin A to protect against the well-known morbidity and mortality of vitamin A deficiency were clearly expressed. The discovery of the sulfa antibiotics and their clinical applications soon overshadowed investigations of vitamin A as "anti-infective" therapy, and there was about a 50-year lull in clinical investigation of vitamin A as an intervention to reduce morbidity and mortality until the late 1980s [160].

In 1950, a joint expert committee on nutrition of the Food and Agricultural Organization (FAO) and the World Health Organization (WHO) recommended that studies be made on the relationship of nutritional status to resistance against intestinal parasites. Further observations made in the ensuing decade suggested that many infectious diseases were associated with malnutrition. A WHO Expert Committee on Nutrition and Infection reviewed the issue of the interaction between nutrition and infection in 1965, and a comprehensive monograph, *Interactions of Nutrition and Infection*, by Nevin Scrimshaw, Carl Taylor, and John Gordon appeared in 1968 [161]. The effect of nutritional status on resistance to diarrheal and respiratory disease, viral, parasitic, and other infections was reviewed, and the present state of knowledge regarding the effects of specific micronutrient deficiencies on immune function was presented. The authors concluded

Infections are likely to have more serious consequences among persons with clinical or subclinical malnutrition, and infectious diseases have the capacity to turn borderline nutritional deficiencies into severe malnutrition. In this way, malnutrition and infection can be mutually aggravating and produce more serious consequences for the patient than would be expected from a summation of the independent effects of the two.

This seminal work served as the foundation for research on nutritional immunology, especially for vitamin A and for zinc research, in the last three decades of the twentieth century. An important detailed review of the effects of single nutrients on immunity was made by William Beisel in 1982 [162]. Tremendous advances in nutritional immunology have been made in the last 20 years, and many of these recent findings regarding the relationship between micronutrients and immunity to infection are presented elsewhere in this book.

Growth in Food Production

In England, growth in food production from 1750 to 1880 was not seen not so much as owing to technological innovation as to increasing soil fertility and crop yield through manuring and sowing of legumes [163]. Improved reaping machines appeared in the early nineteenth century, and cast iron replaced wrought iron and wood in many agricultural implements. Introduction of new fodder crops for winter feeding enabled better animal husbandry. In France, railway construction was considered to be a vital factor improving the agricultural economy in the mid-nineteenth century, and animal breeding, crop rotation, and mechanization contributed to improve agricultural practice [164]. In England, the better road transport increased the market for the dairy producer. Advances in the process by which ammonia could be produced from atmospheric nitrogen allowed more widespread use of fertilizers in the early twentieth century [165]. Increased mechanization with tractors, combined harvesters, automatic hay balers, and seed and fertilizer drills has been noted between 1910 and 1950 in England, and advances in plant breeding brought new cereal and clover varieties [165]. In the United States, technological advances in the plow, reaper, binder, and thresher aided the development of mechanized farming in the nineteenth century. Industrialized agriculture expanded in the beginning of the twentieth century with the development of gasoline-powered tractors.

Long-Term Trends in Diet

Available evidence suggests that the majority of the world's population before 1800 consumed a diet that is below contemporary minimum standards of optimal nutrition [166]. In France, the caloric intake of the average diet increased steadily during the nineteenth century, but the basic composition of the diet did not appear to change much until after about 1880 [167]. Inspired by the French voluntary *Caisses des Écoles*, which fed hungry school children, charities were founded to feed children in England. The Victorian working-class diet was especially poor in quality and quantity [168]. Near the end of the nineteenth century, over 1 in 10 children attending London schools were estimated to be habitually going hungry [169]. Alarm was raised over the problem of inadequate nutrition when the report of the Inter-Departmental Committee on Physical Deterioration was published in 1904 [170]. The committee showed that 40–60% of young men presenting for military service at the time of the South African War were rejected on medical grounds, and much of this physical inadequacy was attributed to malnutrition. This and other reports led to the Education (Provision of Meals) Act of 1906, which mandated national policy for feeding needy children at school. The number of London children receiving meals was about 27,000 in 1907 and by 1909 that number had doubled [171]. When the *Report on the Present State of Knowledge concerning Accessory Food Factors* (*Vitamines*) appeared in 1919, it helped shape dietary recommendations based on newer knowledge of vitamins [172]. The value of milk was emphasized by the report, and a study showed that those provided supplemental milk each day had better weight and height gain than those who were not supplemented [173]. By 1945, about 40% of the school population was taking school meals and 46% were drinking school milk [171].

An association between low socioeconomic level and inadequate diet was known in France [51] and England [174]. In *A Study of the Diet of the Labouring Classes in Edinburgh* (1901), D. Noël Paton and his colleagues showed that many workers did not have the income to obtain a sufficient supply of food and lacked the education to make correct choices of food [175]. A discussion later followed in the *British Medical Journal* [176]:

> Who is responsible for the conditions which lead to the state of poverty and bad nutrition disclosed by this report? Lies the fault with poor themselves—is it because they are thriftless, because they lack training in cooking and in the economical spending of such income as they possess? Or is it that the actual wages which they can command are so low that it is impossible for them to purchase the actual necessities of life?

Whether the problem lay with lack of education or inadequate income was unclear, and each side had its adherents [177]. In 1936, John Boyd Orr (1880–1971) published *Food Health and Income: Report on a Survey of Diet in Relation to Income*, and this report created a sensation in England and was widely publicized around the world. This dietary survey suggested that the poorest of the poor, about four and one half million people, consumed a diet deficient in all dietary constituents examined, and that the next poorest, about nine million people, had a diet adequate in protein, fat, and carbohydrates but deficient in all vitamins and minerals [178]. Only half the population surveyed had a diet that was adequate in all dietary constituents, including all vitamins and minerals. Although the per capita consumption of fruit, vegetables, and dairy products had greatly increased between 1909 and 1934 in Great Britain, there was clearly more that could be done to improve nutrition [178]. Analysis of household budgets suggests that the average daily intakes of vitamin A, vitamin C, and thiamin were mostly inadequate in 1900 but increased to largely sufficient intakes by 1944 among poor, working-class, and middle-class families in Great Britain [174]. Long-term analysis of nutritional status shows that height grew in the United Kingdom from the mid-nineteenth century through the years following World War II [179].

In the United States, there have been large dietary changes over the last 200 years [17, 180]. In the early nineteenth century, many individuals did not consume adequate amounts of fruits, vegetables, and dairy products, and dietary deficiencies were not uncommon among rural and urban dwellers. From about 1830 to 1870, the mean stature of Americans had a prolonged decline, and this may possibly have been due to increased urbanization and poorer nutrition for urban workers during industrialization [181, 182], and from the 1880s to the present, there has been a steady increase in stature. The apparent per capita consumption of dairy products increased in the United States between 1909 and 1930 [183, 184]. The discovery of the vitamins led to a greater awareness of nutrition, and the pharmaceutical and food industries promoted their products to mothers using a combination of fear, hope, and guilt [185]. Fortification of baker's bread with thiamin, riboflavin, niacin, iron, and calcium became mandatory in 1943. When federal wartime legislation ended in 1946, many states continued to require the enrichment of bread [180].

When George Newman, one of the primary architects of public health reform in Great Britain, wrote to a colleague in 1939, he reminisced about the "silent revolution" in Great Britain:

> [They]…who say I am an idealist and wild optimist do not know their history. How can one be otherwise who knew England and English medicine in 1895 and know it now? It is the greatest silent revolution in our time. The opportunity and the quality of human life have, as you truly say, been 'transformed.' They don't know what 'malnutrition' means nowadays. Everybody is undernourished in some degree a way, but prevalent malnutrition is rare, while it used to be common [186].

In *The Building of a Nation's Health* in 1939, Newman identified adequate nutrition as being one of the "most powerful instruments" of preventive medicine [187].

The Decline of Mortality

In *The Modern Rise of Population* (1976), Thomas McKeown (1912–1988) showed that population grew in Europe since the mid-eighteenth century, and he attributed the population growth largely to a reduction in deaths from infectious diseases [1]. The decline of infectious disease mortality was occurring prior to the identification of specific pathogens, the widespread use of immunizations, the development of antibiotics, and the rise of sophisticated, technologically based clinical medicine (Fig. 1.6). Improved nutrition, greater food supplies, purification of water, better sanitation, and improved housing are among the main factors cited in the reduction of infectious disease morbidity and mortality [2]. A close interrelationship between nutrition, infection, and hygiene was acknowledged [2, 3], and McKeown's conclusions were primarily based upon observations of infectious disease mortality rates from the late nineteenth century and later. These views have become orthodox and influential in the debate regarding appropriate strategies for reducing mortality in low- and middle-income countries (LMICs), and scientific findings of the last 20 years from LMICs largely supports McKeown's contention that nutritional status influences infectious disease morbidity and mortality.

Others have disputed some of McKeown's conclusions, citing evidence that population growth from the sixteenth century may have been primarily owing to an increase in fertility rather than decline in mortality [188], or that the relationship between nutrition and infection is "controversial" [189]. There is little question that there has been a general decline in mortality in Europe since the middle of the seventeenth century, but given the close relationship between socioeconomic level, education, housing, food, clean water, sanitation, and hygiene, it has been difficult to separate out specific causal factors [190–192]. During the same period there has been a probable reduction in exposure to pathogenic organisms through changes in man's environment [4], and over the last 200 years, there has been a near disappearance of deficiency diseases that were once commonly

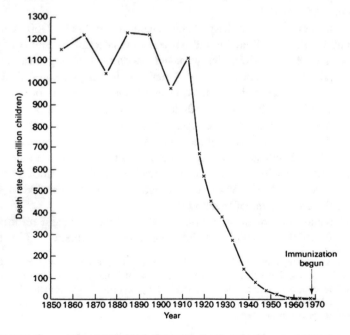

Fig. 1.6 Case fatality rates for measles, 1850–1970. From [1]. Reprinted with permission from Elsevier

reported in Europe, such as goiter, pellagra, rickets, and xerophthalmia [129, 150, 193]. These deficiency diseases cause significant morbidity and mortality but have been relatively neglected in historical demography.

Graduate Education in Public Health

The early sanitary reform efforts in the nineteenth century were dominated by nonmedical personnel in the United States and Europe, as it was often seen as the responsibility of engineers, biologists, and chemists. The appointment of John Simon (1816–1904), a surgeon, to the head of the Medical Department of the Privy Council in 1854 was a visible sign of change where the public health system was dominated by the medical profession [194]. New public health legislation created a need for qualified medical practitioners to serve as officers of health, and programs offering a diploma in public health appeared in Dublin, Edinburgh, and Cambridge. In Vienna, the subjects of "Medical Police" and "Forensic Medicine" were combined under the designation of "State Medicine" at the Vienna Medical School [195]. At first, "Medical Police" was taught largely with emphasis on knowledge of ordinances and sanitary regulations in Austria, which were influenced by Frank's *Medicinische Polizey*, but emphasis slowly changed to scientific investigation and sanitation after cholera and typhoid epidemics struck Vienna.

Courses in public health were taught in some universities in the United States at the turn of the century, but schools of hygiene and public health were not created as a separate entity until the early twentieth century. In 1916, the School of Hygiene and Public Health was established at the Johns Hopkins University with William H. Welch as its director [196] and the School of Public Health opened at Harvard University in 1922 [197]. With endowment of the Rockefeller Foundation, the London School of Hygiene and Tropical Medicine opened in 1929. By 1925, the teaching of hygiene varied enormously, with institutes of hygiene established among medical faculty in Germany and Sweden, hygiene taught through bacteriology in France, and new schools of public health at Johns Hopkins, Harvard, and Pennsylvania in the United States [198]. The number of universities with schools or programs of public health continued to grow in the United States, Great Britain, and Europe [199].

International Organizations

Among the larger institutions involved in scientific research related to public health were the Institut Pasteur, the Lister Institute, the Rockefeller Institute, and the National Institutes of Health. The success of Pasteur in microbiological investigations and rabies immunization led to the establishment of the Institut Pasteur in Paris in 1888. The institute was a model for bacteriological research, and within a few years, other Pasteur Institutes were established in more than 40 places around the world. These institutes scattered around the globe were loosely knit and linked by ideology [200]. The Institut Pasteur made major contributions to preventive medicine with new vaccines and therapies for infectious diseases [201]. In 1891, the Lister Institute was established in London, and research on vitamins was a major part of the research program, with notable emphasis upon rickets [202].

The Rockefeller Foundation established an International Health Commission in 1913, and the commission grew out of early efforts of the Rockefeller Sanitary Commission to eradicate hookworm in the southern United States [203]. The International Health Division, or Health Commission, of the Rockefeller Foundation, expanded efforts to eradicate hookworm overseas, and during the 1920s the focus expanded to malaria, yellow fever, and tuberculosis [204, 205]. The Rockefeller Foundation helped to transform medical education in the United States and tended to emphasize a technological approach to medicine [206].

The National Institutes of Health had its early roots in public health with the establishment of the Hygienic Laboratory of the Marine Hospital Service in 1887 [207]. The laboratory was responsible for bacteriological work, including diagnosis of infectious diseases among immigrants. The scope of the laboratory increased with Progressive Era regulations such as the Biologics Control Act of 1902 and the Pure Food and Drugs Act of 1906. In 1912, the service became known as the U.S. Public Health Service, and among its activities were investigations of pellagra by Joseph Goldberger. The National Institute of Health was formally established by the U.S. Congress in 1930, and by 1948 it consisted of several institutes to become the National Institutes of Health (NIH) [208]. Although the NIH had its roots in hygiene and public health, a shift occurred with the creation of the Communicable Disease Center (CDC) in Atlanta, Georgia in 1946. The CDC soon dealt with epidemics and other public health crises such as influenza outbreaks, polio surveillance, and measles eradication.

International health organizations grew out of efforts to coordinate quarantines and control international epidemics such as cholera and plague. In 1907 the *Office International d'Hygiène Publique* (*International Office of Public Health*) was established in Rome, and the purpose of the organization was to collect and disseminate epidemiological information about smallpox, plague, cholera, and other diseases. The Health Organization of the League of Nations was created in 1923, and its activities included promotion of health, international standardization of biological tests and products, and control of disease. In 1948, the World Health Organisation (WHO) was created after international ratification, and it assumed the activities of the Health Organization of the League of Nations and other offices. The Pan American Sanitary Bureau became the regional office of the WHO for Latin America in 1949, and in 1958 it changed its name to the Pan American Health Organization (PAHO). Treatment campaigns against yaws, smallpox eradication, oral rehydration therapy, and childhood immunizations were among the many achievements of the WHO since its inception.

The United Nations International Children's Emergency Fund (UNICEF) was created in 1946 by resolution of the United Nations General Assembly, and the purpose of UNICEF was to protect the well- being of children around the world. Early activities of UNICEF included shipments of powdered milk for children in Europe, vaccination efforts, support for vector control, and provision of equipment for maternal and child health centers [209]. Most of UNICEF's assistance in Africa in the 1950s went toward malaria eradication.

The Food and Agricultural Organization (FAO) was founded in 1945 in Quebec, Canada, with the purpose of raising the levels of nutrition and standards of living, securing improvements in the production and distribution of food and agricultural products, and improving the condition of rural populations [210]. The first director general of FAO was John Boyd Orr, who brought attention to the relationship between income and diet in England in the 1930s. The FAO, based in Rome, provides assistance for sustainable agriculture, promotes transfer of skills and technology in field projects, offers advice on agricultural policy and planning, and fosters international cooperation on nutrition, biodiversity, and agricultural commodities.

The World Bank originated with reconstruction efforts after World War II, when delegates from 44 nations met in Bretton Woods, New Hampshire, and drew up articles of agreement for the International Bank for Reconstruction and Development in 1944 [211, 212]. The mission of the World Bank shifted from reconstruction to development, especially for economically developing countries. World Bank loans to poor countries in Africa and Asia increased under the tenure of the World Bank's fifth president, Robert McNamara. McNamara was aware of Alan Berg's work on nutrition and health at the Brookings Institution, which later appeared in *The Nutrition Factor* [212, 213], and a nutrition unit was created at the World Bank in 1972. The role of the Bank was to encourage development-oriented work rather than mass food distribution in developing countries, and such projects included identification of populations at high risk for malnutrition, developing food

Table 1.1 Major diseases in Europe, Great Britain, and the United States during the nineteenth century

Infectious diseases	Nutrition deficiency disorder
Diarrheal disease	Rickets
Cholera	Pellagra
Malaria	Goiter/cretinism
Yellow fever	Nutritional blindness
Tuberculosis	
Typhoid	
Typhus	
Measles	

subsidy programs, integrating nutrition assistance with primary care and family planning, nutrition education, promotion of home gardening, improving water and sanitation, and delivering micronutrient supplements [214].

Conclusions

Over the last 200 years in most of Europe and the United States, there has been a major reduction in mortality rates, a virtual elimination of many infectious diseases, an improvement in diet, and virtual disappearance of nearly all nutritional deficiency disorders. Many of the so-called "tropical" diseases such as malaria, yellow fever, and cholera were once endemic or epidemic in industrialized countries and have now disappeared (Table 1.1). Case fatality rates for many infectious diseases dropped tremendously during the late nineteenth century and early twentieth century. New knowledge of nutrition and the characterization of vitamins helped to improve the diet in the early twentieth century, and innovations in agricultural practices helped to increase food production. After World War II, international organizations grew in strength and are addressing basic issues of nutrition, hygiene, and control of infectious diseases in LMICs. Nutrition has played a major role among the developments in public health during the last 200 years and is likely to remain as a major foundation for public health.

Discussion Points

- How did the idea originate regarding progress in public health?
- What are the roots of statistics that are commonly used in public health today?
- How did the idea of contagion replace that of miasmas?
- Who were the major proponents of the social reform movement related to infant mortality?
- When was vitamin A first known to reduce morbidity and mortality of children?
- What were the major changes in diet in industrialized countries in the last 200 years?
- What is main idea of Thomas McKeown in regard to mortality decline in Europe?

References

1. McKeown T. The modern rise of population. London: Edward Arnold; 1976.
2. McKeown T. The role of medicine: dream, mirage, or nemesis?. Princeton: Princeton University Press; 1979.

3. Woods R, Woodward J, editors. Urban disease and mortality in nineteenth-century England. New York, NY: St. Martin's Press; 1984.
4. Riley JC. The eighteenth-century campaign to avoid disease. New York, NY: St. Martin's Press; 1987.
5. Rosen G. A history of public health. New York, NY: MD Publications; 1958.
6. Duffy J. The sanitarians: a history of american public health. Urbana and Chicago: University of Illinois Press; 1990.
7. Fee E, Acheson RM. A history of education in public health: health that mocks the doctors' rules. Oxford and New York: Oxford University Press; 1991.
8. Porter R. The greatest benefit to mankind: a medical history of humanity. New York and London: W. W. Norton; 1997.
9. Winslow CEA. The conquest of epidemic disease: a chapter in the history of ideas. Princeton: Princeton University Press; 1943.
10. Dowling HF. Fighting infection: conquests of the twentieth century. Cambridge, MA: Harvard University Press; 1977.
11. Ackerknecht EH. History and geography of the most important diseases. New York, NY: Hafner; 1965.
12. Carpenter KJ. Protein and energy: a study of changing ideas in nutrition. Cambridge, UK: Cambridge University Press; 1994.
13. Carpenter KJ. The history of scurvy and vitamin C. Cambridge, UK: Cambridge University Press; 1986.
14. Roe DA. A plague of corn: the social history of pellagra. Ithaca and London: Cornell University Press; 1973.
15. Drummond JC, Wilbraham A. The Englishman's food: a history of five centuries of English diet. London: Jonathan Cape; 1939.
16. Tannahill R. Food in history. New York: Stein and Day; 1973.
17. Levenstein HA. Revolution at the table: the transformation of the American diet. New York and Oxford: Oxford University Press; 1988.
18. Newman LF, editor. Hunger in history: food shortage, poverty, and deprivation. Oxford: Blackwell; 1990.
19. Frankel C. The faith of reason: the idea of progress in the French enlightenment. New York, NY: King's Crown Press, Columbia University; 1948.
20. Diderot D, Alembert JLR d', Mouchon P. Encyclopédie, ou dictionnaire raisonné des sciences, des arts et des métiers, par une société de gens de lettres, vol. 17. Paris: Briasson; 1751–1765.
21. de Condorcet Marquis MJANC. Esquisse d'un tableau historique des progrès de l'esprit humain. 2nd ed. Paris: Agasses; 1795.
22. de Condorcet Marquis MJANC. Sketch for a historical picture of the progress of the human mind. Translation by June Barraclough. London: Weidenfeld and Nicholson; 1955.
23. Baker K. Condorcet: from natural philosophy to social mathematics. Chicago: University of Chicago Press; 1975.
24. Godwin W. An enquiry concerning political justice, and its influence on general virtue and happiness. London: G. G. J. and J. Robinson; 1793.
25. Malthus TR. An essay on the principle of population as it affects the future improvement of society, with remarks on the speculations of Mr. Godwin, M. Condorcet, and Other Writers. London: Johnson; 1798.
26. Avery J. Progress, poverty and population: re-reading Condorcet, Godwin and Malthus. London and Portland, Oregon: Frank Cass; 1997.
27. Frank JP. System einer vollständigen medicinischen Polizey. 3rd Rev. ed. Wien; 1786–1817.
28. Sigerist HE. The people's misery: mother of diseases, an address delivered in 1790 by Johann Peter Frank, translated from the Latin, with an introduction. Bull Hist Med. 1941;9:81–100.
29. Sigerist HE. Landmarks in the history of hygiene. London: Oxford University Press; 1956.
30. Greenwood M. Medical statistics from Graunt to Farr. Cambridge, UK: Cambridge University Press; 1948.
31. Pearson ES, editor. The history of statistics in the 17th and 18th centuries against the changing background of intellectual, scientific and religious thought: lectures by Karl Pearson given at University College London during the academic sessions 1921–1933. New York, NY: MacMillan; 1978.
32. Graunt J. Natural and political observations mentioned in a following index, and made upon the bills of mortality. London: J. Martin, J. Allestry and T. Dicas; 1662.
33. Westergaard H. Contributions to the history of statistics. London: P. S. King and Son; 1932.
34. Petty W. Several essays in political arithmetic. London: Robert Clavel and Henry Mortlock; 1699.
35. Halley E. An estimate of the degrees of mortality of mankind, drawn from curious tables of the births and funerals of the city of Breslaw, with an attempt to ascertain the price of annuities upon lives. Phil Trans. 1693;17:596–610.
36. Eyler JM. Victorian social medicine: the ideas and methods of William Farr. Baltimore: Johns Hopkins University Press; 1979.
37. Farr W. Vital statistics, or the statistics of health, sickness, diseases, and death. In: McColloch JR, editor. A statistical account of the British empire: exhibiting its extent, physical capacities, population, industry, and civil and religious institutions. No. 2. London; 1837. P. 567–601.

38. Quetelet A. Sur l'homme et le développement de ses facultés, ou Essai de physique sociale. Paris: Bachelier; 1835.
39. Cullen MJ. The statistical movement in early Victorian Britain: the foundations of empirical social research. New York, NY: Barnes and Noble; 1975.
40. Porter TM. The rise of statistical thinking, 1820–1900. Princeton, NJ: Princeton University Press; 1986.
41. Galton F. Natural inheritance. London and New York: Macmillan; 1889.
42. Pearson K. Mathematical contributions to the theory of evolution, III. Regression, heredity and panmixia. Phil Trans Roy Soc London A. 1896;187:253–318.
43. Stigler SM. The history of statistics: the measurement of uncertainty before 1900. Cambridge, MA and London: Harvard University Press; 1986.
44. Fisher RA. The design of experiments. London: Oliver and Boyd; 1935.
45. Neyman J, Pearson ES. On the use and interpretation of certain test criteria for purposes of statistical inference. Biometrika. 1928;20A (part 1):175–240, (part 2):263–294.
46. Marks HM. The progress of experiment: science and therapeutic reform in the United States, 1900–1990. Cambridge, UK: Cambridge University Press; 1997.
47. Ackerknecht EH. Hygiene in France, 1815–1848. Bull Hist Med. 1948;22:117–55.
48. La Berge A. Mission and method: the early nineteenth-century French Public Health Movement. Cambridge, UK and New York: Cambridge University Press; 1992.
49. Villermé LR. De la famine et ses effets sur la santé dans les lieux qui sont le théâtre de la guerre. J gén méd chir pharm. 1818;65:3–24.
50. Villermé LR. Recherches statistiques sur la ville de Paris et le département de la Seine. Bull Soc méd d'emul. 1822;1–41.
51. Benoiston de Châteauneuf LF. Recherches sur les consommations de tout genre de la ville de Paris en 1817, comparées à ce qu'elles étaient en 1789. Paris: the author; 1820.
52. Coleman W. Death is a social disease: public health and political economy in early industrial France. Madison: University of Wisconsin Press; 1982.
53. Villermé LR. Des epidémies sous les rapportes de l'hygiène publique, de la statistique médicale et de l'économie politique. Paris; 1833.
54. Villermé LR. Tableau de l'état physique et moral des ouvriers employés dans les manufactures de coton, de laine et de soie, vol. 2. Paris: Jules Renouard; 1840.
55. Napoli Archivio di Stato. Statistica del 1811. Ministero dell'Interno, 1% Inventario, 96:1–65.
56. Constantini AM. Ambiente, alimentazione e salute nell'inchiesta murattiana del 1811. Medicina nei Secoli. 1996;8:339–57.
57. Genovesi A. Ragionamento intorno all'agricoltura con applicazione al Regno di Napoli. In: Scrittori Classici Italiani di Economia Politica. Parte Moderna, Tomo IX. Milano: G. G. De Stefanis; 1803. P. 305–325.
58. Bentham J. Traités de législation civile et pénale. Paris: Bossange, Masson and Besson; 1802.
59. Chadwick E. Report to her majesty's principal secretary of state for the home department, from the poor law commissioners, on an inquiry into the sanitary condition of the labouring population of Great Britain. London: W. Clowes and Sons; 1842.
60. Finer SE. The life and times of Sir Edwin Chadwick. London: Methuen; 1952.
61. Shattuck L. Report of a general plan for the promotion of public and personal health, devised, prepared and recommended by the commissioners appointed under a resolve of the legislature of Massachusetts, relating to a sanitary survey of the state. Boston: Dutton and Wentworth; 1850.
62. Cassedy JH. Demography in early America: beginnings of the statistical mind, 1600–1800. Cambridge, MA: Harvard University Press; 1969.
63. Cassedy JH. American medicine and statistical thinking, 1800–1860. Cambridge, MA and London: Harvard University Press; 1984.
64. Hirsch A. Handbook of geographical and historical pathology. London: New Sydenham Society; 1883–1886.
65. Bulloch W. The history of bacteriology. London: Oxford University Press; 1938.
66. Pelling M. Cholera, fever, and English medicine, 1825–1865. Oxford: Oxford University Press; 1978.
67. Panum PL. Iagttagelser, anstillede under Maeslinge-Epidemien paa Faerøerne i Aaret 1846. Bibliothek f. Laeger. 1847;1:270–344.
68. Manicus A. Maeslingerne paa Faeröerne i Sommeren 1846. Ugeskr Laeger. 1847;6:189–210.
69. Snow J. On the mode of communication of cholera. 2nd ed. London: John Churchill; 1855.
70. Budd W. Malignant cholera: its mode of propagation and its prevention. London: John Churchill; 1849.
71. Bruce FE. Water-supply. In: Singer C, Holmyard EJ, Hall AR, Williams TI, editors. A history of technology, vol. V. The late nineteenth century, c. 1850 to c. 1900. New York and London: Oxford University Press; 1958.
72. Goubert JP. The conquest of water: the advent of health in the industrial age. Princeton: Princeton University Press; 1986.

73. Hamlin C. The science of impurity: water analysis in nineteenth century Britain. Berkeley and Los Angeles: University of California Press; 1990.
74. Girette J. La civilisation et le choléra. Paris: L. Hachette; 1867.
75. Bretonneau PF. Des inflammations spéciales du tissu muqueux et en particulier de la diphthérite, ou inflammation pelliculaire. Paris: Crevot; 1826.
76. Budd W. Typhoid fever; its nature, mode of spreading, and prevention. London: Longmans, Green and Company; 1873.
77. Henle FGJ. Pathologische Untersuchungen. Berlin: A. Hirschwald; 1840.
78. Koch R. Untersuchungen über die Aetiologie der Wundinfectionskrankheiten. Leipzig: F. C. W. Vogel; 1878.
79. Koch R. Die Aetiologie der Milzbrand-Krankheit, begründet auf die Entwicklungsgeschichte des Bacillus anthracis. Beitr z Biol d Pflanzen. 1876; Bd. II, Heft 2, 277–310.
80. Laveran CLA. Un nouveau parasite trouvé dans le sang plusieurs malades atteints de fièvre palustre. Bull Soc méd Hôp Paris (Mém). 1881;2 sér. 17:158–164.
81. Koch R. Die Aetiologie der Tuberculose. Berlin klin Wchnschr. 1882;19:221–30.
82. Koch R. Ueber die Cholerabakterien. Dtsch med Wchnschr. 1884;10:725–8.
83. Legge TM. Public health in European capitals: Berlin, Paris, Brussels, Christiania, Stockholm, and Copenhagen. London: Swan Sonnenschein; 1896.
84. Sedgwick WT. Principles of sanitary science and the public health with special reference to the causation and prevention of infectious diseases. New York and London: Macmillan; 1903.
85. Chapin CV. The sources and modes of infection. 2nd ed. New York, NY: Wiley; 1912.
86. Lesch JE. Science and medicine in France: the emergence of experimental physiology, 1790–1855. Cambridge, MA: Harvard University Press; 1984.
87. Magendie F. Précis élémentaire de physiologie. 2nd ed. Paris: Méquignon-Marvis; 1825.
88. Magendie F. Mémoire sur les propriétés nutritives des substances qui ne contiennent pas d'azote. Bulletin des Sciences par la Société philomatique de Paris. 1816;4:137–8.
89. Mulder GJ. Ueber die Zusammensetzung einiger thierischen Substanzen. J prakt Chemie. 1839;16:129–52.
90. von Liebig J. Die Thier-Chemie oder die organische Chemie in ihrer Anwendung auf Physiologie und Pathologie. Braunschweig; 1846.
91. von Voit C. Handbuch der Physiologie des gesammt-Stoffwechsels und der Fortpflanzung. Theil 1. Physiologie des allgemeinen Stoffwechsels und der Ernährung. In: Hermann L, editor. Handbuch der Physiologie. vol, 6. Leipzig: F.C.W. Vogel; 1881. P. 1–575.
92. Atwater WO. Methods and results of investigations on the chemistry and economy of food. No. 21. Washington, U. S. Department of Agriculture, Office of Experiment Stations, Bulletin; 1895.
93. Sée G. Du régime alimentaire. Traitement hygiénique des malades. Paris: Adrien Delahaye and Émile Lescrosnier; 1887.
94. Thompson WG. Practical dietetics with special reference to diet in disease. New York, NY: D. Appleton; 1896.
95. Friedenwald J, Ruhräh J. Diet in health and disease. 2nd ed. Philadelphia and London: W. B. Saunders; 1906.
96. Lusk G. The elements of the science of nutrition. Philadelphia and London: W. B. Saunders; 1906.
97. Chittenden RH. The nutrition of man. New York, NY: Frederick A. Stokes; 1907.
98. Meckel RA. Save the babies: American public health reform and the prevention of infant mortality, 1850–1929. Baltimore and London: Johns Hopkins University Press; 1990.
99. Klaus A. Every child a lion: the origins of maternal infant and health policy in the United States and France, 1890–1920. Ithaca and London: Cornell University Press; 1993.
100. Newman G. Infant mortality: a social problem. London: Methuen and Company; 1906.
101. Peters OH. Observations upon the natural history of epidemic diarrhoea. Cambridge, UK: Cambridge University Press; 1911.
102. Eyler JM. Sir Arthur Newsholme and state medicine, 1885–1943. Cambridge, UK: Cambridge University Press; 1997.
103. Shimazono N, Katsura E. Review of Japanese literature on beriberi and thiamine. Kyoto: Vitamin B Research Committee of Japan; 1965.
104. Takaki K. Prevention of beriberi in the Japanese Navy. Se-i-kai Med J. 1885;4:29–37.
105. Takaki K. Three lectures on the preservation of health amongst the personnel of the Japanese Navy and Army. Lancet. 1906;1:1369–1374, 1451–1455, 1520–1523.
106. Eijkman C. Polyneuritis bij hoenderen. Geneesk Tijdschr nederl Indië. 1890;30:295–334; 1892;32:353–362; 1896;36:214–269.
107. Grijns G. Over polyneuritis gallinarum. Geneesk Tijdschr nederl. Indië. 1901;41:3–110.
108. Steenbock H. A review of certain researches relating to the occurrence and chemical nature of vitamin A. Yale J Biol Med. 1932;4:563–78.
109. Wolf G, Carpenter KJ. Early research into the vitamins: the work of Wilhelm Stepp. J Nutr. 1997;127:1255–9.

110. Lunin N. Über die Bedeutung der anorganischen Salze für die Ernährung des Thieres. Zeitschr physiol Chem. 1881;5:31–9.
111. von Bunge G. Lehrbuch der physiologischen und pathologischen Chemie. Leipzig: FCW Vogel; 1887.
112. Socin CA. In welcher Form wird das Eisen resorbirt? Zeitschr physiol Chem. 1891;15:93–139.
113. Pekelharing CA. Over onze kennis van de waarde der voedingsmiddelen uit chemische fabrieken. Nederlandsch Tijdschr. Geneeskunde. 1905;41:111–24.
114. Stepp W. Experimentelle Untersuchungen über die Bedeutung der Lipoide für die Ernährung. Z Biol. 1911;57:136–70.
115. Hopkins FG. The analyst and the medical man. Analyst. 1906;31:385–404.
116. Funk C. On the chemical nature of the substance which cures polyneuritis in birds induced by a diet of polished rice. J Physiol. 1911;43:395–400.
117. Funk C. The etiology of the deficiency diseases. Beri-beri, polyneuritis in birds, epidemic dropsy, scurvy, experimental scurvy in animals, infantile scurvy, ship beri-beri, pellagra. J State Med. 1912;20:341–68.
118. Needham J, Baldwin E, editors. Hopkins and biochemistry, 1861–1947. Cambridge, UK: W. Hefner and Sons; 1949.
119. Osborne TB, Mendel LB. Feeding experiments with isolated food-substances. No. 156. Washington, DC: Carnegie Institute of Washington, Publication; 1911.
120. Osborne TB, Mendel LB. The relationship of growth to the chemical constituents of the diet. J Biol Chem. 1913;15:311–26.
121. Hopkins FG. Feeding experiments illustrating the importance of accessory factors in normal dietaries. J Physiol. 1912;44:425–60.
122. McCollum EV, Davis M. The necessity of certain lipins in the diet during growth. J Biol Chem. 1913;15:167–75.
123. Mellanby E. The part played by an "accessory factor" in the production of experimental rickets. J Physiol. 1918–1919;52:xi–xii.
124. Mellanby E. A further demonstration of the part played by accessory food factors in the aetiology of rickets. J Physiol. 1918–1919;52:liii–liv.
125. McCollum EV, Simmonds N, Becker JE, Shipley PG. Studies on experimental rickets. XXI. An experimental demonstration of the existence of a vitamin which promotes calcium deposition. J Biol Chem. 1922;53:293–312.
126. Karrer P, Morf R, Schöpp K. Zur Kenntnis des Vitamins-A aus Fischtranen. Helv Chim Acta. 1931;14:1036–40.
127. Karrer P, Morf R, Schöpp K. Zur Kenntnis des Vitamins-A aus Fischtranen II. Helv Chim Acta. 1931;14:1431–6.
128. Holmes HN, Corbet RE. The isolation of crystalline vitamin A. J Am Chem Soc. 1937;59:2042–7.
129. Carpenter KJ, editor. Pellagra. Benchmark papers in biochemistry, vol. 2. Stroudsburg: Hutchinson Ross; 1981.
130. Sambon LW. Progress report on the investigation of pellagra. J Trop Med Hyg. 1910;13:289–300.
131. Etheridge EW. The butterfly caste: a social history of pellagra in the south. Westport, CT: Greenwood; 1972.
132. Searcy GH. An epidemic of acute pellagra. Alabama Med J. 1907;20:387–92.
133. Report of the Pellagra Commission of the State of Illinois, November, 1911. Springfield, IL: State Journal Company; 1912.
134. Siler JF, Garrison PE, MacNeal WJ. The relation of methods of disposal of sewage to the spread of pellagra. Arch Intern Med. 1914;14:453–74.
135. Terris M, editor. Goldberger on pellagra. Baton Rouge: Louisiana State University Press; 1964.
136. Goldberger J, Wheeler GA, Sydenstricker E. A study of the diet of nonpellagrous and of pellagrous households in textile mill communities in South Carolina in 1916. J Am Med Assoc. 1918;71:944–9.
137. Goldberger J, Wheeler GA. Experimental pellagra in the human subject brought about by a restricted diet. Public Health Rep. 1915;30:3336–9.
138. Williams CD. A nutritional disease of childhood associated with a maize diet. Arch Dis Child. 1933;8:423–33.
139. Semba RD. The rise and fall of protein malnutrition in global health. Ann Nutr Metab. 2016;69:79–88.
140. Ruxin J. The United Nations Protein Advisory Group. In: Smith SF, Phillips J, editors. Food, science, policy and regulation in the twentieth century: international and comparative perspective. Routledge: London & New York; 2000. p. 151–66.
141. United Nations. International action to avert the impending protein crisis. New York: United Nations; 1968.
142. McLaren DS. The great protein fiasco. Lancet. 1974;2:93–6.
143. Waterlow JC, Payne PR. The protein gap. Nature (London). 1975;258:113–7.
144. Silverstein AM. A history of immunology. San Diego: Academic Press; 1989.
145. Fox FW. Vitamin A and infection: a review of recent work. East Afr Med J. 1933;10:190–214.
146. Robertson EC. The vitamins and resistance to infection. Medicine. 1934;13:123–206.
147. Clausen SW. The influence of nutrition upon resistance to infection. Physiol Rev. 1934;14:309–50.
148. Blegvad O. Xerophthalmia, keratomalacia and xerosis conjunctivae. Am J Ophthalmol. 1924;7:89–117.
149. Blegvad O. Om xerophthalmien og dens forekomst i Danmark i aarene 1909–1920. København: Gyldendalske Boghandel; 1923.

150. Bloch CE. Blindness and other diseases in children arising from deficient nutrition (lack of fat-soluble A factor). Am J Dis Child. 1924;27:139–48.

151. Bloch CE. Further clinical investigations into the diseases arising in consequence of a deficiency in the fat-soluble A factor. Am J Dis Child. 1924;28:659–67.

152. Green HN, Mellanby E. Vitamin A as an anti-infective agent. BMJ. 1929;2:691–6.

153. Semba RD. The vitamin A story: lifting the shadow of death. Basel: Karger; 2012.

154. Ellison JB. Intensive vitamin therapy in measles. Br Med J. 1932;2:708–11.

155. Semba RD. On Joseph Bramhall Ellison's discovery that vitamin A reduces measles mortality. Nutrition. 2003;19:390–4.

156. Prescott SC, Proctor BE. Food technology. New York: McGraw-Hill Book Company Inc; 1937.

157. Lancet. Parliamentary intelligence. Ottawa and cod-liver oil. Lancet. 1932;2:978–979.

158. British Medical Journal. Medical notes in parliament. Ottawa agreements: cod-liver oil. Br Med J. 1932;2:661.

159. British Medical Journal. Medical notes in parliament. Ottawa agreements: cod-liver oil. Br Med J. 1932;2:819.

160. Beaton GH, Martorell R, L'Abbe KA, Edmonston B, McCabe G, Ross AC, Harvey B. Effectiveness of vitamin A supplementation in the control of young child morbidity and mortality in developing countries. ACC/SCN State-of-the-Art Nutrition Policy Discussion Paper No. 13, United Nations, New York; 1993.

161. Scrimshaw NS, Taylor CE, Gordon JE. Interactions of nutrition and infection. Geneva: WHO; 1968.

162. Beisel WR. Single nutrients and immunity. Am J Clin Nutr. 1982;35(suppl):417–68.

163. Chambers JD, Mingay GE. The agricultural revolution, 1750–1880. New York, NY: Schocken Books; 1966.

164. Price R. The modernization of rural France: communications networks and agricultural market structures in nineteenth-century France. New York, NY: St. Martin's Press; 1983.

165. Holmes CJ. Science and practice in English arable farming, 1910–1950. In: Oddy DJ, Miller DS, editors. Diet and health in modern Britain. London, Sydney, and Dover, New Hampshire: Croom Helm; 1985.

166. Aymard M. Toward the history of nutrition: some methodological remarks. In: Forster R, Ranum O, editors. Food and drink in history. Selections from the annales economies, sociétés, civilisations, vol. 5. Baltimore and London: Johns Hopkins University Press; 1979. P. 1–16.

167. Toutain JC. La consommation alimentaire en France de 1789 à 1964. Geneva: Droz; 1971.

168. Wohl AS. Endangered lives: public health in Victorian Britain. Cambridge, MA: Harvard University Press; 1983.

169. Buckley ME. The feeding of school children. London: G. Bell and Sons; 1914.

170. Great Britain. Inter-Departmental Committee on physical deterioration. Report of the Inter-Departmental Committee on physical deterioration, vol. 3. London: Wyman and Sons; 1904.

171. Burnett J. The rise and decline of school meals in Britain, 1860–1990. In: Burnett J, Oddy DJ, editors. The origins and development of food policies in Europe. London and New York: Leicester University Press; 1994.

172. Medical Research Committee. Report on the present state of knowledge concerning accessory food factors (Vitamines), compiled by a committee appointed jointly by the Lister Institute and Medical Research Committee. London: Her Majesty's Stationery Office; 1919.

173. Mann HCC. Diets for boys during the school age. Medical Research Council Special Report Series, No. 105. London: H. M. Stationery Office; 1926.

174. Nelson M. Social-class trends in British diet, 1860–1980. In: Geissler C, Oddy DJ, editors. Food, diet and economic change past and present. Leicester, London and New York: Leicester University Press; 1993. p. 101–20.

175. Paton DN, Dunlop JC, Inglis E. A study of the diet of the labouring classes in Edinburgh, carried out under the auspices of the town council of the city of Edinburgh. Edinburgh: Otto Schulze; 1901.

176. Editorial. Diet of the labouring classes. BMJ. 1913;1:647.

177. Smith D, Nicolson M. Nutrition, education, ignorance and income: a twentieth-century debate. In: Kamminga H, Cunningham A, editors. The science and culture of nutrition, 1840–1940. Amsterdam and Atlanta: Rodopi; 1995. p. 288–318.

178. Orr JB. Food health and income: report on a survey of the adequacy of diet in relation to income. London: Macmillan; 1936.

179. Floud R, Wachter K, Gregory A. Height, health and history: nutritional status in the United Kingdom, 1750–1980. Cambridge, UK: Cambridge University Press; 1990.

180. McIntosh EN. American food habits in historical perspective. Westport, CT and London: Praeger; 1995.

181. Fogel RW, Engerman SL, Trussell J. Exploring the uses of data on height. Soc Sci History. 1982;6:401–21.

182. Lindert PH, Williamson JG. Three centuries of American inequality. In: Research in economic history, vol. 1. Greenwich, CT: JAI. 1976. P. 69–123.

183. U.S. Bureau of the Census. Historical statistics of the United States, colonial times to 1970. Washington, DC: Government Printing Office; 1975.

184. U.S. Department of Agriculture. Consumption of foods in the United States, 1909–1952. Agricultural Handbook No. 62. Washington, DC: Government Printing Office; 1953.

185. Apple RD. Vitamania: vitamins in American culture. New Brunswick, NJ: Rutgers University Press; 1996.

186. Newman G. Letter to Charles Flemming. July 28, 1939. [Collection of the author].
187. Newman G. The building of a nation's health. London: Macmillan; 1939.
188. Wrigley EA, Schofield RS. The population history of England, 1541–1871. Cambridge, MA: Harvard University Press; 1981.
189. Livi-Bacci M. Population and nutrition: an essay on European demographic history. Cambridge, UK: Cambridge University Press; 1986.
190. Tranter NL. Population and society, 1750–1940: contrasts in population growth. London and New York, NY: Longman; 1985.
191. Schofield R, Reher D, Bideau A, editors. The decline of mortality in Europe. Oxford: Claredon Press; 1991.
192. Corsini CA, Viazzo PP, editors. The decline of infant and child mortality. The European experience: 1750–1990. The Hague: Kluwer Law International; 1997.
193. Hess AF. Rickets including osteomalacia and tetany. Philadelphia: Lea and Febiger; 1929.
194. Fee E, Porter D. Public health, preventive medicine, and professionalization: Britain and the United States in the nineteenth century. In: Fee E, Acheson RM, editors. A history of education in public health. Health that mocks the doctors' rules. Oxford and New York, NY: Oxford University Press; 1991. P. 15–43.
195. Lesky E. The Vienna medical school of the 19th century. Baltimore and London: Johns Hopkins University Press; 1976.
196. Fee E. Disease and discovery: a history of the Johns Hopkins School of Hygiene and Public Health, 1916–1939. Baltimore and London: Johns Hopkins University Press; 1987.
197. Curran JA. Founders of the Harvard School of Public Health, with biographical notes, 1909–1946. New York, NY: Josiah Macy, Jr. Foundation; 1970.
198. Flexner A. Medical education: a comparative study. New York, NY: Macmillan; 1925.
199. Cottrell JD. The teaching of public health in Europe. Geneva: WHO; 1969.
200. Moulin AM. The Pasteur Institutes between the two world wars. The transformation of the international sanitary order. In: Weindling P, editor. International health organizations and movements, 1918–1939. Cambridge: Cambridge University Press; 1995. P. 244–65.
201. Delaunay A. L'Institut Pasteur: des origines a aujourd'hui. Paris: Editions France-Empire; 1962.
202. Chick H, Hume M, Macfarlane M. War on disease: a history of the Lister Institute. London: André Deutsch; 1971.
203. Ettling J. The germ of laziness: Rockefeller philanthropy and public health in the new south. Cambridge, MA and London: Harvard University Press; 1981.
204. Farley J. The international health division of the Rockefeller Foundation: the Russell years, 1920–1934. In: Weindling P, editor. International health organizations and movements, 1918–1939. Cambridge, UK: Cambridge University Press; 1995. p. 203–21.
205. Cueto M. The cycles of eradication: the Rockefeller Foundation and Latin American public health, 1918–1940. In: Weindling P, editor. International health organizations and movements, 1918–1939. Cambridge, UK: Cambridge University Press; 1995. p. 222–43.
206. Brown ER. Rockefeller medicine men: medicine and capitalism in America. Berkeley: University of California Press; 1979.
207. Williams RC. The United States Public Health Service, 1798–1950. Washington, DC: Commissioned Officers Association of the United States Public Health Service; 1951.
208. Harden VA. Inventing the NIH: federal biomedical research policy, 1887–1937. Baltimore and London: Johns Hopkins University Press; 1986.
209. Black M. The children and the nations: the story of UNICEF. Sydney: P.I.C. for Unicef; 1986.
210. Phillips RW. FAO: its origins, formation and evolution, 1945–1981. Rome: Food and Agricultural Organization of the United Nations; 1981.
211. Salda ACM. Historical dictionary of the World Bank. Lanham, MD and London: Scarecrow Press; 1997.
212. Kapur D, Lewis JP, Webb R. The World Bank: its first half century. Washington, DC: Brookings Institution Press; 1997.
213. Berg A. The nutrition factor: its role in national development. Washington, DC: Brookings Institution; 1973.
214. Berg A. Malnutrition what can be done? Lessons from World Bank experience. Baltimore: Johns Hopkins University Press; 1987.

Part II
Contextualizing International Nutrition—Considering Benefit-Cost, Evidence-Base and Capacity

Chapter 2
Economics of Nutritional Interventions

Susan Horton

Keywords Cost-effectiveness · Benefit:cost · Micronutrients · Stunting · Cost · DALYs (disability-adjusted life years)

Learning Objectives

- Identify the economic consequences of undernutrition
- Describe the costs of nutritional interventions
- Prioritize nutritional interventions in terms of cost-effectiveness, and benefit–cost
- Analyze the growing economic burden associated with obesity in low- and middle-income countries
- Develop insights regarding health policy in low- and middle-income countries.

Introduction

Nutrition is a basic need and a key input as well as a desired outcome of economic development. The most important reason for investing in nutrition is to allow individuals to survive and thrive and reach their full potential. Quantifying the economic benefits of nutrition interventions can be a powerful way to advocate for increased resources for nutrition. Economic analysis can also help to decide how best to allocate investments to improve nutrition among competing programs, and how to use public funding most effectively.

Undernutrition is associated with 3.1 million child deaths each year (45% of all child deaths in 2011 [1]). This includes deaths associated with stunting, wasting, suboptimal breastfeeding, fetal growth restriction, and deficiencies of micronutrients including vitamin A and zinc. Estimates of economic losses associated with individual micronutrients can be as large as 1–2% of GDP (Gross Domestic Product, a measure of national income). More recently, studies have attempted to estimate the losses associated with stunting, and these losses can be as large as 8–10% of GDP (see The Costs of Undernutrition section). Stunting is to a large extent a consequence of diets which are chronically inadequate in quantity and quality, and is a good indicator of overall nutritional status. Recent work suggests that breastfeeding has benefits on IQ and income later in life, which is separate from measured nutritional status.

S. Horton (✉)
Balsillie School of International Affairs, University of Waterloo,
200 University Avenue West, Waterloo, ON N2L 6C2, Canada
e-mail: sehorton@uwaterloo.ca

© Springer Science+Business Media New York 2017
S. de Pee et al. (eds.), *Nutrition and Health in a Developing World*,
Nutrition and Health, DOI 10.1007/978-3-319-43739-2_2

There is a whole range of interventions which aim to improve nutritional status. Programs providing a substantial part of the diet tend to be more expensive and difficult to sustain financially, and as such are restricted to vulnerable groups (school feeding programs, food distribution to refugees, and feeding programs during short-term crises for example). There are many low-cost interventions designed to improve nutrition, such as micronutrient interventions and behavior change interventions (breastfeeding promotion being a particularly key behavior change) (see The Costs of Interventions to Reduce Undernutrition section).

It is not enough for a program to be inexpensive: it also needs to be cost-effective (see Cost-Effectiveness and Benefit–Cost of Interventions to Reduce Undernutrition section). Micronutrient interventions have been ranked as either the top or second to top development priority according to three Copenhagen Consensus exercises [2]. Over the last decade, knowledge of how to successfully rehabilitate children suffering from severe-acute malnutrition (SAM) at the community level has advanced considerably. Community care for SAM is not inexpensive, but is very cost-effective.

Benefit:cost analysis can be applied to those nutrition interventions whose main outcome is not to avert deaths, but to improve cognition, which in turn is associated with increased educational attainment. Better education and higher cognitive scores are associated with higher wages, which economists take as a measure of higher productivity. The benefit:cost ratios for selected micronutrient interventions range from 6:1 to 40:1; and the benefit:cost from interventions to reduce stunting are estimated at 8:1. These are all very favorable ratios, and suggest nutrition interventions are a good investment.

Although undernutrition has been until now the primary concern in low and middle-income countries (LMICs), overweight and obesity is of growing concern also in poor countries. Indeed, there may be interactions, in that adults who were in utero or early childhood facing diets of scarcity, are more susceptible to cardiovascular disease and diabetes if faced with diets of abundance later in life (see Chap. 32). Economic studies of the costs of overweight and obesity in LMICs are growing, although fewer in number than such studies for high income countries. The literature on the effectiveness of interventions to reduce overweight and obesity in LMICs is still modest, and the literature on costs and cost-effectiveness of such interventions is more modest still. This is one priority area for future research (see Future Research section). Another priority research area is "implementation science" which is important for nutrition as well as for health to provide guidance on scaling up effective programs. Using economic methods can also be valuable here as described in the following sections.

The Costs of Undernutrition

Undernutrition has a variety of consequences, depending on its severity, and on the particular nutrient (s) which is/are deficient. Economic studies have focused on the costs of at least half-a-dozen nutritional deficiencies, including vitamin A, iron, iodine, folic acid, zinc, and chronic undernutrition as indicated by stunting. Table 2.1 lists some of the functional consequences of deficiencies of these five micronutrients, as well as those associated with stunting, focusing on effects in early life (including effects during pregnancy). While undernutrition in the elderly is also an important topic, it is not covered here. The table also lists consequences of suboptimal breastfeeding. Breastfeeding has impacts on mortality and cognition which are independent of the effects of stunting. According to a review by Horta and Victora [3] there are plausible biological mechanisms for this effect due to the presence of long-chain unsaturated fatty acids in breastmilk, not present to the same degree in breastmilk substitutes, which are associated with cortical development.

Table 2.1 Summary of effects of selected nutritional deficiencies

Nutritional deficiency	Selected functional consequences for which economic effects have been estimated
Folic acid (in women periconception)	Neural tube defects [4] Lower mean birthweight [5]
Iodine	Cognitive impairments for children, if mother was deficient in pregnancy [6] Cognitive impairments in school-age children [7]
Iron	Increased anemia Cognitive impairments (significant in children $\geq$ 8 year) [8] Lower maximal physical work capacity (adults), lower endurance for physical work [9]
Vitamin A	Increased mortality (all-cause and diarrhea) in children [10]
Zinc	Stunting; increased diarrhea; increased pneumonia [11, 12]
Multiple (stunting)	Lower cognitive scores; Lower educational attainment; Lower earnings in adulthood [13]; increased risk of obesity/diabetes/NCDs in later life
Suboptimal breastfeeding	Higher mortality [14, 15]; lower cognitive scores and education [16]

The evidence for micronutrients is from several systematic reviews [4–12] of randomized controlled trials (RCT) involving supplementation, all recently cited by Bhutta et al. in the *Lancet* series [17]. For stunting the evidence cited is from the only major longitudinal follow-up from an RCT in childhood where children in the intervention group received supplements containing both micronutrients and protein/calories [13]. There are also supporting studies including numerous cross-sectional economic studies examining the effect of height on earnings. One study summarized eight studies for industrialized countries [18] and another eight studies for LMICs [19]; they conclude that the median increase in male wages per additional centimeter of height is 0.4% in industrialized countries, and 4% in LMICs. There are studies of natural experiments following droughts, for example, a study examining the effect on height and educational attainment in Zimbabwe [20], as well as studies following famines. A recent literature uses econometric methods to examine the interrelationships among height, cognitive attainment, schooling and earnings, for example a study of Mexico [21], which also contains references to other countries. Together, these studies also support the impact of stunting on cognition, educational attainment, and earnings. For breastfeeding, the evidence comes from systematic reviews of a mix of studies including prospective cohort and case-control studies.

There are two different techniques for incorporating an economic perspective on health and the functional impairments associated with ill health. The first approach is to use cost-effectiveness analysis, and the second is to use cost-benefit analysis (see Drummond et al. [22] for a standard reference which describes these methods in detail). In both approaches, a common outcome measure is used for various health interventions.

For cost-effectiveness analysis the common outcome is a health measure, such as deaths averted, life years saved (LYS), Quality-Adjusted Life Years (QALYs) saved, or Disability-Adjusted Life Years (DALYs) averted. LYS are typically not discounted, whereas for QALYs, and the DALY measure used here, life years saved in the future are discounted by the usual social discount rate of 3% per annum. The significance of discounting is that it makes investments with benefits far in the future (such as improved nutrition for children) less attractive. The higher the discount rate, the less attractive the investment.

For cost–benefit analysis the common outcome is a monetary unit. One frequent benefit of a health intervention is decreased treatment costs, both those incurred by the health sector as well as drug costs incurred by the patient (these two are sometimes referred to as direct costs), and those nontreatment costs borne by households (sometimes referred to as indirect costs) such as cost of caregiver's time, transportation costs to seek treatment, etc. Another benefit is associated with improved human capital.

Better health affects cognitive development, educational attainment and work participation, and hence economic productivity. Thus, the cost–benefit analysis compares the costs of providing an intervention to prevent a certain condition to the benefit in terms of higher earnings and other 'income benefits' resulting from the intervention, as well as future healthcare cost savings.

Some authors attach a monetary value to health outcomes (i.e., deaths and morbidity/disability), in order to combine health and economic costs into a single metric. There are a variety of techniques for doing this, such as using the Value of a Statistical Life or using a human capital approach, e.g., evaluating life by summing up future lost productivity [22]. These calculations involve many assumptions and ethical issues, such that many authors prefer to measure benefits such as mortality reductions separately from economic benefits, and to use cost-effectiveness rather than cost–benefit when examining interventions whose main benefit is saving lives.

When applying cost-effectiveness and cost–benefit methods to micronutrient deficiencies, there is a difficulty of comparing the costs of those deficiencies (vitamin A and zinc, for example) where the outcomes are primarily mortality and morbidity, with those deficiencies (iron and iodine, for example) where cognitive losses and hence economic productivity losses are more significant. Hence we may not be able to readily compare the economic gains associated with improved vitamin A and zinc status, with those of improved iron and iodine status. Similarly, improvements in folate status and reduced stunting have various outcomes both in terms of reduced morbidity/mortality as well as in terms of productivity and reduced treatment costs.

In Table 2.2 we summarize some estimates for costs associated with undernutrition, both in terms of health and economic costs. Later in this chapter we combine these with costs of nutrition interventions (The Costs of Interventions to Reduce Undernutrition section) to present cost-effectiveness and benefit:cost estimates for undernutrition (Cost-Effectiveness and Benefit–Cost of Interventions to Reduce Undernutrition section).

The costs of undernutrition are significant, whether in terms of increased mortality (particularly for vitamin A and zinc), lost cognition and productivity (iodine, iron), or a combination of effects (both mortality/morbidity and large treatment costs for folic acid; both mortality and losses in cognition, educational attainment, and productivity for stunting as well as suboptimal breastfeeding).

Costs measured in terms of losses at the individual level are useful, but not always easy to interpret. Various studies have been done to estimate the losses associated with certain nutritional deficiencies, at the level of a country (Table 2.3). These are obtained from models which rely on coefficients from individual-level studies such as those in Table 2.2.

The losses associated with individual micronutrient deficiencies are up to a couple of percent of GDP in the most severely affected countries. As presented in the next section, the losses are large in relation to the cost of interventions which can successfully reduce these deficiencies.

One problem with the estimates of losses attributable to individual micronutrients is that it is not easy to add up these losses in cases where there are multiple micronutrient deficiencies. For example, countries where iodine deficiency is a public health problem often have other micronutrient deficiencies as well. We would also expect interaction among the outcomes of micronutrient interventions, both in their uptake and in their impact. Some micronutrients interact in a positive way in uptake, for example, improved intake of vitamin C enhances the bioavailability of iron. Some interact in a negative way, for example, depending on amounts provided, supplementation with iron can impede uptake of zinc and vice versa, and similarly iron and calcium interact.

Micronutrients are also likely to interact in their impact on health and on productivity. For example, the effect on mortality or productivity for iron is likely to differ according to whether the individual is deficient or replete in other micronutrients. Effects may also vary according to other differences in the environment. For example, the impact of vitamin A supplementation on mortality also depends on the causes of child mortality and other measures to prevent these, such as immunization.

Table 2.2 Examples of health and economic costs associated with selected nutritional deficiencies

Nutritional deficiency	Examples of cost
Folic acid (in women periconception)	RR = 0.28 of NTDs[a] for supplementation of women of reproductive age [5]; Annual treatment costs per case: US$51,574 (NTD); $11,061–65,177 (spina bifida) $ of 2003; Spain $2734 (spina bifida), $ of 1988; South Africa $12,609 (NTD) $ of 2008 [23]
Iodine	Productivity loss per child born to a mother with goiter estimated as 10% [24]
Iron	17% productivity loss estimated in heavy manual labor; 5% in light manual, 4% in other work, for anemic adults [25]; Standardized mean difference in IQ score >8 years of age: 0.41 [8]
Vitamin A	Reduction of all-cause mortality (RR 0.76); diarrhea-related mortality (RR 0.72), reduced incidence of diarrhea (RR 0.85) and measles mortality (0.50) [10]
Zinc	Preschool children in 24-week preventive supplementation study had greater height gain (0.37 cm), 13% reduction in diarrhea and 19% in pneumonia compared to control [11, 12]
Multiple (stunting)	Children who were not stunted at 36 months, compared to those who were, in adulthood had [13]: – 20% higher hourly earnings (men); 7.2% higher (women) – Almost 20% higher per capita household income – 3.6 more grades completed schooling – 1 standard deviation higher in cognitive scores – 1.86 fewer children (women) 1 cm additional height is associated with 0.55% higher earnings for men in high income countries (median, 8 cross-sectional studies) [18] 1 cm additional height is associated with 4.5% greater earnings for men in low and middle-income countries (median, 8 cross-sectional studies) [19] Stunting in children is associated with increased relative risk of mortality: relative risk is 5.5 for severe stunting and 2.3 for moderate stunting, compared to children who are mildly stunted/not stunted [26]
Suboptimal breastfeeding	In 2011, 804,000 child deaths (11.6% of all child deaths) attributable to suboptimal breastfeeding [1]; breastfeeding associated with an increase in IQ of about 3 points [16]

[a]*NTD* neural tube defects; *RR* relative risk

More recently, several studies have used a broader indicator of nutritional status to model the loss of GDP. The first such studies in Latin America [28, 29] used underweight (weight-for-age) as the measure, which is not ideal, since stunted obese individuals are not classified as underweight. In Latin America considerable progress has been made against undernutrition so in some countries the losses were as low as 1.7% of GDP, while in others as great as 11.4%. A study for sub-Saharan Africa [30], using a similar methodology (but conflating a mixture of indicators including underweight, stunting and low birthweight) found somewhat greater losses than in Latin America, as Sub-Saharan African countries in general have greater levels of undernutrition. Two other studies [19, 31] used stunting alone (a cleaner indicator) and estimated the loss as 11.2% of GDP, with effects via education and cognition underlying a large component of this. One of these studies [19] estimated that between a quarter and a third of the nutrition effect occurs indirectly (through cognition and education); and the other estimated that 73% is due to productivity effects, 11% due to reduced mortality, with the balance due to intergenerational benefits; taller mothers have taller children, but the full benefit of nutritional improvements may take 3–4 generations to fully manifest themselves. This study is conservative since it did not include the long-term effects of stunting on noncommunicable diseases.

Suboptimal breastfeeding imposes significant costs globally. Estimates for the US suggest that the annual benefit for moving from current rates of 12.3% of exclusive breastfeeding at 6 months to 90% would be a savings of US$13 bn and 911 fewer child deaths per annum [32]. For the UK a modest

Table 2.3 Examples of economic cost of undernutrition at a country or regional level

Magnitude of effect[a]	What was modeled?
Iron deficiency	
0.81% GDP[b]: median for 10 LMICs [25]	Used anemia
Iodine deficiency	
0.48% of global GDP [27]	Rough estimate based on 12% prevalence of goiter prior to universal salt iodization
Stunting/underweight[c]	
1.7–11.4% of GDP: range for 7 Latin American/Caribbean countries [28, 29]	Used underweight
1.9–16.5% of GDP: range for 5 African countries [30]	Used a mixture of underweight, stunting and low birthweight
11.2% of GDP: estimate modeled for LMICs using 12 LMICs with good time series data on height to reflect different regions 1900–2000 [19]	Used adult male height
11.2% of GDP: average for 66 LMICs [31]	Used stunting

Notes
[a]Magnitude of effect depends on severity of condition
[b]*GDP* gross domestic product (similar to GNI or gross national income)
[c]Note that impact on NCDs later in life are not included in the cost estimates

improvement in rates (such that 45% of women were to breastfeed exclusively for 4 months as opposed to 7% currently, and 75% of babies in neonatal units were to be breastfed at discharge) would save £17 m annually in costs of treating childhood illnesses (2009–10 prices; US$27 m). For the UK effects on mothers were also modeled, and there were £21 m annually (US$34 m) in cost savings for breast cancer as well as 512 QALYs saved per year [33]. A global study estimates the cost of cognitive losses associated with inadequate breastfeeding (defined as the gap between 100% exclusive breastfeeding to 6 months, compared to current levels) as $302 billion US (2012 $), or 0.49% of world GNI. This is comprised of losses of $230 bn (0.53% of GNI) in high income countries, and $71 bn (0.39% of GNI) in LMICs [34].

The Costs of Interventions to Reduce Undernutrition

If the benefits from improved nutrition are so large, why do parents not invest more in improved nutrition for their children, assuming that they know the benefits? Understanding this can help with evaluating possible interventions. First and foremost, undernutrition is linked to poverty. The poorest households in low-income countries already spend 80% or more of their income on food, and are still unable to purchase sufficient food (and food of appropriate diversity and nutritional quality) to obtain a diet which meets the needs of all household members. Second, households may lack nutritional knowledge, particularly of the specific needs of small children who need to eat more frequently than adults, and who (because of fast growth and metabolic requirements) are especially vulnerable to micronutrient deficiencies. Households can perhaps be educated or incentivized to adopt better behaviors. Furthermore, households may not have access to convenient and nutrient-dense foods appropriate for small children, or may be constrained in their ability to feed children optimally, for example exclusive breastfeeding may not be compatible with the mother's work situation. Poor households also often have poorer living conditions and worse access to clean water and sanitation, such that infections and parasites may impede good nutritional status. Breaking these constraints can vary considerably in cost, as well as in effectiveness: it is more costly to alleviate poverty or provide additional food to a family than to provide nutritional education, but effectiveness may also differ. We will turn to costs of interventions now.

Table 2.4 summarizes estimates of the unit costs of selected nutritional interventions, using two different methodologies. The table presents costs for the two low-income regions of the world with the highest burden of undernutrition, namely sub-Saharan Africa and South and Southeast Asia. (See the original sources for these costs, also for costs for the other LMIC regions). The ingredients method costs utilize the OneHealth [35] tool, a tool which utilizes World Health organization databases for cost of health inputs. Where OneHealth did not already have a cost estimate, lists of "ingredients" were constructed for nutrition interventions (health worker time, drug and other input costs, and an assumed percentage for administration, storage, transport, distribution, and other overhead costs). The SUN estimates were constructed by the author from available country program data both from published studies and gray literature.

Cost of nutrition interventions varies. Interventions that do not involve food (micronutrient interventions, nutrition education) are modest in cost, typically less than $6 per child/pregnant woman per year and in the case of fortification, less than $1 per person per year. The exception is calcium supplementation which costs almost $19 per pregnancy. Programs involving distribution of food are an order of magnitude (ten times) more expensive than micronutrient interventions excluding calcium. Finally, the specialized food involved in community management of severe-acute malnutrition, along with the supervision required, makes these the most costly programs discussed here. Note that the $140 per child estimate for a 4-month treatment is probably more likely than the higher Scaling Up Nutrition (SUN) estimate, which was made earlier when SAM interventions were less well

Table 2.4 Unit costs (cost per child/per mother in US $) of interventions to reduce undernutrition

Intervention	Cost in AFR-E, ingredients method 2010 $ [17]	Cost in SEAR-D, ingredients method 2010 $ [17]	Cost used in SUN estimates for sub-Saharan Africa and South Asia [36]
Salt iodization (per person per year)	0.06[a]	0.06[a]	0.06
Multiple micronutrient supp (per pregnancy)[b]	6.13	5.84	N/a
Calcium supplements (per pregnancy)	18.87	18.59	N/a
Energy/protein supp (per pregnancy)	25.00[b]	25.00[2]	N/a
Vitamin A supplements (per child)	2.82	1.58	1.33
Preventive zinc supplements (per child): SUN estimate is for multiple micronutrient powders	5.88	4.63	7.98
Breastfeeding promotion (per birth)	14.18	11.69	5.82
Complementary feeding education (per child)	5.22	3.54	1.83
Complementary food supplement for 6–23 months olds (per child)	50.00[b]	50.00[b]	40.00–80.00[b]
SAM management (per case—duration 4 months)	146.19	138.72	221.60
Fortification of wheat/similar with iron (per person per year); cost to also include folic acid is negligible	–	–	0.20

N/a means not available; AFR-E refers to those countries in the World Health Organization subregion in sub-Saharan Africa with the poorest demographic profile; and SEAR-D to the corresponding region in Southeast Asia. South Asia estimates are for the region as described by the World Bank. SUN refers to the Scaling Up Nutrition movement
[a]Uses SUN estimates
[b]Author's estimates, since an exact protocol for the amount, duration and composition of such supplements has not been developed

established. We will discuss relative cost-effectiveness of these various programs shortly: however for LMIC governments, affordability of interventions is very important as it requires having access to financial and nonfinancial resources. Any program costing $140 per child in a low-income country is difficult to afford if a significant number of children are involved.

Two sets of unit cost estimates have been used in global costing exercises. The SUN estimates were used for a set of interventions similar (but not identical) to those from a previous *Lancet* nutrition series [37], and the ingredients method estimates for the 2013 *Lancet* nutrition series [17]. In each case, priority countries were picked comprising 90% of world stunting. For the SUN estimates there were 36; for the 2013 *Lancet* series there were 34 (with considerable overlap). In each case, the cost of increasing existing coverage to reach 90% of the population was estimated. The 2013 *Lancet* estimates were that scaling up ten key direct nutrition interventions would cost $9.6 bn annually. While this is a large number, the cost would be likely split between international assistance (in particular for the poorest countries) and domestic resource mobilization. If approximately one-third of the cost was covered by international assistance (i.e., $3 bn) this can be put in context of constituting about 11% of the annual global assistance for health, which was almost $27 bn in 2010 [38].

The total $9.6 bn total was divided up by intervention as shown in Fig. 2.1. Micronutrient interventions (other than calcium) account for around a third of the total (one sixth for calcium alone, and the other sixth for vitamin A, multiple micronutrients in pregnancy, and zinc). Nutrition education programs (around breastfeeding and complementary feeding) account for another $1 bn. Finally, programs involving food account for over half of the total, fairly equally split between targeted food supplements for pregnant women and young children in food-insecure households, and community management of severe-acute malnutrition.

The *Lancet* estimates [17] only cover the costs of "nutrition-specific" interventions—interventions known to directly affect nutrition. In the long run, however, nutrition-sensitive investments are needed to sustain improved nutritional status. These investments in agriculture, women's empowerment, water and sanitation, poverty alleviation, etc., are essential. These will promote human development in the long run, including a diet that is appropriate in quality and quantity to promote human health. Costing for these nutrition-sensitive investments has not yet been undertaken. If sufficient

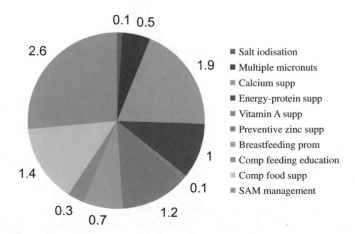

Fig. 2.1 Annual cost of increasing coverage of nutrition interventions identified as effective and cost-effective in US $ billion [1]. Coverage increases from current levels to 90% in 34 priority countries. *Source* Uses data in web appendix for [17]

nutrition-sensitive investments can be made, then some of the shorter term nutrition-specific interventions can be discontinued. High-income countries do not need to provide food supplements except to particular vulnerable populations, and rarely have to treat severe-acute malnutrition.

Cost-Effectiveness and Benefit–Cost of Interventions to Reduce Undernutrition

Just because an intervention is inexpensive, does not make it worth implementing. Similarly, some programs which have significant cost can be worth implementing. This is where cost-effectiveness (and benefit:cost) analysis can assist.

A summary of studies undertaken between 2000 and 2008 [23, 37] suggested the following:

- Cost-effectiveness figures (cost per DALY averted)

  - $5–15 for vitamin A supplements and periodic zinc supplements (in multiple micronutrient powders)
  - $40 for community-based management of SAM
  - $50–150 for behavior change interventions (at scale)
  - $73 for therapeutic zinc
  - $66–115 for iron fortification
  - $90 for folic acid fortification
  - $500–1000 for food supplements for young children

- Benefit:cost ratios were as follows:

  - 6:1 for deworming
  - 8:1 for iron fortification of staples
  - 30:1 for salt iodization
  - 46:1 for folic acid fortification

The highest priorities using the cost-effectiveness metric are the interventions with the lowest cost per DALY averted. For the benefit:cost metric, all four interventions examined are well worthwhile as their benefits (higher future wages or healthcare savings) are considerably higher than their costs. One problem is that it is not simple to compare interventions whose outcomes are DALYs, with those whose outcomes are expressed in benefit:cost terms. Thus iron fortification (where outcomes are primarily cognitive, with some modest lives saved) does not rank high on the cost-effectiveness metric, but ranks high on a benefit:cost metric.

These figures put several micronutrient initiatives at the top amongst the nutritional interventions, because they are effective but inexpensive. Community management of SAM—although costly per child—ranks next, simply because it saves the lives of children who otherwise have a high probability of dying. Effective behavior change interventions come next. Although frequently inexpensive (especially those using radio or other media, rather than one-on-one counseling), these programs vary wildly in their effectiveness often due to differences in the populations being served, including their ability to change their behavior which is linked to their circumstances and to what they can afford, and the intensity of the implementation and oversight that is being built into the programs. Finally, programs involving food supplements are the least cost-effective because providing food is costly.

These cost-effectiveness data for nutritional interventions are comparable to other high-priority health interventions for children in LMICs [39]. Other health interventions costing approximately $10 per DALY saved include, for example: vaccination against TB, DPT, polio, and measles (the traditional "Expanded Program of Immunization" for children); use of insecticide-treated nets against malaria; and residual household spraying against malaria. Health interventions costing around $40 per

DALY include a couple of different counseling programs against HIV/AIDS, plus condom promotion and distribution. Interventions costing $1000 per DALY include antiretroviral treatment for HIV/AIDS, and use of aspirin and beta-blockers to prevent ischemic heart disease. These values indicate that nutrition interventions are of comparable cost-effectiveness as other high-priority public health interventions (and selected medical interventions) in LMICs.

Updated cost-effectiveness estimates are available not for individual interventions, but for components of a recommended nutrition package in the 2013 *Lancet* series, summarized in Table 2.5. In this study, a full epidemiological model was used (LiST: the Lives Saved Tool to examine the combined impact of a variety of recommended nutritional interventions delivered together [40]).

When several interventions are implemented together, or at the same time, we expect the combined impact on averting deaths and illness will be less than the sum of all the individual effects. For example, both measles vaccination and vitamin A reduce measles mortality and morbidity, but the combined effect is smaller (lives can be saved by one or other intervention, but the same life cannot be saved twice). Using a comprehensive model such as LiST avoids the double counting involved when several interventions are used simultaneously.

Note that some of the interventions in Table 2.5 have stronger effects on cognitive development but limited impacts on mortality, for example, salt iodization, iron supplements, and the food supplements both for pregnant women and young children. However, the LiST model does not take account of cognitive benefits.

Although the cost-effectiveness numbers in Table 2.5 are not quite as low as those from earlier studies, the interventions modeled remain attractive as high-priority interventions. Note that the data in Table 2.5 will be somewhat closer to those from SUN [37] once adjusted for inflation. The use of a single tool to model all the interventions when combined is more methodologically sound than separate estimates for individual interventions.

One recent study [41] used the same unit cost data as in the *Lancet* series (presented in Table 2.5) [17] to estimate the benefit:cost of interventions to reduce stunting. This is a different metric than cost-effectiveness shown in Table 2.5, since stunting can be related to improved cognition, hence education and productivity, which the LiST model does not incorporate. This study consisting of 17 LMICs estimated the cost of stunting as presented in Table 2.3, but rather than presenting the losses as a percentage of GDP, it compared the anticipated benefits from reduced stunting, to the costs of

Table 2.5 Cost-effectiveness of a package of nutritional interventions in 34 priority countries[a]

Intervention	Annual cost ($ bn)	Lives saved per year	Cost per life-year saved (DALY saved)
Optimum maternal nutrition in pregnancy[b]	$3.4 bn	102,000	$571 ($1051)
Infant and young child feeding[c]	$2.3 bn	221,000	$175 ($322)
Micronutrient supplementation for children[d]	$1.3 bn	145,000	$159 ($293)
Management of severe-acute malnutrition[e]	$2.6 bn	435,000	$125 ($230)
Total	$9.6 bn	903,000	$179 ($329)

[a]Results are for when entire package of all interventions is scaled up at once to 90% coverage in the 34 priority countries in [17]

[b]Consists of multiple micronutrient supplements to all; calcium supplements to mothers at risk of low intake; maternal balanced energy protein supplements to mothers at risk of low intake and universal salt iodization

[c]Consists of promotion of early and exclusive breastfeeding to 6 months, and continued breastfeeding to 24 months; appropriate complementary feeding education in food-secure environments, and education plus supplements in food-insecure environments

[d]Consists of vitamin A supplementation between 6 and 59 months of age and preventive zinc supplements between 12 and 59 months of age

[e]Community-based management

reducing stunting using SUN and the Lancet series methods [17, 37]. The results suggest that the benefit:cost of reducing stunting in the median country is 18:1, and that the economic benefits (as well as the benefits of saving 900,000 lives) make this a very worthwhile investment.

Future Research

In the preceding sections we have focused on undernutrition, however, it is clear that overweight and obesity in LMICs are also becoming a large issue both for well-being and the associated economic costs. One early study [42] estimated that in 1995, the costs of undernutrition and those of overweight/obesity were about the same for China, while the undernutrition costs still exceeded costs of overweight/obesity in India. However it was also estimated that by 2025, costs of overweight/ obesity would exceed those of underweight for China, and the two sets of costs would be similar in magnitude for India. In this study, the economic costs of overweight/obesity were based on mortality from, and treatment costs of, diet-related noncommunicable diseases.

A more recent study for China [43] provides more detailed estimates of the costs of overweight and obesity. It separates direct costs (for medical treatment) from indirect (lost productivity due to premature mortality, morbidity, and absenteeism from work). Direct costs were estimated to account for 0.48% of GDP in 2000, and were predicted to increase to 0.50% in 2025. Estimates of indirect losses were considerably larger, amounting to 3.58% of GDP in 2000 but predicted to substantially increase to 8.73% by 2025.

A study for Brazil [44] focused only on the direct costs, which were estimated as 0.09% of GDP annually for the 2008–10 period. The authors compared these to similar estimates for Western Europe (ranging from 0.09 to 0.61% of GDP, depending on the country), and Korea (0.22% of GDP). The lower impact in the Brazil study may also have been due to including a narrower range of disease conditions than the study for China, as well as excluding indirect costs.

Even for industrialized countries where there has been intense interest in overweight and obesity, we are still at an early stage in identifying the cost-effectiveness of interventions to prevent or reduce these conditions. There is a broad array of interventions, ranging from individual actions to public health measures, and encompassing behavioral measures, price and regulatory policy, curative measures, etc.

Furthermore, obesity and overweight outcomes are harder to model than those of underweight or stunting. While stunting is largely determined early in life (within the first three years, although some catch-up is possible later), overweight and obesity can change over the life course. Hence it is harder to predict the impact on chronic diseases whose adverse consequences manifest in later life. At the same time, we are aware that dietary and possibly physical activity habits are set early in life, such that it is important to begin policies now to protect against, and reverse, the growing trends in overweight and obesity. This is an area of growing research need, also for LMICs.

Another area where research is needed for LMICs is in "implementation science" for nutritional interventions. As the SUN movement (http://www.scalingupnutrition.org) and related initiatives succeed in drawing attention and resources, it is important that programs are effective and cost-effective. Economics research can assist here too.

Discussion Points

- When can/should we use benefit:cost methods to evaluate nutrition interventions, and when can/should we use cost-effectiveness methods?
- How can economics methods be useful for practitioners and policymakers interested in nutrition?

- Are nutrition interventions good "value for money" for governments in LMICs and why?
- Nutrition education programs cost pennies per child, whereas treatment of severe-acute malnutrition can cost upwards of $200 per child. Does this mean we should give higher priority to nutrition education?
- How do public health policy priorities need to change in response to the "nutritional transition" underway in LMICs?
- How do interactions among nutrition interventions affect their cost-effectiveness/benefit:cost?

References

1. Black RE, Victora CG, Walker SP, Bhutta ZA, Christian P, De Onis M, Essati J, Grantham-McGregor S, Katz J, Martorell R, Uauy R and the Maternal and Child Nutrition Study Group. Maternal and child undernutrition and overweight in low-income and middle-income countries. Lancet. 2013;382:427–51.
2. http://www.copenhagenconsensus.com. Accessed 12 Sept 2014.
3. Horta BL, Victora CG. Long-term effects of breastfeeding: a systematic review. Geneva: WHO; 2013.
4. De-Regil LM, Fernandez-Gaxiola AC, Dowswell T, Pena-Rosas JP. Effects and safety of periconceptional folate supplementation for preventing birth defects. Cochrane Database Sys Rev. 2010;10:CD007950.
5. Lassi ZS, Salam RA, Haider BA, Bhutta ZA. Folic acid supplementation during pregnancy for maternal health and pregnancy outcomes. Cochrane Database Sys Rev. 2013;3:CD006896.
6. Zimmermann MB. The effects of iodine deficiency in pregnancy and infancy. Paediatr Perinat Epidemiol. 2012;26 (supp 1):108–17.
7. Zimmermann MB, Connolly K, Bozo M, Bridson J, Rohner F, Grimci L. Iodine supplementation improves cognition in iodine-deficient schoolchildren in Albania: a randomized, controlled, double-blind study. Am J Clin Nutr. 2006;83:108–14.
8. Sachdev H, Gera T, Nestel P. Effect of iron supplementation on mental and motor development in children: systematic review of randomised controlled trials. Public Health Nutr. 2005;8:117–32.
9. Ross J, Horton S. Economic consequences of iron deficiency. Ottawa: Micronutrient Initiative, Technical Paper; 1998.
10. Imdad A, Herzer K, Mayo-Wilson E, Yakoob MY, Bhutta ZA. Vitamin A supplementation for preventing morbidity and mortality in children from 6 months to 5 years of age. Cochrane Database Syst Rev. 2010;12: CD008524.
11. Imdad A, Bhutta ZA. Effect of preventive zinc supplementation on linear growth in children under 5 years of age in developing countries: a meta-analysis of studies for input to the lives saved tool. BMC Public Health. 2011;11 (suppl3):S22.
12. Yakoob MY, Theodoratou E, Jabeen A, et al. Preventive zinc supplementation in developing countries: impact on mortality and morbidity due to diarrhea, pneumonia and malaria. BMC Public Health. 2011;11(suppl3):S23.
13. Hoddinott J, Maluccio JA, Behrman JR, Flores R, Martorell R. Effect of a nutrition intervention during early childhood on 5 economic productivity in Guatemalan adults. Lancet. 2008;271:411–6.
14. Lamberti LM, Fischer Walker CI, Noiman A, et al. Breastfeeding and the risk for diarrhea morbidity and mortality. BMC Public Health. 2011;11(suppl 3):S15.
15. Lamberti LM, Zakarija-Grkovic I, Fischer Walker CI, et al. Breastfeeding for reducing the risk of pneumonia morbidity and mortality in children under two: a systematic literature review and meta-analysis. BMC Public Health. 2013;13(suppl 3):S18.
16. Horta BL, Victora CG. Long-term effects of breastfeeding: a systematic review. Geneva: WHO; 2013.
17. Bhutta ZA, Das JK, Rizvi A, Gaffey MF, Walker N, Horton S, Webb P, Lartey A, Black RE for Lancet Maternal and Child Nutrition & Interventions Review Group. Evidence based interventions for improving maternal and child nutrition: what can be done and at what cost? Lancet. 2013;382:452–77.
18. Gao W, Smyth R. Health, human capital, height and wages in China. J Dev Stud. 2010;46:466–84.
19. Horton S, Steckel RH. Malnutrition: global economic losses attributable to malnutrition 1900–2000 and projections to 2050. In: Lomborg B, editor. How much have global problems cost the world? Cambridge: Cambridge University Press; 2013.
20. Alderman H, Hoddinott J, Kinsey BH. Long term consequences of early childhood malnutrition. Oxford Economic Papers. 2006;58:450–64.
21. Vogl T. Height, skills, and labor market outcomes in Mexico. J Dev Econ. 2014;107:84–96.

22. Drummond MF, Schulpher MJ, Torrance GW, O'Brien B, Stoddart GI. Methods for the economic evaluation of health care programs. 3rd ed. Oxford: Oxford Medical Publications; 2005.

23. Yi Y, Lindemann M, Colligs A, Snowball C. Economic burden of neural tube defects and impact of prevention with folic acid. Eur J Pediatr. 2011;170(11):1391–400.

24. Ross J. Profiles guidelines: calculating the effects of malnutrition on economic productivity and survival [mimeo.]. Washington DC: Academy for Educational Development; 1997.

25. Horton S, Ross J. The economics of iron deficiency. Food Policy. 2003;28(1):51–75. Also Corrigendum. Food Policy 2006;52:141–143.

26. Olofin I., McDonald CM, Ezzati M, Flaxman S, Black RE, Fawzi WW, Caulfield LE, Danaei G, for the Nutrition Impact Model Study (anthropometry cohort pooling). Associations of suboptimal growth with all-cause and cause-specific mortality in children under five years: a pooled analysis of ten prospective studies. PLoS ONE 2013;8:e64636. Doi:10.1371/journal.pone.0064636, http://www.plosone.org/article/info%3Adoi%2F10.1371%2Fjournal.pone.0064636.

27. Horton S. The economics of nutritional interventions. In: Semba RD, Bloem M, editors. Nutrition and health in developing countries. 2nd ed. Totowa NJ: Humana Press; 2005.

28. Martínez R, Fernández A. Model for analysing the social and economic impact of child undernutrition in Latin America. 52. United Nations. Serie manuals 52. 2007. http://www.eclac.cl/publicaciones/xml/5/35645/Serie_manual_52_eng.pdf.

29. Martinez R, Fernández A. The cost of hunger: social and economic impact of child undernutrition in Central America and the Dominican Republic. United Nations. 2008. http://www.eclac.org/publicaciones/xml/9/32669/DP_CostHunger.pdf.

30. African Union Commission, NEPAD Planning and Coordinating Agency, UN Economic Commission for Africa, and UN World Food Programme, 2013. The cost of hunger in Africa: social and economic impact of child undernutrition in Egypt, Ethiopia, Swaziland and Uganda. Abridged report. Available at http://www.costofhungerafrica.com. Accessed 12 Sept 2014.

31. Stricker S, Beretta-Piccoli N, Horton S. The cost of stunting in low and middle income countries. 2014; Unpublished draft.

32. Bartick M, Reinhold A. The burden of suboptimal breastfeeding in the United States: a pediatric cost analysis. Pediatrics. 2010;125:e1048–56.

33. Renfrew MJ, Pokhrel S, Quigley M, McCormick F, Fox-Rushby J, Dodds R, et al. Preventing disease and saving resources; the potential contribution of increasing breastfeeding rates in the UK: UNICEF; 2012. Available at: http://www.unicef.org.uk/Documents/Baby_Friendly/Research/Preventing_disease_saving_resources.pdf?epslanguage=en. Accessed 12 June 2014.

34. Rollins, N., Bhandari N, Hajeebhoy N, Horton S, Lutter C, Martines JM, Piwoz E, Richter L, Victora C. Breastfeeding in the 21st century: Why invest, and what it will take to improve breastfeeding practices in less than a generation. Lancet Breastfeeding Series Paper 2. 2016;387:491–504.

35. United National OneHealth model. Available at http://www.futuresinstitute.org/onehealth.aspx.

36. Horton S, Shekar M, McDonald C, Mahal A. Scaling-up nutrition: what will it cost? Washington, DC: World Bank Directions in Development; 2009.

37. Bhutta ZA, Ahmed T, Black RE et al, for the Maternal and Child Undernutrition Group. What works? Interventions for maternal and child undernutrition and survival. Lancet 2008;371:417–40.

38. Murray CJL, Anderson B, Burstein R, Leach-Kemon K, Schneider M, Tardif A, Zhang R. Development assistance for health: trends and prospects. Lancet. 2011;378:8–10.

39. Laxminarayanan R, Chow J, Shahid-Salles S. Intervention cost-effectiveness: overview of main messages. In: Jamison DT, Alleyne G, Breman J, Claeson M, Evans DB, Jha P, Measham AR, Mills A, editors. Disease control priorities in developing countries. 2nd ed. Oxford: Oxford University Press; 2006.

40. http://www.jhsph.edu/departments/international-health/centers-and-institutes/institute-for-international-programs/list/index.html. Accessed 12 Sept 2014.

41. Hoddinott J, Alderman H, Behrman JR, Haddad L, Horton S. The economic rationale for investing in stunting. Matern Child Nutr. 2013;9(S2):69–82.

42. Popkin B, Horton S, Kim S, Mahal A, Jin A. Diet-related noncommunicable diseases in China and India: the economic costs of the nutrition transition. Nutr Rev. 2001;59:379–90.

43. Popkin BM, Kim S, Rusev ER, Du S, Zizza C. Measuring the full economic costs of diet, physical activity and obesity-related chronic diseases. Obes Rev. 2006;7:271–93.

44. Bahia L, Freire Coutinho ES, Barufali LA, de Azevedo Abreu G, Malhão, Ribeiro de Souza CP, Araujo DV. The costs of overweight and obesity-related diseases in the Brazilian public health system:cross-sectional study. BMC Public Health. 2012;12:440–6.

Chapter 3
Nutrition Evidence in Context

Saskia de Pee and Rebecca F. Grais

Keywords Evidence-based guidelines · Nutrition science · Impact evaluation · External validity · Systematic review · Context

Learning Objectives

- Explain the concept of evidence-based medicine (EBM).
- Understand the differences between medicine and nutrition science with regard to the type of evidence that is required for choosing an intervention.
- Know which factors affect the external validity of RCTs in nutrition.
- Understand why context plays such an important role in the impact of most nutrition-specific interventions.
- Be able to propose a design for assessing how a specific intervention implemented under real-life circumstances contributes to improving nutritional status of a specific target group.

Introduction

Reducing the burden of malnutrition requires interventions that address its causes in an effective manner. In order to decide which interventions to implement, one requires evidence of what works best and at what cost. This raises the question as to what evidence is suitable. For example, if the aim is to reduce anemia in a population, should one look at evidence of impact of interventions to prevent malaria, delay clamping of the umbilical cord, provide iron/folic acid tablets to pregnant women, micronutrient powders (MNPs) to children aged 6–23 months, deworming, or all of those? And would one require evidence on the specific impact of each of these interventions in the absence or the presence of the other interventions? We would also need to know whether the findings among one target group can be extended to other target groups and whether impact found in one setting, for example in sub-Saharan Africa, will be the same in for example South Asia or Latin America. And, what kinds of

S. de Pee
Nutrition Division, World Food Programme, Rome, Italy
e-mail: Saskia.depee@wfp.org; depee.saskia@gmail.com

S. de Pee
Friedman School of Nutrition Science and Policy, Tufts University, Boston, MA, USA

R.F. Grais (✉)
Epicentre (Medecins sans Frontieres), 8 rue Saint Sabin, 75011 Paris, France
e-mail: rebecca.grais@epicentre.msf.org

© Springer Science+Business Media New York 2017
S. de Pee et al. (eds.), *Nutrition and Health in a Developing World*,
Nutrition and Health, DOI 10.1007/978-3-319-43739-2_3

research designs provide reliable quality of evidence, should they only be individually randomized, double-blind and placebo-controlled, or can observational studies or nutrition surveillance data also provide useful information? Then, apart from evidence of impact, one also needs to factor in the programming costs, coverage of the intended target group, and their adherence to the intervention, when making decisions as to what strategies and programs to implement to improve nutrition.

This chapter puts evidence for nutrition in context, by reviewing the history of EBM and how it is being applied to nutrition, what principle difficulties are of doing that and how to take that into account when interpreting available evidence for impact of nutrition-specific interventions, how to choose interventions and strategies for improving nutrition, and what to monitor and evaluate when implementing nutrition-specific or -sensitive programs.

Evidence-Based Medicine

Conceptually, EBM is the application of the scientific method to medical decision-making. Until relatively recently, research results were incorporated in decision-making through a highly subjective process, sometimes referred to as "the art of medicine." This means that decisions about individual patients depended on each individual physician or medical professional to determine what research evidence, if any, to consider. In the case of decisions that applied to populations, guidelines and policies were usually developed by committees of experts, but there was no formal process for determining the extent to which research evidence should be considered. The assumption was that the practitioners incorporate evidence in their thinking, based on their education, experience, and ongoing study of the applicable literature and therefore this would be sufficient.

However, in the 1970s these assumptions came under critique. Feinstein's publication of Clinical Judgment in 1967 focused attention on the role of clinical reasoning and identified biases that can affect it [1]. In 1972, Cochrane published "Effectiveness and Efficiency," which described the lack of controlled trials supporting many practices that had previously been assumed to be effective [2]. Along with other research looking at clinical judgment and weakness in evidence underlying common practices in medicine, evidence-based methods emerged.

The term "evidence-based" was first used in the context of population-level policies by David M. Eddy. Eddy first published the term "evidence-based" in March 1990, in an article in the Journal of the American Medical Association (JAMA) that laid out the principles of evidence-based guidelines and population-level policies, which Eddy described as *explicitly describing the available evidence that pertains to a policy and tying the policy to evidence. Consciously anchoring a policy, not to current practices or the beliefs of experts, but to experimental evidence. The policy must be consistent with and supported by evidence. The pertinent evidence must be identified, described, and analyzed. The policymakers must determine whether the policy is justified by the evidence. A rationale must be written* [3]. This paper was one of a series of 28 publications in JAMA between 1990 and 1997 on formal methods for designing population-level guidelines and policies [3, 4].

The objective of EBM is to improve decision-making by focusing on the use of evidence generated from well-designed and conducted research. EBM can be applied to medical education, decisions about the clinical care of individuals, international guidelines and policies applied to populations, or administration of health services in general [5]. In essence, EBM advocates that to the greatest extent possible, decisions and policies should be based on evidence, not just the beliefs of patients, clinicians, experts, politicians, or administrators. It thus tries to assure that a clinician's opinion, which may be limited by knowledge gaps or biases, is supplemented with all available knowledge from the scientific literature so that best practice can be determined and applied. It promotes the use of formal, explicit methods to analyze evidence [6].

Although all medicine based on science has some degree of empirical support, EBM classifies evidence by its strengths and considers only the strongest types (coming from meta-analyses, systematic reviews, and RCTs) as yielding strong recommendations. Weaker types (such as from case-control and observational studies) can yield only weak recommendations [5]. In brief, the method for designing evidence-based recommendations and guidelines follows the following process. First, the questions are framed, by specifying population of interest, interventions or a comparison of interventions, desired outcomes, period, and context. Second, the available published peer-reviewed scientific literature is searched to identify studies that address the questions. Third, each of these studies is reviewed to assess whether the study addresses the question and what it reports about it. If several studies address the question, their results are synthesized (meta-analysis or systematic review). Fourth, the results of the review of the literature on the question are then compiled and summarized to draw a conclusion about the question. Finally, recommendations or guidelines are written based on this review [7, 8].

Systematic reviews of peer-reviewed research studies are a major part of the evaluation of particular practices, treatments and preventive measures, among others. The Cochrane Collaboration is one of the best-known programs that conduct systematic reviews. Once all the best evidence is assessed in a Cochrane review, the intervention or practice is categorized as (1) likely to be beneficial, (2) likely to be harmful, or (3) evidence did not support either benefit or harm. In order to make these assessments, the evidence that is available is "graded." Different organizations and groups have different classifications for grading, although there are certain differences, in general the following applies to the majority of grading assessments [9, 10].

The strongest evidence for interventions is provided by a systematic review of multiple, randomized, blinded, placebo-controlled trials with allocation concealment and complete follow-up involving a homogeneous patient population and medical condition (see forthcoming paragraphs for additional information on RCTs). In contrast, patient testimonials, case reports, and expert opinion have little value because of the biases inherent in observation and reporting of outcomes, difficulties in ascertaining who is an expert, and subjectivity [11]. In sum, evidence generated can be classified into the following categories:

- Level I: Evidence obtained from at least one properly designed RCT.
- Level II-1: Evidence obtained from well-designed controlled trials without randomization.
- Level II-2: Evidence obtained from well-designed cohort or case-control analytic studies, preferably from more than one center or research group.
- Level II-3: Evidence obtained from multiple time series designs with or without the intervention.
- Level III: Opinions of respected authorities, based on clinical experience, descriptive studies, or reports of expert committees [12].

Once classified into categories (the above categorization is generally agreed upon), the evidence itself is graded for its quality by the individuals or group(s) performing the evidence-based review. Strong or weak recommendations are then made based on this review. High-quality evidence can be interpreted as there being a very low probability of further research completely changing the conclusions. Moderate quality evidence is such as that further research may completely change the conclusions. Low quality of evidence is such that further research is likely to change the conclusions completely. Very low quality evidence is such that research will most probably change the conclusions completely [13].

In order to understand these classifications and grading, it is important to understand the underlying principles of a RCT. In a RCT, people being studied are randomly allocated to one or several different interventions. The RCT is considered the gold standard for a clinical trial and is often used to test the efficacy or effectiveness of various types of interventions [14, 15]. Random assignment of intervention is done after subjects have been assessed for eligibility and recruited, but before the intervention to be studied begins. Conceptually, the process is like tossing a coin. After randomization, the two (or more) groups of participants are followed in exactly the same way, and the only differences between the care they receive, is the intervention that is being tested. Randomization minimizes allocation bias, balancing both known and unknown characteristics of the participants across the intervention groups. Blinding[1] ensures that there is no subjectivity introduced and use of a placebo (or absence of the intervention) ensures that the study measures the effect of the intervention directly. These design features improve the internal validity of the RCT. The reason RCTs are held as the gold standard in medical research is that the tenets of the design allow for an establishment of causality [16, 17].

The extent to which RCTs' results are applicable outside the trial setting varies (external validity). Factors that can affect RCTs' external validity most applicable to nutrition include: where the RCT was performed (e.g., what works in one setting may not work in another); characteristics of the participants (e.g., an RCT may exclude pregnant women); and the study procedures and follow-up care may be difficult to achieve in the "real world" meaning that the results may not be the same when applied outside of a study.

Further, the information obtained from an explanatory RCT may not be what is most useful for policymaking. Epidemiologists distinguish between the efficacy and the effectiveness of an intervention. Efficacy trials (usually RCTs) are explanatory trials and aim to determine whether an intervention leads to an expected result under ideal conditions. Effectiveness trials aim to measure the degree of effect in the "real world." As such, the study procedures in effectiveness studies resemble programmatic or "normal" practices. These concepts exist on a continuum and their generalizability depends upon the population, the condition, the severity of the illness, and the intervention itself among other factors. As such, the generalizability of findings from one single study may range from low to high depending on how the results are to be used [18]. An RCT may address either efficacy or effectiveness (and sometimes even both in the case of certain interventions like vaccines).

Because RCTs are the gold standard, observational data, historical trends, and certain effectiveness studies are graded much lower. Such a standard is justified by the usually high cost of certain medical treatments, by the risk that therapeutic decisions based on inadequate evidence would shift treatment away from possibly more efficacious therapies, and from the need to balance benefits against the risks that accompany pharmacotherapy. RCTs are comparatively very expensive, can be challenging from an ethical perspective (see Chap. 36 by Doherty and Chopra), often long to conduct and with a delay between study completion and publication, and before the results lead to (modification of) guidelines and implementation in practice. Due to these limitations, relying on evidence generated from RCTs alone limits the scope and applicability of research for public health programming. Furthermore, by their very nature, programming considerations are rarely incorporated into RCTs, and in many cases, questions about nutritional programming may not lend themselves to an RCT design thereby excluding these questions from consideration. It is important to note that use of RCTs is not limited to specific interventions, but can also be used in impact evaluations. In this case, different nutritional programs are the interventions and the primary objective of the trial is to measure the impact of different programs. Like RCTs in the medical paradigm, these impact evaluation RCTs do not lend well to evaluating nutritional programming. This is due to the often long period of time needed to measure impact, particularly with respect to nutrition-sensitive programming.

For the reasons discussed above, decisions about nutritional interventions also need to draw heavily on studies with designs other than RCTs. These other types of evaluations are particularly important when an intervention is complex, or is implemented amidst a complex set of other interventions that also affect the main outcome indicator(s), such that the results of an RCT will be

---

[1]A blind(ed) study is one where information about the intervention is masked from the participant, to reduce or eliminate bias, until after the study result outcome is known. In double-blind studies, both the participants and investigators are blinded to which participants received which intervention. Triple-blind studies have participants, investigators and the safety committee, which reviews results, masked to intervention groups.

unacceptably artificial (not applicable to the real world); when an intervention has been established as efficacious at a small scale, but its effectiveness at scale needs to be assessed, which is often the case in nutritional interventions; and there are also cases when ethical concerns preclude the use of an RCT [19].

Nutrition Science

Nutrition science deals with food and nourishment, especially in humans and also includes the study of human behaviors related to food choices [20, 21]. A person's nutritional status is affected by food intake and by disease, which are recognized as the two direct (or immediate) causes of malnutrition [22, 23]. Disease affects food intake, by lowering appetite, affects how food intake supports nutritional status by affecting nutrient utilization, i.e., disease leads to nutrient losses and less efficient absorption, and increases the body's nutrient needs. Nutrition focuses on maintaining or improving health by focusing on the diet [24].

An essential nutrient is a nutrient that the body cannot synthesize on its own—or not to an adequate amount—and must be provided by the diet. These nutrients are necessary for the body to function properly. The six categories of essential nutrients include carbohydrates, protein, fat, vitamins, minerals, and water. Nutrients are required for metabolic processes that provide energy, support growth and tissue replacement, affect cellular and humoral immune systems, neural and cognitive development, etc. [25]. Results of deficiencies of nutrients are many, some of which are specific (e.g., signs of deficiency of specific vitamins) while others are systemic and involve several nutrients (e.g., reduced growth or increased morbidity).

Semba's chapter 'Historical Perspective' (Chap. 1) provides a thorough overview of how modern medicine and nutritional science evolved over the last two centuries [26] and a recent article by Semba focuses specifically on the history around discovery and provision of single micronutrients and the introduction of multi-micronutrient supplements and fortified foods, through the health and the food system, respectively [27]. The roots of modern nutritional science are in experimental physiology in France at the beginning of the nineteenth century. Gradually during the nineteenth century, the different substances in food, and the fact that they are essential for the body, were discovered. Proteins, carbohydrates, fats, salts and water, foods such as milk, whey and egg yolk were recommended for certain diseases, and the protection of infant health by breastfeeding was realized. Late in the nineteenth and early in the twentieth century, vitamin theory and characterization of vitamins were established. Specific deficiency signs, such as beriberi for thiamin, scurvy for vitamin C, and pellagra for niacin, triggered the investigations and lead to the discovery of the specific vitamins.

Between 1920 and 1940, different trials were done that found that nutrition and immunity were closely related. Vitamin A was a nutrient of particular interest and became known as the anti-infective vitamin. The practice of consuming cod liver oil, a very good source of vitamins A and D, became widespread in the US and Europe in the late 1920s and remained popular for several decades, for the prevention of illness among children. A relationship between quality of the diet and tuberculosis incidence was also observed as British prisoners of war in Germany, during the Second World war, who received a supplementary food ration from the Red Cross consisting of meat, butter, cheese, milk powder and other foods had a 15 times lower TB incidence as compared to Russian prisoners of war who were housed under the same circumstances, but did not receive such food rations [28]. As medicine advanced in the 1940s and 1950s, especially with the treatment of infections using antibiotics, the role of nutrition was not prominently recognized anymore. At the same time, special courses and curricula on nutrition were developed which took a more comprehensive approach, by also looking at underlying and basic causes of malnutrition, and addressing these as well as cultural aspects. As the focus on the latter became more important, the medical approach to nutrition was de-emphasized.

By now, the medical focus is back in nutrition with advances in science and the increased ability to identify and measure physiological and biological processes. However, nutrition has specificities that are essentially different from medical science, especially in the following ways:

a. Intervening to improve nutrition, e.g. with nutrient or food supplements, is different from a drug or vaccine, as it does not fit the paradigm of one causative pathogen that can be cured or prevented. High-dose, single-nutrient supplements come closest, but even then, they are provided to 'cure' a deficiency state of the specific nutrient, which causes dysfunction [29]. It is also important to recognize that as knowledge progresses, our understanding of the causal pathways, even for infectious organisms, are becoming increasingly complex.

b. Testing before use/consumption. New molecules (drugs) are subject to a series of tests before they can be explored for their potentially beneficial effects. These tests start in the lab and end, if they were proven effective in clinical trials, with continued monitoring of benefits and side effects when it is has become available on the market as prescription drug. However, for nutrients, it is the lack of them that causes dysfunction or disease, so the question about harm may arise when rather high doses are given, but not when they are consumed at levels that are close to recommended intakes [30]. For individuals with specific conditions that involve sensitivity to specific food components, such as Crohn's disease, peanut allergy, etc., specific dietary advice is formulated, based on a positive response/absence of illness when certain foods are avoided.

c. Risk–benefit analyses in medicine and nutrition are very different. In medicine, drugs are prescribed in order to treat or prevent a condition in a specific individual, whereas nutrient intakes and population-wide distribution of specific nutrient supplements are provided to an entire population or target group, based on the prevalence of deficiencies in the population and the risks associated with these deficiencies. The risk–benefit analysis for the individual focuses on the benefit of treating a diagnosed condition or preventing a health-threatening condition, e.g., by giving a polio vaccination. Risks, such as side effects of the drug or vaccination, are therefore compared against known benefits at the individual level. When dietary supplements are provided to complement a diet that is likely deficient for a substantial proportion of the population, however, the benefits for a specific individual are not known, unless his/her deficiency state is confirmed and already resulted in a recognized dysfunction. This makes it sometimes difficult to assess the benefit–risk ratio, as the risk tends to be overestimated when the benefit is not properly understood [31, 32]. However, in fact, looking at it from the perspective of the required level of confidence to decide to act, i.e. implement an intervention to treat a disease or to prevent a nutrient deficiency, as a function of certainty that the intervention has an effect and its benefit–risk ratio, the required level of confidence should be higher for drugs to treat disease than for nutrient interventions to prevent disease [29, 31].

d. Everyone has a certain nutrient intake, provided by their diet. Nutrition interventions add to or partially replace these intakes. Unless megadoses are provided such as in the case of a high-dose vitamin A capsule, nutrition interventions tend to achieve a modest increase of nutrient intake and the magnitude of the net increase varies within the target population, because nutrient needs and intakes vary among individuals.

Evidence for Nutrition-Specific Interventions and Programs

Can the Evidence-Based Medicine Paradigm Be Applied to Nutrition?

As mentioned above, the paradigm of EBM is also being applied for evidence-based nutrition where efficacy of commodities, for treating or preventing specific conditions, is to be proven before they are being recommended for wider use. For example, WHO publishes evidence-based guidelines that are commodity specific, e.g. on MNP, for which systematic reviews of existing evidence are done. Such systematic reviews first specify which outcomes are of interest and for which target group(s). In the case of MNP this may, for example, include anemia, specific micronutrient deficiencies, linear growth, diarrhea, and mortality. However, what is ultimately included in the systematic review depends on the published evidence that is available. In the case of MNP, this may mean that only the impact on iron deficiency, anemia, and vitamin A deficiency can be reviewed among 6–23-month-old children, for the specific formulations of MNP that were used for the studies.

Some drawbacks of applying the paradigm of EBM to nutrition are the following:

a. The focus is often intervention instead of problem-based. Rather than focusing on a combination of interventions for reducing or preventing a condition (e.g., anemia or stunting), the focus is on the impact of a single commodity on selected outcomes. Recently packages of interventions have begun to be explored, but this is a relatively new approach and different studies examine other combinations of nutrition-specific and medical interventions (for example, vaccination, malaria, and nutritional interventions as a package).
b. While a nutrition intervention may have several impacts, often only a few specific ones are the primary outcomes in a study. Due to that, the impact on other outcomes is either not assessed or not with enough statistical power to conclude whether it has an impact on these outcomes [29]. This particularly applies to interventions with a combination of nutrients, such as special nutritious food supplements.
c. Even though there are different formulations and different uses of a specific commodity and they are used in different contexts, they are often taken together in systematic reviews. For example, MNP may contain 3, 5, 15, or another number of micronutrients and in different dosages, or fortified blended foods (FBF) can contain different ingredients such as with or without milk powder or they may be fortified with different vitamin and mineral mixes. Furthermore, they may be provided at different dosages or frequencies (e.g., one sachet of MNP per day every day vs. 10 sachets per month, or 50 g/d vs. 200 g/d of FBF). Also, as existing diets as well as the composition and intake of the commodities differ, the difference that they make can vary greatly, e.g. the intervention may increase existing nutrient intake by 30% versus 200%, which is basically the difference of just topping up an intake that is already almost adequate versus really correcting a deficiency, and hence they will have a different impact. If a systematic review assesses the impact of a commodity without distinguishing different formulations that were used or without assessing the difference made to existing intake in the specific studies, the findings are not very useful for guiding programs in specific settings among specific populations.
d. Individual-level benefits may be masked when looking at the population-level benefits of certain nutritional interventions. For example, pooled analysis of studies that compared the impact of prenatal multiple micronutrient supplements versus Fe/FA supplements found an average increase of birthweight of 22 g, which appears to be quite small. However, among women with a BMI of 20 kg/m^2 or higher, birth weight increased 39 g, compared to 6 g in mothers with BMI under 20 kg/m^2 [33]. The fact that there was a subgroup that benefitted substantially more has a number of implications. First of all, the findings are not generalizable to any group of pregnant women.

Secondly, when intervening among women with a low BMI, there is a need for additional interventions to increase their weight gain simultaneously with increasing their micronutrient intake. And, thirdly, in order to avoid complications during delivery of a heavier baby to a potentially stunted woman with a smaller pelvis, availability of quality obstetric care should also be ensured.

Choosing a Control Group for a Nutrition Intervention Study

As mentioned above, the gold standard in intervention study design is an RCT, which includes one or more intervention groups and a control group (with or without placebo), and the groups are comparable in all other regards. When studying the impact of nutrient supplements that provide nutrients at a dosage level of several times the recommended intake, this design can quite easily be applied.

However, when a food is the intervention, and even when groups are comparable on all other measured characteristics, for example a flour for a cereal porridge in order to prevent stunting, this is more difficult. First of all, there cannot be a placebo, i.e. there is no porridge that provides no nutrients, and if there was, it would not be ethical to provide it, which makes the inclusion of a control/comparison group more complex. Secondly, in the intervention group, the porridge may replace other foods that would have otherwise been consumed and these will continue to be consumed in the comparison group. Thus, the difference between the diets of the two groups is not just that the intervention group has the special porridge whereas the other one does not, because the comparison group eats other foods in place of the porridge. This means that such a study can assess the difference in nutritional status when one group receives a porridge of a certain composition, but that the difference that is found is not simply explained by the additional nutrient intake from the porridge, but by the difference of total daily nutrient intake between the two groups, which should hence be carefully assessed. Furthermore, this difference of nutrient intake between the two groups is context-specific, i.e. in one location the comparison group may predominantly consume a watery gruel, whereas in another location the comparison group may have access to more nutrient dense foods such as fruits and animal source foods. In the first scenario, the special porridge is likely to make a substantial difference to daily nutrient intake, whereas the difference may be much smaller in the second scenario where it would also replace some nutrient-dense foods (Fig. 3.1). Although theoretically possible to control for these differences when analyzing the results of studies using food, in reality these differences are often not assessed and therefore cannot be accounted for. Thus, when different effectiveness of interventions with certain products is observed, it is important to explore differences in terms of programmatic effectiveness and contextual factors.

Sometimes, it is not possible to assign no intervention to a comparison group, for example in the case of treatment of a condition for which a certain treatment is already being provided, such as moderate acute malnutrition. In that case, the comparison group may get the standard of care, whereas the intervention group receives the new treatment of which the impact needs to be assessed. Or, one may have a 'positive control group' that receives an optimal intervention, which for resource or feasibility reasons could not be provided at large scale, but serves as a kind of 'gold standard' comparison for the more realistic/feasible intervention(s). The latter is similar to the approach in animal nutrition, where the optimal nutrient intake and diet is known, and for cost, environmental impact or other reasons, modifications of the diet are tested for impact on nutritional status, growth or health of the animals. In human nutrition for resource-limited settings, the approach is the opposite, i.e. we know that the diet is not adequate, and we try to improve nutrition through behavior change

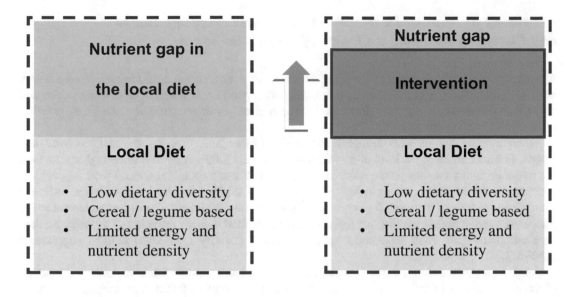

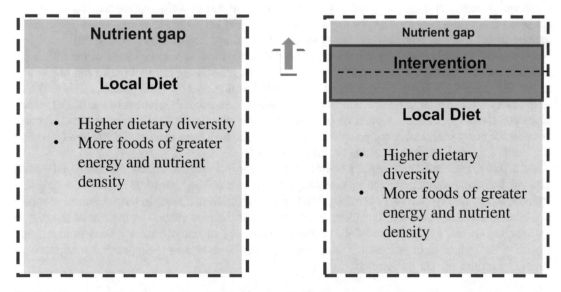

Fig. 3.1 The extent to which a nutritious food adds essential nutrients to the total nutrient intake (i.e., fills a nutrient intake gap) varies depending on the prevailing diet, which varies across contexts and among individuals

communication/providing special nutritious commodities/giving cash to the household, etc., not because these have been designed to provide the full recommended nutrient intake, but because this is what is affordable for the public sector (i.e., government/donors) or is preferred for other reasons (i.e., cash as safety net type support that provides decision autonomy to the household) and we like to assess whether that modification makes enough of a difference.

Magnitude of Nutrient Intervention in Relation to Existing Intake and Chance of Detecting a Change of Nutritional Status

It is important to think quantitatively when designing or interpreting a nutrition intervention study, both with regard to the magnitude of the intervention as well as with regard to existing intake and how much difference, in absolute terms, the intervention makes in comparison to the intake prior to, or in absence of, the intervention.

When nutrient supplements are provided, such as vitamin A capsules or multi-micronutrient tablets, dosage may be at the level of the recommended daily intake or several times higher than that, but normal/existing nutrient intake is unlikely to change. When a special nutritious food is provided, this may be a food that is meant to replace all other food that is consumed, except breast milk, for example in the case of treatment for severe acute malnutrition, but it may also be a complement to the daily diet, such as in the case of a fortified complementary food that can provide 1–2 servings per day, or a complementary food supplement such as a small quantity lipid-based nutrient supplement (LNS-SQ, <120 kcal/serving).

As also mentioned above, the difference made to the person's nutrient intake is not only a function of the composition of the food supplement, but also of the amount of it that is consumed, and what it replaces. In the case of a fortified complementary food, the nutrient content is often chosen such that those who consume a relatively large number of servings of the product do not have a too high intake, for example, one serving provides 1/3 of RNI, so that 3 servings would provide 100% of the RNI. However, as many children, especially when the household has to self-purchase the food, may not consume more than one serving per day or even just a few servings per week, recent recommendations from GAIN as well as WFP are to provide 50% of the RNI per serving [34, 35].

Being able to achieve an impact with the intervention depends on the magnitude of the difference that is made to a person's nutrient intake, as well as on the preexisting nutrient intake and nutritional status. For example, when existing nutrient intake is deficient, e.g. at 30–50% of RNI, adding 30% of RNI makes a substantial difference and may well result in detectable differences in nutritional status. However, if existing intake is around 70–90%, adding 30% may not result in a measurable difference, because for many individuals, the preexisting level of intake may have been sufficient already, so that additional intake of nutrients is either stored or excreted.

And lastly, nutrients have impacts beyond specific and nonspecific effects on nutritional status, e.g., on functional outcomes such as morbidity. For these reasons, assessing impact of a nutrition intervention should be done very carefully. First of all, the difference made in terms of nutrient intake needs to be carefully assessed, including an assessment of the contribution of the rest of the diet to nutrient intake and actual intake of the nutrient supplement or complementary food product, and secondly, the outcomes of interest and sample size need to be chosen carefully, such that impact on a variety of indicators can be detected.

Outcome Focused Interventions, Collecting and Interpreting the 'Right' Evidence

In the section above, we have discussed why the level and achieved change of nutrient status are very important to consider when conducting a nutrition intervention study that provides extra nutrients in one way or another. This is particularly relevant when the primary outcome to assess the intervention is also affected by other factors. For example, stunting may be aggravated by morbidity, which can be due to suboptimal hygiene and sanitation practices. This can modify the effect of the nutritional intervention under study. For example, not finding an impact on morbidity when providing daily

MNP in a study may be because the hygiene and sanitation situation is so poor that increasing nutrient intake does not improve immune system performance because nutrients are not utilized well (excreted due to diarrhea for example). However, had the study been conducted among a population with a better hygiene and sanitation situation, the increased nutrient intake would have improved nutritional status which could have resulted in a lower morbidity incidence. Similarly, if the situation in terms of hygiene changes for the better or for worse during the study, in both intervention and control groups, this can also affect the ability to detect a difference due to the intervention.

Differences in nutrient intake, nutritional status and effect modifiers across different contexts vary by an order of magnitude that can be similar to the difference made by a particular nutrition intervention. This substantially limits the external validity of findings of nutrition intervention studies and this can be further exacerbated with poor study design and implementation. This also makes systematic reviews of impact of nutritious commodities challenging to interpret and problematic to generalize across contexts. This has implications for program managers and policymakers with regard to deciding which interventions are most appropriate to improve nutrition in a specific country or area (see Box 3.1) and for assessing whether the implemented package has the desired impact (see Box 3.2).

Box 3.1. Evidence Needed for Designing and Implementing Nutrition Strategies and Programs in a Country

The links between direct, underlying, and basic causes of undernutrition have been clear from the time of the introduction of the UNICEF conceptual framework in the 1980s, and the role of different types of nutrition-specific and nutrition-sensitive interventions have been clearly identified and shown by the framework published in the Lancet series 2013. However, making a judicious choice among the possible interventions and ascertaining that implementing them in a specific way in a particular context will achieve the desired impact, and in a cost-effective way, is the challenge faced by the nutrition field today.

To design programs and strategies for improving nutrition in a particular country, the global knowledge and recommendations need to be applied locally and for doing so, the following kinds of information and evidence are required:

1. **Which nutrition problems exist in a specific country**
   Evidence of what nutrition problems exist (e.g., stunting, anemia, low birth weight, overweight), amongst whom (age, sex, socioeconomic status) and where.
2. **Thorough situation analysis to identify the main causes of malnutrition in the country**
   It is important to identify the main, or most likely, causes of the nutritional problems in the particular context, i.e. what is the contribution of the different direct causes (dietary intake, disease and inflammation, caring practices) and which underlying causes are particularly important. For example, if micronutrient intake is not adequate, is that because micronutrient-rich foods are not available, not affordable, or awareness of the importance to consume them is lacking; or if many births are small for gestational age, is there a large proportion of births among adolescent girls, do women not eat enough during pregnancy to avoid having a large baby, and/or to widespread food insecurity?
3. **Evidence on how the causes of malnutrition can potentially be addressed**
   Evidence is required on which specific interventions have the potential to improve nutritional status by impacting the direct and underlying causes that are most important in the specific context. This is where evidence based guidelines are important.

Box 3.2. Evidence to be Gathered on Impact of Implementing Nutrition Strategies and Programs in a Specific Context

While much of the nutrition research focuses on assessing impact of specific interventions under well-controlled circumstances, for example through (cluster) RCTs, real-life circumstances mean that several nutrition-specific and nutrition-sensitive interventions are often implemented at the same time and that coverage, uptake and adherence is subject to quality of program implementation and beneficiary/consumer interest and demand. This means that an intervention that works well in one area, may not work well in another, because programme implementation varies, the intervention is not well adapted to the specific target population and therefore uptake and adherence are low, other circumstances are very different, e.g. hygiene and sanitation is not a major cause of malnutrition in one area while it is in the other, etc. Furthermore, several other factors also impact on the outcome of interest, i.e., nutritional status or functional outcomes such as morbidity.

Therefore, the key areas of evidence that should be used and contributed by programs that aim to improve nutrition, either directly (i.e., nutrition-specific programs that address direct causes) or indirectly (i.e., nutrition-sensitive programs that address underlying causes) are the following (see also Chap. 27 by Olney, Leroy & Ruel):

1. **Programme design, implementation and monitoring**

    The specific interventions need to be delivered and received by the intended beneficiaries and should be used/implemented as recommended. A qualitative assessment, using formative research methods, is required to inform program design. This should address questions such as who are trusted authorities that can deliver and/or support the intervention, what influences caretakers' child feeding practices, what is an appropriate design for the packaging of the special nutritious food. Once the program has been designed, its implementation and achievements needs to be monitored, through programme monitoring, process evaluations and coverage surveys, the results of which can be used to improve programme design and implementation.

2. **Programme's impact on nutrition outcomes and intermediate pathways**

    When the programme is implemented, it needs to be ascertained that the programme is received as intended and impacts points along the pathway to improved nutritional status, and, ultimately, that nutritional status improves. This is addressed by programme evaluations.

3. **Magnitude of impact of specific intervention package in context X under circumstances Y amongst whom, how, why, at what cost**

    This is the ultimate question, i.e. does the specific programme, conducted in context X (e.g., low income country, high prevalence of food insecurity), experiencing circumstances Y (e.g., increased food prices and floods) achieve the desired impact on nutritional outcomes, which components may have had the most impact, and what are the reasons for having/not having an impact? This question is addressed by a very comprehensive programme evaluation/operational research and can use specific research designs including one or more comparison groups that receive other interventions or serve as a control who may receive the intervention at a later stage (step-wedge design).

Assessing Impact of Programs for Improving Nutrition

The main focus of this chapter has so far been on assessing impact of specific nutrition interventions, especially those that use nutritious commodities (supplements or special foods). However, preventive health and nutrition programs rarely provide just one intervention, as their aim is to reduce morbidity and mortality in the short term and improve nutrition, health and development for the longer term, even for life. Ideally, a combination of nutrition-specific interventions, preventive health interventions such as immunization and malaria control, as well as nutrition-sensitive interventions such as improving water and sanitation, diversifying crops and village garden produce, and increasing access to education, are implemented. Ultimately, one would like to know the impact of such a 'package' of interventions and strategies, delivered by different sectors, on nutrition, health, development, morbidity and mortality, and preferably also which components made the biggest difference and at the lowest cost.

These questions are very difficult to disentangle into sub questions that focus on specific interventions or strategies, because individuals are exposed to several interventions at the same time. For example, if one is interested in assessing the impact of social behavior change communication (SBCC) on the diversity of children's diets and on their nutritional status and conducts a study where two groups both participate in a food security program of an NGO that also provides health care services, one of which receives the SBCC, and a third group only receives the health care services, one can assess how the combination of SBCC and food security intervention improves dietary diversity as compared to neither intervention, or how SBCC improves dietary diversity when added to a food security intervention. The food security intervention may have improved access to specific, self-produced foods, but may also have increased purchasing power, which may lead to earlier health care seeking, purchasing of specific nutritious foods, etc. Therefore, one will not know whether SBCC alone, without concurrent intervention for food security, could have improved dietary diversity and nutritional status in the particular setting.

In such a situation, one possible design is a RCT of several packages of interventions, which will have to be allocated to clusters instead of to individuals, because of the way some of the intervention components are implemented. Another, more pragmatic, approach would be to monitor program implementation, key outcome indicators and other relevant factors that can affect the intervention and/or the outcome over time as programs and strategies evolve (see Box 3.2 and Chap. 27). This is especially relevant when all components of the package have already independently, in other settings, been shown to be effective, such as is the case for the nutrition-specific interventions recommended by the 2013 Lancet series.

Nutrition surveillance is a very good way of collecting comprehensive information on implementation, coverage and adherence to nutrition-specific and -sensitive programs as well as underlying and basic causes of malnutrition and as such enables comprehensive plausibility analyses for impact of nutrition interventions and strategies under real-life circumstances [36] (see also the chapter on Health and Nutrition Surveillance by Bloem, de Pee and Semba in the 2nd edition of this book [37]).

Can Stunting Be the Indicator of Need for Nutrition Interventions and the Indicator of Their Impact?

For monitoring the undernutrition situation within a country over time and across countries, stunting is the preferred indicator because it reflects the cumulative impact of nutrition insults, i.e. inadequate nutrient intake and disease across a period of 1000 days, starting at conception and lasting until the child's second, or even third, birthday, and it also reflects the impact of underlying and basic causes of malnutrition. Furthermore, it reflects other consequences of undernutrition as well, i.e., a stunted individual also suffers from micronutrient deficiencies which have consequences for performance of the immune system, cognitive development and hence schooling performance and income earning later in life. Stunting is also a good indicator for monitoring improvements of a population's nutritional status over a longer period of time, i.e. at least a few years, as related to the cumulative exposure to nutrition-specific and -sensitive policies and strategies, including pro-poor safety nets and changes of the economic situation.

However, stunting may not be the best primary outcome indicator of a specific intervention, for two reasons. First of all, stunting accumulates over a substantial period of time that covers pre-pregnancy, affecting nutritional status at conception, pregnancy, early lactation and the complementary feeding period, and is affected, positively and negatively, by many different factors. Therefore, while a specific intervention may make a contribution to improving nutrition, it may not cover a long enough period of the first 1000 days or be insufficient on its own to lead to substantial change of stunting without other conditions also being in place. Secondly, as stunting is defined as inadequate linear growth (being too short for one's age), specific nutrients are required to prevent stunting, i.e. allow adequate growth of bones and muscles [38]. While these nutrients are provided by a diverse diet that includes plant source foods, animal source foods and fortified foods, specific nutrition interventions may be a better source of certain nutrients, for example micronutrients, than of the nutrients required for linear growth. In that case, the intervention may have a limited impact on stunting but still affect other outcomes that are also caused by an inadequate diet, such as micronutrient deficiencies, cognitive development and morbidity. It is thus very important that interventions for reducing undernutrition in a population are not only judged by their impact on stunting, but also by their impact on other forms and consequences of undernutrition.

Importance of Trends and Context

As discussed above, applying the evidence-based medical paradigm to nutrition, as well as the evolution of nutritional science over the last two centuries, has led to a major focus on individual nutrients and their short—to medium-term impacts, and on mixtures of individual nutrients often in the form of supplements. However, for interventions that aim to change dietary intake using foods, whether naturally available foods or special nutritious foods such as FBF or MNP, the existing evidence-grading paradigm has additional limitations. For example:

- changing dietary behavior, even when it involves consumption of a special food, is different from taking a drug.
- dosage of nutrients is modest compared to existing nutrient intake.
- the key outcomes are affected by many other factors in addition to the one specific nutrition intervention that is tested, and controlling for these differences is often problematic.
- the role of the context in determining the extent of change that can potentially be achieved as well as presence of facilitating or hindering factors is much greater, which leads to difficulties in generalizing study results.

Therefore, the emphasis in nutrition science on the causal paradigm that is used in infectious disease research is arguably often counterproductive with respect to programming for nutrition. Adding to the complexity with regard to nutritional interventions in emergencies is the emphasis on mortality reduction as the primary outcome used for establishing benefits, whereas there are many additional factors determining mortality risk as well as other, longer term, benefits of nutrition interventions.

Facing the limitations of the evidence-grading paradigm for nutrition, what other evidence can be referred to? While observational data are typically rated as low quality evidence, because one has not controlled the situation that has been observed, nor intervened in any particular way, much can be learned from observational data, such as those collected by a surveillance system or spanning a long period of time (historical data). An example of observational data covering a long period of time is the increase of height of Dutch men in the decades after the Second World War, when sanitation and access to clean water were already optimized and public health service provision was good [39]. Of the two direct causes of improved nutrition, dietary intake was hence the most important, and this indeed improved with better access to a diverse diet, with an increasing share of animal source foods and processed, fortified foods as the economy improved. This relationship could not have been tested with a suitable experimental design.

Also, by comparing trends over time across different contexts, one can identify factors that are likely related to these differences. Similarly, while the immediate, underlying, and basic causes of malnutrition are known, their importance in different contexts varies, and identifying which ones are most important where is important for tailoring interventions. For example, stunting is caused by maternal factors, including age of the mother at the time of the pregnancy and nutrition during pregnancy as well as complementary feeding practices. In some settings, maternal factors are more important than in others, for example in South Asia as compared to Africa, so that in those settings interventions that delay age at marriage and first child birth and that improve adolescent and maternal nutritional status should be of high priority.

Ascertaining and Monitoring Impact of Measures to Improve Nutrition in a Target Population

The nutrition interventions that are provided are often selected from evidence-based recommendations that are based on efficacy studies that were carefully controlled and implemented under certain, context-specific, circumstances. While these contexts vary among different studies, the fact that coverage of and compliance with the intervention, as well as other factors that can interfere with the intervention or its effects, were carefully controlled means that their results cannot be translated one-to-one to real-life programmatic circumstances. This also applies to the monitoring of their impact, which is far more complex, and should not be done in a way that evaluates the impact of the intervention as such, but rather evaluates change of nutritional status in relation to all factors that may impact it, including coverage and adherence to relevant interventions. However, before even contemplating trying to assess change of nutritional status, the focus should be on the choice and implementation of the intervention.

Especially when the intervention is food-based, i.e. modifies the diet, either with specific nutritious foods or by recommending dietary changes possibly accompanied by homestead food production or other food security interventions, it is very important to think [40]:

- Quantitatively, i.e., about the magnitude of the difference that needs to be made in order to achieve recommended nutrient intakes;
- Biologically, i.e., nutrients will need to be released from the foods during digestion and become available for absorption (i.e., the nutrient need to be bioavailable and the consumer in good health);
- Behavior, i.e., consumers need to obtain, like and consume the food and at the recommended frequency and amount; and
- Programming, i.e., how to ensure that the food(s) are produced or manufactured, become available for the intended consumers, are purchased or distributed to the beneficiaries, etc.?

For choosing the intervention, it is important to note that evidence of efficacy is not required for every new application of a tested intervention. For example, the evidence of impact of MNP on iron status and anemia can be extended to school children, provided that they receive it in similar dosing and mixed with similar foods with regard to content of iron absorption inhibitors; the recommendations for fortification of wheat flour, which were based on several studies, were extended to maize flour because of its great similarity to wheat flour [41] and can to a large extent also be extended to rice [42].

Let us consider the case where it is decided to improve nutrient intake of 6–23 months old children through the distribution of a fortified blended food, for example Super Cereal Plus or a locally produced equivalent product, in order to reduce nutrient intake gaps and hence contribute to prevention of undernutrition, including micronutrient deficiencies and stunting. The food contains 1 RNI of 20 nutrients per 50 g of powder (200 kcal), which makes 300 g of porridge. In this case the following considerations are important:

a. Nutrient contribution from the food needs to be substantial enough in comparison to the nutrient intake gap. For example, if the full dose is consumed every day, the child will have an intake of 1 RNI/d. However, if the child eats approximately half of that, because she/he is still small, breast feeding and/or also eats some food from the family pot, the nutrient intake from the specific food will be less (but total nutrient intake may still be close to the target, depending on the nutritional value of the rest of the diet).

b. The food/commodity needs to be nutritious, efficacious and safe. In the case of the fortified blended food, it should contain nutrient forms that have good bioavailability and are stable within the food (i.e., not interacting with the other nutrients). There is good guidance available for which forms of micronutrients have good bioavailability and can be used for which types of food [43, 44] so that one does not require results from efficacy studies for each formulation of a specific food. Manufacturing should be done according to specifications and while adhering to good manufacturing practices, including Hazard Analysis and Critical Control Points (HACCP). Shelf life should be as desired (i.e., product remains stable during the period stated on the label) and the manufacturer and its product(s) need to be audited by independent firms.

c. The consumption of the food should be as desired, for example 1–2 servings/day. This requires that:

- the commodity is available to the intended consumers (distributed/purchased) and acquired by them
- the commodity is accepted by the consumers (i.e., product type is acceptable, packaging is appreciated, appearance, smell and taste are good)
- it is consumed as recommended (target group, amount consumed per serving, number of servings per day/week).

These are all aspects related to design and implementation of the appropriate delivery of the intervention, including that the target population accepts/desires to acquire and consume it.

A common pitfall when assessing effectiveness or impact of interventions that use specific nutritious products under programmatic circumstances, is that there is too much emphasis on assessing biological impact (i.e., is anemia reduced when MNP is added to school meals or is stunting prevalence less when FBF are introduced), while inadequate attention is paid to ensuring and monitoring the above factors that determine the actual difference of nutrient intake that this intervention achieves. Also, it often happens that other factors that affect the biological indicator, e.g. helminth infection, or deworming, or iron supplement consumption, are not adequately monitored or assessed before and during the intervention. In fact, implementing and assessing the nutritional intervention itself is the easy part (and most clear), the rest is far harder.

Therefore, a lot of attention should go toward:

- the design of the intervention, along the lines of the above example;
- its implementation, which is not just limited to delivery of a specific commodity, but stretches along the entire chain from manufacturing a quality food, packaging it in appropriate packaging that maintains the quality and is attractive to the consumer, to SBCC about a nutritious diet, fed in a responsive manner and including the special nutritious food, and ensuring availability of product at the appropriate time and place;
- monitoring implementation, to check whether implementation happens as intended and to be able to detect and act when something does not go well; and
- monitoring confounders and outcome, i.e., factors that are relevant for program implementation and intervention delivery (e.g., changes of purchasing power when consumers should buy the product) as well as for intended outcome (e.g., implementation of public health interventions and access to health care).

The importance of good intervention implementation, its complexity, and the inadequate emphasis that this has received in general has lead to the recent formation of the Society for Implementation Science in Nutrition [45].

In summary, this means that in our specific example the focus of the program should be on ensuring that nutrient intake increases as desired, as that should lead, over time and provided that other nutrition-specific as well as sensitive are also implemented, to improvement of the nutritional status of the population over time.

To be able to assess that, one should thus not only ensure and monitor the appropriate implementation of the intervention and the intermediate (product availability, acceptance and consumption) and ultimate outcomes (nutrient intake, nutritional status) that are of direct interest, but also the factors that can modify, i.e. strengthen or weaken, these outcomes. The chapter by Olney, Leroy and Ruel provides a good description of how program impact pathway frameworks can be used to design program evaluations that take many of these other factors into consideration. And the Chapter in the second edition, by Bloem, de Pee and Semba describes how nutrition surveillance can be used to monitor ongoing implementation of strategies and programs and for example assess variation of exposure among different subgroups and relate this to attenuating or enhancing influences and related outcomes.

Finally, it is important to remember that if the introduction of a specific intervention is not accompanied by the desired/anticipated change of nutritional status, this may be because it is poorly adapted, does not make enough of a difference, i.e. the intake gap is larger than anticipated, and/or other factors negate the impact of the intervention, such as disease or simultaneously reduced access to previously consumed nutritious foods. When dietary deficiencies are very likely, as shown by dietary intake surveys or specific or proxy indicators of nutritional status, there is no reason to question whether interventions that fill a gap between actual and recommended nutrient intake are necessary. Rather, the question should be whether the total combinations of interventions that the population is subjected too, were effectively delivered and make enough of a difference, under prevailing circumstances, including other nutrition-specific or -sensitive programming and modifying factors.

Conclusion

Applying the evidence-based medical paradigm to nutrition, as well as the evolution of nutritional science over the last two centuries, has led to a major focus on individual nutrients and their short- to medium-term impacts, and on mixtures of individual nutrients often in the form of supplements.

However, for interventions that aim to change dietary intake using foods, whether naturally available foods or specific, fortified, nutritious foods, the evidence-based medical paradigm has several limitations, as follows: (a) the approach is intervention- rather than problem-based, (b) the intervention is superimposed on an already existing food and nutrient intake which affects the net difference it makes, (c) the focus is on just a few of many outcomes, (d) generalization across interventions disregards potentially important differences (e.g., complementary foods are taken together without recognizing their different nutrient content and energy density as well as acceptability by the target population), and (e) external validity of RCTs is low as effect size is limited (unless megadoses are provided) and context affects nutrient needs, acceptance and compliance with the intervention, and presence and influence of effect modifiers (e.g., sanitation, hygiene and subclinical infection).

Therefore, the emphasis on the causal paradigm is often counterproductive for guiding policy and programming decisions for nutrition. Choice of interventions should be guided by a thorough situation analysis of the most likely causes of the specific nutrition problems among different subgroups of the population, as well as a good understanding of what can be delivered to and accepted by the target population, and include both nutrition-specific and nutrition-sensitive interventions. Analysis of observational and surveillance data, including for concurrent trends overtime and across different contexts, can provide important insights into what could work where, how and for whom.

Evaluating nutrition strategies and programs can be done in many ways and different designs should be used for collecting evidence on implementation and impact, with special emphasis on characterizing and assessing the role of context, which is a key to understanding the results.

Discussion Points

- Why can the evidence-based paradigm from medicine not be equally applied to nutrition?
- How can systematic reviews take the role of context into account?
- What evidence should governments require for choosing which set of nutrition-specific and -sensitive interventions to implement to reduce stunting prevalence, and how should the impact of an intervention package be assessed?
- If context plays such an important role in determining the impact of nutrition-specific and -sensitive interventions, how can learnings from nutrition programs inform programming and strategies in other countries and regions?

References

1. Feinstein A. Clinical judgment. Baltimore: Williams & Wilkins; 1967.
2. Cochrane A. Effectiveness and efficiency: random reflections on health services. London: Nuffield Provincial Hospitals Trust; 1972.
3. Eddy DM. Practice policies—guidelines for methods. JAMA 1990;263(13):1839–41. Doi:10.1001/jama.1990. 03440130133041.
4. Eddy DM. Clinical decision making: from theory to practice: a collection of essays. Am Med Assoc. 1996. ISBN 0763701432.
5. Evidence-Based Medicine Working Group. Evidence-based medicine. a new approach to teaching the practice of medicine. JAMA. 1992;268(17):2420–5. Doi:10.1001/jama.268.17.2420.
6. Rosenberg W, Donald A. Evidence based medicine: an approach to clinical problem-solving. BMJ. 1995;310 (6987):1122–6. Doi:10.1136/bmj.310.6987.1122.
7. Eddy DM. Variations in physician practice the role of uncertainty. Health Aff. 1984;3(2):74–89. Doi:10.1377/ hlthaff.3.2.74.

8. Dawes M, Summerskill W, Glasziou P, et al. Sicily statement on evidence-based practice. BMC Med Educ. 2005;5 (1):1. Doi:10.1186/1472-6920-5-1.
9. Higgins JPT, Green S, editors. Cochrane handbook for systematic reviews of interventions. Version 5.1.0 [updated March 2011]. The Cochrane collaboration, 2011. Available from www.cochrane-handbook.org.
10. "EBM: Levels of Evidence". Essential evidence plus.
11. Tonelli MR. In defense of expert opinion. Acad Med. 1999;74(11):1187–92. Doi:10.1097/00001888-199911000-00010.
12. U.S. Preventive Services Task Force. Guide to clinical preventive services: report of the U.S. Preventive Services Task Force. US: DIANE Publishing; 1989. p. 24. ISBN 978-1-56806-297-6.
13. Balshem H, Helfand M, Schünemann HJ, et al. GRADE guidelines: 3. Rating the quality of evidence. J Clin Epidemiol. 2011;64(4):401–6.
14. Sackett DL, Straus SE, Richardson WS, Rosenberg W, Haynes RB. Evidence-based medicine: how to practice and teach EBM. 2nd ed. Edinburgh, United Kingdom: Churchill Livingstone; 2000. p. 173–7.
15. Stanley K. Design of randomized controlled trials. Circulation. 2007;115(9):1164–9. Doi:10.1161/CIRCULATIONAHA.105.594945.
16. Chalmers TC, Smith H Jr, Blackburn B, Silverman B, Schroeder B, Reitman D, et al. A method for assessing the quality of a randomized control trial. Doi:10.1016/0197-2456(81)90056-8.
17. Moher D, Hopewell S, Schulz KF, Montori V, Gøtzsche PC, Devereaux PJ, et al. CONSORT 2010 explanation and elaboration: updated guidelines for reporting parallel group randomised trials. Br Med J. 2010;340:c869. Doi:10.1136/bmj.c869. PMC 2844943.
18. Gartlehner G, Hansen RA, Nissman D, Lohr KN, Carey TS. Criteria for distinguishing effectiveness from efficacy trials in systematic reviews. Technical review 12 (Prepared by the RTI-International-University of North Carolina Evidence-based Practice Center under Contract No. 290-02-0016.) AHRQ Publication No. 06-0046. Rockville, MD: Agency for Healthcare Research and Quality; Apr 2006.
19. Victora CG, Habicht J-P, Bryce J. Evidence-based public health: moving beyond randomized trials. Am J Public Health. 2004;94(3):400–5.
20. Beauman C, Cannon G, Elmadfa I, Glasauer P, Hoffmann I, Keller M, et al. The principles, definition and dimensions of the new nutrition science. Public Health Nutr. 2005;8(6a). Doi:10.1079/phn2005820.
21. The Giessen Declaration. Public health nutrition. 2005;8(6a). Doi:10.1079/phn2005768.
22. Black R, Allen L, Bhutta Z, Caulfield L, de Onis M, Ezzati M, et al. Maternal and child undernutrition: global and regional exposures and health consequences. Lancet. 2008;371(9608):243–60. Doi:10.1016/s0140-6736(07)61690-0.
23. United Nations Children's Fund. The care initiative: assessment, analysis and action to improve care for nutrition. New York: Nutrition Section, UNICEF; Apr 1997.
24. Blackburn G. Presidential address: interaction of the science of nutrition and the science of medicine. J Parenter Enteral Nutr. 1979;3(3):131–6.
25. Mahan L, Escott-Stump S, Raymond J, Krause M. Krause's food & the nutrition care process. St. Louis, Mo.: Elsevier/Saunders; 2012.
26. Semba R. Nutrition and development: a historical perspective. In: Taren D, de Pee S, Bloem MW, editors. Nutrition and health in developing world. 3rd ed. Totowa, NJ: Humana Press; 2016.
27. Semba RD. The historical evolution of thought regarding multiple micronutrient nutrition. J Nutr. 2012;142:143S–56S.
28. Leyton GB. Effects of slow starvation. Lancet. 1946;2:73–9.
29. Blumberg J, Heaney R, Huncharek M, et al. Evidence-based criteria in the nutritional context. Nutr Rev. 2010;68 (8):478–84. Doi:10.1111/j.1753-4887.2010.00307.x.
30. Mann J. Discrepancies in nutritional recommendations: the need for evidence based nutrition. Asia Pac J Clin Nutr. 2002;11(s3):S510–5. Doi:10.1046/j.1440-6047.11.supp3.1.x.
31. Kraemer K, de Pee S, Badham J. Evidence in multiple micronutrient nutrition: from history to science to effective programs. J Nutr. 2011;142(1):138S–142S. Doi:10.3945/jn.111.142414.
32. Allen L. To what extent can food-based approaches improve micronutrient status? Asian Pac J Clin Nutr. 2008;17 (S1):103–5.
33. Fall C, Fisher D, Osmond C, Margetts B. Multiple micronutrient supplementation during pregnancy in low-income countries: a meta-analysis of effects on birth size and length of gestation. Food Nutr Bull. 2009;30(4S):S533–46.
34. Global Alliance for Improved Nutrition. Nutritional guidelines for complementary foods and complementary food supplements supported by GAIN. Global Alliance for Improved Nutrition; 2014.
35. WFP. Technical specifications for the manufacture of super cereal plus—corn soya blend. http://documents.wfp.org/stellent/groups/public/documents/manual_guide_proced/wfp262697.pdf.
36. Habicht JP, Victora CG, Vaughan JP. Evaluation designs for adequacy, plausibility and probability of public health programme performance and impact. Int J Epidem. 1999;28:10–8.

37. Bloem M, de Pee S, Semba R. How much do data influence programs for health and nutrition? Experience from health and nutrition surveillance systems. In: Semba R, Bloem M, editors. Nutrition and health in developing countries. 2nd ed. Totowa, NJ: Humana Press; 2008. p. 831–57.

38. Golden M. Proposed nutrient requirements of moderately malnourished populations of children. Food Nutr Bull. 2009;30(3):S267–343.

39. Larnkjær A, Schrøder SA, Schmidt IN, et al. Secular change in adult stature has come to a halt in northern Europe and Italy. Acta Paediatr. 2006;95:754–5.

40. De Pee S. Special nutritious solutions to enhance complementary feeding. Editorial. Matern Child Nutr. 2015;11: i–viii.

41. WHO. Recommendations on wheat and maize flour fortification meeting report: interim consensus statement. Geneva: World Health Organization; 2009.

42. De Pee S. Proposing nutrients and nutrient levels for rice fortification. Ann N Y Acad Sci. 2014;1324:55–66.

43. World Health Organization and Food and Agricultural Organization of the United Nations. Allen L, de Benoist B, Dary O, Hurrell R, editors. Guidelines on food fortification with micronutrients. Geneva: World Health Organization; 2006.

44. World Health Organization. Technical note: supplementary foods for the management of moderate acute malnutrition in infants and children 6–59 months of age. Geneva: World Health Organization; 2012.

45. Implementationsciencesociety.org. Society for Implementation Science in Nutrition (SISN). Retrieved from http://www.implementationsciencesociety.org/ (2015). Visited 4 Sept 2015.

Chapter 4
Developing Capacity in Nutrition

Jessica C. Fanzo and Matthew M. Graziose

Keywords Capacity development · Nutrition · Workforce · Training · Education

Learning Objectives

- Define capacity development in the context of nutrition service delivery.
- Understand why developing capacity in nutrition is necessary in the post-2015 development era.
- Understand the capacity gaps in global nutrition workforce at the individual, institutional, and systemic levels.
- Describe the pros and cons of using competencies in education and training of the nutrition workforce.
- Analyze key issues in monitoring and evaluating nutrition capacity development.

Building a Case for Nutrition Capacity Development

The Burden of Malnutrition

Despite remarkable progress, the world is still struggling to address the burden of malnutrition, which is alarming in both scale and scope. Nearly every country is facing this burden, yet it is not evenly distributed. In 2014, over half of all stunted children lived in Asia and over one-third lived in Africa [1]. And, while several regions have halted the increase in childhood stunting, the Africa region has seen the number of stunted children increase by nearly one quarter [1]. Even within countries there are geographic and wealth disparities in the rates of malnutrition, with rural and poor children at increased risk [2, 3].

Portions of this chapter were originally published in the journal *Advances in Nutrition*. 2015;6:639–647.

J.C. Fanzo (✉)
Berman Institute of Bioethics and School of Advanced International Studies, Johns Hopkins University, 1717 Massachusetts Avenue, #730, Washington, DC 20036, USA
e-mail: jfanzo1@jhu.edu

M.M. Graziose
Health and Behavior Studies, Teachers College Columbia University, 525 West 120th Street, Box 137, New York, NY 10027, USA
e-mail: mattgraziose@gmail.com

© Springer Science+Business Media New York 2017
S. de Pee et al. (eds.), *Nutrition and Health in a Developing World*,
Nutrition and Health, DOI 10.1007/978-3-319-43739-2_4

The prevalence of overweight, obesity, and diet-related non-communicable diseases (NCDs) is also increasing in nearly every region of the globe [4–9]. In the United States and the United Kingdom, the rate of adult obesity has tripled over the past three decades and today, obesity affects nearly a third of the populations in these countries [4]. Between 1990 and 2014, the rate of childhood overweight has increased drastically in Asia (22% increase and 4.9% prevalence) and Africa (91% increase and 5.2% prevalence), and these regions now have nearly 30 million overweight children [1]. In addition, consumption of high-fat and high-sugar foods and beverages has increased in many regions of the world [10], contributing to an epidemic of diabetes and other related NCDs [5, 6]. No country has yet to reverse the increasing trend in overweight and obesity [7]. The new normal is undernutrition and obesity coexisting within the same country, community, or even household [11–13]. A concurrent, related challenge is that micronutrient deficiencies are also widespread, affecting approximately one-third of the world's population.

A Complex Nexus of Contributing Factors

The conceptual framework we use for understanding malnutrition categorizes causes as immediate, underlying, or basic [2, 3]. In the coming decades, protecting nutrition will more than ever require attention to the basic and underlying causes of malnutrition. Contributing to the already demanding challenge of addressing malnutrition are several current and forecasted challenges including: climate change; population growth; extreme poverty; energy-intensive dietary patterns; water scarcity; land and natural resource degradation; rising prices of food, fuel and fertilizer; and political instability [14–16]. These factors will contribute to a shift in the global burden of disease, both in type and locus, and an increase in food insecurity in many parts of the world if we continue with business as usual.

There is growing recognition of the bidirectional relationship between climate variability and agriculture, which affect health and nutritional status, commonly called the "diet–environment–health trilemma" [17]. The links between climate change and nutrition can no longer be ignored and represent a serious threat to food and nutrition security. Under these circumstances, the approaches we use to improve nutritional status must also consider knock-on effects for the environment and vice versa. Thus, the world's greatest future challenge lies in ensuring access to healthy and nutritious food for the world's population, while concurrently reconciling environmentally sustainability [18].

Capacity Is Essential to Achieving International Goals and Targets

While the problem of malnutrition is complex, it is not intractable. There is a substantial scientific evidence base describing the effectiveness of several nutrition-specific interventions that target the immediate causes of malnutrition [19]. Although the global nutrition community still strives to better understand the underlying and basic causes of malnutrition, a host of potential nutrition-sensitive interventions have been proposed that, through affecting the direct causes of malnutrition, also contribute to improving nutritional status through sectors such as agriculture, education, social protection, and sanitation [20]. Similarly, a series of potential policies and programs have been proposed as priority actions for addressing overweight, obesity, and NCDs [21].

A growing momentum for scaling up nutrition is built on back of this collection of scientific evidence. Nutrition enjoys a high level of attention, committed funding, and recognition from donors, country governments, businesses, and academia [22]. Several recent reports, including the 2008 and 2013 Lancet Series on Maternal and Child Nutrition, the annual Global Nutrition Report [23, 24], and the Copenhagen Consensus outcomes on Malnutrition, and high-level meetings such as the Nutrition for Growth Summit in London (2013) and the Second International Conference on Nutrition (2014) have solidified the consensus on the importance of and means to alleviate malnutrition. They have also led to innovative investments and approaches such as the Scaling Up Nutrition (SUN) movement and the 1000 days partnership.

Yet there is a lack of capacity to deliver on the promises that improved nutrition holds for the world's citizens, which has, to date, received scant attention. The growing political, institutional, and organizational commitment in nutrition must be leveraged to develop *capacities* to deliver, scale-up, and sustain interventions on the ground. We do not solely need "more studies and more data," but more and improved capacity to coordinate the successful interventions we have already identified [25]. As the world begins to prioritize approaches to meet the Sustainable Development Goals (SDGs)—a set of 17 goals and indicators adopted by world leaders in September 2015—there is a need to re-think and re-work how capacities to advance nutrition can be built to support policy, research, programming, financing, and delivering of services to improve the livelihoods of people around the world [26–28].

The post-2015 development era is anticipating a "grand convergence" whereby new technology, increased investment, and a solid evidence-base informs the scale-up of interventions to reach universal low rates of infant and maternal mortality [29]. Experts have cautioned that the grand convergence is only possible by narrowing the delivery gap—the divide between the types of interventions known to be effective and those actually being delivered [30]—with attention to the major challenges ahead and the growing burden of obesity and diet-related NCDs [31]. Closing the gap and addressing emerging complex challenges of the food environment and obesity pandemic will take keen attention to the capacities of those at the frontline of interventions. The global nutrition community now finds itself in a critical inflection point, with donors, governments, civil society, and the private sector focused on using momentum to significantly expand the host of evidence-based nutrition interventions, yet this expansion cannot happen or will fail if it is not accompanied by attention to the capacities of individuals and institutions to support the targets, programs, and agendas that have been put in motion.

Defining Capacity Development

The definitions for capacity development are numerous and the term is oftentimes used interchangeably with others such as "capacity building," "training," "institutional building" "institutional development," or "organizational development." A common element of most definitions is the act of achieving stated objectives [32–43].

Throughout this chapter, we use a simplified definition for capacity development: *the process through which individuals, organizations, and societies obtain, strengthen, and maintain the skills and capabilities to set and achieve their own development objectives over time.*

Capacity development in nutrition refers to strengthening the *delivery of essential nutrition services*, which is defined as "the encounter between individuals who require nutrition services and those tasked with delivering them" [44]. However, it is widely acknowledged that this process goes beyond simply the training of those individuals, requiring supportive structures and systems for service delivery. Inherent to this definition are the three levels of capacity development [36]:

1. *Individual*: the knowledge, attitudes, tools, and skills necessary to perform nutrition-related work;
2. *Institutional/organizational*: the staff, infrastructure, access to information, and support necessary to manage the delivery of nutrition services;
3. *Systemic*: the structure, frameworks, sector policies, and roles within which nutrition services are delivered.

In the next section, we summarize the existing sources of data, both quantitative and qualitative, regarding the current status of nutrition capacity.

Assessing Nutrition Capacity

Our ability to characterize nutrition capacity is limited by the lack of formal assessment methods. While several frameworks have been proposed, few authors have utilized these in a systematic manner to identify capacity gaps [23, 32, 35, 42, 43]. Given that these frameworks have not been consistently operationalized, there is limited ability to compare and contrast capacity across disparate contexts and before- and after-training interventions. There is also is a lack of information on the relationship between the three levels of capacity and how they relate to service delivery [43].

Global Health Workforce and Capacity to Deliver Nutrition Services

Health workers are a major component of human resources for health and are essential for the delivery of most, if not all, health and nutrition interventions. Broadly defined, health workers are individuals who are "engaged in actions whose primary intent is to enhance health" [45]. While there is no agreed upon definition as to what constitutes the nutrition workforce, for the purpose of this chapter we similarly define nutrition workers as those who are involved in the delivery of nutrition services. Multiple approaches have been used to estimate current capacity gaps in the broader healthcare workforce (Table 4.1) that can likewise be used to estimate requirements for a nutrition workforce, each with their own advantages and disadvantages. However, the lack of a consistent definition for the nutrition workforce remains a challenge for accurately characterizing capacity to deliver nutrition services and most of the existing data is focused on the traditional health workforce.

Determining the size of the workforce is an integral first step to assessing capacity. The World Health Organization (WHO) currently maintains estimates of the global health workforce, including physicians, dentists, nurses, midwives, and other healthcare workers, as part of its Global Health Workforce Statistics [45]. For example, there are currently an estimated 1.3 million community health workers across the globe, though this is likely an underestimate given the gaps in the number of countries reporting data [38]. Besides data gaps, these estimates are also subject to several limitations, such as disparate data collection methods used across countries and different definitions for health occupations.

Yet it is currently impossible to determine the size of the global nutrition workforce, as these data do not exist across all countries. Within the WHO database, the numbers of nutritionists per country are aggregated and categorized within "other health service providers," which include many disparate health occupations, such as ambulance workers, medical assistants, and medical imaging technicians, among others. The Service Availability and Readiness Assessment (SARA), also collected by the WHO, quantifies the number of health facilities and the healthcare workforce within a country. However, relatively few of these assessments disaggregate the number of nutritionists (for example, the 2013 report for Kenya shows that there are a total of 496 nutritionists in the country, or 0.12 per 10,000 citizens). Even the number of rural workers rooted in the agriculture sector (i.e., extension agents), who are increasingly involved in delivering nutrition services, is not well characterized [47].

Despite these data gaps, there is good reason to believe that access to human resources are a valuable proxy for nutrition capacity, given that many of the nutrition-specific interventions are incorporated into the traditional healthcare model. A previous cross-country analysis has found that access to health services is among one of the strongest predictors of nutritional status [48]. Additionally, in an ecological study of 118 countries, researchers have estimated that increasing the density of health workers by 1% is associated with a 0.47% reduction in maternal mortality and a 0.23% reduction in infant mortality [49]. In Fig. 4.1, we present the relationship between health

Table 4.1 Approaches to estimate workforce requirements in the nutrition sector

Approach	Description	Data requirements	Pros	Cons
Demand-based	An estimate of workforce requirements is obtained after accounting for projected population growth and demographic shifts and the associated burden of malnutrition	Epidemiological and demographic trends	Potentially independent of the way nutrition services are currently delivered	Often nutrition needs are determined by experts and may not reflect needs perceived by the population
Supply-based	An estimate of workforce requirements is quantified based on the current burden of malnutrition in the population and the programs in which workers are educated and trained	Number of education/training programs and their graduation/completion rates	Can consider productivity and skill-mixes of the workforce	Assumes a consistent demand for nutrition services
Worker-to-population ratio	Using a reference country or region, an adequate nutrition worker: population ratio is estimated and used as the criterion	Census of nutrition workforce	Easy to understand and use as an advocacy tool	Ignores changes in workforce quality, performance or distribution
Service targets	An estimate of workforce requirements is obtained based on what is considered necessary for the delivery of essential nutrition services	Nutrition-specific intervention coverage data	Identifies necessary competencies for the workforce	Likely to result in unrealistic targets

Adapted from Amorim Lopes et al. (2015) [46]

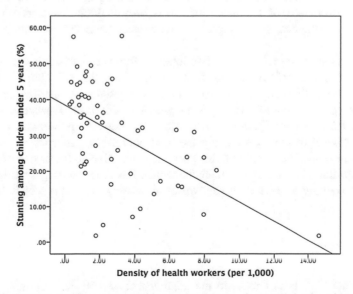

Fig. 4.1 Relationship between stunting among children under 5 years of age and density of health workers (nurses, physicians, community health workers, and other health workers [includes nutritionists]). *Source* the authors analysis of 2014 World Health Organization data

worker density and rates of stunting among children less than 5 years of age for the 56 countries reporting both indicators in the WHO database.

Using a demand-based approach to estimate workforce requirements, many experts agree that the world is experiencing a massive shortage of health workers, potentially in excess of 4 million individuals [50]. Among countries in sub-Saharan Africa, the estimate of the gap is 800,000 health professionals (including doctors, nurses, and midwives), at a cost of $2.6 billion in wages, to meet projected demands [51]. Using a worker-to-population ratio in Bangladesh to approximate demand, it was estimated that 1.28 million community health workers would be required to expand coverage for nutrition services across the nation [52]. Although investments in human resources are crucially needed, they cannot happen without systematic assessments of the health needs of the population and subsequent examinations of the quality and efficiency of health workers to determine where, why, and when they are needed.

A service-target approach can also be used to estimate workforce requirements. This approach relies on an indicator of coverage—or the proportion of individuals reached by a service or program. Although these data are scarce, the most expansive set of nutrition-specific coverage indicators, amassed in the *2014 Global Nutrition Report*, provides further evidence of the delivery gap [23]. The report tracks the coverage of several nutrition-specific interventions and prevalence rates of certain nutrition practices including: early initiation of breastfeeding, exclusive breastfeeding rates up to 6 months, continued breastfeeding at 12 months, vitamin A supplementation for preschool-age children and iron-folic acid supplementation for pregnant women. Only one country in the world exceeded 50% coverage for all interventions/practices among the intended target populations. While coverage data characterizes the prioritization of nutrition services, it does not tell us whether the capacity is external—funded by donors—or internal, and likely more sustainable, to a country. The service-target approach may result in unrealistic estimates and, while it may highlight priority areas for action, it does not identify the optimal strategies for use across disparate contexts to promote nutrition practices or provide essential services.

Workforce size and intervention coverage also tell us nothing about the quality of service delivery. Effective coverage must be the end goal, where those in need have not only the access to essential nutrition services, but also access to *effective* essential nutrition services [23]. This can only be achieved through a high-quality workforce. There are several factors that are likely to contribute to the quality and performance of the healthcare workforce including balanced workload, proper supervision, adequate supplies, and equipment, and respect from the community and the health system [53].

Several other indicators are relevant to describing performance of health workers including the workforce distribution and skill-mix. The draft report of the 2030 Global Strategy on Human Resources for Health identifies gaps in the size, quality, and geographic distribution of the healthcare workforce as one of the primary challenges to global health [54]. Presently, the workforce is unequally distributed across rural and urban locations and between public and private institutions [50]. As a result, several regions, particularly the rural poor areas, suffer the worst effects of inadequate or no access to care. Distribution of the workforce also refers to the proper mix of skills within an individual and within the team in which she/he works. Ensuring the proper skill-mix results in an improvement in the quality of service delivery while minimizing the cost at which they are delivered.

Assessments of Multi-country Nutrition Initiatives

Capacity development has been central to the approach of several multi-country nutrition scaling initiatives, yet recent evaluations have identified capacity as a key bottleneck.

- The SUN movement has been successful in providing opportunities for coordination and collaboration in-country on the delivery of nutrition services [55]. Notwithstanding the successes, the issue of weak capacity was noted several times in a consultation with stakeholders from six exemplar SUN countries—Bangladesh, Nepal, Indonesia, Ethiopia, Nigeria, and Kenya. Weak capacity was often caused by inadequately qualified personnel and front-line staff, with high employee turnover [43].
- The Mainstreaming Nutrition Initiative—a three-year project funded by the World Bank from 2006–2009 to raise the profile of nutrition in Bangladesh, Vietnam, Bolivia, Peru, and Guatemala —identified several factors which are likely to hamper the delivery of nutrition services, including staff and supervisory workload, poor remuneration and job satisfaction, lack of mastery of tools and skills for new interventions, and limited financial resources. Several of these countries have sought multi-sectoral approaches to address malnutrition, yet are constrained by: underdeveloped staff and infrastructure; weakness in horizontal coordination and vertical coordination; and poor performance and workload capacity for basic program planning, management, and monitoring and evaluation [56].
- The United Nations REACH program combines the expertise of the World Food Programme (WFP), United Nations Children's Fund (UNICEF), Food and Agricultural Organization (FAO), and the World Health Organization (WHO) to develop human and institutional capacities for nutrition services in the countries in which it works. Between 2008 and 2015, the program had been operating in 20 countries, yet an external evaluation found that the program was undefined in its theory of change regarding capacity, conflicted between a focus on exclusively mobilizing partners to provide technical capacity inputs or to itself playing a direct role in addressing capacity gaps [57].
- In order to understand capacity to deliver behavior-change communication interventions to promote infant and young child feeding practices, Pelto et al. (2015) surveyed international organizations currently operating in developing countries (including CARE, HKI, Alive and Thrive, JSI, CRS, World Bank, UNICEF) [58]. In terms of institutional support for such interventions, the authors found that less than half of organizations provided technical or financial support for evaluation activities and only a third routinely offered re-training opportunities for their workforce. In addition, few organizations had ongoing activities to communicate with or directly influence policymakers.

In the following sections, we focus specifically on what is known about capacity among countries in Africa and Asia because of the high burden of malnutrition with modest progress and the pervasiveness of outdated educational curricula and training schemes. These regions thus require new and innovative approaches to build capacity.

Nutrition Capacity in African Countries

Africa is experiencing a health paradox: it has the highest burden of disease per capita, yet simultaneously has the lowest ratio of health workers to its population. While the health challenges for Africa are broad, recent assessments of health facilities in Africa highlight the lack of capacity for delivering essential nutrition services, especially essential maternal, newborn, and child health services. A survey of health service facilities in Burkina Faso, Mozambique, and Niger found that, across all three countries, there were gaps in the nutrition and dietary assessments of prenatal women, counseling on breastfeeding, and monitoring of child growth [59]. A more recent situation analysis examining infant and young child nutrition services in Burkina Faso, Chad, Mali, Mauritania, Niger, and Senegal found that the majority of programs in these countries had targeted vulnerable populations but had not yet reached a national level of coverage [60]. There was also a lack of institutional support for the capacity of community health workers, including inadequate and out-of-date training materials.

A major concern for the African region is that the education and training of the nutrition workforce has not kept pace with the health needs of its population [61]. Across the region, there is limited readiness to scale-up nutrition services and an insufficient human resource capacity for public health nutrition, with a shortage of staff, lack of degree programs, and poorly focused nutrition training [62]. In a landscape analysis of existing academic training programs within 16 West African countries, Sodjinou et al. (2014) identified a total of 83 programs at the undergraduate, masters, and doctoral level, which were confined to 10 countries [63]. Half of the countries surveyed do not have any existing undergraduate nutrition degree-granting programs. Within the existing academic programs there is a failure to provide a comprehensive approach to teaching all aspects of nutrition, with little focus on public health nutrition or obesity and NCDs, and few opportunities for practical experiences [63–65]. Several of the countries surveyed currently offer training programs, yet they are often narrowly focused and short in duration [65]. Even the countries with adequate training programs fail to produce enough graduates in the field of nutrition to support their needs; for example, in 2012 the region graduated about 517 individuals at the undergraduate level, which is well below a conservative estimated requirement of 2028 [63]. The shortage of a workforce and the lack of up-to-date curricula are not isolated to the nutrition field; it also appears pervasive throughout the health sector [66, 67].

Academic research output is also indicative of nutrition capacity in Africa. Two recent bibliometric assessments of literature originating from Africa have found that, overall, there is a dearth of publications originating from institutions in Africa and few that examine key topics in public health nutrition [68, 69]. In addition, less than 40 articles per year are published from the West African region and a majority of publications are co-authored or have a lead-author from an academic institution from outside of the continent. An additional challenge to supporting homegrown nutrition research is the lack of institutional review boards to govern the ethical review process [69]. Although publications are merely one product of research that may not accurately characterize the process of training researchers and practitioners, it belies an institutional failure to provide adequate funding and training to sustain homegrown leaders in the field of nutrition [70, 67].

Nutrition Capacity in Asian Countries

The Asia region, too, is devoid of a developed workforce that is adept at delivering essential nutrition services. Shrimpton et al. (2013) describe the findings of three recent assessments of nutrition capacity in Bangladesh, Nepal, and Indonesia for the UNICEF East Asia and Pacific Regional Office [52]. None of these countries are implementing behavior change communication on infant and young child feeding interventions at a national scale, which is due in large part to a shortage of a workforce to deliver these essential services. At the workforce level there is a critical need for competencies, preparation, on-the-job training, and materials (assessment materials, instruments, and curricula). At the organizational level, there is limited coordination, sensitivity to nutrition, and access to nutrition epidemiological information. Across these countries there are few nutrition champions who are trained to spearhead projects, inspire others, and work as part of a team.

India suffers a huge deficit of healthcare workers, including nurses and doctors. According to a recent census of healthcare personnel, more than a third of the health workforce, and up to two-thirds of workers in rural areas, was deemed unqualified [71], although this census was not sensitive enough to determine the extent of nutrition workers [71]. A potential contributing factor is a poor focus on training and educating a workforce for nutrition. In a survey of 190 institutions in India, Khandelwal et al. (2012) found that few higher education institutions are focused on nutrition. Nutrition has historically been tied to home science (e.g., home economics) and, while most offered food and nutrition science degrees, only 4 institutions within the country offered a public health nutrition degree. Presently, India allocates little financial support to education (3.2% of GDP) and there is a lack of institutional research funding for public health nutrition [72].

One study examined the institutional research capacity in India, Pakistan, Bangladesh—three countries participating in the Leveraging Agriculture for Nutrition in South Asia initiative, a research consortium [73]. One of the main challenges to delivering nutrition services experienced in India was the high turnover rate of bureaucrats in government, leading to a lack of capacity on nutrition. Similarly, a lack of integration between nutrition programs within different ministries was noted as a barrier in Pakistan. Across all countries, there was a lack of understanding of nutrition among policymakers and inefficient knowledge transfers between levels of government for implementing nutrition services. Individual leadership represents an important means to raise the profile of nutrition within countries and to advocate for attention to the problem.

A situation analysis of the graduate-level academic training for nutrition in Iran [74] found that the nutrition community was small and narrowly focused, unable to appropriately address the nutrition needs of the nation. In addition, the authors conclude that the training programs that do exist are not properly focused on the breadth of technical expertise necessary to develop effective program managers who can successfully participate in intersectoral programming.

Capacity for Addressing Obesity and Non-communicable Diseases

While capacity to alleviate undernutrition has received some attention, as the above reviewed liter-ature shows, capacity to address overweight, obesity, and NCDs has also been the subject of some assessments. In 2010, the WHO conducted a survey to assess capacity to prevent and control NCDs within 185 countries [75]. While most countries reported having a unit or branch dedicated to NCDs, 12% had no funding stream and cited concerns about the number and quality of staff. Low-income countries, particularly those in West Africa, were more likely to report gaps in funding of NCD prevention and control [76]. International donors were cited by 56% of countries as a major funding stream. The key to addressing the challenge of NCDs includes the ability to conduct effective surveillance of the population-level risk factors of NCDs—only 25% of countries have conducted surveys of blood lipids and only 36% have conducted surveys of diet since 2007.

The WHO 2016 *Global Report on Diabetes* examines the world's capacity to respond to the diabetes epidemic [77]. Although 85% of countries have existing policies and plans for diabetes (stand-alone or integrated with those for NCDs generally), there is a huge disparity in the types of countries that are implementing these policies. For example, just over 30% of low-income countries reported fully implementing diabetes guidelines as compared to over 60% of high-income countries. Only half of low-income countries reported an availability of blood glucose monitoring equipment, an essential technology for diagnosing and managing diabetes. Across all countries surveyed, less than half had a proper national surveillance system to track epidemiological trends in disease rates and/or assess the impact of large–scale interventions.

The *Lancet Series on Obesity* confirms that the education and training of medical professionals and heath sector personnel are poor with respect to the prevention and treatment of obesity [78]. The authors conclude that clinical treatments currently in use for obesity will not be effective unless accompanied by community-based initiatives that promote supportive environments and sustain weight loss. In other words, prevention of overweight and obesity is not just a matter of the health care sector and nutritionists, but also of professionals involved in physical activity, city design, food industry, etc. Especially among low- and middle-income countries, there is little attention to nutrition education of medical professionals and the creation of multi-sectoral teams focused on prevention and management of overweight, obesity, and associated NCDs [78–80].

Developing Capacity in Nutrition

Building on What We Know

The assessments summarized in the previous section provide evidence of a failure to systematically examine and address nutrition capacity. The recognition that the world lacks capacity in the nutrition workforce is important to provide rationale and motivation for change, but it does not in itself identify the appropriate strategies to remediate the problem. Likewise, the calls for attention to capacity in nutrition are not new; the inability to effectively translate scientific knowledge from the field of nutrition to action on the ground was identified by Alan Berg, who in 1993 suggested that the nutrition field requires an "engineer"-type position that has a varied skill-set and is able to troubleshoot nutrition problems on the ground [81]. The notion that the field of nutrition lacks a focus on problem solving in multiple, diverse settings still holds true today. Across the globe, there are several commonalities in the types of nutrition capacity gaps experienced.

First, there is a dearth of high-quality training for those on the frontline of service delivery [82, 83]. Gillespie et al. (2013) argue that it is no coincidence that the regions with insufficient nutrition service delivery are those that lack appropriate academic curricula and high-quality training programs [43]. Africa and Asia, in particular, suffer from outdated training and assessment materials, lack of practical, hands-on training, and poor academic focus on public health nutrition. There is no authoritative source of information pertaining to the education of the workforce globally, and, in institutions that offer nutrition education programs, what is being taught is often poorly or narrowly focused [70].

Second, there is a lack of leadership and advocacy skills training [43]. There are few in-service training programs for nutrition graduates, especially ones that focus on building advocacy skills to challenge ministers and policymakers to create supportive policies and funding streams [52]. Nutrition professionals are not taught how and when to engage champions and policymakers, what tactics to use, and how to balance potential conflicts of interest. If this training and learning does take place, it is often ad hoc, taught by managers on-the-job without direct incentives to do so.

Third, there is a lack of understanding how to foster multi-sectoral collaborations [56], which stem in part from poor training of the nutrition workforce to work as part of a multidisciplinary team. The complex challenge of addressing malnutrition and the interrelated and forecasted issues requires different skills sets than the ones on hand to today. There is a need to draw upon multiple areas of expertise and to engage other sectors like agriculture, social protection, infrastructure, and sanitation. With the understanding that challenges to nutrition can be mediated by actions from the private sector, greater collaboration between public and private sector actors should be encouraged, with keen attention to the role of regulatory bodies.

Because nutrition is an issue with massive implications for the health of populations and the development of all nations, it is imperative that attention and investment in nutrition capacity development be advanced so that the world may reach post-2015 era goals and targets. Discussions about capacity development, however, cannot take place in isolation; the individual cannot be considered separately from the institutions and organizations to which the responsibility of educating and training fall or, more importantly, the policies, structures and systems that govern the process. Central to this challenge is the need to foster an appropriate "skill-mix" among the nutrition workforce, both within individuals and the teams in which they work. In the following sections, we describe approaches to develop capacity at the three previously defined levels, which are informed by what is currently known about nutrition capacity gaps.

Approaches to Develop Individual Capacity

The very existence of this book, and indeed this chapter, is evidence of the attention to developing individual-level capacity in nutrition. The importance of this level of capacity cannot be overstated, as those who operate on the frontlines of intervention delivery often are the primary contact with nutritionally vulnerable populations. This includes those who are providing nutrition services directly, such as community health workers, doctors, nurses, midwives and nutrition educators, and also those who are operating within nutrition-sensitive approaches, including agricultural extension agents, child development practitioners, and social protection liaisons. Addressing individual capacity will take innovative approaches keen to the needs and desires of those at the frontline.

The emphasis on developing a front-line nutrition workforce, distinct from the clinically orientated workforce, is an implicit recognition that preventive, population-based approaches are required to address malnutrition in all its forms [38, 84]. To ensure that individuals are successful in this work, we need to thoroughly define what it entails, as well as how it complements existing clinical practice, and the required competencies, knowledge, skills, and attitudes [38, 84]. To maximize the impact of current and future investments in nutrition, a comprehensive, multidisciplinary approach to education and training of the workforce is necessary, embedded within a supportive organizational and systemic capacity to forecast and address new challenges. In the sections below, we summarize the strategies to develop individual-level capacities in the post-2015 development era.

New Knowledge and Skills to Address Post-2015 Challenges

There is broad agreement on several ongoing and future challenges requiring a highly skilled workforce for nutrition, including a growing burden of overweight, obesity, and NCDs; industrialization of the food chain; population growth; and climate change. These challenges necessitate a host of new knowledge and skills, particularly for those responsible for implementing and delivering high-quality nutrition interventions and services. This "program manager" position requires technical knowledge or hard skills in nutrition (e.g., basic nutrition science, climate change, quantitative analysis) as well as soft skills (e.g., communication, advocacy, management, and team-building skills across disciplines).

A new cadre of program managers in the post-2015 era will need to understand and apply systems thinking to all facets of nutrition-related programming (e.g., intervention design, implementation, monitoring and evaluation). They must draw on expertise and best practice to assess epidemiological changes, trends in urbanization, and risks of climate shocks or price changes. Program managers will be faced with seemingly competing demands, such as the need to address both the challenges of undernutrition and of overweight and obesity within the same geography. They must understand how to better link the current health systems for treatment of diet-related diseases such as diabetes and hypertension, while simultaneously addressing a food environment that may yet provide limited access to safe and nutritious foods.

New Ways of Working with Other Disciplines

The modern day nutrition challenges will require multi-sectoral solutions suited to the local context and include close collaboration with actors from many sectors, such as agriculture, food science, health, education, social protection, anthropology, engineering, and sanitation [85]. In this transdisciplinary space, nutrition professionals need to be fluent in discussing the concepts and constructs of other disciplines in order to effectively engage with decision-makers in other sectors, and seize opportunities to influence policies and programs. Creating mutual understanding towards an aligned commitment takes openness, dialogue and time to develop.

Program managers will have to facilitate both horizontal (e.g., across sectors) and vertical (e.g., from national to district and community levels) coordination in order to effectively deliver nutrition services [86]. For this, they will need to be adept at building and guiding multidisciplinary teams and ensuring that nutrition outcomes and impacts are prioritized or included, as is relevant, for the program and desired outcome. One example of a country that has sustained a successful multi-sectoral approach is Nepal, where attention to the organizational structure has allowed for the creation of cross sector teams who work on nutrition-sensitive approaches [38].

The nutrition workforce is increasingly tasked with collaborating with the traditional health system. To ensure that the work of frontline nutritionists is valued, there is a need to revise the existing training and education schemes of doctors, nurses and other medical professionals to be more aware and pro-active about nutrition [87]. This approach will give rise to teams who work together on the design, implementation and evaluation of nutrition interventions and thus have an appropriate mix of skills to address post-2015 challenges.

Curriculum and Credentials for Development Needs

By defining the knowledge, skills, and attitudes necessary to be effective in a given profession, competencies provide a framework for developing a workforce [84, 88]. Assumptions associated with the use of competencies are that they have broad applicability and that they represent aspirations for the field, reflecting the work needed rather than what already exists [84, 88]. We summarize several competencies that may govern the capacity development of the nutrition workforce.

- Hughes et al. (2012) identified a competency framework for effective public health nutrition practice. The authors identified several enabling knowledge and skills that are likely necessary for this type of work: biological, economic, political, behavioral, environmental, and social sciences [84, 88, 89].
- The Society for Nutrition Education and Behavior (SNEB) proposed a set of competencies that define an effective nutrition educator. These encompass: food and nutrition knowledge; nutrition across the lifecycle; food science; physical activity; food and nutrition knowledge; agricultural production and food systems; program design, implementation and evaluation; behavior and education theory; written, oral, social media communication; and research methods [90].
- Meeker et al. (2013) developed a competency framework to describe the skills required for emergency nutrition preparedness, response and recovery, which has since been adopted by several international non-governmental organizations including Concern Worldwide, World Vision, Valid International and International Medical Corps [91].
- Competency-based approaches have been sought for the education and training of medical professionals to include a focus on nutrition science and practice [79, 80]. These include topics and skills likely to complement existing medical practice, such as diet/physical activity assessment; critical care; referrals to a registered dietitian; and/or nutrition in health promotion [92].

Competency-based training and education are not without controversy. We highlight the debate around competency-based approaches in Table 4.2. A primary concern lies in the priority of local knowledge for local solutions—where institutions guide the development of training and education programs with the recognition that effective solutions may come from already existing wisdom and that there is no one-size-fits-all approach. One way to ensure that programs are guided by the needs of society and are continually updated to reflect new nutrition challenges is to provide students with practical and hands-on training through direct exposure to ongoing nutrition interventions occurring on the ground (e.g., "learning by doing").

Table 4.2 Arguments for and against the use of competencies in education and training programs for nutrition workers

Supporters say that competencies…	Detractors say that competencies…
Individual-level	
Foster accountability and consistency in the delivery of services	Lead to a "race to the bottom" in that workers will only meet prespecified competencies and no more
Enable transdisciplinary teams where workers complement each other based on their defined competencies	Cannot capture much of what makes workers successful in teams (e.g., how do we define leadership?)
Prevent overlap across disciplines/sectors by using clearly defined roles	May result in a "checklist" form of work, where workers create routines do not stray from them
Institutional-level	
Lead to clear, student-centered learning goals	Create a "teaching to the test" mentality in education
Create clarity in role/job specifications	Lead to simplistic assessments of learning/mastery in roles
Create equity across the discipline for learners of all backgrounds	Leave little room for innovation, diversity or contextual adaptation

Adapted from Hughes et al. (2012) [88]

Regardless of the use of competencies, there is consensus on the need for revised program curricula for training and credentialing the nutrition workforce. For those enrolled in formal pre-service nutrition education programs, several areas of study appear necessary, including nutritional biology and biochemistry, nutrition assessment, epidemiology, statistics, program management, analysis and writing, leadership and advocacy and negotiation, behavioral science, communication, and ethics. To foster multi-sectoral engagement and teamwork, those in formal nutrition programs should be required to include courses in agriculture, food systems, environment, toxicology, ethnography, economics, climate change, and/or urbanization.

Informal education and vocational training of the nutrition workforce is important for those outside the net of formal education programs. Vocational and community schools can offer certificates and short course trainings, but more frequent and more in-depth opportunities to build both applied program and teamwork skills should also be provided. This could take the form of expanded in-service (or "on-the-job") trainings, network meetings to build skills, massive open online courses (MOOCs) or case studies. Certified refresher courses and employment-links could also be offered to the workforce. Community health workers and other front-line workers would be more likely to take on the shorter trainings and enroll in local vocational schools. A continuing challenge is the development of course material that is relevant, well-managed and maintained.

Advocacy and Leadership

Leaders within the nutrition community currently struggle with how to use narratives and storytelling to transfer knowledge and skills that both motivates and assists community leaders and potential nutrition champions to effectively influence policymaking. Skills, such as relationship management, giving compelling presentations, communications, and advocacy, are needed in order to effectively influence policymaking and should be institutionalized and incorporated into education/training programs at universities. Communicating for influence and advocacy is often more art than science, and is developed over time through repeated experiences. Mentoring appears one promising approach that could support the transfer and development of these soft skills necessary for the frontline workforce.

Potential training components for high impact communications, influencing and obtaining stakeholder buy-in might include: (a) preparation: policy and stakeholder analysis and assessment and understanding implications of policies on nutritional outcomes (positive, negative, or neutral); (b) understanding of the political economy and languages of other sectors; (c) understanding target audience needs, incentives, and rewards so as to proactively guide them in making nutrition-related decisions; (d) building and delivering influential presentations; and (e) leveraging partners to deliver and reinforce messages and creating buy-in and ownership of nutrition-sensitive actors.

One example of a highly regarded leadership program is the African Nutrition Leadership Programme (ANLP)—a 10-day intensive program that develops transformational leadership capabilities aimed at improving the delivery of programs and services and at accelerating the impact of nutrition interventions. To date the ANLP has 325 alumni networked across 34 African countries. Content covered by the program includes, among others: change leadership; self-awareness; communication; value-driven teamwork; team effectiveness; managing resistance to change; advocacy; results-oriented action planning; gaining stakeholder commitment; and continued personal and institutional growth and development [93].

Innovative Approaches to Education and Training

Training programs can be broadly distinguished as "in-service" or "pre-service." While an appropriate mix of both types of training is necessary, in-service training represents an opportunity to increase the skills and knowledge of those at the periphery of the health sector, who have not had formal pre-service education and training prior to working in a position that focuses on nutrition [84]. A 2013 systematic review of in-service nutrition training programs for community health workers concluded that such programs increase the knowledge, competence and self-efficacy of those delivering interventions [94]. Although little is known about the optimal duration or delivery platform for training programs, a practical approach appears to be providing a series of booster sessions at fixed intervals to augment and refresh the training content [95].

Below, we provide several examples of training programs for nutrition professionals that utilize novel platforms or innovative content.

- The eNutrition Academy is a global training platform founded by the African Nutrition Society, the American Society for Nutrition, the Federation of African Nutrition Societies, IUNS and the Nutrition Society of the UK and Ireland. The academy aims to build the capacity of institutions by providing access to high-quality education and training resources. For example, the academy provides access to several MOOCs through its website [96].
- The UK Department for International Development and Irish Aid have supported the London School of Hygiene & Tropical Medicine to deliver two masters-level open-access online training modules called: Programming for Nutrition Outcomes and Agriculture, Nutrition and Health. By June 2015, these modules had been accessed by over 30,000 people in over 150 countries [97].
- The Food and Agriculture Organization (FAO) has recently developed the ENACT course which introduces participants to the principles and practice of "education for effective nutrition in action." It is designed for undergraduate students and professionals in agriculture, nursing, health services, or related nongovernmental organizations. The course provides skills to encourage long-term improvements in diet through an active approach that accounts for needs of the audience and environmental constraints [98].
- One training program administered via the Aga Khan Development Network (AKDN) is designed to improve the delivery of integrated nutrition and early child development interventions [95]. The five-day training for community health workers provides experience and best practices regarding strategies that encourage families to adopt behaviors that support both the physical growth and cognitive development of children. This represents a paradigm shift from trainings that have

historically been delivered via only one sector and did not take advantage of synergies in an integrated delivery mechanism.

- The mHealth or mobile-health revolution has also engendered novel approaches to training and education using new technologies as the delivery platform, including the Internet, mobile phones, and MOOCs [99]. Many examples are rooted in the traditional health system, such as the use of SMS messages to deliver medical abstracts to practitioners, or the use of technologies primarily as data gathering instruments.

Approaches to Develop Institutional Capacity

Given that it is unlikely that investment in knowledge is all that is required for capacity development [100], institutional capacity is needed to sustain the momentum in nutrition capacity, so that training and education initiatives are institutionalized and sustained [101]. Approaches to develop institutional capacity focus on the staff, infrastructure, access to information, and supports necessary to manage the delivery of nutrition services.

Coordinating bodies for education and training are necessary to support and sustain new initiatives, which are necessary not only at the international level but also at the provincial, district, and community levels. United Nations agencies can meet a crucial need by establishing normative guidelines and providing technical support for such programs. Institutions such as World Food Programme, United Nations Children's Fund, and Helen Keller International also have the potential to institutionalize trainings on certain topics and skills. The SUN movement and other cross-national initiatives should include investments in continuing education for nutrition. The SUN, by facilitating cross-sector engagement, also has a unique opportunity to foster networks for program managers and frontline staff for sharing experiences and best practices.

One recommendation to build institutional capacity that has reached widespread consensus is the establishment of a North–South and South–South consortium of universities [102]. This consortium could meet, discuss, and formulate a universal core set of competencies and curricula for the nutritional professional who does research and development in the context of future challenges and opportunities. This would involve an exercise to map current gaps and to predict future needs of a nutrition professional workforce so that training institutions start to offer courses and revised curricula that will support these needs.

Those entering the nutrition workforce desire to be valued by their institutions, and need to be confident that they will have a career with opportunities for advancement and remuneration. As many positions within the nutrition field are temporary consultancies, this may be a challenge. Institutions can focus on ensuring that salaries meet expectations and providing nonmonetary incentives and benefits that are responsive to the desires of their workers, including a focus on health promoting activities for their own employees. This may also require thinking about nutrition careers beyond nongovernment organizations and academia, and also to engage the private sector, as a potential area of growth for many working in food, agriculture, and nutrition.

For institutions to support capacity development it must be explicit in their mission statement, not conflict with other priorities or financial commitments and be aligned with existing incentives provided by institutions [32, 35]. Performance-based incentives are increasingly used to increase the productivity of the health workforce. These approaches provide explicit incentives to act, such as cash provided based on prespecified performance outcomes. Several development agencies have adopted this approach, including the World Bank and the United Kingdom Department for International Development (DFID) [24]. In Bangladesh, programs led by BRAC and Alive and Thrive have provided incentives to frontline workers linked to breastfeeding and complementary feeding behavior-change outcomes, which resulted in increased coverage rates and adoption of target behaviors [103]. Incentives can similarly be provided to individuals who attain additional credentials or participate in in-service training programs.

Approaches to Develop Systemic Capacity

The goal of developing systemic capacity is to define a set of structures, frameworks, sector policies, and roles that are ultimately supportive of nutrition services and contribute to their sustainability. Building a workforce for nutrition is not only a technical challenge; the series of decisions that govern the capacity development of individuals is inherently a political process. The ability to carry out stated objectives—in this case the evidence-based solutions to malnutrition—relies on focused attention to capacity development by stakeholders in civil society, UN organizations, foundations, development banks, businesses, and academia.

Systemic capacity is akin to creating an enabling environment for nutrition—one that supports and sustains momentum for the effective implementation of actions that alleviate malnutrition [43, 104, 105]. This is a nascent area of work, which only recently has been subject to coordinated approaches. There are several indicators of systemic capacity that can be used to assess progress in this area [106]. First, capacity development must be a stated commitment of those in leadership positions, with transparency in the use of financial, human, and physical resources. Second, there must be a cohesive set of policies that support the development of capacity, without unnecessary administrative or bureaucratic burden. Third, there must be intersectoral forums created for decision-making across sectors with public, private, and nongovernmental institutional involvement. These three factors are indicative of progress in systemic support for nutrition capacity and, although there are hints of progress in this area, there is much more work to be done.

More broadly, the approaches we suggest for training and education require a system that prioritizes monitoring and evaluating capacity development outcomes. Discourse about capacity is often hidden because it fails to reach priority among funding organizations, and is undervalued and unrecognized as compared to the stated, official purposes of grants and contracts [83, 107]. In practice, monitoring and evaluating capacity development often comes as an afterthought to satisfy donor accountability requirements [40]. To establish a supportive system, there must continue to be reporting requirements in grants and contracts for nutrition service delivery, but there must be an explicit value proposition for conducting this type of capacity development research, such that the findings are shared with relevant stakeholders and be used to adapt and improve future capacity development activities. Prioritizing capacity development will ensure that governments and institutions can continue to deliver nutrition services in the absence of external development aid [100].

Monitoring and Evaluating Nutrition Capacity

Nutrition is currently experiencing a data revolution—the number and types of indicators collected to assess nutrition status is larger than ever [24]. However, as this chapter has argued, there is a lack of attention to one of the most important indicators: capacity. The *Global Nutrition Report*, an authoritative collection of all existing nutrition indictors, identifies a glaring gap in the collection of capacity-related indicators [23, 24]. Properly understanding capacity gaps requires more research on intervention implementation, including the barriers to effective delivery of services at the individual, organizational, and systemic levels.

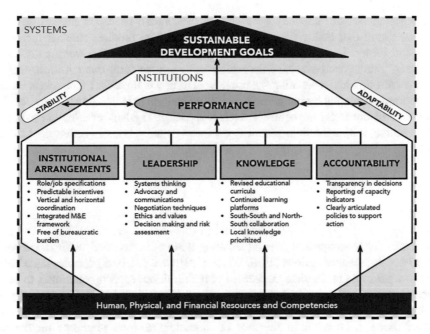

Fig. 4.2 A framework for monitoring and evaluating capacity development in nutrition. Adapted from (UNDP 2009) [34]

How do we monitor and evaluate capacity? Often, monitoring of capacity is being neglected because the outcomes are less tangible and challenging to measure. The choice of capacity assessment methods largely depends on types of interventions for which developed capacities are sought. Two questions should be considered when examining capacity development: *capacity for what?* and *capacity for whom?* [41].

In Fig. 4.2, we present a monitoring and evaluation framework for understanding nutrition capacity development considering the three aforementioned levels and four core domains that may encompass the breadth of capacity development work (institutional arrangements, knowledge, leadership, and accountability) [34, 40]. Central to this framework is the recognition these domains are governed by the existing competencies and the human, physical, and financial inputs. An additional consideration is that performance, at the individual-level and institutional-level, must be both stable and adaptable.

Monitoring and evaluating approaches to develop capacity is no different from that of any other intervention. Previous authors have proposed using standard public health intervention planning cycle, with explicit mention of how each stage of the cycle can be adapted with capacity in mind [32, 34]. This cycle may follow the following steps: (1) engage stakeholders; (2) assess capacity; (3) formulate a response or intervention; (4) implement intervention; and (5) evaluate. At each assessment stage, there are emerging methods that can be used to assess the less obvious dimensions of capacity, such as surveys of individual opinions and behaviors; focus-groups with frontline workers; observations of interactions between groups; and examinations of institutional protocols for decision-making [41]. In addition, there are indicators that can be used to assess performance at each level of capacity, from the individual to the system. While it is important that monitoring and evaluation plans are prespecified prior to the intervention, with outputs that are part of a clearly hypothesized pathway, they also need to be flexible and adaptable with the understanding that capacity development is a nonlinear process [40], with quick-wins coupled with longer battles [34].

Although monitoring and evaluating nutrition capacity is necessary, the data collection, analyses, and interpretation activities do not come without a cost. Who should be responsible for financing the monitoring and evaluation of capacity development outcomes? There are several obvious sugges-tions. First, we argue that donor driven aid include dedicated funding streams for both capacity development and its monitoring and evaluation. Second, we argue that governments take a pivotal role in educating, training, and assessing the performance of their front-line nutrition workers—while subsequently monitoring and evaluating the progress. Third, we argue that researchers build the body of research on implementation by including process evaluations in their studies with specific attention to how interventions are likely to require and affect capacity. The lack of attention to capacity as its own area of research, within the field of nutrition as well as more broadly across the health field, has failed to produce a body of knowledge that is actionable.

Conclusions

Nutrition is increasingly recognized as a crosscutting issue with massive implications for the social and economic development of nations [108]. While experience and best practices have been amassed with respect to what to do to alleviate the burden of malnutrition, capacity continues to be the critical limiting factor for the scale-up—in both coverage and impact—and sustainability of programs to address malnutrition. Calls for investment in capacity development in nutrition are not new, but are the subject of renewed attention in the face of mounting external pressures on the delivery of successful nutrition-specific and -sensitive services. Contributing to the already demanding challenge of addressing malnutrition are the current and anticipated issues that will cause a shift in the global burden of disease, both in type and locus, leading to an increase in food insecurity, changing food environments, and new pressures on the health system.

Capacity development will remain a critical feature of nutrition and development agendas in the coming decades. The SDGs offer an opportunity to excite, inspire, and guide the world in the post-2015 era; it is critical that advancing good nutrition be recognized as an underlying and crosscutting prerequisite to promote sustainable development. To maximize the impact of investments in nutrition, we must intensify efforts to develop the capacities of the future workforce for nutrition; failure to do so will render the well-meaning goals and targets of the future unattainable [109].

Discussion Points

- Define capacity development. Provide examples of actions at the individual, institutional, and systemic levels that demonstrate capacity for delivering nutrition services.
- How will the forecasted challenges for the post-2015 era make providing essential nutrition services more difficult? Think about each of the three levels of capacity.
- What do the current gaps in nutrition capacity tell us about equity both within and between countries?
- Distinguish between the pros and cons of using a competency-based approach. What are some examples of competencies you have been expected to meet in your education?
- What types of indicators could be used to monitor and evaluate nutrition capacity? When is capacity development finished?

References

1. United Nations Children's Fund, World Health Organization, The World Bank Group. Levels and trends in child malnutrition (2015). http://www.who.int/nutgrowthdb/estimates2014/en/. Retrieved 25 Mar 2016.
2. Black RE, Victora CG, Walker SP, et al. Maternal and child undernutrition and overweight in low-income and middle-income countries. Lancet. 2013;382:427–51.
3. United Nations Children's Fund. Improving child nutrition: the achievable imperative for global progress. New York, NY, USA (2008).
4. Finucane MM, Stevens GA, Cowan MJ, et al. National, regional, and global trends in body-mass index since 1980: systematic analysis of health examination surveys and epidemiological studies with 960 country-years and 9·1 million participants. Lancet. 2011;377:557–67.
5. Ng M, Fleming T, Robinson M, et al. Global, regional, and national prevalence of overweight and obesity in children and adults during 1980–2013: a systematic analysis for the global burden of disease study 2013. Lancet. 2014;384:766–81.
6. Ramachandran A, Snehalatha C. Rising burden of obesity in Asia. J Obes. 2010;1–8.
7. Roberto C, Swinburn B, Hawkes C, et al. Patchy progress on obesity prevention: emerging examples, entrenched barriers, and new thinking. Lancet. 2015;385(9985):2400–9.
8. Swinburn BA, Sacks G, Hall KD, et al. The global obesity pandemic: shaped by global drivers and local environments. Lancet. 2011;378:804–14.
9. Sweety P. Public health: India's diabetes time bomb. Nature. 2012;485:S14–6.
10. Imamura F, Micha R, Khatibzadeh S, et al. Dietary quality among men and women in 187 countries in 1990 and 2010: a systematic assessment. Lancet. 2015;3:e132–42.
11. Caballero B. A nutrition paradox—underweight and obesity in developing countries. NEJM. 2005;352:1514–6.
12. Malik VS, Willet W, Hu FB. Global obesity: trends, risk factors and policy implications. Nat Rev Endocrinol. 2013;9:13–27.
13. Popkin BM, Adair LS, Ng SW. Global nutrition transition and the pandemic of obesity in developing countries. Nutr Rev. 2012;70:3–21.
14. Foresight. The future of food and farming. Final Project Report. London: Government Office for Science; 2011.
15. Godfray HCJ, Beddington JR, Crute IR, et al. Food security: the challenge of feeding 9 billion people. Science. 2010;327:812–8.
16. Chicago Council on Global Affairs. Healthy food for a healthy world: leveraging agriculture and food to improve global nutrition. Chicago, IL: 2015.
17. Tilman D, Clarke M. Global diets link environmental sustainability and human health. Nature. 2014;515:518–22.
18. Johnston JL, Fanzo JC, Cogill B. Understanding sustainable diets: a descriptive analysis of the determinants and processes that influence diets and their impact on health, food security, and environmental sustainability. Adv Nutr. 2014;5:418–29.
19. Bhutta ZA, Das JK, Rizvi A, et al. Evidence-based interventions for improvement of maternal and child nutrition: what can be done and at what cost? Lancet. 2013;382(9890):452–77.
20. Ruel MT, Alderman H. Nutrition-sensitive interventions and programmes: how can they help to accelerate progress in improving maternal and child nutrition? Lancet. 2013;382:536–51.
21. Beaglehole R, Bonita R, Horton R, et al. Priority actions for the non-communicable disease crisis. Lancet. 2011;377:1438–47.
22. Development Initiatives. The aid financing landscape for nutrition. London: Development Initiatives; 2013.
23. International Food Policy Research Institute. Global nutrition report 2014: actions and accountability to accelerate the world's progress on nutrition. Washington, DC; 2014.
24. International Food Policy Research Institute. Global nutrition report 2015: actions and accountability to advance nutrition and sustainable development. Washington, DC; 2015.
25. Heikens GT, Amadi BC, Manary M, Rollins N, Tomkins A. Nutrition interventions need improved operational capacity. Lancet. 2008;371:181–2.
26. Horton R, Lo S. Nutrition: a quintessential sustainable development goal. Lancet. 2013;382:371–2.
27. Grosse S, Roy K. Long-term economic effect of early childhood nutrition. Lancet. 2008;371:365–6.
28. World Bank. Repositioning nutrition as central to development: a strategy for large-scale action. Washington, DC: The World Bank; 2006.
29. Jamison DT, Summers LH, Alleyne G, et al. Global health 2035: a world converging within a generation. Lancet. 2013;382.1898–955.
30. Kruk ME, Yamey G, Angell SY, Beith A, et al. Transforming global health by improving the science of scale-up. PLoS Biol. 2016;14(3):e1002360.

31. Global Burden of Disease Study. Global, regional, and national incidence, prevalence, and years lived with disability for 301 acute and chronic diseases and injuries in 188 countries, 1990–2013: a systematic analysis for the Global Burden of Disease Study 2013. Lancet. 2013;386(9995):743–800.

32. Baillie E, Bjarnholt C, Gruber M, Hughes R. A capacity-building framework for public health nutrition practice. Publ Health Nutr. 2008;12:1031–8.

33. United Nations Development Programme. Capacity assessment and development in a systems and strategic management context. Technical advisory paper no. 3. Management Development and Governance Division, Bureau of Development Policy, New York; 2000.

34. United Nations Development Programme. Capacity development: a UNDP primer. New York, NY: Bureau for Development Policy Capacity Development Group; 2009.

35. Gillespie S, Margetts B. Strengthening capacities for enhancing the nutrition sensitivity of agricultural policy and practice. SCN News. 2013;40:53–8.

36. Gillespie SR. Strengthening capacity for nutrition. IFPRI discussion paper no. 106. Washington, DC: IFPRI; 2001.

37. Shrimpton R, Hughes R, Recine E, Mason JB, Sander D, Marks GC, Margetts B. Nutrition capacity development: a practice framework. Public Health Nutr. 2011;17.

38. Shrimpton R, du Plessis LM, Delisle H, Blaney S, Atwood ST et al. Public health nutrition capacity: assuring the quality of workforce preparation for scaling up nutrition programmes. Public Health Nutr. 2015.

39. Potter C, Brough R. Systemic capacity building: a hierarchy of needs. Health Policy Plan. 2004;19:336–45:682–8.

40. Ortiz A, Taylor P. Learning purposefully in capacity development: why, what and when to measure?. Paris, France: International Institute for Educational Planning; 2009.

41. Food and Agriculture Organization. FAO approaches to capacity development in programming: process and tools. Rome, Italy: Office of Knowledge Exchange, Research and Extension; 2012.

42. LaFond AK, Brown L, Macintyre K. Mapping capacity in the health sector: a conceptual framework. Int J Health Plann Mgmt. 2002;17:3–22.

43. Gillespie S, Haddad L, Mannar V, Nisbett N, Menon P. The politics of reducing malnutrition: building commitment and accelerating progress. Lancet. 2013;382:552–69.

44. Frenk J, Bhutta ZA, Cohen J, Crisp N, Evans T, Fineberg H, Garcia P, Ke Y, Kelly P, Kistnasamy B, et al. Health professionals for a new century: transforming education to strengthen health systems in an interdependent world. Lancet. 2010;376:1923–58.

45. Dal Poz MR, Kinfu Y, Drager S, Kunjumen. Counting health workers: definitions, data, methods and global results. Geneva, Switzerland: Human Resources for Health World Health Organization; 2007.

46. Amorim Lopes M, Santos Almeida A, Almada-Lobo B. Handling healthcare workforce planning with care: where do we stand? Hum Resour Health. 2015;13:38.

47. Fanzo J, Marshall Q, Dobermann D, Wong J, et al. Integration of nutrition into extension and advisory services: a synthesis of experiences, lessons, and recommendations. Food Nutr Bull. 2015;36(2):120–37.

48. Headey DD. Developmental drivers of nutritional change: a cross-country analysis. World Dev. 2013;42:76–88.

49. Anand S, Barnighausen T. Human resources and health outcomes: a cross-country econometric study. Lancet. 2004;364:1603–9.

50. Chen L, Evans T, Anand S, et al. Human resources for health: overcoming the crisis. Lancet. 2004;364:1984–90.

51. Scheffler RM, Mahoney CB, Fulton B, Dal Poz MR, Preker AS. Estimates of health care professional shortages in sub-Saharan Africa by 2015. Health Affairs; 2009.

52. Shrimpton R, Atwood SJ, Sanders D, Mason JB. An overview and regional perspective on the assessment of nutrition capacity of national and mid-level personnel carried out in three Asian countries. Prepared for UNICEF East Asia and Pacific Regional Office 07 June 2013.

53. Jaskiewicz W, Tulenko K. Increasing community health worker productivity and effectiveness: a review of the influence of the work environment. Hum Resour Health. 2012;10:38.

54. World Health Organization. Global strategy on human resources for health: workforce 2030. Accessed April 2016 from http://apps.who.int/gb/ebwha/pdf_files/EB138/B138_36-en.pdf?ua=1.

55. Nbarro D. Global child and maternal nutrition—the SUN rises. Lancet. 2012;382:666–7.

56. Pelletier D, Frongillo EA, Gervais S, et al. Nutrition agenda setting, policy formulation and implementation: lessons from the mainstreaming nutrition initiative. Health Policy Plann. 2012;27:19–31.

57. World Food Programme. Summary report of the joint evaluation of the REACH initiative (2011–2015).

58. Pelto GH, Matin SL, Van Liere M, Fabrizio CS. The scope and practice of behavior change communication to improve infant and young child feeding in low- and middle-income countries: results of a practitioner study in international development organizations. Mater Child Nutr. 2016;12(2):229–44.

59. Hampshire RD, Aguayo VM, Harouna H, Roley JA, Tarini A, Baker S. Delivery of nutrition services in health systems in sub-Saharan Africa: opportunities in Burkina Faso, Mozambique and Niger. Publ Health Nutr. 2004;7:1047–53.

60. Wuehler SE, Hess SY, Brown KH. Situational analysis of infant and young child nutrition activities in the Sahel —executive summary. Matern Child Nutr. 2011;7(S1):1–185.

61. Aryeetey RO, Laar A, Zotor F, Ghana SUN Academic Platform. Capacity for scaling up nutrition: a focus on pre-service training in West Africa and a Ghanaian case study. Proc Nutr Soc. 2015;74:533–7.

62. Trubswasser U, Nishida C, Engesveen K, Coulibaly-Zerbo F. Landscape analysis: assessing countries' readiness to scale up actions in the WHO African region. Afr J Food Agric Nutr Dev. 2012;12:6260–73.

63. Sodjinou R, Fanou N, Deart L, et al. Regional Nutrition Working Group. Region-wide assessment of the capacity for human nutrition training in West Africa: current situation, challenges, and way forward. Glob Health Action 2014;7:23247.

64. Sodjinou R, Bosu WK, Fanou N, et al. Nutrition training in medical and other health professional schools in West Africa: the need to improve current approaches and enhance training effectiveness. Glob Health Action. 2014;7:24827.

65. Sodjinou R, Bosu WK, Fanou N, et al. A systematic assessment of the current capacity to act in nutrition in West Africa: cross-country similarities and differences. Glob Health Action. 2014;7:24763.

66. Eichbaum Q, Nyarango P, Ferrao J, et al. Challenges and opportunities for new medical schools in Africa. Lancet Glob Health. 2014;2:e689–90.

67. Chu KM, Jayaraman S, Kyamanywa P, Ntakiyiruta G. Building research capacity in Africa: equity and global health collaborations. PLoS Med. 2014;11(3):e1001612.

68. Aaron GJ, Wilson SE, Brown KH. Bibliographic analysis of scientific research on selected topics in public health nutrition in West Africa: review of articles published from 1998 to 2008. Glob Publ Health. 2010;5(Suppl 1):S42–57.

69. Lachat C, Nago E, Roberfroid D, Holdsworth M, et al. Developing a sustainable nutrition research agenda in sub-Saharan Africa—findings from the SUNRAY project. PLoS Med. 2014;11(1):e1001593.

70. Brown KH, McLachlan M, Cardosa P, Tchibindat F, Baker SK. Strengthening public health nutrition research and training capacities in West Africa: report of a planning workshop convened in Dakar, Senegal, 26–28 March 2009. Glob Publ Health. 2010;5(Suppl 1):S1–19.

71. Rao KD, Bhatnagar A, Berman P. So many, yet few: human resources for health in India. Hum Resour Health. 2012;10:9.

72. Khandelwal S, Dayal R, Jha M, Zodpey S, Reddy KS. Mapping of nutrition teaching and training initiatives in India: the need for public health nutrition. Publ Health Nutr. 2012;15:2020–5.

73. Gillespie S, van den Bold M, Hodge J, Herforth A. Leveraging agriculture for nutrition in South Asia and East Africa: examining the enabling environment through stakeholder perceptions. Food Sec. 2015;7:463–77.

74. Sheikholeslam R, Ghassemi H, Galal O, Djazayery A, Omidvar N, Nourmohammadi I, Tuazon A. Graduate level training in nutrition: an integrated model for capacity building—a national report. Iran J Publ Health. 2015;44 (3):388–95.

75. World Health Organization. Assessing national capacity for the prevention and control of noncommunicable diseases: report of the 2010 global survey. Geneva, 2010.

76. World Health Organization. Noncommunicable diseases in the South-East Asia region. Switzerland, Geneva: World Health Organization; 2011.

77. World Health Organization. Global report on diabetes. Switzerland: World Health Organization Geneva; 2016.

78. Dietz WH, Baur LA, Hall K, et al. Management of obesity: improvement of health-care training and systems for prevention and care. Lancet. 2015;2521–33.

79. Ebrahim S, Squires N, di Fabio JL, et al. Radical changes in medical education needed globally. Lancet Glob Health. 2015;3:e128.

80. Kris-Etherton PM, Akabas SR, Douglas P, et al. Nutrition competencies in health professionals' education and training: a new paradigm. Adv Nutr. 2015;6:83–7.

81. Berg A. Sliding toward nutrition malpractice: time to reconsider and redeploy. Annu Rev Nutr. 1993;13:1–15.

82. Pepping F. The current capacity for training in public health nutrition in West Africa. Glob Publ Health. 2010;5: S20–41.

83. Pepping F. UNU/IUNS nutrition capacity building efforts in Africa. SCN News. 2006;33:39–42.

84. Hughes R, Shrimpton R, Recine E, Margetts B. A competency framework for global public health nutrition workforce development. A background paper. World Public Health Nutrition Association; 2011.

85. Garrett J, Natalicchio M. Working multisectorally in nutrition: principles, practices, and case studies. Washington, DC: IFPRI; 2011.

86. Mejia Acosta A, Fanzo JC. Fighting maternal and child malnutrition: analysing the political and institutional determinants of delivering a national multisectoral response in six countries: a synthesis paper. Institute of Development Studies; 2012.

87. DiMaria-Ghalilli RA, Mirtallo JM, Tobin BW, Hark L, Van Horn L, Palmer CA. Challenges and opportunities for nutrition education and training in the health care professions: intraprofessional and interprofessional call to action. Am J Clin Nutr. 2014;99(5S):1184S–93S.

88. Hughes R, Shrimpton R, Recine E, Margetts B. Empowering our profession. [Commentary] World Nutr. 2012;3:33–54.
89. Hughes R, Margetts R. The public health nutrition intervention management bi-cycle: a model for training and practice improvement. Publ Health Nutr. 2011;15(11):1981–8.
90. Society for Nutrition Education and Behavior (SNEB). Nutrition educator competencies for promoting healthy individuals, communities, and food systems. http://www.sneb.org/documents/SNEB_Nutrition_Education_ Competencies.pdf. Accessed Apr 2016.
91. Meeker J, Perry A, Dolan C, Emary C, Golden K, Abla C, Walsh A, Maclaine A, Seal A. Development of a competency framework for the nutrition emergencies sector. Public Health Nutr. 2013;17:689–99.
92. Kushner RF, Van Horn L, Rock CL, Edwards MS, Bales CW, Kohlmeier M, Akabas SR. Nutrition education in medical school: a time of opportunity. Am J Clin Nutr. 2014;99(5 Suppl):1167S–73S.
93. African Nutrition Leadership Programme. Accessed May 2016 from http://www.africanutritionleadership.org.
94. Sunguya BF, Poudel KC, Mlunde LB, et al. Nutrition training improves health workers nutrition knowledge and competence to manage child undernutrition: a systematic review. Front Public Health. 2013;1:37.
95. Yousafzai AK, Rasheed MA, Daelmans B, et al. Capacity building in the health sector to improve care for children nutrition and development. Ann NY Acad Sci. 2014;1308:172–82.
96. Geissler C, Amuna P, Kattelmann KK, Zotor FB, Donovan S. The eNutrition Academy: supporting a new generation of nutritional scientists around the world. Adv Nutr. 2016;7:190–8.
97. London School of Hygiene & Tropical Medicine. Programming for nutrition outcomes module. http://www. lshtm.ac.uk/eph/dph/research/nutrition/programming_nutrition_outcomes_module.html. Accessed 26 Apr 2016.
98. Food and Agriculture Organization. The ENACT course in nutrition education. http://www.fao.org/nutrition/ education/professional-training/enact/en/. Accessed 26 Apr 2016.
99. Hall CS, Fottrell E, Wilkison S, Byass P. Assessing the impact of mHealth interventions in low- and middle-income countries what has been shown to work. Glob Health Action. 2014;7:25606.
100. Potter C, Brough R. Systemic capacity building: a hierarchy of needs. Health Policy Plann. 2004;19:336–45.
101. Geissler C. Capacity building in public health nutrition. Proc Nutr Soc. 2015;74:430–6.
102. Lachat C, Roberfr[io]d D, van den Broeck L, van den Briel N, et al. A decade of nutrition research in Africa: assessment of the evidence base and academic collaboration. Publ Health Nutr. 2014;18(10):1890–7.
103. Martin L, Haque MR. Performance-based cash incentives for volunteers in BRAC's community-based alive & thrive infant and young child feeding program in Bangladesh. November 2013.
104. Haddad L. Building an enabling environment to fight undernutrition: some research tools that may help. Eur J Dev Res. 2012;25:13–20.
105. Nisbett N, Gillespie S, Haddad L, Harris J. Why worry about the politics of childhood under nutrition? World Dev. 2014;64:420–33.
106. Otoo S, Agapitova N, Behrens J. The capacity development results framework: a strategic and results-oriented approach to learning for capacity development. World Bank; June 2009.
107. Hawe P, King L, Noort M, Gifford SM, Lloyd B. Working invisibly: health workers talk about capacity-building in health promotion. Health Promot Int. 1998;13:285–95.
108. Hoddinott J, Alderman H, Behrman JR, Haddad L, Horton S. The economic rationale for investing in stunting reduction. Matern Child Nutr. 2013;9:69–82.
109. Horton R. Offline: why the sustainable development goals will fail. Lancet. 2011;383:2196.

Part III
Malnutrition, Nutrients and (Breast)Milk Explained

Chapter 5
The Spectrum of Malnutrition

Douglas Taren and Saskia de Pee

Keywords Malnutrition · Undernutrition · Overweight/obesity · Anthropometry · Micronutrients · Biomarkers

Learning Objectives

- Identify the stages of the malnutrition spectrum.
- Describe how various indicators of nutritional status can be used to determine the spectrum of malnutrition.
- Compare regional differences for the indicators of malnutrition.
- Explain how stages of nutritional status affect estimates of malnutrition.
- Analyze which specific indicators of nutritional status can be used to assess need for and impact of different nutrition policies and programs.

Introduction

The purpose of this chapter is to provide a foundation on how to determine the nutritional status of individuals and the types and prevalence of malnutrition in a population. The spectrum of malnutrition includes both undernutrition and so-called "overnutrition," which is actually "unbalanced" nutrition indicated by overweight and obesity. Indicators of the spectrum of malnutrition provide important insights on where to focus interventions and how to assess change and results of nutrition interventions with regards to changes in nutritional status. Diet, age, infections, chronic diseases, and genetic variation directly affect nutritional status and its indicators in an individual. Assessing the spectrum of malnutrition at a national or community level uses the prevalence of indicators of nutritional status used for individuals and additional measures of underlying and basic causes of malnutrition such as food insecurity, socioeconomic status, and environmental factors at individual, household, regional, or national level.

D. Taren (✉)
Mel and Enid Zuckerman College of Public Health, University of Arizona,
1295 North Martin Avenue, Tucson, AZ 85724, USA
e-mail: taren@email.arizona.edu

S. de Pee
Nutrition Division, World Food Programme, Rome, Italy
e-mail: Saskia.depee@wfp.org; depee.saskia@gmail.com

S. de Pee
Friedman School of Nutrition Science and Policy, Tufts University, Boston, MD, USA

© Springer Science+Business Media New York 2017
S. de Pee et al. (eds.), *Nutrition and Health in a Developing World*,
Nutrition and Health, DOI 10.1007/978-3-319-43739-2_5

The stages that constitute the spectrum of malnutrition become evident as one considers nutritional status moving away from an optimal homeostasis of nutrient balance. There are also many functional outcomes of malnutrition. There are several types and combinations of malnutrition that can occur within a nation/community or within a household and even for an individual (Table 5.1).

The spectrum of malnutrition for energy balance ranges from severe undernutrition to severe overnutrition leading to morbid obesity. Simultaneously, an individual can show signs of chronic undernutrition with a short height but also be overweight suggesting varying nutritional status during the lifespan. In middle and high income countries, overweight/obesity is more prevalent among food insecure households, because processed high-fat and high-sugar foods tend to be cheaper than fresh, nutritious foods, and women are most affected [1–7]. See Chap. 7 by Doak and Popkin for further discussion on overweight and obesity.

Single micronutrient malnutrition can range from severe clinical signs of deficiencies to toxicity. Because of the dietary origin of most micronutrient deficiencies, most people suffer from multiple micronutrient deficiencies rather than single ones, and it occurs both among people with undernutrition as well as people with overweight/obesity, due to the fact that foods high in energy are not

Table 5.1 Community, household and individual measures of malnutrition

Term	Definition	Example of indicator
Food insecurity	A combination of factors that lead to households to have an unstable and/or insufficient amounts of safe and nutritious food and can be chronic, seasonal or transitory	Questionnaire based on four domains of food security: availability, access, stability, and utilization of food; integrated food security scale
Undernourishment	Proportion of a population that is not meeting their energy requirements	Estimated from food balance sheets, including import and export
Undernutrition	A measure of inadequate nutrient intake compared to needs (can be acute or chronic and also affected by disease)	Anthropometric measures of stunting, wasting, underweight
Overweight/obese, sometimes referred to as 'overnutrition'	A measure of positive energy balance	Anthropometric measures of overweight (BMI, WHZ, waist circumference, waist/hip ratio)
Stunted and plump	Overnutrition on top of previous chronic undernutrition	Simultaneous state of (previously acquired) stunting and (current) overweight
Micronutrient deficiency	An inadequate amount of a vitamin or essential mineral in the body	One or more biomarker that relates to amount of nutrients in body, clinical signs of deficiency (e.g., xerophthalmia for vitamin A deficiency)
Multiple micronutrient deficiencies	An inadequate amount of two or more vitamins or essential minerals in the body	Multiple biomarkers indicating amounts of micronutrients in body or clinical signs of deficiencies
Double-burden of malnutrition: population	Excessive prevalence of both undernutrition and overweight/obesity, note that micronutrient deficiencies are often found to co-occur with both forms of malnutrition	Anthropometric measures of undernutrition (stunting, wasting) and overweight/obesity
Double-burden of malnutrition: household	One or more household members who have undernutrition while other member(s) is (are) overweight/obese (micronutrient deficiencies may occur among both)	Anthropometric measures of household members who are overweight/obese and others, often children, who have undernutrition, e.g., stunting
Double-burden of malnutrition: individual	Stunted and overweight/obese, in addition the individual may suffer from micronutrient deficiencies	Anthropometric measures of being stunted and overweight, and possibly also a biomarker indicating a micronutrient deficiency

necessarily good sources of micronutrients. Within a family, undernutrition, micronutrient deficiencies, and overweight/obesity may occur, sometimes all in the same person, sometimes as different combinations among different people [8, 9]. As countries go through the nutrition transition, the spectrum of malnutrition, which was initially dominated by wasting, stunting, and micronutrient deficiencies, see a rise of overweight and obesity, first among adults, while micronutrient deficiencies remain prevalent and stunting and wasting in young children may decline, but only gradually. This transition leads to a national double-burden of malnutrition in both children and adults [10, 11]. Due to the fact that children who are stunted are at an increased risk of overweight and obesity as they become older and that food consumption in a population goes from and inadequate amount and quality of food to an increase of energy intake but still an inadequate dietary quality, overweight and micronutrient deficiencies co-exist in most populations that go through the nutrition transition. This can be seen in rural settings but appear to have a greater impact in urban settings as described by Ruel et al. in Chap. 32. When economic development continues, people have more choices to improve dietary diversity, and leisure time increases and more time is spend on physical activity, both the energy balance and dietary quality improve among the population, resulting in a lower prevalence of both overweight/obesity and micronutrient deficiencies.

Diet, anthropometrics, biomarkers, gene modifications, functional changes, and clinical signs are indicators that can be used to measure the current or past nutritional status of individuals. Nutrition indicators are influenced by natural genetic variations in the population as to what is a homeostatic stage of health of an individual. Infections and various disease states can directly affect the nutritional status of individuals. Additionally, other physiological factors perturb normal physiological responses, such as inflammation that modifies the level of biomarkers of nutritional status [12–15]. Thus, there are many occasions when using a single cut point for identifying malnourished individuals result in both false positives and false negative classifications of malnutrition. Nonetheless, using standardized cut points to identify the stage of malnutrition is useful when classifying individuals and when comparing the prevalence of malnutrition between nations and between communities and over time in the same population.

Indicators of undernutrition also suggest different levels of severity of deficiency in addition to the prevalence of deficiencies. There are indicators that suggest low storage levels of a micronutrient before there are functional and clinical signs of a deficiency. It is also possible to assess a nutritional deficiency based on changes in response to increasing the intake of a nutrient, and subsequent changes in the level of indicators that are linked to the status of the nutrient such as for linear growth with zinc supplementation and the retinol dose response test to determine if vitamin A stores are sufficient. Alternatively, a change in hemoglobin values without measures of iron status following a regimen of iron supplementation can indicate whether a person had iron deficiency anemia.

The reported prevalence of malnutrition depends on what stages of malnutrition are being measured. The prevalence decreases when indicators of more severe deficiency are being measured. At the same time, how indicators respond to intervention measures will depend on what type of indicators are being measured. Changes in dietary intake may be measured before changes occur in biomarkers for a nutrient. While at the same time, where prevalence of severe deficiency is still high, the biomarkers that measure the greater severity of deficiency may be the indicators that are most responsive to nutrition interventions compared with other biomarkers.

It is important to realize that the indicators of nutritional status may not be linearly related to degrees of nutritional status and can vary from person to person. This variation is also a reason that multiple indicators of nutritional status are often needed to determine the stage of malnutrition. Indicators of nutritional status also take varying times to change. In some cases, providing a supplement or fortified food can result in a rapid change for an indicator such as giving a high-dose vitamin A supplement to a child with a Bitot's spot. However, it may take more than a month for hemoglobin to increase after iron supplementation when a person has iron deficiency anemia.

Biomarkers that measure stores may suggest a greater deficiency compared with biomarkers that indicate some functional change in metabolism. Nutrient rich diets can also change nutritional status but may require more time to lead to change of indicators of nutritional status.

Using Specific Indicators of Nutritional Status to Determine the Stage of Malnutrition

Food and Available Energy

The amount of food available for human consumption is the basis for determining the prevalence of undernourishment in countries. The availability, access, stability, and utilization of food are primary domains that determine food security [16]. Food balance sheets at the national level account for food production, food loss, food imports, and food export for a country. The focus of the food balance sheets is on energy and is modeled from national level data on food production, import and export, and population composition. The amount of energy from foods as accounted for in the food balance sheets is compared with the mean dietary energy requirements (MDER) for a country based on a country's population size, and the energy needed related to the stature, sex, ages, and physical activity level of the population, and assuming a certain distribution of food across the population, to account for the fact that access to food is not equally distributed. Simply put, the difference between the amount of food available within a country and the amount needed to meet the MDER and taking distribution into account is used to determine what proportion of a population likely consumes less than the calorie requirement for an active and healthy life [16]. This is the statistic used for the hunger indicator, i.e., the number of "undernourished" people.

Food balance sheets and data on production of each food item by season with food prices are also used to determine the risk of future food shortages and the onset of famine conditions [17, 18]. Food balance sheets can also be used do to identify specific crops whose increased cultivation could help alleviate micronutrient deficiencies [19, 20]. However, food balance sheets may overestimate dietary intake because they are based on food availability and do not account for acquisition, use and losses at household level [21]. Furthermore, not all foods that are produced and consumed are included on food balance sheets. This is particularly the case for small-scale production of fruits, vegetables, and small livestock at household and community level for own consumption or selling at small markets, which is not captured by the data that are collected for food balance sheets.

While the prevalence of undernourishment is estimated at population level, food insecurity, mainly focusing on adequacy of energy intake, can also be assessed at sub-national level. The Integrated Food Security Scale classifies populations into five stages of security: (1) generally food secure, (2) borderline food insecurity, (3) acute food and livelihood crises, (4) humanitarian emergency, and (5) famine/humanitarian catastrophe [22].

Several other indicators have also been used as measures of food security [23]. The Global Hunger Index is based on undernourishment, child underweight, and child mortality, and is used to compare low income and middle income nations and categorize their food security and nutrition situation as low, moderate, serious, alarming, and extremely alarming [24]. The Global Food Security Index uses affordability, availability, and utilization and allows for comparisons between countries [25]. The Poverty and Hunger Index is a multidimensional index that uses the percent of the population living on less than one dollar per day, the poverty gap, the percent share of income/consumption for a country's poorest quintile, the percent of underweight children and the percent of the population that is undernourished [26]. These indices provide various ways to compare countries regarding the level of food security and malnutrition that exist in the world.

For assessment of food security at household level, specific questionnaires have been developed, of which the household food insecurity access scale (HHFIAS) is one of the most widely used [27]. As food security is achieved when all people, at all times, have physical and economic access to sufficient, safe, and nutritious food to meet their dietary needs and food preferences for an active and healthy life, the focus should not only be on meeting energy requirements, but also of other nutrients. This needs to be assessed through other measures, including dietary intake, data on which needs to be collected at household or individual level.

Diet

Measuring dietary intake can estimate macro and micronutrient intake when linked to food composition databases. Dietary data can also provide information on the consumption of foods that promote or inhibit nutrient absorption. Measuring the diet of individuals provides information about energy intake, but there may be substantial misreporting as suggested by studies that compared dietary intake data to findings on energy expenditure or protein intake using doubly labeled water and urinary nitrogen excretion techniques [28, 29]. Factors that have been found to be associated with misreporting of dietary intake include disease state, lifestyle, nutritional status, dietary factors, age, sex, psychological factors, and behavioral health [30–32].

The most commonly used methods for measuring diet include one day or multiple days of 24-h recalls. Other methods are based on collecting dietary history, having people keep a diet diary or using a food frequency questionnaire (FFQ). Collecting dietary intake on multiple days provides a better indication of usual diet compared with one day of intake. Where diets are relatively monotonous, a one day recall reflects usual intakes at population level better than it does in situations where dietary diversity is higher. When dietary intake measurements are collected for individual days it is important to take into account factors such as the normality of the day's diet, the day of the week, week of the month, holidays, and season. FFQs on the other hand provide an estimate of the average food and nutrient intake during a specific period of time. However, asking frequency of intake of too many foods may result in overestimation.

Collecting dietary data also can also be used to measure dietary diversity, and dietary patterns that affect nutritional status. Dietary patterns provide information on what types of foods are being consumed and when foods are being consumed together. The FAO has proposed using 24 h recalls to calculate dietary diversity scores (DDS) at the household level and for individuals. The household DDS categorizes the reported foods consumed by all household members into 12 food groups. An individual DDS is based on 9 categories [33]. There is no specific cut point for determining what is a low or high DDS. Comparisons can be made within and between populations based on the distribution of the food groups (e.g., Z-scores or quartiles) or with predetermined cut points. For example, individual DDS could be grouped as low (0–3 food groups), medium (4–6 food groups), and high (≥7 food groups). The WHO has determined that having consumed less than four food groups in the previous 24-h for children between 6 and 23 months of age classifies as not having adequate diversity, which is a proxy for being unlikely to meet nutrient intake recommendations [34]. The Food Consumption Score (FCS) is a more detailed household level DDS that also incorporates a measure of nutrient density, by assigning a higher multiplication factor to certain food groups such as animal source foods [20].

When dietary data are converted to nutrient intake it is possible to use the Dietary Reference Intakes (DRIs) to estimate the adequacy of consuming specific nutrients [35]. The DRIs are composed of four values to estimate nutrient adequacy. The Recommended Dietary Allowance (RDA) is the individual's average daily dietary intake level that is sufficient to meet the nutrient requirement of 97–98% of healthy individuals in a particular life stage and gender group. Thus, if one consumes the

RDA for a nutrient, the likelihood of an inadequate intake is low. The calculation for Adequate Intake (AI) is the recommended intake based on the nutrient intake by a group of healthy people that are assumed to be adequate whether it is measured by observation or with an experiment. The AI is used when an RDA cannot be determined. The third method to determine the adequacy of a diet is based on the Estimated Average Requirement (EAR). The EAR is the daily nutrient intake level that is estimated to meet the requirement for 50% of healthy individuals in a specific life stage (age, pregnancy) and gender. The proportion of people in a country or community that is consuming less than the EAR is defined as the proportion of the population that has an inadequate intake for specific nutrients, except for when the consumption of the nutrient is skewed [36]. Finally, the tolerable upper intake level (UL) is the level that should not be exceeded by far for a long period of time in order to avoid the risk of adverse health effects [35]. The UL has been set based on toxicity data, from observations or case reports among humans or animal experiments, to which a generous safety margin has been applied. Using the DRI metrics allows for an assessment of nutrient intakes at population level, ranging from likely deficient to excess and toxicity. Additional information on how these values are used in practices are presented by de Pee in Chap. 8. Another good resource for the dietary recommendations for micronutrients is available at the Linus Pauling Institute website (http://lpi. oregonstate.edu). It also provides information on the function, functional changes and clinical deficiency signs for micronutrients.

Anthropometric Measurements

Weight, height/length, and mid-upper arm circumference are the basic anthropometric measures used to monitor growth and to determine the presence of malnutrition. Other anthropometric measurements include waist and hip circumferences, head circumference, and skinfold measurements. The underlying assumption of these is that they are assessments of body composition related to the amount of fat mass and non-fat mass (lean body mass) for a person.

More direct measures of body composition are also available. Hydrostatic (underwater) weighing uses the buoyance of fat to measure the difference between fat mass and lean body mass. The use of more advance methods such as bioelectrical impedance and deuterated water utilize the amount of body water to estimate a body's fat mass and non-fat mass. More recently, air displacement plethysmography (ADP) technology is used to determine body volume on the basis of the pressure/volume relationship to estimate body composition derived from body density. The present gold standard for determining body composition is whole body dual-energy X-ray absorptiometry (DEXA) scan that uses a 4-component model (fat, water, minerals, and protein) to assess nutritional status by distinguishing lean body mass, fat mass, and bone mass. These methods are mostly used for research studies or in higher income countries as part of clinical assessments of nutritional status.

Anthropometric Measures for Adults and Aging

Weight and height measures are used to determine the body mass index (BMI). Adult BMI values that are used to classify nutritional status are based of four major classifications: underweight, normal, overweight, and obese. These can be further broken down to more specific cut points (Table 5.2). The cut point for these classifications are based on their association with different health outcomes, e.g., maternal underweight being associated with poor pregnancy outcomes, and a decreased immune response to infections, and an increased risk for chronic diseases as BMI values increase from normal to overweight to obese [37]. However, the role that BMI has on predicting adiposity may decrease with age as the proportion body fat and muscle mass changes even though the same BMI cut points

Table 5.2 Adult weight classifications

Weight category for individuals	BMI range (kg/m^2)
Underweight	<18.5
Severe underweight	<16.0
Moderate underweight	16.0–<17.0
Mild underweight	17.0–<18.5
Normal range	18.5–<25.0
Overweight	≥25.0
Obese	≥30.0
Mild obesity	30.00–<35.0
Moderate obesity	35.00–<40.0
Severe obesity	≥40.0
Additional categories: public health action and reporting[a]	
Overweight	≥23.0
Obesity	≥27.5
Obesity class I	27.5–<32.5
Obesity class II	32.5–<37.5
Obesity class III	≥37.5

[a]Action points along the spectrum of BMI at which countries could make decisions regarding risks for their population [42]

are also used to classify people older than 60 years of age, as being overweight or obese [38]. BMI is also used to monitor the growing prevalence of obesity worldwide [39]. One issue that currently plagues international standards are data that indicates Asians and Asian Americans have a higher prevalence of diabetes at the same BMI values compared with whites implying that lower BMI values may be appropriate as cut points for overweight and obesity in this population [40, 41]. WHO [42] has suggested that for many Asian populations, a BMI of 23.0 or higher represents an increased risk comparable with 25.0 for overweight in other populations and a BMI of 27.5 or higher represents high risk comparable to a BMI of 30.0 for obese. An analysis of the Malaysian National Health and Morbidity Survey that included a sample of 32,703 adults of multiple Asian ethnicities suggested that the classification of overweight in men should start with a BMI of 23.0 and a BMI of 24.0 for women [43].

As the global prevalence of obesity is increasing, waist circumference is becoming recognized as an important measure of abdominal fat with its association with adiposity and an increased risk for type 2 diabetes, cardiovascular disease, and mortality [44, 45]. Recommendations for what are appropriate cut points for waist circumference are not consistent. Optimal cut points for waist circumference has varied tremendously across studies [46]. A waist circumference of >88 cm (>35 in) for women and >102 cm (>40 in) for men has been used in the United States [37]. However, lower cut points of 80 cm for women and 94 cm for men have been recommended by the International Diabetes Federation [47]. Lower cut points of 80 and 90 cm for women and men, respectively, have even been recommended for South Asians and Eastern Asians [48].

However, there are several nuances with regard to how waist circumference is related to chronic disease. It appears that the determination of cut points may be related to the mean waist circumference measures of a population raising the issue of whether there should be specific cut points for different populations [46]. For example, in a meta-analysis that incorporated 58 studies, waist circumference as an estimate of adiposity, had a greater association with hypertension in studies in which the study population had a mean BMI of <22.0 compared with studies in which mean BMI was >22.0, suggesting that the risk of hypertension associated with adiposity is greater in lean than in non-lean populations [49].

Waist-to-hip ratios have also been shown to have a strong association with an increased risk for chronic diseases and various cut points have been used across studies. The WHO has identified a ratio >0.90 and >0.85 as cut points for men and women, respectively, which substantially increase the risk of metabolic complications [50]. However, unlike waist circumference, there is not a recommendation to have separate cut points based on ethnicity or geographic region as there is less variability between populations for waist-to-hip ratios compared with waist circumference.

Anthropometric Measures for Birth Outcomes and Pregnancy

Infant birth weight is the standard anthropometric measure that indicates infant health. Infants with birth weights <2500 g are identified as low birth weight (LBW) infants and birth weights <1500 g identify infants with very low birth weight (VLBW). Infants with a birth weight >4000 g are identified as having a high birth weight (HBW). Given birth weight and gestational age are correlated there is also a need to know if low birth weights are due to a premature delivery (births before 37 weeks gestation) and/or because a new born had intrauterine growth restriction (IUGR). IUGR is one of the main reasons for having a small-for-gestational age infant (SGA). Sex specific fetal growth curves by Fenton and Kim provide weight-for-gestational age percentiles that can be used to classify newborns as SGA infants [51]. A weight-for-gestational age less than the 10th percentile is used to define SGA while other infants are considered to be average for gestational age (AGA). Percentiles are also available for length and head circumference for gestational age. See Chap. 6 by de Onis for further information on reference curves for birth outcomes. Babies born at term and without LBW have the lowest risk for morbidity and mortality. Risk increases for term infants born SGA but without LBW. The risk for morbidity and mortality increases more for preterm infants who are AGA. The trajectory of risk continues to increase for term SGA infants with LBW, and for preterm AGA with LBW and the greatest risk is for preterm SGA babies who have LBW [52]. SGA infants have significantly greater risk for death, bronchopulmonary dysplasia, necrotizing enterocolitis, and retinopathy of prematurity and the risk increases more for children who have a weight-for-gestational age < the 3rd percentile [53, 54]. Christian et al. [55] reported that the long-term effect of being born SGA was greater on decreasing cognitive development in Nepali children 7–9 years of age compared with being born preterm AGA. Cognitive scores increased for children with greater head circumference at birth. Chapter 23 by Gonzalez-Casanova, Ramakrishnan, and Martorell, provides a more comprehensive review of the issues related to methods to identify SGA infants, its epidemiology and association with future child health.

SGA infants can be further classified as having asymmetrical or symmetrical IUGR, where the former is more common and reflects restriction of growth mainly in the third and/or late second trimester, whereas the latter is defined as restricted growth throughout pregnancy. Maternal prenatal anemia was reported to have an association with symmetrical IUGR while tobacco use was associated with asymmetrical IUGR [56]. These results suggest that smoking affects weight gain during the later part of pregnancy by potentially decreasing blood volume expansion and increasing the risk for placental infarcts later in pregnancy leading to poor placental perfusion. Furthermore, asymmetric IUGR was related to greater mortality compared with symmetric IUGR in a cohort of Mexican infants, possibly due to the lower birth weights for the asymmetric infants [57].

Infants who are born with a weight-for-gestational age above the 90th percentile are classified as large for gestational age (LGA). Mothers giving birth to an LGA infant are at an increased risk for prolonged labor, birth trauma, and delivering by caesarean sections [58]. LGA infants are at a greater risk for fetal hypoxia and having postnatal hypoglycemia. Long-term health effects for LGA infants include a greater risk for chronic diseases including obesity, diabetes, and asthma [59].

Pre-pregnancy anthropometric measures are an important indicator for birth outcomes as a low pre-pregnancy weight is related to LBW and a high pre-pregnancy weight is related to a high birth weight infant [60], which may be mediated by gestational glucose intolerance or diabetes. A pre-pregnancy BMI <18.5 or a height of <145 cm have been identified as measures that relate to poor pregnancy outcomes [61, 62]. Pregnant women with a MUAC <22 or 23 cm are defined as having malnutrition and greater risk for having a poor pregnancy outcome based on infant birth weight, preterm birth, and reduced fetal growth for both African and Asian women [63]. Similarly in a cohort of 14,040 singleton births, the risk for having a LBW infant was higher among women who had a height of <145 cm (OR = 1.93) or who had a MUAC <23.5 cm (OR = 1.47). The greatest risk for having a LBW infant was among women who were both thin and short (OR = 2.8) [64]. A higher MUAC was also associated with a higher birth weight and a lower risk for having a LBW infant in HIV positive women [65]. Additionally, on the other tail of the malnutrition spectrum for birth weight, women who themselves were born as LGA had a significantly greater risk of giving birth to a LGA infant. Furthermore, women born as SGA and who became overweight (BMI >30.0) had the greatest risk for giving birth to a LGA infant, adding to the important literature on the generational effects of malnutrition [66].

Weight gain during pregnancy is an important antenatal indicator of nutritional status that is related to birth outcomes due to its association with blood volume expansion and greater placental perfusion [67]. Underweight women should gain more weight than women with higher BMI values. The Institute of Medicine recommendation for weight gain are 12.5–18 kg for underweight women (BMI <18.5), 11.5–16 kg for normal weight women (BMI: 18.5–24.9), 7–11.5 kg for overweight women (BMI 25–29.9) and only 5–9 kg for obese women (BMI >30.0) [68]. Maternal weight gain throughout pregnancy is positively associated with fetal growth (femur length and abdominal circumference) and birth weight [69]. Insufficient weight gain in underweight and normal weight women during the later part of pregnancy are associated with low birth weight infants, premature births, and SGA infants [70].

Given the global increase in obesity, there is now a greater focus on the birth outcome of overweight women. Prenatal obesity, excessive weight gain, and gestational diabetes are major risk factors for having a LGA infant [59, 66, 71, 72]. A systematic review of Brazilian studies indicated that overweight women are at greater risk for excessive weight gain, gestational diabetes, large for gestational age infants and greater rates of caesarean sections [73]. A meta-analysis that included nine prospective studies and three retrospective studies indicated that excessive gestational weight gain beyond those recommended by the IOM was also associated with a greater increase in post-partum weight retention in studies that had 1, 9 and up to 15 years of follow up data [74]. In a cohort study of 456,711 Swedish women, women who increased their pre-pregnancy BMI by four points after their first pregnancy had a greater relative risk for having a stillbirth with their subsequent pregnancy. The risk for neonatal mortality was also increased during a second pregnancy for normal weight women who increased their BMI after their first pregnancy. On the other hand, weight loss between the first and second pregnancy decreased the risk of neonatal mortality for overweight women but increased the risk for infant mortality for women who had a healthy weight in their first pregnancy [71].

Anthropometric Measures for Children

The development and use of weight and height/length curves are described in detail by de Onis in Chap. 6. Weight and height measurements can be used independently or converted to z-scores based on age and sex. The standard converted measures are height-for-age z-scores (HAZ), weight-for-height/length z-scores (WHZ), and weight-for-age z-scores (WAZ). The sex specific percentile for body mass index (BMI) is used for children 2–18 years of age. The percentile accounts for the changes in body composition during childhood and adolescence. The mid-upper arm circumference (MUAC) is used extensively to screen for undernutrition and to determine if children are well enough to be discharged after nutritional rehabilitation. It is also important to note that WHZ and MUAC do not measure the same group of children and this is further elaborated below [75].

With regards to overnutrition, various percentiles for weight-for-length and BMI-for-age are used to classify children as being overweight or obese, respectively. In the United States, a weight-for-recumbent length at or above the 95th percentile on the CDC's 2000 growth charts is considered to be overweight for children less than 2 years of age. Children, 2–19 years of age who have a BMI for age that is between the 85 and 95th percentiles are classified as being overweight and children who have a BMI for age > the 95th percentile are classified as being obese [76]. The WHO classifies children (2 years and older) as being normal weight when their BMI for age Z-score is between −2.0 and <+1.0 z-score, overweight children have z-scores between +1.0 z-score and +2.0 z-scores and children with a z-score of >+2.0 are classified as being obese. Children classified as being overweight or obese have been shown to have an increase risk for hypertension, insulin resistance, and increased LDL cholesterol [77].

Anthropometric measures are also used to screen for undernutrition and triage children for nutritional rehabilitation. WHZ is the standard for determining wasting and when edema is present, a child is automatically considered to have severe wasting. Derrick and Patrice Jelliffe [78] were also the first to recommend using the MUAC in 1966 even in the presence of oedema. The popularity for using MUAC took off after a report by Shakir and Morely [79] in a *Lancet* article in 1974 using a tricolor cord. They proposed to use this method for screening because reliable weighing scales were not available and birth dates were not known prohibiting the calculation of weight for age percentiles. MUAC can use a fixed cut-off for 12–59 month old children, which greatly facilitates use of the measure at community level. Currently, a MUAC of <11.5 cm is used to identify children aged 12–59 months eligible for SAM treatment and MUAC measurements between 11.5 and 12.5 cm for MAM treatment, as a low MUAC is a strong risk factor for death as it will select more younger children who have a greater risk of mortality [80]. MUAC may also be a better indicator of under-nutrition in children with diarrhea compared with WAZ or WHZ measures based on classifications either before or after rehydration [81]. A MUAC of 12.5 cm can be used to discharge children after treating SAM or MAM and this cut point may support longer treatment regimens compared with a percent weight gain especially for more severely malnourished children [82].

Using either MUAC <11.5 cm or WHZ <−3.0 partially identify the same groups of children suffering from malnutrition [75]. A study in Nigeria suggested that the MUAC is more sensitive for identifying SAM as compared to using anthropometric z-scores, which may lead to underreporting of SAM [83]. A secondary analysis showed that using a MUAC of 11.5 cm for screening for SAM missed over 90% of children with a WHZ <−3.0. Conversely, using a WHZ <−3.0 missed 80% of children with a MUAC <11.5 cm. MUAC may also be a better predictor for identifying children at risk for death in Asian populations where many children are considered to be thin but fat due to an increased abdominal circumference [84]. Furthermore, MUAC may be more responsive to treatment for SAM and MAM as it is related to changes in muscle mass before additional fat mass is accumulated [85]. Some authors suggested to use MUAC for screening in the community and then use both MUAC and WHZ for admission criteria at the primary health care unit [86]. However, MUAC has better predictability of death and using the MUAC within community management of acute malnutrition is also preferred because of the ease of measurement, it is more age independent for children less than 6 years of age and there is not a need for a lot of equipment [87].

It is of interest to note that the MUAC was merged with height measures to create a ratio by Quaker Service Team during the Biafra war in Nigeria and they termed the adjusted values as the QUACK Stick [88]. This adjustment was done due to concerns about not knowing the age of children, and therefore they used height as a substitute for age. A validation study conducted of the QUACK Stick indicated that the smallest MUAC ratio (<10th percentile) related to a relative risk of about 4.0 for mortality compared with children >50th percentile [89]. However, later studies have not been able to confirm that adjusting MUAC for length increased the prediction of risk of death [90].

Additionally, MUAC is still more commonly used since increased leg length is mostly associated with healthy children [91].

Moderate wasting includes children with a WHZ that is <−2.0 z-score and > or equal to −3.0 z-score without the presence of edema. Severe wasting is a WHZ z-score that is <−3.0 z-score or the presence of edema. A HAZ that is <−2.0 z-score is an indication of stunting due to chronic under-nutrition and <−3.0 z-score indicates severe stunting. Multiple anthropometric measurements over time provide a better understanding of what stage of malnutrition exists for an individual. Changes in z-scores can indicate a worsening of nutritional status if a child's z-score is decreasing but has not yet reached <−2.0 z-score. Increases in z-scores can indicate that there is catch up growth occurring in children who suffered from undernutrition or can indicate a risk for developing overweight.

Clinical Signs of Malnutrition

Conducting a systematic medical history and physical exam are essential for correctly assessing a person for clinical signs of malnutrition. A medical history should include obtaining information about changes in recent health status, the use of medications, other herbs and tonics that may have been used, exposure to violence, changes in body weight, adequacy of diet, factors that may increase metabolic stress, and other clinically appropriate illnesses, diseases, and syndromes [92–94]. A physical exam from head to toe includes palpating and visually assessing skin, mucosal tissue, teeth, eyes, skinfolds, and joints. A pediatric subjective Global Nutritional Assessment has been described for children [95]. The mini-nutritional assessment can be used for elderly that includes additional measures of functional impairment for changes in daily activities and psychiatric screening [96, 97]. Clinical signs of malnutrition occur when there is a severe deficit in nutritional status for both under and overnutrition and for micronutrient deficiencies. The most common clinical signs of malnutrition have been well documented in a color atlas by McLaren [98].

Some clinical signs are mostly associated with a single nutrient due to the specific physiological role of the nutrient and because the nutrient is usually the nutrient that is most often deficient, such as the causal role of vitamin A deficiency in conjunctival xerosis. However, it is also possible to have a clinical outcome that can be related to multiple nutritional deficiencies such as the association that dermatitis has with niacin, essential fatty acids, zinc, and protein deficiencies. Impaired wound healing is another clinical sign that is associated with multiple nutrients that are involved with protein synthesis such as protein, zinc, and vitamin C. Furthermore, while pallor is most commonly associated with iron deficiency it may also occur due to other causes of anemia including folate and vitamin B12 deficiency.

The reasons for and the timeline associated with the occurrence of clinical signs are important for understanding their association or lack thereof with nutritional status and what should be the expected outcomes from nutritional interventions. Clinical signs of malnutrition can occur quickly in response to acute changes in nutritional status when the tissue turnover occurs during a short period of time such as with the formation of a Bitot's spots due to vitamin A deficiency. Additionally, Bitot's spots can quickly become full blown xerophthalmia due to an increased demand for vitamin A during an infection. Dehydration is one of the signs of malnutrition that occurs the fastest during acute and protracted diarrheal episodes in infants and young children. Prolonged skinfolds, sunken eyes, and dry oral mucosa are signs of dehydration that can appear quickly after the onset of diarrhea. Additionally, children who have a high demand for nutrients can also develop signs of malnutrition quickly such as with the case with preterm infants who start off with a low level of nutrient stores and who have an increased requirements for nutrients [99]. Other clinical signs develop over a long period of time while physiological and anatomical adjustments can be made in response to malnutrition.

For example, the changes in bone structure with rickets take time to develop in response to vitamin D deficiency.

Clinical signs of malnutrition can occur not only because of an imbalance in nutrient intake but also because of how infections and other environmental conditions unmask nutritional deficiencies. Biotin deficiency can lead to fungal infections which in turn causes discoloration of the nail plate. B12 deficiency can be caused by tapeworm infections and other diseases that affect intrinsic factor required for vitamin B12 absorption. Zinc deficiency can occur as a result of burns which increases the requirement for Zinc for protein synthesis for wound healing.

Clinical signs of malnutrition can be transient and can disappear within hours or days after appropriate nutritional intervention. For example, Bitot's spots may disappear within days after a child received a therapeutic dose of vitamin A. However, clinical signs may also just transform or remain after a nutritional intervention has occurred. For example, goiters may not disappear after iodine treatment due to the fibrous growth that occurred in response to iodine deficiency and which remains after iodine status has returned to normal levels. Similarly, it may take months or years to have acanthosis nigricans regress and it may never disappear in response to weight loss and improved insulin resistance [100, 101].

There are several signs of vitamin and mineral deficiencies that have been described for centuries and remain of important public health significance. Although the prevalence of several of these deficiencies has decreased over the past half a century, they do occur when food resources become extremely limited, when populations and families have monotonous diets and when infections occur in populations with marginal nutritional status. Table 5.3 provides the summary of the signs and diseases associated with micronutrient deficiencies.

In terms of protein-energy malnutrition (PEM), the salient features include loss of subcutaneous tissue, muscle wasting, and the presence of edema. However, the mechanisms related to a loss in fat and muscle mass differs based on the underlying causes such as the cachexia that is associated with inflammation and metabolic disturbances that occur with cancer and that are not reversed with additional caloric intake. Similarly, sarcopenia, the muscle loss that occurs with aging is different from the protein-energy malnutrition that is seen in young children [102]. Thus, the signs of PEM may not by definition relate to an imbalance between intake of protein and energy compared to energy expenditure.

The most classical outcomes of PEM in children results in marasmus and kwashiorkor. Williams [103], a Jamaican physician working at the Children's Hospital in Accra on the Gold Coast Colony first described kwashiorkor in a 1933 article in the *Archives of Diseases of Childhood*. She described it as syndrome that consisted first mostly of edema and then wasting, diarrhea, irritability, various sores of the mucous membranes, thin, sparse, brittle hair that is easily pulled out and that turns a dull brown or reddish color and a consistent pattern of specific desquamation of the skin. In a later *Lancet* article she provided a differential diagnosis of kwashiorkor from beriberi (thiamin deficiency) and vitamin A deficiency [104]. Additional clinical signs of PEM appeared as a substantial decrease in subcutaneous tissue that is apparent along the legs, arms, buttocks, and face. Skin changes include dermatitis, sores, and hyper pigmented plagues, and in the oral area, cheilosis, angular stomatitis, and papillary atrophy. A physical exam will reveal abdominal distention secondary to a decrease in abdominal musculature and hepatomegaly due to fatty infiltration. Also, finger and toe nails were reported to become fissured with ridged nails.

Later, the results of a Wellcome Trust meeting in Jamaica developed a two-by-two classification scheme to differentiate the signs of marasmus and kwashiorkor [105]. Simply, a child with severe deficit of weight and a loss of subcutaneous fat tissue was considered to have marasmus and the presence of edema identified a person as having kwashiorkor and when present together a child was identified as having marasmic kwashiorkor [106].

Table 5.3 Deficiency signs and symptoms

Selected nutrients	Deficiency signs and symptoms
Vitamin A (retinol)	• Night blindness • Various stages of xerophthalmia • Hair follicle blockage with a permanent "goose-bump" appearance, follicular hyperkeratosis • Dry, rough skin
Vitamin D (calciferol)	• Rickets • Osteomalacia and osteoporosis • Epiphyseal swelling
Vitamin K (phylloquinone)	• Small hemorrhages in the skin or mucous membranes (petechia) • Intraocular hemorrhage
Vitamin B1 (thiamin)	• Beriberi (cardiac and neurologic) • Wernicke and Korsakov syndromes (alcoholic confusion and paralysis) • Sensory loss, blurred vision • Dyspnea • Muscular wasting • Sometimes edema (wet beriberi) • Malaise • Ataxia • Reduced tendon jerks (reflex) • Mental confusion • Tense calf muscles • Distended neck veins • Jerky movement of eyes • Staggering gait and difficulty walking • Infants may develop cyanosis • Round, swollen (moon) face • Foot and wrist drop
Vitamin B2 (riboflavin)	• Redness and scaling of nasolabial folds • Diffuse depigmentation • Non specific—fatigue, eye changes, dermatitis, brain dysfunction, impaired iron absorption • Tearing, burning, and itching of the eyes • Fissuring in the corners of the eyes • Soreness and burning of the lips, mouth, and tongue with fissuring and/or cracking of the lips and corners of the mouth • Purple swollen tongue • Seborrhea of the skin in the nasolabial folds, scrotum, or vulva • Capillary overgrowth around the corneas
Vitamin B3 (niacin)	• Pellagra identified by the four Ds: dermatitis, dementia, diarrhea and death if not treated. The dermatitis from niacin deficiency has classical presentation of dermatitis that is symmetrical and occurs at pressure points (e.g., buttocks) and on sun exposed skin • Sensory loss • Tremors • Sore tongue • Amblyopia • Anorexia • Indigestion
Vitamin B6 (pyridoxine)	• Dermatitis • Neurological disorders, convulsions • Anemia • Inflammation of the lining of the mouth, tongue inflammation • Fissures in the corners of the mouth

(continued)

Table 5.3 (continued)

Selected nutrients	Deficiency signs and symptoms
Vitamin B9 (folic Acid)	• Glossitis • Neural tube defects • Weakness, fatigue, and depression • Pallor • Dermatologic lesions
Vitamin B12 (cobalamin)	• Lemon-yellow tint to the skin and eyes • Smooth, red, thickened tongue • Pallor • Ataxia
Vitamin C (ascorbic acid)	• Scurvy (fatigue, hemorrhages, low resistance to infection, anemia) • Edema • Swollen, bleeding, and/or retracted gums or tooth loss; mottled teeth; enamel erosion • Painful subperiosteal haematoma • Lethargy and fatigue • Skin lesions • Small red or purplish pinpoint discolorations on the skin or mucous membranes (petechiae) • Intraocular hemorrhage • Darkened skin around the hair follicles, • Corkscrew hair or spiral and unemerged hairs
Calcium	• Decreased bone mineralization, rickets, osteoporosis
Chromium	• Corneal lesions
Copper	• Hair and skin depigmentation • Pallor
Fluoride	• Increased dental decay, affects on bone health
Iodine	• Goiter • Developmental delay • Mental retardation • Hypothyroidism
Iron	• Fatigue • Decreased cognitive function • Headaches • Glossitis • Nail changes, koilonychias, thin, concave nails with raised edges • Skin pallor • Pale conjunctiva • Fatigue
Magnesium	• Tremors, muscle spasms, and tetany • Personality changes
Selenium	• Cutaneous alterations can occur including xerosis, erythematous scaly papules
Zinc	• Dwarfism and hypogonadism • Hepatosplenomegaly • Hyperpigmentation • Acrodermatitis enteropathica • Alopecia (hair loss) • Acral rash • Skin and eye lesions • Nasolabial seborrhea • Decubitus ulcers

Adapted from: Overview_of_micronutrient_deficiency_disorders_and_clinical_signs.ppt. www.micronutrient.org/nutritiontoolkit/ModuleFolders/3.Indicators%5CClinical%5CTools%5C
Gallagher [136]
Marks [137]
Allen et al. [138]
Tulchinsky [139]

Biomarkers

Nutrient deficiencies were classically associated with the clinical signs and symptoms described in the previous section. However, it is now known that there are physiological and functional consequences related to nutritional deficiencies before clinical signs appear. Biomarkers include direct measures of a nutrient in blood or tissue or can be a product of nutrient metabolism. Urinary levels of thiamin can be a measure of current thiamin intake while thyroid hormone can be a consequence of long-term iodine deficiency. However, even direct measures of a nutrient may fail to reflect overall nutritional status as is the case the with blood calcium which can remain normal in patients with osteoporosis. Biomarkers can also include functional markers as part of indirect tests of nutritional status. There are biomarkers for metabolic consequences of nutritional status such as the result of an oral glucose tolerance test that would be used to screen for type 2 Diabetes [107].

Although not always in the same sequential fashion for all nutrients, biomarkers indicate different stages of nutrient deficiency [108]. The earliest changes include biomarkers that measure a decrease in body stores, followed by measures of DNA damage and altered gene expression. Additional decreases in nutritional status result in disturbed immune functions and a decrease in storage proteins and then an increase in the concentration of nutrient transporters. Eventually, as the deficiency for some nutrients becomes more severe, there will be a decrease in their plasma concentration and a decrease in specific enzyme activities and ultimately clinical signs and symptoms associated with deficiency.

The sensitivity and specificity of biomarkers are affected by their turnover rate and non-nutritional factors such as genetic variations between people and their interactions with non-nutritional factors such as inflammation [108]. Inflammation can either decrease or increase biomarkers used to assess nutritional status [109]. For example, inflammation can depress serum retinol concentrations but increase serum ferritin and serum transferrin receptor concentrations. The most common markers of inflammation include c-reactive protein (CRP) and alpha(1)-acid glycoprotein (AGP) to determine an active incubation period when a person has recently been exposed (CRP elevated and AGP not changed), early convalescence (CRP still elevated but declining and AGP elevated), or late convalescence with only AGP elevated [110, 111]. Thus, the inferences made regarding vitamin A and iron status should be adjusted based on these stages of inflammation. This means that these markers of inflammation should also be assessed when assessing vitamin A and iron status indicators.

Biomarkers and Environmental Factors

Some indicators of nutritional status also have to be adjusted for environmental factors and the stage of life. Hemoglobin levels vary with altitude. The reference value has been set for people living at <1000 m above sea level and it increases with additional altitude. Smoking values also increases what should be a normal hemoglobin value. Hemoglobin values are also adjusted for the trimester of pregnancy. Normal values for biomarkers may also depend on a person's age [112].

Often multiple biomarkers need to be used at the same time to provide an indication of nutritional status. BMI, more direct measures of fat free mass, and changes of body weight can be combined to give a better indication of malnutrition in older individuals [113]. Although, WHO uses serum B12 to identify adequate (>221 pmol/L), low (148–221 pmol/L) and deficient B12 status (<148 pmol/L), these values may not be sensitive for identifying early stages of B12 deficiency [112]. Methylmalonic acid and homocysteine have therefore been used as indirect measures of B12 status due to the fact that their concentrations result from B12-dependent enzymes. However, because their concentrations are also dependent on folate a better indicator of B12 deficiency may be to use four indicators of B12 status (total B12, holo-transcobalamin, methylmalonic acid, and total homocysteine) [112].

Biomarkers and Time

Assessment of selenium status is an example of how the advancements of biomarkers has improved the ability to identifying both short- and long-term nutritional status. Hair and toenail selenium have been used to estimate long-term intake but do not reflect a person's current selenium status. Several selonoproteins, glutathione peroxidase and Se-transporter selenoprotein P can be used together to determine if a person is nutritionally adequate for selenium. Buccal cells offer the possibility of a minimally invasive biomarker but it is a laboratory intensive method to measure current selenium status given their turnover rate [114, 115]. Blood samples and enzyme status also relate to the functional outcomes of selenium status. Overall tissue values help determine total body selenium concentration and relate to function. Selenium toxicity can be determined using selenium concentrations in plasma, erythrocyte, hair, nail, and urine [116].

Fatty acids also provide a good example of how various biomarkers can be used to measure current and long-term nutrient intake based on tissue turnover. Measures of the fatty acid composition of the phospholipid membrane of red blood cells (RBCs) are an indicator of fatty acid intake during the past couple of months based on the 128-day lifespan of RBCs. While the fatty acid composition of adipose tissue provides a better estimation of what has been the long-term distribution for intake fatty acids over a longer period of time [107].

Biomarkers and Obesity

Several biomarkers that are associated with obesity can be modifiable indicators regarding the severity of obesity in an individual or population. Also, the obesity-associated biomarkers can have an effect on the indicators for other nutrients. For example, inflammatory biomarkers that are increased with obesity can affect the ferritin concentration and the release of retinol binding protein. Additionally, adipokines (leptin, interleukin-6 and tumor necrosis factor-alpha), and gut hormones such as ghrelin produced in the stomach also increase with obesity and are also associated with decreased memory and general cognitive measures that could modify the associations between other nutrients and cognitive development [117]. Measures of telomeres (repeated tandem TTAGGG) of DNA related to aging also can modify their length with weight reduction in adolescents [118].

In the context of obesity, certain studies aim to measure factors associated with energy balance. In addition to using questionnaires to measure energy intake and expenditures more precise measures can be used. For energy expenditure, direct calorimetry and the use of double-labeled water provide accurate measures but are expensive and can only be used by a few laboratories in the world, which limits their use to studies. For wider use, various motion monitors and heart rate monitors can provide more precise estimates of energy expenditure [119].

Biomarkers Proteomics

Proteomics, the comprehensive study of the amount, variation, and modification of an organism's proteins has the potential to identify biomarkers related to nutritional status and identify who are responders and non-responders to nutrition interventions [120]. Identifying specific proteomes may support the measures of multiple protein-nutrition associations that can be used to determine if deficiencies exist for vitamin A, D, E, copper, and selenium with their associated circulating blood proteins [121, 122]. It has been suggested that the measure of six proteins—(ApoC-III; ApoB; pyruvate kinase; forkhead box 04; Unc5 homolog; Regulator of G-protein signaling 8) may be able to be used as biomarkers for Vitamin E status [122].

Biomarkers and Dietary Intake

Metabolomics, the gut microbiota, and skin scans are more recent methods used to measure dietary patterns. Metabolomics has been used to sparse out the endogenous, drug and food metabolomes to assess dietary patterns and are able to provide important measures for different fruits and vegetables, cereal products, soy, meats, dairy, fish, and various beverages including tea, coffee, wine, and total alcohol intake [123]. For example, heat map analysis of urine using 1H nuclear magnetic resonance (NMR) spectral identified formate, citrulline, taurine, and isocitrate as appropriate biomarkers for the consumption of sugar sweetened beverages [124]. Also, carbon stable isotope techniques using Carbon 13 has been used to measure consumption of simple sugars [125].

Using the gut microbiota and genes associated with the microbes has the potential as measures of dietary patterns. The microbiota appears to be different between western and non-western diets, between breastfed and non-breastfed infants, and between well nourished an malnourished children [126]. Improvements in the nutritional status and maturity of the microbiota in children with kwashiorkor compared with their discordant twin have been shown to occur after intervention using a peanut-based ready to use therapeutic food [127]. Additionally, non-invasive skin scans using Resonance Raman Spectroscopy (RRS) is a potential method for measuring carotenoid status and differences in fruit and vegetable intake and to validate dietary assessment methods successful in children. Plasma and skin carotenoids had an R^2 equal to 0.62 and skin and dietary carotenoids had an R^2 equal to 0.42 in children 5–17 years of age [128, 129].

Functional Outcomes

Throughout this chapter, there have been references to functional outcomes of nutritional status. These functional measures can be specific to the classical signs of malnutrition (e.g., night blindness with vitamin A deficiency), related to metabolic changes that occur with malnutrition (e.g., abnormal oral glucose tolerance tests due to type 2 diabetes as a result of obesity), and the numerous biomarkers that are available to assess the stages of nutritional status. However, there are numerous functional outcomes of nutritional status that provide insight to the spectrum of malnutrition that may be present but only determined specifically to a nutritional deficit after nutritional supplementation. Improvements in hemoglobin values after iron supplementation is one example that directly relates to a specific nutrient. However, other functional changes in cognitive ability, aerobic capacity, growth, and immune responses can also be functional outcomes that change with improving nutritional status of a single or group of nutrients. These functional measures are important measures along the spectrum of nutritional status that relate to activities of daily living, quality of life, and future morbidity and mortality.

Global Measures of Malnutrition

Prevalence measures of malnutrition are provided for the world, regions, and countries. They provide information about the types, scale, and range of malnutrition that exists, which is valuable information for comparisons. These global measures are used to monitor worldwide changes over time and are important for monitoring the Sustainable Development Goals. Both the number of malnourished people and the prevalence of malnutrition need to be considered when determining the spectrum of malnutrition, whether between regions or countries and between regions within countries.

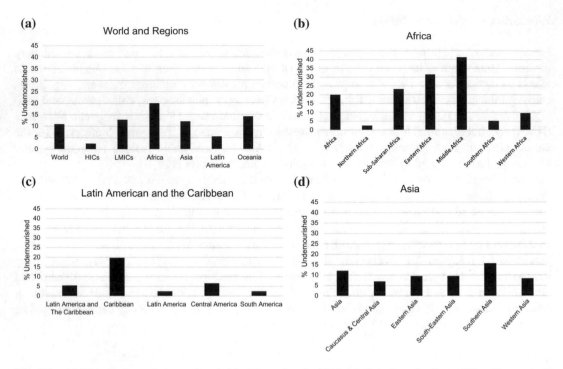

Fig. 5.1 **a–d** Percent of population undernourished by region for 2014–16. Data from the *State of Food Insecurity in the World* (FAO [16])

Undernourishment

The number of undernourished people has gone down from 1010.7 million in 1991 to 792.5 million in 2015 [130]. The percent of undernourishment within countries for the 114 countries that had provisional data from 2014 to 16, a quarter of the countries were estimated to have less than 2.5% of its population undernourished, the median was 9.45% [16]. The top quarter had more than 20.7% of their population undernourished and six countries had greater than 40% of their population undernourished (Sudan, Zambia, Central African Republic, Namibia, Republic of Korea and Haiti). The prevalence of undernourished people by region was greatest in Africa (20%) followed by Oceania (14.2%) and Asia (12.1%). For example, in Africa, Middle Africa has the greatest prevalence (41.3%) compared to Northern Africa with a prevalence of 2.5% (Fig. 5.1). However, the level of undernourished populations in Asia are relative consistent.

Low Birth Weight and Small-for-Gestational Age

It is estimated that there are more than 18 million low birth weight infants born each year. However, there are more than 32 million infants born SGA, accounting for 27% of all live births [52]. The prevalence of low birth weight is almost nine times greater in South Asia (26%) compared with East Asia, which has the lowest prevalence (3%). Regional differences for the prevalence of SGA in LMICs ranges from a low of 7.0% for East Asia to 45% for South Asia (Fig. 5.2). These values translate to having a 6.4 times difference between the highest and lowest regional prevalence rate for SGA and an 8.7 times difference for low birth weight. However even though these are the best

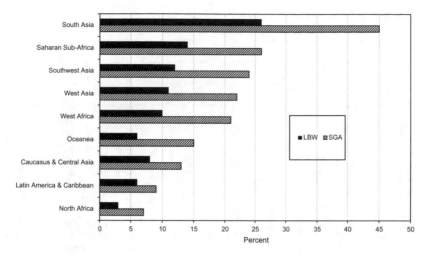

Fig. 5.2 Prevalence of low birth weight and small-for-gestational age infants. Adapted from Lee et al. [52]. *LBW* low birth weight; *SGA* small-for-gestational age

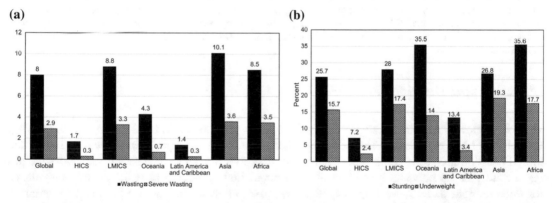

Fig. 5.3 a, b Regional prevalence rates for undernutrition. *HICS* high income countries; *LMICS* low and middle income countries; stunting: height-for-age z-score <−2.0; underweight: weight-for-age z-score <−2.0; wasting: weight-for-height z-score <−2.0; severe wasting: weight-for-height z-score <−3.0. Adapted from Black et al. [132]

estimates possible, they need to be assessed with care as they are based on several cohort studies that may not be representative [131].

Undernutrition

The prevalence of undernutrition can be less than one percent (severe wasting in high income countries) to greater than 35% (stunting in both Africa and Oceania) depending on the indicator used and the region of the world [132]. Globally, regional rates for stunting have the greatest prevalence at 25.7% followed by underweight (15.7%), total wasting (8.0%) and severe wasting (2.9%). At the low end, severe wasting by region usually remains less than five percent in LMICs (Fig. 5.3). However, this still means that there may be a 300% difference between regions. However, the range for the prevalence of stunting and underweight are significantly less between regions for LMICs.

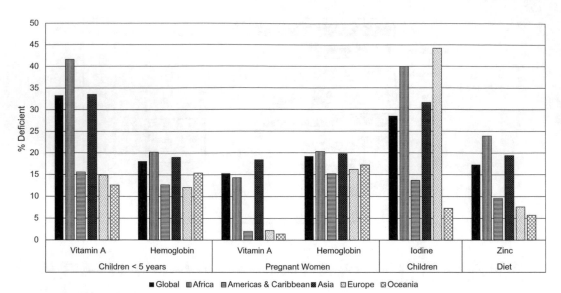

Fig. 5.4 Regional prevalence of micronutrient deficiencies. Vitamin A: serum retinol <0.70 μmol/L; hemoglobin: <11 mg/dl; iodine: urinary iodine concentration <100 μg/L for school age children, see [134]; zinc: based FAO food balance data sheets using the IZINCG physiological requirements using the Miller equation to estimate zinc absorption and an assumed 25% interindividual variation in zinc intake. Data are for the time frame 2003–2007, see [135]. Adapted from Black et al. [132]

Micronutrient Deficiencies

The four major micronutrient deficiencies in LMICs are for vitamin A, iron, iodine, and zinc [132]. Globally for LMICs, vitamin A deficiency in children has the greatest prevalence based on low serum retinol concentrations with 33.3% of children less than five years with low serum values. Iodine has the second greatest prevalence (28.5%). African populations generally have the greatest prevalence for micronutrient deficiencies (Fig. 5.4). However, exceptions to this include the rate of vitamin A deficiency for pregnant women in Asia and the highest prevalence of low urinary iodine concentrations which is found in Europe.

It is also possible to determine the ranges that exist in the United States for multiple vitamins, minerals, carotenoids, and fatty acids using the 5, 50, and 95th percentiles from NHANES based on age, race, and sex [133]. The CDC report also provides the percent of people who have been identified as having deficient concentrations for RBC folate, serum levels for vitamins B6, B12, D, E, and low serum ferritin concentrations. Additionally, the percent with high concentrations for Vitamin D and ferritin are presented.

Overweight/Obesity

While the prevalence for undernourishment, undernutrition, and for many micronutrient deficiencies has declined, the prevalence of overweight has increased since 1990 in LMICs [39]. The greatest percent change has occurred in East Asia and the Pacific followed by Latin America and the Caribbean. Recent regional prevalence rates for overweight are lowest in South Asia (16.9%) compared with 70.6% for the Middle East and North Africa (Fig. 5.5).

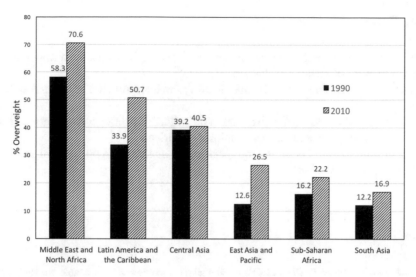

Fig. 5.5 Overweight Prevalence by Region. Adapted from Popkin and Slining [39]

The Spectrum of Malnutrition Across Regions

Measuring malnutrition across regions illustrates that there is a distribution for each measure used to determine the prevalence of malnutrition and the absolute estimate for the prevalence of malnutrition depends on the indicator used to measure nutritional status. While some measures of malnutrition may have a smaller prevalence as seen with wasting and severe wasting, they are not less important as it represents a group with a greater risk for future morbidity and mortality. On the other hand, the prevalence for obesity is increasing throughout the world and in some regions and countries it is the measure of malnutrition with the greatest prevalence. It also should be noted that the prevalence of vitamin A deficiency in children and anemia in both children and pregnant women are consistently present in all the regions.

Conclusion

This chapter presents the indicators that are used to measure the spectrum of malnutrition. It provides information on how to use indicators of food security, dietary intake, anthropometry, and biomarkers to assess the nutritional status at the global, national, household, and individual level. It highlights new areas of research regarding nutritional assessment such as metabolomics and gut microbiota that can help determine differences in nutritional status and dietary patterns. These indicators of nutritional status have significant variation across regions of the world and are used to assess global and national prevalence of different forms of malnutrition as well as to track progress toward improving nutrition. These indicators are also used to assess the impact of nutrition interventions, whether in research studies or for public health programs. When selecting indicators for these purposes it is important to take into account what they indicate, how responsive they are likely to be to the specific intervention(s) and to note that indicators are also affected by a person's age, sex, and non-nutritional factors.

Discussion Points

- How would you differentiate whether a biomarker is an indicator of nutritional status or an indicator for disease or metabolic changes?
- Discuss factors, at individual level, that may modify the interpretation of biomarkers of nutritional status.
- Compare different indicators of nutritional with regards to how they represent the stages of malnutrition for energy, macronutrients, and micronutrients.
- What measures are used to determine the spectrum of malnutrition on a global scale and how are they different from each other?

References

1. Atalah E, Amigo H, Bustos P. Does Chile's nutritional situation constitute a double burden? Am J Clin Nutr. 2014;100(6):1623S–7S.
2. Cheung HC, Shen A, Oo S, Tilahun H, Cohen MJ, Berkowitz SA. Food insecurity and body mass index: a longitudinal mixed methods study, Chelsea, Massachusetts, 2009–2013. Preventing Chronic Dis. 2015;12:E125.
3. Dubois L, Francis D, Burnier D, Tatone-Tokuda F, Girard M, Gordon-Strachan G, et al. Household food insecurity and childhood overweight in Jamaica and Quebec: a gender-based analysis. BMC Public Health. 2011;11:199.
4. Kac G, Velasquez-Melendez G, Schlussel MM, Segall-Correa AM, Silva AA, Perez-Escamilla R. Severe food insecurity is associated with obesity among Brazilian adolescent females. Public Health Nutr. 2012;15(10):1854–60.
5. Kaur J, Lamb MM, Ogden CL. The association between food insecurity and obesity in children—the National Health and Nutrition Examination Survey. J Acad Nutr Diet. 2015;115(5):751–8.
6. Rosas LG, Guendelman S, Harley K, Fernald LC, Neufeld L, Mejia F, et al. Factors associated with overweight and obesity among children of Mexican descent: results of a binational study. J Immigr Minor Health. 2011;13 (1):169–80.
7. Santos LM. Obesity, poverty, and food insecurity in Brazilian males and females. Cadernos de Saude Publica. 2013;29(2):237–9.
8. Freire WB, Silva-Jaramillo KM, Ramirez-Luzuriaga MJ, Belmont P, Waters WF. The double burden of undernutrition and excess body weight in Ecuador. Am J Clin Nutr. 2014;100(6):1636S–43S.
9. Abdollahi M, Abdollahi Z, Sheikholeslam R, Kalantari N, Kavehi Z, Neyestani TR. High occurrence of food insecurity among urban Afghan refugees in Pakdasht, Iran 2008: a cross-sectional study. Ecol Food Nutr. 2015;54 (3):187–99.
10. Motadi SA, Mbhenyane XG, Mbhatsani HV, Mabapa NS, Mamabolo RL. Prevalence of iron and zinc deficiencies among preschool children ages 3 to 5 y in Vhembe district, Limpopo province South Africa. Nutrition. 2015;31(3):452–8.
11. Tzioumis E, Adair LS. Childhood dual burden of under- and overnutrition in low- and middle-income countries: a critical review. Food Nutr Bull. 2014;35(2):230–43.
12. Becker C, Orozco M, Solomons NW, Schumann K. Iron metabolism in obesity: how interaction between homoeostatic mechanisms can interfere with their original purpose. Part I: underlying homoeostatic mechanisms of energy storage and iron metabolisms and their interaction. J Trace Elem Med Biol. 2015;30:195–201.
13. Cherayil BJ. Pathophysiology of iron homeostasis during inflammatory states. J Pediatr. 2015;167(4 Suppl): S15–9.
14. Osterholm EA, Georgieff MK. Chronic inflammation and iron metabolism. J Pediatr. 2015;166(6):1351–7.
15. Schmidt PJ. Regulation of iron metabolism by hepcidin under conditions of inflammation. J Biol Chem. 2015;290 (31):18975–83.
16. FAO, IFAD, WFP. The state of food insecurity in the world. Meeting the 2015 international hunger targets: taking stock of uneven progress. Rome: Food and Agriculture Organization of the United Nations; 2015.
17. Jones AD, Ngure FM, Pelto G, Young SL. What are we assessing when we measure food security? A compendium and review of current metrics. Adv Nutr. 2013;4:481–505.
18. Lizumi T, Sakuma H, Yokozawa M, Luo JJ, Challinor AJ, Brown ME, et al. Prediction of seasonal climate-induced variations in global food production. Nat Clim Change. 2013;3:904–8.

19. Arsenault JE, Hijmans RJ, Brown KH. Improving nutrition security through agriculture: an analytical framework based on national food balance sheets to estimate nutritional adequacy of food supplies. Food Secur. 2015;7: 693–707.
20. World Food Program. Vulnerability analysis and mapping. Food consumption analysis: calculation and use of the food consumption score in food security analysis. Rome: World Food Program; 2008.
21. Del Gobbo LC, Khatibzadeh S, Imamura F, Micha R, Peilin S, Smith M, et al. Assessing global dietary habits: a comparison of national estimates from the FAO and the Global Dietary Database. Am J Clin Nutr. 2015;101:1038–46.
22. IPC Global Partners. Integrated food security phase classification technical manual, version 1.1. Rome; 2008.
23. Pangaribowo EH, Gerber N, Torero M. Food and nutrition security indicators: a review. Bonn: University of Bonn; 2013.
24. von Grebmer K, Bernstein J, Prasai N, Yin S, Yohannes Y. Global hunger index. Armed conflict and the challenge of hunger. Bonn, Washington DC, and Dublin: Welthungerhilfe, International Food Policy Research Institute, and Concern Worldwide; 2015.
25. Economist Intelligence Unit. Global food security index 2012: an assessment of food affordability, availability and quality. London: Economist; 2011.
26. Masset E. A review of hunger indices and methods to monitor country commitment to fighting hunger. Food Policy. 2011;36:S102–8.
27. Coates J, Swindale A, Bilinsky P. Household food insecurity access scale (HFIAS) for measurement of household food access: indicator guide. Washington DC: Food and Nutrition Technical Assistance (FANTA) Project, Academy for Educational Development, Project FaNTAF; 2007.
28. Livingstone MBE, Black A. Markers of the validity of reported energy intake. J Nutr. 2003;133:895S–920S.
29. Taren DL, Tobar M, Hill A, Howell W, Shisslak C, Bell I, et al. The association of energy intake bias with psychological scores of women. Eur J Clin Nutr. 1999;53:570–8.
30. Mendez MA. Invited commentary: dietary misreporting as a potential source of bias in diet-disease associations: future directions in nutritional epidemiology research. Am J Epidemiol. 2015;181(4):234–6.
31. Lutomski JE, Broeck J, Harrington J, Shiely F, Perry IJ. Sociodemographic, lifestyle, mental health and dietary factors associated with direction of misreporting of energy intake. Public Health Nutr. 2010;14(3):532–41.
32. Broyles ME, Harris R, Taren DL. Diabetics under report energy intake in NHANES III greater than non-diabetics. Open Nutr J. 2008;2:54–62.
33. Kennedy G, Ballard T, Dop MC. Guidelines for measuring household and individual dietary diversity. Rome: Food and Agriculture Organization, Nutrition and Consumer Protection Division; 2013.
34. WHO. Indicators for assessing infant and young child feeding practices. Part 2: measurement. Geneva: World Health Organization; 2010.
35. IOM. Dietary DRI reference intakes: the essential guide to nutrient requirements. In: Otten JJ, Hellwig J, Meyers L, editors. Washington DC: National Academies Press; 2006.
36. Trumbo PR, Barr SI, Murphy SP, Yates AA. Dietary reference intakes: cases of appropriate and inappropriate uses. Nutr Rev. 2013;71(10):657–64.
37. The Obesity Expert Panel 2013. Executive summary: guidelines (2013) for the management of overweight and obesity in adults. A report of the American College of Cardiology/American Heart Association Task Force on Practice Guidelines and The Obesity Society. Obesity. 2014;22(Suppl 2):S5–39.
38. Mathus-Vliegen EMH. Obesity and the elderly. J Clin Gastroenterol. 2012;46(7):533–44.
39. Popkin BM, Slining MM. New dynamics in global obesity facing low- and middle-income countries. Obes Rev. 2013;14(Suppl 2):11–22.
40. Hsu W, Araneta MRG, Kanaya AM, Chiang JL, Fujimoto W. BMI cut points to identify at-risk Asian Americans for type 2 diabetes screening. Diab Care. 2015;38:150–8.
41. Bhardwaj S, Misra A. Obesity, diabetes and the Asian phenotype. World Rev Nutr Diet. 2015;111:116–22.
42. WHO Expert Consultation. Appropriate body-mass index for Asian populations and its implications for policy and intervention strategies. Lancet. 2004;363:157–63.
43. Cheong KC, Yusoff AF, Ghazali SM, Lim KH, Selvarajah S, Haniff J, et al. Optimal BMI cut-off values for predicting diabetes, hypertension and hypercholesterolaemia in a multi-ethnic population. Public Health Nutr. 2011;16(3):453–9.
44. Bays H. Central obesity as a clinical marker of adiposopathy; increased visceral adiposity as a surrogate marker for global fat dysfunction. Curr Opin Endocrinol Diab Obes. 2014;21:345–51.
45. Cameron AJ, Magliano DJ, Soderberg S. A systematic review of the impact of including both waist and hip circumference in risk models for cardiovascular diseases, diabetes and mortality. Obes Rev. 2013;14:86–94.
46. Wang Z, Ma J, Si D. Optimal cut-off values and population means of waist circumference in different populations. Nutr Res Rev. 2010;23:191–9.
47. International Diabetes Federation. International Diabetes Federation (IDF) worldwide definition of the metabolic syndrome. Brussels: Belgium; 2006.

48. Lear SA, James PT, Ko GT, Kumanyika S. Appropriateness of waist circumference and waist-to-hip ratio cutoffs for different ethnic populations. Eur J Clin Nutr. 2010;64:42–61.
49. Arabshahi S, Busingye D, Subasinghe AK, Evans RG, Riddell MA, Thrift AG. Adiposity has a greater impact on hypertension in lean than not-lean populations: a systematic review and meta-analysis. Eur J Epidemiol. 2014;29:311–24.
50. WHO. Waist circumference and waist-hip ratio. In: Report of a WHO Expert Consultation, Geneva, 8–11 Dec 2008. Geneva: World Health Organization; 2011.
51. Fenton TR, Kim JH. A systematic review and meta-analysis to revise the Fenton growth chart for preterm infants. BMC Pediatr. 2013;13.
52. Lee ACC, Katz J, Blencowe H, Cousens S, Kazuki N, Vogel JP, et al. National and regional estimates of term and preterm babies born small for gestational age in 138 low-income and middle-income countries in 2010. Lancet Glob Health. 2013;1:e26–36.
53. Grisaru-Granovsky S, Reichman B, Lerner-Geva L, Boyko V, Hammerman C, Samueloff A, et al. Mortality and morbidity in preterm small-for-gestational-age infants: a population-based study. Am J Obstet Gynecol. 2012;150:e1-d7.
54. Regev RH, Lusky A, Dolan T, Litmanovitz I, Arnon S, Reichman B, et al. Excess mortality and morbidity among small-for-gestational-age premature infants: a population-based study. J Pediatr. 2003;143:186–91.
55. Christian P, Murray-Kolb LE, Tielsch JM, Katz J, LeClerq SC, Khatry SK. Associations between preterm birth, small-for gestational age, and neonatal morbidity and cognitive function among school-age children in Nepal. BMC Pediatr. 2014;14.
56. Delpisheh A, BrabinL, Drummond S, Brabin B. Prenatal smoking exposure and asymmetric fetal growth restriction. Ann Human Biol. 2008;35(6):573–83.
57. Zepeda-Monreal J, Rodriquez-Balderrama I, Ochoa-Correa EC, de la O-Cavazos ME, Ambriz-Lopez R. Crecimiento intrauterino. Factores para su restricción. Rev Med Inst Mex Seguro Soc. 2012;50(2):173–81.
58. Pasupathy D, McCowan LME, Poston L, Kenny LC, Dekker GA, North RA, et al. Perinatal outcomes in large infants using customised birthweight centiles and conventional measures of high birthweight. Paediatr Perinat Epidemiol. 2012;26:543–52.
59. Kim SY, Sharma AJ, Sappenfield W, Wilson HG, Salihu HM. Association of maternal body mass index, excessive weight gain, and gestational diabetes mellitus with large-for-gestational-age births. Obstet Gynecol. 2014;123(4):737–44.
60. Yu Z, Han S, Zhu J, Sun X, Ji C, Guo X. Pre-pregnancy body mass index in relation to infant birth weight and offspring overweight/obesity: a systematic review and meta-analysis. PLoS One. 2013;8(4).
61. Li N, Liu E, Guo J, Pan L, Li B, Wang P, et al. Maternal prepregnancy body mass index and gestational weight gain on pregnancy outcomes. PLoS ONE. 2013;8(12).
62. Kozuki N, Katz J, Lee ACC, Vogel JP, Silveira MF, Sania A, et al. Short maternal stature increases risk of small for-gestational-age and preterm births in low and middle-income countries: individual participant data meta-analysis and population attributable fraction. J Nutr. 2015;145:2542–50.
63. Ververs M, Antierens A, Sackl A, Staderini N, Captier V. Which anthropometric indicators identify a pregnant woman as acutely malnourished and predict adverse birth outcomes in the humanitarian context? PLOS Curr Disasters [Internet]. 2013;1:15p.
64. Sebayang SK, Dibley MJ, Kelly PJ, Shanker AV, Shanker AJ. The summit study group. Determinants of low birthweight, small-for-gestational-age and preterm birth in Lombok, Indonesia: analyses of the birthweight cohort of the SUMMIT trial. Trop Med Int Health. 2012;17(8):938–50.
65. Ramlal RT, Tembo M, Soko A, Chigwenembe M, Ellington S, Kayira D, et al. Maternal mid-upper arm circumference is associated with birth weight among HIV-infected Malawians. Nutr Clin Pract. 2012;27(3):416–21.
66. Cnattingius S, Villamor E, Lagerros YT, Wikstrom A-K, Granath F. High birth weight and obesity—a vicious circle across generations. Int J Obes. 2012;36:1320–4.
67. Siega-Riz AM, Gray GL. Gestational weight gain recommendations in the context of the obesity epidemic. Nutr Rev. 2013;71:S26–30.
68. IOM. Weight gain during pregnancy: reexamining the guidelines. Washington DC: Guidelines NRCCtRIPWG; 2009.
69. Hinkle SN, Johns AM, Albert PS, Kim S, Grantz K. Longitudinal changes in gestational weight gain and the association with intrauterine fetal growth. Eur J Obstet Gynecol Reprod Biol. 2015;190:41–7.
70. Sharma AJ, Vesco KK, Bulkley J, Callaghan WM, Bruce FC, Staab J, et al. Associations of gestational weight gain with preterm birth among underweight and normal weight women. Matern Child Health J. 2015;19:2066–73.
71. Cnattingius S, Villamor E. Weight change between successive pregnancies and risks of stillbirth and infant mortality: a nationwide cohort study. Lancet. 2016;387:558–65.

72. Ferraro ZM, Barrowman N, Prud'homme D, Walker M, Wen SW, Rodger M, et al. Excessive gestational weight gain predicts large for gestational age neonates independent of maternal body mass index. J Matern-Fetal Neonatal Med. 2012;25(5):538–42.

73. Godoy AC, do Nascimento SL, Surita FG. A systematic review and meta-analysis of gestational weight gain recommendations and related outcomes in Brazil. Clinics. 2015;70(11):758–64.

74. Mannan M, Doi SAR, Mamun AA. Association between weight gain during pregnancy and postpartum weight retention and obesity: a bias-adjusted meta-analysis. Nutr Rev. 2013;71(6):343–52.

75. Briend A, Maire B, Fontaine O, Garenne M. Mid-upper arm circumference and weight-for-height to identify high-risk malnourished under-five children. Matern Child Nutr. 2012;8(1):130–3.

76. Ogden CL, Carroll MD, Kit BK, Flegal KM. Prevalence of obesity and trends in body mass index among US children and adolescents, 1999–2010. JAMA. 2012;307(5):483–90.

77. de Onis M, Martinez-Costa C, Nunez F, Nguefack-Tsague G, Montal A, Brines J. Association between WHO cut-offs for childhood overweight and obesity and cardiometabolic risk. Public Health Nutr. 2012;16(4):625–30.

78. Burgess HJL, Burgess AP. The arm circumference as a public health index of protein-calorie malnutrition of early childhood. J Trop Pediatr. 1969:189–92.

79. Shakir A, Morley D. Measuring malnutrition. Lancet. 1974:758–9.

80. Briend A. Use of MUAC for severe acute malnutrition. CMAM Forum [Internet]. 2012. Available from: http://www.cmamforum.org/Pool/Resources/FAQ-1-Use-of-MUAC-Briend-Eng-June-2012(1).pdf.

81. Modi P, Nasrin S, Hawes M, Glavis-Bloom J, Alam NH, Hossain MI, et al. Midupper arm circumference outperforms weight-based measures of nutritional status in children with diarrhea. J Nutr. 2015;145:1582–7.

82. Dale NM, Myatt M, Proudhon C, Briend A. Using mid-upper arm circumference to end treatment of severe acute malnutrition leads to higher weight gains in the most malnourished children. PLoS ONE. 2013;8(2):e55404.

83. Ojo O, Deane R, Amuna P. The use of anthropometric and clinical parameters for early identification and categorisation of nutritional risk in pre-school children in Benin City, Nigeria. J R Soc Promot Health. 2000;120(4):230–5.

84. D'Angelo S, Yajnik CS, Kumaran K, Joglekar C, Lubree H, Crozier SR, et al. Body size and body composition: a comparison of children in India and the UK through infancy and early childhood. J Epidemiol Commun Health. 2015;69(12):1147–53.

85. Briend A, Khara T, Dolan C. Wasting and stunting—similarities and differences: policy and programmatic implications. Food Nutr Bull. 2015;36(1):S15–23.

86. Laillou A, Prak S, de Groot R, Whitney S, Conkle J, Horton L, et al. Optimal screening of children with acute malnutrition requires a change in current WHO guidelines as MUAC and WHZ identify different patient groups. PLoS ONE. 2014;9(7).

87. Garenne M, Maire B, Fontaine O, Briend A. Adequacy of child anthropometric indicators for measuring nutritional stress at population level: a study from Niakhar, Senegal. Public Health Nutr. 2012;16(9):1533–9.

88. Arnhold R. The QUAC stick: a field measure use by the Quaker service team in Nigeria. J Trop Pediatr. 1969;15:243–6.

89. Sommer A, Loewenstein MS. Nutritional status and mortality: a prospective validation of the QUAC stick. Am J Clin Nutr. 1975;28:287–92.

90. Briend A, Zimicki S. Validation of arm circumference as an indicator of risk of death in one to four year old children. Nutr Res. 1986;6:249–61.

91. Bogin B, Varela-Silva MI. Leg length, body proportion, and health: a review with a note on beauty. Int J Environ Res Public Health. 2010;7(3):1047–75.

92. Ball TM, Taren D. Use of arm circumference (AC) measurements and maternal reporting of illness. J Trop Pediatr. 1995;41:250–2.

93. Jensen GL, Hsiao PY, Wheeler D. Adult nutrition assessment tutorial. J Parenter Enteral Nutr. 2012;2012(3):267–74.

94. Secker DJ, Jeejeebhoy KN. How to perform a subjective global nutritional assessment in children. J Acad Nutr Diet. 2012;112(3):424–31.

95. Detsky AS, McLaughlin JR, Baker JP. What is subjective global assessment of nutritional status. JPEN. 1994;11:8.

96. Guigoz Y, Vellas B, Garry PJ. Mini nutritional assessment: a practical assessment tool for grading the nutritional status of elderly patients. Facts Res Gerontol. 1994;4(Suppl 2):15.

97. Kaiser MJ, Bauer JM, Ramsch C, Uter W, Guigoz Y, Ceerholm T, et al. Frequency of malnutrition in older adults: a multinational perspective using the mini nutritional assessment. J Am Geriatr Soc. 2010;58:1734–8.

98. McLaren D. Color atlas of nutritional disorders. Chicago: Year Book Medical Publishers; 1981.

99. Finch CW. Review of trace mineral requirements for preterm infants: what are the current recommendations for clinical practice? Nutr Clin Pract. 2015;30(1):44–58.

100. Kapoor S. Diagnosis and treatment of acanthosis nigricans. SkinMed. 2010;8(3):161–5.

101. Kutlubay Z, Engin B, Bairamov O, Tuzun Y. Acanthosis nigricans: a fold (intertriginous) dermatosis. Clin Dermatol. 2015;33:466–70.
102. Ter Beek L, Vanhauwaert E, Slinde F, Orrevall Y, Henriksen C, Johansson M, et al. Unsatisfactory knowledge and use of terminology regarding malnutrition, starvation, cachexia and sarcopenia among dietitians. Clin Nutr. 2016.
103. Williams CD. A nutritional disease of childhood associated with a maize deit. Arch Dis Child. 1933;8:423–33.
104. Williams CD, Oxon BM, Lond H. Kwashiorkor. A nutritional disease of children associated with a maize diet. Lancet. 1935:1151–2.
105. Anonymous. Classification of infantile malnutrition. Lancet. 1970:302–3.
106. Waterlow JC. Classification and definition of protein-calorie malnutrition. Br Med J. 1972;3:566–9.
107. Potischman N, Freudenheim JL. Biomarkers of nutritional exposure and nutritional status: an overview. J Nutr. 2013;133(3):873S–45.
108. Elmadfa I, Myere AL. Developing suitable methods of nutritional status assessment: a continuous challenge. Adv Nutr. 2014;5:590S–8S.
109. Raiten DJ, Ashour FAS, Ross AC, Meydani SM, Dawson HD, Stephensen CB, et al. Inflammation and nutritional science for programs/policies and interpretation of research evidence (INSPIRE). J Nutr. 2015;145:1039S–108S.
110. Thurnham DI, Northrop-Clewes CA, Knowles J. The use of adjustment factors to address the impact of inflammation on vitamin A and iron status in humans. J Nutr. 2015;145:1137S–43S.
111. Thurnham DI. Inflammation and biomarkers of nutrition. Sight Life. 2015;29(1):51–9.
112. Fedosov SN, Brito A, Miller JW, Green R, Allen LH. Combined indicator of vitamin B 12 status: modification for missing biomarkers and folate status and recommendations for revised cut-points. Clin Chem Lab Med. 2015;53 (8):1215–25.
113. Cederholm T, Bosaeus I, Barazzoni R, Bauer J, Van Gossum A, Klek S, et al. Diagnostic criteria for malnutrition. An ESPEN consensus statement. Clin Nutr. 2015;34:335–40.
114. Combs GF, Trumbo PR, McKinley MC, Milner J, Studenski S, Kimura T, et al. Biomarkers in nutrition: new frontiers in research and application. Ann NY Acad Sci. 2013;1278:1–10.
115. Combs GF. Biomarkers of selenium status. Nutrients. 2015;7:2209–36.
116. Martens IBG, Cardoso BR, Hare DJ, Niedzwiecki MM, Lajolo FM, Martens A, et al. Selenium status in preschool children receiving a Brazil nut—enriched diet. Nutrition. 2015;31:1339–43.
117. Miller AL, Lee HJ, Lumeng JC. Obesity-associated biomarkers and executive function in children running title: obesity and executive function. Pediatr Res. 2015;77(1–2):143–7.
118. Garcia-Calzon S, Moleres A, Marcos A, Campoy C, Moreno LA, Azcona-Sanjulian MC, et al. Telomere length as a biomarker for adiposity changes after a multidisciplinary intervention in overweight/obese adolescents: the EVASYON study. PLoS ONE. 2014;9(2):e89828.
119. Plasqui G, Bonomi AG, Westerterp KR. Daily physical activity assessment with accelerometers: new insights and validation studies. Obes Rev. 2013;14:451–62.
120. de Roos B, McArdle HJ. Proteomics as a tool for the modelling of biological processes and biomarker development in nutrition research. Br J Nutr. 2008;99(Suppl 3):S66–71.
121. Cole RN, Ruczinski I, Schulze K, Christian P, Herbrich S, Wu L, et al. The plasma proteome identifies expected and novel proteins correlated with micronutrient status in undernourished Nepalese children. J Nutr. 2013;143:1540–8.
122. West KP, Cole RN, Shrestha S, Schulze KJ, Lee SE, Betz J, et al. A plasma a-tocopherome can be identified from proteins associated with vitamin E status in school-aged children of Nepal. J Nutr. 2015;145:2646–56.
123. Scalbert A, Brennan L, Manach C, Andres-Lacueva C, Dragsted LO, Draper J, et al. The food metabolome: a window over dietary exposure. Am J Clin Nutr. 2014;99:1286–308.
124. Gibbons H, McNulty BA, Nugent AP, Walton J, Flynn A, Gibney MJ, et al. A metabolomics approach to the identification of biomarkers of sugar-sweetened beverage intake. Am J Clin Nutr. 2015;101:471–7.
125. Jahren AH, Bostic JN, Davy BM. The potential for a carbon stable isotope biomarker of dietary sugar intake. J Anal At Spectrom. 2014;29:795–816.
126. Subramanian S, Blanton LV, Frese SA, Charbonneau M, Mills DA, Gordon JI. Cultivating healthy growth and nutrition through the gut microbiota. Cell. 2015;161:36–48.
127. Smith MI, Yatsunenko T, Manary MJ, Trehan I, Mkakosya R, Cheng J, et al. Gut microbiomes of Malawian twin pairs discordant for kwashiorkor. Science. 2013;339:548–54.
128. Aguilar SS, Wengreen HJ, Lefevre M, Madden GJ, Gast J. Skin carotenoids: a biomarker of fruit and vegetable intake in children. J Acad Nutr Diet. 2014;114:1174–80.
129. Nguyen LM, Scherr RE, Linnell JD, Ermakov IV, Gellermann W, Jahns L, et al. Evaluating the relationship between plasma and skin carotenoids and reported dietary intake in elementary school children to assess fruit and vegetable intake. Arch Biochem Biophys. 2015;572:73–80.
130. FAOSTAT [Internet]. Food and Agriculture Organization of the United Nations. 2016 [cited 15 Mar 2016]. Available from: http://faostat3.fao.org/home/E.

131. Stoltzfus R, Rasmussen KM. The dangers of being born too small or too soon. Lancet. 2013;382:380–1.
132. Black RE, Victora CG, Walker SP, Bhutta ZA, Christian P, de Onis M, et al. Maternal and child undernutrition and overweight in low-income and middle-income countries. Lancet. 2013;382(9890):427–51.
133. National Center for Environmental Sciences. Second national report on biochemical indicators of diet and nutrition in the U.S. population. Atlanta: United States Centers for Disease Control and Prevention, Division of Laboratory Sciences; 2012.
134. Andersson M, KarumbunathanV, Zimmermann MB. J Nutr. 2012;142:744–50.
135. Wessells KR, Brown KH. PLoS One. 2012;7:e50568.
136. Gallagher ML. Intake: the nutrients and their metabolism. In: Mahan LK, Escott-Stump S, Raymond JL, editors. Krause's food and the nutrition care process, 13th ed. St. Louis: Elsevier Saunders; 2012. p. 32–128.
137. Marks J. The vitamins: their role in medical practice. Boston: Springer MTP Press Limited; 1985.
138. Allen L, de Benoist B, Dary O, Hurrell R. Guidelines on food fortification with micronutrients. Geneva: World Health Organization and Food and Agricultural Organization of the United Nations; 2006.
139. Tulchinsky TH. Micronutrient deficiency conditions: global health issues. Public Health Rev. 2010;32:243–55.

Chapter 6
Child Growth and Development

Mercedes de Onis

Keywords Anthropometry · Malnutrition · Infant and child growth · Child development · Growth retardation · Infant nutrition · Child health · Adolescents · Interventions · Stunting · Overweight · Wasting

Learning Objectives

- Review concepts, indicators, and standards for anthropometric measurements to describe the nutritional status of a community or nation.
- Describe the differences between developing growth standards versus growth references and the rationale for using a single international growth standard for all children.
- Describe the magnitude and geographical distribution of growth retardation in developing countries.
- Outline the main consequences of impaired growth in terms of morbidity, mortality, child development, and adult life health outcomes.
- Review interventions aimed at promoting healthy growth and development.

Introduction

The growth and development of infants and young children, as opposed to mere survival, is of paramount importance. Most developing countries have experienced dramatic decreases in their infant and under-five mortality rates over the last three decades. As greater numbers of children survive it becomes critical to pay closer attention to children's ability to develop their full physical and mental potentials. This will in turn have important consequences in adult life.

Child growth is internationally recognized as the best global indicator of physical well-being in children because poor feeding practices—both in quantity and quality—and infections, or more often a combination of the two, are major factors that affect physical growth and mental development in children [1]. Poor child growth is the consequence of a range of factors that are closely linked to the overall standard of living and whether a population can meet its basic needs, such as access to food, housing, and health care. Child growth assessment thus not only serves as a means for evaluating the health and nutritional status of children but also provides an excellent measurement of the inequalities in health faced by populations. Based on this principle, internationally set health goals for 2025

M. de Onis (✉)
Department of Nutrition, World Health Organization, Avenue Appia 20, 1211 Geneva, Switzerland
e-mail: deonism@who.int

© Springer Science+Business Media New York 2017
S. de Pee et al. (eds.), *Nutrition and Health in a Developing World*,
Nutrition and Health, DOI 10.1007/978-3-319-43739-2_6

include global targets related to stunting, wasting, and overweight among children younger than 5 years [2, 3].

There is strong evidence that poor physical growth is usually associated with deficient or delayed mental development [4], and a number of studies have demonstrated a relationship between growth status and school performance and intellectual achievement [5, 6]. The precise mechanism linking impaired growth and poor mental development is not known. The association cannot be regarded as a simple causal relationship because of the complex environmental factors that affect both growth and development; many socioeconomic disadvantages that coexist with stunting may also detrimentally affect mental development. It is possible that more than one mechanisms act together. For example, nutritionally deprived children are often described as lethargic, possibly because they reduce their activity as a protective measure to conserve energy or due to lack energy to be active [7]. This reduced activity limits the child's ability for exploration and interaction, and thus may have negative consequences for children's motor and cognitive development. Children who do not practice their existing skills may be less likely to acquire new skills. At the same time, the apathy these children exhibit could lead adults to treat them differently from non-lethargic children. Undernutrition could also have a direct effect on children's central nervous system. These complex relationships make it difficult to disentangle the exact mechanisms of the association between deficits in growth and poor mental development.

Impaired growth is ultimately a response to limited nutrient availability and/or utilization at the cellular level. Although in the past most of the attention has been directed toward the negative consequences associated with inadequate protein-energy intake, there is increasing recognition of the important role that micronutrient deficiencies plays in children's growth and development. At severe levels of protein-energy deficiency, linear growth probably stops and body reserves are used as energy and protein sources to maintain vital functions. At less severe stages, however, it may be possible to cope by simply slowing the rate of linear growth and other compensatory mechanisms such as reduced activity. The negative consequences of micronutrient deficiencies range from altered immunity and increased risk of infectious diseases and death to reduced growth and mental development [8].

Nutritional deficiencies in turn are deeply rooted in poverty and deprivation. Poverty breeds undernutrition, which, in turn, generates poverty in a vicious cycle that perpetuates across generations. The intrinsic links between poverty and nutrition have been reviewed in detail elsewhere [9]. Based on national level data, Fig. 6.1 shows the effect of socioeconomic status on stunting (i.e., low height-for-age) for four countries in Asia and Latin America. These associations are consistent across those countries with a similar dose-response relationship.

Regardless of the origin, the consequences of impaired growth and development in children can be long-lasting and compromise educational performance and the ability to contribute to society. Most growth retardation occurs very early in life; the two periods of highest vulnerability are during intrauterine development and during the transition from reliance on breast milk to addition of other foods to the diet. In fact, as shown in Fig. 6.2, almost all of the growth retardation documented in studies carried out in developing countries has its origin in the first 2–3 years of life [10]. Once present, growth retardation usually remains for life as growth deficits are generally not recuperated nor are the developmental deficits that co-occur with them [11].

This chapter reviews concepts, indicators, and growth standards for assessing impaired fetal and child growth; describes the magnitude and geographical distribution of growth retardation in developing countries; outlines the main health and social consequences of impaired growth in terms of morbidity, mortality, child development, and adult life consequences; and reviews interventions aimed at promoting healthy growth and development.

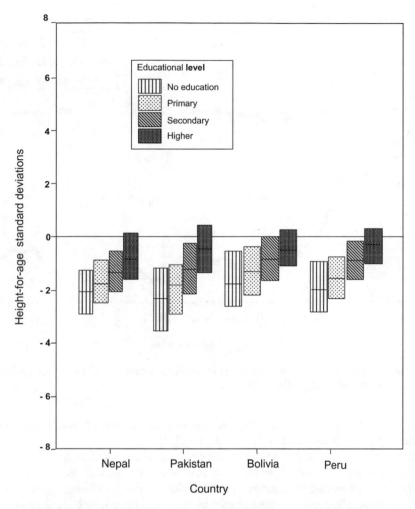

Fig. 6.1 Variation of height-for-age according to educational level. Data from DHS surveys from Nepal, Pakistan, Bolivia, Peru, is combined sexes

Measuring Impaired Growth: Concepts and Indicators

Fetal Growth

Growth failure is a cumulative process that often begins in utero. Many populations across the world, particularly in sub-Saharan Africa and South Asia, are exposed to adverse environmental and nutritional conditions that negatively affect growth and development in the first 1000 days of life (e.g., from conception to the age of 2 years) [12, 13] increasing the risk of early death and chronic adult diseases [4].

Differentiating between healthy and impaired growth in early life is crucial if cost-effective preventive strategies are to advance. Thus, fetal and newborn body size and gestational age at birth need to be measured accurately. This remains a challenge in most parts of the world as early antenatal care is not the norm and the tools to assess fetal growth adequately are not readily available. However, when size and gestational age at birth are measured accurately and are supported by serial ultrasound

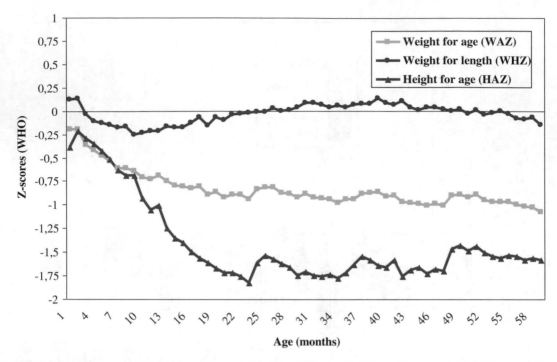

Fig. 6.2 Mean anthropometric Z-scores by age relative to the WHO standard. From Victora et al. [10]. Reprinted with permission from American Academy of Pediatrics

fetal growth patterns in high-risk pregnancies, they become strong predictors of long-term morbidity, mortality, and cognitive development of a population [12].

Close monitoring of pregnancy and birth events can only be delivered by a health care system that is able to incorporate appropriate technology and with the human resources to support it. Unfortunately, such systems are uncommon in those regions of the world where growth impairment is most prevalent. Thus, clinicians and researchers traditionally have relied on simpler indicators of newborn size as a proxy for fetal growth, without considering gestational age.

The low birth weight (LBW) rate, i.e., the number of newborns with a birth weight below 2500 g, is the most commonly used indicator to make comparisons across populations, propose actions and define targets for improvement. However, it is now increasingly accepted that LBW is an inadequate term because the traditional definition (birth weight <2500 g) fails to account for gestational age at birth or acknowledge that LBW is a complex syndrome with multiple aetiologies and not a single phenotype [14, 15].

The 2500 g cut-off selects an heterogeneous group composed of preterm newborns (<37 weeks' gestation), small for gestational age (SGA) newborns at term, and the overlap between these two entities, i.e., preterm SGA newborns who typically have the worst outcomes [14]. These phenotypes have their own subgroups with individual components linked almost certainly to different etiological factors and long-term effects, and distributions across populations that are dependent on the prevalence of the underlying causal factors [16]. They also have substantially different morbidity and mortality rates and long-term outcomes, requiring different preventive and therapeutic interventions. Understanding and differentiating the various phenotypes and their subgroups is thus essential [17].

Notably, the <2500 g definition fails to include a large number of term SGA and severely SGA newborns, whose birth weight is 2500 g or higher, but below the 10th percentile of the anthropometric standards for their gestational age [14], who are also at higher risk of morbidity, mortality and long-term sequelae. Worldwide, there are an estimated 14–17 million newborns in this group annually [8, 14]. However, they are typically excluded from priority interventions during the early postnatal period, as they are not acknowledged as being at risk. It is important to note that, strictly speaking, SGA newborns are not synonymous to intrauterine growth retardation (IUGR); some SGA newborns may merely represent the lower tail of the normal fetal growth distribution. In individual cases, however, it is usually very difficult to determine whether an observed birth weight that is low for gestational age is the result of true in utero growth restriction or represents a "normally small" newborn. Classification of IUGR is therefore based on the established cut-off for small-for-gestational-age. The higher the prevalence of SGA in a given population, the greater the likelihood that SGA is a result of IUGR [1].

The issue of which reference curve to use in assessing growth at birth has been a cause of debate. Based on the observation that children of well-off populations in developing countries experience similar growth patterns as those of healthy, well-nourished children in developed countries, and that children of the same genetic background show differing growth performance depending on the environment in which they grow up, there is prevailing international consensus that children of all races have the same growth potential, and that country- or race-specific growth references are not advised [1, 18]. Growth curves should certainly not be adjusted for factors that may be a cause of growth retardation. For example, making adjustments for the height of stunted parents in deprived populations could reinforce the wrong impression that children from these populations are born small for genetic reasons and that not much can be done about this. On this basis, a group of international experts recommended that an international fetal growth reference curve should be developed based on pooled data from countries in different geographical regions where fetal growth is believed to be optimal [19, 20]. The challenge was taken by the INTERGROWTH-21st Consortium that designed a multi-country study to complement the World Health Organization (WHO) growth standards by providing comparable international standards for fetal growth from 9 weeks of gestation to birth and newborn size (weight, length, and head circumference) according to gestational age and sex. The INTERGROWTH-21st Project included three complementary components. A cross-sectional study of all newborns in eight study sites (Brazil, China, India, Italy, Kenya, Oman, the United Kingdom, and the United States). A cohort of healthy women was also enrolled in a longitudinal component in the same centers to monitor fetal growth with ultrasound scans from 9 to 14 weeks of gestation to birth. In addition, in the third component, the postnatal growth of those infants in the longitudinal cohort who were born prematurely was monitored. Nearly 60,000 children and their families have been enrolled in the three study components, with the same eligibility criteria as those used to develop the WHO growth standards. These international anthropometric standards to evaluate fetal and newborn growth have been made recently available for international use [21–23].

High socioeconomic level populations receiving adequate health care in low-middle income countries are as well-nourished and healthy as those in high-income countries, with similar pregnancy and infant outcomes including preterm birth and LBW. Hence, identifying populations at greatest risk, as well as those that are most likely to respond to health and nutrition interventions, is a global priority and fundamental for the success of large-scale programs. Reducing the burden of death and disability resulting from poor maternal health and the consequences of a poor intrauterine environment, such as stunting and poor cognitive development, is achievable in most countries as long as efforts are targeted to address the health and nutrition needs of the majority of the people.

In fact, data recently published by WHO [24] provide strong evidence that even short-term nutritional improvement (during intrauterine life and childhood) can result, in just one generation, in a mean gain in adult height that is up to 8 cm greater than the mean parental height. In other words, in developing countries, trans-generational improvements in height are achievable faster than expected if women of reproductive age have adequate health and nutrition, and their children receive adequate breastfeeding and complementary feeding and have good access to evidence-based health care.

Child Growth Indicators and Their Interpretation

In children the three most commonly used indicators to assess growth status are weight-for-height, height-for-age, and weight-for-age. Table 6.1 shows the WHO classification of nutrition conditions in children and adolescents based on weight and length/height (recumbent length is measured up to 2 years of age and standing height from 2 years onwards) [25]. Weight-for-height and height-for-age are key indicators because they permit the distinction of stunted, wasted, and overweight children, allowing the appropriate targeting of interventions [26–29]. The routine collection of length and height measurements is important because this enables not only the assessment of weight-for-height but also body mass index (i.e., ratio of weight in kilograms to the square of height in meters), a valuable indicator for monitoring the public health problem of overweight and obesity in childhood [30, 31]. Weight-for-age, on the other hand, is still a commonly used indicator [32]; however, it lacks the biological specificity necessary to separate weight- from height-related deficits or excesses in growth.

The interpretation of the most commonly used anthropometric indicators is as follows:

Low height-for-age: Stunted growth reflects a process of failure to reach linear growth potential as a result of suboptimal health and/or nutritional conditions. On a population basis, high levels of stunting are associated with poor socioeconomic conditions (Fig. 6.1, which uses education level of parent as proxy for socioeconomic status) and increased risk of frequent and early exposure to adverse conditions such as illness and/or suboptimal feeding practices. Similarly, a decrease in the national

Table 6.1 WHO classification of nutrition conditions in children and adolescents based on anthropometry

Condition	Age: Birth to 60 months[a,c] Indicator and cut-off	Age: 61 months to 19 years[b,c] Indicator and cut-off
Obese	BMI-for-age (or weight-for-length/height) > 3SD	BMI-for-age > 2SD (2SD approximates BMI 30 kg/m[b] at 19 years)
Overweight	BMI-for-age (or weight-for-length/height) > 2SD to 3SD	BMI-for-age >1SD to 2SD (1SD approximates BMI 25 kg/m[b] at 19 years)
Possible risk of overweight	BMI-for-age (or weight-for-length/height) > 1SD to 2SD	Not applicable
Moderately underweight	Weight-for-age < −2SD to −3SD	Weight-for-age (up to 10 y) < −2SD to −3SD
Severely underweight	Weight-for-age < −3SD	Weight-for-age (up to 10 years) < −3SD
Moderately wasted	Weight-for-length/height (or BMI-for-age) < −2SD to −3SD	BMI-for-age < −2 to −3SD
Severely wasted	Weight-for-length/height (or BMI-for-age) < −3SD	BMI-for-age < −3SD
Moderately stunted	Length/height-for-age < −2SD to −3SD	Height-for-age < −2SD to −3SD
Severely stunted	Length/height-for-age < −3SD	Height-for-age < −3SD

[a]WHO Child Growth Standards: http://www.who.int/childgrowth/en/index.html
[b]WHO Growth Reference for school-aged children and adolescents: http://www.who.int/growthref/en/
[c]Z-score and percentile equivalence
−3 = 0.1
−2 = 2.3
−1 = 15.9
+1 = 84.1
+2 = 97.7
+3 = 99.9

stunting rate is usually indicative of improvements in overall socioeconomic conditions of a country [33]. The worldwide variation of the prevalence of low height-for-age is considerable, ranging from 5% to over 60% in low-income countries [34, 35]. In many such settings, growth restriction starts from birth (or even intrauterus) until about 24-36 months of age, after which mean heights run parallel to the current international reference [10]. Thus, age modifies the interpretation of findings: for children in the age group below 2–3 years, low height-for-age probably reflects an active process of "failing to grow" or "stunting;" while for older children, it reflects a state of "having failed to grow" or "being stunted." From the point of view of interventions, it is important to differentiate between these two groups.

Low weight-for-height: Wasting or thinness indicates in most cases a recent and severe process of weight loss, which is often associated with acute starvation and/or severe disease. However, wasting also may be the result of chronic unfavorable conditions. Provided there is no severe food shortage, the prevalence of wasting is usually below 5%, even in poor countries [35]. The Indian subcontinent, where a higher prevalence of wasting is found, is an important exception. On the severity index, prevalences between 10 and 14% are regarded as serious, and 15% or above as critical [1]. Typically, the prevalence of low weight-for-height shows a peak in the second year of life [35]. Lack of evidence of wasting in a population does not imply the absence of current nutritional problems: stunting and other deficits, such as of micronutrients, may be present [36].

Low weight-for-age: Weight-for-age reflects body mass relative to chronological age. It is influenced by both the height of the child (height-for-age) and his/her weight (weight-for-height), and its composite nature makes interpretation complex. For example, weight-for-age fails to distinguish between short children of adequate body weight and tall, thin children. However, in the absence of significant wasting in a community, similar information is provided by weight-for-age and height-for-age, unless there is a substantial proportion of children who are stunted but overweight, in which case underweight prevalence is lower than stunting prevalence. Short-term change, especially reduction in weight-for-age, reveals changes in weight-for-height. In general terms, the worldwide variation of low weight-for-age and its age distribution are similar to those of low height-for-age [35].

High weight-for-height: Overweight is the preferred term for describing high weight-for-height [1]. Even though there is a strong correlation between high weight-for-height and obesity as measured by adiposity, greater lean body mass (e.g., muscles) can also contribute to high weight-for-height. On an individual basis, therefore, "fatness" or "obesity" should not be used to describe high weight-for-height. However, on a population-wide basis, high weight-for-height (i.e., above +2SD of the WHO Child Growth Standards median) can be considered as an adequate indicator of overweight, because the majority of children with high weight-for-height are overweight. Strictly speaking, the term obesity should be used only in the context of adiposity measurements, for example skinfold thickness.

Other available anthropometric indicators that are used to describe growth status during childhood include mid-upper arm circumference (MUAC), body mass index (BMI), skinfolds, and head circumference. MUAC is frequently used in the identification and management of children with severe and moderate acute malnutrition (SAM and MAM) [26, 37]. In the context of SAM programs, MUAC is used with a fixed cut-off (less than 115 mm), however, its proper application would require the use of age-specific cut-offs based on the WHO Child Growth Standards [38]. This implies the need to determine age, an important drawback of using MUAC-for-age under difficult field conditions (e.g., refugee crises, draughts). The use of a fixed cut-off for MUAC identifies children at a greater risk of mortality as young children are more likely to be identified.

For some of these measurements, like skinfolds, technical difficulties result in high intra- and inter-individual variation and require skilled individuals to perform the measurements accurately and precisely. A full description of standardized protocols for accurately taking and interpreting anthropometric measurements can be found elsewhere [39].

International Anthropometric Standards

The designation of a child as having impaired growth implies some means of comparison with a "reference" child of the same age and sex. Thus, in practical terms, anthropometric values need to be compared across individuals or populations in relation to an acceptable set of reference values. This need has made the choice of a growth reference population an important issue that has received considerable attention in the last decades as the correct interpretation of accurate and reliable anthropometric measurements is heavily dependent on the use of appropriate growth curves to compare and interpret anthropometric values [10, 40].

This section presents the growth charts the WHO developed for preschool age children (WHO Child Growth Standards) and school-aged children and adolescents (WHO Growth Reference for School-aged Children and Adolescents).

WHO Child Growth Standards (0–60 Months)

In April 2006 the WHO released new standards for assessing the growth and development of children from birth to 5 years of age [38, 41]. The new standards were developed to replace the National Center for Health Statistics (NCHS)/WHO international growth reference [42], whose limitations have been described in detail elsewhere [1, 43].

The origin of the Child Growth Standards dates from the early 1990s when WHO conducted a comprehensive review of anthropometric references. The review showed that the growth pattern of healthy breastfed infants deviated significantly from the NCHS/WHO international reference [44, 45]. In particular, the reference was inadequate for assessing the growth pattern of healthy breastfed infants [46]. An expert group recommended the development of new standards, adopting a novel approach that would describe how children should grow when free of disease and receiving care that followed healthy practices such as breastfeeding and non-smoking [47]. This approach would permit the development of a normative standard as opposed to a reference that merely described how children grew in a particular place and time. Although standards and references both serve as a basis for comparison, each enables a different interpretation. Since a standard defines how children should grow, deviations from the pattern it describes are evidence of abnormal growth. A reference, on the other hand, does not provide as sound a basis for making such value judgments, although in practice references often are mistakenly used as standards.

Following the World Health Assembly's endorsement of these recommendations in 1994, the WHO Multicentre Growth Reference Study (MGRS) [48] was launched in 1997 to collect primary growth data that would allow the construction of new growth charts consistent with best health practices. The MGRS, whose goal was to describe the growth of healthy children, was a population-based study conducted in six countries from diverse geographical regions: Brazil, Ghana, India, Norway, Oman, and the USA [48]. The study combined a longitudinal follow-up from birth to 24 months with a cross-sectional component of children aged 18–71 months. In the longitudinal component, mothers and newborns were enrolled at birth and visited at home a total of 21 times at weeks 1, 2, 4, and 6; monthly from 2–12 months; and bimonthly in the second year [48].

The study populations lived in socioeconomic conditions favorable to growth. The individual inclusion criteria were: no known health or environmental constraints to growth (based on site-specific education and income criteria), mothers willing to follow MGRS feeding recommendations (i.e., exclusive or predominant breastfeeding for at least 4 months, introduction of complementary foods by 6 months of age, and continued breastfeeding to at least 12 months of age), no maternal smoking during pregnancy and lactation, single and term birth, and absence of significant

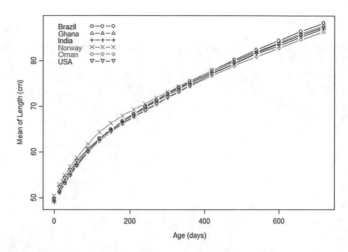

Fig. 6.3 Mean length (cm) from birth to 2 years for the six WHO Multicentre Growth Reference Study sites. From WHO Multicentre Growth Reference Study Group [18]. Copyright © 2007, Wiley, reprinted with permission

morbidity. Rigorously standardized methods of data collection and procedures for data management across sites yielded high-quality data [38, 48]. The length of children was strikingly similar among the six sites (Fig. 6.3), with only about 3% of variability in length being due to intersite differences compared to 70% for individuals within sites [18]. The multi-country study Intergrowth-21st has also found similar results for the fetus and newborn [49]. The similarity in growth during early childhood across human populations means either a recent common origin as some suggest [50] or a strong selective advantage associated with the current pattern of growth and development across human environments. Data from all sites were pooled to construct the standards, following state-of-the-art statistical methodologies [38].

Weight-for-age, length/height-for-age, weight-for-length/height, and body mass index (BMI)-for-age percentile and z-score values were generated for boys and girls aged 0–60 months [38]. Standards for head circumference, mid-upper arm circumference, and triceps and subscapular skinfolds were released in 2007 [51]; and growth velocity standards for weight, length, and head circumference were issued in 2009 [52]. Figure 6.4 presents a generic growth chart for body mass index-for-age in percentile values for girls aged 0–60 months. The full set of tables and charts is available at the growth standards website (www.who.int/childgrowth/en) together with tools like software, macros, and training materials that facilitate application. The disjunction observed at 24 months in the length/height-based charts represents the change from measuring recumbent length (i.e., lying down) to standing height in children below and above 2 years of age, respectively. Windows of achievement for six gross motor development milestones were also constructed (Fig. 6.5) [53].

Detailed evaluation of the WHO standards as part of their introduction has provided an opportunity to assess their impact on child health programs. Since their release in 2006, the standards have been widely implemented globally, with over 130 countries thus far having adopted them [54]. Reasons for adoption include: (1) providing a more reliable tool for assessing growth that is consistent with the Global Strategy for Infant and Young Child Feeding; (2) protecting and promoting breastfeeding; (3) enabling monitoring of malnutrition's double burden, stunting and overweight; (4) promoting healthy growth and protecting the right of children to reach their full genetic potential; and (5) harmonizing national growth assessment systems. In adopting the WHO growth standards, countries have harmonized best practices in child growth assessment and established the breastfed infant as the norm against which to assess compliance with the right of children to achieve their full genetic growth potential.

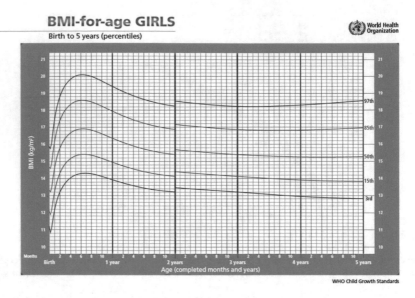

Fig. 6.4 Body mass index-for-age in percentile values for girls aged 0–60 months

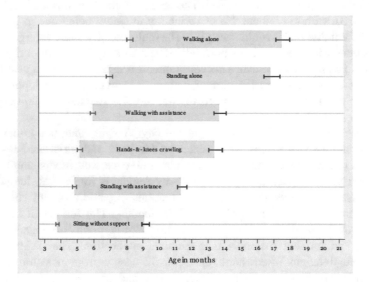

Fig. 6.5 Windows of achievement for six gross motor milestones in the WHO Child Growth Standards. From WHO Multicentre Growth Reference Study Group [53]. Copyright © 2007, Wiley, reprinted with permission

The WHO standards provide an improved tool for monitoring the rapidly changing rate of growth in early infancy [55]. They also demonstrate that healthy children from around the world who are raised in healthy environments and follow recommended feeding practices have strikingly similar patterns of growth. The ancestries of the children included in the WHO standards were widely diverse. They included people from Europe, Africa, the Middle East, Asia, and Latin America. In this regard, they are similar to growing numbers of populations with increasingly diverse ethnicities. These results indicate that we should expect the same potential for child growth in any country. They also imply that deviations from this pattern must be assumed to reflect adverse conditions that require correction, e.g., inadequate or lack of breastfeeding, nutrient-poor or energy-excessive complementary foods, unsanitary environments, deficient health services, and/or poverty.

Technical and scientific research has validated the robustness of the WHO standards and improved understanding of the broad benefits of their use:

- The WHO standards identify more children as severely wasted [56]. Besides being more accurate for predicting mortality risk [57–59], using these standards results in shorter duration of treatment, higher rates of recovery, fewer deaths, and reduced loss to follow-up or need for inpatient care [60].
- The WHO standards confirm the dissimilar growth patterns for breastfed and formula-fed infants, and they provide an improved tool for correctly assessing the adequacy of growth in breastfed infants [61, 62]. They thereby reduce considerably the risk of unnecessary supplementation or breastfeeding cessation, which are major sources of morbidity and mortality in poor-hygiene settings.
- In addition to confirming the importance of the first 2 years of life as a window of opportunity for promoting growth, the WHO standards demonstrate that intrauterine retardation in linear growth is more prevalent than previously thought [10, 40], thereby making a strong case for starting interventions early in pregnancy and even before, including interventions to delay the age at marriage and first pregnancy to late in adolescence or in early adulthood.
- Another important feature of the WHO standards is that they demonstrate that undernutrition during the first six months of life is a considerably more serious problem than previously thought [40, 63], thereby reconciling the rates of undernutrition observed in young infants and the prevalence of low birth weight and early abandonment of exclusive breastfeeding.
- Using the WHO standards results in a greater prevalence of overweight that varies by age and the nutritional status of the index population [40]. The WHO standards also improve early detection of excess weight gain among infants and young children [64, 65], showing that obesity often begins in early childhood, as indeed should measures to tackle this global public health menace.
- Lastly, the WHO standards are an important means for ensuring the right to health of all children and achieving their full growth potential. They provide sound scientific evidence that, on average, young children everywhere experience similar growth patterns when their health and nutrition needs are met. For this reason the WHO standards can be used to assess compliance with the UN Convention on the Rights of the Child, which recognizes the duties and obligations to children that cannot be met without attention to normal human development.

WHO Growth Reference for School-Aged Children and Adolescents (61 Months–19 Years)

Much less is known about the growth and nutritional status of school-age children and adolescents. Reasons for this lack of knowledge include the rapid changes in somatic growth, problems of dealing with variations in maturation, and difficulties in separating normal variations from those associated with health risks.

The release of the WHO standards for preschool children and increasing public health concern over childhood obesity stirred interest in developing appropriate growth curves for school-age children and adolescents. As countries proceeded to implement WHO growth standards for preschool children, the gap between these standards and existing growth references for older children became a matter of concern. The 1977 NCHS reference [42] and more recent examples such as the CDC 2000 reference [66, 67], the IOTF cut-off points [68] and other contemporary references [69, 70] all suffer from a biological drawback characterized by weight-based curves, such as the BMI, that are markedly skewed to the right, thereby redefining overweight and obesity as "normal" [71, 72]. The upward skewness of these references results in an underestimation of overweight and obesity and an over-estimation of undernutrition (e.g., prevalence of thinness or children below the third percentile) [73, 74]. The latter is worrisome as it might prompt the overfeeding of healthy, constitutionally small children.

A potential approach to overcoming this flaw would be to use lower cut-offs to screen for overweight and obesity [72]. However, better still would be to use growth curves based on data from populations who have achieved expected linear growth while not being affected by excessive weight gain relative to linear growth [75]. The case made for using a national reference has traditionally been that it is more representative of a given country's children than any other reference could possibly be. But given the child obesity epidemic, this is no longer valid for weight or BMI. No sooner is a new reference produced than it is out of date.

The need to harmonize growth assessment tools, conceptually and pragmatically, prompted evaluation of the feasibility of developing a single international growth reference for school-aged children and adolescents [73]. Recognizing the limitations of existing reference curves (e.g., the NCHS/WHO growth reference, the CDC 2000 growth charts, and the IOTF cut-offs) for assessing childhood obesity, the expert group recommended that appropriate growth curves for these age groups be developed for clinical and public health applications. It also agreed that a multicenter study, similar to that leading to the development of the WHO Child Growth Standards from birth to 5 years of age, would not be feasible for older children because it would be impossible to control the dynamics of their environment. It was thus decided that a growth reference should be constructed for this age group using available historical data [75].

Following the expert group recommendations, WHO proceeded to reconstruct the 1977 NCHS/WHO growth reference for the period 5–19 years. It used the original sample (a non-obese sample with expected heights), supplemented with data from the WHO Child Growth Standards (to facilitate a smooth transition at 5 years), and applied state-of-the-art statistical methods [76]. The new curves are closely aligned with the WHO Child Growth Standards at 5 years, and the recommended adult cut-offs for overweight and obesity at 19 years (BMI of 25 and 30, respectively). The full set of tables and charts released in April 2006 for height, weight, and BMI can be found at: www.who.int/growthref/en, including application tools such as software for clinicians and public health specialists [77].

The WHO reference for school-age children and adolescents provides a suitable reference for the 5–19 years age group to be used in conjunction with the WHO Child Growth Standards from 0 to 5 years. Since its release in 2007 many countries have switched to using these charts including high-income countries, for example Canada, Switzerland, [78] and several others in Europe [79].

Issues in the Interpretation of Growth Data

One essential consideration is the appropriate use of the reference data. The way in which a reference is interpreted and the clinical and public health decisions that will be based upon it are as important as the choice of the reference. The reference should be used as a general guide for screening and monitoring and not as a fixed standard that can be applied in a rigid fashion to individuals from different ethnic, socioeconomic, and nutritional and health backgrounds. For clinical or individual-based application, reference values should be used as a screening tool to detect individuals at greater risk of health or nutritional disorders; and they should not be viewed as a self-sufficient diagnostic tool. For population-based application, the reference values should be used for comparison and monitoring purposes. In a given population, a high prevalence of anthropometric deficit will be indicative of significant health and nutritional problems, however, it is not only those individuals below the cut-off point who are at risk; the entire population is at risk, and the cut-off point should be used only to facilitate the application of the indicator.

There are two systems by which a child or a group of children can be compared to the reference population: percentiles and Z-scores (standard deviation [SD] scores). For population-based assessment (including surveys and nutritional surveillance), the Z-score is widely recognized as the best system for analysis and presentation of anthropometric data because of its advantages compared to the other methods [1]. A major advantage of the Z-score system for population-based applications is that a group of Z-scores can be subjected to summary statistics such as the mean and SD. The mean Z-score, though less commonly used, has the advantage of describing the nutritional status of the entire population directly without resorting to a subset of individuals below a set cut-off. A mean Z-score significantly lower than zero (the expected value for the reference distribution) usually means that the entire distribution has shifted downward, suggesting that most, if not all, individuals have been affected. Using the mean Z-score as an index of severity for health and nutrition problems results in increased awareness that, if a condition is severe, an intervention is required for the entire community, not just those who are classified as "undernourished" by the cut-off criteria [80, 81]. In addition, the observed SD value of the Z-score distribution is very useful for assessing data quality [1]. At the individual level, however, although there is substantial recognition that Z-score is the most appropriate descriptor of malnutrition, clinicians, and health and nutrition centers (e.g., supplementary feeding programs in refugee camps) have been in practice reluctant to adopt its use for individual assessment. A detailed description of the percentile and Z-score systems, including a discussion of their strengths and weaknesses, can be found elsewhere [82].

In clinical applications, children are commonly classified using a cut-off value, often <-2 and $>+2$ Z-scores. The rationale for this is the statistical definition of the central 95% of a distribution as the "normal" range, which is not necessarily based on the optimal point for predicting functional outcomes. A better approach to classifying individual children would be to base the cut-offs on the relationship between growth deficits and health outcomes, such as mortality, morbidity, and child development. The difficulty of this approach is that these relationships differ according to the prevalence of health and nutritional disorders, and cut-offs would have to be developed locally taking account of local circumstances, something that is not advisable. The cut-offs in Z-scores and percentiles currently recommended by WHO for the different nutrition conditions classified based on anthropometry are presented in Table 6.1.

Lastly, experience with population surveillance has contributed to emphasizing the usefulness of identifying prevalence ranges to assess the severity of a situation as the basis for making public health decisions. For example, when 10% of a population is below the $-2SD$ cut-off for weight-for-height, is that too much, too little, or average? The intention of the so-called "trigger-levels" is to assist in answering this question by giving some kind of guideline for the purpose of establishing levels of public health importance of a situation. Such classifications are very helpful for summarizing prevalence data and can be used for targeting purposes when establishing intervention priorities. It is important to note that the trigger-levels vary according to the different anthropometric indicators. The prevalence ranges shown in Table 6.1 are those currently recommended [1] to classify levels of stunting, underweight, and wasting, noting that in the reference population, 2.5% is below $-2SD$, by definition, and this is considered "normal" i.e., within normal biological variation.

Prevalence of Growth Retardation in Developing Countries

A recent comprehensive review estimated that 32 million babies are born SGA, 27% of births in LMICs, and that about 800,000 neonatal deaths and 400,000 post-neonatal infant deaths can be attributed to the increased risk associated with having fetal growth restriction [8]. This finding contradicts the widespread assumption that SGA infants, by contrast with preterm babies, are not at a substantially increased risk of mortality. Additionally, babies who are SGA have an increased risk of growth faltering in the first 2 years of life, and the same study suggests that 20% of stunting might be attributable to fetal growth restriction [8]. These estimates confirm that fetal growth restriction is a major public health problem and emphasize the need for interventions before and during pregnancy. Although there is considerable variation in SGA prevalence across regions, the prevalence is highest in South-Central Asia followed by sub-Saharan Africa. There are also large intra-country variation rates.

Stunted linear growth has become the main indicator of childhood undernutrition because it is highly prevalent in all developing countries and has important consequences for health and development [34]. It should replace underweight as the main anthropometric indicator for children [8]. Linear growth assessment in primary care is an essential component of country efforts to reduce childhood stunting and achieve healthy weight gain. More experience is needed in the operational aspects of the assessment and interpretation of linear growth and the relationship between weight and height by health workers and in the effective intervention responses (see below).

The most recent analyses indicate that in 2011, there were an estimated 165 million under-five stunted children, a 35% decrease from an estimated 253 million in 1990 [3] (Table 6.2). Globally, the prevalence decreased from an estimated 40% in 1990 to 26% in 2011. At regional level, there was very little decline in Africa (from 42 to 36%) compared to Asia (from 48 to 27%). At present, Eastern and Western Africa and South-central Asia have the highest prevalence estimates among UN subregions (42% in East Africa and 36% in both West Africa and South-central Asia). The largest number of children affected by stunting, 69 million, live in South-central Asia (Table 6.2). Oceania, has a very high rate of stunting (36% in 2011), nonetheless contributes little in numbers affected due to its relatively small population [3].

Nationally, there is great variation in rates of childhood stunting. Figure 6.6 maps countries according to their latest national stunting prevalence estimate. Rates are categorized by severity levels

Table 6.2 Prevalence and numbers of stunted[a] children under 5 years by UN region—1990 to 2025

UN regions and subregions	1990		2011		2025	
	%	Millions	%	Millions	%	Millions
Africa	**41.6**	**45.7**	**35.6**	**56.3**	**32.0**	**60.6**
	38.5–44.6	42.3–49.0	33.3–38.0	52.5–60.0	28.2–35.8	53.4–67.8
Eastern	**50.6**	**18.0**	**42.1**	**22.8**	**36.7**	**24.9**
	44.2–57.0	15.7–20.3	38.9–45.4	21.0–24.6	32.4–41.1	22.0–27.9
Middle	**47.2**	**6.4**	**35.0**	**7.8**	**27.8**	**7.3**
	36.4–58.2	5.0–7.9	29.1–41.4	6.5–9.2	16.5–42.8	4.4–11.3
Northern	**28.6**	**6.3**	**21.0**	**5.0**	**16.9**	**4.0**
	22.3–35.8	4.9–7.9	14.6–29.4	3.5–7.0	9.9–27.4	2.3–6.4
Southern	**36.2**	**2.2**	**30.8**	**1.8**	**27.5**	**1.5**
	32.9–39.7	2.0–2.4	25.2–37.0	1.5–2.2	20.8–35.3	1.2–2.0
Western	**39.1**	**12.8**	**36.4**	**18.9**	**34.6**	**22.9**
	35.4–42.9	11.5–14.0	31.7–41.2	16.5–21.5	27.1–42.9	17.9–28.4
Asia[b]	**48.4**	**188.7**	**26.8**	**95.8**	**17.1**	**56.5**
	45.6–51.1	178.1–199.3	23.2–30.5	82.8–108.8	12.6–21.6	41.6–71.4
Eastern[b]	**36.8**	**47.9**	**8.5**	**7.5**	**2.7**	**2.0**
	34.9–38.6	45.5–50.3	7.9–9.2	7.0–8.1	2.5–2.9	1.8–2.1
South-central	**59.3**	**107.5**	**36.4**	**68.8**	**23.5**	**42.3**
	54.4–64.0	98.6–116.1	30.1–43.2	57.0–81.7	16.5–32.4	29.7–58.3

(continued)

Table 6.2 (continued)

UN regions and subregions	1990		2011		2025	
	%	Millions	%	Millions	%	Millions
South-eastern	**47.3**	**27.0**	**27.4**	**14.6**	**17.5**	**8.7**
	38.1–56.6	21.7–32.3	21.8–33.7	11.6–18.0	11.7–25.3	5.8–12.6
Western	**29.2**	**6.3**	**18.0**	**4.8**	**12.6**	**3.5**
	22.7–36.6	4.9–7.9	10.4–29.5	2.8–7.9	5.4–26.7	1.5–7.4
Latin America and Caribbean	**24.6**	**13.7**	**13.4**	**7.1**	**8.5**	**4.2**
	19.3–29.9	10.8–16.7	9.0–17.7	4.8–9.4	4.8–12.2	2.4–6.1
Caribbean	**16.5**	**0.7**	**6.7**	**0.2**	**3.5**	**0.1**
	9.4–27.2	0.4–1.1	3.1–13.7	0.1–0.5	1.5–8.3	0–0.3
Central America	**34.0**	**5.4**	**18.6**	**3.0**	**11.8**	**1.8**
	23.9–45.8	3.8–7.2	11.6–28.5	1.9–4.6	6.8–19.5	1.0–3.0
South America	**21.4**	**7.7**	**11.5**	**3.9**	**7.4**	**2.3**
	15.5–28.8	5.6–10.4	6.9–18.6	2.3–6.2	3.6–14.5	1.1–4.6
Oceania[c]	**40.4**	**0.4**	**35.5**	**0.5**	**32.4**	**0.5**
	26.8–55.7	0.3–0.5	16.0–61.4	0.2–0.8	7.7–73.4	0.1–1.1
Developing countries	**44.6**	**248.4**	**28.0**	**159.7**	**21.3**	**121.8**
	42.6–46.7	237.0–259.9	25.6–30.4	145.9–173.4	18.4–24.2	105.1–138.5
Developed countries	**6.1**	**4.7**	**7.2**	**5.1**	**8.1**	**5.7**
	3.3–11.0	2.5–8.5	4.1–12.6	2.9–8.9	4.5–14.2	3.2–9.9
Global	**39.9**	**253.1**	**25.7**	**164.8**	**19.9**	**127.4**
	38.1–41.8	241.4–264.9	23.5–27.9	150.8–178.8	17.2–22.5	110.5–144.4

Reproduced from de Onis et al. [3] with permission from Wiley
[a]Height-for-age below −2SD from the WHO Child Growth Standards
[b]Excluding Japan
[c]Excluding Australia and New Zealand

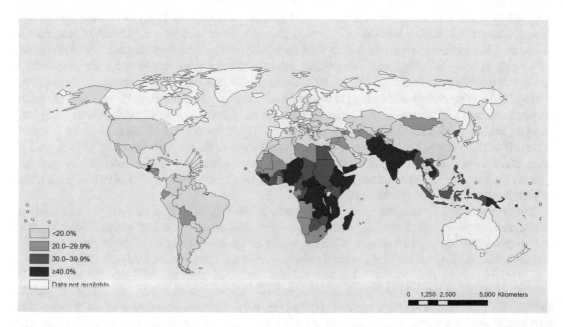

Fig. 6.6 Stunting among children under 5 years of age—latest national prevalence estimates Reproduced from de Onis et al. [3] with permission from Wiley

[1], ranging from low (below 20%) to very high ($\geq 40\%$). Extremely high levels appear in countries like Afghanistan, Burundi and Yemen, with levels above 50% in most recent surveys. Other countries of sub-Saharan Africa, South-central, and South-eastern Asia also present high or very high stunting rates. Rates are consistently higher in rural than in urban areas, and can vary considerably by age and region within countries. Country-specific prevalence data, disaggregated by age group, sex, urban/rural residence and region, are available from the *WHO Global Database on Child Growth and Malnutrition* [www.who.int/nutgrowthdb].

Health and Social Consequences of Impaired Growth

The health and social consequences of the current high prevalences of fetal and child growth retardation in developing countries are severe [4, 8]. Fetuses who suffer from growth retardation have higher perinatal morbidity and mortality [8, 83–85], are at an increased risk of sudden infant death syndrome (SIDS) [86], and have higher infant mortality and childhood morbidity [8, 87]. During childhood they are more likely to have poor cognitive development [88, 89] and neurologic impairment [90–92]; in adulthood they are at increased risk of cardiovascular disease [93], high blood pressure [94], obstructive lung disease [95], diabetes [96], high cholesterol concentrations [97] and renal damage [98].

During childhood, the major outcomes of poor growth can be classified in terms of mortality, morbidity (incidence and severity), and psychological and cognitive development. There are also important consequences in adult life in terms of body size, work and reproductive performances, and risk of chronic diseases [4].

A number of studies have demonstrated the association between increasing severity of anthropometric deficits and mortality [99, 100] which, in turn, has important implications for policy and programs addressing child survival [99]. Stunted, underweight, and wasted children have an increased risk of death from diarrhea, pneumonia, measles, and other infectious diseases [101]. The most recent analysis estimated that more than 1 million annual child deaths can be attributed to stunting and about 800,000 to wasting (about 60% of which are attributable to severe wasting) [8]. These attributable deaths cannot be added because of the overlap of these and other nutritional conditions. Undernutrition in the aggregate (including fetal growth restriction, stunting, wasting, and deficiencies of vitamin A and zinc along with suboptimum breastfeeding) was estimated to be the cause of 3.1 million child deaths annually or 45% of all child deaths in 2011 [8]. The majority of deaths were owing to the potentiating effect of mild-to-moderate levels of undernutrition as opposed to severe undernutrition. Thus, strategies that focus only on severely undernourished children will be insufficient to improve child survival in a meaningful way. The most significant impact can be expected when all grades of severity are targeted. Similarly, children suffering from impaired growth tend to have more severe diarrhoeal episodes and are more susceptible to several infectious diseases frequently seen in developing countries, such as malaria or meningitis [102, 103]. The risk of pneumonia is also increased in these children [104].

There is strong evidence that poor fetal growth or stunting in the first 2 years of life leads to irreversible damage, including shorter adult height, lower attained schooling, reduced adult income, and decreased offspring birthweight [4]. This results in an intergenerational effect since low birth weight babies are themselves likely to have anthropometric deficits at later ages [105, 106]. These low birth weight babies, born to stunted mothers, contribute to closing the intergenerational cycle by which low maternal size and anemia, predispose to LBW babies, which in turn predisposes to growth failure of children, leading back to small adults (Fig. 6.7). Also the occurrence of early pregnancy will contribute both in terms of LBW and inducing premature cessation of growth in the adolescent

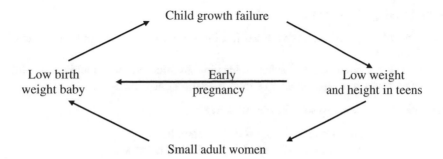

Fig. 6.7 Intergenerational cycle of growth failure

mother. The implications of this vicious cycle are enormous for the human and socioeconomic development of the affected populations.

In summary, the magnitude of the problem and the severity of the health and social consequences associated with impaired growth cannot be overemphasized. Child growth is a major determinant of human development. Thus, there is an urgent need to develop and/or identify effective interventions for improving child growth and development. Population-wide interventions aimed at preventing intrauterine growth retardation are also urgently required, given the strong association between pre- and postnatal growth and the widespread incidence of fetal growth retardation in developing countries.

Interventions Aimed at Promoting Healthy Growth and Development

It is widely recognized that the "window of opportunity" for reducing stunting and promoting healthy growth and development is the ~1000 days from conception until 2 years of age [10], although assuring adequate maternal nutrition prior to conception, including delaying the age at marriage and first pregnancy to beyond adolescence, is also likely to be important [107, 108]. It is also agreed that nutrition interventions alone are insufficient, and hence recent efforts to foster nutrition-sensitive development, including nutrition-sensitive agriculture to improve household food security; maternal education and women's empowerment in support of their own health and their capacity to care for their children; improved hygiene, sanitation and water quality to reduce infections; and social protection programs to increase purchasing power and access to services and amenities are also being prioritized [109].

A comprehensive review of the evidence regarding efficacy and effectiveness of prenatal and postnatal nutrition interventions identified a set of ten proven nutrition-specific interventions, which if scaled up from present population coverage to cover 90% of the need, would eliminate about 900,000 child deaths in the 34 high nutrition-burden countries, where 90% of the world's stunted children live [107]. These interventions are classified into four packages:

- **Optimum maternal nutrition during pregnancy**

  - Maternal multiple micronutrient supplementation to all
  - Maternal calcium supplementation to mothers at risk of low intake
    Maternal balanced energy protein supplements as needed
  - Universal salt iodisation

- **Infant and young child feeding**

  - Promotion of early and exclusive breastfeeding for 6 months and continued breastfeeding for up to 24 months
  - Appropriate complementary feeding education in food secure populations and additional complementary food supplements in food insecure populations

- **Micronutrient supplementation in children at risk**

  - Vitamin A supplementation between 6 and 59 months of age
  - Preventive zinc supplements between 12 and 59 months of age

- **Management of acute malnutrition**

  - Management of moderate acute malnutrition
  - Management of severe acute malnutrition

Analysis of these nutrition-specific packages showed that the most lives could be saved by the therapeutic feeding for severe acute malnutrition, followed by the infant and young child nutrition package [107].

In addition to nutrition-specific interventions, acceleration of progress in nutrition will also require increases in the nutritional outcomes of effective, large-scale, nutrition-sensitive development programs [109]. Nutrition-sensitive programs address key underlying determinants of nutrition such as poverty, food insecurity, and scarcity of access to adequate care resources. They can therefore help enhance the effectiveness, coverage, and scale of nutrition-specific interventions.

Poor growth is part of a vicious cycle that includes poverty and disease. These three factors are interlinked in such a way that each contributes to the presence and permanence of the others. The future of human societies relies on children being able to achieve their optimal physical growth and mental development. Never before has there been so much knowledge to assist families and societies in their desire to raise children to reach their full potential. A fundamental need is to focus the attention of policy-makers on nutritional status as one of the main indicators of development, and as a precondition for the socioeconomic advancement of societies in any significant long-term sense. A good start in life will pay off, both in terms of human capital and economic development.

Discussion Points

- Describe the implications of SGA, IUGR and LBW on the current health and future nutritional status and health of individuals.
- Provide reasons for using stunting rather than underweight as a universal indicator for undernutrition.
- Discuss the importance and practical implications of regularly assessing children's length/height and weight, as opposed to just weight.
- How do growth standards differ from growth references?
- Why is growth considered the key nutritional indicator for children in low-income countries?
- How should anthropometric measures be used to determine the short-term and long-term impact of nutritional interventions?

References

1. World Health Organization. Physical status: the use and interpretation of anthropometry. Technical Report Series No. 854. Geneva, WHO; 1995.
2. WHO. Resolution WHA65.6. Maternal, infant and young child nutrition. In: Sixty-fifth World Health Assembly, Geneva, 21–26 May. Resolutions and decisions, annexes. World Health Organization: Geneva; 2012. (WHA65/2012/REC/1). http://apps.who.int/gb/ebwha/pdf_files/WHA65/A65_11-en.pdf. Accessed 7 May 2014.
3. de Onis M, Dewey KG, Borghi E, Onyango AW, Blössner M, Daelmans B, Piwoz E, Branca F. The World Health Organization's global target for reducing childhood stunting by 2025: rationale and proposed actions. Matern Child Nutr. 2013;9(Suppl. 2):6–26.
4. Victora CG, Adair L, Fall C, et al., for the maternal and child undernutrition study group. Maternal and child undernutrition: consequences for adult health and human capital. Lancet 2008;371:340–57.
5. Martorell R, Rivera J, Kaplowitz H, Pollitt E. Long-term consequences of growth retardation during early childhood. In: Hernandez M, Argente J, editors. Human growth: basic and clinical aspects. Amsterdam: Elsevier Science Publishers; 1992. p. 143–9.
6. Adair L.S., Fall C.H.D., Osmond C., Stein A.D., Martorell R., Ramirez-Zea M., et al. for the COHORTS Group. (2013) Associations of linear growth and relative weight gain during early life with adult health and human capital in countries of low and middle income: findings from five birth cohort studies. Lancet 2013;382:525–34.
7. Spurr GB. Physical activity and energy expenditure in undernutrition. Prog Food Nutr. 1990;14:139–92.
8. Black RE, Victora CG, Walker SP, Bhutta ZA, Christian P, de Onis M et al., and the Maternal and Child Nutrition Study Group. Maternal and child undernutrition and overweight in low-income and middle-income countries. Lancet 2013;382:427–51.
9. Administrative Committee on Coordination-Subcommittee on Nutrition (ACC-SCN). Nutrition and Poverty. Nutrition Policy Paper #16. Geneva: ACC-SCN; 1997.
10. Victora CG, de Onis M, Hallal PC, Blössner M, Shrimpton R. Worldwide timing of growth faltering: revisiting implications for interventions using the World Health Organization growth standards. Pediatrics. 2010;125: e473–80.
11. Martorell R, Kettel Khan L, Schroeder DG. Reversibility of stunting: epidemiological findings in children from developing countries. Eur J Clin Nutr. 1994;48(Suppl 1):S45–57.
12. Katz J, Lee ACC, Kozuki N, Lawn JE et al., and the CHERG Small-for-Gestational-Age-Preterm Birth Working Group. Mortality risk in preterm and small-for-gestational-age infants in low-income and middle-income countries: a pooled country analysis. Lancet 2013;382:417–25.
13. Liu L, Johnson HL, Cousens S, et al. Global, regional, and national causes of child mortality: an updated systematic analysis for 2010 with time trends since 2000. Lancet. 2012;379:2151–61.
14. de Onis M, Blössner M, Villar J. Levels and patterns of intrauterine growth retardation in developing countries. Eur J Clin Nutr. 1998;52(S1):S5–15.
15. Lee ACC, Katz J, Blencowe H et al., for the CHERG SGA-Preterm Birth Working Group. National and regional estimates of term and preterm babies born small for gestational age in 138 low-income and middle-income countries in 2010. Lancet Glob Health 2013;1:e26–36.
16. Villar J, Abalos E, Carroli G, et al. Heterogeneity of perinatal outcomes in the preterm delivery syndrome. Obstet Gynecol. 2004;104:78–87.
17. Kramer MS, Papageorghiou A, Culhane J, et al. Challenges in defining and classifying the preterm birth syndrome. Am J Obstet Gynecol. 2012;206:108–12.
18. WHO Multicentre Growth Reference Study Group. Assessment of differences in linear growth among populations in the WHO multicentre growth reference study. Acta Paediatr Suppl. 2006;450:56–65.
19. Bakketeig LS, Butte N, de Onis M, Kramer M, O'Donnell A, Prada JA, Hoffman HJ. Report of the IDECG Working Group on definitions, classifications, causes, mechanisms and prevention of IUGR. Eur J Clin Nutr. 1998;52(S1):S94–6.
20. Villar J, Knight HE, de Onis M, Bertino E, Gilli G, Papageorghiou AT, Ismail LC, Barros FC, Bhutta ZA. International Fetal and Newborn Growth Consortium (INTERGROWTH-21st). Conceptual issues related to the construction of prescriptive standards for the evaluation of postnatal growth of preterm infants. Arch Dis Child. 2010;95:1034–8.
21. Villar J, Altman DG, Purwar M, et al. The objectives, design and implementation of the INTERGROWTH-21st project. BJOG. 2013,120(Suppl 2).9–26.
22. Villar J, Cheikh Ismail L, Victora CG, Ohuma EO, Bertino E, Altman DG et al., for the International Fetal and Newborn Growth Consortium for the 21st Century (INTERGROWTH-21st). International standards for newborn weight, length, and head circumference by gestational age and sex: the Newborn Cross-Sectional Study of the INTERGROWTH-21st Project. Lancet 2014;384:857–68.

23. Papageorghiou AT, Ohuma EO, Altman DG, Todros T, Cheikh Ismael L, Lambert A, et al., for the International Fetal and Newborn Growth Consortium for the 21st Century (INTERGROWTH-21st). International standards for fetal growth based on serial ultrasound measurements: the Fetal Growth Longitudinal Study of the INTERGROWTH-21st Project. Lancet 2014;384:869–79.
24. Garza C, Borghi E, Onyango AW, de Onis M, for the WHO Multicentre Growth Reference Study Group. Parental height and child growth from birth to 2 years in the WHO multicentre growth reference study. Matern Child Nutr 2013;9(Suppl 2):58–68.
25. World Health Organization. Training course on child growth assessment. Geneva, World Health Organization; 2008. From: http://www.who.int/childgrowth/training/en/. Accessed 6 May 2014.
26. WHO. WHO child growth standards and the identification of severe acute malnutrition in infants and children. A joint statement by the World Health Organization and the United Nations Children's Fund, 2009. (http://www.who.int/nutrition/publications/severemalnutrition/9789241598163/en/index.html).
27. WHO. Updates on the management of severe acute malnutrition in infants and children. Geneva, World Health Organization; 2013.
28. de Onis M, Blössner M, Borghi B. Global prevalence and trends of overweight and obesity among preschool children. Am J Clin Nutr. 2010;92:1257–64.
29. Uauy R, Kain J. The epidemiological transition: need to incorporate obesity prevention into nutrition programmes. Public Health Nutr. 2002;5:223–9.
30. Lobstein T, Baur L, Uauy R. Obesity in children and young people: a crisis in public health. Obes Rev. 2004;5:4–104.
31. Dietz WH. Health consequences of obesity in youth: childhood predictors of adult disease. Pediatrics. 1998;101:518–25.
32. de Onis M, Wijnhoven TMA, Onyango AW. Worldwide practices in child growth monitoring. J Pediatr. 2004;144:461–5.
33. Frongillo EA Jr, de Onis M, Hanson KMP. Socioeconomic and demographic factors are associated with worldwide patterns of stunting and wasting of children. J Nutr. 1997;127:2302–9.
34. de Onis M, Blössner M, Borghi E. Prevalence and trends of stunting among preschool children, 1990–2020. Public Health Nutr. 2011;15:142–8.
35. United Nations Children's Fund, World Health Organization, The World Bank. UNICEF-WHO-The World Bank: 2012 Joint child malnutrition estimates - Levels and trends. UNICEF, New York; WHO, Geneva; The World Bank, Washington, DC; 2014. http://www.who.int/nutrition/publications/childgrowthstandards_estimates2011/en/.
36. Martorell R, Young MF. Patterns of stunting and wasting: potential explanatory factors. Adv Nutr. 2012;3:227–33.
37. World Health Organisation, World Food Programme, United Nations Standing Committee on Nutrition, United Nations Children's Fund. Community-based management of severe acute malnutrition, 2007 (http://www.who.int/nutrition/publications/severemalnutrition/9789280641479/en/index.html).
38. WHO: Multicentre Growth Reference Study Group. WHO Child Growth Standards: Length/Height-for-Age, Weight-for-Age, Weight-for-Length, Weight-for-Height and Body Mass Index-for-Age: Methods and Development. Geneva, WHO; 2006.
39. de Onis M, Onyango AW, Van den Broeck J, Cameron WC, Martorell R, for the WHO Multicentre Growth Reference Study Group. Measurement and standardization protocols for anthropometry used in the construction of a new international growth reference. Food and Nutrition Bulletin 2004;25 (Suppl 1):S27-S36.
40. de Onis M, Onyango AW, Borghi E, Garza C, Yang H and the WHO Multicentre Growth Reference Study Group. Comparison of the WHO Child Growth Standards and the NCHS/WHO international growth reference: implications for child health programmes. Public Health Nutr 2006;9:942–47.
41. de Onis M, Garza C, Onyango AW, Martorell R, editors. WHO Child Growth Standards. Acta Paediatr Suppl 2006;450:1–101.
42. Dibley MJ, Goldsby JB, Staehling NW, Trowbridge FL. Development of normalized curves for the international growth reference: historical and technical considerations. Am J Clin Nutr. 1987;46:736–48.
43. de Onis M, Yip R. The WHO growth chart: historical considerations and current scientific issues. Bibl Nutr Dieta. 1996;53:74–89.
44. de Onis M, Habicht JP. Anthropometric reference data for international use: recommendations from a World Health Organization Expert Committee. Am J Clin Nutr. 1996;64:650–8.
45. de Onis M, Garza C, Habicht JP. Time for a new growth reference. Pediatrics. 1997;100(5):E8.
46. WHO Working Group on Infant Growth. An evaluation of infant growth: the use and interpretation of anthropometry in infants. Bull World Health Organ. 1995;73:165–74.
47. Garza C, de Onis M. WHO multicentre growth reference study group: rationale for developing a new international growth reference. Food Nutr Bull. 2004;25(suppl 1):S5–14.

48. de Onis M, Garza C, Victora CG, Bhan MK, Norum KR, editors. WHO multicentre growth reference study (MGRS): rationale, planning and implementation. Food Nutr Bull 2004;25 (Suppl 1):S1–89.

49. Villar J, Papageorghiou AT, Pang R, Ohuma EO, Cheikh Ismail L, Barros FC, et al., for the International Fetal and Newborn Growth Consortium for the 21st Century (INTERGROWTH-21st). The likeness of fetal growth and newborn size across non-isolated populations in the INTERGROWTH-21st Project: the Fetal Growth Longitudinal Study and Newborn Cross-Sectional Study. Lancet Diab Endocrinol 2014; 2:781–92.

50. Rosenberg NA, Pritchard JK, Weber JL, et al. Genetic structure of human populations. Science. 2002;298:2381–5.

51. World Health Organization. WHO child growth standards: head circumference-for-age, arm circumference-for-age, triceps skinfold-for-age and subscapular skinfold-for-age: methods and development. Geneva: World Health Organization; 2007.

52. World Health Organization. WHO child growth standards: growth velocity based on weight, length and head circumference: methods and development. Geneva: World Health Organization; 2009.

53. WHO Multicentre Growth Reference Study Group. WHO motor development study: windows of achievement for six gross motor development milestones. Acta Paediatr. 2006;95(Suppl 450):86–95.

54. de Onis M, Onyango A, Borghi E, Siyam A, Blössner M, Lutter CK, for the WHO Multicentre Growth Reference Study Group. Worldwide implementation of the WHO child growth standards. Public Health Nutr 2012;15:1603–10.

55. de Onis M, Siyam A, Borghi E, Onyango AW, Piwoz E, Garza C. Comparison of the World Health Organization growth velocity standards with existing US reference data. Pediatrics. 2011;128:e18–26.

56. Dale NM, Grais RF, Minetti A, Miettola J, Barengo NC. Comparison of the new World Health Organization growth standards and the National Center for Health Statistics growth reference regarding mortality of malnourished children treated in a 2006 nutrition program in Niger. Arch Pediatr Adolesc Med. 2009;163:126–30.

57. Lapidus N, Luquero FJ, Gaboulaud V, Shepherd S, Grais RF. Prognostic accuracy of WHO growth standards to predict mortality in a large-scale nutritional program in Niger. PLoS Med. 2009;6:c1000039.

58. Vesel L, Bahl R, Martines J, Penny M, Bhandari N, Kirkwood BR and WHO Immunization-linked Vitamin A Supplementation Study Group. Use of new World Health Organization child growth standards to assess how infant malnutrition relates to breastfeeding and mortality. Bull World Health Organ 2010;88:39–48.

59. O'Neill S, Fitzgerald A, Briend A, Van den Broeck J. Child mortality as predicted by nutritional status and recent weight velocity in children under two in rural Africa. J Nutr. 2012;142:520–5.

60. Isanaka S, Villamor E, Shepherd S, Grais RF. Assessing the impact of the introduction of the World Health Organization growth standards and weight-for-height z-score criterion on the response to treatment of severe acute malnutrition in children: secondary data analysis. Pediatrics. 2009;123:e54–9.

61. Saha KK, Frongillo EA, Alam DS, Arifeen SE, Persson LA, Rasmussen KM. Use of the new World Health Organization child growth standards to describe longitudinal growth of breastfed rural Bangladeshi infants and young children. Food Nutr Bull. 2009;30:137–44.

62. Bois C, Servolin J, Guillermot G. Usage comparé des courbes de l'Organisation mondiale de la santé et des courbes françaises dans le suivi de la croissance pondérale des jeunes nourrissons. Arch Pediatr. 2010;17:1035–41.

63. Kerac M, Blencowe H, Grijalva-Eternod C, McGrath M, Shoham J, Cole TJ, Seal A. Prevalence of wasting among under 6-month-old infants in developing countries and implications of new case definitions using WHO growth standards: a secondary data analysis. Arch Dis Child. 2011;96:1008–13.

64. van Dijk CE, Innis SM. Growth-curve standards and the assessment of early excess weight gain in infancy. Pediatrics. 2009;123:102–8.

65. Maalouf-Manasseh Z, Metallinos-Katsaras E, Dewey KG. Obesity in preschool children is more prevalent and identified at a younger age when WHO growth charts are used compared with CDC charts. J Nutr. 2011;141:1154–8.

66. National Center for Health Statistics. 2000 CDC growth charts: United States. Available from: http://www.cdc.gov/growthcharts/. Accessed 26 Feb 2014.

67. Flegal KM, Wei R, Ogden CL, Freedman DS, Johnson CL, Curtin LR. Characterizing extreme values of body mass index-for-age by using the 2000 centers for disease control and prevention growth charts. Am J Clin Nutr. 2009;90:1314–20.

68. Cole TJ, Lobstein T. Extended international (IOTF) body mass index cut-offs for thinness, overweight and obesity. Pediatr Obes. 2012;7:284–94.

69. Khadilkar VV, Khadilkar AV, Cole TJ, Sayyad MG. Cross sectional growth curves for height, weight and body mass index for affluent Indian children, 2007. Indian Pediatr. 2009;46:477–89.

70. Carrascosa A, Fernández JM, Fernández C, Ferrández A, López-Siguero JP, Rueda C, Sánchez E, Sobradillo B, Yeste D. Estudio Transversal Español de Crecimiento 2008: II. Valores de talla, peso e índice de masa corporal in

32.064 sujetos (16.607 varones, 15.457 mujeres) desde el nacimiento hasta alcanzar la talla adulta. An Pediatr (Bar) 2008;68:552–69.

71. de Onis M. The use of anthropometry in the prevention of childhood overweight and obesity. Int J Obes. 2004;28: S81–5.

72. de Onis M. Growth curves for school-age children and adolescents. Indian Pediatr. 2009;46:463–5.

73. Butte NF, Garza C, de Onis M. Evaluation of the feasibility of international growth standards for school-aged children and adolescents. J Nutr. 2007;137:153–7.

74. Turck D, Michaelsen KF, Shamir R, Braegger C, Campoy C, Colomb V, Decsi T, Domellöf M, Fewtrell M, Kolacek S, Mihatsch W, Moreno LA, van Goudoever J. World Health Organization 2006 child growth standards and 2007 growth reference charts: a discussion paper by the committee on Nutrition of the European Society for Paediatric Gastroenterology, Hepatology, and Nutrition. J Pediatr Gastroenterol Nutr. 2013;57:258–64.

75. Butte NF and Garza C, editors. Development of an international growth standard for preadolescent and adolescent children. Food Nutr Bull 2006;27(suppl):S169–326.

76. de Onis M, Onyango AW, Borghi E, Siyam A, Nishida C, Siekmann J. Development of a WHO growth reference for school-aged children and adolescents. Bull World Health Organ. 2007;85:660–7.

77. WHO AnthroPlus for personal computers Manual: Software for assessing growth of the world's children and adolescents. Geneva, World Health Organization, 2009. From: http://www.who.int/growthref/tools/. Accessed 26 Feb 2014.

78. Courbes de croissance validées par la Société suisse de pédiatrie. Kinderspital Zürich, 2014.

79. WHO European Regional Office. Country profiles on nutrition, physical activity and obesity in the 53 WHO European Region Member States. Copenhagen: WHO Regional Office for Europe; 2014.

80. Yip R, Scalon K. The burden of malnutrition: a population perspective. J Nutr. 1994;124:2043S–6S.

81. de Onis M. Measuring nutritional status in relation to mortality. Bull World Health Organ. 2000;78:1271–4.

82. Gorstein J, Sullivan K, Yip R, de Onis M, Trowbridge F, Fajans P, et al. Issues in the assessment of nutritional status using anthropometry. Bull World Health Organ. 1994;72:273–83.

83. Villar J, de Onis M, Kestler E, Bolaños F, Cerezo R, Berendes H. The differential neonatal morbidity of the intrauterine growth retardation syndrome. Am J Obstet Gynecol. 1990;163:151–7.

84. Williams RL, Creasy RK, Cunningham GC, Hawes WE, Norris FD, Tashiro M. Fetal growth and perinatal viability in California. Obstet Gynecol. 1982;59:624–32.

85. Balcazar H, Haas JD. Retarded fetal growth patterns and early neonatal mortality in a Mexico city population. Bull Pan Am Health Organ. 1991;25:55–63.

86. Øyen N, Skjaerven R, Little R, Wilcot A. Fetal growth retardation in Sudden Infant Death Syndrome (SIDS) babies and their siblings. Am J Epidemiol. 1995;142:84–90.

87. Ashworth A. Effects of intrauterine growth retardation on mortality and morbidity in infants and young children. Eur J Clin Nutr. 1998;52(S1):S34–42.

88. Paz I, Gale R, Laor A, Danon YL, Stevenson DK, Seidman DS. The cognitive outcome of full term small for gestational age infants at late adolescence. Obstet Gynecol. 1995;85:452–6.

89. Low J, Handley-Derry M, Burke S, et al. Association of intrauterine fetal growth retardation and learning deficits at age 9 to 11 years. Am J Obstet Gynecol. 1992;167:1499–505.

90. Parkinson CE, Wallis S, Harvey DR. School achievement and behaviour of children who are small-for-dates at birth. Dev Med Child Neurol. 1981;23:41–50.

91. Taylor DJ, Howie PW. Fetal growth achievement and neurodevelopmental disability. Br J Obstet Gynaecol. 1989;96:789–94.

92. Villar J, Smeriglio V, Martorell R, Brown CH, Klein RE. Heterogenous growth and mental development of intrauterine growth-retarded infants during the first three years of life. Pediatrics. 1984;74:783–91.

93. Osmond C, Barker DJ, Winter PD, Fall CH, Simmonds SJ. Early growth and death from cardiovascular disease in women. BMJ. 1993;307:1519–24.

94. Williams S, George I, Silva P. Intrauterine growth retardation and blood pressure at age seven and eighteen. J Clin Epidemiol. 1992;45:1257–63.

95. Barker DJP. The intrauterine origins of cardiovascular and obstructive lung disease in adult life: The Mark Daniels lecture 1990. J R Coll Phys Lond. 1991;25:129–33.

96. Hales CN, Barker DJ, Clark PM, et al. Fetal and infant growth and impaired glucose tolerance at age 64. BMJ. 1991;303:1019–22.

97. Barker DJ, Martyn CN, Osmond C, Hales CN, Fall CH. Growth in utero and serum cholesterol concentrations in adult life. BMJ. 1993;307:1524–7.

98. Hinchliffe SA, Lynch MR, Sargent PH, Howard CV, Van Velzen D. The effect of intrauterine growth retardation on the development of renal nephrons. Br J Obstet Gynaecol. 1992;99:296–301.

99. Pelletier D, Frongillo EA, Habicht JP. Epidemiologic evidence for a potentiating effect of malnutrition on child mortality. Am J Public Health. 1993;83:1130–3.

100. Caulfield LE, de Onis M, Blössner M, Black RE. Undernutrition as an underlying cause of child deaths associated with diarrhea, pneumonia, malaria, and measles. Am J Clin Nutr. 2004;80:193–8.

101. Black RE, Allen LH, Bhutta ZA, Caulfield LE, de Onis M, Ezzati M, Mathers C, Rivera J, for the Maternal and Child Undernutrition Study Group. Maternal and child undernutrition: global and regional exposures and health consequences. Lancet 2008;371:243–60.

102. Tomkins A, Watson F. Malnutrition and infection: a review. ACC/SCN State-of-the-Art Series, Nutrition Policy Discussion Paper No. 5. Geneva: Administrative Committee on Coordination/Subcommittee on Nutrition; 1989.

103. Man WDC, Weber M, Palmer A, Schneider G, Wadda R, Jaffar S, Mulholland EK, Greenwood BM. Nutritional status of children admitted to hospital with different diseases and its relationship to outcome in The Gambia, West Africa. Trop Med Int Health. 1998;3:1–9.

104. Victora CG, Fuchs SC, Flores A, Fonseca W, Kirkwood BR. Risk factors for pneumonia in a Brazilian metropolitan area. Pediatrics. 1994;93(6 Pt 1):977–85.

105. Klebanoff MA, Yip R. Influence of maternal birth weight on rate of fetal growth and duration of gestation. J Pediatr. 1987;111:287–92.

106. Binkin NJ, Yip R, Fleshood L, Trowbridge FL. Birthweight and childhood growth. Pediatrics. 1988;82:828–34.

107. Bhutta ZA, Das JK, Rizvi A, Gaffey MF, Walker N, Horton S, Webb P, Lartey A, Black RE. Lancet nutrition interventions review group; maternal and child nutrition study group. Evidence-based interventions for improvement of maternal and child nutrition: what can be done and at what cost? Lancet. 2013;382:452–77.

108. Prentice AM, Ward KA, Goldberg GR, Jarjou LM, Moore SE, Fulford AJ, et al. Critical windows for nutritional interventions against stunting. Am J Clin Nutr. 2013;97:911–8. doi:10.3945/ajcn.112.052332.

109. Ruel MT, Alderman H, and the Maternal and Child Nutrition Study Group. Nutrition-sensitive interventions and programmes: how can they help to accelerate progress in improving maternal and child nutrition? Lancet; 2013. Published online June 6, doi:10.1016/S0140-6736(13)60937-X.

Chapter 7
Overweight and Obesity

Colleen M. Doak and Barry M. Popkin

Keywords Nutrition transition · Obesity · Overweight · BMI · Trends

Learning Objectives

- To show the prevalence of adult overweight and obesity in low and middle income countries by region.
- To document the trends in increasing (or decreasing) overweight and obesity prevalence in low and middle income countries by region.
- Within each of the regions, to compare urban versus rural differences in overweight and obesity prevalence in low and middle income countries.
- Within each region, to compare the gender differences prevalence and trends of overweight and obesity prevalence in lower and middle income countries.
- To look for subregional patterns in order to identify the geographic areas of high and/or rapidly emerging overweight and obesity prevalences.

Introduction

The last century witnessed a remarkable change in patterns of disease. The control of infectious disease, together with changing life styles, led to longer life expectancies and the emergence of chronic disease as a primary cause of death. This change from infectious to chronic disease, first described by Omran [1] is known as the epidemiologic transition. However, as a result of the occurrence of HIV and related drug resistant infections some countries have witnessed a reversal in the expected trends [2]. In spite of HIV and related rises in the prevalences of infectious disease, obesity and chronic disease prevalences are still emerging at an accelerated rate in many developing

C.M. Doak (✉)
Department of Health Sciences, VU University, De Boelelaan 1083, W&N Building,
Room U-437, 1081 HV Amsterdam, The Netherlands
e-mail: c.m.doak@vu.nl

B.M. Popkin
Department of Nutrition, University of North Carolina at Chapel Hill, Carolina Population Center,
CB # 8120 University Square, Chapel Hill, NC 27516-3997, USA
e-mail: popkin@unc.edu

© Springer Science+Business Media New York 2017   143
S. de Pee et al. (eds.), *Nutrition and Health in a Developing World*,
Nutrition and Health, DOI 10.1007/978-3-319-43739-2_7

countries [3–5]. In 2005, prevalences of overweight/obesity exceeded undernutrition in a majority of 37 developing countries studied in both urban and rural areas [6]. Popkin and Slining [7] showed continuing rapid increase in overweight prevalence even in recent years in spite of a global food and economic crisis [7].

The high prevalence of overweight and obesity in developing countries are a result of continued changes to lifestyle patterns, such as diet and physical activity, leading to an accelerated increase in overweight, obesity, and related chronic diseases in many countries. This transition in diet and physical activity patterns, associated with an energy dense diet and a sedentary lifestyle, has been described as the nutrition transition [8]. The nutrition transition as a global phenomenon has been documented including the industrialized nations of Europe and North America as well as lower and middle income countries of Asia, Latin America, the Caribbean, Africa, and the Middle East [9]. Previously, we reported on data based on adults available from a number of countries in each region of the world [4, 10]. Elsewhere, we show that there are equally important concerns of overweight and obesity emerging among children and adolescents in lower income countries. However, we focus our attention here on adults due to the methodological issues of documenting adolescent trends in overweight and obesity. Namely, in adolescents overweight and obesity, as measured by BMI, are influenced by population differences in height and maturation [11]. Thus, in comparing countries over time, it is difficult to disentangle emerging overweight and obesity trends from documented population changes in growth (height) and maturation.

Before the global food and economic crises, trends showed an accelerated obesity prevalence emerging in even more countries. Those earlier results showed that, in low income countries experiencing the nutrition transition, obesity is usually observed first in urban areas and in the high income, elite. Urban lifestyles were also related to diet and activity patterns associated with the nutrition transition, contributing further to obesity [6]. Although the urban elite are usually the first to experience obesity, the epidemic is also shifting to the middle and lower classes. Previous articles by Monteiro et al. [12–14] show that as GNP increases, the burden of obesity tends to shift toward lower socioeconomic groups.

The shift of the burden of obesity toward the poor is also accompanied by different risks by age and gender. Low income women are at greater risk than low income men at lower levels of economic development [12]. Other studies also show high prevalences of overweight/obesity in women, even in communities where there are also high prevalences of undernutrition for children [15]. Detailed analysis comparing the obesity trends in multiple countries shows a pattern in which adults experience higher absolute increases in the rates of obesity as compared to children [16]. Further evidence for differences in obesity risk is illustrated by studies showing overweight/obese adults clustering together with undernourished children [17, 18].

In the next section, we outline the methods used in this chapter. Large nationwide surveys are used for determining trends in obesity prevalence. Then we focus briefly on some of the public health effects related to the ongoing epidemic of overweight and obesity.

Methods

Measures

Body mass index (BMI) is the standard measure of overweight and obesity status used in large-scale surveys of nutritional status in adults. The World Health Organization cutoffs for adults are used to delineate obesity: less than 18.5 for thinness (chronic energy deficiency), 18.5–24.99 for normal,

25.0–29.99 for overweight Grade I, 30.0–39.99 for overweight Grade II, and 40.0 and above for overweight Grade III [19]. For this chapter, Grades II and III are combined and due to limitations of space the prevalences of underweight and normal weight will not be included in figures and tables.

Survey Design and Sample

Results are updated from the previous edition [17] with new data from Popkin [7] Jones-Smith et al. [20–23] and Ng et al. [24]. Results reported here are based on data from published surveys conducted in low and middle income countries. We focus mainly on large representative samples of adults used in the previous edition, adding in information from publications comparing overweight and obesity prevalences globally by region. Our selection criteria for presenting data from other surveys were size, sampling design, and geographic area. If a study were representative of a region or country, it was always used. If it came from a country with few studies and did not fit our criteria of national representativeness, we used it if the sample size were large and it seemed reasonably representative of the population being sampled. We are now at a point where the Demographic Health Surveys (DHS) surveys have been repeated in many countries and in other countries additional nationally representative surveys exist, in many instances with multiple survey years. Thus, since the previous edition, numerous additional surveys have been added and publications with trends data are available. Thus, we are able to focus in depth on trends using existing published data. Regional comparisons are made based on nationally representative surveys of women aged 19–49 of overweight (BMI ≥ 25), with data weighted by each country's population. Additional publications will be selected based on their inclusion of results from both males and females. This additional process will ensure comparisons of the prevalence of overweight and above in men and in women and also gender differences in the comparisons of trends by region and over time [7].

Comparative Approach

Given the quantity and quality of information available for adult females, we will first explore differences of overweight and above in adult females, by region. Additionally, the results will be further stratified by urban and rural residence to confirm whether the prevalences are higher in urban areas, as is expected. Next, results will show overweight and above prevalences stratified by urban and rural residence to clarify whether regional patterns observed for national prevalences remain true for both urban and rural areas. Finally, available trends data will be shown to identify countries and regions with the most rapidly increasing trends in overweight and obesity.

Ideally, we would use the same approach for males as taken for females, however, regional results for males [24] are reported broken into smaller subregions than the results reported for females [7]. Using this information, we will first clarify subregional patterns by making use of the different definitions used for identifying and classifying global regions. Next, the results for males and females will be used to clarify gender differences by region [24]. Thus analysis will focus on prevalences for males in comparison to the females, to first identify whether there are gender differences in overweight and obesity prevalences by region. More specifically, gender differences will be explored to clarify the regional patterns in adult males vis-à-vis those found in adult females. These results also include information separately for obesity and/or stratified by urban and rural residence. These data will be shown where possible, to clarify the patterns and trends of overweight and obesity in men and women living in low and middle income countries.

Results

Elsewhere, we present some information on comparable trends in higher income countries [10]. This chapter focuses on lower income countries.

The Prevalence in Lower and Middle Income Countries

Prevalence

Figure 7.1 shows regional comparisons of female overweight (Grade I and above) using nationally representative surveys. The highest prevalences of overweight and above occur in the Middle East and North Africa Latin America and the Caribbean and in Central Asia. In contrast, countries in South Asia and sub-Saharan Africa have the lowest prevalences for overweight and obesity. Figure 7.2 shows these same regional comparisons, stratified by urban and rural residency, showing identical regional patterns in both urban and rural areas.

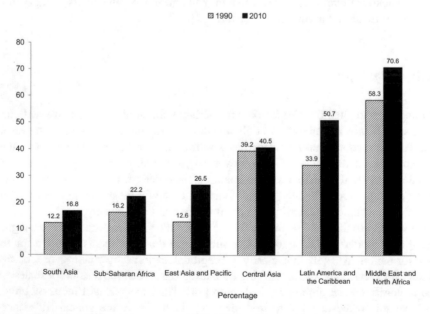

Fig. 7.1 Female % overweight by region across, 1990–2010* (*Data are weighted by each country's population. Based on nationally representative surveys of women aged 19–49 ($n = 815,609$). Overweight BMI ≥ 25. Data from the year closest to 1990 and 2010 for each country)

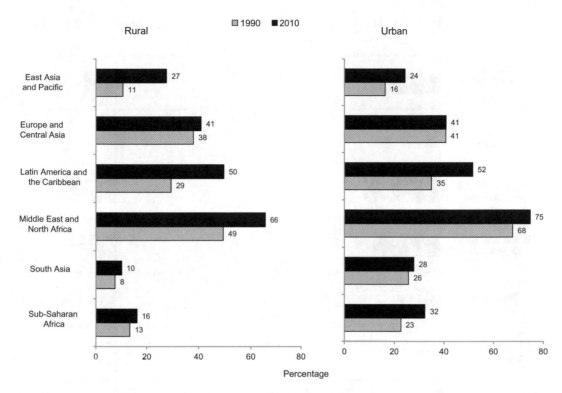

Fig. 7.2 Trends in female % overweight by region, 1990–2010* (*Data are weighted by each country's population. Based on nationally representative surveys of women aged 19–49 ($n = 815,609$). Overweight BMI $\geq$ 25. Data from the year closest to 1990 and 2010 for each country)

Obesity Trends in Lower and Middle Income Countries

We have excellent data on trends in overweight in women, these trends are shown by region in Fig. 7.3. These results show increasing prevalences in overweight and above in all regions except for Europe and Central Asia, in which there is a very small reduction of 0.1% per year. Figure 7.4 shows the results per country and organized according to country GDP and stratified by urban and rural residence. Overall there is a pattern of increasing overweight and above both in urban and in rural areas, with the notable exceptions of Kazakhastan and rural Nigeria. Smaller reductions in overweight and obesity are also seen in Losotho (both urban and rural), in urban Morocco and Senegal, and in rural Mozambique.

Figure 7.5 shows the regional prevalences of overweight and obesity separately for males and females. These results are based on national surveys for 2013 and are age standardized and are organized by regional classifications that are different from the definitions shown in Figs. 7.1, 7.2, 7.3, and 7.4. In all regions, except for East Asia, females have a higher prevalence of overweight and above (BMI $\geq$ 25) than males. Even in East Asia the prevalence of overweight in males is not substantially different. However, the regional comparisons in Fig. 7.5 show that, in spite of the gender differences, both male and females have the highest prevalence of overweight and above (BMI $\geq$ 25) in North Africa and the Middle East followed by Eastern Europe and Central Asia. However, gender

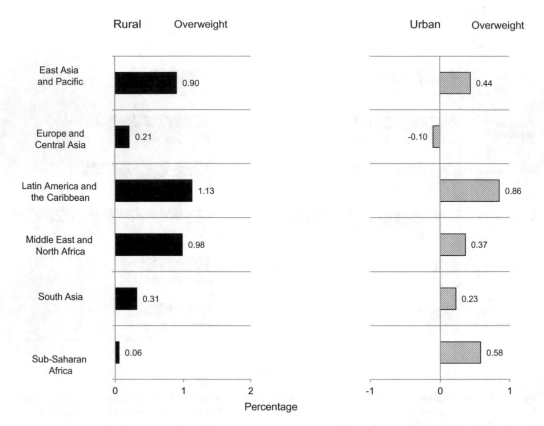

Fig. 7.3 Urban/rural comparisons: Female % overweight, annualized change regional population-weighted percent—1990s–2000s* (*Data are weighted by each country's population. Based on nationally representative surveys of women aged 19–49 (n = 815,609). Overweight is BMI ≥ 25. Data from the year closest to 1990 and 2010 for each country)

differences contribute to diverging patterns for regional comparisons for two regions, namely Southern sub-Saharan Africa and Andean Latin America. In these regions, female overweight and obesity is as high or even higher than in North Africa although for males it is substantially (>20% difference in prevalence) different. In both of these regions, the 95% confidence intervals for the regional prevalences reported by Ng et al. [24] show that the lower prevalence found males is statistically (p < 0.05) lower than that of females.

In addition to gender comparisons, Fig. 7.5 provides information on subregional definitions, allowing for identification of subregions where overweight/obesity is highest. In the broader region of Asia, it is Central Asia where the overweight and above prevalence is highest, and exceeds 50% for males and females alike. Although most European countries are not shown, the prevalence of overweight and above in Eastern Europe is also high, again exceeding 50% for males as well as females. In North Africa and the Middle East the prevalence of overweight and above is high, exceeding 50% for both males and females. By contrast, in sub-Saharan Africa, it is only in females of the Southern sub-Saharan Africa region where overweight and obesity prevalence exceeds 50%. The subregional classifications for Latin America and the Caribbean are particularly illuminating given the gender differences. In both males and females, Central Latin America shows high regional

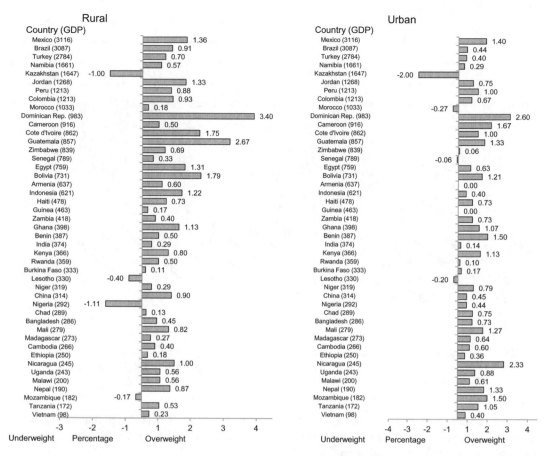

Fig. 7.4 By GNP: Annualized change in female % overweight, 1990s–2000s* (*Based on nationally representative surveys of women aged 19–49 (*n* = 815,609). Overweight is BMI ≥ 25. Data from the year closest to 1990 and 2010 for each country)

prevalences for overweight and above. However, the highest prevalence is in Andean Latin America for females but in Southern Latin America in males.

Table 7.1 shows the results for larger surveys with data available for males as well as females. Results are stratified by urban and rural residence where possible. The results from figures and tables show in most countries prevalences of overweight and obesity is less in men than it is in women [15, 25–47]. However, it is important to note that in some countries the gender differences deviate when separately considering overweight grades I versus II and III. For example, in Table 7.1, Malaysian females have lower prevalences of grade I, but a higher prevalence of grade II and III. In Kuwait, the pattern is the opposite, in which females show higher prevalences of obesity (grades II and III overweight) but lower prevalences of grade I overweight. However, in most regions the highest prevalences for overweight (grade I) and obesity (grade II and III overweight) occur in females. Table 7.1 also shows that these patterns hold true after stratification by urban and rural residence.

Table 7.2 shows the results for countries with surveys collected over multiple time points, to show trends reported from 2005 and earlier. These data show that obesity and overweight have been

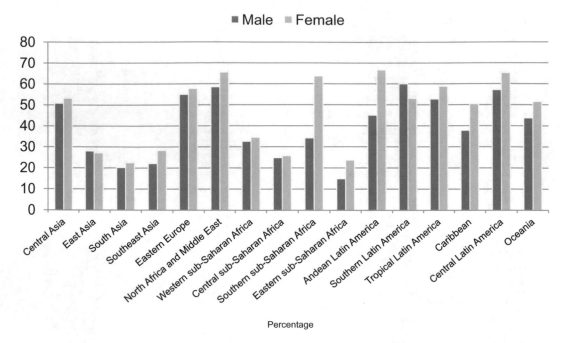

Fig. 7.5 % overweight and obese by region, males versus females (Data are weighted by each country's population. Based on nationally representative surveys of women aged 19–49 (*n* = 815,609). Overweight is BMI ≥ 25. Data from the year closest to 1990 and 2010 for each country)

increasing in nearly all regions. The trends shown here are consistent with the reported results shown in Fig. 7.3. These results show increasing overweight prevalences for both overweight and obesity in males as well as females for all countries.

Implications for Public Health

The obesity epidemic is linked with rapid shifts in adult-onset diabetes and many other noncommunicable diseases [48]. Adult-onset diabetes and many other comorbidities of obesity are increasing rapidly in many lower income countries [49, 50]. The most relevant comorbidities are hypertension, dyslipidemia, and atherosclerosis. The epidemiological prevalence data are spotty but indicate serious and high levels of these conditions, in particular adult-onset diabetes. A study from 1997 provided a strong basis for linking diet, activity, and body composition trends discussed above to increased rates of prevalence for several types of cancer [51].

A clear literature has shown that in terms of mechanisms and epidemiology, obesity and activity are closely linked to adult-onset diabetes. Several reviews lay out the case for these factors. Zimmet and his colleagues [34, 49, 52, 53] have been particularly earnest in exploring these issues at the population level in lower income and transitional societies. Some basic characteristics of adult-onset diabetes may provide a clear basis for linking key components of the nutrition transition—increases in obesity and reductions in activity—to the rapid increases in adult-onset diabetes in lower income countries.

Table 7.1 Obesity patterns in lower and middle income countries (Adults and studies with large sample size)

Country	Year	Sample (n)	Overweight/obesity criteria		% Overweight or obese		
			Criteria	Age group	Males	Females	Total
L. America							
Brazil [25]	2003	59,204	≥25	≥18	38.2	38.1	38.1
Mexico [26]	1995	2042 (U)	≥25	≥18	50.0	58.0	–
Caribbean							
Cuba [27]	1982	30,063	≥25	20–59	31.5	39.4	36.4
	1982	20,539 (U)	≥25	20–59	36.0	41.8	39.7
	1982	9513 (R)	≥25	20–59	22.6	33.9	29.4
Asia							
China [28]	1992	54,006	≥25	>20 years	11.9	17.0	14.6
	1992	18,472 (U)	≥25	>20 years	20.8	25.1	23.1
	1992	35,534 (R)	≥25	>20 years	7.4	12.7	10.2
China [25]	2000	4722	≥25	≥18	22.1	24.6	23.4
China	2000	4046	≥25	20–45	20.2	19.3	–
India [29]	1989	1784 (U)	≥25	15–76	36.9	44.1	40.9
Indonesia [25]	2000	22,725	≥25	≥18	11.4	22.1	17.0
Kyrgy Republic	1993	4053	≥30	18–59	4.2	10.7	–
	1993	4053	25–<30	18–59	26.4	24.3	–
Malaysia [30]	1990	4747	25–30	18–64	24.0	18.1	21.4
	1990	4747	≥30	18–64	4.7	7.9	6.1
Philippines [31]	1993	9585	≥30	20 years	1.7	3.4	–
	1993	9585	25–30	20 years	11.0	11.8	–
Thailand [32]	1985	3495 (U)	≥25	35–54	25.5	21.4	24.6
	1985	3495 (U)	≥30	35–54	2.2	3.0	2.4
West Pacific							
Fiji, Fijians [33]	1993	1190	≥27	>18	26.6	47.4	37.8
Fiji, Fijians [33]	1993	1226	≥25	>18	18	33.9	25.9
Nauru [34]	1994	1344	≥30	25–69	80.2	78.6	79.4
New Caledonia [35]	1992–94	6503 (R)	25 (F) 27 (69)	30–59	44.6	71.4	59.0
	1992–94	641 (U)	≥25 (F) ≥27 (69)	30–59	59.1	79.6	72.7
American Samoa [36]	1994	345	>25	25–58	63.8	96.9	83.5
	–	–	>30	25–58	45.9	87.8	70.8
Western Samoa [36]	1995	475	>25	25–58	83.8	92.2	88.2
	–	–	>30	25–58	37.1	66.2	52.2
Tonga [37]	1986	654	>32 (69) >30 (F)	20–49	10	39.1	–
	–	–	>26 (69) >24 (F)	20–49	47.6	77.9	–
No. Africa/Mid East							
Bahrain [38]	1991/2	290	>30	>20	26.3	29.4	27.9
Egypt [39]	1983–85	433 (R)	NCHS OB	15–74	6.8	10.1	9.0
Egypt [39]	1983–85	433 (R)	NCHS OVE	15–74	12.9	25.1	21.0
Jordan [40]	1994–6	2836	>30	>25 years	32.7	59.8	49.7
Kuwait [41]	1993–94	3435	>30	18	32.3	40.6	36.4
	1993–94	3435	>25–30	18	35.2	32.3	33.8

(continued)

Table 7.1 (continued)

Country	Year	Sample (n)	Overweight/obesity criteria		% Overweight or obese		
			Criteria	Age group	Males	Females	Total
Saudi Arabia [42]	1996	13,177	>30	15–95	16.0	24.0	19.8
	1996	13,177	25–30	15–95	29.0	27.0	28.0
Tunisia [43]	1990	8611	>30	Adults	2.4	8.3	5.3
	1990	8611	25	Adults	20.0	32.7	26.3
Sub-Sahara Africa							
South Africa [44]	1979	7187	>30	15–64	14.7	18.0	16.5
	1979	7187	25–30 (M) 24–30 (F)	15–64	41.9	38.8	40.3
South Africa [15]	1990	986 (Bl)	30	15–64	7.9	44.4	28.0
Mauritius [34]	1992	5111	>30	25–74	5.3	15.1	10.6
	1992	5111	>25	25–74	35.7	47.7	42.2

BL Black; *U* Urban; *R* Rural

Obesity

It is clear that obesity, and more particularly, the upper-body distribution of body fat, is a key parameter in the etiology of adult-onset diabetes. A vast literature has shown significant direct obesity relationships with adult-onset diabetes and animal studies support this relationship. The work on abdominal obesity and its effects is more recent but appears to be promising in explaining more precisely the role that body composition plays. In addition, there is a strong relationship between weight gain and risk of developing diabetes. The odds of getting diabetes are considerable with a weight gain of 5–8 kg for adults and the strength of association is even higher with greater weight gain [54].

Physical Activity

It is understood that exercise may help to prevent adult-onset diabetes in an obese patient. Exercise may offset the hyper-insulinemia that is associated with obesity and reduces the likelihood that a person will display the signs that allow him/her to be categorized as having adult-onset diabetes, after controlling for a given level of obesity. Because exercise is associated with lower insulin levels, it may help to offset (or prevent) the hyper-insulinemia which is common among obese persons, and consequentially the development of insulin resistance. Zimmet [52] reviews these relationships and notes other critical studies on this topic.

Interactions of Obesity and Activity

Physical activity and obesity have independent effects on serum insulin, but together they interact such that the impact of physical activity differs according to the level of obesity. For example studies show that for each level of BMI or waist–hip ratio, there is a different effect of physical activity on serum insulin level.

Table 7.2 Obesity trends among adults in lower and middle income countries

Country	Year	Sample (*n*)	Obesity Criteria	% obese Males	Females	Total
South America						
Brazil [25]	1975	88,625	≥25	15.7	24.0	20.0
	1989	13,350	≥25	25.7	39.5	31.8
	2003	59,204	≥25	38.2	38.1	38.1
Brazil [45]	1974/75	94,699	25	19.6	27.2	23.5
	1989	23,544	25	31.1	50.8	38.9
	1996	3179	25	–	35.8	–
Brazil [45]	1974/75	94,699	25–29.99	16.8	20.1	18.5
Brazil [45]	1989	23,544	25–29.99	24.9	37.6	29.9
Brazil [46]	1974	94,699	>30	3.1	8.2	5.7
	1989	23,544	>30	5.9	13.3	9.6
Mexico [26]	1995	2042 (U)	25–<30	39.0	35.0	–
	1996	203 (R)	25–<30	20.0	26.0	–
Mexico [26]	1988	19,022	>27	–	15.0	–
	1995	2042 (U)	>30	11.0	23.0	–
	1996	203 (R)	>30	4.0	19.0	–
South Pacific						
Nauru [47]	1975/76	–	>30	63.2	72.4	–
	1982	–	>30	70.7	75.8	–
Nauru [47]	1987	–	>30	67.2	69.8	–
	1994	1344	>30	80.2	78.6	79.4
Rural W. Samoa [47]	1978	745	>30	18.7	37.9	29.7
	1991	960	>30	34.8	52.1	44.1
Urban W. Samoa [47]	1978	744	>30	38.2	60.3	50.0
	1991	769	>30	48.4	72.1	61.9
Fiji (Ethnic Fijian) [33]	1958–70	1947	≥26	34.7	57.8	46.7
	1980	–	≥25	32	64	49
	1993	–	≥27	26.8	47.4	37.8
	1993	–	≥25	–	64.4	46.9
Fiji (Ethnic Indian) [33]	1958–70	485	≥26	3.6	22.1	14.4
	1980	1288	≥27 (≥25 M)	11	38	26
	1993	1226	≥27	9	–	21.4
	1993	1226	≥25	18	33.9	25.9
American Samoa, age 25–39 [36]	1990	–	>25	98.4	94.4	–
	1994	–	>25	100	95.7	–
	1990	–	>30	76.6	78.7	–
	1994	–	>30	80.3	86.1	–
American Samoa, age 40–58 [36]	1990	–	>25	97.9	95.7	–
	1994	–	>25	97.5	97.8	–
Western Samoa, age 25–39 [36]	1991	–	>25	88	87.3	–
	1995		≥25	84.9	89	
Western Samoa, age 40–58 [36]	1991	–	>25	83.9	93.6	–
	1995	–	>25	82.5	95.8	–

(continued)

Table 7.2 (continued)

Country	Year	Sample (*n*)	Obesity Criteria	% obese Males	Females	Total
Asia						
China [25]	1991	8680	≥25	10.3	15.2	12.9
	2000	9570	≥25	22.1	24.6	2304
China	1989	5056	25–30	5.9	10.3	8.2
	1991	5353	25–30	9.5	11.4	9.5
	1993	4920	25–30	8.3	11.3	9.9
	1989	5056	>30	0.3	0.6	0.5
	1991	5353	>30	0.5	0.8	0.7
	1993	4920	>30	0.7	0.7	0.7
Indonesia [25]	1993	13,827	≥25	7.9	15.3	12.0
	2000	22,725	≥25	11.4	22.1	17.0
Vietnam [25]	1992	6545	≥25	1.0	2.2	1.6
	1997	16,270	≥25	2.9	5.4	4.3
	2002	92,484	≥25	4.3	6.5	5.5
Africa						
Mauritius (32)	1987	5021	<25–30	22.7	27.5	25.2
	1992	5111	<25–30	30.4	32.6	31.6
	1987	5021	>30	3.4	10.4	7.1
	1992	5111	>30	5.3	15.1	10.6
Europe						
Russia	9/1992	7305	30–45	8.4	23.2	–
	2/1993	9058	30–45	9.7	25.8	–
	8/1993	9238	30–45	9.2	25.7	–
	11/1993	8278	30–45	10.0	25.7	–
	12/1994	6967	30–45	9.5	26.6	–
	10/1995	6528	30–45	9.3	27.2	–
	10/1996	6231	30–45	10.8	27.9	–
	9/1992	7305	25–30	33.5	33.1	–
	2/1993	9058	25–30	34.4	32.5	–
	8/1993	9238	25–30	34.1	32.6	–
	11/1993	8278	25–30	34.4	32.2	–
	12/1994	6967	25–30	35.4	31.6	–
	10/1995	6528	25–30	31.8	31.4	–
	10/1996	6231	25–30	33.4	30.5	–
	2004	7077	≥25	47.4	58.4	53.4

Genetic Component

Zimmet and others who have focused on this issue as it relates to lower income countries have suggested that the highest genetic susceptibility for adult-onset diabetes was for Pacific Islanders, American Indians, Mexican Americans and other Hispanics, and Asian Indians [52]. Those with modest genetic susceptibility include Africans, Japanese, and Chinese. McGarvey et al. [36, 55] and O'Dea et al. [56] have thoroughly explored the same issues among Australian Aborigines and other South Pacific groups and have provided careful documentation of this linkage of the nutrition transition with adult-onset diabetes.

Research and Policy Implications

It is clear that the nutrition transition is closely linked with rapid increases in obesity. It is also clear that there is great potential for serious adverse public health consequences from the nutrition transition and the resultant large increase in obesity. These trends in obesity are not limited to one region, country, or racial/ethnic grouping. The overall levels that we find in selected countries such as Mexico, Brazil, Egypt, South Africa, China, Malaysia, and most nations from both the Middle East and the Western Pacific are indicative of major public health problems. These changes appear to be occurring across many countries which underscores the urgent need to better understand the underlying environmental causes. International studies can help to better understand the cultural, environmental, and behavioral determinants that contribute to the universal trends towards rising overweight and obesity.

Clearly excess body fat develops when dietary energy intake exceeds energy expenditure. Excess energy intake and insufficient physical activity are major direct determinants of energy imbalance. Diet and activity patterns have shifted in comparable ways in many countries and as such, diet and activity may contribute to the obesity epidemic in a similar way across all populations. Other contributors, such as metabolic differences, inactivity, and macronutrient composition such as percentage energy from fat, are unknown [57]. Clearly diet and activity do contribute to overweight and obesity as shown by longitudinal studies in lower income countries [58–61]. Although there will be large differences in the underlying socioeconomic and behavioral factors related to obesity in each country, the policies and programs that alter these patterns may be best understood by examining settings around the world.

There is a major new shift in the way low and middle income countries are addressing the rapid increases in obesity and the related changes in the structure of diet and activity. The proceedings of a Bellagio 2013 conference on large-scale regulatory and other efforts to address global obesity, focusing on food system changes, highlighted some critical changes for selected countries [7]. Whereas the Western Pacific Islands used taxation and trade policies to begin to address the issue [62], Mexico created the most comprehensive prevention approach [63]. Mexico instituted a 10% sugar-sweetened beverage tax, an 8% junk food tax, and marketing controls on selective television programming. Other Latin American countries within the year will institute far more complex controls with higher taxation levels and negative logos on front of the packages for foods identified as being particularly high in added sugar, sodium, or unhealthy saturated fats. Chile was the first to begin to address this topic but other efforts are now far along in Peru and Ecuador [64]. Countries in Asia are considering adopting jointly the Choices healthy front of the package profiling system [65]. Several countries in Asia are considering taxation on sugar-sweetened beverages and others are instituting other types of innovative programs to address food system shifts [66].

The challenge we face in lower income countries is in determining how to arrest this rapid increase in obesity before the health system is overwhelmed with obesity-related problems. Effective prevention requires that obesity and chronic disease appear on the national agenda in the earliest stages. Evidence shows that obesity occurs in adults before it occurs in children, and that obesity occurs first in women and then in men. Thus, in the context of economic growth, it is important to have monitoring systems in place. To the extent that monitoring is not possible, low and middle income countries should emphasize economic growth in the context of ensuring a healthy food supply and an active lifestyle. While no countries have been able to reverse existing trends, there are examples of countries such as South Korea [67, 68] that have experienced a less severe epidemic in obesity due to government programs promoting healthful, traditional, foods. A new generation of efforts in low and middle income countries to reduce intake of less healthful and more obesity-promoting foods is one step forward but careful evaluation is needed to understand the impact of such policies.

Discussion Points

- What are possible explanations for the regional differences in adult overweight and obesity?
- In many European countries, overweight and obesity is higher in males than in females. What are possible explanations for the high prevalence of female overweight and obesity in low and middle income countries?
- Why is overweight and obesity higher in urban versus rural areas of low and middle income countries?
- What are possible explanations for the global increasing in overweight and obesity prevalences? What global changes could explain these trends emerging in the past 2 decades?

Acknowledgments The authors thank the following staff of the Carolina Population Center, University of North Carolina at Chapel Hill: Tom Swasey for his work on the graphics and Frances Dancy for administrative assistance.

References

1. Omran AR. The epidemiologic transition. A theory of the epidemiology of population change. Milbank Mem Fund Q. 1971;49(4):509–38.
2. McGuire AL, et al. There and back again: the impact of adult HIV prevalence on national life expectancies. HIV Med. 2005;6(2):57–8.
3. Popkin B. The nutrition transition in the developing world. Dev Policy Rev. 2003.
4. Popkin BM. An overview on the nutrition transition and its health implications: the Bellagio meeting. Public Health Nutr. 2002;5(1A):93–103.
5. Popkin B. The nutrition transition: nutritional change in the developing world is most rapid. Annu Rev Nutr. 2005.
6. Mendez MA, Monteiro CA, Popkin BM. Overweight exceeds underweight among women in most developing countries. Am J Clin Nutr. 2005;81(3):714–21.
7. Popkin BM, Slining MM. New dynamics in global obesity facing low- and middle-income countries. Obes Rev. 2013;14:11–20.
8. Popkin BM, Lu B, Zhai F. Understanding the nutrition transition: measuring rapid dietary changes in transitional countries. Public Health Nutr. 2002;5(6A):947–53.
9. Popkin BM, Adair LS, Ng SW. Global nutrition transition and the pandemic of obesity in developing countries. Nutr Rev. 2012;70(1):3–21.
10. Popkin BM, Doak CM. The obesity epidemic is a worldwide phenomenon. Nutr Rev. 1998;56(4 Pt 1):106–14.
11. Doak CM, Hoffman DJ, Norris SA, Campos Ponce M, Polman K, Griffiths PL. Is body mass index an appropriate proxy for body fat in children? Glob Food Secur. 2013;2(2):65–138.
12. Monteiro CA, et al. Obesity and inequities in health in the developing world. Int J Obes Relat Metab Disord. 2004;28(9):1181–6.
13. Monteiro CA, Conde WL, Popkin BM. The burden of disease from undernutrition and overnutrition in countries undergoing rapid nutrition transition: a view from Brazil. Am J Public Health. 2004;94(3):433–4.
14. Monteiro CA, et al. Socioeconomic status and obesity in adult populations of developing countries: a review. Bull World Health Organ. 2004;82(12):940–6.
15. Steyn K, et al. Anthropometric profile of a black population of the Cape Peninsula in South Africa. East Afr Med J. 1998;75(1):35–40.
16. Nielsen SJ, Siega-Riz AM, Popkin BM. Trends in energy intake in U.S. between 1977 and 1996: similar shifts seen across age groups. Obes Res. 2002;10(5):370–8.
17. Doak CM, et al. The dual burden household and the nutrition transition paradox. Int J Obes Relat Metab Disord. 2005;29(1):129–36.
18. Garrett JL, Ruel MT. Stunted child-overweight mother pairs: prevalence and association with economic development and urbanization. Food Nutr Bull. 2005;26(2):209–21.
19. WHO Expert Committee on Physical Status. Physical status: the use and interpretation of anthropometry. In: WHO, editor. Technical Report Series 854. Geneva: World Health Organization; 1995
20. Popkin BM. Does global obesity represent a global public health challenge? Am J Clin Nutr. 2011;93(2):232–3.

21. Jones-Smith JC, et al. Cross-national comparisons of time trends in overweight inequality by socioeconomic status among women using repeated cross-sectional surveys from 37 developing countries, 1989–2007. Am J Epidemiol. 2011;173(6):667–75.
22. Jones-Smith JC, et al. Is the burden of overweight shifting to the poor across the globe? Time trends among women in 39 low- and middle-income countries (1991–2008). Int J Obes (Lond). 2012;36(8):1114–20.
23. Jones-Smith JC, et al. Emerging disparities in overweight by educational attainment in Chinese adults (1989–2006). Int J Obes (Lond). 2012;36(6):866–75.
24. Ng M, et al. Global, regional, and national prevalence of overweight and obesity in children and adults during 1980–2013: a systematic analysis for the global burden of disease study 2013. Lancet. 2014;384(9945):766–81.
25. Popkin BM, Conde W, Hou N, Monteiro C. Why the lag globally in obesity trends for children as compared to adults? Unpublished manuscript. 2005.
26. Rivera JA, et al. Epidemiological and nutritional transition in Mexico: rapid increase of non-communicable chronic diseases and obesity. Public Health Nutr. 2002;5(1A):113–22.
27. Berdasco A. Body mass index values in the Cuban adult population. Eur J Clin Nutr. 1994;48(Suppl 3):S155–63; discussion S164.
28. Ge K, Zhai F, Yan H. The dietary and nutritional status of Chinese population: 1992 National Nutrition Survery, vol. 1. Beijing: People's Medical Publishing House; 1996.
29. Dhurandhar NV, Kulkarni PR. Prevalence of obesity in Bombay. Int J Obes Relat Metab Disord. 1992;16(5):367–75.
30. Ismail M, et al. Prevalence of obesity and chronic energy deficiency (CED) in adult Malaysians. Malay J Nutr. 1995;1(19).
31. Solon F. Nutrition related chronic diseases in the Philippines. In: N.C.o.t. Philippines, editor. Nutrition Center of the Philippines Report Series. Makati City, Philippines; 1997.
32. Tanphaichitr V, et al. Prevalence of obesity and its associated risks in Urban Thais. In: Oomura YTS, Inoue S, Shimazu T, editors. Progress in obesity research 1990. London: Libbey; 1991. p. 649–53.
33. Saito S. National Nutrition Survey. In: Suva F., R.o.F. National Food and Nutrition Committee, editor. Main Report. 1995.
34. Hodge AM, et al. Incidence, increasing prevalence, and predictors of change in obesity and fat distribution over 5 years in the rapidly developing population of Mauritius. Int J Obes Relat Metab Disord. 1996;20(2):137–46.
35. Tassie JM, et al. Nutritional status in adults in the pluri-ethnic population of New Caledonia. The CALDIA Study Group. Int J Obes Relat Metab Disord. 1997;21(1):61–6.
36. McGarvey S, Quested C, Tufa J. Correlates and predictors of cross-sectional and longitudinal adiposity in adults from Samoa and American Samoa. Providence, RI: Department of Medicine, Brown University; 1998.
37. Kingdom of Tonga National Food and Nutrition Committee. The 1986 National Nutrition Survey of the Kingdom of Tonga., N.C.S.P. Commission, editor. 1987.
38. al-Mannai A, et al. Obesity in Bahraini adults. J R Soc Health, 1996;116(1):30–2, 37–40.
39. Khorshid A, Galal O. National agricultural research project. In: Final Technical Report. 1 Oct 1995, 31 Aug 1992; 1995.
40. Ajlouni K, Jaddou H, Batieha A. Obesity in Jordan. Int J Obes Relat Metab Disord. 1998;22(7):624–8.
41. al-Isa AN. Prevalence of obesity among adult Kuwaitis: a cross-sectional study. Int J Obes Relat Metab Disord. 1995;19(6):431–3.
42. al-Nuaim AR, et al. High prevalence of overweight and obesity in Saudi Arabia. Int J Obes Relat Metab Disord. 1996;20(6):547–52.
43. Shetty PS, James WP. Body mass index. A measure of chronic energy deficiency in adults. FAO Food Nutr Pap. 1994;56:1–57.
44. Jooste PL, et al. Prevalence of overweight and obesity and its relation to coronary heart disease in the CORIS study. S Afr Med J. 1988;74(3):101–4.
45. Monteiro CA, et al. Shifting obesity trends in Brazil. Eur J Clin Nutr. 2000;54(4):342–6.
46. Monteiro CA, et al. The nutrition transition in Brazil. Eur J Clin Nutr. 1995;49(2):105–13.
47. Hodge AM, et al. Dramatic increase in the prevalence of obesity in western Samoa over the 13 year period 1978–1991. Int J Obes Relat Metab Disord. 1994;18(6):419–28.
48. Beaglehole R, Yach D. Globalisation and the prevention and control of non-communicable disease: the neglected chronic diseases of adults. Lancet. 2003;362(9387):903–8.
49. Zimmet PZ, McCarty DJ, de Courten MP. The global epidemiology of non-insulin-dependent diabetes mellitus and the metabolic syndrome. J Diabetes Complications. 1997;11(2):60–8.
50. King H, Aubert RE, Herman WH. Global burden of diabetes, 1995–2025: prevalence, numerical estimates, and projections. Diabetes Care. 1998;21(9):1414–31.
51. Fund WCR. Food, nutrition and the prevention of causes: a global perspective. World Cancer Research Fund in association with the American Institute for Cancer Research. Washington, DC. 1997

52. Zimmet PZ. Kelly west lecture 1991. Challenges in diabetes epidemiology—from West to the rest. Diabetes Care. 1992;15(2):232–52.
53. Dowse GK, et al. Changes in population cholesterol concentrations and other cardiovascular risk factor levels after five years of the non-communicable disease intervention programme in Mauritius. Mauritius non-communicable disease study Group. Bmj. 1995;311(7015):1255–9.
54. Ford ES, Williamson DF, Liu S. Weight change and diabetes incidence: findings from a national cohort of US adults. Am J Epidemiol. 1997;146(3):214–22.
55. Parra E, et al. Genetic variation at 9 autosomal microsatellite loci in Asian and Pacific populations. Hum Biol. 1999;71(5):757–79.
56. O'Dea K, et al. Obesity, diabetes, and hyperlipidemia in a central Australian aboriginal community with a long history of acculturation. Diabetes Care. 1993;16(7):1004–10.
57. Bray GA, Popkin BM. Dietary fat intake does affect obesity! Am J Clin Nutr. 1998;68(6):1157–73.
58. Jahns L, Baturin A, Popkin BM. Obesity, diet, and poverty: trends in the Russian transition to market economy. Eur J Clin Nutr. 2003;57(10):1295–302.
59. Paeratakul S, et al. Changes in diet and physical activity affect the body mass index of Chinese adults. Int J Obes Relat Metab Disord. 1998;22(5):424–31.
60. Paeratakul S, et al. Measurement error in dietary data: implications for the epidemiologic study of the diet-disease relationship. Eur J Clin Nutr. 1998;52(10):722–7.
61. Bell AC, Ge K, Popkin BM. Weight gain and its predictors in Chinese adults. Int J Obes Relat Metab Disord. 2001;25(7):1079–86.
62. Snowdon W, Thow A. Trade policy and obesity prevention: challenges and innovation in the Pacific Islands. Obes Rev. 2013;14(Suppl 2):150–8.
63. Barquera S, Campos I, Rivera J. Mexico attempts to tackle obesity: the process, results, push backs and future challenges. Obes Rev. 2013;14 (Suppl 2):69–78.
64. Corvalán C, Reyes M, Garmendia ML, Uauy R. Structural responses to the obesity and non-communicable diseases epidemic: the Chilean Law of Food Labeling and Advertising. Obes Rev. 2013;14(Suppl 2):79–87.
65. Roodenburg A, Popkin B, Seidell J. Development of international criteria for a front of package food labelling system: the international choices programme. Eur J Clin Nutr. 2011;65(11):1190–200.
66. Foo L, et al. Obesity prevention and management: Singapore's experience. Obes Rev. 2013;14(Suppl 2):106–13.
67. Kim S, Moon S, Popkin BM. The nutrition transition in South Korea. Am J Clin Nutr. 2000;71(1):44–53.
68. Lee MJ, Popkin BM, Kim S. The unique aspects of the nutrition transition in South Korea: the retention of healthful elements in their traditional diet. Public Health Nutr. 2002;5(1A):197–203.

Chapter 8
Nutrient Needs and Approaches to Meeting Them

Saskia de Pee

Keywords RNI · RDA · DRI · EAR · UL · Energy density · Nutrient density · Dietary diversity · Fortification · Biofortification · Amylase · Supplementation

Learning Objectives

- Understand how nutrient intake recommendations have been established and how they are applied.
- Understand energy density and nutrient density, how they can be increased and for which subgroups of the population they are most important.
- Be able to explain the different level of risk associated with an intake below the estimated average requirement (EAR) and at or above the tolerable upper intake level (UL).
- Be able to distinguish different strategies for improving nutrient intake and understand their roles, limitations, and complementarity.

Introduction

People's diets need to provide the nutrients required for growth, development, and health. While there are several direct, underlying, and basic causes of malnutrition, meeting nutrient requirements is one of the prerequisites for achieving optimal health and nutrition. Essential nutrients are those that the body cannot synthesize on its own—or not to an adequate amount—and must be provided by the diet. Nutrients are required for metabolic processes that provide energy, support growth, and tissue replacement, affect cellular and humoral immune systems, neural and cognitive development among others. Six categories of essential nutrients can be distinguished, which include three groups of macronutrients, i.e., carbohydrates, protein, and fat, two groups of micronutrients, i.e., vitamins and minerals, and water. In total, these encompass approximately 40 individual nutrients that are required in different quantities to meet people's needs.

Nutrient needs vary throughout the life cycle, by age, sex, physiological state, activity level, health, and nutritional status. Furthermore, nutrient needs also vary among physiologically comparable individuals. As an individual's specific needs are unknown, an estimate is used based on age,

S. de Pee (✉)
Nutrition Division, World Food Programme, Rome, Italy
e-mail: Saskia.depee@wfp.org; depee.saskia@gmail.com

S. de Pee
Friedman School of Nutrition Science and Policy, Tufts University,
Boston, MD, USA

© Springer Science+Business Media New York 2017
S. de Pee et al. (eds.), *Nutrition and Health in a Developing World*,
Nutrition and Health, DOI 10.1007/978-3-319-43739-2_8

sex, physiological state, and activity level. Nutrient needs are particularly high during growth, e.g., early childhood, adolescence, pregnancy, and when recovering from illness (i.e., during convalescence) or malnutrition. Older people also have increased needs due to less efficient utilization of nutrients (see also Chap. 26 by Bermudez and Solomons).

This chapter discusses nutrient needs from a public health nutrition, i.e. population, perspective. It describes how nutrient intake recommendations are established and how this is translated into food-based dietary guidelines. It explains how likelihood of nutrient deficiencies can be assessed and what strategies and commodities can be used to prevent or fill nutrient intake gaps among different subgroups in a population, in particular young children, including considerations for their use.

Nutrient Intake Recommendations—Terminology and Concepts

Dietary Reference Intakes

For normal, healthy people, Dietary Reference Intakes (DRI), have been formulated, including the RDA (or RNI), EAR, AI, and UL [1, 2], which are discussed below.

RNI and RDA

The Recommended Nutrient Intake (RNI, established by FAO/WHO, for use anywhere in the world) [3], or Recommended Dietary Allowance (RDA, established by the Food and Nutrition Board of the Institute of Medicine, for North America) [2], specifies the amount of a nutrient that would meet the needs of 97.5% of healthy individuals of a specific population subgroup. The RNI and RDA are usually established based on the same data and are virtually the same for most nutrients, except when one committee has recently considered new evidence, whereas the other committee has not yet done so.

EAR

The Estimated Average Requirement (EAR) is the daily intake value of a nutrient that is estimated to meet the nutrient requirement of half the healthy individuals in a life stage and gender group (Fig. 8.1). Before setting the EAR, a specific criterion of adequacy is selected, based on a careful review of the literature. When selecting the criterion, preventing deficiency or reducing disease risk is considered. Thus, it is not based on achieving optimal status or performance, which would be difficult to define and typically occurs across a range of status and hence intake.

The EAR is used to set the RDA by adding two standard deviations (SD) to the EAR, when the SD is known. When data about variability of requirements are insufficient to calculate an SD, the RDA is set at 1.2 times the EAR [1].

As the EAR represents the point at which the needs of 50% of the population are met, the proportion of the population with a lower intake is assumed to have a deficient intake and the proportion with a higher intake to have an adequate intake. However, since we do not know individual requirements, having an intake below or above the EAR cannot be used to estimate adequacy at individual level. The RNI/RDA should be used for that instead, as at that level almost everyone (97.5%) would meet their needs. At population level, the aim is for all individuals to have an intake above the EAR as that means that the proportion with an inadequate intake would be 0.

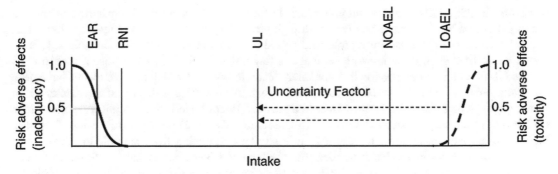

Fig. 8.1 The risks of adverse health effects from decreasing intakes and the risks of adverse health effects with increasing intakes. The estimated average requirement (EAR) reflects the intake where 50% of a population group is at risk of inadequacy, whereas the tolerable upper intake level (UL) is set an uncertainty factor lower than the no observed adverse effect level (NOAEL) or lowest observed adverse effect level (LOAEL). The recommended nutrient intake (RNI) is set at two standard deviations above the EAR and reflects the intake level at which 2.5% of a population group is at risk of inadequacy. © 2015 Bruins et al. [7], Open Access

Besides using the EAR to estimate the proportion of a population that is likely to have an inadequate intake, the EAR is also used for setting fortification levels. In this case, the target is for all fortified foods, together, to provide the EAR of the particular nutrient(s) that the food vehicles are fortified with, as this would shift the intake of the population, including nutrients consumed from the rest of the diet, to above the EAR level [4]. Nutrients for which the proportion of the population that has an intake below the EAR is small would not be considered for fortification.

The EARs that are used for setting the fortification level are those of the general population, i.e., adult males and females. The EAR in combination with the amount of the food vehicle that is typically consumed determines the fortification level. For example, the EAR for thiamin (vitamin B1) is 0.9 mg for women and 1.0 mg for men. For populations with an average rice consumption among adults of <75 g/d, a level of 2.0 mg thiamin per 100 g of fortified rice is recommended, whereas for populations with a rice intake of 150–300 g/d it is 0.5 mg/100 g [5]. Subgroups with comparable nutrient needs but lower intakes of the fortified food will not fully meet their EAR from consuming the fortified food. This includes groups such as young children who consume smaller amounts of food or small-holder farmers who do not consume much of the fortified vehicle when they mostly consume self-produced foods.

AI

When the EAR cannot be set, because of insufficient information on disease or health risks, the Adequate Intake level (AI) is set instead of the RNI and RDA [1]. This is for example the case for young infants (0–5 mo) for whom the AI is based on the composition of breastmilk consumed by healthy, full-term, exclusively breastfed infants. Like the RDA/RNI, the AI is the goal for the nutrient intake of individuals as it should meet the needs of almost every normal, healthy individual in the specific group.

UL

While the RNI/RDA specifies the desired intake, for normal healthy people, the UL, which stands for *Tolerable Upper Intake Level*, is the highest level of daily nutrient intake that is likely to pose no risk of adverse health effects to almost all individuals in the general population of a specific age and sex group [1]. It is a level of intake that can, with high probability, be tolerated biologically. The UL is not to be exceeded by far and for a prolonged period of time. For almost all nutrients, the UL is far above the RNI/RDA, thus an intake level that is a few times the RNI does not pose a problem.

The UL is set based on applying an uncertainty factor to levels at which adverse events have been observed, either in humans, based on case reports (e.g., accidental overdosing of supplements), or from animal studies (LOAEL: Lowest Observed Adverse Event Level), or the highest level at which no adverse effect was observed (NOAEL: No Observed Adverse Event Level) (see Fig. 8.1). The higher the level of uncertainty, for example in case of extrapolating from animals to humans, the higher the uncertainty factor that is applied [6]. The type of adverse event that is referred to differs. For example, in the case of zinc, an inhibitory effect on copper absorption has been the basis for setting the UL, and for this, a common intake level of copper has been assumed. In the case of multi-micronutrient supplements or specific fortified food complements that contain copper, zinc and other micronutrients, zinc intake can be somewhat higher than the UL.

It should also be noted that in terms of risk, the EAR and UL are very different. The EAR is the midpoint of required intake, i.e., at this level the risk of inadequacy is 50% and the consequences of too low (micro)nutrient intakes are well-known. The risk of an intake close to the UL, however, is negligible as it is set an uncertainty factor lower than the intake at and above which adverse effects may be expected [7]. Also, due to absence of adequate safety data a high uncertainty factors is applied for a couple of micronutrients, which results in the EAR and usual intakes being quite close to the UL. This is the case for vitamin A, calcium, copper, fluoride, iodine, iron, manganese, and zinc [7].

Furthermore, in addition to considering the risks of well-known levels of too low intake versus the much less certain and hence conservative level of too high intake at which adverse health effect may occur, it is also important to note that the UL applies to chronic intakes of normal, healthy people. In fact, the recommended intakes for specific groups, such as children undergoing treatment for moderate or severe acute malnutrition (MAM or SAM), are above the UL for certain nutrients in order to rebuild body tissues and nutrient stores [8].

Groups and Circumstances with Higher Nutrient Needs

Some groups have higher nutrient needs, such as people who are suffering from (chronic) infection (e.g., HIV or TB) [9], or people who are recovering from malnutrition, including children with severe or moderate acute malnutrition (SAM or MAM) [8]. Their needs are higher due to clinical vulnerabilities, the high needs for rebuilding fat and muscle tissue, replenishing of their bodies' nutrient stores, and, for children, catching up on lost growth opportunity [8–10].

For SAM and MAM, recommended nutrient intakes have been proposed [8, 11], which are generally higher for SAM than for MAM, except for the so-called "type 2 nutrients," since linear growth had not yet been taken into consideration when the recommendations for SAM were put together. Type 2 nutrients are particularly important for linear growth and include for example Phosphorus, Zinc, Magnesium, and sulfur amino acids [12]. For type 1 nutrients, which include most vitamins and minerals, biochemical tests can be used to determine whether someone has deficient, marginal, adequate, or too high levels. However, the status of type 2 nutrients cannot be determined, because they are not stored but either used for bone and muscle growth, or excreted when there is a surplus for some but no further supply of another nutrient [12]. Which nutrient(s) constrain linear growth in a particular population can only be determined by assessing the response to supplementation of specific type 2 nutrients that can be chosen based on what is suspected based on intake levels.

For people living with HIV (PLHIV), several studies have assessed the impact of different interventions, using different combinations of (micro)nutrients. However, since all studies used a different set and amounts of micronutrients, and some were conducted before antiretroviral treatment became available and others after, it has not yet been possible to recommend specific micronutrient intake levels [13, 14] and Chap. 20 by Paranandi and Wanke). WHO recommends ensuring that the RNI for normal healthy people is achieved by PLHIV [15]. Meanwhile, the Academy of Science of South Africa recommends a nutrient intake between 1–2 times the RNI, especially where PLHIV may already have low intakes prior to becoming infected [16].

Treatment of adults with malnutrition in resource-limited settings is often done with products that are used for treating children, such as F100 (therapeutic milk), ready-to-use therapeutic food (RUTF) or fortified blended food (FBF). However, for some nutrients absolute intake becomes rather high in case these foods provide most of the energy the adult requires [13] and the food and taste preferences of adults are different from children, as for example documented for PLHIV in Malawi [17].

Furthermore, while the RNI has been formulated to meet the needs of 97.5% of normal, healthy individuals, it may not be sufficient for people who frequently suffer from infections or subclinical inflammation (such as endemic enteric dysfunction) [18, 19].

With regard to growth, the dietary reference values for children are based on estimates that assume continuous, steady growth. However, growth occurs in a saltatory manner, i.e., in spurts followed by periods of slow or no growth. Saltatory growth may be more intense when there is more morbidity or other periods of growth shortfall (e.g., seasonal dietary inadequacies) and require nutrient intakes above the RNI [10].

Meeting Nutrient Requirements from the Diet

Can We Tell Whether Diets Meet Nutrient Requirements?

As mentioned above, people's individual nutrient requirements are not known. For energy, one can estimate whether intake is in balance with expenditure by monitoring weight, or whether pants or skirts become tighter or looser.

For individual nutrients, one may only know that intake is deficient or excessive when specific signs of deficiency or toxicity are observed, or by doing specific biochemical tests. Furthermore, for some nutrients there are no specific signs of deficiency or excess, just systemic signs, e.g., increased morbidity or lack of linear growth (resulting in stunting) in the case of zinc deficiency. Therefore, and because people do not select nutrients for consumption, but foods, unless they take a supplement, dietary intake recommendations should be such that when they are followed, it is likely that all nutrient requirements will be met.

The prevalence of undernutrition, as shown by indicators such as stunting and anemia, or of overnutrition, such as overweight and obesity, indicates whether, at group level, nutrient intake appears to meet needs. It is important to note that inadequate nutrient intake is one of the direct causes of undernutrition, while disease and inflammation as well as inadequate caring practices are the other direct causes. Thus, meeting nutrient requirements is a prerequisite for being free of malnutrition, but an adequate nutrient intake alone cannot guarantee being free from undernutrition. Disease and inflammation, including endemic enteric dysfunction (EED), can interfere with nutrient intake (anorexia), absorption (e.g., diarrhea and EED) and utilization (higher needs).

Which Single Foods Meet (Almost) All Nutrient Intake Recommendations?

There are very few foods that provide all nutrients that people require, with the exception of breastmilk (for exclusively breastfed 0–5 months old infants born at-term with normal birth weight of well-nourished mothers, except for vitamins D and K (see Chap. 16)), F100 and RUTF for SAM patients, clinical nutrition used in hospitals, and some specifically formulated foods or meals such as army rations.

Some food products are particularly developed to provide enough energy and nutrients to sustain people for a couple of days if necessary, such as high energy biscuits (HEB) that are distributed in case of emergencies, bars for mountaineers, and sports bars and drinks for athletes. However, these foods usually do not meet all individual nutrient needs, because (a) they are distributed to different target groups that do not all have the same nutrient needs and (b) they are not meant to be the only food someone consumes, or are meant to be replaced by a more complete offering of foods within a few days (in the case of HEBs).

Similarly, some foods are formulated to be a major complement to the existing diet, such as foods for treatment of MAM. In the case of those foods, the recommended nutrient composition is such that they can supply 70% of the macronutrient needs, assuming that the MAM child will also consume some family foods and may also consume breast milk, while providing close to 100% of the needs for other (micro)nutrients that may not be supplied in adequate amounts by the prevailing diet [8, 20].

Selecting Foods that Can Meet Nutrient Requirements

For most people, locally available foods should meet their nutrient requirements. For some nutrients though, meeting requirements from a diet based on local, unfortified, foods is very challenging. This is particularly true for iodine, which is leeched out of many soils, making seafood the only good natural source (see Chap. 12). In several countries milk is also a good source of iodine, but that is related to the feed of the cattle and the iodine containing tincture that is used to clean their udders. For some other nutrients, meeting the requirements of specific subgroups of the population is very challenging, e.g., iron, zinc, and calcium are generally recognized as key "problem" nutrients for children aged 6–23 months [21–25] and depending on context other nutrients may also be difficult to meet by this group, such as vitamin B12, preformed vitamin A and essential amino acids, for which animal-source foods are the only (B12) or main source [22–25].

In order to consume the recommended amounts of different nutrients, such as essential amino acids, essential fatty acids, vitamins and minerals, foods from different food groups need to be consumed (see Table 8.1 from [26]). Also, from within these food groups, different foods need to be chosen. For example, all animal-source foods provide high quality protein [27] that contains essential amino acids in good amounts. However, while fish is a good source of essential fatty acids (see Chap. 14), red meat has a high content of minerals, in particular iron, with high bioavailability, and dairy products are a good source of calcium, phosphorus and contain insulin-like growth factor. Hence, consumption of a diverse diet is essential for achieving an adequate intake of all required nutrients.

Country-specific food-based dietary guidelines (FBDG) are formulated to guide people's choice of foods toward a diverse diet that matches local food availability and preferences, and that is likely to meet the needs of most nutrients [28, 29]. FBDG also recommend limiting the intake of "empty calorie" foods, i.e., those that are just a source of energy (fat and/or sugar) but do not contain much, if any, essential nutrients, and of foods that contain harmful components (e.g., alcohol, trans-fatty acids, etc.). They often also recommend consumption of specific nutrient-rich foods, such as iodized salt or milk fortified with vitamins A and D. Many FBDG also promote drinking water and engaging in

Table 8.1 Essential nutrients and active compounds and their dietary sources, adapted from [26]

Nutrients and active compounds of concern	Dietary sources	Comments
Vitamins, plant origin	Vegetables and fruits, grains	Bioavailability (due to anti-nutrient content of plant foods) as well as absolute quantity of foods to be consumed to meet nutrient intake recommendations are of concern
Vitamins, animal origin (especially B6, B12, retinol)	Breast milk, animal milk, organ meat, red meat, poultry, fish, eggs, butter (retinol)	No single animal-source food (ASF) provides all the micronutrients that are required from ASF in adequate amounts[a]. Thus, a variety of ASF is required
Minerals	Animal-source foods and plant foods	When largely relying on plant foods, intake has to be high (can for example be increased by using a dried leaf concentrate) and bioavailability has to be improved, particularly by reducing content of phytate and polyphenols, and/or adding vitamin C. For example, bioavailability of iron is much higher from meat than from vegetables (see Chap. 10)
Iodine	Sea food, incl algae, and iodized salt	The use of iodized salt contributes greatly to the prevention of iodine deficiency disorders (see Chap. 12)
Proteins, to result in a diet with high PDCAAS[b] or DIAAS[c] value	Soy beans, peanuts, legumes, breast milk, animal milk, organ meat, red meat, poultry, fish, eggs	Same comment as for vitamins from ASF, a mixture of foods is required to ensure adequate intake of all essential amino acids
Essential fatty acids, especially a favorable n−6:n −3 ratio (∼6)	Fatty fish or their products, soy bean oil, rapeseed oil (also known as canola oil)	Only fatty fish and a few vegetable oils have the preferred fatty acid profile (see also Chap. 14) and these are not generally consumed in large amounts in LMICs
Linear growth stimulating factors in milk[d]	Dairy products (breast milk, animal milk, yogurt, cheese)	Dried skimmed milk (DSM) when reconstituted with water is not appropriate for young children because of the lack of fat. Full cream milk powder is usually DSM to which, powdered, vegetable fat has been added. Cow's milk is not appropriate for children below 12 months of age (see also Chap. 15)
Enzymes, that break down phytate (phytase), and complex carbohydrates (α-amylase)	Phytate is present in grains themselves and released when germinating (requires soaking for 24 h) or fermenting. Amylase is present in saliva and in malt	Intrinsic enzyme activity can be stimulated through specific home-processing or exogenous enzymes can be added during industrial processing to work either during the food production process or while food is being prepared by the consumer

[a]Even breast milk is a poor source for certain micronutrients, in particular iron, vitamins D and K (see also Chap. 16). When a child is born with adequate iron stores, these stores in combination with exclusive breast milk consumption for the first 6 months of life will ensure that iron needs are met. Introducing complementary foods early reduces bioavailability of some micronutrients, particularly minerals, from breast milk and could thus increase the risk of deficiencies when the complementary foods are not of appropriate composition

[b]Protein Digestibility Corrected Amino Acid Score (PDCAAS) is based on an estimate of crude protein digestibility determined over the total digestive tract, and values stated using this method generally overestimate the amount of amino acids absorbed

[c]Digestible Indispensable Amino Acid Score (DIAAS), which is based on amino acid digestibility at the end of the small intestine, provides a more accurate measure of the amounts of amino acids absorbed by the body and the protein's contribution to human amino acid and nitrogen requirements. Some food products may claim high protein content, but since the small intestine does not absorb all amino acids the same, they are not providing the same contribution to a human's nutritional requirements. DIAAS will gradually replace PDCAAS as measure of protein quality as results of in vivo measurements of bioavailability become available

[d]Different components of milk, including phosphorus and insulin-like growth factor, have been linked to linear growth (see Chap. 15)

physical activity to promote healthy lifestyles and prevent overweight. Some FBDG distinguish recommendations for children and for adults, whereas others are formulated for the general population. Recently, some FBDG also take environmental footprint and sustainability of food production aspects into consideration.

Nutrition education for the general public often focuses on explaining FBDG, with limited attention to constraints and enablers for making appropriate food choices. Dietary advice for specific subgroups of the population and dietary counseling for individuals take specific needs and constraints relating to food choice, food access, preparation, and consumption into consideration [30] and is often provided by specifically trained professionals, such as community health workers or dieticians.

Energy Density and Nutrient Density

Energy density and nutrient density are two most important characteristics of food, because they determine how much energy and nutrients are contained in a specific amount of food. For example, a glass of water provides no energy and no nutrients, and a handful of nuts contain macronutrients and micronutrients in a greater amount than an apple.

Energy Density

Energy density is the amount of energy in a particular quantity of food, expressed as kcal (or kJ) per gram. Food labels specify energy density for the food as packaged. However, in the case of dry foods that need to be reconstituted or prepared, such as porridge, the energy density of the food as consumed is more relevant from a nutritional point of view.

For example, a porridge flour in dry form typically contains around 4 kcal/g, while the porridge that is made from it may contain 0.3–1.2 kcal/g, depending on the ingredients, how they have been processed, and how it is prepared, i.e., how much water is added to reach a desired viscosity (thickness) of the porridge. If the energy density of a porridge is low, one can feel full while only having consumed a limited amount of energy, and hence a larger number of servings is required in order to meet energy needs as compared to when energy density would have been higher. Foods with high energy density are particularly important for young children (aged 6–23 months) with limited stomach capacity and relatively high energy and nutrient needs to sustain their rapid growth and development.

Feeding recommendations for 6–23 months old children therefore specify a different number of meals and snacks per day, depending on the energy density of the main complementary foods provided and whether they are breastfed [31] or not breastfed [32]. The Codex standard for processed cereal-based foods for infants and young children specifies a minimum energy density of the porridge of 0.8 kcal/g [33]. This same level is recommended in the WHO technical note for foods for MAM treatment [20] and is also in-line with the guidelines for feeding of the breastfed [31] and non-breastfed [32] 6–23 months old child. Many home-prepared staple-based spoonable porridges have a lower energy density, due their high content of complex carbohydrates (starch) and low viscosity.

Energy density can be increased by predigestion of the starchy portion of the grain, i.e., breaking the complex carbohydrates into smaller chains, which reduces the bulk so that energy content can be increased while maintaining the same viscosity. Amylase is an enzyme that catalyzes the hydrolysis of starch, i.e., it breaks down complex carbohydrates, and is contained in saliva of humans and some mammals as well as in some plants. Predigestion by natural amylases can be achieved by inducing germination of seeds by soaking or humidifying [34, 35]. This can be done at home or at industrial level. In either case, it is important to ensure that growth of mycotoxin producing microorganisms does not occur while moisture content is high. Industrial processing can also predigest the starch, by pre-cooking or using amylase. Amylase is also used for brewing beer and producing bread.

While amylase can be applied during industrial processing, it can also be added to flour in order to "act" while the porridge is being prepared. For this application the porridge flour and water should be mixed and then warmed up together, as the amylase will "act" while the temperature gradually increases and will then be inactivated when it reaches >90 °C [36].

The addition of amylase to flour has, for example, been found to increase energy density of Supercereal Plus porridge from 0.7 to 1.1 kcal/g [37]. The same study found that porridge volumes consumed by 12–23 months old children were comparable between Supercereal Plus porridges with and without amylase and that, due to the difference in energy density, energy, and nutrient intake per meal was approximately 67% higher from the porridges with amylase.

For comparison, lipid-based nutrient supplements (LNS), which have a very low water and high-fat and sugar content and can be consumed without further preparation, contain approximately 5.3 kcal/g [11, 38]. It is good to note that children will likely want to drink more, whether breastmilk, water or other liquids, when consuming LNS as compared to porridge.

Increasing energy density of porridge by adding oil and sugar should, however, be done cautiously, because it will lower nutrient density.

Nutrient Density

Nutrient density is expressed as the amount of a nutrient per unit of energy, for example 3 mg iron/100 kcal. Certain subgroups of the population require foods with high nutrient densities as their energy intake is low compared to their nutrient needs. For example, during early childhood, the need for essential nutrients, such as iron, zinc, and essential amino acids is very high due to growth, while the energy requirement is relatively low as body size is still small. Per 100 kcal of food, a 6–8 month-old breastfed infant needs more than four times as much zinc and nine times as much iron as an adult male [39]. This means that foods provided to infants need to be more nutrient-dense, in addition to also having to be more energy-dense, than foods consumed by older children and adults.

Concurrently Increasing Energy and Nutrient Density

Let us look at what happens to nutrient density when energy density is increased by adding oil or sugar. A 50 g serving of porridge that contains 40 kcal and 1.2 mg of iron (equal to an iron density of 3 mg/100 kcal), will contain 60 kcal when 5 g of sugar or 2.2 g of oil is added, but its iron density will decrease from 3 to 2 mg/100 kcal. Thus, in order to achieve the same iron intake, the child would need to consume 1.5 times as much kcal of the porridge. Alternatively, the iron content of the porridge would need to be increased in a way that does not reduce energy density. Adding more flour or vegetables are not good options, because flour would increase thickness of the porridge, which will be compensated by adding more water and hence it would negate the energy density increasing effect of the sugar or oil, and adding leafy vegetables will increase volume and reduce energy density.

Home-processing methods that hydrolyse phytate and hence decrease its inhibitory effect on mineral absorption, such as sprouting, malting, and fermentation, can increase bioavailability of minerals [40] while also increasing energy density through enabling endogenous amylase action. The use of these methods, while effective, is not widespread, they take time and mycotoxin producing organisms may grow in the moist environment. Other ways to increase nutrient density without reducing energy density include adding some meat, which already has a high energy- and nutrient-density itself, or adding micronutrient premix. Premix can be included in the fortified flour, or be added to the meal in the form of so-called "home-fortification," where a micronutrient powder [41–43] or small amount of fortified spread (e.g., small-quantity lipid-based nutrient supplement, SQ-LNS) is added to the porridge [44, 45].

High Energy Foods with Low or High Nutrient Density

The low density, or absence, of essential nutrients in high-fat and high-sugar foods, such as chips, cookies, and sugar-sweetened beverages, is why these are called "empty-calorie" foods, i.e., they have a high caloric content but provide not much if anything of other nutrients. In order to prepare meals with adequate and balanced nutrient content, nutrient-dense foods should be selected, such as fruits, vegetables, animal-source foods, as well as fortified foods, and the intake of high-fat and high-sugar foods should be limited.

The high nutrient and high energy needs of children with SAM, for example, can be met with RUTF, which is a lipid-based product that has a high energy density due its high content of sugar and vegetable oil, and its high nutrient density is achieved through fortification.

How to Determine (Risk of) Nutrient Deficiencies, at Population Level?

Given that there are specific recommended nutrient intakes for normal, healthy people, and that public health nutrition is concerned with ensuring that most people in a population meet their requirements, indicators are required to determine whether intakes are meeting needs and whether specific measures are required to increase intake, by the general population or specific subgroups.

In terms of indicators, there are those that assess nutrient intake, those that assess nutritional status, for example, in blood, urine, hair, or saliva, and those that assess specific or unspecific clinical signs of deficiency or excess.

Let us look at the history of vitamin A deficiency control and how different indicators were used to guide decisions about the need and strategies for increasing vitamin A status. In the 1990s, vitamin A supplementation among children under-five using high-dose capsules gradually increased in scale as several studies, and the meta-analysis of these studies, had shown its impact on preventing child mortality (see Chap. 9 by Palmer, Darnton-Hill and West). Fortification, for example of vegetable oil, and dietary diversification, including home gardening, were also promoted, for longer term sustainability as well as for addressing deficiency in other target groups that were not eligible for vitamin A supplementation. However, the question that policy makers and scientists grappled with was "What should be the basis for deciding to implement a vitamin A deficiency control program, including vitamin A supplementation?"

Initially, the guidance from the International Vitamin A Consultative Group (IVACG) was to assess the prevalence of vitamin A deficiency, using two or three indicators that included dietary intake of vitamin A, vitamin A status and/or clinical signs of deficiency (night blindness and xerophthalmia). However, collecting these data, preferably at national scale and among different target groups, requires financial resources, time and expertise such as food composition tables, laboratory capacity, etc. These requirements proved to be a considerable bottleneck and delayed decision-making. Then, at the twentieth IVACG meeting in Hanoi in 2001, it was decided that rather than proving that there was a vitamin A deficiency problem by focusing on indicators specific for vitamin A deficiency, mortality rates should be used to assess the likelihood that vitamin A deficiency was a problem. Under-five mortality rate (U5MR) above 50/1000 live births was considered sufficient "evidence of need" to implement a vitamin A supplementation program among children aged 6–59 months [46], because vitamin A supplementation addresses a cause of child mortality that is very likely to play a role where child mortality is above that level. The evidence requirement was thus turned around: based on U5MR > 50 a vitamin A deficiency problem should be assumed requiring immediate or continuing action, and also for U5MR between 20 and 50 it should be assumed unless indicators of vitamin A status could show that this was not the case [46]. This change of guidance markedly increased the number of countries that started, and still implement, vitamin A supplementation programs.

For prevention of undernutrition, including micronutrient deficiencies, programming is also often based on estimating the likelihood of inadequate intake using proxy indicators. For example, the home-fortification technical advisory group (HF-TAG) has listed the following indicators for determining whether micronutrient deficiencies are likely among young children (6–59 or 6–23 months old) in a publication endorsed by Centre for Disease Control, Atlanta (CDC), Global Alliance for Improved Nutrition (GAIN), Helen Keller International (HKI), Micronutrient Initiative, Sight and Life, Sprinkles Global Health Initiative, UC Davis, UNICEF, and WFP [41]:

- anemia prevalence, as indicator of micronutrient deficiencies more broadly;
- stunting prevalence as indicator of likely dietary inadequacies;
- frequent infections, as indicator of higher (micro)nutrient needs;
- nightblindness during pregnancy as indicator of dietary micronutrient deficiencies more broadly;
- lack of dietary diversity, in particular low consumption of animal-source foods and fortified foods;
- inadequate nutrient density of typical complementary foods, which is common where children eat from the family pot and do not receive foods that are specifically prepared for them;
- food insecurity.

In settings where deficiencies of micronutrients and other essential nutrients are likely, and likely related to inadequate nutrient content of complementary foods, the HF-TAG recommends to use home-fortification (explained in next section) for improving the essential nutrient content of complementary foods. The following indicators are proposed by HF-TAG to determine whether low nutrient intake from complementary food is likely:

- low dietary diversity due to limited availability and/or affordability of foods from different food groups;
- insufficient nutrient content and density of complementary foods, e.g., predominant consumption of watery porridges;
- poor bioavailability of micronutrients in case of largely plant-source based meals (e.g., phytate in plant foods limits absorption of minerals such as iron and zinc).

Thus, for population level interventions that aim to improve intake of essential nutrients, including micronutrients, proxy indicators of risk of deficiency rather than evidence of deficiency of individual nutrients, which would require data on their actual intake and/or status, often suffices. Furthermore, since dietary deficiencies rarely apply to single micronutrients, HF-TAG recommends providing a combination of 15 vitamins and minerals. Some of these micronutrients, i.e., minerals and fat-soluble vitamins, can be stored by the body, while water soluble vitamins cannot. The home-fortificant should hence be consumed on a regular basis, as opposed to daily for one or two months followed by a couple of months without supplementation, to ensure a continuous addition to daily nutrient intake.

While the above concerns the evidence required to implement a home-fortification program, for which likelihood of dietary deficiency suffices, the commodity that is provided should be chosen based on data that show that it has good shelf-life and is efficacious for improving micronutrient status. This can apply to the specific formulation as a whole, or to its individual components, i.e., the forms of the micronutrients that are included. For micronutrient powder, evidence of impact on micronutrient status is available for a number of its micronutrients [42, 43] and for the other ones chemical forms have been chosen that are known to have good stability and bioavailability.

However, in specific situations more information is required in addition to proxy indicators of likely dietary deficiencies, including:

- Where there are concerns about excessive intake of specific nutrients, for example, in situations where fortification and supplementation are taking place concurrently, it is important to collect nutrient intake data, especially among the subgroups that might reach higher intake levels than intended. When good intake data are available, specific software such as IMAPP [47] can be used to simulate how different food vehicles and micronutrient addition levels would change the prevalence of micronutrient intakes below the EAR and above the UL in different population groups. See also Bruins et al. for a further discussion about the traditional cut-point method to set fortification levels and a stepwise approach that considers risk-benefit in greater detail with examples from mostly high-income countries where nutrient intakes are higher and multiple foods are fortified, and good quality intake data are available [7]. In addition, biochemical indicators can be used to assess whether too high circulating levels of specific nutrients affect a proportion of the population, e.g., of iodine or vitamin A (see also Chap. 5 on Malnutrition spectrum).
- Among populations with specific conditions, such as high prevalence of thalassemia who may have increased iron absorption and storage [48], or who prepare their food in iron pots due to which their iron intake may already be adequate, it could be decided to add no, or a low level, of iron. If such specific conditions are suspected, this needs to be investigated and included in the risk-benefit assessment.

Ways to Correct Inadequate Nutrient Intake at Population Level

Population level interventions for increasing (micro)nutrient intake can target (a) the population in general, (b) specific subgroups with a higher risk of inadequate intakes, such as children aged 6–23 months, and/or (c) groups with a higher risk of deficiencies, such as those with low socio-economic status who do not consume an adequately diverse diet.

There are basically three ways to increase nutrient intake: (1) by increasing intake of natural, unprocessed, foods that are a good source of specific nutrients, (2) by increasing consumption of foods of which micronutrient levels have been increased through fortification, and (3) by nutrient supplementation. It is important to note that these strategies are complementary, because they may be applied to different target groups, increase the intake of different nutrients, reach different individuals, etc.

Dietary approaches for increasing (micro)nutrient intake encompass both increasing intake of nutrient-dense, unprocessed foods, such as animal-source foods, vegetables, and fruits, as well as increasing consumption of fortified foods.

Increasing Contribution from Nutrient-Rich, Unprocessed, Foods

Increasing intake of naturally nutrient-rich foods is preferred wherever possible, and greater dietary diversity increases the likelihood that nutrient needs are being met. Table 8.1 shows which types of foods contribute which type of nutrients. As mentioned before, dietary diversity is essential for meeting nutrient requirements, and this includes choosing foods from different food groups and also different foods from within these food groups. Social behavior change communication (SBCC) typically focuses on good infant and young child feeding practices, including breastfeeding practices, introduction of complementary foods, which foods to choose and how to prepare them, number and size of meals and snacks, hygiene practices for food preparation and storage, etc., and also addresses constraints to being able to implement the advice [30].

Preserving nutrient content and reducing losses, during food storage, processing and preparation, can also contribute to increasing nutrient intake. The choice of a specific combination of foods and ways of processing can also be used to improve bioavailability of micronutrients, such as avoiding having tea with meals (as tannins inhibit iron absorption) and adding fruit (as vitamin C enhances iron absorption), or germination of seeds to release phytase, which breaks down phytate, an important inhibitor of iron and zinc absorption.

However, it is important to assess and manage constraints related to meeting nutrient requirements from locally available, unfortified, foods by different groups in the population. For example, availability and affordability of foods limit the extent to which dietary diversity can be increased [49, 50], some nutrients are required in very high amounts by specific population groups (e.g., pregnant women), some nutrients are only contained in sufficient amounts in animal-source foods (vitamin B12, preformed vitamin A, minerals with good bioavailability such as iron and zinc), and some nutrients cannot be obtained from natural foods (e.g., iodine only occurs naturally in seafood).

Fortification

Fortification refers to the addition of micronutrients to foods to restore levels to the levels prior to processing, or to enrich foods because of the population's need for the micronutrient(s) and the opportunity to add it, e.g., as food is being processed (grain is milled to flour, salt is processed and packaged, etc.). The provision of micronutrients was ranked as one of the most cost-effective interventions for economic development according to the 2012 Copenhagen Consensus, and adding them in the form of fortification is particularly cost-effective because it can piggyback on already existing distribution channels for the food vehicles. The following forms of fortification can be distinguished:

Biofortification

Biofortification refers to breeding crops, conventionally or using genetic modification, to contain a higher level of micronutrients, such as provitamin A rich orange-flesh sweet potatoes, rice and cassava, high iron beans, and pearl millet, rice and wheat with increased zinc content [51]. This form of fortification is comparable to staple food fortification, with the advantage that the crop can be harvested, prepared and consumed without any specific, industrial processing. This makes biofortification very suitable for population groups that do not access processed foods, provided that they will accept the biofortified crop, also for its growing properties such as drought and pest resistance and yield, and access it [52]. Another important difference is that biofortification usually focuses on 1–3 micronutrients per crop, whereas industrial fortification can add a larger number of micronutrients.

Industrial Fortification of Foods for the General Population

Foods that are fortified for the general population can include wheat and maize flour, vegetable oil, salt, sugar, margarine, breakfast cereals, milk powder, fish sauce, soy sauce, etc. [53]. Fortification of commonly consumed foods started almost 100 years ago in Europe and North America, and is still an important strategy in those countries and beyond for preventing deficiencies of specific micronutrients. For example, to prevent iodine deficiency, many countries have now introduced iodized salt (see Chap. 12). Foods such as flour and rice are, for example, fortified with folic acid, to prevent neural tube defects, with iron to prevent iron deficiency and iron deficiency anemia, and with B-vitamins to prevent anemia, weakness, fatigue, and other consequences [5, 54]. Foods containing fat, such as milk and margarine, are often fortified with vitamins A, D and E.

One of the earliest stories of fortification with vitamin A is from Denmark. When margarine replaced butter in Denmark, between 1911 and 1917, a gradual increase of keratomalacia, which had just been recognized as a clinical sign of vitamin A deficiency at that time, was noted. This incidence dropped in 1918–19 when a German submarine blockade prevented Denmark from exporting its butter and it was rationed at a price that was more affordable to the poor. When the blockade was lifted in May 1919, keratomalacia re-occurred [55, 56]. Physicians treated the disease with milk, butter and cod liver oil. In 1937, Denmark mandated that margarine be fortified with vitamin A and the United States and Great Britain also introduced it around the same time [56].

Industrial Fortification of Foods for Specific Target Groups

Foods fortified for the general population cannot address the whole gap of micronutrient(s) in the diet of groups with relatively high needs, such as young children who consume small amounts of these foods that are fortified at a level that meets the requirements of adults (as described before, young children need foods of higher nutrient density). Infant cereals are a good example of a special nutritious food for young children.

Home-Fortification or Point-of-Use Fortification

Instead of adding fortificants during industrial processing, they can also be added manually to prepared foods, just before consumption. This can be applied to individuals' meals at home (home-fortification) or to group meals such as in a school's kitchen (point-of-use fortification). The best-known commodity for this form of fortification is micronutrient powder (MNP), which is used for fortifying meals with micronutrients, often 15 vitamins and minerals at a level of 1 RNI [41–43]. For young children (6–23 or 6–59 months), a single dose sachet of 1 g is used, while for school children a multi-serving sachet of 8 g has been developed for adding to a meal of 20 children. Another commodity that can be used for home-fortification is a small-quantity LNS (LNS-SQ), often 20 g/d, which can be added to a child's porridge or might also be eaten straight out of its sachet [44, 45]. LNS contains micronutrients, as well as macro-minerals (e.g., Ca, P, Mg), milk powder and essential fatty acids. As it contains a wider range of essential nutrients than MNP, it is typically used where the nutrient intake gap of the target population is estimated to be larger, for example, as indicated by not only a high prevalence of anemia, but also of stunting.

Considerations for Fortification

Foods fortified for the general population, such as flour, salt, sugar, and vegetable oil, piggyback on already existing food distribution systems and consumption practices. However, when fortification is not mandatory, consumers need to make a conscious choice for a fortified product, which is often also somewhat more expensive. Thus, informing consumers about the benefits and encouraging consumption of the fortified option is very important and should be done by both the public sector ("select fortified options because of health benefits") and the private sector ("this food is fortified with the following micronutrients"). Special nutritious foods, as opposed to foods fortified for the general population, are designed to meet the requirements of specific groups, who need to be specifically reached and encouraged to consume the specific product, whether it is a fortified complementary food or a product for home-fortification such as micronutrient powder.

The choice between different commodities for home-fortification and specialized nutritious foods such as infant cereals can be made based on the estimated nutrient gap, food consumption practices such as familiarity and acceptance of specific commodities, who will be targeted using which distribution channel and modality, ability to pay, whether it is the consumer or the public sector paying, etc. For example, in a relatively small country where micronutrient deficiencies are the main problem, where the health system appears best placed to distribute a nutritious product to all children aged 6–23 months, and the budget is limited, MNP may be selected. In a larger LMIC where a segment of the population already purchases infant cereals, the government can promote those infant cereals that meet well-defined nutritional and safety standards. This will assist the population as they make choices for self-purchasing, and the government can ensure access to these "approved" products by poorer segments of the population through a subsidy or voucher scheme that could for example be linked to social safety net support. Such an approach is comparable to that of the Special Supplemental Nutrition Program for Women, Infants, and Children (WIC) that provides Federal grants to States in the US for specific supplemental foods, health-care referrals, and nutrition education for low-income pregnant, breastfeeding, and non-breastfeeding postpartum women, and to infants and children up to age five [57, 58].

Whichever commodity is selected to improve the nutrient content of the complementary feeding diet, it should be promoted and distributed in a way that supports breastfeeding, promotes a healthy, diverse complementary feeding diet based on locally available and affordable foods, and respects local dietary habits. The introduction of new foods or commodities for home-fortification should be carefully planned, starting with assessment of local practices and values around foods and health, in order to design appropriate strategies and communication messages, including on optimizing use of locally available foods and good feeding practices [59–61]. In general, a combination of communication channels will need to be used, including interpersonal with trusted people, such as health-care workers and community volunteers, messages on the packaging, and mass media. The specific information on the commodity should cover different aspects, including why consumption of the commodity is recommended, which should link to values that the target group has, by whom it should be consumed, how, in what amount, how frequently, etc. Furthermore, these specific commodities should be promoted and distributed as part of a wider strategy or program on good infant and young child feeding and health. In fact, they are best distributed using platforms that already provide information or interventions for nutrition and health to the target group, such as child-health days [62].

The fact that food systems are accessed differently by different groups can also be used to target the distribution of foods fortified for the general population to groups that need it the most. Some examples: rice fortification in Bangladesh has started with fortifying the rice that is distributed through the social safety net scheme in a particular part of the country [63]; in Gujapati, India, fortified rice is included in the midday meal program that is provided to school children; and in Indonesia, a soy sauce producer decided to fortify the soy sauce that is sold in single meal sachets and is preferentially bought by the poor, whereas the richer buy soy sauce sold in glass bottles and smaller plastic bottles that was not fortified. Prior to its distribution through commercial channels, the iron fortified soy sauce had already been used in the Tsunami relief operation in Aceh [64].

Setting the Nutrient Level for Fortification

When fortifying foods, there should be a good balance between benefit, i.e., correcting intake and preventing deficiency and associated disorders, and risk, i.e., providing too much to certain individuals who already have high intakes or have special conditions that interfere with nutrient needs or utilization such as thalassemia [48].

As explained above, the EAR, RNI, and UL should guide setting the level for fortification. The EAR of adult males and females is the target level that the fortified food(s) should provide at common levels of consumption of the fortified vehicle. This level is around 70% of the RNI and the RNI is several times lower than the UL. By setting the level in this way, consuming too much of a nutrient that is added to a food consumed by the general population is virtually impossible. For example, if flour is fortified to provide the EAR of folic acid, i.e., 200 µg/d, at an average flour consumption level of 250 g/d, one would have to consume 1.2 kg of the fortified flour every day over a prolonged period of time to consistently exceed the UL of 1 mg.

From this example, it follows that a too high micronutrient intake mainly comes from supplements, which generally have a higher micronutrient content and can therefore more easily be overdosed. However, directions for use specify the recommended dose and overdosing on supplements is rare. Specialized fortified products, such as micronutrient powder and LNS-SQ, could potentially also be overdosed, but since they contain approximately 1 RNI per dose, are packaged in single-serving sachets, carry clear instructions on consuming not more than one serving per day, and are usually provided in limited numbers at a time (10–30 servings per month), the risk of excessive intake is also very low for this type of commodity.

To set the (micro)nutrient level for complementary foods or complementary food supplements for home-fortification (LNS-SQ, MNP), the following considerations are important:

- The target is to reach the RNI for a wide variety of nutrients from the total diet, including the specific additional commodity.
- The requirement of the group with the largest nutrient intake gap is most important.
- The frequency at which the commodity will be consumed, i.e., if consumption is likely to be a few days per week, the micronutrient content may have to be set at 1 RNI, whereas it can be lower if consumption will likely be daily.
- Will people purchase the commodity or will it be distributed for free, in which case the number of dosages provided can be more controlled.

Complementary foods in Europe are typically fortified at a level of one-third of the RNI per serving, because children are more likely to receive more than one serving of this kind or other fortified products, such as powdered milk or formula, per day. However, where few fortified foods are available for this target group and consumption frequency is generally still low, a higher level of fortification is recommended, to ensure that they are likely to make a substantial enough contribution to micronutrient intake, also when they are not consumed every day. For example, GAIN recommends that a serving of complementary food contains 50% of the RNI [65] and similarly, Supercereal Plus for complementary feeding that is supported by the World Food Programme contains 1 RNI per 50 g of porridge flour that makes 200–300 g of porridge [66].

Standards, Specifications and Quality Control for Fortified Foods

Food standards specify the required quality and nutrient content of foods, in order to provide clarity and protection for both manufacturers and consumers. The FAO/WHO Codex Alimentarius Commission develops harmonized international standards, guidelines, and codes of practice and countries often use these as the basis for national legislation. Fortification levels are typically set in specifications, which are developed for foods with a specific purpose or for a specific target group and are more specific than standards, which usually apply to broader categories of foods.

Compliance of final products with standards and specifications needs to be ensured by manufacturers while the public sector, i.e., government and non-governmental organizations, should independently monitor manufacturing practices and final products. Conducting tests for nutrient content and safety, in terms of microbiology, toxins, external matter, etc., at various points during the production chain requires specific expertise, both within and outside of manufacturing facilities.

Field tests have become available to assess, quantitatively or semi-quantitatively, the nutrient levels of fortified foods at household or sales points [67]. Such tests are very helpful to monitor implementation of fortification programs.

Supplementation

Supplementation is mainly indicated when nutrient intake should be substantially increased or can be given at a high dose with long time intervals in-between, such as in the case of fat-soluble vitamins that will be stored by the body, or when food fortification cannot reach specific target groups, for example when people use self-produced salt or sugar, which is hence not fortified with iodine or vitamin A, respectively. Most supplementation is in the form of tablets or capsules and hence often targeted at older children and adults, such as pregnant and lactating women. Some supplements are in the form of syrup or oil. For public health programming, syrup is not very practical because of its large volume and cost, which hinders use at scale. Possibly, the best example of a supplement in oil is vitamin A, which is distributed in capsules that are cut open and the content squeezed into the child's mouth at biannual vitamin A supplementation days (see Chap. 9).

Ascertaining Impact of Measures to Correct Dietary Deficiencies

The impact of interventions for increasing (micro)nutrient intake should primarily be evaluated for their impact on nutrient intake. For this, several aspects need to be ensured and assessed, as follows [68]:

- The food/commodity is nutritious, efficacious, and safe. In the case of fortification that means that it contains nutrient forms that have good bioavailability and stability as included in the commodity (i.e., not interacting with the other nutrients). For production, it means that this is done according to specification and shelf-life is confirmed (i.e., content of vitamins remains within the range specified on the label).

  - The commodity is available to the intended consumers, whether distributed for free or to be purchased.
  - The commodity is accepted by the consumers (i.e., product type is acceptable, packaging is appreciated, appearance, smell and taste are good).
  - The target group obtains the commodity as intended.
  - The commodity is consumed as expected or recommended (amount consumed per serving, number of servings per day/week).
  - Intake of (micro)nutrients from other sources remains the same, so that the specific fortified commodity complements the existing (micro)nutrient intake from other foods.

For all these "conditions" to be met, they should be well planned, implemented, assessed, and adjusted where necessary. This requires good planning and continuous coordination among all stakeholders involved, whether it concerns a specific project or a strategy that is implemented nationwide. The larger and more complex the strategy, and the more stakeholders of different disciplines (e.g., health, education, agriculture, and social protection) and constituencies (private sector, government, civil society, and academia) are involved, the better the coordination should be. Integration into existing systems is likely to work best and is more cost-efficient.

For monitoring implementation, coverage, and compliance as well as trends of dietary diversity, total nutrient intake, nutritional status, and health over time, existing data collection systems should be used as much as possible. For example, national standard of living survey data can be used to assess food expenditure patterns, DHS data can be used to monitor dietary diversity and consumption frequency among young children, and specific questions can be added to either of these data collection system that, for example, assess penetration and consumption of specific fortified foods.

As mentioned above, while nutrient intake needs to be adequate in order to avoid deficiencies, adequate intake of specific (micro)nutrients alone may not be enough to achieve a good nutritional status, for example as assessed by the prevalence of stunting or anemia. This can be related to suboptimal intake of other nutrients as well as to other direct causes of undernutrition such as disease, helminthes infections, subclinical inflammation, and environmental enteric dysfunction. For example, recent proteomics and metabolomics research has found that stunted children have lower circulating levels of essential amino acids, which may mean that their intake of good quality protein is limiting their linear growth [69]. Increasing these children's intake of micronutrients will improve micronutrient status and may reduce problems associated with micronutrient deficiencies, such as morbidity, but may have a limited intake on stunting reduction if their protein intake is not adequate, or on anemia if they also suffer from malaria. Chapter 3 discusses in more detail the difficulties of assessing impact of a modest increase of nutrient intake, for example, from fortified foods, on nutritional status and functional outcomes that are also influenced by many other factors.

The interest to assess impact on indicators such as prevalence of anemia and stunting is driven by the fact that their prevalence is often what prompts action as well as by the fact that evidence-based guidelines are intervention rather than problem focused (see Chap. 3). However, while stunting and anemia are indeed related to inadequate nutrient intake, that is not their only cause. The success of interventions to improve nutrient intake should therefore not be assessed based on their impact on these composite outcome indicators but rather from impact on what it directly aims to addresses, i.e., nutrient intake and whether that is increased enough.

Instead of evaluating the impact of a specific intervention that addresses one of the causes of stunting or anemia, comprehensive assessments over time are required. These assessments do not have to be undertaken exclusively for this purpose, but can also be conducted by adding specific questions or modules to other systems (see above). It is important that multiple factors are covered that relate both to dietary and health aspects and their related factors, to enable an understanding of whether progress is being made, and what the main limiting factors for further progress are that may need further action [70, 71] (See also Chap. 3 by de Pee and Grais and Chap. 27 by Olney, Leroy, and Ruel).

Conclusion

Dietary reference intakes have been established for normal, healthy people of different age, sex, physiological state and physical activity groups. The EAR (estimated average requirement) specifies the level at which 50% of the population would meet their needs and the RNI (recommended nutrient intake) the level at which 97.5% would meet their needs. People who suffer from malnutrition or frequent or chronic infections have higher nutrient needs, and for some of these groups specific intake recommendations have been proposed. Meeting nutrient intake recommendations requires consumption of a diverse diet. Groups with high nutrient needs, relative to body size and/or energy intake, such as young children, should consume foods with high energy and nutrient densities (i.e., energy per g of food as consumed, and amount of nutrients per unit of energy, respectively). Proxy indicators of likely (in)adequacy of nutrient intake, such as dietary diversity and food insecurity, or of malnutrition, such as anemia and stunting, can be used to determine whether (micro)nutrient intakes are likely to be adequate or not. Many groups require some fortified commodities, at a minimum iodized salt for non-seafood consuming populations and iron and zinc in foods or food supplements for many 6–23 months old children. Options for fortification include biofortification (i.e., breeding crops with higher nutrient content), fortification of staple foods or foods for specific groups, and home-fortification. One can target nutrient interventions to specific groups, in terms of stage of the lifecycle as well as socioeconomic status (affordability issues) or geographic area (accessibility issues) and use different channels, including health programs, commercial channels, and social safety nets. When measures are taken to increase nutrient intake, these should be evaluated for their impact on nutrient intake. Over time changes of nutritional status can be monitored, but it is important to acknowledge that nutritional status is also affected by other factors, which should all be monitored as well.

Discussion Points

- Which food processing and preparation methods can be used at home to increase (a) energy density and (b) nutrient density?
- What should be the nutrient intake target for a specific population group, their EAR or their RNI?
- What are the advantages and difficulties of mandatory fortification, from public health, food manufacturers and consumers perspectives?
- How should the targeted nutrient intake contribution of a specific fortified commodity be decided, i.e., which target group's needs should guide setting of the level, and what information is required to be able to propose a level?
- How can the public sector and the private sector, including both food and non-food sectors, contribute to improving nutrient intake among the most vulnerable, including specific age as well as socioeconomic groups?

References

1. Institute of Medicine (US) Food and Nutrition Board. Dietary reference intakes: a risk assessment model for establishing upper intake levels for nutrients. Washington (DC): National Academies Press (US); 1998.
2. Institute of Medicine. Dietary reference intakes: the essential reference for dietary planning and assessment. Washington, DC: IOM; 2006.
3. World Health Organization/Food and Agriculture Organization. Vitamin and mineral requirements in human nutrition. 2nd ed. Geneva, Switzerland: World Health Organization; 2004.
4. Allen L, de Benoist B, Dary O, Hurrell R, editors. Guidelines on food fortification with micronutrients. Geneva: World Health Organization (WHO) and Food and Agriculture Organization (FAO) of the United Nations; 2006.
5. De Pee S. Proposing nutrients and nutrient-levels for rice fortification. Ann NY Acad Sci. 2014. doi:10.1111/nyas. 12478.
6. Renwick AG. Toxicology of micronutrients: adverse effects and uncertainty. J Nutr. 2006;136:493S–501S.

7. Bruins MJ, Mugambi G, Verkaik-Kloosterman J, Hoekstra J, Kraemer K, Osendarp S, Melse-Boonstra A, Gallagher AM, Verhagen H. Addressing the risk of inadequate and excessive micronutrient intakes: traditional versus new approaches to setting adequate and safe micronutrient levels in foods. Food Nutr Res. 2015;59:26020.
8. Golden MH. Proposed recommended nutrient densities for moderately malnourished children. Food Nutr Bull. 2009;30:S267.
9. Scrimshaw NS. Effect of infection on nutrient requirements. Am J Clin Nutr. 1977;30(9):1536–44.
10. Garza C. Commentary: please sir, I want some more (and something else). Int J Epidemiol. 2015. doi:10.1093/ije/dyv299.
11. World Health Organization/World Food Program/Standing Committee on Nutrition/United Nations Children's Fund. Community-based management of severe malnutrition. A joint statement by the World Health Organization, the World Food Programme, the United Nations System Standing Committee on Nutrition, and the United Nations Children's Fund. Geneva: World Health Organization; 2007.
12. Golden MH. Specific deficiencies versus growth failure: type I and type II nutrients. SCN News. 1995;12:15–21.
13. De Pee S, Semba RD. Role of nutrition in HIV infection: review of evidence for more effective programming in resource-limited settings. Food Nutr Bull. 2010;31:S313–44.
14. Forrester JE, Sztam KA. Micronutrients in HIV/AIDS: is there evidence to change the WHO 2003 recommendations? Am J Clin Nutr. 2011;94(6):1683S–9S.
15. World Health Organization. Nutrient requirements for people living with HIV/AIDS. WHO, Geneva, Switzerland. 2003. (http://www.who.int/nutrition/publications/Content_nutrient_requirements.pdf. Accessed 1 Apr 2016).
16. Academy of Sciences of South Africa (ASSAf). HIV/AIDS, TB and nutrition. Scientific inquiry into the nutritional influences on human immunity with special reference to HIV infection and active TB in South Africa. Pretoria, South Africa: AssAf; 2007.
17. Rodas-Moya S, Kodish S, Manary M, Grede N, de Pee S. Preferences for food and nutritional supplements among adult people living with HIV in Malawi. Publ Hlth Nutr. 2015. doi:10.1017/S1368980015001822.
18. Dewey KG, Mayers DR. Early child growth: how do nutrition and infection interact? Matern Child Nutr. 2011;7:129–42.
19. Mbuya MNN, Humphrey JH. Preventing environmental enteric dysfunction through improved water, sanitation and hygiene: an opportunity for stunting reduction in developing countries. Matern Child Nutr. 2016;12.
20. World Health Organization. Technical note: supplementary foods for the management of moderate acute malnutrition in infants and children 6–59 months of age. Geneva, Switzerland: WHO; 2012.
21. Dewey KG. The challenge of meeting nutrient needs of infants and young children during the period of complementary feeding: an evolutionary perspective. J Nutr. 2013;143:2050–4.
22. Fahmida U, Santika O, Kolopaking R, Ferguson E. Complementary feeding recommendations based on locally available foods in Indonesia. Food Nutr Bull. 2014;35:S174–9.
23. Hernandez L, Campos R, Enneman A, Soto-Mendez MJ, Vossenaar M, Solomons NW. Contribution of complementary food nutrients to estimated total nutrient intakes for urban Guatemalan infants in the second semester of life. Asia Pac J Clin Nutr. 2011;20:572–83.
24. Osendarp S, Broersen B, van Liere MJ, De-Regil L, Bahirathan L, Klassen E, Neufeld LM. Complementary feeding diets made of local foods can be optimized, but additional interventions will be needed to meet iron and zinc requirements in 6–23 month old children in low and middle income countries. Submitted for publication.
25. De Carvalho IST, Granfeldt Y, Dejmek P, Hakansson A. From diets to foods: using linear programming to formulate a nutritious, minimum-cost porridge mix for children aged 1 to 2 years. Food Nutr Bull. 2015;36 (75–85):51.
26. De Pee S, Bloem MW. Current and potential role of specially formulated foods and food supplements for preventing malnutrition among 6–23 month-old children and for treating moderate malnutrition among 6–59 month-old children. Food Nutr Bull Suppl. 2009;30:S434–63.
27. Dror DK, Allen LH. The importance of milk and other animal-source foods for children in low-income countries. Food Nutr Bull. 2011;32:227–43.
28. World Health Organisation European Region. Food based dietary guidelines in the WHO European Region. Copenhagen, Denmark, Europe: WHO; 2003.
29. Gibney MJ, Sandstrom B. A framework for food-based dietary guidelines in the European Union. Public Health Nutr. 2001;4:293–305.
30. Lamstein S, Koniz-Booher P, Beall K, Aakesson A, Anson M. SBCC pathways for improved infant and young child nutrition practices. Spring working paper. Spring, Washington, DC. 2014. Available from: http://www.jsi.com/JSIInternet/Inc/Common/_download_pub.cfm?id=15116&lid=3. Accessed 1 Apr 2016.
31. Pan American Health Organization/World Health Organization. Guiding principles for complementary feeding of the breastfed child. Washington, DC: Pan American Health Organization; 2003.
32. World Health Organization. Guiding principles for feeding non-breastfed children 6–24 months of age. Geneva, Switzerland: WHO; 2005.

33. FAO/WHO. Codex Alimentarius. Standard for processed cereal-based food for infants and young children, STAN 074-1981, Rev 1-2006.
34. Van Hoan N, Van Phu P, Salvignol B, Berger J, Trèche S. Effect of the consumption of high energy dense and fortified gruels on energy and nutrient intakes of 6–10-month-old Vietnamese infants. Appetite. 2009;53(2):233–40.
35. Moursi M, Mbemba F, Trèche S. Does the consumption of amylase-containing gruels impact on the energy intake and growth of Congolese infants? Public Health Nutr. 2003;6(03):249–57.
36. Apar DK, Ozbek B. α-Amylase inactivation by temperature during starch hydrolysis. Process Biochem. 2004;39:1137–44.
37. Kampstra AN, Van Hoan N, Koenders DJPC, Schoop R, Broersen BC, Mouquet-Rivier C, Traoré T, Bruins MJ, de Pee S. Energy and nutrient intake increased by 47–67% when amylase was added to fortified blended foods—a study among 12–35 months old Burkinabè children. Submitted for publication.
38. Manary MJ, Ndekha MJ, Ashorn P, Maleta K, Briend A. Home based therapy for severe malnutrition with ready-to-use food. Arc Dis Child. 2004;89:557–61.
39. Dewey KG, Vitta BS. Strategies for ensuring adequate nutrient intake for infants and young children during the period of complementary feeding. Alive and thrive technical brief, issue 7, Nov 2013. Available from: http://picn.ucdavis.edu/resources/a-and-t/insight_issue_7_ensuring_adequate_nutrition.pdf. Accessed 1 Apr 2016.
40. Hotz C, Gibson RS. Traditional food-processing and preparation practices to enhance the bioavailability of micronutrients in plant-based diets. J Nutr. 2007;137:1097–100.
41. De Pee S, Timmer A, Martini E, Neufeld L, Van Hees J, Schofield D, Huffman S, Siekmann J, Kraemer K, Zlotkin S, Osei A, Dewey K. Programmatic guidance brief on use of micronutrient powders (MNP) for home fortification, a document of the home fortification. Technical advisory group (HF-TAG). Geneva, Switzerland, 2011. Available at: http://www.hftag.org/resource/hf-tag_program-brief-dec-2011-pdf/. Accessed 1 Apr 2016.
42. World Health Organization. Guideline: use of multiple micronutrient powders for home fortification of foods consumed by infants and children aged 6–23 months of age. Geneva, Switzerland: WHO; 2011.
43. Dewey KG, Yang ZY, Boy E. Systematic review and meta-analysis of home fortification of complementary foods. Matern Child Nutr. 2009;5:283–321.
44. Dewey KG, Arimond M. Lipid-based nutrient supplements: how can they combat child malnutrition? PLoS Med. 2012;9:e1001314.
45. Arimond M, Zeilani M, Jungjohann S, Brown KH, Ashorn P, Allen LH, Dewey KG. Considerations in developing lipid-based nutrient supplements for prevention of undernutrition: experience from the international lipid-based nutrient supplements (iLiNS) Project. Matern Child Nutr. 2015;2015(11):31–61.
46. Schultink W. Use of under-five mortality rate as an indicator for vitamin A deficiency in a population. J Nutr. 2002;132:1881S–3S.
47. Iowa State University. Software for intake distribution estimation. www.side.stat.iastate.edu/. Accessed 3 Mar 2016.
48. Mishra AK, Tiwari A. Iron overload in beta thalassaemia major and intermedia patients. Maedica. 2013;8:328–32.
49. Baldi G, Martini E, Catharina M, Muslimatun S, Fahmida U, Jahari AB, Hardinsyah, Frega R, Geniez P, Grede N, Minarto, Bloem MW, de Pee S. Cost of the diet (CoD) tool: first results from Indonesia and applications for policy discussion on food and nutrition security. Food Nutr Bull. 2013 Jun;34(2 Suppl):S35–42.
50. Geniez P, Mathiassen A, de Pee S, Grede N, Rose D. Integrating food poverty and minimum cost diet methods into a single framework: a case study using a Nepalese household expenditure survey. Food Nutr Bull. 2014;35:151–9.
51. Saltzman A, Birol E, Bouis HE, Boyd E, de Moura FF, IslamY, et al. Biofortification: progress toward a more nourishing future. Glob Food Sec. 2013;2:9–17.
52. Tumuhimbise GA, Namutebi A, Turyashemererwa F, Muyonga J. Provitamin A crops: acceptability, bioavailability, efficacy and effectiveness. Food Nutr Sci. 2013;4:430–5.
53. Moench-Pfanner R, Laillou A, Berger J. Introduction: large-scale fortification, an important nutrition-specific intervention. Food Nutr Bull. 2012;33:S255–9.
54. World Health Organization. Recommendations on wheat and maize flour fortification report: interim consensus statement. Geneva: World Health Organization; 2009.
55. Bloch CE. Clinical investigation of xerophthalmia and dystrophy in infant and young children (xerophthalmia et dystrophia aliogenetica). J Hyg. 1921;19:283–304.
56. Semba RD. The vitamin A story: lifting the shadow of death (Chap. 6). In: Koletzko B, editor. Milk, butter, and early steps in human trials (vol. 104, p. 106–31). World review of nutrition and dietetics. Basel, Switzerland: Karger; 2012.
57. Schultz DJ, Shanks CB, Houghtaling B. The impact of the. special supplemental nutrition program for women, infants, and children food package revisions on participants: a systematic review. J Acad Nutr Diet. 2009;2015 (115):1832–46.
58. Pomeranz JL, Chriqui JF. The supplemental nutrition assistance program. Analysis of program administration and food law definitions. Am J Prev Med. 2015;49:428–36.

59. Pelto GH, Armar-Klemesu M, Siekmann J, Schofield D. The focused ethnographic study 'assessing the behavioral and local market environment for improving the diets of infants and young children 6 to 23 months old' and its use in three countries. Matern Child Nutr. 2013;9:35–46.

60. Kodish S, Rah JH, Kraemer K, de Pee S, Gittelsohn J. Understanding low usage of micronutrient powder in the Kakuma Refugee Camp, Kenya: findings from a qualitative study. Food Nutr Bull. 2011;32:292–303.

61. Kodish SR, Aburto NJ, Hambayi MN, Dibari F, Gittelsohn J. Patterns and determinants of small-quantity LNS utilization in rural Malawi and Mozambique: considerations for interventions with specialized nutritious foods. Matern Child Nutr. 2016;12. doi:10.1111/mcn.12234.

62. Mirkovic KR, Perrine CG, Subedi GR, Mebrahtu S, Dahal P, Jefferds MED. Micronutrient powder use and infant and young child feeding practices in an integrated pilot program. Asia Pac J Clin Nutr. 2016;25. doi:10.6133/apjcn.2016.25.2.19.

63. Ebbing H, Rosenzweig J, Karim R. Case study: Bangladesh. In: Codling K, Fabrizio C, Ghoos K, Rosenzweig J, Smit J, Yusufali R, editors. Scaling up rice fortification in Asia. Kaiseraugst, Switzerland: Sight and Life & WFP; 2015. p. 79–83.

64. De Pee S, Moench-Pfanner R, Bloem MW. The Indian Ocean Tsunami of 26 December 2004. In: Semba RD, Bloem MW, editors. Nutrition and health in developing countries. 2nd ed. Totowa, NJ: Humana Press; 2008.

65. Global Alliance for Improved Nutrition (GAIN). Nutritional guidelines for complementary foods and complementary food supplements supported by GAIN. Geneva, Switzerland: GAIN; (undated).

66. De Pee S, Kiess L, Moench-Pfanner R, Bloem MW. Providing access to nutrient-rich diets for vulnerable groups in low- and middle-income settings. In: Sharing the apple: global perspectives on nutrition (in press).

67. Laillou A, Renaud C, Berger J, Moench-Pfanner R, Fontan L, Avallone S. Assessment of a portable device to quantify vitamin A in fortified foods (flour, sugar, and milk) for quality control. Food Nutr Bull. 2014;35:449–57.

68. De Pee S. Special nutritious solutions to enhance complementary feeding. Editorial. Matern Child Nutr. 2015;11:i–viii.

69. Semba RD, Shardell M, Ashour FA, Moaddel R, Trehan I, Maleta KM, Ordiz MI, Kraemer K, Khadeer MA, Ferrucci L, Manary MJ. Child stunting is associated with low circulating essential amino acids. EBioMedicine. 2016;3. doi:10.1016/j.ebiom.2016.02.030.

70. Bloem MW, de Pee S, Semba RD. How much do data influence programs for health and nutrition?—experience from health and nutrition surveillance systems. In: Semba RD, Bloem MW, editors. Nutrition and health in developing countries. 2nd ed. Totowa, NJ: Humana Press; 2008.

71. Bloem MW, de Pee S, Hop le T, Khan NC, Laillou A, Minarto, Moench-Pfanner R, Soekarjo D, Soekirman, Solon JA, Theary C, Wasantwisut E. Key strategies to further reduce stunting in Southeast Asia: lessons from the ASEAN countries workshop. Food Nutr Bull. 2013 Jun;34(2 Suppl):S8–16.

Chapter 9
Vitamin A Deficiency

Amanda C. Palmer, Ian Darnton-Hill and Keith P. West Jr.

Keywords Vitamin A · Xerophthalmia · Epidemiology · Prevention · Treatment

Learning Objectives

- Describe the two major functions of vitamin A that underscore the nutrient's public health importance.
- Identify dietary sources of preformed vitamin A and provitamin A carotenoids.
- Describe how vitamin A is absorbed and metabolized.
- Describe the consequences of vitamin A deficiency for ocular health and survival of infants, children, and reproductive aged women.
- Describe the epidemiology and the clinicopathologic features of vitamin A deficiency in childhood and during the reproductive years.
- Evaluate the current approaches for the prevention of vitamin A deficiency.

Introduction

According to the World Health Organization (WHO), vitamin A deficiency affects an estimated 190 million preschool-aged children and 10 million pregnant women in low-income countries [1]. Prevalent cases of preschool xerophthalmia are believed to number ~5 million, of which 10% can be considered potentially blinding, continuing to make this ocular condition the leading cause of preventable pediatric blindness in the developing world [2]. Recent analyses suggest a decline in the prevalence of vitamin A deficiency over the past quarter of a century, from 39% in 1991 to 29% in 2013 [3]. The greatest progress has been achieved in Southeast Asia and Latin American and the Caribbean, whereas prevalence estimates exceed 40% in both sub-Saharan Africa and South Asia [3].

A.C. Palmer · K.P. West Jr. (✉)
Department of International Health, Johns Hopkins University,
615 N. Wolfe Street, W2041, Baltimore, MD 21205, USA
e-mail: kwest1@jhu.edu

A.C. Palmer
e-mail: apalme17@jhu.edu

I. Darnton-Hill
Institute of Obesity, Nutrition & Exercise, University of Sydney,
Sydney, NSW 2006, Australia
e-mail: ian.darnton-hill@sydney.edu.au

© Springer Science+Business Media New York 2017
S. de Pee et al. (eds.), *Nutrition and Health in a Developing World*,
Nutrition and Health, DOI 10.1007/978-3-319-43739-2_9

Even with these reductions, vitamin A deficiency remains an underlying cause of at least 157,000 early childhood deaths due to diarrhea, measles, malaria and other infections each year [4]. Deficiency is also recognized as a problem among women of reproductive age in many developing countries [5–10], appearing to reflect a chronicity of dietary deficiency that may extend from early childhood into adolescence [11] and adulthood.

This chapter provides a brief orientation to the vitamin itself, including its chemical structure, dietary sources, absorption, metabolism, and functions followed by discussions of the ocular, health, and survival consequences of vitamin A deficiency, its epidemiology in childhood and during the reproductive years, its clinicopathologic features, diagnosis, treatment, and approaches to prevention through dietary improvement, supplementation, fortification, and biofortification.

The Nutrient: Vitamin A

Vitamin A is essential in regulating numerous key biologic processes in the body, including those involved in morphogenesis, growth, maturation, vision, reproduction, immunity, and more broadly, cellular differentiation and proliferation throughout life. Neither humans nor animals can synthesize or survive without vitamin A. Thus, it must be provided from the diet in sufficient amounts to meet all physiologic needs. Excellent, comprehensive reviews exist on the structure, absorption, metabolism, and functions of vitamin A [12, 13].

Structure and Nomenclature

The term vitamin A generically refers to compounds with biologic activity of all-*trans* retinol (R–OH) that, as depicted in Fig. 9.1, also include retinaldehyde (retinal) (R–CHO), various retinyl esters (the dominant form in food) (R–OO), and retinoic acids (R–OOH), among other vitamin A-active metabolic intermediates [12, 13]. Geometric isomers, in *trans* (straight-chained) and *cis* (bent-chained) configuration, are known to occur with retinal (e.g., in the visual cycle) and retinoic acid (e.g., that interact with nuclear receptors to activate gene transcription). Naturally occurring vitamin A compounds are considered to be a subset of a much larger family of "retinoids" that share a common, monocyclic, double-bonded chemical structure with various functional terminal groups. The vast majority of retinoids, however, are synthetic, investigative compounds that are not found in the diet and do not possess vitamin A activity [13, 14].

Lipid-soluble, yellow, and orange pigments known as carotenoids, found mostly in plants, provide the precursor form of vitamin A to all mammalian diets. There are ~ 600 known carotenoids in nature, most of which have the general chemical structure of $C_{40}H_{56}O_n$, where n, the number of oxygen molecules, can vary from 0 to 6. The colors of carotenoids derive from their extensive double-bond structures that absorb light. Carotenoids lacking oxygen in their chemical make-up are termed hydrocarbon carotenoids or "carotenes" (e.g., β-carotene, α-carotene, and lycopene) while those containing oxygen within their polar functional group are known as "xanthophylls" (e.g., β-crpytoxanthin). Among the many carotenoids, ~ 50 have been shown to possess biological activity of vitamin A, though far fewer are considered of nutritional importance in the human diet [13, 15]. Beta-carotene is the most ubiquitous carotenoid in foods and most efficient in its bioconversion to vitamin A, with a structure that, when centrally cleaved by enzyme action in the intestine yields two identical molecules of retinal that can be reduced to retinol [16]. Asymmetric (or eccentric) cleavage of β-carotene may also occur, generating molecules of different chain length called β-apocarotenals,

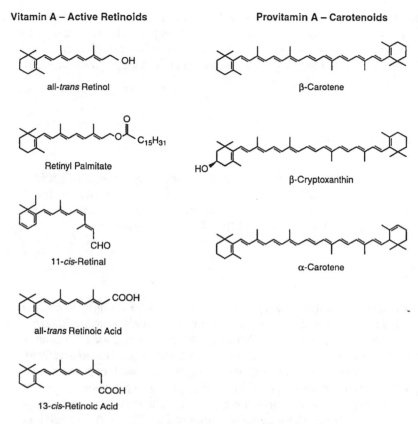

Fig. 9.1 Chemical structure of vitamin A-active retinoids and some of the most common provitamin A carotenoids. Ring and side-chain structures to which end groups are attached are referred in the text as "R" (adapted from [13, 15])

the longer of which can still be shortened to form a molecule of either retinal or retinoic acid (Fig. 9.1) [17]. Chemical structures of all-*trans* β-carotene, α-carotene, and β-cryptoxanthin comprising the most abundant provitamin A carotenoids are depicted in Fig. 9.1.

Absorption and Transport

As fat-soluble compounds, vitamin A and its precursor carotenoids are digested and absorbed by mechanisms common to lipids, and thus require the presence of dietary fat. Approximately 5–10 g of fat in a meal appears to be sufficient to assure absorption [13]. Preformed vitamin A esters are hydrolyzed to retinol by pancreatic and brush border enzymes, mixed with micelles and absorbed by diffusion, though protein carriers may also facilitate uptake [18]. Within the enterocyte, most retinol from preformed and provitamin A sources is re-esterified, incorporated into chylomicrons with other lipophilic molecules (including β-carotene), and secreted through intestinal lymph into portal circulation. A small proportion of unesterified retinol is also released into general circulation that can nourish tissues directly [13, 18]. Prior to reaching the liver, chylomicrons are reduced in size to remnants that, because of their lipophilic nature, retain most of the vitamin A. On reaching the liver, deposited retinyl esters are hydrolyzed to retinol and transferred to stellate cells to be stored as esters.

Fifty to 80% of the stored vitamin A in the body resides in the liver, from where it is released into circulation in association with retinol-binding protein (RBP) and transthyretin, a protein complex that transports the vitamin to tissue sites where it is delivered to cells via RBP receptors located on the cell surface [13]. Within the cell, binding proteins escort retinoids to their cytoplasmic and nuclear sites of action.

Metabolism and Functions

Among numerous cellular mechanisms influenced by vitamin A, at least two reveal its essentiality, and underscore its public health importance: one, as an optical sensor in the visual cycle, the description of which earned George Wald the Nobel Prize in 1964 [19], and the other as a regulator of gene transcription which affects cellular differentiation and function.

Visual Cycle

Participation of vitamin A in the visual cycle enables vision under conditions of dim light. Inadequate vitamin A nutriture can sufficiently deprive rod cells to such an extent that it impairs night vision and leads to "night blindness," a well-known disorder and clinical indicator of vitamin A deficiency [2]. In the cascade of events that enable low-light vision, vitamin A, in its aldehyde form (11-*cis* retinal), acts as a light-absorbing component (chromophore) of the visual pigment rhodopsin (known as "visual purple"), a protein which resides at the outer segments of rod photoreceptor cells in the retina [20, 21]. The initial step in vision occurs when light strikes photoreceptors and causes 11-*cis* retinal to isomerize to its all-*trans* form. The reaction induces a change in the conformation of rhodopsin that activates another protein, transducin, which initiates a change in cell membrane potential and a cascade of neurochemical reactions that transmit signals along the optic nerve to the brain, creating a visual image [21, 22]. As all-*trans* retinal dissociates from rhodopsin, the visual pigment becomes colorless at which point it is said to be "bleached." The open protein remains deactivated until it reattaches another molecule of 11-*cis* retinal to form rhodopsin and regain its photoreactive potential [21, 22]. The 11-*cis* retinal required to react with opsin comes from retinol that is either delivered to the retinal pigment epithelium (RPE) of the eye via choroidal circulation or has been recycled via the visual (or retinoid) cycle [21], depicted in Fig. 9.2. In this cycle, the all-*trans* retinal released from rhodopsin after bleaching is reduced to all-*trans* retinol and escorted by an interphotoreceptor retinoid binding protein (IRBP) from the rod through an interstitial matrix to the RPE, where it is esterified, hydrolyzed and isomerized, and finally oxidized to 11-*cis* retinal. A parallel, light-induced pathway also exists in the RPE that forms 11-*cis* from all-*trans* retinal [21, 22]. The retinoid cycle is completed when the 11-*cis* isomer of retinal is escorted by the IRBP back from the pigment epithelium to the rod outer segment where it attaches to opsin to form rhodopsin.

Gene Regulation

A second major function of vitamin A involves its ability to regulate gene transcription, representing the pathways by which vitamin A is likely to mediate most, though not all, of its effects on embryonic development, organogenesis (e.g., lung, heart, vasculature, central nervous system, kidney, and limbs), immune function, tissue epithelialization (including the corneal and conjunctival surfaces of the eye) and homeostasis, hematopoiesis, and bone growth and development [13, 23, 24]. In the

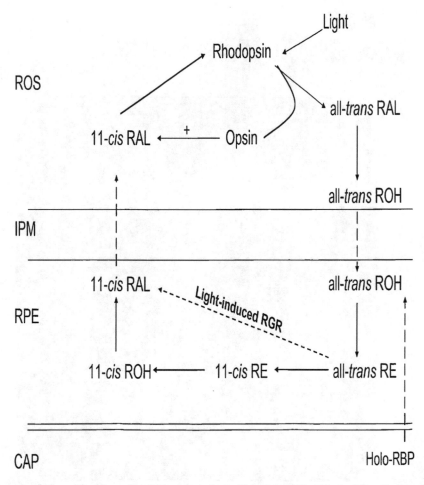

Fig. 9.2 The visual (or retinoid) cycle. *RAL* retinal (retinaldehyde); *ROL* retinol; *RE* retinyl ester; *ROS* rod photoreceptor outer segment; *IPM* interphotoreceptor matrix; *RPE* retinal pigment epithelium; *CAP* choriocapillaris; *RGR* retinal G-protein-linked receptor. Heavy *dashed lines* represent retinoid binding transport of vitamin A. The *lighter dashed line* represents a light-induced conversion pathway to 11-*cis* retinal in the RPE

nucleus of the cell, all-*trans* and 9-*cis* retinoic acids complex with, and activate, retinoid acid (RAR) and retinoid X (RXR) receptors that bind to short sequences of deoxyribonucleic acid (DNA) known as retinoic acid response elements (RARE) that are located within or near target genes. These interactions signal the process of gene transcription by ribonucleic acid (RNA) (Fig. 9.3), a process that leads to translation and synthesis of regulatory proteins that regulate cell differentiation, signaling, and apoptosis [13, 23, 25, 26]. Over 500 genes are thought to respond to retinoic acid, either via the direct, activated RARE pathway or, other indirect transcriptional mechanisms [13, 26]. Depletion in vitamin A nutriture alters molecular dynamics that can lead to pathological changes in cell phenotype, which are most observable in rapidly dividing cells, such as those of the epithelial linings and the immune system. During vitamin A depletion, columnar and mucous-secreting goblet cells of the respiratory tract undergo reversible squamous metaplasia and keratinization [27, 28]. When these changes occur on the ocular surface, xerosis (drying) of the conjunctival or cornea ensues, which can lead to xerophthalmia [29].

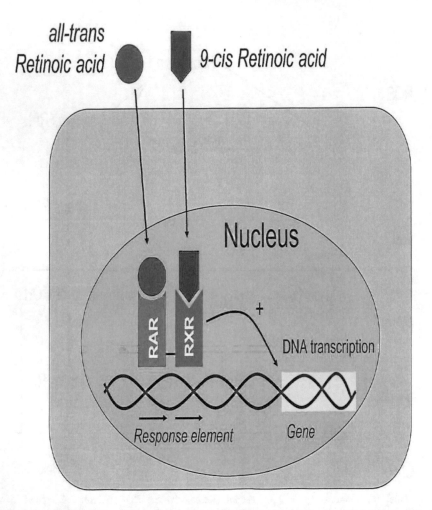

Fig. 9.3 Vitamin A mechanisms in gene regulation. Retinoic acids activate retinoic acid (*RAR*) or retinoid X (*RXR*) receptors that induce response elements on a DNA strand to signal gene transcription by messenger RNA (adapted from [459])

Dietary Sources and Intake Recommendations

Dietary vitamin A is consumed in the human diet as preformed retinyl esters, from animal sources or fortified food items, or as provitamin A carotenoids obtained primarily from plant sources.

Preformed vitamin A activity can be estimated from food composition tables, wherein one μg of retinol is the standard, defined as 1 μg of retinol activity equivalent (RAE) [30]. If the retinol content is reported as an ester, the molecular weight is factored in: for example, 1.83 μg of retinyl palmitate (the most common vitamin A ester in food) = 1 μg RAE. It is generally held that 70–90% of preformed vitamin A from esters in the diet is absorbed and utilized [13]. Animal sources of preformed vitamin A include liver, fish liver oils, butter, cheese, milk fat, other dairy products, and egg yolk [31]. Animal liver typically provides 5000–20,000 μg RAE, cod liver oil ∼30,000 μg RAE, whole cow or goat milk ∼50 to 60 μg RAE, and cheeses ∼300 μg RAE per 100 g edible portion [32]. Fortified foods provide another major dietary source of preformed vitamin A which include ready-to-eat cereals, snack foods, beverages, margarine, and processed dairy products [33]. Vitamin A-fortified foods are increasingly available in developing countries, including sugar [34–36], cereal flours [37], edible oils [37–40]. Approximately 25–75% of the total vitamin A intake is preformed in high-income countries, with North America being at the upper end of this range [41]. In many low-middle income countries (LMICs), preformed vitamin A intake typically lies at the lower end or below this range [42].

Breast milk provides in many poor settings the sole reliable source of vitamin A for the first 6 months of life or longer. Over 90% of its vitamin A content derives from highly bioavailable esters. Among healthy women, mature breast milk contains ∼600 to 700 μg of vitamin A per liter [43] which, at an intake of ∼725 ml per day, provides a breastfed infant with ∼435 to 500 μg of dietary vitamin A [43], an amount considered to be adequate during infancy [30]. In food insecure settings, breast milk can contain half this concentration [43, 44] but still provides clinically protective amounts to infants and toddlers [45, 46].

Provitamin A carotenoids represent the major source of dietary vitamin A in the developing world, among which β-carotene is the most ubiquitous and bioavailable [15, 16]. Food sources of provitamin A carotenoids include dark green leafy vegetables, egg yolk, and deeply colored yellow and orange vegetables and fruits, including carrot, ripe mango and papaya, yellow-orange sweet potato, pumpkin, winter squash, apricot, and a number of indigenous fruits and plants [47]. The β-carotene content typically ranges from ∼5 to 60 μg per 100 g edible portion in these foods [47]. However, absorption and bioconversion of dietary β-carotene and other provitamin A carotenoids into retinol (i.e., bio-efficacy) is a complex process that is influenced by numerous factors captured by the mnemonic "SLAMENGHI" [48–50]; a term that reflects the effects of *s*pecies of carotenoid and its molecular *l*inkage, the *a*mount of carotenoid consumed in a meal, the source food *m*atrix (a dominant influence), *e*ffectors that may enhance or impair digestion, absorption and bioconversion, including intestinal parasites, the *n*utritional status, *g*enetic make-up and *h*ealth status of the host, and nutrient *i*nteractions. Table 9.1 provides examples of these influences, several of which (i.e., food matrix and effectors) can be modified by food choices and the ways food is processed. For example, yellow fruit, cooked yams, added dietary fat, such as red palm oil, reduced fiber in meals, and various processes of

Table 9.1 SLAMENGHI mnemonic on factors that affect carotenoid bioavailability and bioconversion to vitamin A (modified from [48–50])

	Factors	Examples
S	Species of carotenoid	All-*trans* β-carotene may be better absorbed than 9-*cis* β-carotene [49, 450]
L	Molecular linkage	Carotenoids in esters may be absorbed differently than in free form [49]
A	Amount of carotenoid	Proportion absorbed may decrease with amount eaten at a meal [451]
M	Matrix in which carotenoid sits	β-carotene is better absorbed from soft yellow fruit than dark green leaves [51]; cooking, mincing or pureeing improves bioavailability [52–54]
E	Effectors of absorption and bioconversion	Intestinal parasitic infections, including those that decrease fat absorption, decrease β-carotene bioavailability [452, 453]; Fibre, pectin, cellulose, chlorophyll, type of fat and other carotenoid in food affect β-carotene bioavailability [55, 450]; 5–10 g of fat in meals improve β-carotene bioavailability [56, 57, 354]
N	Nutritional status of host	Low vitamin A status enhances enzyme cleavage and bioavailability of β-carotene [58]; low protein and zinc status may reduce β-carotene bioavailability [450]
G	Genetic make-up of host	May partly explain differences in β-carotene response to host dietary interventions (i.e., carotenoid "responders" vs. "non-responders") [454, 455], or gender differences in serum β-carotene responses [50]
H	Health status of host	Carotenoid absorption may be reduced in intestinal and malabsorptive diseases [50, 450]
I	Interactions (biological) with other nutrients	Supplementation with one carotenoid may increase or decrease plasma concentrations of other carotenoids [50]

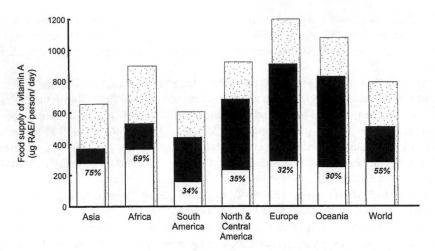

Fig. 9.4 Vitamin A activity in the regional and world food supplies as provitamin A carotenoids with their percent of total (based on a 12:1 β-carotene:retinol conversion ratio, *white segments*), and as preformed retinyl esters (*black segments*). *Stippled bar* represents the previous estimate of total vitamin A using a 6:1 conversion ratio, reflecting a 55% overestimate globally (based, in part, on [63])

cooking, mincing, or pureeing (e.g., of carrots and spinach) are all factors that favor bioavailability [51–57].

Historically, the molar retinol equivalency of dietary β-carotene and other provitamin A carotenoids was assumed to be 6:1 and 12:1, respectively [42, 58]. These ratios were called into question by research carried out in Indonesia showing differential bioefficacy when β-carotene was delivered in the form of stir-fried vegetables versus an enriched wafer [59]. Subsequent work revealed equivalency ratios of 12:1 for β-carotene in a fruit matrix and 26:1 from leafy vegetables and carrots [60]. In 2001, based on accumulating evidence from bioefficacy studies [61], the Institute of Medicine doubled equivalency ratios to 12:1 for dietary β-carotene and 24:1 for other provitamin A carotenoids [30, 62]. Halving the retinol activity equivalency of provitamin A carotenoids in food had two immediate effects. First, it revealed a previous 55% overestimate of the vitamin A content in the global food supply (Fig. 9.4) [63], amplifying concern for populations that are largely dependent on vegetables and fruits to meet dietary vitamin A requirements [48]. Second, the change made clear the virtual impossibility for most poor, young children to meet their vitamin A requirements through vegetable and fruit intake alone [7]. The problem is illustrated in Table 9.2, where gram amounts of a provitamin A-containing food basket needed to meet the Recommended Dietary Allowances (RDA) [30, 62] or the Recommended Nutrient Intake (RNI) [31] are given by age, according to a 12:1 bioconversion ratio (for β-carotene), in a typical poor setting where an estimated 25% of the RDA is consumed as preformed vitamin A. In this setting, a 4- to 6-year-old child needs to consume 120 g of vegetables and fruit daily to meet his/her RDA, depending on the ratio adopted. This is equivalent to at least a 40 g serving of such foods 3 times a day. Where less preformed vitamin A is typically consumed, the required intakes of vegetables and fruits increase further.

Public Health Significance of Vitamin a Deficiency

Public health consequences that can be attributed to vitamin A deficiency are defined as "vitamin A deficiency disorders" or VADD [64], which include the specific ocular manifestations of xerophthalmia and its blinding sequelae as well as nonspecific consequences, such as anemia, immune

Table 9.2 Dietary reference intakes [62] (DRI), recommended nutrient intakes [31] (RNI) and dietary requirements for vitamin A for children and adults by age and gender

Age group	Gender	DRI (34-IOM, 2001) μg RAE per day	RNI (FAO, 2002) μg RE per day	Amount of β-Carotene-rich Food (g) required to meet RDA	
				Conversion ratio	
		RDA	RNI	12:1	24:1
1–3 year	M & F	300	400	90	180
4–6 year	M & F	400	450	120	240
7–8 year	M & F	400	500	120	240
9 year	M & F	600	500	180	360
Adolescents					
10–13 year	M/F	600/600	400/600	180	360
14–18 year	M/F	900/700	400/600	240	480
Adults					
19–65 year	M/F	900/700	600/500	240	480
Pregnancy		~760	850	228	456

Food items include an illustrative mixture of dark green leaves (spinach, kangkong or swamp cabbage, mustard greens) and one fruit (mango), providing a mean β-carotene content of 3 mg per 100 g [278], equal to 250 μg retinol activity equivalents (RAE) at a 12:1 β-carotene:retinol equivalency ratio or 125 μg RAE at a conversion ratio of 24:1 [62]. Amounts required to meet the RDA assumes that 25% of the allowance is already being met by dietary sources of preformed vitamin A. An average RDA of 800 μg RAE represents the dietary target for ages 14–18 and 19–65 year. RNI values are provided for comparison; these were set by the FAO/WHO assuming a bioconversion factor of 6 μg β-carotene to 1 μg retinol and are expressed in terms of retinol equivalents (RE) [63].

dysfunction, increased susceptibility to infection, poorer growth, and mortality (Fig. 9.5). VADD may also include consequences in adult life that might be causally linked to early life exposure to vitamin A deficiency (discussed below). At present, VADD are known to occur in children and women of reproductive age.

Prevalence

The extent of vitamin A deficiency can be assessed based on the clinical stages of xerophthalmia (Gr. *xeros = drying; ophthalmia = of the eye*) [29]. Earlier, antecedent stages of squamous metaplasia, detectable by impression cytology, or the impaired dark adaptation that precedes outright night blindness [65], serve both as physiologic indicators of deficiency and health consequences, or disorders, of vitamin A deficiency.

While not a disorder per se, low vitamin A status defined by biochemical indicators is most commonly used to determine the prevalence of vitamin A deficiency. Serum or plasma retinol concentrations, measured by high performance liquid chromatography, serve as the primary basis for global prevalence estimates [1]. Retinol-binding protein (RBP), which theoretically circulates in a 1:1 molar ratio with retinol, is increasingly measured as an alternate indicator for reasons of cost, stability under field conditions, and laboratory capabilities [66]. However, questions remain regarding appropriate cutoffs for RBP, as molar ratios of retinol to RBP vary in the literature from 0.70 to 1.79 [67]. As retinol-binding protein is an acute phase reactant, concentrations of both retinol and its binding protein may be negatively influenced by the inflammatory response to an infection or other insult [68–71]. This can result in the misclassification of individuals with adequate status and potentially overestimate the prevalence of deficiency in a population. Methods have been proposed to assess and account for inflammation [68, 72, 73]; however, both adjusted and unadjusted

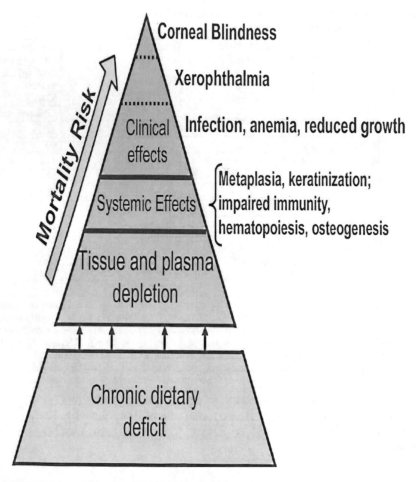

Fig. 9.5 Vitamin A deficiency disorders (VADD) (adapted from [5])

concentrations should be reported. Other status measures have been described in detail and will be increasingly necessary as population status improves in order to be informative across a broader range of the vitamin A status continuum [74].

Preschool-Aged Children

The WHO estimates that ∼33% of preschool-aged children, or 190 million, are vitamin A-deficient (Table 9.3) [1]. The estimate is based on proportions of surveyed children with a serum retinol concentration below the conventional cut-off of 0.70 µmol/L [66]. A prevalence of deficiency of ≥15% among preschool-aged children 6–71 months of age is considered to represent a public health problem [64, 66] (Table 9.4). Nearly 5.2 million preschoolers residing in LMICs, or nearly 1%, are thought to have xerophthalmia [1]. Highest risk populations are in periequatorial regions of the world [5]. The combined prevalence of xerophthalmia and serum retinol concentration <0.70 µmol/L is depicted in Fig. 9.6. The lower threshold of 0.5% for xerophthalmia represents the WHO cutoff for Bitot's spots, while the 1.5% cutoff represents the sum of both thresholds for Bitot's spots (0.5%) and night blindness (1.0%) [64]. The resultant geographic pattern roughly parallels broad ecological indices of poverty and undernutrition. Findings of more recent vitamin A status assessments generally

Table 9.3 Global prevalence and burden of preschool child and maternal gestational vitamin A deficiency (serum retinol < 0.70 μmol/L), by region

WHO region	Preschool-aged children (<5 year)		Pregnant women	
	Prevalence (%)[a]	Burden (millions)	Prevalence (%)	Burden (millions)
Africa	44.4 (41.3–47.5)[b]	56.4 (52.4–60.3)	13.5 (8.9–18.2)	4.18 (2.73–5.63)
Americas	15.6 (6.6–24.5)	8.68 (3.70–13.7)	2.0 (0.4–3.6)	0.23 (0.04–0.41)
South East Asia	49.9 (45.1–54.8)	91.5 (82.6–100)	17.3 (0.0–36.2)	6.69 (0.00–14.0)
Europe	19.7 (9.7–29.6)	5.81 (2.87–8.75)	11.6 (2.6–20.6)	0.72 (0.16–1.29)
Eastern Mediterranean	20.4 (13.2–27.6)	13.2 (8.54–17.9)	16.1 (9.2–23.1)	2.42 (1.38–3.47)
Western Pacific	12.9 (12.3–13.5)	14.3 (13.6–14.9)	21.5 (0.0–49.2)	4.90 (0.00–11.2)
Global	33.3 (31.1–35.4)	190 (178–202)	15.3 (7.4–23.2)	19.1 (9.30–29.0)

Reprinted with permission from WHO. Global prevalence of vitamin A deficiency in populations at risk 1995–2005. WHO Global Database on Vitamin A Deficiency. Geneva, World Health Organization, 2009. www.who.int/entity/nutrition/publications/micronutrients/vitamin_a_deficiency/9789241598019/en/
[a]Excludes countries with a 2005 Gross Domestic Product ≥ USD15,000
[b]95% Confidence intervals

Table 9.4 IVACG/WHO xerophthalmia classification and minimum indicator prevalence criteria for vitamin A deficiency to be a public health problem [64]

Definition (Code)	Minimum prevalence
Children 24–59 months	
History of night blindness (XN)	>1.0%
Conjunctival xerosis (X1B)	–
Bitot's spots (X1B)	>0.5%
Corneal xerosis (X2)	–
Corneal ulceration/keratomalacia (X3)	>0.01%
Xerophthalmic corneal scars (XS)	>0.05%
Serum retinol concentrations <0.35 μmol/L	>5%
Serum retinol concentrations <0.70 μmol/L	>15%
Women of child-bearing age	
History of night blindness	≥5%

uphold the WHO data published in 2009, showing an estimated 29% prevalence of vitamin A deficiency [1, 3]. Sub-Saharan Africa and South Asia had the highest prevalence, at 48 and 44% of children, respectively.

Newborns and Neonates

Early infancy is a precarious period as limited materno-fetal transfer of retinol endows infants with only a 2-weeks to 2-months hepatic supply of vitamin A and low circulating retinol concentrations [75–77]. Whereas body vitamin A stores rise toward normal during infancy in well-nourished

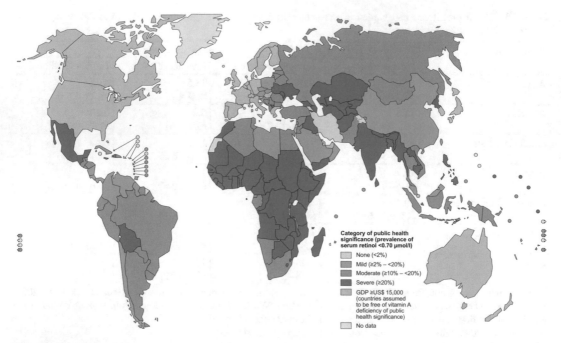

Fig. 9.6 Global distribution of preschool child vitamin A deficiency defined by deficient serum retinol concentration (<0.70 μmol/L)

societies [77, 78], the status of infants reared under vitamin A-deprived and infection-exposed conditions tends to remain depressed [77, 79] which may increase risks of morbidity and mortality in the first 6–12 months of life (discussed below). Prematurity exacerbates the vitamin A-depleted state at birth [80]. However, poor access to newborns and their high mortality in the developing countries, coupled with difficulties in drawing blood and uncertainty about the plasma retinol cutoff have left the extent and severity of neonatal vitamin A deficiency unknown at this time.

School-Aged Children

In undernourished populations, vitamin A deficiency may extend into the peri-adolescent years. While limited surveys exist in this age group, data from South East Asia suggest that 23% of children 5–15 years of age, or ~83 million, may have serum retinol concentrations below 0.70 μmol/L and nearly 3% to have non-blinding, mild xerophthalmia (night blindness or Bitot's spots) [11]. Recent surveys from Ethiopia [81] and Brazil [82], as well as a summary report on nutritional status in this age group covering the period 2002–2009 [83], reveal similar estimates of hyporetinolemia. While risk factors and health consequences of deficiency at this age are unknown, poor adolescent vitamin A nutriture may predispose girls to chronic vitamin A deficiency in adult life that could exacerbate deficiency during pregnancy and lactation [84].

Women of Reproductive Age

Vitamin A deficiency afflicts women of child-bearing ages in food insecure societies, especially in the second half of pregnancy when nutritional demands are high, circulating vitamin A is relatively low, and risk of developing night blindness greatest [84]. Population data on serum retinol distributions during and following pregnancy, however, remains sparse. The current best estimate is that ~7–23% of pregnant women in low-income countries have deficient serum retinol concentrations (<1.05 μmol/L), with the average prevalence being 15%, or ~19 million affected gravida in a given year [1] (Table 9.3). On the other hand, because a history of night blindness can be reliably ascertained [85], a number of surveys have elicited a history of maternal night blindness, yielding an overall prevalence estimate of ~8%, with estimates generally ranging from 10 to 20% where malnutrition and childhood vitamin A deficiency are known to exist [1]. A provisional cutoff of ≥5% has been set for classifying night blindness during pregnancy as a public health problem (Table 9.4) [64, 85].

Effects on Child Morbidity and Mortality

Vitamin A deficiency has long been known as the "anti-infective" vitamin [86, 87]. Decades of animal experiments show that progressive vitamin A depletion leads to poor growth, weight loss, infection, and death, usually before eye signs develop [88]. The regulatory roles of vitamin A in maintaining epithelial cell differentiation and function and immune competence [68] provide biologic plausibility to its importance in decreasing severity and mortality from infectious diseases [2]. A modern era of epidemiologic investigation into the role of vitamin A deficiency in child mortality was launched with community-based studies of Sommer and colleagues in the late seventies that found Indonesian children with mild xerophthalmia, but no other obvious nutritional stress, to be two to three times more likely to develop diarrhea or respiratory infection [89] and more likely, in a dose-responsive fashion, to die [90] than children without eye signs (Fig. 9.7). Additional longitudinal studies in India [91] and Thailand [92] have generally corroborated increased risks of incident morbidity among children with mild xerophthalmia or hyporetinolemia, respectively.

Between 1986 and 1992, six of eight population-based, intervention trials that enrolled more than 165,000 children in Southeast Asia [93, 94], South Asia [95–98] and Africa [99, 100] found that vitamin A supplementation, achieved by periodic high-dose supplementation (e.g., 200,000 IU if >12 month of age, half-doses below 12 month), weekly low-dose supplementation (15,000 IU) or via food fortification, could reduce child mortality by 6–54% (Fig. 9.8). Meta-analyses of findings from these early trials have shown that, in areas of endemic vitamin A deficiency, all-cause preschool

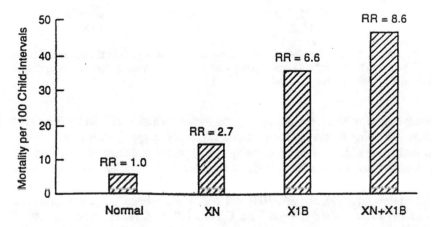

Fig. 9.7 Mortality rates of Indonesian preschool children without xerophthalmia (normal) and by severity of "mild" xerophthalmia (XN < X1B < XN + X1B) (adapted from [90])

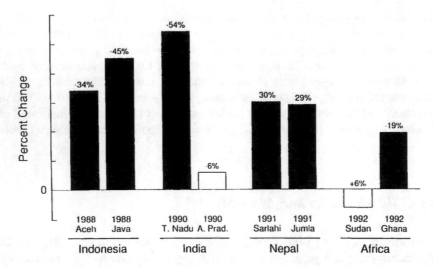

Fig. 9.8 Percent changes in mortality rates of children between ∼6 or 12 months to <84 months of age receiving vitamin A compared to children receiving control supplements while participating in community intervention trials in Southeast Asia (Aceh [93] and Java [94], Indonesia), South Asia (Tamil Nadu [95], and Andhra Pradesh [96], India and Sarlahi [97] and Jumla [98], Nepal), and Africa (Ghana [99] and Sudan [100]). Total number of enrolled children >165,000 [2]

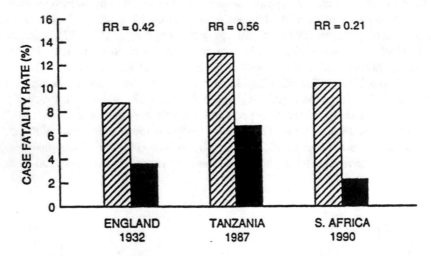

Fig. 9.9 Fatality rates of children hospitalized with severe measles who participated in clinical vitamin A trials in England [105], Tanzania [106], and South Africa [107]. Risk of mortality among vitamin A recipients is <50% that of controls in each study (from [110])

child mortality can be reduced, on average, by 23–34% by vitamin A interventions [101–104], with the effect size depending on the studies included and analytic approaches taken.

The remarkably consistent effect on mortality can be partly explained by an ability of vitamin A to lower case fatality from measles by ∼50%, as observed in field trials and hospital-based treatment trials [2, 105–107] (Fig. 9.9). Vitamin A can be expected to lower risk of fatality from severe diarrhea and dysentery by ∼40% [95, 97, 98, 108] and possibly *Plasmodium falciparum* malaria as well, based on findings from a trial in Papua New Guinea [109]. A recent WHO-sponsored analysis to calculate global and regional burdens of disease estimated ∼50% reductions in case fatality from diarrhea and measles among vitamin A recipients [110]. Similarly, high-dose vitamin A supplementation of HIV-infected children in several African trials has reduced adverse outcomes by 50% or more, including all-cause and diarrhea-associated mortality [111, 112], diarrhea incidence or duration [112, 113] and stunting [114] over 18–24 month periods of follow-up. Notwithstanding these protective effects against several potentially fatal infectious diseases, vitamin A supplementation has had little influence on risk of mortality from acute lower respiratory infections, unrelated to measles, for reasons that remain poorly understood [115].

Subsequent program effectiveness analyses, based on nonexperimental designs, continue to support a favorable impact of vitamin A on child survival. In the Yemen, admissions and case fatality for severe, dehydrating diarrhea among preschoolers presenting to four major hospitals in Sana'a were reduced by 25% and ~50%, respectively, after the first year of semi-annual vitamin A supplementation [116]. In Nepal, the 2001 Demographic and Health Survey, conducted after several years of national supplementation activities, estimated vitamin A receipt to be consistent with a ~50% decline in 1–4 year-old child mortality [117]. The magnitude of decline, which exceeds estimates from efficacy trials, may result from additional promotion activities delivered in tandem with vitamin A capsules. Analysis of population-based surveys also supports the effect of vitamin A supplementation on reducing child mortality in both Ghana [118] and Niger [119]. The largest assessment of program effectiveness to date was carried out in northern India to test the impact of "deworming and enhanced vitamin A," or "DEVTA," delivered by village anganwadi child-care centers [120]. While reductions in the prevalence of xerophthalmia and poor vitamin A status (serum retinol <0.70 μmol/L) were evident, this study reported no beneficial effect of supplementation on mortality [120]. However, the study has been widely criticized in the literature [121–125], in particular for the lack of rigorous vital events tracking necessary to accurately measure the study's primary outcome.

Effects on Infant Morbidity and Mortality

Vitamin A may favor infant survival in undernourished populations, depending on the age dosed, "route" of supplementation, nutritional status, and dominant disease patterns. In both Nepal [126] and Tanzania [127], reaching the fetus and infant via routine maternal supplementation with vitamin A or/and β-carotene during pregnancy and lactation had no overall effect on infant mortality, except for a subset of infants born to night blind women in Nepal who were more likely to survive following maternal vitamin A supplementation [128]. Direct dosing trials in South Asia and Africa, where infants were periodically given oral vitamin A (ranging from 25,000 to 100,00 IU per dose) from ~1 to 5 months of age, also failed to benefit infant survival [129, 130].

A series of randomized, double-blinded, placebo-controlled trials have considered the impact of supplementing newborns (Table 9.5). The first of these was carried out by Humphrey et al. in Indonesia, where researchers provided 50,000 IU of vitamin A or a placebo at birth and followed infants through their first birthday [131]. Newborn dosing in this setting reduced infant mortality by 64%, with the effect seemingly stronger in males compared to females [131]. Subsequent trials conducted in Asia have reported significant reductions of 23% [132], 16% [133], and 10% [134] in infant mortality. Effects did not differ by infant sex, but the effect reported from Tamil Nadu, India appeared to be limited to low birthweight infants [132]. While causal paths uniquely responsive to early neonatal (vs later) high-dose vitamin A receipt remain poorly understood, diseases in early infancy that could plausibly respond include respiratory infections (e.g., from *Streptococcus pneumoniae*) [135], diarrhea, sepsis and necrotizing enterocolitis [77].

The first newborn vitamin A trial in Africa was conducted in an urban population in Zimbabwe where mothers were otherwise normal in their vitamin A status (i.e., <1% with a serum retinol concentration below 0.70 μmol/L). In this setting a 50,000 IU oral dose of vitamin A given to either

Table 9.5 Efficacy trials of newborn vitamin A supplementation in Asia and Africa

Location	Sample description	Dosage	Follow-up period (months)	Risk ratio (95% CI)
Asia				
Indonesia [131]	2067 neonates	50,000 IU administered at birth (88% reached within 24 h)	12	0.39 (0.15–1.01)
TamilNadu, India [132]	11,619 neonates	50,000 IU administered at birth (46% reached within 24 h)	6	0.78 (0.62–0.98)
Bangladesh [133]	15,937 neonates in 596 clusters	50,000 IU administered at birth (79% reached within 24 h)	6	0.85 (0.72–1.01)
Haryana, India [134]	44,984 neonates	50,000 IU administered at birth (65% reached within 24 h)	6	0.90 (0.81–1.00)
Africa				
Zimbabwe [136]	9208 HIV- neonates	50,000 IU administered within 96 h	12	1.12 (0.80–1.57)
Guinea-Bissau [138]	4345 neonates	50,000 IU administered at birth (median: 16 d)	12	1.13 (0.77–1.65)
Guinea-Bissau [139]	1717 low birthweight neonates	25,000 IU administered at birth (51% reached within 48 h)	12	1.01 (0.72–1.42)
Guinea-Bissau [140]	6048 neonates	25,000 or 50,000 IU administered at birth	6	1.28 (0.91, 1.81)
Ghana [141]	22,955 neonates	50,000 IU administered at birth (73% reached within 48 h)	6	1.12 (0.95–1.33)
Tanzania [142]	30,892 neonates	50,000 IU administered at birth (78% reached within 24 h)	6	1.10 (0.95–1.26)

HIV-positive [136] or negative [137] infants at birth failed to confer a survival benefit during infancy. Maternal receipt of 400,000 IU of vitamin A immediately after birth also failed to improve infant survival in this population [136, 137]. Smaller trials conducted in Guinea-Bissau similarly reported no impact of newborn vitamin A dosing [138–140], although treatment regimens for two of these differed in that infants were reached later in the neonatal period [138] or with a lower 25,000 IU dose [139]. While nonsignificant, the investigators called attention to effect modification by sex, with point estimates in the direction of being protective in males and suggesting adverse effects in girls [138–140]. These somewhat controversial findings prompted three additional trials. The first of these, cited above, confirmed the previously reported survival benefit in South Asia [134]. The latter two were conducted in Ghana and Tanzania and reported no beneficial impact of supplementation nor any differences by sex [141, 142].

Overall, trials of newborn dosing with vitamin A show a consistent protective effect in South and South East Asian populations [131–134], but no survival benefit in sub-Saharan Africa [136, 138–142]. This differential effect has been attributed primarily to the underlying nutritional status of the study populations, with very little evidence of maternal vitamin A deficiency in the studies carried out in Africa [143, 144]. This suggests that newborn dosing would be justified in populations with evidence of an elevated prevalence of maternal vitamin A deficiency [144]. However, WHO guidelines are established at a global, as opposed to a regional, level and therefore, the Organization does not currently recommend neonatal vitamin A supplementation as a public health intervention [145].

Effects on Maternal Morbidity and Mortality

In chronically undernourished populations, vitamin A deficiency can pose a health risk to women during pregnancy and lactation. In rural South Asia [6, 9, 146] and sub-Saharan Africa [5], and in poor, urban areas of Latin America [5, 147], 10–20% of women have reported night blindness in pregnancy. Maternal night blindness is likely due to maternal vitamin A deficiency as it often develops late in pregnancy [84] when serum retinol is low [148], and then typically resolves within days after childbirth. The condition is associated with a poor diet, anemia, wasting, and increased occurrence of diarrhea and other morbid symptoms [9, 84, 146]. In Nepal, women who developed night blindness during pregnancy were at a $\sim$4-fold higher risk of dying during pregnancy through the first two years after parturition (3600 per 100,000 person-years) than mothers who reported not having the condition. Most often, causes of death among women who were night blind were associated with infection [149].

Under such high-risk conditions, such as in southern Nepal where maternal mortality rates exceed 600 per 100,000, once-weekly supplementation with either vitamin A or β-carotene at dosages that approximated a 7-day RDA (7000 μg RAE or 42 mg, respectively), reduced all-cause pregnancy-related mortality by 40 and 49%, respectively [150]. Given the plethora of physiologic effects of vitamin A, it is plausible that several potentially fatal causal paths could have responded to improved vitamin A (or β-carotene) nutriture, such as puerperal sepsis, other infections, anemia-involved causes, hypertensive-diseases, and hemorrhage [151]. Notably, the value of late-gestational vitamin A therapy for prophylaxis against puerperal sepsis was recognized in humans and animals as early as the 1930s [152]. Higher maternal serum retinol concentration and vitamin A supplement receipt were recently shown to be associated with improved proinflammatory cytokine responses to infection among Ghanaian gravida [153]. Replicate trials conducted in Bangladesh [154] and Ghana [155], which showed no beneficial effect of supplementation, suggest that there may be thresholds, or plateaus, at which populations may respond to vitamin A. Maternal mortality in these two settings was less than half that of Nepal, and less likely to have been infectious in nature and thus plausibly reduced by a vitamin A intervention. Furthermore, in contrast to Nepal [149], there was limited evidence of severe vitamin A deficiency in either Bangladesh or Ghana [154, 155].

In HIV-positive populations, vitamin A deficiency is clearly associated with adverse pregnancy health. A strong, dose-risk gradient has been demonstrated between maternal serum retinol concentration and risk of vertical transmission of HIV [156]. Cervicovaginal shedding of HIV DNA [157], genital tract infections [158], and, more variably, clinical mastitis [159, 160] have also been associated with poor maternal vitamin A status. The strength and consistency of the evidence of association suggests that vitamin A interventions could improve maternal health, infant survival, and reduce HIV transmission [161]. However, randomized controlled trials of vitamin A and related interventions in HIV settings do not support an anti-HIV role for maternal vitamin A use. Overall, the majority of studies have not demonstrated any impact on transmission of HIV from mother to infant [137, 162, 163], nor any benefit in terms of perinatal or infant mortality [136, 162, 164]. One trial reported an increased risk of both genital HIV shedding [165] and HIV transmission [127]; however, the supplement used in that trial contained both preformed vitamin A (5000 IU) and high-dose β-carotene (30 mg). Thus, the observed risk cannot be attributed to vitamin A alone [166].

Effects of Early Life Exposure

A large body of the literature supports the role of vitamin A during embryonic and fetal development [24, 167, 168], and highlights the consequences of vitamin A inadequacy during this critical period [169–171]. Until recently, however, there have been limited opportunities to address questions regarding the effects of early life exposure to vitamin A deficiency in humans. From 2006 to 2008, researchers working in Nepal recontacted participants of two major vitamin A supplementation trials [97, 150] and their offspring to measure a number of health outcomes that could plausibly be altered by random exposure to supplemental vitamin A in this chronically deficient population.

Subjects from the first trial (1989–1991) received vitamin A (200,000 IU) or placebo capsules every four months as preschool-aged children and were 14–23 years of age at the time of follow-up [97]. Outcomes of interest in this age group included hearing loss and asthma. Hearing loss among children in low-income countries is most commonly the result of repeated ear infections [172]. Given the role of vitamin A in immune defense [68], deficient preschool-aged children may have more frequent and severe ear infections [173, 174]. Researchers hypothesized that this could lead to an increased risk for hearing loss. While periodic vitamin A supplementation did not reduce ear discharge, as an indicator of otitis media, during early childhood, supplementation reduced the risk of hearing loss in these children by 42% [175]. Asthma was also considered as an outcome in this cohort given the role of vitamin A in lung development and in the regeneration of epithelial lung tissue [176, 177], as well as evidence showing airway hyperresponsiveness in deficient animals that could be reversed with vitamin A [178, 179]. While there was a 6.6% prevalence of wheezing in this population, there were no differences between children who had been randomly assigned to receive vitamin A or the placebo during their preschool years [180].

Women enrolled in the second trial (1994–1997) were randomized to receive weekly supplements of 7000 μg RAE as either vitamin A or β-carotene, or a placebo capsule, from pre-pregnancy through the period of lactation [150]. Their offspring were 9–13 years of age at the time of follow-up. Outcomes included lung function, asthma, cognition, and immune markers. The inclusion of respiratory outcomes was driven by a large literature on the role of vitamin A in the maturation of the respiratory system [177, 181–183] and impairments linked with vitamin A inadequacy [24, 177, 181]. Nepali children exposed to vitamin A supplementation while in utero and via breast milk had significantly better lung function than those whose mothers received β-carotene or a placebo [184]. Supplementation had no effect, however, on the prevalence of asthma (4.8% overall) or indices of airway obstruction [180]. Improved cognitive and motor ability of children whose mothers were supplemented was hypothesized based on the role of vitamin A in neural tube formation, neural development, and synaptic signaling [185–191] and human studies that indicated a potential linkage between improved status in early life and motor skills during the preschool years [192, 193]. Among children in the Nepali cohort, however, maternal vitamin A or β-carotene supplementation had no impact on cognitive or motor ability [194], potentially due to the relative protection of the central nervous system to early life insults. Given the layered development of the immune system, where the fetal and neonatal progenitors that give rise to innate-like lymphocytes are progressively replaced by products of adult stem cells, protection of lymphopoiesis from insult may be less crucial [195]. Vitamin A is known to be important for early lymphopoiesis [196] and data from the animal literature show significantly lower counts of innate-like B1a and B1b cells in offspring whose dams were fed a vitamin A-restricted diet [197]. This reduction could be ameliorated by retinoic acid [197]. Although cells were unavailable for immunophenotyping, researchers found that Nepali children whose mothers were in the vitamin A treatment group had significantly greater natural antibody concentrations [198], which are the unique protein product of the innate-like B1a cell population [199].

Historical Background

Several rich, historical accounts have been published detailing the diverse paths to the discovery of vitamin A and its functions by scientific pioneers, especially in the modern era of the nineteenth and twentieth centuries [87, 200–203]. Vitamin A deficiency, manifest as xerophthalmia, has plagued humankind for at least 3500 years. Night blindness, and its treatment with foods now known to be rich in preformed vitamin A esters, such as roasted ox, ass or beef liver, was reported from ancient Assyria, Egypt, and Greece [200] (Table 9.6). Medical treatises from Europe, China, the Middle East, and Southeast Asia throughout the first and second millennia documented the occurrence of night blindness and therapeutic value of animal liver. Clinical descriptions of corneal xerophthalmia first appeared in England in the eighteenth century, followed by additional reports in the nineteenth and early twentieth centuries of its occurrence, in association with infection and poor growth, and its cure with animal and fish liver and oil products [200]. Characterization of conjunctival xerosis with superficial accumulation of keratinized cells and bacilli, named a "Bitot's Spot," was described as early as 1860 by von Huebbenet and then by its namesake, Bitot, in France in 1863.

Table 9.6   Historical benchmarks in the discovery of vitamin A, its deficiency and prevention

Antiquity		Night blindness recognized in Egypt, Greece, Assyria
460-325 BC		Ancient Egyptians and Greeks cured night blindness with roasted ox liver [200]
Nineteenth century		Magendie reports corneal xerophthalmia in dogs following dietary manipulation von Hubbenet and Bitot describe conjunctival xerosis with "Bitot's Spots" [223]
		Boll discovers in frogs that light bleaches the retina; Kuhne refines observations and discovers "visual purple" [202]
		Budd, in England, describes corneal xerophthalmia in East Indians, and Livingston notes (xerophthalmic) corneal lesions in Africans subsisting on manioc diet [200]
		Guggenheim reports night blindness with keratomalacia in Russian children during Great Lenten Fast [200]
		Lunnin points to other indispensable survival factors in whole milk (than those known at the time) [87]
Twentieth century	1904	Mori reports "Hikan" in Japanese children which responds to dietary intervention with liver, and especially cod liver oil [204]
	1912	Hopkins postulates "accessory factors" necessary for life; Funk names these factors "vitamines" [87]
	1913	McCollum and Davis [206], and Osborne and Mendell [207] discover "fat-soluble A"
	1919	Bloch finds xerophthalmia in Danish orphans subsisting on milk-fat free, oatmeal diet [208]
	1928	Green and Mellanby coin term "anti-infective" for vitamin A [210]
	1931	Green and Pindar show cod liver oil reduces puerperal fever [152]
	1932	Ellison reports that vitamin A reduces measles fatality [105]
	1935	Wald describes "the visual cycle" [213]
	1948	Ramalingaswami relates "nutritional diarrhea" to vitamin A deficiency [212]
	1960	Gopalan draws global attention to endemic vitamin A deficiency in India [218]
	1966	McLaren publishes detailed photo accounts of xerophthalmia [219]
	1964	Wald wins the Nobel Prize for describing the visual cycle [202]
		Oomen, McLaren and Escapini publish "Epidemiology and Public Health Aspects of Hypovitaminosis A" [220]
	1974	The International Vitamin A Consultative Group is established [222]
	1983 −84	Sommer and colleagues in Indonesia report mild xerophthalmia is associated with increased risk of incident child morbidity [89] and mortality [90]
	1986– 1993	Sommer and colleagues report that vitamin A can reduce child mortality in Indonesia [93]; this initial report is replicated in five trials carried out in Asia [94, 95, 97, 98] and Africa [99]
	1989	UNICEF World Summit for Children considers vitamin A essential for child survival [377]

(continued)

Table 9.6 (continued)

1992	At the International Conference on Nutrition in Rome, countries commit to preventing vitamin A deficiency [456]
1995	Bioavailability of provitamin A carotenoids in vegetables challenged by Clive West and coworkers in Indonesia [59, 60, 457, 458]
1998	Christian and colleagues in Nepal reveal maternal night blindness as indicator of maternal vitamin A deficiency, poor health, and survival [84, 149]
1999	West and coworkers in Nepal report vitamin A or β-carotene supplementation can lower maternal mortality [150]. These results are not replicated however in trials carried out in Ghana or Bangladesh [154]
2001	Institute of Medicine in the United States revises the β-carotene:retinol conversion ratio from 6:1 to 12:1, and the ratio for other provitamin A carotenoids from 12:1 to 24:1 [62]
2002	Annecy Accords define "vitamin A deficiency disorders," add maternal night blindness as an indicator of deficiency, and recognize inability of young children to eat adequate amounts of vitamin A from vegetables alone [64]
2003	Ramathullah et al. report from India a 23% reduction in infant mortality by giving newborns a single ~ 50,000 IU oral dose of vitamin A [132], affirming earlier work by Humphrey et al. in Indonesia [131].
2009	WHO reports that 190 million children and 10 million pregnant women are affected by vitamin A deficiency worldwide [1]
2010–15	Evidence accumulates on long-term effects of vitamin A deficiency, including hearing loss [175], impaired lung function [184], and lower circulating concentrations of natural antibodies [198]
2005–16	Efficacy trials support the introduction of biofortified staple crops as a vitamin A deficiency control strategy [429–433]

In the 1870s, the foundation for understanding the visual cycle was laid by Franz Boll and Willy Kuhne in Germany. Working with frog eyes, they observed that light bleached the purple pigment (they termed "visual purple") in retinal rod cells and that its regeneration required interaction with the retinal pigment epithelium [202]. Recognition of the existence of indispensable, accessory nutritional factors emerged in the late nineteenth century. In Japan, in 1904, Mori drew attention to the inadequacy of rice and barley-based diets of children with "Hikan" (a disease that included keratomalacia), and the condition's rapid clinical response to cod liver oil [204]. Interestingly, the therapeutic or preventive value of dark green leaves (rich dietary β-carotene source) against xerophthalmia was not reported in the early literature. Indeed, Westhoff working in Indonesia in 1911 drew attention to more frequent occurrence of xerophthalmia in areas where green leafy vegetables were often consumed [205].

The dawning of modern, experimental animal nutrition in the early twentieth century led to the discovery of "vitamines" [87]. McCollum and Davis [206] and, at nearly the same time, Osborne and Mendel [207] showed that the addition of an ether-soluble extract from butter, egg yolk, or milk to the diets of young rats could promote growth, reduce morbidity, and enhance survival. McCollum called the extract "fat-soluble A" which was shortly thereafter renamed "Vitamine A." The clinical relevance of the animal findings became quickly apparent. Bloch, a Danish pediatrician during World War I, observed how orphans subsisting on a fat-free milk, oatmeal, and barley soup diet were at greater risk of keratomalacia, infection and poor growth, similar to McCollum's vitamin A-deficient animals, compared to children whose diet included a modest amount of whole milk [208]. He surmised vitamin A deficiency to be the underlying cause of "Dystrophia Alipogenetica." With Wolbach and Howe's classic description in 1923 of metaplasia and keratinization of epithelial linings in vitamin A-depleted animals [209], loss of the "barrier function" of epithelial linings became a plausible explanation for their decreased resistance to infection.

Animal experiments in the twenties led Green and Mellanby to coin vitamin A as an "anti-infective" factor [87, 210], while seminal clinical studies in humans through the forties continued to relate vitamin A deficiency or xerophthalmia to infectious disease risk [211, 212]. The 1930s found George Wald piecing together the many components of the "visual cycle" that earned him a Nobel Prize in 1966 [213]. During this time observations emerged of an inverse relationship between febrile illness and plasma vitamin A concentration [214] and urinary excretion of vitamin A during disease [215], both now understood to be part of the acute phase response to inflammation [70, 216, 217]. Successful therapeutic applications of vitamin A were also reported in those years, for example, in reducing childhood fatality from measles [105], puerperal fever in mothers [152], and other infectious conditions [87].

Epidemiologic studies since the 1950s have guided our understanding of the public health consequences of vitamin A deficiency, and benefits of its prevention in human populations. Clinical investigations by Gopalan in India [218] and McLaren in Jordan [219] provided photographic and clinical detail of conjunctival and corneal xerophthalmia and its interactions between vitamin A and protein-energy deficiencies. In 1964, Oomen, McLaren and Escapini's 46-country FAO/WHO "survey" of national health and nutrition institutions from extant reports on xerophthalmia revealed the global extent of this problem throughout the developing world [220]. While, the lack of population-based data and biases inherent in this type of data were appreciated, the report mobilized further surveys, research and commitment to prevent vitamin A deficiency and served as the forerunner of the current WHO micronutrient deficiency information system [221]. By 1974 the International Vitamin A Consultative Group (IVACG) was formed, which provided essential global scientific and policy leadership in vitamin A deficiency prevention for over a quarter of a century [222].

The modern era of understanding the public health consequences of childhood vitamin A deficiency, and the impact of its prevention, was ushered in with a national survey, longitudinal study, and a series of hospital-based clinical studies of xerophthalmia by Sommer and colleagues in Indonesia in the late nineteen seventies [223]. Most notable from this work were reports that children with non-blinding, mild xerophthalmia (night blindness and Bitot's spots) were at higher risks of death (Fig. 9.7) [90], diarrhea and respiratory infections [89] than children without these eye signs, and that an estimated 5 million potentially blinding cases of corneal xerophthalmia occurred each year [224]. The dose-response nature of mortality risk with mild eye signs suggested a causal association, prompting intervention trials that came to reveal that vitamin A could reduce child mortality (Fig. 9.8). Subsequent research from Nepal showed that improving maternal vitamin A status could reduce pregnancy-related mortality by ~44% [150]. However, these results were not replicated in Bangladesh [154] or Ghana [155], where the baseline risk of infection and vitamin A deficiency were lower. Similar disparities in underlying nutritional and infectious exposures are also likely to explain the results of newborn vitamin A dosing trials [143], which have shown survival benefits in Asia [131–134] but not in Africa [136, 138, 139, 141, 142]. Beyond the question of survival, emerging research is highlighting the potential long-term implications of early vitamin A inadequacy [175, 184, 194, 198].

Epidemiology

Our understanding of the epidemiology of vitamin A deficiency derives largely from studies of the mild and more frequent stages of xerophthalmia [night blindness (XN) and Bitot's spots (X1B)], and evidence of association with low serum retinol concentrations. The distribution of deficiency by location, person, and time can identify risk factors that may be proximal and causal (e.g., diet, care, and morbidity), less proximal but having causal influence (e.g., socioeconomic status [SES], seasonal food availability), or that reflect indirect association. Knowledge of risk factors can influence the design and targeting of interventions and provide the "context" within which vitamin A deficiency exists.

Location

Vitamin A deficiency is characterized as a moderate or severe public health problem in approximately 122 LMICs [1] largely spanning periequatorial regions of the world (Fig. 9.6) [5], where rural and urban poor are exposed to frequent infections and depend heavily on plant sources of vitamin A [63]. Vitamin A deficiency tends to cluster within countries, providing insight into causation and groups for targeting. Where national surveys or surveillance data exist [225–227], it is clear that regions with a high prevalence of xerophthalmia share common dietary and other ecologic exposures (e.g., poverty, high levels of infectious diseases, poor development and health infrastructures, and strong seasonal fluctuation in food availability). Clustering of risk appears to intensify within smaller, disadvantaged groupings. Population-based surveys in Africa (Malawi and Zambia), South Asia (Bangladesh and Nepal) and Southeast Asia (Indonesia) reveal a consistent 1.5 to 2.0-fold risk of xerophthalmia among children in villages where other children have the condition [228, 229]. More striking is a 7- to 13-fold higher risk of having, or developing, xerophthalmia among children whose siblings have the condition, compared to children whose siblings are non-xerophthalmic [228]. A similar parent-child intensity of clustering has been observed in Cambodia, where young children were 4–5 times more likely to have xerophthalmia when the mother was night blind who, in turn, was 9-times more likely to be being night blind if one of her children had xerophthalmia [230]. This high level of shared risk of vitamin A deficiency is likely due to common exposures to a chronic, poor diet [231, 232], and inadequate care, malnutrition, and disease that characterize mothers [9] and children in high-risk families.

Persons at Risk

Age

Xerophthalmia follows rather consistent patterns with respect to age, gender, and socioeconomic factors. Based on hospital admissions data from Indonesia [223], and Nepal [233] the incidence of corneal xerophthalmia, which rarely affects more than 0.1% of a population even in high-risk areas [223], appears to peak at 2–3 years of age. Acute onset of corneal disease may follow any combination of recent weaning from the breast with sole dependence on a poor household diet, an episode of severe measles, persistent diarrhea, other severe febrile illness, or wasting malnutrition, coupled with poor child care [2, 223]. Although the incidence of corneal disease declines beyond age three, the prevalence of healed, corneal scarring (XS), which represents permanent, potentially blinding sequella, continues to rise among survivors [2, 223]. The prevalence of mild xerophthalmia (XN and X1B) typically, though not always [234], rises with age through the fifth year of life and often beyond, irrespective of area of the world or age-specific rates of deficiency [7, 226, 235–243].

The relationship between subclinical vitamin A deficiency (based on serum retinol concentration) and age is less consistent [7, 244–246]. However, even where data suggest a declining prevalence over the preschool years [7, 83, 246] there is evidence of an elevated prevalence of marginal-to-deficient vitamin A status in school-aged years [11, 83, 247]. It is plausible that chronic deficiency could persist into the reproductive years of women [5, 248–251], thereby raising the risk of night blindness during pregnancy [84, 149]. This pattern may be reflecting a rise seen over time as children in high-risk populations continue to be exposed to a poor diet, lacking breast milk [45, 252, 253], and insufficient vegetables, fruits, and animal products with adequate vitamin A content [254–257].

Gender

Boys tend to show a higher prevalence of mild xerophthalmia than girls throughout the preschool and early school-aged years [2, 7, 244, 258–261]. Animal experiments also often reveal increased vulnerability of male versus female risks to vitamin A depletion with respect to growth, vitamin A status and survival [262], suggesting there may be, in part, a genetic basis to this risk difference. The gender bias is less apparent for subclinical (biochemical) deficiency [244] and has not been observed in severe, corneal xerophthalmia [223].

Socioeconomic Status (SES)

In general, socioeconomic disadvantage covaries inversely with the risk of vitamin A deficiency, presumably by influencing both availability and accessibility to an adequate diet, and appropriate hygiene and care that can lead to less illness among poorer children. Low household socioeconomic status is typically associated with xerophthalmia in young children, reflected by less parental education [46, 223, 225, 238, 245, 255, 261–265] and landholding [46, 223, 225, 261, 266], poorer housing quality [46, 223, 255], and hygiene [46, 223, 264], fewer small assets [46, 238, 262] and draft animals [231, 238, 261] owned, and a more frequent history of child mortality in the family [46, 223, 255]. Not surprisingly, women with night blindness also come from socioeconomically disadvantaged families, exhibiting a poor diet, less asset ownership, and increased risks of anemia and infection [9, 84]. Typically, odds ratios for xerophthalmia lie between 1.5 and 2.5 when comparing risks among families with lower versus higher SES. Socioeconomic influence on variation in serum retinol has been less consistently observed [239, 244, 267–269], perhaps related to homeostatic mechanisms that maintain serum retinol across a wide range of status making this association more difficult to detect when serum retinol is expressed on a continuous scale. At the community level, high-risk villages, marked by the presence of ≥ 1 child with xerophthalmia, tend to be poorer than those where no children have xerophthalmia [255]. Differentials in SES cannot be relied on to predict risk of vitamin A deficiency but do provide the context in which vitamin A deficiency occurs and, in part, a basis for understanding how vitamin A deficiency clusters within households and communities.

Periodicity

Periodicity in risk of vitamin A deficiency is captured mostly by the influence of season and long-term trends on incidence or prevalence. Spring peaks in xerophthalmia were widely noted in early twentieth century China, Europe, and Japan, variably coinciding with the spring growth spurt, changes in diet and the diarrhea season [2]. Drought increases risk of xerophthalmia [270, 271]. In rural South Asia, the incidence of xerophthalmia follows a predictable seasonality, waxing during the hot, dry season (March–June), and waning during the monsoon period (July–August) to a low level that is sustained beyond the major rice harvest months of November and December [272]. This annual cycle has been best depicted by Sinha who clinically examined 300 preschool children in the Village of Ichag, West Bengal each month for over 2 years (Fig. 9.10) [273]. The seasonal peak of

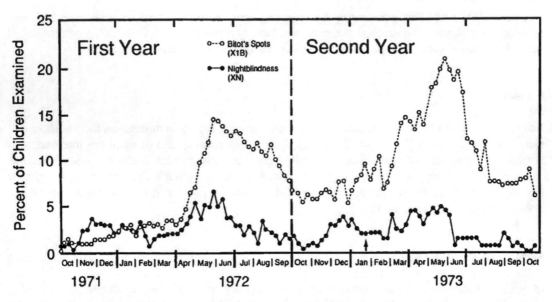

Fig. 9.10 Seasonality of prevalence of mild xerophthalmia in Ichag Village, West Bengal, India over a two-year period. Data to right of *arrow* represent control group only among children who participated in a placebo-controlled vitamin A trial [273]

night blindness and Bitot's spots was preceded by a period of high growth that followed the major harvest, which presumably draws down vitamin A reserves, and coincides with a period of low intake of fruits and vegetables and high incidence of diarrhea and measles [272]. Appearance of the mango season coupled with slowed growth may partly explain the decrease in xerophthalmia late in the monsoon period. Seasonal patterns provide insight into appropriate timing and nature of interventions, which should aim to mute the seasonal peak (e.g., distributing high-dose vitamin A prior to the highest risk season) and, wherever feasible, address dietary, and morbidity-related causes (e.g., promoting gardens or vegetable marketing, assuring high measles vaccine coverage), wherever feasible [29, 274, 275].

Risk of vitamin A deficiency can also shift over long periods of time that likely reflect gradual improvements in economic development, food security, and health services [275]. Though time trend data are absent, the past century witnessed the virtual disappearance of xerophthalmia from industrialized Western Europe, North America, and Japan. More recently, in Indonesia, the risk of potentially blinding vitamin A deficiency markedly decreased from the late 1970s to the early 1990s, reflected by a 75% reduction in the national prevalence of xerophthalmia [241] and a well-documented decline in xerophthalmia admissions to the Cicendo Eye Hospital in Bandung (Fig. 9.11) [276]. Such progress, however, can be reversed in the presence of political and economic turmoil, as when xerophthalmia began to reappear in Indonesia following its economic collapse in the late 1990s [277].

Proximal Causes

Vitamin A deficiency, as a public health problem, results from a chronic, dietary insufficiency of vitamin A, either preformed or from precursor carotenoids. It often occurs in association with protein-energy malnutrition, other micronutrient deficiencies and, as part of a "vicious cycle" with infection, in which one exacerbates and increases susceptibility to the other.

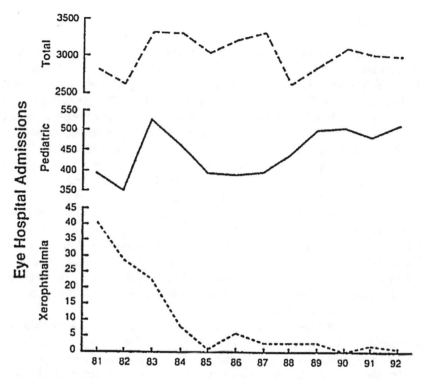

Fig. 9.11   Number of admissions at the Cicendo Eye Hospital, Bandung, Indonesia between 1981 and 1992 [276]. The decline in xerophthalmia admissions likely reflected a true decrease (*bottom line*), given rising pediatric admissions (*middle line*) and stable total admissions (*top line*) over the same time period

Breastfeeding

In affluent populations, newborns are born with low liver stores of vitamin A that increase rapidly thereafter throughout the preschool years [77], presumably reflecting dietary sufficiency from breast milk and complementary foods that promote storage of vitamin A in relation to normal requirements for growth and other needs. In food insecure settings, liver vitamin A stores may fail to accumulate beyond early infancy [77, 278]. This may be due, in part, to a combination of low breast milk vitamin A concentration, which can often be half that of breast milk from well-nourished populations of women [43, 44]. Still, breast milk provides a critical dietary source of vitamin A [279] that may protect children from xerophthalmia. In many populations, breastfeeding through the third year of life is associated with age-adjusted odds ratios of 0.1–0.5, representing 50–90% reductions in the probability of having xerophthalmia compared to children who have ceased breastfeeding [223, 252, 253, 280–283]. In Malawi, accelerated weaning, involving both premature introduction of complementary foods (at 3 vs. 4 months of age) and early cessation of breastfeeding were associated with increased risk of preschool xerophthalmia [45]. A dose-response association was observed in Nepal: children who were breast fed up to ten times per day or greater than 10 times per day were 68 and 88%, respectively, less likely to have xerophthalmia than children of the same age who had ceased breastfeeding [46]. When protracted diarrhea, measles or severe respiratory infections co-occur with xerophthalmia, however, increased demands for and losses of vitamin A lessen the protective benefit of breastfeeding on xerophthalmia [252].

Complementary Feeding

The mix of foods offered to young children can modify or even eliminate the excess risk of xerophthalmia associated with the progressive removal of breast milk from the diet. In Indonesia, where no association existed between breastfeeding and xerophthalmia in the preschool years, children not routinely given milk, egg, yellow fruits and vegetables, dark green leaves, or meat/fish in the first 12 months following breastfeeding cessation were ~3 times more likely to be xerophthalmic than matched-control children given these foods [255]. Similarly, in Nepal, protective odds ratios against xerophthalmia in the preschool years ranged from 0.09 to 0.41 for regular ($\geq 3 \times$ per week) consumption of meat, fish, egg, and mango in the first 2 years of life [46]. Feeding histories of younger siblings in the first 2 years of life were similar to the cases and controls in the study (Table 9.7) [232], reflecting a chronically poor diet in high-risk households.

Numerous epidemiologic studies provide the basis for a progression of complementary feeding that appears to guard children from xerophthalmia through the preschool years. Intake of sweet, yellow fruit (mango and papaya) are strongly protective in the second and third years of life, denoted by a solid line in Fig. 9.12. As the influence of breastfeeding weakens, dark green leafy vegetables appear strongly protective from the third year onward. Finally, after infancy routine consumption of animal foods with preformed vitamin A (egg, dairy products, fish, and liver) appears to be highly protective [2, 223, 226, 255, 280, 282–286].

How and with whom children eat their meals may affect their risk of vitamin A deficiency. Detailed ethnographic studies in Nepal have shown that rural children are twice as likely to consume vegetables, fruits, pulses, meat or fish, and dairy products when they share a plate with another relative during meals than when left to eat alone. Among plate sharers, however, chronically vitamin A-deficient children (i.e., those with a known history of xerophthalmia) were 1.7 times (OR, 95% CI: 1.0–2.8) more likely to share a plate at meal time with an adult male than lower risk children residing in non-xerophthalmic households [287]. Sharing a plate at mealtime with a female of any age, on the other hand, was "protective" against xerophthalmia (OR = 0.6; 95% CI: 0.4–0.9), possibly reflecting female behavior that is more nurturing toward younger children.

Table 9.7 Correlations in sibling feeding patterns and reported frequencies of intake of foods ($n = 67$ focus child and younger sibling pairs[a]) [231]

Specific food items	Correlation between siblings	
	Spearman's rank correlation	P value
Preformed vitamin A sources		
Meat	0.38	<0.002
Fish	0.39	<0.002
Traditional tonic	0.38	<0.002
Animal milk	0.66	<0.001
Other breast milk	0.50	<0.001
Eggs	0.53	<0.001
Carotenoid sources		
Mango	0.54	<0.001
Dark green leaves	0.33	<0.001
Papaya	0.14	0.27

[a]Only younger siblings who were >24 months at time of interview used in analysis

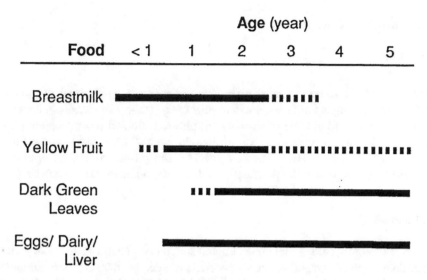

Fig. 9.12 Composite depiction of age-specific protection against xerophthalmia conferred by food sources of vitamin A based on epidemiologic studies in Southern Asia and Africa. *Solid bar* denotes strong, consistent evidence of protection; *dash* indicates weaker epidemiologic evidence [460]

Infectious Disease Morbidity

Vitamin A deficiency and infection interact within a "vicious cycle" [88], whereby one exacerbates and increases susceptibility to the other. The bidirectional relationship complicates frequent cross-sectional evidence of depressed plasma retinol levels with diarrhea, acute respiratory infections, measles, malaria, HIV/AIDS, and other infectious illnesses which can be attributed in part to an acute phase response [68]. However, prospective studies show that infection can induce vitamin A deficiency through a variety of ways, depending on the cause, duration, and severity of infection and vitamin A status of the host at onset. Serum retinol may be depressed because of decreased dietary intake or malabsorption due to diarrhea or intestinal pathogens [288–290], impaired release or accelerated depletion of hepatic retinol reserves [291], increased retinol utilization by target tissues or increased urinary losses [217, 292–294]. Hyporetinolemia may adversely affect immune competence, which could exacerbate or predispose children to infection [68].

Urinary retinol loss, reflecting losses in body stores, can vary greatly by type and severity of infection. In a Bangladesh study [217], 6, 19, 17, and 65% of children hospitalized with dysentery, watery diarrhea, pneumonia, or sepsis excreted more than 0.07 μmol (20 μg) of retinol in urine per day, corresponding to 10% of a preschool child's estimated metabolic requirement. Total urinary excretion of retinol per episode of sepsis was 6.0 μmol, amounting to ∼20% of an average young child's (3-month) liver reserve of 35 μmol, or 75% of a marginally vitamin A-nourished child's much lower liver reserve (e.g., 8 μmol) [217]. This suggests that severe infection acutely decompensates vitamin A nutriture which could precipitate xerophthalmia. Indeed, in a prospective study in Indonesia, preschoolers with either diarrhea or acute respiratory disease were twice as likely to have developed xerophthalmia in a subsequent 3-month period then healthier children [22]. Severe diarrhea, dysentery, measles, and other severe, febrile illnesses are frequently reported to precede corneal xerophthalmia [2].

Clinicopathological Features

Xerophthalmia

Conjunctival and corneal xerosis, corneal ulceration and necrosis, and retinal dysfunction causing poor dark adaptation and night blindness, are the ocular consequences of vitamin A deficiency. Active "xerophthalmia" includes all of these clinical stages, plus less studied and understood lesions in the retinal pigment epithelium, described as "xerophthalmic fundus" [223, 295]. These fundal changes are not considered further here. Healed corneal scars resulting from corneal xerophthalmia are not considered "active" but represent the potentially blinding sequellae of xerophthalmia [29, 223].

Night Blindness (XN)

Night blindness is the earliest, specific clinical manifestation of vitamin A deficiency and is usually the most prevalent stage of xerophthalmia. Its occurrence reflects a failure in rod photoreceptor cells in the retina to maintain peripheral vision under dim light which can be detected by dark adaptometry. Impaired dark adaptation occurs in the presence of depressed serum retinol concentrations [296, 297] and is responsive to vitamin A supplementation [298]. Typically, a history of night blindness can be elicited using a local term for the condition, often translated as "chicken eyes" (domestic fowl lack rods and, thus, night vision) or "twilight" or "evening" blindness [2, 29, 223]. A history of night blindness is associated with low-to-deficient serum retinol concentrations in preschool-aged children [2, 223, 265, 299, 300] and pregnant women [84] compared to individuals without the condition. Night blindness during pregnancy can be reliably elicited by history which can serve as an indicator of individual and community risk of vitamin A deficiency [10]. Objective methods are also available that can detect impairments in night vision prior to the onset of night blindness [297, 301].

Conjunctival Xerosis with Bitot's Spots (X1B)

Vitamin A deficiency leads to a keratinizing metaplasia of mucosal surfaces of the body, including the bulbar conjunctiva. In chronic deficiency, xerosis of the conjunctiva appears as a dry, nonwettable, rough, or granular surface, best seen on oblique illumination from a hand-light [29, 223, 295]. On the ocular surface, the tear film breaks up, revealing a xerotic surface that has been likened to "sandbanks at the receding tide" [219]. Histologically, the lesions represent a transformation of normal, surface, columnar epithelium, with abundant mucous-secreting goblet cells, to a stratified, squamous epithelium that lacks goblet cells [29, 295]. In advanced xerosis, gray-yellow patches of keratinized cells and saprophytic bacilli, called "Bitot's spots," may aggregate on the surface, temporal to the limbus and, in more severe cases, on nasal surfaces as well (Fig. 9.13). The lesions may be bubbly, foamy, or cheese-like in appearance [295].

Corneal Xerosis (X2), Ulceration and Necrosis (X3)

Corneal xerophthalmia represents acute decompensation of the cornea, representing a sight-threatening medical emergency [29, 223, 295] that is also associated with high case fatality [223]. Mild xerosis ("drying") presents as superficial punctate erosions that lend a hazy, non-wettable and irregular appearance to the cornea on handlight examination. Usually both eyes are involved. With increased severity the cornea becomes edematous and takes on a dry, granular appearance, described like the "peel of an orange" [223]. Vitamin A therapy successfully treats corneal xerosis,

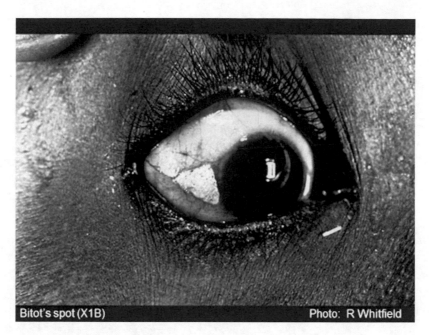

Bitot's spot (X1B)   Photo: R Whitfield

Fig. 9.13 Bitot's spot (X1B) [29, 223]

though in advanced disease, thick plaques of cornified epithelium form that may slough off. Ulceration can be round or oval in appearance, shallow or deep to the stroma, usually sharply demarcated and often peripheral to the visual axis. Usually, only one ulcer forms in the affected eye. Vitamin A treatment will heal the tissue leaving an opaque stromal scar, or leukoma. Ulcers that perforate the entire cornea (through Descemet's membrane) and are plugged with iris will, on healing, form an adherent leukoma. These are often at the periphery of the cornea, and leave central vision of a healed eye intact [29, 295]. Keratomalacia ("corneal melting or softening") refers to necrosis of cornea, forming initially opaque localized lesions that can expand rapidly to cover and blind the cornea (Fig. 9.14). Therapy with vitamin A leaves a densely scarred cornea, often with resultant phthisis (shrunken globe) or staphyloma (protuding cornea) [295].

Infection

Vitamin A deficiency predisposes individuals to severe infection [89] and a higher risk of mortality in infants and young children [101–104]. In populations with a high infectious burden, this risk may extend to pregnant and lactating women [149, 150]. Multiple roles of vitamin A in maintaining epithelial barrier function, supporting innate immune cells, and regulating both cellular and antibody-mediated immunity [68] provide biologic plausibility for vitamin A deficiency as a cause of morbidity.

Poor Growth

Experimental vitamin A depletion in animals causes a deceleration in weight gain to a "plateau," as hepatic retinol reserves become exhausted, and eventual weight loss [206, 207, 262]. This dynamic is difficult to observe in children. Corneal xerophthalmia is associated with severe stunting of linear

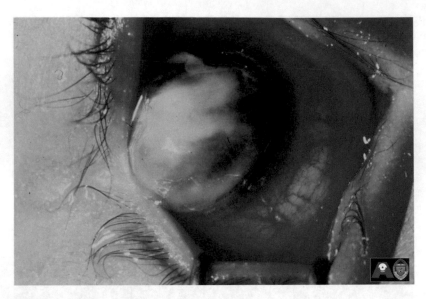

Fig. 9.14 Corneal xerophthalmia/keratomalacia (X3) [29, 223]

growth and acute wasting, likely due to a combination of protein-energy malnutrition, infection, and multiple micronutrient deficiencies [2, 223]. Mild xerophthalmia (XN or X1B) is associated with moderate stunting and mild wasting in children [2, 223, 255, 286] and wasting in pregnant women [84]. Spontaneous recovery from xerophthalmia, likely due to dietary improvement, has been associated with gain in weight but less noticeable catch-up in linear growth over a six-month period [302].

In general, vitamin A supplementation cannot be expected to measurably improve weight or height gain in a population [303–308], although it may lead to measurable increases in lean body mass reflected by incremental upper arm muscle area [306, 309] and there may be growth responses in subsets of a population [309] or on a seasonal basis [306, 310]. The latter may represent direct effects, or may be mediated by factors such as morbidity [306]. In some settings, vitamin A may result in accelerated linear growth [311–313], particularly among children who are moderately to severely vitamin A deficient and for whom the deficiency may be growth-limiting [306, 312, 313]. Repeated bouts of infection may blunt the growth response [314], an effect that may also explain seasonal growth responses to vitamin A [315]. Moderately ill (e.g., children recovering from severe measles), wasted or clinically vitamin A-deficient children may show marked ponderal and apparent lean body gains following vitamin A supplementation [306, 316, 317].

Anemia

There is considerable observational evidence to support the inclusion of anemia as a vitamin A deficiency disorder. Anemia is prevalent among children with night blindness [318]. As first reported by Hodges et al. in 1978, there are also strong correlations between serum retinol and hemoglobin concentrations among children, adolescents, and reproductive-aged women [318–322]. These observations may be explained, in part, by infection-related anemia [323]. However, early animal research on vitamin A and anemia indicated that vitamin A deficiency could alter hematopoietic tissue in the bone marrow, reduce hematopoietic cell counts, and lead to hemosiderosis of the spleen and liver [209, 324]. Since those initial reports, mechanistic studies have demonstrated numerous alterations in iron metabolism and reduced erythrocytosis resulting from vitamin A deficiency [318, 325–328].

A number of vitamin A intervention trials have shown improvements in hematological indices among children [322]. These include the impact evaluations of fortified monosodium glutamate in Indonesia [94] and fortified sugar in Guatemala [329], as well as trials of low-dose supplementation on either a daily or weekly basis [330–332], and, of relevance to existing vitamin A programs, periodic high-dose supplementation [328, 333–335]. The effects of high-dose supplementation appear to be transient [334] and are likely limited to children with moderate to low iron and vitamin A status [318, 335]. Vitamin A supplementation of reproductive-aged women has also proven efficacious in improving hemoglobin status when delivered alone [336], or, to a greater extent, in combination with iron [336–340]. Although some studies have reported no additional benefit of vitamin A in this high-risk group, their findings may be explained by the relative vitamin A adequacy of study subjects [341] or the failure of the intervention to improve vitamin A status [342, 343].

Treatment

Children with any stage of xerophthalmia should be treated with vitamin A according to WHO treatment guidelines [344]; i.e., with high-dose vitamin A at presentation, the next day and 1–4 weeks later (Table 9.8). Supportive nutritional and antibiotic therapy should be considered, as indicated by the patient's condition, along with dietary counseling. Children with measles should always receive vitamin A (Table 9.7) as they are very likely to be benefit from such therapy both in terms of saving sight and reducing case fatality [2].

Night blindness responds within 24–48 h of high-dose vitamin A treatment leading to a return to normal scotopic (night time) vision [29, 299]. The efficacy of the treatment guidelines for night blind women is presumed. In Nepal, long-term, weekly supplementation with ~23,000 IU only prevented about two-thirds of maternal night blindness cases [146], suggesting that a higher, more frequent or sustained dosage may be needed in some food insecure settings to resolve this symptom. Bitot's spots (X1B) in preschool children generally respond to high-dose vitamin A within 2–5 days, becoming smaller in size and disappearing within 2 weeks. A small percentage of lesions may persist as smaller aggregates on the conjunctival surface for months [29, 223]. In older children, X1B may be more refractory to vitamin A. Although similar in clinical appearance, factors associated with responsive and nonresponsive X1B differ: the latter are more frequent with age, associated with localized versus

Table 9.8 WHO/UNICEF schedule for use of vitamin A supplements (adapted from [344, 374])

Age group	Recommended dosage
For prevention of vitamin A deficiency disorders	
Infants and children	
6–11 months of age	100,000 IU orally
12–59 months of age	200,000 IU orally, every 4–6 months
For treatment of xerophthalmia, measles and severe protein-energy malnutrition	
Infants and children	
<6 months of age	50,000 IU @ 1, 2, and 14 days
6–11 months of age	100,000 IU @ 1, 2, and 14 days
12+ months of age	200,000 IU @ 1, 2, and 14 days (dosing @ days 1 and 2 for measles treatment and @ day 1 for kwashiorkor or weight-for-height <3 standard deviations is sufficient)
Reproductive age women	10,000 IU daily or 25,000 IU weekly for at least 3 months
Reproductive age women with severe, active xerophthalmia	200,000 IU @ 1, 2, and 14 days

more generalized metaplasia and goblet cell loss, less often associated with night blindness, and observed at higher serum retinol concentrations than responsive X1B [345–347].

Corneal xerophthalmia can rapidly lead to blindness without immediate vitamin A treatment. Corneal xerosis quickly responds to vitamin A, usually within 2–5 days of therapy, with the cornea returning to normal without permanent sequelae within 1–2 weeks [29, 223]. Shallow, small corneal ulcers, that usually form peripheral to the visual axis, heal with minimal structural damage or risk of visual loss. Ulcers will form an opaque stromal scar or leukoma. Corneal necrosis (keratomalacia) must be treated immediately with standard vitamin A therapy, coupled with topical antibiotics and other nutritional measures [29, 223]. Healing may induce large lesions to slough, forming decemetoceles [295].

Prevention

The main cause of vitamin A deficiency is an insufficient dietary intake of vitamin A, likely compounded by poor bioavailability of provitamin A carotenoids from the vegetable-based diets [48] that dominate in many low-income countries (Fig. 9.4). Other important contributing factors include infections, which increase both the demand for and urinary losses of vitamin A [217, 348], as well as increased requirements for vitamin A at certain stages in the life cycle (i.e., growth, pregnancy, and lactation) [62]. Sociocultural factors, such as intra-household distribution and gender preference and other economic constraints to achieving an adequate diet and health provide the context within which deficiency occurs and prevention must take place [349–351]. Preventive measures can be categorized into these approaches [352]:

  (i)   **Dietary diversification**: increasing vitamin A intake from available and accessible foods, achieved through nutrition education, social marketing, home or community garden programs, and other measures to improve food security;
 (ii)   **Supplementation**: delivery of vitamin A supplements to high-risk groups, typically preschool-aged children, on a periodic basis;
(iii)   **Fortification**: addition of preformed vitamin A to commonly consumed foods such as oil, sugar, or flour to increase regular dietary vitamin A intakes; and,
(iv)   **Biofortification**: increasing the provitamin A carotenoid concentrations in staple crops via conventional plant breeding techniques or genetic modification.

Dietary Diversification

Improving dietary intake of high-risk groups requires an adequate, affordable, and diverse supply of food sources of vitamin A, which preferably includes preformed sources of vitamin A throughout the year, consumed in sufficient amounts, especially by those at highest risk: infants, young children, adolescent girls and women of reproductive age. A first-line, dietary intervention to protect infants and young children from vitamin A deficiency is extended breastfeeding which consistently exhibits a protective association against xerophthalmia even through the fourth year of life [2, 45, 252, 253, 280–282], although effectiveness data are lacking to show a change in vitamin A status from breastfeeding promotion. Although it has been possible to demonstrate increased retinol levels in the breast milk for 2–8 months after maternal postpartum vitamin A supplementation [79, 251, 353], the effects of this intervention have not been evaluated with respect to infant survival and the strategy is no longer included as part of global recommendations [344]. With weaning, soft yellow fruits and vegetables, dark green leaves, eggs and other food sources of vitamin A should routinely be provided [2, 223, 250, 255, 280] which, in controlled studies, have been shown to raise low serum retinol concentrations in children [2]. Some dietary fat should also be part of the meal to allow absorption of provitamin A carotenoids [56, 57, 354].

Where food sources of vitamin A are inadequate, homestead gardening that combines horticultural, credit, and nutrition education or social marketing services [355] has raised vitamin A intakes [274], improved household economic return and, therefore, improved food security [356]. Further, food-based interventions that promote participation of women and rally community support through creative social marketing appear capable of changing behavior and enhancing vitamin A intake [349, 357–359] and, in some instances, have been shown to improve vitamin A status [349]. Given evidence of poor bioavailability of green leafy vegetables and other vegetable-based provitamin A carotenoids [48, 62], it remains unclear to what extent dietary diversification alone can provide for adequate dietary vitamin A intakes and sustained adequate status.

Approaches to improve the effectiveness of dietary interventions will likely need to include the promotion of food sources of preformed vitamin A (animal and fortified foods), a wider variety of carotenoid-containing foods [274, 284, 360] and that promote food preparation methods that enhance carotenoid absorption, including the consumption of dietary fat (Table 9.1). Understanding local diets will also be crucial to guide dietary diversification efforts [256, 361, 362]. This research may inform, for example, education efforts regarding the use of *crude* red palm oil [363–365] or the use of drying technologies to enable year-round consumption of fruits such as mango or papaya [366]. Dietary data can also be used for the purposes of linear programming [367–369], which can guide diversification strategies by identifying culturally acceptable foods that may be promoted to increase the nutrient density of diets without exceeding cost constraints [370].

Supplementation

Periodic, high-dose vitamin A supplementation remains the most widely practiced, direct means to prevent the health consequences of deficiency by governments throughout the world [371–373]. The rationale for periodic supplementation with a high dose of vitamin A rests on the assumption that, as a fat-soluble nutrient, it is stored in the body, principally in the liver, and released in association with transport proteins to meet demands of body tissues, as required. Thus, a theoretical four- to six-month supply (usually 100,000–200,000 IU or $\sim$30–60 mg RAE) provided at one time can establish a nutritional reserve for use during periods of reduced dietary intake or increased need [344], despite a likely dosage absorption of only 30–50% under prevalent conditions of morbidity and malnutrition often found in targeted populations [2, 371] and intercurrent infection that can diminish liver stores [291]. The World Health Organization first called for universal vitamin A supplementation in 1997 [374] and has recently reissued its recommendation for supplementation of all infants and children aged 6–59 months in areas with a vitamin A deficiency public health problem [344]. Specifically, one 100,000 IU dose delivered between 6 and 11 months of age is recommended, followed by doses of 200,000 IU delivered every four to six months from 12 to 59 months of age [344]. Supplements are typically provided in the form of a gelatinous capsule or oily syrup delivered with a spoon [344]. High-dose vitamin A is well tolerated by children, although up to $\sim$10% of preschoolers may experience transient side effects (nausea, vomiting, headache, diarrhea, or fever have been reported) following receipt of 200,000 IU [375].

The efficacy of periodic, high-dose vitamin A supplementation in preventing mortality among preschool-aged children has been detailed above and supported by multiple meta-analyses over the past 20 years [101–104, 376]. Supplementation is also efficacious ($\sim$90%) in preventing any stage of xerophthalmia for a period of approximately 6 months [2], with community-based periodic vitamin A

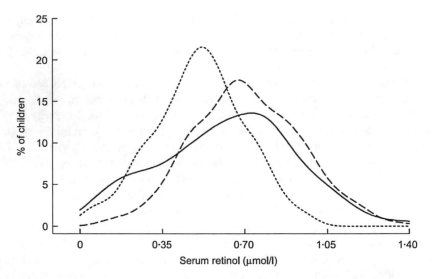

Fig. 9.15 Distribution of serum retinol concentrations at initial contact, 1 month and 4 months following a mass vitamin A supplementation campaign among Indian children in Orissa State (1–4 years) (from [378], © 2012 *Cambridge University Press*, Reprinted with permission)

delivery proving ∼75% effective in high-risk populations [2, 273, 371, 372, 377]. The protective effect of supplementation against hyporetinolemia (i.e., serum retinol <20 µg/dl or <0.70 µmol/L) is limited [378]. Two quasi-experimental studies carried out by Pereira and Begum in the late 1960s suggest that high-dose supplements can prevent hyporetinolemia for a period of roughly 8–10 weeks [379, 380]. The protective period is likely to be shorter in populations with lower dietary vitamin A intakes [380] or poorer vitamin A status [381]. This effect is illustrated in Fig. 9.15 using data from a prospective cohort of children in Orissa State, India who were supplemented in accordance with WHO guidelines [382]. The baseline prevalence of hyporetinolemia in this population was 64% just prior to dosing [382]. Prevalence had declined to 46% at one month following capsule receipt, but, by four months post-dosing, an estimated 86% of children had serum retinol concentrations <0.70 µmol/L [382]. In sum, supplementation is an essential strategy for protecting against xerophthalmia and excess mortality caused by vitamin A deficiency. However, it cannot sustainably improve vitamin A status in a population [378].

Each year UNICEF procures and distributes over 400 million vitamin A supplements to nearly 80 countries [383]. Supplements are included on the list of essential medicines [344], to be managed via regular supply chain mechanisms for maternal and child health services. The "fixed site" delivery of capsules is generally integrated with immunization services [384]. Depending on health system functionality therefore, coverage is likely to be much higher for younger children [385]. Capsules are commonly given in tandem with the measles immunization at nine months of age. Reliance on this contact, as opposed to the recommended dosing at six months of age [344], may limit the survival benefit of supplementation during infancy [386]. Reliance on fixed site delivery alone can severely limit coverage in areas with ineffectual health systems [383]. As supplementation was scaled up as a child survival intervention, the linkage of capsule delivery with National Immunization Day campaigns for polio eradication enabled a rapid increase in coverage with at least one annual dose [387]. This strategy was eventually overtaken by what became semi-annual delivery of vitamin A supplements with other child health interventions, such as deworming or insecticide-treated bednet distribution, termed Child Health Days or Weeks [388]. Child Health Days have ensured high supplement coverage [389] and remain the most common delivery strategy at this time [378, 390].

Fortification

Fortification represents an increasingly important food-based approach to control vitamin A and other micronutrient deficiencies in LMICs [33], drawing on experiences from high-income countries, where food production and marketing systems are highly industrialized, integrated, and readily reach the consumer [391, 392]. Fortification is likely to be most effective when one or more food "vehicles" are widely consumed by high-risk groups, processing and distribution are centralized (i.e., in a limited number of facilities to enable quality control), organoleptic change from addition of vitamin A is imperceptible over time under ambient conditions, and costs of fortification are both small relative to the product itself, and absorbable by the consumer [33]. Data on usual vitamin A intakes, ideally from repeated 24 h dietary recalls, is crucial in identify potential food vehicles and to set appropriate fortification levels [33], as illustrated by reports from Cameroon [40, 393], Vietnam [394], and Uganda [395]. Data collection on usual intake of potentially fortifiable food vehicles can be aided by tools such as the Fortification Rapid Assessment Tool, or FRAT [396].

Efficacy trials designed and powered to test the impact of fortified foods on health outcomes are limited in number. However, one large-scale trial in Indonesia provides strong evidence of a survival benefit, reporting an 11% reduction in infant mortality and 45% reduction in child mortality [94]— exceeding the child survival benefit of high-dose vitamin A supplementation [93, 95, 97–99]. This trial, as well as research carried out in the Philippines, also showed significant reductions in xerophthalmia among young children [94, 397, 398]. Most efficacy trials and large-scale effectiveness studies reported in the literature have focused on serum retinol concentration as a primary outcome. Studies of both monosodium glutamate [311, 397] and household sugar fortification [399–401] have demonstrated significant improvements in vitamin A status. Given the fat-soluble nature of vitamin A, products such as oil would serve as an ideal food vehicle [33]. Two studies from the Philippines have considered fat-based vehicles [398, 402]. The first of these, which tested the impact of fortified margarine, significantly improved serum retinol status of children [398]. The latter trial of fortified coconut oil failed to improve vitamin A status, but serum retinol concentrations among children in this study were already adequate [402]. Staples such as flour, rice, and salt offer the opportunity for fortification with multiple micronutrients that could lead to the prevention of several micronutrient deficiencies [403]. Studies of wheat flour [404, 405], maize meal [406], and salt [407, 408] support both the feasibility and potential efficacy of this strategy for vitamin A deficiency control.

As a preventive strategy, industrial-scale food fortification has the potential to sustainably improve vitamin A intakes and, therefore, status. This rightward shift in population vitamin A status is most clearly illustrated by population-level data from Nicaragua (Fig. 9.16), which initiated its national sugar fortification program in 1999 [400]. Cross-sectional assessments carried out over subsequent years exemplify the stable, low prevalence of vitamin A deficiency that can be achieved with this intervention [401]. Fortification has been fundamental to the success of several other Latin American countries as well in effectively eliminating vitamin A deficiency [409]. While scale-up has been slower in other LMICs, largely due to a lack of production and market potential for fortifiable foods in many economies [391], fortification of sugar, oil, wheat flour, maize meal, and other commodities is moving beyond the pilot phase in all high-risk regions [34, 37–40, 410, 411]. Additional vehicles for vitamin A fortification supported by existing technology include margarine or other spreads, milk or milk powder, instant noodles, salt, and infant formulas [33]. Fortified rice premixes made from extruded rice flour and resembling natural milled grains have also been developed and are awaiting expanded testing and use [412]. As programs are taken to scale, the assessment of vitamin A content of fortified foods at different points in the supply chain (factory, market, and point of use), as well as periodic dietary and biochemical assessments of target populations are recommended [33, 378], with a particular focus to ensure that fortified foods penetrate into poor, geographically remote markets [413].

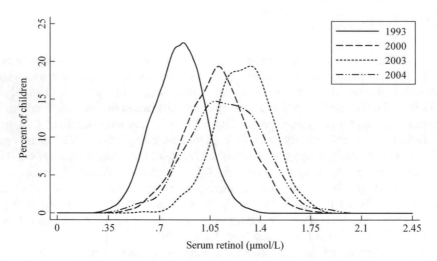

Fig. 9.16 Distribution of serum retinol concentrations prior to and at 1, 4, and 5 years following implementation of a vitamin A sugar fortification program among Nicaraguan children (1–5 years) (from [378], © 2012 *Cambridge University Press*, Reprinted with permission)

Biofortification

Biofortification is an emerging strategy developed to reach small-scale, subsistence farmers with staple crops that can significantly increase provitamin A carotenoid intakes [414]. The broad goal in developing biofortified crops is to fill a nutritional gap (e.g., 50% of the estimated average requirement) under varying assumptions of staple crop consumption, bioconversion, and carotenoid retention during storage and cooking [415]. Conventional plant breeders have employed methods, such as marker-assisted selection, to identify and improve on staple crop varieties with naturally higher micronutrient content [416, 417]. To date, these methods have yielded improved cultivars of maize and cassava at or above a targeted 15 μg β-carotene per gram [418, 419], as well as sweet potato varieties providing ∼ 30 to 100 μg β-carotene per gram [420]. There is inadequate variability in the trait for provitamin A carotenoid content of rice grain to rely on conventional breeding methods alone [421]. Potrykus and Beyer developed the first transgenic rice cultivar by introducing genes from daffodil (*Narcissus pseudonarcissus*) and bacteria (*Erwinia uredovora*), enabling β-carotene biosynthesis in the rice endosperm [422]. The most advanced cultivars of "Golden Rice" provide up to 70 μg β-carotene per gram [423].

Nutrition research on biofortification published over the past decade supports the bioavailability [424], effective bioconversion [425–428], and adequate retention of provitamin A carotenoids from these crops [418]. Orange-fleshed sweet potato, the first of the provitamin A carotenoid-rich crops to be released, has been tested in Mozambique and South Africa, showing that consumption of this crop could significantly increase serum retinol among high-risk groups [429] and vitamin A liver stores [430], as measured by the modified-relative-dose-response test. Biofortified maize at the 15 μg β-carotene per gram target has been tested in trials enrolling preschool-aged children in rural Zambia. Regular consumption significantly improved total body vitamin A, as measured by retinol isotope dilution, in a three-month trial enrolling ∼ 150 children [431]. A larger trial of ∼ 1200 children reported significant improvements in serum β-carotene concentration, but not serum retinol, in a population with marginal vitamin A status [432]. That same trial found improvements in eye function among children with serum retinol concentration <1.05 μmol/L at the outset of the intervention (AC Palmer et al., unpublished data, 2016). A third trial, which provided biofortified maize over a three-week period to lactating mothers, suggested a reduced prevalence of low breast milk retinol (AC Palmer et al., unpublished data, 2016).

One cultivar of cassava with a β-carotene content of ∼5 µg/g has been tested in Kenya in 2012 among deficient school-aged children, where the authors demonstrated a significant impact on both β-carotene and retinol concentration in serum after a ∼4.5 month feeding period [433].

Even while breeders continue to improve available varieties and scientists continue to assess nutritional efficacy, conventionally bred biofortified staple crops have been released and are being scaled-up in countries throughout sub-Saharan Africa [434, 435]. A number of studies have documented good consumer acceptability of these varieties [429, 436–440], despite important differences in organoleptic properties, as well as willingness to pay on the part of farmers [441, 442] and consumers [443]. While there have been challenges in terms of achieving adequate adoption and identifying appropriate and cost-effective delivery strategies [434], data have begun to accumulate from Mozambique and Uganda to support the effectiveness of orange-fleshed sweet potatoes as a means to increase vitamin A intakes among at risk populations [444, 445] and, in one setting, to reduce the prevalence of marginal vitamin A status among preschool-aged children and women of reproductive age [444]. While there has been progress with the conventionally bred biofortified crops [434], the acceptability of transgenic varieties continues to be challenged at multiple levels [446]. At present, the roll-out of Golden Rice is largely halted by political and regulatory hurdles [447].

Conclusion

Vitamin and mineral deficiencies rarely occur alone, rarely have a single cause, and always occur in a wider ecological, social and political environment. Poor quality diets low in micronutrients are invariably a consequence of poverty, itself a consequence of local, national, and global inequities. Increasingly, it is recognized that vitamin A supplementation programs, while highly efficacious at controlling the excess mortality and xerophthalmia resulting from vitamin A deficiency, have only a transient impact on a population's vitamin A status [378]. While nations have been successful at achieving high coverage with this intervention, less attention has been paid to sustainably improve dietary intakes and status, which will be a prerequisite for any scale-back of universal vitamin A supplementation [378]. Countries need to be simultaneously looking to reinforce approaches to diversify diets, including through the initiation and/or strengthening of industrial food fortification and the introduction of biofortified staple crops [390]. Guidance is increasingly available on the selection of an appropriate mix of interventions [390, 448, 449]. These preventive strategies must be supported by continued investment in women's education and development programs aimed at improving social inequities.

Discussion Points

- Using the acronym SLAMENGHI, which strategies might you recommend to improve the effectiveness of dietary diversification in improving vitamin A status?
- What are the justifications for vitamin A deficiency control among preschool-aged children, infants, and women of reproductive-age? How would you judge the strength of the evidence in each case?
- What socio-demographic and health conditions may predispose children to vitamin A deficiency?
- What are the major clinical features of severe vitamin A deficiency? Even in less severe deficiency, what types of disorders can be attributed to inadequate vitamin A nutriture?
- What types of information would you need in order to guide a comprehensive program for vitamin A deficiency control in a given country? How would you judge the effectiveness of that program?

References

1. World Health Organization. Global prevalence of vitamin A deficiency in populations at risk 1995–2005. WHO Global Database on Vitamin A Deficiency. Geneva, Switzerland: World Health Organization; 2009.
2. Sommer A, West KP Jr. Vitamin A deficiency: health, survival and vision. New York: Oxford University Press; 1996.
3. Stevens GA, Bennett JE, Hennocq Q, Lu Y, De-Regil LM, Rogers L, et al. Trends and mortality effects of vitamin A deficiency in children in 138 low-income and middle-income countries between 1991 and 2013: a pooled analysis of population-based surveys. Lancet Glob Health. 2015;3(9):e528–36.
4. Black RE, Victora CG, Walker SP, Bhutta ZA, Christian P, de Onis M, et al. Maternal and child undernutrition and overweight in low-income and middle-income countries. Lancet. 2013;382(9890):427–51.
5. West KP Jr. Extent of vitamin A deficiency among preschool children and women of reproductive age. J Nutr. 2002;132(9):2857S–66S.
6. Katz J, Khatry SK, West KP, Humphrey JH, Leclerq SC, Kimbrough E, et al. Night blindness is prevalent during pregnancy and lactation in rural Nepal. J Nutr. 1995;125(8):2122–7.
7. Gorstein J, Shreshtra RK, Pandey S, Adhikari RK, Pradhan A. Current status of vitamin A deficiency and the National Vitamin A Control Program in Nepal: results of the 1998 National Micronutrient Status Survey. Asia Pac J Clin Nutr. 2003;12(1):96–103.
8. Ahmed F, Azim A, Akhtaruzzaman M. Vitamin A deficiency in poor, urban, lactating women in Bangladesh: factors influencing vitamin A status. Public Health Nutr. 2003;6(5):447–52.
9. Semba RD, de Pee S, Panagides D, Poly O, Bloem MW. Risk factors for nightblindness among women of childbearing age in Cambodia. Eur J Clin Nutr. 2003;57(12):1627–32.
10. Saunders C, do Carmo Leal M, Gomes MM, Campos LF, dos Santos Silva BA, Thiapo de Lima AP, et al. Gestational nightblindness among women attending a public maternity hospital in Rio de Janeiro, Brazil. J Health Popul Nutr. 2004;22(4):348–56.
11. Singh V, West KP Jr. Vitamin A deficiency and xerophthalmia among school-aged children in Southeastern Asia. Eur J Clin Nutr. 2004;58(10):1342–9.
12. O'Byrne SM, Blaner WS. Retinol and retinyl esters: biochemistry and physiology. J Lipid Res. 2013;54(7):1731–43.
13. Blomhoff R, Blomhoff HK. Overview of retinoid metabolism and function. J Neurobiol. 2006;66(7):606–30.
14. Dawson MI, Hobbs PD. The synthetic chemistry of retinoids. In: Sporn MB, Roberts MA, Goodman DS, editors. The retinoids: biology, chemistry, and medicine. 2nd ed. New York: Raven Press, Ltd.; 1994. p. 5–178.
15. Krinsky NI, Johnson EJ. Carotenoid actions and their relation to health and disease. Mol Aspects Med. 2005;26(6):459–516.
16. Nagao A. Absorption and metabolism of dietary carotenoids. BioFactors. 2011;37(2):83–7.
17. Eroglu A, Harrison EH. Carotenoid metabolism in mammals, including man: formation, occurrence, and function of apocarotenoids. J Lipid Res. 2013;54(7):1719–30.
18. Harrison EH. Mechanisms involved in the intestinal absorption of dietary vitamin A and provitamin A carotenoids. Biochim Biophys Acta. 2012;1821(1):70–7.
19. Wald G. Molecular basis of visual excitation. Science. 1968;162(3850):230–9.
20. Hargrave PA. Rhodopsin structure, function, and topography: the Friedenwald lecture. Invest Ophthalmol Vis Sci. 2001;42(1):3–9.
21. Lamb TD, Pugh EN Jr. Dark adaptation and the retinoid cycle of vision. Prog Retin Eye Res. 2004;23(3):307–80.
22. Pepperberg DR, Crouch RK. An illuminating new step in visual-pigment regeneration. Lancet. 2001;358(9299):2098–9.
23. Huang P, Chandra V, Rastinejad F. Retinoic acid actions through mammalian nuclear receptors. Chem Rev. 2014;114(1):233–54.
24. Zile MH. Function of vitamin A in vertebrate embryonic development. J Nutr. 2001;131(3):705–8.
25. Omori M, Chytil F. Mechanism of vitamin A action. Gene expression in retinol-deficient rats. J Biol Chem. 1982;257(23):14370–4.
26. Balmer JE, Blomhoff R. Gene expression regulation by retinoic acid. J Lipid Res. 2002;43(11):1773–808.
27. McDowell EM, Keenan KP, Huang M. Effects of vitamin A-deprivation on hamster tracheal epithelium. A quantitative morphologic study. Virchows Arch B Cell Pathol Incl Mol Pathol. 1984;45(2):197–219.
28. McDowell EM, Keenan KP, Huang M. Restoration of mucociliary tracheal epithelium following deprivation of vitamin A. A quantitative morphologic study. Virchows Arch B Cell Pathol Incl Mol Pathol. 1984;45(2):221–40.
29. Sommer A. Vitamin A deficiency and its consequences: a field guide to detection and control. Geneva, Switzerland: World Health Organization; 1995.
30. Otten JJ, Hellwig JP, Meyers LD, editors. Dietary reference intakes: the essential guide to nutrient requirements. Washington, D.C.: National Academies Press; 2006.

31. FAO/WHO. Human Vitamin and Mineral Requirements. Report of joint FAO/WHO expert consultation. Rome: Food and Agriculture Organization; 2002.
32. USDA National Nutrient Database for Standard Reference, Release 28. Available from: https://ndb.nal.usda.gov/ndb/.
33. World Health Organization, Food and Agriculture Organization. Guidelines on food fortification with micronutrients. Geneva, Switzerland: WHO/FAO; 2006.
34. Fiedler JL, Lividini K. Managing the vitamin A program portfolio: a case study of Zambia, 2013–2042. Food Nutr Bull. 2014;35(1):105–25.
35. Dary O, Mora JO. Food fortification to reduce vitamin A deficiency: International Vitamin A Consultative Group recommendations. J Nutr. 2002;132(9 Suppl):2927S–33S.
36. Sablah M, Klopp J, Steinberg D, Touaoro Z, Laillou A, Baker S. Thriving public-private partnership to fortify cooking oil in the West African Economic and Monetary Union (UEMOA) to control vitamin A deficiency: Faire Tache d'Huile en Afrique de l'Ouest. Food Nutr Bull. 2012;33(4 Suppl):S310–20.
37. Bhagwat S, Gulati D, Sachdeva R, Sankar R. Food fortification as a complementary strategy for the elimination of micronutrient deficiencies: case studies of large scale food fortification in two Indian States. Asia Pac J Clin Nutr. 2014;23(Suppl 1):S4–11.
38. Rohner F, Raso G, Ake-Tano SO, Tschannen AB, Mascie-Taylor CG, Northrop-Clewes CA. The effects of an oil and wheat flour fortification program on pre-school children and women of reproductive age living in Cote d'Ivoire, a malaria-endemic area. Nutrients. 2016;8(3).
39. Sandjaja, Jus'at I, Jahari AB, Ifrad, Htet MK, Tilden RL, et al. Vitamin A-fortified cooking oil reduces vitamin A deficiency in infants, young children and women: results from a programme evaluation in Indonesia. Public Health Nutr. 2015;18(14):2511–22.
40. Engle-Stone R, Nankap M, Ndjebayi AO, Brown KH. Simulations based on representative 24-h recall data predict region-specific differences in adequacy of vitamin A intake among Cameroonian women and young children following large-scale fortification of vegetable oil and other potential food vehicles. J Nutr. 2014;144 (11):1826–34.
41. U.S. Department of Agriculture ARS, Beltsville Human Nutrition Research Center, Food Surveys Research Group and U.S. Department of Health and Human Services, Centers for Disease Control and Prevention, National Center for Health Statistics. What we eat in America, NHANES 2009-2010. Available from https://www.ars.usda.gov/SP2UserFiles/Place/80400530/pdf/0910/tables_1-40_2009-2010.pdf.
42. Solomons N, Vitamin A. In: Bowman BA, Russell RM, editors. Present knowledge in nutrition. 9th ed. Washington, D.C.: International Life Sciences Institute; 2006. p. 157–83.
43. Haskell MJ, Brown KH. Maternal vitamin A nutriture and the vitamin A content of human milk. J Mammary Gland Biol Neoplasia. 1999;4(3):243–57.
44. Wallingford JC, Underwood BA. Vitamin A deficiency in pregnancy, lactation, and the nursing child. In: Bauernfeind JC, editor. Vitamin A deficiency and its control. New York: Academic Press; 1986. p. 101–52.
45. West KP Jr, Chirambo M, Katz J, Sommer A. Breast-feeding, weaning patterns, and the risk of xerophthalmia in Southern Malawi. Am J Clin Nutr. 1986;44(5):690–7.
46. Khatry SK, West KP Jr, Katz J, LeClerq SC, Pradhan EK, Wu LS, et al. Epidemiology of xerophthalmia in Nepal. A pattern of household poverty, childhood illness, and mortality. The Sarlahi Study Group. Arch Ophthalmol. 1995;113(4):425–9.
47. Rodriquez-Amaya DB. A guide to carotenoid analysis in foods. Washington, D.C.: International Life Sciences Institute; 1999.
48. West CE, Eilander A, van Lieshout M. Consequences of revised estimates of carotenoid bioefficacy for dietary control of vitamin A deficiency in developing countries. J Nutr. 2002;132(9 Suppl):2920S–6S.
49. West CE, Castenmiller JJ. Quantification of the "SLAMENGHI" factors for carotenoid bioavailability and bioconversion. Int J Vitam Nutr Res. 1998;68(6):371–7.
50. Castenmiller JJ, West CE. Bioavailability and bioconversion of carotenoids. Annu Rev Nutr. 1998;18:19–38.
51. de Pee S, West CE, Permaesih D, Martuti S. Muhilal, Hautvast JG. Orange fruit is more effective than are dark-green, leafy vegetables in increasing serum concentrations of retinol and β-carotene in schoolchildren in Indonesia. Am J Clin Nutr. 1998;68(5):1058–67.
52. Rock CL, Lovalvo JL, Emenhiser C, Ruffin MT, Flatt SW, Schwartz SJ. Bioavailability of β-carotene is lower in raw than in processed carrots and spinach in women. J Nutr. 1998;128(5):913–6.
53. Castenmiller JJ, West CE, Linssen JP, van het Hof KH, Voragen AG. The food matrix of spinach is a limiting factor in determining the bioavailability of β-carotene and to a lesser extent of lutein in humans. J Nutr. 1999;129 (2)1349 55.
54. Ncube TN, Greiner T, Malaba LC, Gebre-Medhin M. Supplementing lactating women with pureed papaya and grated carrots improved vitamin A status in a placebo-controlled trial. J Nutr. 2001;131(5):1497–502.
55. Riedl J, Linseisen J, Hoffmann J, Wolfram G. Some dietary fibers reduce the absorption of carotenoids in women. J Nutr. 1999;129(12):2170–6.

56. Takyi EE. Children's consumption of dark green, leafy vegetables with added fat enhances serum retinol. J Nutr. 1999;129(8):1549–54.

57. Drammeh BS, Marquis GS, Funkhouser E, Bates C, Eto I, Stephensen CB. A randomized, 4-month mango and fat supplementation trial improved vitamin A status among young Gambian children. J Nutr. 2002;132(12):3693–9.

58. van Vliet T, van Vlissingen MF, van Schaik F, van den Berg H. Beta-carotene absorption and cleavage in rats is affected by the vitamin A concentration of the diet. J Nutr. 1996;126(2):499–508.

59. de Pee S, West CE, Muhilal, Karyadi D, Hautvast JG. Lack of improvement in vitamin A status with increased consumption of dark-green leafy vegetables. Lancet. 1995;346(8967):75–81.

60. de Pee S, Bloem MW, Gorstein J, Sari M, Satoto Yip R, et al. Reappraisal of the role of vegetables in the vitamin A status of mothers in Central Java, Indonesia. Am J Clin Nutr. 1998;68(5):1068–74.

61. Van Loo-Bouwman CA, Naber TH, Schaafsma G. A review of vitamin A equivalency of β-carotene in various food matrices for human consumption. Br J Nutr. 2014;111(12):2153–66.

62. Institute of Medicine: Food and Nutrition Board. Dietary Reference Intakes for Vitamin A, Vitamin K, Arsenic, Boron, Chromium, Copper, Iodine, Iron, Manganese, Molybdenum, Nickel, Silicon, Vanadium, and Zinc. Washington, D.C.: National Academy Press; 2001. xxii, 773 pp.

63. FAO/WHO. Requirements of Vitamin A, Iron, Folate and Vitamin B12, Report of a Joint FAO/WHO Expert Consultation. Rome: FAO; 1988.

64. Sommer A, Davidson FR. Assessment and control of vitamin A deficiency: the Annecy Accords. J Nutr. 2002;132(9 Suppl):2845S–50S.

65. Congdon NG, West KP Jr. Physiologic indicators of vitamin A status. J Nutr. 2002;132(9 Suppl):2889S–94S.

66. de Pee S, Dary O. Biochemical indicators of vitamin A deficiency: serum retinol and serum retinol binding protein. J Nutr. 2002;132(9 Suppl):2895S–901S.

67. Engle-Stone R, Haskell MJ, Ndjebayi AO, Nankap M, Erhardt JG, Gimou MM, et al. Plasma retinol-binding protein predicts plasma retinol concentration in both infected and uninfected Cameroonian women and children. J Nutr. 2011;141(12):2233–41.

68. Raiten DJ, Sakr Ashour FA, Ross AC, Meydani SN, Dawson HD, Stephensen CB, et al. Inflammation and Nutritional Science for Programs/Policies and Interpretation of Research Evidence (INSPIRE). J Nutr. 2015;145 (5):1039S–108S.

69. Stephensen CB, Gildengorin G. Serum retinol, the acute phase response, and the apparent misclassification of vitamin A status in the third National Health and Nutrition Examination Survey. Am J Clin Nutr. 2000;72 (5):1170–8.

70. Thurnham DI, Mburu AS, Mwaniki DL, De Wagt A. Micronutrients in childhood and the influence of subclinical inflammation. Proc Nutr Soc. 2005;64(4):502–9.

71. Smith FR, Suskind R, Thanangkul O, Leitzmann C, Goodman DS, Olson RE. Plasma vitamin A, retinol-binding protein and prealbumin concentrations in protein-calorie malnutrition. III. Response to varying dietary treatments. Am J Clin Nutr. 1975;28(7):732–8.

72. Thurnham DI, McCabe GP, Northrop-Clewes CA, Nestel P. Effects of subclinical infection on plasma retinol concentrations and assessment of prevalence of vitamin A deficiency: meta-analysis. Lancet. 2003;362 (9401):2052–8.

73. Larson LM, Addo OY, Sandalinas F, Faigao K, Kupka R, Flores-Ayala R, et al. Accounting for the influence of inflammation on retinol-binding protein in a population survey of Liberian preschool-age children. Matern Child Nutr. 2016.

74. Tanumihardjo SA, Russell RM, Stephensen CB, Gannon BM, Craft NE, Haskell MJ, et al. Biomarkers of nutrition for development (BOND)-Vitamin A review. J Nutr 2016;146(9):1816S–48S.

75. Olson JA, Gunning DB, Tilton RA. Liver concentrations of vitamin A and carotenoids, as a function of age and other parameters, of American children who died of various causes. Am J Clin Nutr. 1984;39(6):903–10.

76. Gebre-Medhin M, Vahlquist A. Vitamin A nutrition in the human foetus. A comparison of Sweden and Ethiopia. Acta Paediatr Scand. 1984;73(3):333–40.

77. West KP, Jr. Public health impact of preventing vitamin A deficiency in the first six months of life. In: Delange FM, West KP, Jr., editors. Micronutrient deficiencies in the first months of life. Nestle nutrition workshop series pediatric program, vol 52. Vevey/S. Karger; 2003. p. 103–27.

78. Lindblad BS, Patel M, Hamadeh M, Helmy N, Ahmad I, Dawodu A, et al. Age and sex are important factors in determining normal retinol levels. J Trop Pediatr. 1998;44(2):96–9.

79. Humphrey JH, Rice AL. Vitamin A supplementation of young infants. Lancet. 2000;356(9227):422–4.

80. Mactier H, Weaver LT. Vitamin A and preterm infants: what we know, what we don't know, and what we need to know. Arch Dis Child Fetal Neonatal Ed. 2005;90(2):F103–8.

81. Herrador Z, Sordo L, Gadisa E, Buno A, Gomez-Rioja R, Iturzaeta JM, et al. Micronutrient deficiencies and related factors in school-aged children in Ethiopia: a cross-sectional study in Libo Kemkem and Fogera districts, Amhara Regional State. PLoS ONE. 2014;9(12):e112858.

82. Custodio VI, Daneluzzi JC, Custodio RJ, Del Ciampo LA, Ferraz IS, Martinelli CE Jr, et al. Vitamin A deficiency among Brazilian school-aged children in a healthy child service. Eur J Clin Nutr. 2009;63(4):485–90.
83. Best C, Neufingerl N, van Geel L, van den Briel T, Osendarp S. The nutritional status of school-aged children: why should we care? Food Nutr Bull. 2010;31(3):400–17.
84. Christian P, West KP Jr, Khatry SK, Katz J, Shrestha SR, Pradhan EK, et al. Night blindness of pregnancy in rural Nepal–nutritional and health risks. Int J Epidemiol. 1998;27(2):231–7.
85. Christian P. Recommendations for indicators: night blindness during pregnancy–a simple tool to assess vitamin A deficiency in a population. J Nutr. 2002;132(9 Suppl):2884S–8S.
86. Mellanby E, Green HN. Vitamin A as an anti-infective agent: its use in the treatment of puerperal septigaemia. Br Med J. 1929;1(3569):984–6.
87. Semba RD. Vitamin A as "anti-infective" therapy, 1920–1940. J Nutr. 1999;129(4):783–91.
88. Scrimshaw NS, Taylor CE, Gordon JE. Interactions of nutrition and infection. Geneva, Switzerland: World Health Organization; 1968.
89. Sommer A, Katz J, Tarwotjo I. Increased risk of respiratory disease and diarrhea in children with preexisting mild vitamin A deficiency. Am J Clin Nutr. 1984;40(5):1090–5.
90. Sommer A, Tarwotjo I, Hussaini G, Susanto D. Increased mortality in children with mild vitamin A deficiency. Lancet. 1983;2(8350):585–8.
91. Milton RC, Reddy V, Naidu AN. Mild vitamin A deficiency and childhood morbidity—an Indian experience. Am J Clin Nutr. 1987;46(5):827–9.
92. Bloem MW, Wedel M, Egger RJ, Speek AJ, Schrijver J, Saowakontha S, et al. Mild vitamin A deficiency and risk of respiratory tract diseases and diarrhea in preschool and school children in northeastern Thailand. Am J Epidemiol. 1990;131(2):332–9.
93. Sommer A, Tarwotjo I, Djunaedi E, West KP Jr, Loeden AA, Tilden R, et al. Impact of vitamin A supplementation on childhood mortality. A randomised controlled community trial. Lancet. 1986;1(8491):1169–73.
94. Muhilal, Permeisih D, Idjradinata YR, Muherdiyantiningsih, Karyadi D. Vitamin A-fortified monosodium glutamate and health, growth, and survival of children: a controlled field trial. Am J Clin Nutr. 1988;48(5):1271–6.
95. Rahmathullah L, Underwood BA, Thulasiraj RD, Milton RC, Ramaswamy K, Rahmathullah R, et al. Reduced mortality among children in southern India receiving a small weekly dose of vitamin A. N Engl J Med. 1990;323 (14):929–35.
96. Vijayaraghavan K, Radhaiah G, Prakasam BS, Sarma KV, Reddy V. Effect of massive dose vitamin A on morbidity and mortality in Indian children. Lancet. 1990;336(8727):1342–5.
97. West KP Jr, Pokhrel RP, Katz J, LeClerq SC, Khatry SK, Shrestha SR, et al. Efficacy of vitamin A in reducing preschool child mortality in Nepal. Lancet. 1991;338(8759):67–71.
98. Daulaire NM, Starbuck ES, Houston RM, Church MS, Stukel TA, Pandey MR. Childhood mortality after a high dose of vitamin A in a high risk population. BMJ. 1992;304(6821):207–10.
99. Ghana VAST Study Team. Vitamin A supplementation in northern Ghana: effects on clinic attendances, hospital admissions, and child mortality. Lancet. 1993;342(8862):7.
100. Herrera MG, Nestel P, el Amin A, Fawzi WW, Mohamed KA, Weld L. Vitamin A supplementation and child survival. Lancet. 1992;340(8814):267–71.
101. Tonascia JA. Meta-analysis of published community trials of the impact of vitamin A on mortality. New York, NY: Helen Keller International; 1993.
102. Beaton GH, Martorell R, Aronson KJ, Edmonston B, McCabe G, Ross AC, et al. Effectiveness of vitamin A supplementation in the control of young child morbidity and mortality in developing countries. Geneva, Switzerland: Administrative Committee on Coordination–Subcommittee on Nutrition (ACC/SCN); 1993.
103. Fawzi WW, Chalmers TC, Herrera MG, Mosteller F. Vitamin A supplementation and child mortality. A meta-analysis. JAMA. 1993;269(7):898–903.
104. Glasziou PP, Mackerras DE. Vitamin A supplementation in infectious diseases: a meta-analysis. BMJ. 1993;306 (6874):366–70.
105. Ellison JB. Intensive vitamin therapy in measles. Br Med J. 1932;2:708–11.
106. Barclay AJ, Foster A, Sommer A. Vitamin A supplements and mortality related to measles: a randomised clinical trial. Br Med J (Clin Res Ed). 1987;294(6567):294–6.
107. Hussey GD, Klein M. A randomized, controlled trial of vitamin A in children with severe measles. N Engl J Med. 1990;323(3):160–4.
108. Arthur P, Kirkwood B, Ross D, Morris S, Gyapong J, Tomkins A, et al. Impact of vitamin A supplementation on childhood morbidity in northern Ghana. Lancet. 1992;339(8789):361–2.
109. Shankar AH, Genton B, Semba RD, Baisor M, Paino J, Tamja S, et al. Effect of vitamin A supplementation on morbidity due to Plasmodium falciparum in young children in Papua New Guinea: a randomised trial. Lancet. 1999;354(9174):203–9.

110. Rice AL, West KP, Jr., Black RE. Vitamin A deficiency. In: Ezzati M, Lopez AD, Rodgers A, Murray CJL, editors. Comparative quantification of health risks global and regional burden of disease attributable to selected major risk factors, vol. 1. Geneva: World Health Organization; 2004. p. 211–56.

111. Fawzi WW, Mbise RL, Hertzmark E, Fataki MR, Herrera MG, Ndossi G, et al. A randomized trial of vitamin A supplements in relation to mortality among human immunodeficiency virus-infected and uninfected children in Tanzania. Pediatr Infect Dis J. 1999;18(2):127–33.

112. Semba RD, Ndugwa C, Perry RT, Clark TD, Jackson JB, Melikian G, et al. Effect of periodic vitamin A supplementation on mortality and morbidity of human immunodeficiency virus-infected children in Uganda: a controlled clinical trial. Nutrition. 2005;21(1):25–31.

113. Coutsoudis A, Bobat RA, Coovadia HM, Kuhn L, Tsai WY, Stein ZA. The effects of vitamin A supplementation on the morbidity of children born to HIV-infected women. Am J Public Health. 1995;85(8 Pt 1):1076–81.

114. Villamor E, Mbise R, Spiegelman D, Hertzmark E, Fataki M, Peterson KE, et al. Vitamin A supplements ameliorate the adverse effect of HIV-1, malaria, and diarrheal infections on child growth. Pediatrics. 2002;109(1): E6.

115. The Vitamin A and Pneumonia Working Group. Potential interventions for the prevention of childhood pneumonia in developing countries: a meta-analysis of data from field trials to assess the impact of vitamin A supplementation on pneumonia morbidity and mortality. Bull World Health Organ. 1995;73(5):609–19.

116. Banajeh SM. Is 12-monthly vitamin A supplementation of preschool children effective? An observational study of mortality rates for severe dehydrating diarrhoea in Yemen. S Afr J Clin Nutr. 2003;16(4):137–42.

117. Thapa S, Choe MK, Retherford RD. Effects of vitamin A supplementation on child mortality: evidence from Nepal's 2001 Demographic and Health Survey. Trop Med Int Health. 2005;10(8):782–9.

118. David P. Evaluating the vitamin A supplementation programme in northern Ghana: has it contributed to child survival? Boston, Massachusetts: John Snow International; 2003.

119. Amouzou A, Habi O, Bensaid K. Niger Countdown Case Study Working Group. Reduction in child mortality in Niger: a Countdown to 2015 country case study. Lancet. 2012;380(9848):1169–78.

120. Awasthi S, Peto R, Read S, Clark S, Pande V, Bundy D, et al. Vitamin A supplementation every 6 months with retinol in 1 million pre-school children in north India: DEVTA, a cluster-randomised trial. Lancet. 2013;381 (9876):1469–77.

121. Mannar V, Schultink W, Spahn K. Vitamin A supplementation in Indian children. Lancet. 2013;382(9892):591–2.

122. Sommer A, West KP Jr, Martorell R. Vitamin A supplementation in Indian children. Lancet. 2013;382 (9892):591.

123. Habicht JP, Victora C. Vitamin A supplementation in Indian children. Lancet. 2013;382(9892):592.

124. Mayo-Wilson E, Imdad A, Herzer K, Bhutta ZA. Vitamin A supplementation in Indian children. Lancet. 2013;382(9892):594.

125. Sloan NL, Mitra SN. Vitamin A supplementation in Indian children. Lancet. 2013;382(9892):593.

126. Katz J, West KP Jr, Khatry SK, Pradhan EK, LeClerq SC, Christian P, et al. Maternal low-dose vitamin A or β-carotene supplementation has no effect on fetal loss and early infant mortality: a randomized cluster trial in Nepal. Am J Clin Nutr. 2000;71(6):1570–6.

127. Fawzi WW, Msamanga GI, Hunter D, Renjifo B, Antelman G, Bang H, et al. Randomized trial of vitamin supplements in relation to transmission of HIV-1 through breastfeeding and early child mortality. AIDS. 2002;16 (14):1935–44.

128. Christian P, West KP Jr, Khatry SK, LeClerq SC, Kimbrough-Pradhan E, Katz J, et al. Maternal night blindness increases risk of mortality in the first 6 months of life among infants in Nepal. J Nutr. 2001;131(5):1510–2.

129. West KP Jr, Katz J, Shrestha SR, LeClerq SC, Khatry SK, Pradhan EK, et al. Mortality of infants <6 mo of age supplemented with vitamin A: a randomized, double-masked trial in Nepal. Am J Clin Nutr. 1995;62(1):143–8.

130. WHO/CHD Immunisation-Linked Vitamin A Supplementation Study Group. Randomised trial to assess benefits and safety of vitamin A supplementation linked to immunisation in early infancy. Lancet. 1998;352(9136):1257–63.

131. Humphrey JH, Agoestina T, Wu L, Usman A, Nurachim M, Subardja D, et al. Impact of neonatal vitamin A supplementation on infant morbidity and mortality. J Pediatr. 1996;128(4):489–96.

132. Rahmathullah L, Tielsch JM, Thulasiraj RD, Katz J, Coles C, Devi S, et al. Impact of supplementing newborn infants with vitamin A on early infant mortality: community based randomised trial in southern India. BMJ. 2003;327(7409):254.

133. Klemm RD, Labrique AB, Christian P, Rashid M, Shamim AA, Katz J, et al. Newborn vitamin A supplementation reduced infant mortality in rural Bangladesh. Pediatrics. 2008;122(1):e242–50.

134. Mazumder S, Taneja S, Bhatia K, Yoshida S, Kaur J, Dube B, et al. Efficacy of early neonatal supplementation with vitamin A to reduce mortality in infancy in Haryana, India (Neovita): a randomised, double-blind, placebo-controlled trial. Lancet. 2015;385(9975):1333–42.

135. Coles CL, Rahmathullah L, Kanungo R, Thulasiraj RD, Katz J, Santhosham M, et al. Vitamin A supplementation at birth delays pneumococcal colonization in South Indian infants. J Nutr. 2001;131(2):255–61.

136. Malaba LC, Iliff PJ, Nathoo KJ, Marinda E, Moulton LH, Zijenah LS, et al. Effect of postpartum maternal or neonatal vitamin A supplementation on infant mortality among infants born to HIV-negative mothers in Zimbabwe. Am J Clin Nutr. 2005;81(2):454–60.

137. Humphrey JH, Iliff PJ, Marinda ET, Mutasa K, Moulton LH, Chidawanyika H, et al. Effects of a single large dose of vitamin A, given during the postpartum period to HIV-positive women and their infants, on child HIV infection, HIV-free survival, and mortality. J Infect Dis. 2006;193(6):860–71.

138. Benn CS, Diness BR, Roth A, Nante E, Fisker AB, Lisse IM, et al. Effect of 50,000 IU vitamin A given with BCG vaccine on mortality in infants in Guinea-Bissau: randomised placebo controlled trial. BMJ. 2008;336 (7658):1416–20.

139. Benn CS, Fisker AB, Napirna BM, Roth A, Diness BR, Lausch KR, et al. Vitamin A supplementation and BCG vaccination at birth in low birthweight neonates: two by two factorial randomised controlled trial. BMJ. 2010;340: c1101.

140. Benn CS, Diness BR, Balde I, Rodrigues A, Lausch KR, Martins CL, et al. Two different doses of supplemental vitamin A did not affect mortality of normal-birth-weight neonates in Guinea-Bissau in a randomized controlled trial. J Nutr. 2014;144(9):1474–9.

141. Edmond KM, Newton S, Shannon C, O'Leary M, Hurt L, Thomas G, et al. Effect of early neonatal vitamin A supplementation on mortality during infancy in Ghana (Neovita): a randomised, double-blind, placebo-controlled trial. Lancet. 2015;385(9975):1315–23.

142. Masanja H, Smith ER, Muhihi A, Briegleb C, Mshamu S, Ruben J, et al. Effect of neonatal vitamin A supplementation on mortality in infants in Tanzania (Neovita): a randomised, double-blind, placebo-controlled trial. Lancet. 2015;385(9975):1324–32.

143. Haider BA, Bhutta ZA. Neonatal vitamin A supplementation: time to move on. Lancet. 2015;385(9975):1268–71.

144. Christian P, Mullany LC, Hurley KM, Katz J, Black RE. Nutrition and maternal, neonatal, and child health. Semin Perinatol. 2015;39(5):361–72.

145. World Health Organization. Guideline: neonatal Vitamin A supplementation. Geneva: World Health Organization; 2011.

146. Christian P, West KP Jr, Khatry SK, Katz J, LeClerq S, Pradhan EK, et al. Vitamin A or β-carotene supplementation reduces but does not eliminate maternal night blindness in Nepal. J Nutr. 1998;128(9):1458–63.

147. Saunders C, Ramalho RA, de Lima AP, Gomes MM, Campos LF, dos Santos Silva BA, et al. Association between gestational night blindness and serum retinol in mother/newborn pairs in the city of Rio de Janeiro, Brazil. Nutrition. 2005;21(4):456–61.

148. Sivakumar B, Panth M, Shatrugna V, Raman L. Vitamin A requirements assessed by plasma response to supplementation during pregnancy. Int J Vitam Nutr Res. 1997;67(4):232–6.

149. Christian P, West KP Jr, Khatry SK, Kimbrough-Pradhan E, LeClerq SC, Katz J, et al. Night blindness during pregnancy and subsequent mortality among women in Nepal: effects of vitamin A and β-carotene supplementation. Am J Epidemiol. 2000;152(6):542–7.

150. West KP Jr, Katz J, Khatry SK, LeClerq SC, Pradhan EK, Shrestha SR, et al. Double blind, cluster randomised trial of low dose supplementation with vitamin A or β-carotene on mortality related to pregnancy in Nepal. The NNIPS-2 Study Group. BMJ. 1999;318(7183):570–5.

151. Faisel H, Pittrof R. Vitamin A and causes of maternal mortality: association and biological plausibility. Public Health Nutr. 2000;3(3):321–7.

152. Green HN, Pindar D, Davis G, Mellanby E. Diet as a prophylactic agent against puerperal sepsis. Br Med J. 1931;2(3691):595–8.

153. Cox SE, Arthur P, Kirkwood BR, Yeboah-Antwi K, Riley EM. Vitamin A supplementation increases ratios of proinflammatory to anti-inflammatory cytokine responses in pregnancy and lactation. Clin Exp Immunol. 2006;144(3):392–400.

154. West KP Jr, Christian P, Labrique AB, Rashid M, Shamim AA, Klemm RD, et al. Effects of vitamin A or β-carotene supplementation on pregnancy-related mortality and infant mortality in rural Bangladesh: a cluster randomized trial. JAMA. 2011;305(19):1986–95.

155. Kirkwood BR, Hurt L, Amenga-Etego S, Tawiah C, Zandoh C, Danso S, et al. Effect of vitamin A supplementation in women of reproductive age on maternal survival in Ghana (ObaapaVitA): a cluster-randomised, placebo-controlled trial. Lancet. 2010;375(9726):1640–9.

156. Semba RD, Miotti PG, Chiphangwi JD, Saah AJ, Canner JK, Dallabetta GA, et al. Maternal vitamin A deficiency and mother-to-child transmission of HIV 1. Lancet. 1994;343(8913):1593 7.

157. Mostad SB, Overbaugh J, DeVange DM, Welch MJ, Chohan B, Mandaliya K, et al. Hormonal contraception, vitamin A deficiency, and other risk factors for shedding of HIV-1 infected cells from the cervix and vagina. Lancet. 1997;350(9082):922–7.

158. Belec L, Mbopi-Keou FX, Roubache JF, Mayaud P, Paul JL, Gresenguet G. Vitamin A deficiency and genital tract infections in women living in Central Africa. J Acquir Immune Defic Syndr. 2002;29(2):203–4.
159. Semba RD, Kumwenda N, Taha TE, Hoover DR, Lan Y, Eisinger W, et al. Mastitis and immunological factors in breast milk of lactating women in Malawi. Clin Diagn Lab Immunol. 1999;6(5):671–4.
160. Nussenblatt V, Lema V, Kumwenda N, Broadhead R, Neville MC, Taha TE, et al. Epidemiology and microbiology of subclinical mastitis among HIV-infected women in Malawi. Int J STD AIDS. 2005;16(3):227–32.
161. Dorosko SM. Vitamin A, mastitis, and mother-to-child transmission of HIV-1 through breast-feeding: current information and gaps in knowledge. Nutr Rev. 2005;63(10):332–46.
162. Kennedy CM, Coutsoudis A, Kuhn L, Pillay K, Mburu A, Stein Z, et al. Randomized controlled trial assessing the effect of vitamin A supplementation on maternal morbidity during pregnancy and postpartum among HIV-infected women. J Acquir Immune Defic Syndr. 2000;24(1):37–44.
163. Kumwenda N, Miotti PG, Taha TE, Broadhead R, Biggar RJ, Jackson JB, et al. Antenatal vitamin A supplementation increases birth weight and decreases anemia among infants born to human immunodeficiency virus-infected women in Malawi. Clin Infect Dis. 2002;35(5):618–24.
164. Fawzi WW, Msamanga GI, Spiegelman D, Urassa EJ, McGrath N, Mwakagile D, et al. Randomised trial of effects of vitamin supplements on pregnancy outcomes and T cell counts in HIV-1-infected women in Tanzania. Lancet. 1998;351(9114):1477–82.
165. Fawzi W, Msamanga G, Antelman G, Xu C, Hertzmark E, Spiegelman D, et al. Effect of prenatal vitamin supplementation on lower-genital levels of HIV type 1 and interleukin type 1β at 36 weeks of gestation. Clin Infect Dis. 2004;38(5):716–22.
166. de Pee S, Semba RD. Role of nutrition in HIV infection: review of evidence for more effective programming in resource-limited settings. Food Nutr Bull. 2010;31(4):S313–44.
167. Clagett-Dame M, DeLuca HF. The role of vitamin A in mammalian reproduction and embryonic development. Annu Rev Nutr. 2002;22:347–81.
168. Sharma HS, Misra UK. Postnatal distribution of vitamin A in liver, lung, heart and brain of the rat in relation to maternal vitamin A status. Biol Neonate. 1986;50(6):345–50.
169. Matthews KA, Rhoten WB, Driscoll HK, Chertow BS. Vitamin A deficiency impairs fetal islet development and causes subsequent glucose intolerance in adult rats. J Nutr. 2004;134(8):1958–63.
170. Chailley-Heu B, Chelly N, Lelievre-Pegorier M, Barlier-Mur AM, Merlet-Benichou C, Bourbon JR. Mild vitamin A deficiency delays fetal lung maturation in the rat. Am J Respir Cell Mol Biol. 1999;21(1):89–96.
171. Lelievre-Pegorier M, Vilar J, Ferrier ML, Moreau E, Freund N, Gilbert T, et al. Mild vitamin A deficiency leads to inborn nephron deficit in the rat. Kidney Int. 1998;54(5):1455–62.
172. Olusanya BO, Newton VE. Global burden of childhood hearing impairment and disease control priorities for developing countries. Lancet. 2007;369(9569):1314–7.
173. Elemraid MA, Mackenzie IJ, Fraser WD, Brabin BJ. Nutritional factors in the pathogenesis of ear disease in children: a systematic review. Ann Trop Paediatr. 2009;29(2):85–99.
174. Ogaro FO, Orinda VA, Onyango FE, Black RE. Effect of vitamin A on diarrhoeal and respiratory complications of measles. Trop Geogr Med. 1993;45(6):283–6.
175. Schmitz J, West KP Jr, Khatry SK, Wu L, Leclerq SC, Karna SL, et al. Vitamin A supplementation in preschool children and risk of hearing loss as adolescents and young adults in rural Nepal: randomised trial cohort follow-up study. BMJ. 2012;344:d7962.
176. Wilson JG, Roth CB, Warkany J. An analysis of the syndrome of malformations induced by maternal vitamin A deficiency. Effects of restoration of vitamin A at various times during gestation. Am J Anat. 1953;92(2):189–217.
177. Chytil F. Retinoids in lung development. FASEB J. 1996;10(9):986–92.
178. McGowan SE, Smith J, Holmes AJ, Smith LA, Businga TR, Madsen MT, et al. Vitamin A deficiency promotes bronchial hyperreactivity in rats by altering muscarinic M(2) receptor function. Am J Physiol Lung Cell Mol Physiol. 2002;282(5):L1031–9.
179. McGowan SE, Holmes AJ, Smith J. Retinoic acid reverses the airway hyperresponsiveness but not the parenchymal defect that is associated with vitamin A deficiency. Am J Physiol Lung Cell Mol Physiol. 2004;286(2):L437–44.
180. Checkley W, West KP Jr, Wise RA, Wu L, LeClerq SC, Khatry S, et al. Supplementation with vitamin A early in life and subsequent risk of asthma. Eur Respir J. 2011;38(6):1310–9.
181. Sharma HS, Misra UK. Biochemical development of the rat lung: studies on cellular DNA, RNA and protein content in relation to maternal vitamin A status. Z Ernahrungswiss. 1987;26(2):116–24.
182. Zachman RD. Role of vitamin A in lung development. J Nutr. 1995;125(6 Suppl):1634S–8S.
183. Massaro GD, Massaro D. Postnatal treatment with retinoic acid increases the number of pulmonary alveoli in rats. Am J Physiol. 1996;270(2 Pt 1):L305–10.
184. Checkley W, West KP Jr, Wise RA, Baldwin MR, Wu L, LeClerq SC, et al. Maternal vitamin A supplementation and lung function in offspring. N Engl J Med. 2010;362(19):1784–94.

185. Rosenquist TH, van Waes JG, Shaw GM, Finnell R. Nutrient effects upon embryogenesis: folate, vitamin A and iodine. Nestle Nutr Workshop Ser Pediatr Program. 2005;55:29–40.
186. Chiang MY, Misner D, Kempermann G, Schikorski T, Giguere V, Sucov HM, et al. An essential role for retinoid receptors RAR-β and RXR-γ in long-term potentiation and depression. Neuron. 1998;21(6):1353–61.
187. Cocco S, Diaz G, Stancampiano R, Diana A, Carta M, Curreli R, et al. Vitamin A deficiency produces spatial learning and memory impairment in rats. Neuroscience. 2002;115(2):475–82.
188. Misner DL, Jacobs S, Shimizu Y, de Urquiza AM, Solomin L, Perlmann T, et al. Vitamin A deprivation results in reversible loss of hippocampal long-term synaptic plasticity. Proc Natl Acad Sci USA. 2001;98(20):11714–9.
189. Etchamendy N, Enderlin V, Marighetto A, Pallet V, Higueret P, Jaffard R. Vitamin A deficiency and relational memory deficit in adult mice: relationships with changes in brain retinoid signalling. Behav Brain Res. 2003;145 (1–2):37–49.
190. Jacobs S, Lie DC, DeCicco KL, Shi Y, DeLuca LM, Gage FH, et al. Retinoic acid is required early during adult neurogenesis in the dentate gyrus. Proc Natl Acad Sci USA. 2006;103(10):3902–7.
191. Luo T, Wagner E, Crandall JE, Drager UC. A retinoic-acid critical period in the early postnatal mouse brain. Biol Psychiatry. 2004;56(12):971–80.
192. Chen K, Zhang X, Wei XP, Qu P, Liu YX, Li TY. Antioxidant vitamin status during pregnancy in relation to cognitive development in the first two years of life. Early Hum Dev. 2009;85(7):421–7.
193. Humphrey JH, Agoestina T, Juliana A, Septiana S, Widjaja H, Cerreto MC, et al. Neonatal vitamin A supplementation: effect on development and growth at 3 y of age. Am J Clin Nutr. 1998;68(1):109–17.
194. Buckley GJ, Murray-Kolb LE, Khatry SK, Leclerq SC, Wu L, West KP, Jr., et al. Cognitive and motor skills in school-aged children following maternal vitamin A supplementation during pregnancy in rural Nepal: a follow-up of a placebo-controlled, randomised cohort. BMJ open. 2013;3(5).
195. Montecino-Rodriguez E, Dorshkind K. B-1 B cell development in the fetus and adult. Immunity. 2012;36(1):13–21.
196. Fahlman C, Jacobsen SE, Smeland EB, Lomo J, Naess CE, Funderud S, et al. All-trans- and 9-cis-retinoic acid inhibit growth of normal human and murine B cell precursors. J Immunol. 1995;155(1):58–65.
197. Chen X, Welner R, Kincade P. A possible contribution of retinoids to regulation of fetal B lymphopoiesis. Eur J Immunol. 2009;39(9):2515–24.
198. Palmer AC, Schulze KJ, Khatry SK, De Luca LM, West KP Jr. Maternal vitamin A supplementation increases natural antibody concentrations of preadolescent offspring in rural Nepal. Nutrition. 2015;31(6):813–9.
199. Baumgarth N, Tung JW, Herzenberg LA. Inherent specificities in natural antibodies: a key to immune defense against pathogen invasion. Springer Semin Immunopathol. 2005;26(4):347–62.
200. Wolf G. A history of vitamin A and retinoids. FASEB J. 1996;10(9):1102–7.
201. Wolf G, Carpenter KJ. Early research into the vitamins: the work of Wilhelm Stepp. J Nutr. 1997;127(7):1255–9.
202. Wolf G. The discovery of the visual function of vitamin A. J Nutr. 2001;131(6):1647–50.
203. Semba RD. The vitamin A story: lifting the shadow of death. New York: Karger; 2012.
204. Mori M. Uber den sog Hikan (Xerosis conjunctivae infantum ev. Keratomalacie). Jahrb Kinderheilk. 1904;1904 (59):175–94.
205. Westhoff CHA. Eenige opmerkingen omtrent oogziekten op Java. Feestbundel Geneesk Tijdschr Ned Indie. 1911:141.
206. McCollum EV, Davis M. The necessity of certain lipins in the diet during growth. J Biol Chem. 1913;15:167–75.
207. Osborne TB, Mendel LB. The influence of butter-fat on growth. J Biol Chem. 1913;16:423–37.
208. Bloch CE. Clinical investigation of xerophthalmia and dystrophy in infants and young children (xerophthalmia et dystropia alipogenetica). J Hyg (Lond). 1921;19:283–304.
209. Wolbach SB, Howe PR. Tissue changes following deprivation of fat-soluble A vitamin. J Exp Med. 1925;42 (6):753–77.
210. Green HN, Mellanby E. Vitamin A as an anti-infective agent. BMJ. 1928;20:691–6.
211. Blackfan KD, Wolbach SB. Vitamin A deficiency in infants. A clinical and pathological study. J Pediatr. 1933;3:679–706.
212. Ramalingaswami V. Nutritional diarrhoea due to vitamin A deficiency. Indian J Med Sci. 1948;2:665–74.
213. Wald G. Carotenoids and the visual cycle. J Gen Physiol. 1935;19(2):351–71.
214. Clausen SW, McCoord AB. The carotenoids and vitamin A of the blood. J Pediatr. 1938;13:635–50.
215. Lawrie NR, Moore T, Rajagopal KR. The excretion of vitamin A in urine. Biochem J. 1941;35(7):825–36.
216. Filteau SM, Morris SS, Abbott RA, Tomkins AM, Kirkwood BR, Arthur P, et al. Influence of morbidity on serum retinol of children in a community-based study in northern Ghana. Am J Clin Nutr. 1993;58(2):192–7.
217. Mitra AK, Alvarez JO, Stephensen CB. Increased urinary retinol loss in children with severe infections. Lancet. 1998;351(9108):1033–4.
218. Gopalan C, Venkatachalam PS, Bhavani B. Studies of vitamin A deficiency in children. Am J Clin Nutr. 1960;8:833–40.

219. McLaren DS, Oomen HA, Escapini H. Ocular manifestations of vitamin-A deficiency in man. Bull World Health Organ. 1966;34(3):357–61.
220. Oomen HA, McLaren DS, Escapini H. Epidemiology and Public Health Aspects of Hypovitaminosis A. A Global Survey on Xerophthalmia. Trop Geogr Med. 1964;16:271–315.
221. World Health Organization. Micronutrient Deficiency Information System: Global database on vitamin A deficiency: World Health Organization; 2007. Available from http://www.who.int/whosis/database/menu.cfm?path=whosis,mn,mn_vitamina,mn_vitamina_data&language=english.
222. Reddy V. History of the International Vitamin A Consultative Group 1975–2000. J Nutr. 2002;132(9 Suppl):2852S–6S.
223. Sommer A. Nutritional Blindness: Xerophthalmia and Keratomalaca. Oxford: Oxford University Press; 1981.
224. Sommer A, Tarwotjo I, Hussaini G, Susanto D, Soegiharto T. Incidence, prevalence, and scale of blinding malnutrition. Lancet. 1981;1(8235):1407–8.
225. Cohen N, Rahman H, Mitra M, Sprague J, Islam S, Leemhuis de Regt E, et al. Impact of massive doses of vitamin A on nutritional blindness in Bangladesh. Am J Clin Nutr. 1987;45(5):970–6.
226. Cohen N, Rahman H, Sprague J, Jalil MA, Leemhuis de Regt E, Mitra M. Prevalence and determinants of nutritional blindness in Bangladeshi children. World Health Stat Q. 1985;38(3):317–30.
227. Wolde-Gebriel Z, Demeke T, West CE. Xerophthalmia in Ethiopia: a nationwide ophthalmological, biochemical and anthropometric survey. Eur J Clin Nutr. 1991;45(10):469–78.
228. Katz J, Zeger SL, Tielsch JM. Village and household clustering of xerophthalmia and trachoma. Int J Epidemiol. 1988;17(4):865–9.
229. Katz J, Zeger SL, West KP Jr, Tielsch JM, Sommer A. Clustering of xerophthalmia within households and villages. Int J Epidemiol. 1993;22(4):709–15.
230. Semba RD, de Pee S, Panagides D, Poly O, Bloem MW. Risk factors for xerophthalmia among mothers and their children and for mother-child pairs with xerophthalmia in Cambodia. Arch Ophthalmol. 2004;122(4):517–23.
231. Gittelsohn J, Shankar AV, West KP Jr, Ram R, Dhungel C, Dahal B. Infant feeding practices reflect antecedent risk of xerophthalmia in Nepali children. Eur J Clin Nutr. 1997;51(7):484–90.
232. Gittelsohn J, Shankar AV, West KP Jr, Faruque F, Gnywali T, Pradhan EK. Child feeding and care behaviors are associated with xerophthalmia in rural Nepalese households. Soc Sci Med. 1998;47(4):477–86.
233. Hennig A, Foster A, Shrestha SP, Pokhrel RP. Vitamin A deficiency and corneal ulceration in south-east Nepal: implications for preventing blindness in children. Bull World Health Organ. 1991;69(2):235–9.
234. Bloem MW, Wedel M, Egger RJ, Speek AJ, Chusilp K, Saowakontha S, et al. A prevalence study of vitamin A deficiency and xerophthalmia in northeastern Thailand. Am J Epidemiol. 1989;129(6):1095–103.
235. Solon FS, Popkin BM, Fernandez TL, Latham MC. Vitamin A deficiency in the Philippines: a study of xerophthalmia in Cebu. Am J Clin Nutr. 1978;31(2):360–8.
236. Klemm RD, Villate EE, Tuason CS, Bayugo G, Mendoza OM. A prevalence study of xerophthalmia in the Philippines: implications for supplementation strategies. Southeast Asian J Trop Med Public Health. 1993;24(4):617–23.
237. Rosen DS, al Sharif Z, Bashir M, al Shabooti A, Pizzarello LD. Vitamin A deficiency and xerophthalmia in western Yemen. Eur J Clin Nutr. 1996;50(1):54–7.
238. Tielsch JM, West KP Jr, Katz J, Chirambo MC, Schwab L, Johnson GJ, et al. Prevalence and severity of xerophthalmia in southern Malawi. Am J Epidemiol. 1986;124(4):561–8.
239. Danks J, Kaufman D, Rait J. A clinical and cytological study of vitamin A deficiency in Kiribati. Aust N Z J Ophthalmol. 1992;20(3):215–8.
240. Katz J, West KP Jr, Khatry SK, Thapa MD, LeClerq SC, Pradhan EK, et al. Impact of vitamin A supplementation on prevalence and incidence of xerophthalmia in Nepal. Invest Ophthalmol Vis Sci. 1995;36(13):2577–83.
241. Muhilal, Tarwotjo I, Kodyat B, Herman S, Permaesih D, Karyadi D, et al. Changing prevalence of xerophthalmia in Indonesia, 1977-1992. Eur J Clin Nutr. 1994;48(10):708–14.
242. Santos LM, Dricot JM, Asciutti LS, Dricot-d'Ans C. Xerophthalmia in the state of Paraiba, northeast of Brazil: clinical findings. Am J Clin Nutr. 1983;38(1):139–44.
243. Fawzi WW, Herrera MG, Willett WC, el Amin A, Nestel P, Lipsitz S, et al. Vitamin A supplementation and dietary vitamin A in relation to the risk of xerophthalmia. Am J Clin Nutr. 1993;58(3):385–91.
244. Kjolhede CL, Stallings RY, Dibley MJ, Sadjimin T, Dawiesah S, Padmawati S. Serum retinol levels among preschool children in Central Java: demographic and socioeconomic determinants. Int J Epidemiol. 1995;24(2):399–403.
245. Rosen DS, Sloan NL, del Rosario A, de la Paz TC. Risk factors for vitamin A deficiency in rural areas of the Philippines. J Trop Pediatr. 1994;40(2):82–7.
246. Khan NC, Ninh NX, Van Nhien N, Khoi HH, West CE, Hautvast JG. Sub clinical vitamin A deficiency and anemia among Vietnamese children less than five years of age. Asia Pac J Clin Nutr. 2007;16(1):152–7.
247. Pant I, Gopaldas T. Effect of mega doses of vitamin A on the vitamin A status of underprivileged school-age boys (7-15 yr). Indian J Med Res. 1987;86:196–206.

248. Stoltzfus RJ, Hakimi M, Miller KW, Rasmussen KM, Dawiesah S, Habicht JP, et al. High dose vitamin A supplementation of breast-feeding Indonesian mothers: effects on the vitamin A status of mother and infant. J Nutr. 1993;123(4):666–75.

249. Ahmed F, Hasan N, Kabir Y. Vitamin A deficiency among adolescent female garment factory workers in Bangladesh. Eur J Clin Nutr. 1997;51(10):698–702.

250. Ahmed F. Vitamin A deficiency in Bangladesh: a review and recommendations for improvement. Public Health Nutr. 1999;2(1):1–14.

251. Rice AL, Stoltzfus RJ, de Francisco A, Chakraborty J, Kjolhede CL, Wahed MA. Maternal vitamin A or β-carotene supplementation in lactating Bangladeshi women benefits mothers and infants but does not prevent subclinical deficiency. J Nutr. 1999;129(2):356–65.

252. Mahalanabis D. Breast feeding and vitamin A deficiency among children attending a diarrhoea treatment centre in Bangladesh: a case-control study. BMJ. 1991;303(6801):493–6.

253. Bloem MW, Hye A, Wijnroks M, Ralte A, West KP Jr, Sommer A. The role of universal distribution of vitamin A capsules in combatting vitamin A deficiency in Bangladesh. Am J Epidemiol. 1995;142(8):843–55.

254. Tarwotjo I, Tilden R, Pettiss S, Sommer A, Soedibjo S, Hussaini G, et al. Interactions of community nutritional status and xerophthalmia in Indonesia. Am J Clin Nutr. 1983;37(4):645–51.

255. Mele L, West KP Jr, Kusdiono Pandji A, Nendrawati H, Tilden RL, et al. Nutritional and household risk factors for xerophthalmia in Aceh, Indonesia: a case-control study. The Aceh Study Group. Am J Clin Nutr. 1991;53 (6):1460–5.

256. Khan NC, Mai LB, Minh ND, Do TT, Khoi HH, West CE, et al. Intakes of retinol and carotenoids and its determining factors in the Red River Delta population of northern Vietnam. Eur J Clin Nutr. 2008;62(6):810–6.

257. Hussain A, Kvale G. Serum vitamin A in relation to socio-economic, demographic and dietary characteristics in Bangladeshi children. Acta Paediatr. 1996;85(8):971–6.

258. Schemann JF, Malvy D, Zefack G, Traore L, Sacko D, Sanoussi B, et al. Mapping xerophthalmia in Mali: results of a national survey on regional distribution and related risk factors. J Am Coll Nutr. 2007;26(6):630–8.

259. Cohen N, Jalil MA, Rahman H, Leemhuis de Regt E, Sprague J, Mitra M. Blinding malnutrition in rural Bangladesh. J Trop Pediatr. 1986;32(2):73–8.

260. Djunaedi E, Sommer A, Pandji A, Kusdiono, Taylor HR. Impact of vitamin A supplementation on xerophthalmia. A randomized controlled community trial. Arch Ophthalmol. 1988;106(2):218–22.

261. Tielsch JM, Sommer A. The epidemiology of vitamin A deficiency and xerophthalmia. Annu Rev Nutr. 1984;4:183–205.

262. West KP Jr. Dietary vitamin A deficiency: effects on growth, infection, and mortality. Food Nutr Bull. 1991;13:119–31.

263. Darnton-Hill I. Vitamin A in the third world. Proc Nutr Soc Aust. 1989;14:13–23.

264. Nestel P, Herrera MG, el Amin A, Fawzi W, Mohammed KA, Weld L. Risk factors associated with xerophthalmia in northern Sudan. J Nutr. 1993;123(12):2115–21.

265. Hussain A, Kvale G, Ali K, Bhuyan AH. Determinants of night blindness in Bangladesh. Int J Epidemiol. 1993;22(6):1119–26.

266. Cohen N, Jalil MA, Rahman H, Matin MA, Sprague J, Islam J, et al. Landholding, wealth and risk of blinding malnutrition in rural Bangladeshi households. Soc Sci Med. 1985;21(11):1269–72.

267. Al-Mekhlafi MH, Azlin M, Aini UN, Shaik A, Sa'iah A, Norhayati M. Prevalence and predictors of low serum retinol and hypoalbuminaemia among children in rural Peninsular Malaysia. Trans R Soc Trop Med Hyg. 2007;101(12):1233–40.

268. Laxmaiah A, Nair MK, Arlappa N, Raghu P, Balakrishna N, Rao KM, et al. Prevalence of ocular signs and subclinical vitamin A deficiency and its determinants among rural pre-school children in India. Public Health Nutr. 2012;15(4):568–77.

269. Ahmed F, Mohiduzzaman M, Barua S, Shaheen N, Margetts BM, Jackson AA. Effect of family size and income on the biochemical indices of urban school children of Bangladesh. Eur J Clin Nutr. 1992;46(7):465–73.

270. Oomen HAPC, ten Doesschate J. The periodicity of xerophthalmia in South and East Asia. Ecol Food Nutr. 1973;2(3):207–17.

271. Desai NC, Desai S, Desai R. Xerophthalmia clinics in rural eye camps. Int Ophthalmol. 1992;16(3):139–45.

272. Sinha DP, Bang FB. Seasonal variation in signs of vitamin-A deficiency in rural West Bengal children. Lancet. 1973;2(7823):228–30.

273. Sinha DP, Bang FB. The effect of massive doses of vitamin A on the signs of vitamin A deficiency in preschool children. Am J Clin Nutr. 1976;29(1):110–5.

274. Bloem MW, Huq N, Gorstein J, Burger S, Kahn T, Islam N, et al. Production of fruits and vegetables at the homestead is an important source of vitamin A among women in rural Bangladesh. Eur J Clin Nutr. 1996;50 (Suppl 3):S62–7.

275. Bloem MW, De Pee S, Darnton-Hill I. New issues in developing effective approaches for the prevention and control of vitamin a deficiency. Food Nutr Bull. 1998;19(2):137–48.

276. Semba RD, Susatio B, Muhilal, Natadisastra G. The decline of admissions for xerophthalmia at Cicendo Eye Hospital, Indonesia, 1981–1992. Int Ophthalmol. 1995;19(1):39–42.

277. Soewarta K, Bloem MW. The role of high-dose vitamin A capsules in preventing a relapse of vitamin A deficiency due to Indonesia's current crisis. Indonesia Crisis Bull. 1999;1:1–4.

278. Miller M, Humphrey J, Johnson E, Marinda E, Brookmeyer R, Katz J. Why do children become vitamin A deficient? J Nutr. 2002;132(9 Suppl):2867S–80S.

279. Brown KH, Black RE, Becker S, Nahar S, Sawyer J. Consumption of foods and nutrients by weanlings in rural Bangladesh. Am J Clin Nutr. 1982;36(5):878–89.

280. Tarwotjo I, Sommer A, Soegiharto T, Susanto D, Muhilal. Dietary practices and xerophthalmia among Indonesian children. Am J Clin Nutr. 1982;35(3):574–81.

281. Cohen N, Measham C, Khanum S, Khatun M, Ahmed N. Xerophthalmia in urban Bangladesh. Implications for vitamin A deficiency preventive strategies. Acta Paediatr Scand. 1983;72(4):531–6.

282. Stanton BF, Clemens JD, Wojtyniak B, Khair T. Risk factors for developing mild nutritional blindness in urban Bangladesh. Am J Dis Child. 1986;140(6):584–8.

283. Schaumberg DA, O'Connor J, Semba RD. Risk factors for xerophthalmia in the Republic of Kiribati. Eur J Clin Nutr. 1996;50(11):761–4.

284. Shankar AV, West KP Jr, Gittelsohn J, Katz J, Pradhan R. Chronic low intakes of vitamin A-rich foods in households with xerophthalmic children: a case-control study in Nepal. Am J Clin Nutr. 1996;64(2):242–8.

285. De Sole G, Belay Y, Zegeye B. Vitamin A deficiency in southern Ethiopia. Am J Clin Nutr. 1987;45(4):780–4.

286. Hussain A, Lindtjorn B, Kvale G. Protein energy malnutrition, vitamin A deficiency and night blindness in Bangladeshi children. Ann Trop Paediatr. 1996;16(4):319–25.

287. Shankar AV, Gittelsohn J, West KP Jr, Stallings R, Gnywali T, Faruque F. Eating from a shared plate affects food consumption in vitamin A-deficient Nepali children. J Nutr. 1998;128(7):1127–33.

288. Sivakumar B, Reddy V. Absorption of labelled vitamin A in children during infection. Br J Nutr. 1972;27(2):299–304.

289. Reddy V, Sivakumar B. Studies on vitamin A absorption in children. Indian Pediatr. 1972;9(6):307–10.

290. Salazar-Lindo E, Salazar M, Alvarez JO. Association of diarrhea and low serum retinol in Peruvian children. Am J Clin Nutr. 1993;58(1):110–3.

291. Campos FA, Flores H, Underwood BA. Effect of an infection on vitamin A status of children as measured by the relative dose response (RDR). Am J Clin Nutr. 1987;46(1):91–4.

292. Stephensen CB, Alvarez JO, Kohatsu J, Hardmeier R, Kennedy JI Jr, Gammon RB Jr. Vitamin A is excreted in the urine during acute infection. Am J Clin Nutr. 1994;60(3):388–92.

293. Alvarez JO, Salazar-Lindo E, Kohatsu J, Miranda P, Stephensen CB. Urinary excretion of retinol in children with acute diarrhea. Am J Clin Nutr. 1995;61(6):1273–6.

294. Semba RD, Muhilal West KP Jr, Natadisastra G, Eisinger W, Lan Y, et al. Hyporetinolemia and acute phase proteins in children with and without xerophthalmia. Am J Clin Nutr. 2000;72(1):146–53.

295. Wittpenn J, Sommer A. Clinical aspects of vitamin A deficiency. In: Bauernfeind JC, editor. Vitamin A deficiency and its control. Orlando, FL: Academic Press; 1986. p. 177–206.

296. Wondmikun Y. Dark adaptation pattern of pregnant women as an indicator of functional disturbance at acceptable serum vitamin A levels. Eur J Clin Nutr. 2002;56(5):462–6.

297. Taren DL, Duncan B, Shrestha K, Shrestha N, Genaro-Wolf D, Schleicher RL, et al. The night vision threshold test is a better predictor of low serum vitamin A concentration than self-reported night blindness in pregnant urban Nepalese women. J Nutr. 2004;134(10):2573–8.

298. Congdon NG, Dreyfuss ML, Christian P, Navitsky RC, Sanchez AM, Wu LS, et al. Responsiveness of dark-adaptation threshold to vitamin A and β-carotene supplementation in pregnant and lactating women in Nepal. Am J Clin Nutr. 2000;72(4):1004–9.

299. Sommer A, Hussaini G, Muhilal, Tarwotjo I, Susanto D, Saroso JS. History of nightblindness: a simple tool for xerophthalmia screening. Am J Clin Nutr. 1980;33(4):887–91.

300. Hussain A, Kvale G, Odland M. Diagnosis of night blindness and serum vitamin A level: a population-based study. Bull World Health Organ. 1995;73(4):469–76.

301. Haskell MJ, Pandey P, Graham JM, Peerson JM, Shrestha RK, Brown KH. Recovery from impaired dark adaptation in nightblind pregnant Nepali women who receive small daily doses of vitamin A as amaranth leaves, carrots, goat liver, vitamin A-fortified rice, or retinyl palmitate. Am J Clin Nutr. 2005;81(2):461–71.

302. Tarwotjo I, Katz J, West KP Jr, Tielsch JM, Sommer A. Xerophthalmia and growth in preschool Indonesian children. Am J Clin Nutr. 1992;55(6):1142–6.

303. Rahmathullah L, Underwood BA, Thulasiraj RD, Milton RC. Diarrhea, respiratory infections, and growth are not affected by a weekly low-dose vitamin A supplement: a masked, controlled field trial in children in southern India. Am J Clin Nutr. 1991;54(3):568–77.

304. Fawzi WW, Herrera MG, Willett WC, Nestel P, el Amin A, Mohamed KA. The effect of vitamin A supplementation on the growth of preschool children in the Sudan. Am J Public Health. 1997;87(8):1359–62.

305. Kirkwood BR, Ross DA, Arthur P, Morris SS, Dollimore N, Binka FN, et al. Effect of vitamin A supplementation on the growth of young children in northern Ghana. Am J Clin Nutr. 1996;63(5):773–81.
306. West KP, LeClerq SC, Shrestha SR, Wu LS, Pradhan EK, Khatry SK, et al. Effects of vitamin A on growth of vitamin A-deficient children: field studies in Nepal. J Nutr. 1997;127(10):1957–65.
307. Lie C, Ying C, Wang EL, Brun T, Geissler C. Impact of large-dose vitamin A supplementation on childhood diarrhoea, respiratory disease and growth. Eur J Clin Nutr. 1993;47(2):88–96.
308. Ramakrishnan U, Latham MC, Abel R. Vitamin A supplementation does not improve growth of preschool children: a randomized, double-blind field trial in south India. J Nutr. 1995;125(2):202–11.
309. West KP Jr, Djunaedi E, Pandji A. Kusdiono, Tarwotjo I, Sommer A. Vitamin A supplementation and growth: a randomized community trial. Am J Clin Nutr. 1988;48(5):1257–64.
310. Bahl R, Bhandari N, Taneja S, Bhan MK. The impact of vitamin A supplementation on physical growth of children is dependent on season. Eur J Clin Nutr. 1997;51(1):26–9.
311. Muhilal, Murdiana A, Azis I, Saidin S, Jahari AB, Karyadi D. Vitamin A-fortified monosodium glutamate and vitamin A status: a controlled field trial. Am J Clin Nutr. 1988;48(5):1265–70.
312. Donnen P, Brasseur D, Dramaix M, Vertongen F, Zihindula M, Muhamiriza M, et al. Vitamin A supplementation but not deworming improves growth of malnourished preschool children in eastern Zaire. J Nutr. 1998;128 (8):1320–7.
313. Hadi H, Stoltzfus RJ, Dibley MJ, Moulton LH, West KP Jr, Kjolhede CL, et al. Vitamin A supplementation selectively improves the linear growth of Indonesian preschool children: results from a randomized controlled trial. Am J Clin Nutr. 2000;71(2):507–13.
314. Hadi H, Stoltzfus RJ, Moulton LH, Dibley MJ, West KP Jr. Respiratory infections reduce the growth response to vitamin A supplementation in a randomized controlled trial. Int J Epidemiol. 1999;28(5):874–81.
315. Hadi H, Dibley MJ, West KP Jr. Complex interactions with infection and diet may explain seasonal growth responses to vitamin A in preschool aged Indonesian children. Eur J Clin Nutr. 2004;58(7):990–9.
316. Coutsoudis A, Broughton M, Coovadia HM. Vitamin A supplementation reduces measles morbidity in young African children: a randomized, placebo-controlled, double-blind trial. Am J Clin Nutr. 1991;54(5):890–5.
317. Donnen P, Dramaix M, Brasseur D, Bitwe R, Vertongen F, Hennart P. Randomized placebo-controlled clinical trial of the effect of a single high dose or daily low doses of vitamin A on the morbidity of hospitalized, malnourished children. Am J Clin Nutr. 1998;68(6):1254–60.
318. Semba RD, Bloem MW. The anemia of vitamin A deficiency: epidemiology and pathogenesis. Eur J Clin Nutr. 2002;56(4):271–81.
319. Fishman SM, Christian P, West KP. The role of vitamins in the prevention and control of anaemia. Public Health Nutr. 2000;3(2):125–50.
320. Hodges RE, Sauberlich HE, Canham JE, Wallace DL, Rucker RB, Mejia LA, et al. Hematopoietic studies in vitamin A deficiency. Am J Clin Nutr. 1978;31(5):876–85.
321. Hashizume M, Chiba M, Shinohara A, Iwabuchi S, Sasaki S, Shimoda T, et al. Anaemia, iron deficiency and vitamin A status among school-aged children in rural Kazakhstan. Public Health Nutr. 2005;8(6):564–71.
322. West KP Jr, Gernand AD, Sommer A. Vitamin A in nutritional anemia. In: Kraemer K, Zimmerman MB, editors. Nutritional Anemia. Basel, Switzerland: Sight and Life; 2007. p. 133–54.
323. Beisel WR, Black RE, West KP Jr. Micronutrients in infection. In: Guerrant RL, Walker DH, Weller PF, editors. Tropical infectious diseases: principles, pathogens and practice. Philadelphia: Churchill Livingstone; 1999. p. 76–87.
324. Findlay GM, Mackenzie R. Opsonins and diets deficient in vitamins. Biochem J. 1922;16(5):574–7.
325. Bloem MW. Interdependence of vitamin A and iron: an important association for programmes of anaemia control. Proc Nutr Soc. 1995;54(2):501–8.
326. Fisher JW. Erythropoietin: physiology and pharmacology update. Exp Biol Med (Maywood). 2003;228(1):1–14.
327. Jelkmann W, Pagel H, Hellwig T, Fandrey J. Effects of antioxidant vitamins on renal and hepatic erythropoietin production. Kidney Int. 1997;51(2):497–501.
328. Zimmermann MB, Biebinger R, Rohner F, Dib A, Zeder C, Hurrell RF, et al. Vitamin A supplementation in children with poor vitamin A and iron status increases erythropoietin and hemoglobin concentrations without changing total body iron. Am J Clin Nutr. 2006;84(3):580–6.
329. Mejia LA, Arroyave G. The effect of vitamin A fortification of sugar on iron metabolism in preschool children in Guatemala. Am J Clin Nutr. 1982;36(1):87–93.
330. Mejia LA, Chew F. Hematological effect of supplementing anemic children with vitamin A alone and in combination with iron. Am J Clin Nutr. 1988;48(3):595–600.
331. Mwanri L, Worsley A, Ryan P, Masika J. Supplemental vitamin A improves anemia and growth in anemic school children in Tanzania. J Nutr. 2000;130(11):2691–6.
332. Smith JC, Makdani D, Hegar A, Rao D, Douglass LW. Vitamin A and zinc supplementation of preschool children. J Am Coll Nutr. 1999;18(3):213–22.

333. Bloem MW, Wedel M, van Agtmaal EJ, Speek AJ, Saowakontha S, Schreurs WH. Vitamin A intervention: short-term effects of a single, oral, massive dose on iron metabolism. Am J Clin Nutr. 1990;51(1):76–9.
334. Bloem MW, Wedel M, Egger RJ, Speek AJ, Schrijver J, Saowakontha S, et al. Iron metabolism and vitamin A deficiency in children in northeast Thailand. Am J Clin Nutr. 1989;50(2):332–8.
335. Semba RD, Muhilal, West KP, Winget M, Natadisastra G, Scott A, et al. Impact of vitamin A supplementation on hematological indicators of iron metabolism and protein status in children. Nutr Res. 1992;12(4–5):469–78.
336. Suharno D, West CE, Muhilal, Karyadi D, Hautvast JG. Supplementation with vitamin A and iron for nutritional anaemia in pregnant women in West Java, Indonesia. Lancet. 1993;342(8883):1325–8.
337. Muslimatun S, Schmidt MK, Schultink W, West CE, Hautvast JA, Gross R, et al. Weekly supplementation with iron and vitamin A during pregnancy increases hemoglobin concentration but decreases serum ferritin concentration in Indonesian pregnant women. J Nutr. 2001;131(1):85–90.
338. Chawla PK, Puri R. Impact of nutritional supplements on hematological profile of pregnant women. Indian Pediatr. 1995;32(8):876–80.
339. Ahmed F, Khan MR, Jackson AA. Concomitant supplemental vitamin A enhances the response to weekly supplemental iron and folic acid in anemic teenagers in urban Bangladesh. Am J Clin Nutr. 2001;74(1):108–15.
340. Ahmed F, Khan MR, Islam M, Kabir I, Fuchs GJ. Anaemia and iron deficiency among adolescent schoolgirls in peri-urban Bangladesh. Eur J Clin Nutr. 2000;54(9):678–83.
341. Kolsteren P, Rahman SR, Hilderbrand K, Diniz A. Treatment for iron deficiency anaemia with a combined supplementation of iron, vitamin A and zinc in women of Dinajpur, Bangladesh. Eur J Clin Nutr. 1999;53 (2):102–6.
342. Semba RD, Kumwenda N, Taha TE, Mtimavalye L, Broadhead R, Garrett E, et al. Impact of vitamin A supplementation on anaemia and plasma erythropoietin concentrations in pregnant women: a controlled clinical trial. Eur J Haematol. 2001;66(6):389–95.
343. van den Broek NR, White SA, Flowers C, Cook JD, Letsky EA, Tanumihardjo SA, et al. Randomised trial of vitamin A supplementation in pregnant women in rural Malawi found to be anaemic on screening by HemoCue. BJOG. 2006;113(5):569–76.
344. World Health Organization. Guideline: vitamin A supplementation for infants and children 6-59 months of age. Geneva: World Health Organization; 2011.
345. Emran N, Tjakrasudjatma S. Clinical characteristics of vitamin A responsive and nonresponsive Bitot's spots. Am J Ophthalmol. 1980;90(2):160–71.
346. Semba RD, Wirasasmita S, Natadisastra G, Muhilal, Sommer A. Response of Bitot's spots in preschool children to vitamin A treatment. Am J Ophthalmol. 1990;110(4):416–20.
347. Sovani I, Humphrey JH, Kuntinalibronto DR, Natadisastra G, Muhilal, Tielsch JM. Response of Bitot's spots to a single oral 100,000- or 200,000-IU dose of vitamin A. Am J Ophthalmol. 1994;118(6):792–6.
348. West CE. Vitamin A and measles. Nutr Rev. 2000;58(2 Pt 2):S46–54.
349. de Pee S, Bloem MW, Satoto Yip R, Sukaton A, Tjiong R, et al. Impact of a social marketing campaign promoting dark-green leafy vegetables and eggs in central Java, Indonesia. Int J Vitam Nutr Res. 1998;68(6):389–98.
350. Darnton-Hill I, Webb P, Harvey PW, Hunt JM, Dalmiya N, Chopra M, et al. Micronutrient deficiencies and gender: social and economic costs. Am J Clin Nutr. 2005;81(5):1198S–205S.
351. Webb P, Nishida C, Darnton-Hill I. Age and gender as factors in the distribution of global micronutrient deficiencies. Nutr Rev. 2007;65(5):233–45.
352. Ramakrishnan U, Darnton-Hill I. Assessment and control of vitamin A deficiency disorders. J Nutr. 2002;132 (9):2947S–53S.
353. Rice AL, Stoltzfus RJ, de Francisco A, Kjolhede CL. Evaluation of serum retinol, the modified-relative-dose-response ratio, and breast-milk vitamin A as indicators of response to postpartum maternal vitamin A supplementation. Am J Clin Nutr. 2000;71(3):799–806.
354. Ribaya-Mercado JD. Influence of dietary fat on β-carotene absorption and bioconversion into vitamin A. Nutr Rev. 2002;60(4):104–10.
355. Talukder A, Kiess L, Huq N, de Pee S, Darnton-Hill I, Bloem M. Increasing the production and consumption of vitamin A-rich fruits and vegetables: Lessons learned in taking the Bangladesh homestead gardening programme to a national scale. Food Nutr Bull. 2000;21(2):165–72.
356. Marsh R. Building on traditional gardening to improve household food security. Food Nutr Agric. 1998;22(4):4–14.
357. Hagenimana V, Oyunga MA, Low J, Njoroge SM, Gichuki ST, Kabira J. The effects of women farmers' adoption of orange-fleshed sweet potatoes: raising vitamin A intake in Kenya. Washington, D.C.: International Center for Research on Women; 1999.
358. Ayalew W, Wolde Gebriel Z, Kassa H. Reducing vitamin A deficiency in Ethiopia: linkages with a women-focused dairy goat farming project. Washington, D.C.: International Center for Research on Women/Opportunities for Micronutrient Interventions; 1999.

359. Smitasiri S, Attig GA, Dhanamitta S. Participatory action for nutrition education: Social marketing vitamin A-rich foods in Thailand. Ecol Food Nutr. 1992;28(3):199–210.

360. Devadas RP, Saroja S, Murthy NK. Availability of β-carotene from papaya fruit and amaranth in preschool children. Indian J Nutr Diet. 1980;17(2):41–4.

361. Adegboye OR, Smith C, Anang D, Musa H. Comparing and contrasting three cultural food customs from Nigeria and analyzing the nutrient content of diets from these cultures with the aim of proffering nutritional intervention. Crit Rev Food Sci Nutr. 2015.

362. Nana CP, Brouwer ID, Zagre NM, Kok FJ, Traore AS. Community assessment of availability, consumption, and cultural acceptability of food sources of (pro)vitamin A: toward the development of a dietary intervention among preschool children in rural Burkina Faso. Food Nutr Bull. 2005;26(4):356–65.

363. Oguntibeju OO, Esterhuyse AJ, Truter EJ. Red palm oil: nutritional, physiological and therapeutic roles in improving human wellbeing and quality of life. Br J Biomed Sci. 2009;66(4):216–22.

364. Souganidis E, Laillou A, Leyvraz M, Moench-Pfanner R. A comparison of retinyl palmitate and red palm oil β-carotene as strategies to address Vitamin A deficiency. Nutrients. 2013;5(8):3257–71.

365. Canfield LM, Kaminsky RG, Taren DL, Shaw E, Sander JK. Red palm oil in the maternal diet increases provitamin A carotenoids in breastmilk and serum of the mother-infant dyad. Eur J Nutr. 2001;40(1):30–8.

366. Muoki PN, Makokha AO, Onyango CA, Ojijo NK. Potential contribution of mangoes to reduction of vitamin A deficiency in Kenya. Ecol Food Nutr. 2009;48(6):482–98.

367. Frega R, Lanfranco JG, De Greve S, Bernardini S, Geniez P, Grede N, et al. What linear programming contributes: World Food Programme experience with the "cost of the diet" tool. Food Nutr Bull. 2012;33(3 Suppl):S228–34.

368. Santini A, Novellino E, Armini V, Ritieni A. State of the art of Ready-to-Use Therapeutic Food: a tool for nutraceuticals addition to foodstuff. Food Chem. 2013;140(4):843–9.

369. Briend A, Ferguson EL, Darmon N. Local food price analysis by linear programming: a new approach to assess the economic value of fortified food supplements. Food Nutr Bull. 2001;22:184–9.

370. Parlesak A, Geelhoed D, Robertson A. Toward the prevention of childhood undernutrition: diet diversity strategies using locally produced food can overcome gaps in nutrient supply. Food Nutr Bull. 2014;35(2):191–9.

371. West KP, Jr., Sommer A. Delivery of oral doses of vitamin A to prevent vitamin A deficiency and nutritional blindness: a state-of-the-art review. Geneva, Switzerland: Administrative Committee on Coordination–Subcommittee on Nutrition (ACC/SCN); 1987.

372. Darnton-Hill I, Sibanda F, Mitra M, Ali MM, Drexler AED, Rahman H, et al. Distribution of vitamin-A capsules for the prevention and control of vitamin-A deficiency in Bangladesh. Food Nutr Bull. 1988;10(3):60–70.

373. Dalmiya N, Palmer A, Darnton-Hill I. Sustaining vitamin A supplementation requires a new vision. Lancet. 2006;368(9541):1052–4.

374. WHO/UNICEF/IVACG. Vitamin A supplements: a guide to their use in the treatment and prevention of vitamin A deficiency and xerophthalmia. Geneva: WHO/UNICEF/IVACG; 1997.

375. Florentino RF, Tanchoco CC, Ramos AC, Mendoza TS, Natividad EP, Tangco JB, et al. Tolerance of preschoolers to two dosage strengths of vitamin A preparation. Am J Clin Nutr. 1990;52(4):694–700.

376. Imdad A, Yakoob MY, Sudfeld C, Haider BA, Black RE, Bhutta ZA. Impact of vitamin A supplementation on infant and childhood mortality. BMC Public Health. 2011;11(Suppl 3):S20.

377. United Nations. World Declaration on the Survival, Protection and Development of Children; and Plan of Action for Implementing the World Declaration on the Survival, Protection and Development of Children in the 1990s. World Summit for Children; 30 Sept 1990; New York, NY: United Nations; 1990.

378. Palmer AC, West KP Jr, Dalmiya N, Schultink W. The use and interpretation of serum retinol distributions in evaluating the public health impact of vitamin A programmes. Public Health Nutr. 2012;15(7):1201–15.

379. Pereira SM, Begum A. Prevention of vitamin A deficiency. Am J Clin Nutr. 1969;22(7):858–62.

380. Pereira SM, Begum A. Failure of a massive single oral dose of vitamin A to prevent deficiency. Arch Dis Child. 1971;46(248):525–7.

381. Humphrey JH, West KP, Jr., Muhilal, See LC, Natadisastra G, Sommer A. A priming dose of oral vitamin A given to preschool children may extend protection conferred by a subsequent large dose of vitamin A. J Nutr. 1993;123(8):1363–9.

382. Gorstein J, Bhaskaram P, Khanum S, Hossaini R, Balakrishna N, Goodman TS, et al. Safety and impact of vitamin A supplementation delivered with oral polio vaccine as part of the immunization campaign in Orissa, India. Food Nutr Bull. 2003;24(4):319–31.

383. Palmer AC, West KP, Jr. A quarter of a century of progress to prevent vitamin A deficiency through supplementation. Food Rev Int. 2010;26(3).

384. International Vitamin A Consultative Group. Report of the XXII International Vitamin A Consultative Group meeting. Vitamin A and the common agenda for micronutrients; 15–17 Nov 2004; Lima, Peru: International Vitamin A Consultative Group; 2004. p. 102.

385. International Vitamin A Consultative Group. Report of the XXI International Vitamin A Consultative Group meeting. Improving the vitamin A status of populations, 3–5 Feb 2003, Marrakech, Morocco; 2003. p. 84.

386. Kupka R, Nielsen J, Nyhus Dhillon C, Blankenship J, Haskell MJ, Baker SK, et al. Safety and mortality benefits of delivering vitamin A supplementation at 6 months of age in Sub-Saharan Africa. Food Nutr Bull. 2016.

387. United Nations Children's Fund. Vitamin A supplementation: a decade of progress. New York, NY: UNICEF, April 2007.

388. Palmer AC, Diaz T, Noordam AC, Dalmiya N. Evolution of the Child Health Day strategy for the integrated delivery of child health and nutrition services. Food Nutr Bull. 2013;34(4):412–9.

389. Sesay FF, Hodges MH, Kamara HI, Turay M, Wolfe A, Samba TT, et al. High coverage of vitamin A supplementation and measles vaccination during an integrated Maternal and Child Health Week in Sierra Leone. Int Health. 2015;7(1):26–31.

390. Klemm RD, Palmer AC, Greig A, Engle-Stone R, Dalmiya N. A changing landscape for vitamin A programs: implications for optimal intervention packages, program monitoring, and safety. Food Nutr Bull. 2016;37(2 Suppl):S75–86.

391. Darnton-Hill I, Nalubola R. Fortification strategies to meet micronutrient needs: successes and failures. Proc Nutr Soc. 2002;61(2):231–41.

392. Bauernfeind JC, Arroyave G. Control of vitamin A deficiency by the nutritification of food approach. In: Bauernfeind JC, editor. Vitamin A deficiency and its control. Orlando, FL: Academic Press; 1986.

393. Engle-Stone R, Ndjebayi AO, Nankap M, Brown KH. Consumption of potentially fortifiable foods by women and young children varies by ecological zone and socio-economic status in Cameroon. J Nutr. 2012;142(3):555–65.

394. Laillou A, le Mai B, le Hop T, Khan NC, Panagides D, Wieringa F, et al. An assessment of the impact of fortification of staples and condiments on micronutrient intake in young Vietnamese children. Nutrients. 2012;4 (9):1151–70.

395. Kyamuhangire W, Lubowa A, Kaaya A, Kikafunda J, Harvey PW, Rambeloson Z, et al. The importance of using food and nutrient intake data to identify appropriate vehicles and estimate potential benefits of food fortification in Uganda. Food Nutr Bull. 2013;34(2):131–42.

396. Hess SY, Brown KH, Sablah M, Engle-Stone R, Aaron GJ, Baker SK. Results of Fortification Rapid Assessment Tool (FRAT) surveys in sub-Saharan Africa and suggestions for future modifications of the survey instrument. Food Nutr Bull. 2013;34(1):21–38.

397. Solon F, Fernandez TL, Latham MC, Popkin BM. An evaluation of strategies to control vitamin A deficiency in the Philippines. Am J Clin Nutr. 1979;32(7):1445–53.

398. Solon FS, Solon MS, Mehansho H, West KP Jr, Sarol J, Perfecto C, et al. Evaluation of the effect of vitamin A-fortified margarine on the vitamin A status of preschool Filipino children. Eur J Clin Nutr. 1996;50(11):720–3.

399. Arroyave G, Mejia LA, Aguilar JR. The effect of vitamin A fortification of sugar on the serum vitamin A levels of preschool Guatemalan children: a longitudinal evaluation. Am J Clin Nutr. 1981;34(1):41–9.

400. MOST/USAID. Summary of Mandatory and Voluntary Staple Food Fortification in Developing Countries 2000 [updated 28 April 2000]. Available from http://www.mostproject.org/PDF/fortificationritu.PDF.

401. Gurdián M, Kontorovsky I, Alvarado E, Ramírez SA, Hernández R. Integrated surveillance system for nutrition interventions. Progress report. Managua, Nicaragua: Ministerio de Salud; 2005 (in Spanish).

402. Candelaria LV, Magsadia CR, Velasco RE, Pedro MR, Barba CV, Tanchoco CC. The effect of vitamin A-fortified coconut cooking oil on the serum retinol concentration of Filipino children 4–7 years old. Asia Pac J Clin Nutr. 2005;14(1):43–53.

403. Klemm RD, West KP Jr, Palmer AC, Johnson Q, Randall P, Ranum P, et al. Vitamin A fortification of wheat flour: considerations and current recommendations. Food Nutr Bull. 2010;31(1 Suppl):S47–61.

404. Solon FS, Klemm RD, Sanchez L, Darnton-Hill I, Craft NE, Christian P, et al. Efficacy of a vitamin A-fortified wheat-flour bun on the vitamin A status of Filipino schoolchildren. Am J Clin Nutr. 2000;72(3):738–44.

405. Rahman AS, Ahmed T, Ahmed F, Alam MS, Wahed MA, Sack DA. Double-blind cluster randomised controlled trial of wheat flour chapatti fortified with micronutrients on the status of vitamin A and iron in school-aged children in rural Bangladesh. Matern Child Nutr. 2015;11(Suppl 4):120–31.

406. Nesamvuni AE, Vorster HH, Margetts BM, Kruger A. Fortification of maize meal improved the nutritional status of 1-3-year-old African children. Public Health Nutr. 2005;8(5):461–7.

407. Zimmermann MB, Wegmueller R, Zeder C, Chaouki N, Biebinger R, Hurrell RF, et al. Triple fortification of salt with microcapsules of iodine, iron, and vitamin A. Am J Clin Nutr. 2004;80(5):1283–90.

408. Pinkaew S, Wegmuller R, Wasantwisut E, Winichagoon P, Hurrell RF, Tanumihardjo SA. Triple-fortified rice containing vitamin A reduced marginal vitamin A deficiency and increased vitamin A liver stores in school-aged Thai children. J Nutr. 2014;144(4):519–24.

409. Cediel G, Olivares M, Brito A, Lopez de Romana D, Cori H, La Frano MR. Interpretation of serum retinol data from Latin America and the Caribbean. Food Nutr Bull. 2015;36(2 Suppl):S98–S108.

410. Nyumuah RO, Hoang TC, Amoaful EF, Agble R, Meyer M, Wirth JP, et al. Implementing large-scale food fortification in Ghana: lessons learned. Food Nutr Bull. 2012;33(4 Suppl):S293–300.

411. van Jaarsveld PJ, Faber M, van Stuijvenberg ME. Vitamin A, iron, and zinc content of fortified maize meal and bread at the household level in 4 areas of South Africa. Food Nutr Bull. 2015;36(3):315–26.
412. Li YO, Lam J, Diosady LL, Jankowski S. Antioxidant system for the preservation of vitamin A in Ultra Rice. Food Nutr Bull. 2009;30(1):82–9.
413. Darnton-Hill I, Bloem M, De Benoist B, Brown LR. Micronutrient restoration and fortification: Communicating change, benefits and risks. Asia Pac J Clin Nutr. 2002;11(s6):s184–96.
414. Bouis HE, Hotz C, McClafferty B, Meenakshi JV, Pfeiffer WH. Biofortification: a new tool to reduce micronutrient malnutrition. Food Nutr Bull. 2011;32(1 Suppl):S31–40.
415. Hotz C, McClafferty B. From harvest to health: challenges for developing biofortified staple foods and determining their impact on micronutrient status. Food Nutr Bull. 2007;28(2 Suppl):S271–9.
416. Toenniessen GH. Crop genetic improvement for enhanced human nutrition. J Nutr. 2002;132(9 Suppl):2943S–6S.
417. Harjes CE, Rocheford TR, Bai L, Brutnell TP, Kandianis CB, Sowinski SG, et al. Natural genetic variation in lycopene epsilon cyclase tapped for maize biofortification. Science. 2008;319(5861):330–3.
418. De Moura FF, Miloff A, Boy E. Retention of provitamin A carotenoids in staple crops targeted for biofortification in Africa: cassava, maize and sweet potato. Crit Rev Food Sci Nutr. 2015;55(9):1246–69.
419. Sayre R, Beeching JR, Cahoon EB, Egesi C, Fauquet C, Fellman J, et al. The BioCassava plus program: biofortification of cassava for sub-Saharan Africa. Annu Rev Plant Biol. 2011;62:251–72.
420. Islam SN, Nusrat T, Begum P, Ahsan M. Carotenoids and β-carotene in orange fleshed sweet potato: A possible solution to vitamin A deficiency. Food Chem. 2016;199:628–31.
421. Beyer P. Golden Rice and 'Golden' crops for human nutrition. N Biotechnol. 2010;27(5):478–81.
422. Beyer P, Al-Babili S, Ye X, Lucca P, Schaub P, Welsch R, et al. Golden Rice: introducing the β-carotene biosynthesis pathway into rice endosperm by genetic engineering to defeat vitamin A deficiency. J Nutr. 2002;132 (3):506S–10S.
423. Ilg A, Yu Q, Schaub P, Beyer P, Al-Babili S. Overexpression of the rice carotenoid cleavage dioxygenase 1 gene in Golden Rice endosperm suggests apocarotenoids as substrates in planta. Planta. 2010;232(3):691–9.
424. La Frano MR, de Moura FF, Boy E, Lonnerdal B, Burri BJ. Bioavailability of iron, zinc, and provitamin A carotenoids in biofortified staple crops. Nutr Rev. 2014;72(5):289–307.
425. Muzhingi T, Gadaga TH, Siwela AH, Grusak MA, Russell RM, Tang G. Yellow maize with high β-carotene is an effective source of vitamin A in healthy Zimbabwean men. Am J Clin Nutr. 2011;94(2):510–9.
426. Li S, Nugroho A, Rocheford T, White WS. Vitamin A equivalence of the β-carotene in β-carotene-biofortified maize porridge consumed by women. Am J Clin Nutr. 2010;92(5):1105–12.
427. La Frano MR, Woodhouse LR, Burnett DJ, Burri BJ. Biofortified cassava increases β-carotene and vitamin A concentrations in the TAG-rich plasma layer of American women. Br J Nutr. 2013;110(2):310–20.
428. Zhu C, Cai Y, Gertz ER, La Frano MR, Burnett DJ, Burri BJ. Red palm oil-supplemented and biofortified cassava gari increase the carotenoid and retinyl palmitate concentrations of triacylglycerol-rich plasma in women. Nutr Res. 2015;35(11):965–74.
429. Low JW, Arimond M, Osman N, Cunguara B, Zano F, Tschirley D. A food-based approach introducing orange-fleshed sweet potatoes increased vitamin A intake and serum retinol concentrations in young children in rural Mozambique. J Nutr. 2007;137(5):1320–7.
430. van Jaarsveld PJ, Faber M, Tanumihardjo SA, Nestel P, Lombard CJ, Benade AJ. Beta-carotene-rich orange-fleshed sweet potato improves the vitamin A status of primary school children assessed with the modified-relative-dose-response test. Am J Clin Nutr. 2005;81(5):1080–7.
431. Gannon B, Kaliwile C, Arscott SA, Schmaelzle S, Chileshe J, Kalungwana N, et al. Biofortified orange maize is as efficacious as a vitamin A supplement in Zambian children even in the presence of high liver reserves of vitamin A: a community-based, randomized placebo-controlled trial. Am J Clin Nutr. 2014;100(6):1541–50.
432. Palmer AC, Siamusantu W, Chileshe J, Schulze KJ, Barffour M, Craft NE, et al. Provitamin A-biofortified maize increases serum β-carotene, but not retinol, in marginally nourished children: a cluster-randomized trial in rural Zambia. Am J Clin Nutr 2016;104(1):181–90.
433. Talsma EF, Brouwer ID, Verhoef H, Mbera GN, Mwangi AM, Demir AY, et al. Biofortified yellow cassava and vitamin A status of Kenyan children: a randomized controlled trial. Am J Clin Nutr. 2016;103(1):258–67.
434. Gilligan DO. Biofortification, agricultural technology adoption, and nutrition policy: some lessons and emerging challenges. Cesifo Econ Stud. 2012;58(2):405–21.
435. Jenkins M, Byker Shanks C, Houghtaling B. Orange-fleshed sweet potato: successes and remaining challenges of the introduction of a nutritionally superior staple crop in Mozambique. Food Nutr Bull. 2015;36(3):327–53.
436. Low JW, Arimond M, Osman N, Cunguara B, Zano F, Tschirley D. Ensuring the supply of and creating demand for a biofortified crop with a visible trait: lessons learned from the introduction of orange-fleshed sweet potato in drought-prone areas of Mozambique. Food Nutr Bull. 2007;28(2 Suppl):S258–70.
437. Low J, Arimond M, Osman N, Osei AK, Zano F, Cunguara B, et al. Towards sustainable nutrition improvement in rural Mozambique: addressing macro- and micronutrient malnutrition through new cultivars and new behaviors; 2005. Available from http://www.aec.msu.edu/fs2/tsni/.

438. Carvalho I, Tivana L, Granfeldt Y, Dejmek P. Improved energy and sensory properties of instant porridge made from a roasted mixture of grated orange-fleshed sweet potatoes and flour made from shredded sun dried cassava. Food Nutr Sci. 2014;5(14):1428–38.

439. Tomlins K, Ndunguru G, Stambul K, Joshua N, Ngendello T, Rwiza E, et al. Sensory evaluation and consumer acceptability of pale-fleshed and orange-fleshed sweetpotato by school children and mothers with preschool children. J Sci Food Agric. 2007;87(13):2436–46.

440. Talsma EF, Melse-Boonstra A, de Kok BP, Mbera GN, Mwangi AM, Brouwer ID. Biofortified cassava with pro-vitamin A is sensory and culturally acceptable for consumption by primary school children in Kenya. PLoS ONE. 2013;8(8):e73433.

441. Mazuze F. Analysis of adoption of orange-fleshed sweet potatoes: the case study of Gaza Province in Mozambique. Maputo: Institute of Agricultural Research of Mozambique; 2007.

442. de Brauw A, Eozenou P. Measuring risk attitudes among Mozambican farmers. J Dev Econ. 2014;111:61–74.

443. Naico A, Lusk J. The value of a nutritionally enhanced staple crop: Results from a choice experiment conducted with orange-fleshed sweet potatoes in Mozambique. J Afr Econ. 2010;19(4):536–58.

444. Hotz C, Loechl C, Lubowa A, Tumwine JK, Ndeezi G, Nandutu Masawi A, et al. Introduction of β-carotene-rich orange sweet potato in rural Uganda resulted in increased vitamin A intakes among children and women and improved vitamin A status among children. J Nutr. 2012;142(10):1871–80.

445. Hotz C, Loechl C, de Brauw A, Eozenou P, Gilligan D, Moursi M, et al. A large-scale intervention to introduce orange sweet potato in rural Mozambique increases vitamin A intakes among children and women. Br J Nutr. 2012;108(1):163–76.

446. Moghissi AA, Pei S, Liu Y. Golden rice: scientific, regulatory and public information processes of a genetically modified organism. Crit Rev Biotechnol. 2016;36(3):535–41.

447. Dubock A. The politics of Golden Rice. GM Crops Food. 2014;5(3):210–22.

448. Brown KH, Engle-Stone R, Kagin J, Rettig E, Vosti SA. Use of optimization modeling for selecting national micronutrient intervention strategies: an example based on potential programs for control of vitamin A deficiency in Cameroon. Food Nutr Bull. 2015;36(3 Suppl):S141–8.

449. Vosti SA, Kagin J, Engle-Stone R, Brown KH. An economic optimization model for improving the efficiency of vitamin A interventions: an application to young children in Cameroon. Food Nutr Bull. 2015;36(3 Suppl):S193–207.

450. de Pee S, West CE. Dietary carotenoids and their role in combating vitamin A deficiency: a review of the literature. Eur J Clin Nutr. 1996;50(Suppl 3):S38–53.

451. Parker RS, Swanson JE, You CS, Edwards AJ, Huang T. Bioavailability of carotenoids in human subjects. Proc Nutr Soc. 1999;58(1):155–62.

452. Taren DL, Nesheim MC, Crompton DW, Holland CV, Barbeau I, Rivera G, et al. Contributions of ascariasis to poor nutritional status in children from Chiriqui Province, Republic of Panama. Parasitology. 1987;95(Pt 3):603–13.

453. Taren DL, Crompton DWT. Mechanisms for interactions between parasitism and nutritional status. Clin Nutr. 1990;8:227–38.

454. Leung WC, Hessel S, Meplan C, Flint J, Oberhauser V, Tourniaire F, et al. Two common single nucleotide polymorphisms in the gene encoding β-carotene 15,15′-monoxygenase alter β-carotene metabolism in female volunteers. Faseb J. 2009;23(4):1041–53.

455. Lietz G, Oxley A, Leung W, Hesketh J. Single nucleotide polymorphisms upstream from the β-carotene 15,15'-monoxygenase gene influence provitamin A conversion efficiency in female volunteers. J Nutr. 2012;142(1):161S–5S.

456. Food and Agriculture Organization, World Health Organization, editors. World Declaration and Plan of Action for Nutrition (ICN/92/2). International Conference on Nutrition, Dec 1992. Rome, Italy: FAO/WHO.

457. van Lieshout M, de Pee S. Vitamin A equivalency estimates: understanding apparent differences. Am J Clin Nutr. 2005;81(4):943–5; author reply 5–6.

458. West CE. Meeting requirements for vitamin A. Nutr Rev. 2000;58(11):341–5.

459. West CE, editor Recent advances in vitamin A research: improving the vitamin status of populations. XXI IVACG meeting; 3–5 Feb 2003.

460. West KP, Jr., McLaren DS. The epidemiology of vitamin A deficiency disorders. In: Johnson GJ, Minassian DC, Weale R, West S, editors. Epidemiology of eye disease, vol. 15. 2nd ed. London: Medical & Health Sciences Publishing; 2003. p. 240–59.

Chapter 10
Iron

Melissa Fox Young and Usha Ramakrishnan

Keywords Iron · Anemia · Micronutrient · Nutrition · Public health

Learning Objectives
By the end of this chapter the reader should be able to:

- Explain the regulation of iron metabolism
- Define iron deficiency and explain at least three methods of assessment
- Describe the epidemiology and main causes of iron deficiency in developing countries
- Explain and substantiate the functional outcomes of iron deficiency
- Explain key strategies to combat iron deficiency

Introduction

Iron is one of the most extensively investigated essential nutrients, which continues to be a dynamic area of research. Just in the past decade our views of iron homeostasis have been completely revolutionized. Despite these advances, iron deficiency remains one of the most common nutrition disorders worldwide, affecting a large proportion of children and women in the developing world. It also remains as a key nutrient deficiency of significant prevalence in virtually all developed countries. Although the burden and causes of iron deficiency are well documented, ensuring adequate prevention and control of iron deficiency remains a challenge especially in resource-poor settings that demand greater efforts to promote and sustain public health measures that are feasible and cost-effective [1].

Role of Iron in Biological Functions

Iron is element 26 in the periodic table and has an atomic weight of 55.85. Iron is found in all living cells. In aqueous solution, iron exists in two oxidation states, either Fe^{2+}, the ferrous form, or Fe^{3+}, the ferric form. Iron changes between these forms, enabling it to serve as a catalyst in redox reactions

M.F. Young (✉) · U. Ramakrishnan
Hubert Department of Global Health, Rollins School of Public Health,
Emory University, 30322 Atlanta, GA, USA
e-mail: melissa.young@emory.edu

U. Ramakrishnan
e-mail: uramakr@emory.edu

© Springer Science+Business Media New York 2017
S. de Pee et al. (eds.), *Nutrition and Health in a Developing World*,
Nutrition and Health, DOI 10.1007/978-3-319-43739-2_10

by donating or accepting electrons. This property lends itself to having numerous vital roles in immune function, neurological function, cognitive development, and energy metabolism. Iron's essential roles in key iron-containing proteins are described below.

Hemoglobin

Hemoglobin has a molecular weight of 68,000 and is composed of four heme units. It plays an essential role in oxygen transport from the lungs to tissues in erythrocytes. It combines with oxygen in the pulmonary circulation and becomes largely deoxygenated in the capillary circulation of tissues. In severe anemia, the hemoglobin content of erythrocytes is reduced, decreasing oxygen delivery to tissues and leading to chronic tissue hypoxia.

Myoglobin

Myoglobin is found in muscle where it transports and stores oxygen needed for muscle contraction. The structure of myoglobin is a single heme group with a single globin chain. Myoglobin accounts for about 10% of the total body iron.

Cytochromes

Cytochromes contain heme and are essential to respiration and energy metabolism. Cytochromes a, b, and c are involved in oxidative phosphorylation and the production of cellular energy. Cytochromes serve as electron carriers in transforming adenosine disphosphate (ADP) to adenosine triphosphate (ATP), the primary energy storage compound. Cytochrome P450 is found in microsomal membranes of liver and intestinal mucosal cells.

Other Iron-Containing Enzymes

NADH dehydrogenase and succinate dehydrogenase are two nonheme iron-containing enzymes involved in energy metabolism. Hydrogen peroxidases also contain iron and protect against the accumulation of hydrogen peroxide. Catalase and peroxidase are two heme-containing enzymes that convert hydrogen peroxide into water and oxygen. Other iron-containing enzymes include aconitase, phosphoenolpyruvate carboxykinase, and ribonucleotide reductase.

Metabolism and Regulation of Iron

The average total body iron is about 3.8 g in men and 2.3 g in women. The iron-containing compounds in the body are grouped into functional iron (in which iron serves a metabolic or enzymatic function), transport iron (bound to transferrin), and storage iron (ferritin and hemosiderin).

Functional Iron

The most functional iron is in the form of heme proteins, i.e., proteins which contain an iron porphyrin prosthetic group. The basic structure of heme is a protoporphyrin-9 molecule with one iron atom. About two-thirds of the iron in the body is functional iron, mostly in the form of hemoglobin within erythrocytes. Other functional iron includes myoglobin and iron-containing enzymes.

Transport of Iron

Iron is transported from the intestine to the tissues by a plasma transport protein, transferrin. Transferrin has an extremely high affinity for Fe^{3+} (ferric state) and can bind two atoms of iron per molecule. Transferrin transports iron from the intestine, storage sites, and hemoglobin breakdown sites and delivers it to other cells through surface receptors specific for transferrin, i.e., transferrin receptor [2]. The receptors bind to the transferrin–iron complex at the cell surface and carry the complex into the cell, where iron is released. The iron supply of the body is reflected in the iron saturation of transferrin. A low transferrin saturation indicates undersupply of iron or deficiency, and a high transferrin saturation indicates oversupply of iron. Transferrin saturation can also be reduced during inflammatory conditions such as a febrile response. Transferrin receptors are found in high concentrations on tissues that have a high uptake of iron, including erythroid precursors, placenta, and liver. The expression of transferrin receptors on tissues is highly regulated in response to the availability of iron. In an iron-rich environment, the number of transferrin receptors decreases. In an iron-poor environment or when iron demand increases, the number of transferrin receptors increases. The concentration of circulating plasma or serum transferrin receptors is proportional to the expression of transferrin receptors on cell surfaces, and this is the basis for the use of circulating transferrin receptors as an indicator of iron status.

Storage of Iron

In men, about one-third of the total body iron is in the form of iron stores, compared to only one-eighth in women. The major iron storage compounds are **ferritin** and **hemosiderin**, which are found primarily in the liver, spleen, reticuloendothelial cells, and bone marrow. In the liver, iron is stored mainly in parenchymal cells or hepatocytes, and iron is also stored in reticuloendothelial cells or Kupffer cells. In the bone marrow and spleen, iron is stored mainly in reticuloendothelial cells. Stored iron is used primarily for the production of hemoglobin and for meeting other cellular needs for iron. Ferritin is also located in the serum in trace amounts in proportion to body iron stores and is a useful indicator of iron status. However, ferritin is also an acute phase protein and increases with inflammation. Wide variations in the amount of storage iron can occur without any apparent effect on body functions. Storage iron is usually almost entirely depleted before the development of iron deficiency anemia. Full-term infants are born with a substantial store of iron, which usually can meet the infant's iron needs until 6 month of age [3]. Preterm and low birth weight (LBW) infants generally have reduced iron stores compared to full-term infants, and as a consequence, these infants may deplete their iron stores as early as 2–3 month of age. Once infants have exhausted their body stores of iron, it is difficult to build up substantial iron stores because of the rapid growth and high iron requirement that occurs up to 24 month of age. After 24 month of age, the growth rate slows and iron stores usually begin to accumulate [4]. Since the first 2 years of life represent a critical period when iron plays a key role in brain development, infant iron stores may be improved through the timely introduction of appropriate sources of iron that include animal source foods, home fortification or fortified complementary foods and/or iron-containing supplements, as described in later sections.

Iron Turnover and Loss

The production and destruction of erythrocytes accounts for most of the turnover of iron in the body and is essential for maintaining iron homeostasis [5]. The average life span of erythrocytes is about 120 d, and in an adult, the daily iron turnover is about 20–25 mg. Most of the iron from degraded erythrocytes is recaptured for the synthesis of hemoglobin. Iron losses in the feces are about 0.6 mg/d from bile, desquamated mucosal cells, and minute amounts of blood [6]. Other routes of iron loss include desquamated skin and sweat (0.2–0.3 mg/d) and urine (<0.1 mg/d). The average daily iron loss from adult men is 1.0 mg/d (range 0.5–2.0 mg/d). Premenopausal women need to replace the iron in menstrual blood loss, which accounts for 0.4–0.5 mg/d, combined with other iron losses for a total average iron loss of 1.3 mg/d [7].

Absorption of Iron

While iron has numerous essential functions it is important to note that iron may also be very toxic given iron's ability to participate in redox reactions and generate free radicals. For example, in certain genetic conditions (hereditary hemochromatosis) iron overload can lead to organ dysfunction and failure. Iron's dual essential yet toxic effects in the body lend to a tightly regulated system. Since the body has no mechanism for the regulated excretion of iron, homeostasis depends on finely regulated dietary iron absorption.

Dietary iron consists primarily of either nonheme iron or heme iron, and these are absorbed by different mechanisms [8]. Heme iron sources include hemoglobin and myoglobin where iron is tightly bound within a porphyrin ring structure. Key dietary sources are meat, poultry, and fish. Nonheme iron includes all other iron sources and comes from both plant and animal sources and is also the form of iron in supplements.

Over the past decade, there have been immense advances in our knowledge of intestinal nonheme iron absorption and regulation [9]. Dietary nonheme iron in the ferrous state (Fe^{2+}) enters the enterocyte from the gut lumen through a divalent metal transporter (DMT1). Iron that reaches the gut in the ferric state can also be transported across the enterocyte but must first be reduced ($Fe^{3+} \rightarrow Fe^{2+}$) by duodenal cytochrome B (DCYTB) on the brush border (apical) membrane before it is transported by DMT1. Nonheme iron that enters the enterocyte is either stored as ferritin or exported across the basolateral membrane through ferroportin (FP-1), also previously referred to as iron-regulated transporter protein-1. This export process involves hephaestin (Hp), a ferroxidase, which oxidizes ferrous iron to ferric (Fe^{3+}) iron in order for it to be exported across the basolateral membrane via FP-1 and subsequently incorporated into serum transferrin (Tf).

Intestinal uptake of heme Fe differs markedly from that of nonheme Fe. The elusive heme transporter was thought to be discovered (heme carrier protein, HCP1) [10]; however, upon further investigation, Qui et al. [11] demonstrated that HCP1 was actually a proton-coupled folate transporter (PCFT) and a poor heme transporter at best, which leaves the primary heme transporter in both the intestine and placenta yet to be fully characterized. It has also been hypothesized that heme iron is taken up by receptor-mediated endocytosis; however, the mechanisms have not been worked out for this pathway either [12]. Furthermore, it is currently unknown if once heme iron enters the intestinal

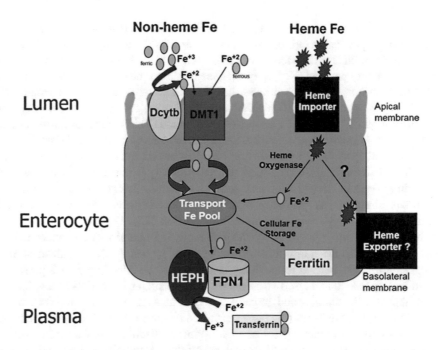

Fig. 10.1 Heme and nonheme iron absorption. Acronyms: divalent metal transporter (*DMT1*), duodenal cytochrome B (*DCYTB*), ferroportin (*FPN1*), hephaestin (*HEPH*)

cell if it is transported across the basolateral membrane intact via one of the recently identified heme transporters, BCRP (breast cancer resistance protein, also known as ABCG2) or FLVCR (feline leukaemic virus receptor C) [13, 14]. Alternatively, heme may be catabolized by heme oxygenase (HO) within the enterocyte so that it can then enter a common inorganic iron pool with nonheme iron (Fig. 10.1) [15].

Iron absorption is primarily influenced by the biochemical form of iron in the gut lumen (heme or nonheme), the iron status of the individual, and the bioavailability of the iron source (based on iron form, meal composition, and the presence of enhancers or inhibitors such as ascorbic acid and phytic acid, respectively) [16]. Although heme iron comprises a smaller proportion of iron in the diet, the absorption of heme iron is significantly greater than nonheme iron and is less affected by the overall composition of the diet and iron status of the individual. On the other hand, iron status of the individual and iron bioavailability have been reported to alter nonheme iron absorption up to 10–15 fold [17]. Thus, individuals with little or no iron stores absorb a greater fraction of nonheme iron from the diet, whereas individuals with sufficient iron stores absorb less iron from the diet. The process of selective absorption is an essential mechanism for regulating iron balance.

Regulation of Iron Homeostasis

There are multiple pathways through which iron homeostasis regulation occurs but two key mechanisms are (1) *iron regulator proteins* (IRPs) which is essential for *cellular regulation* [18, 19] and (2) *hepcidin* which is essential for *systemic regulation* [20, 21].

Cellular iron homeostasis is finely regulated in response to iron status by the coordinated up or down regulation of key proteins involved in iron uptake, export, storage, and utilization through iron regulatory proteins (IRP-1 and IRP-2) [18, 19]. These IRPs bind to specific iron response elements

(IREs) located in the 3′ or 5′ untranslated regions (UTR) of mRNAs that encode for key iron transport proteins and allow for posttranscriptional, iron-dependent regulation. Depending on whether the IRE is located in the 3′ (as found for transferrin receptor, TfR) or 5′ (as found for ferritin) end of the UTR, binding of iron regulatory proteins (IRP) may stabilize or inhibit the translation of key iron proteins in response to cellular iron status. In conditions when the cell is iron-loaded, IRP-1 assembles an iron–sulfur cluster (4Fe–4S) preventing IRE binding and IRP-2 undergoes proteasomal degradation. This up or down regulation of target genes allows for coordinated shifts from production of either iron storage proteins or iron transport or export proteins in response to cellular iron needs.

Hepcidin is a small cysteine-rich peptide hormone that has recently emerged as a key regulator of systemic iron homeostasis (Fig. 10.2) [22]. In normally healthy persons, hepcidin levels are thought to decrease during iron deficiency and increase in states of iron sufficiency. Hepcidin, initially referred to as LEAP-1, was discovered as an urinary antimicrobial peptide synthesized in the liver [23, 24] that could be induced by both high iron status and inflammation [25]. This could serve as a protective mechanism both against iron excess/toxicity and potentially in immunity as the reduced availability of extracellular iron can limit the multiplication rate of invading microbes, though these mechanisms require further examination. Further research has also demonstrated that hepcidin expression may also be diminished in response to increased erythroid drive, hypoxia, and iron deficiency. Transcriptional regulation of hepcidin is complex and remains an open area of research. Hepcidin regulates iron absorption by binding to ferroportin (the basolateral iron export protein) leading to its internalization and degradation within lysosomes. The loss of ferroportin effectively blocks iron export from the enterocyte, leading to a reduction in intestinal absorption. Hepcidin is believed to impact iron metabolism through four primary pathways: regulation of iron absorption in the gut; iron recycling from macrophages; control of hepatic iron storage; and regulation of placental iron transport to the fetus during pregnancy [26].

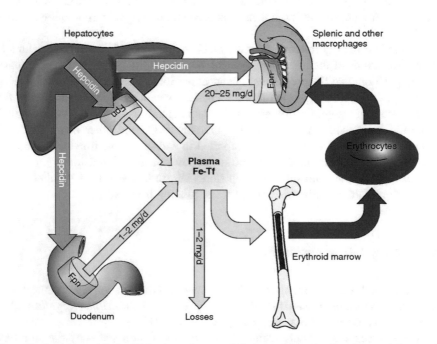

Fig. 10.2 Systemic iron homeostasis. Major iron flows and their regulation by hepcidin and ferroportin. Iron in transferrin is indicated in *blue*, and iron in erythrocytes is in *red*. Hepcidin controls the iron flow into plasma by inducing the endocytosis and proteolysis of the iron exporter ferroportin (*brown*). From Ganz [22]

Assessment of Anemia and Iron Deficiency

Anemia is a commonly used indicator to screen for iron deficiency in clinical settings, or to define the burden of iron deficiency in population-based surveys. Although anemia in itself is not specific for iron deficiency, especially in areas where other conditions such as malaria are common, there is a close association between anemia and iron deficiency. Iron deficiency is the most common cause of anemia in most parts of the world; recent estimates suggest 50% of anemia in nonpregnant and pregnant women and 42% of anemia in children are amendable to iron supplementation [27]. Iron deficiency anemia represents the severe end of the spectrum of iron deficiency and requires the fulfillment of both the definition of anemia and iron deficiency [28]. Iron deficiency without anemia represents a moderate form of iron deficiency where iron-dependent function is impaired and may result in functional consequences. Depleted iron stores represent the mildest form of iron deficiency when there are no functional impairments or anemia. Anemia is defined as hemoglobin concentration below −2 standard deviations (SD) of the age- and sex-specific normal reference. The most commonly used cutoff for anemia is hemoglobin <110 g/L for under five children and pregnant women, <120 g/L for nonpregnant women, and <130 g/L for men. Severe anemia is defined as hemoglobin <70 g/L in pregnant women and children under 5 and <80 g/L for men and nonpregnant women [29].

Iron Deficiency

A number of hematologic and biochemical tests enable the characterization of iron status. Often, iron deficiency is defined by one or more abnormal iron biochemical tests: serum ferritin, transferrin saturation, transferrin receptor, and erythrocyte protoporphyrin (Table 10.1). Iron deficiency anemia is defined as meeting the criteria for both iron deficiency and anemia based on hemoglobin testing. Low serum ferritin per se is regarded as low or depleted iron stores. Even though all iron-related tests respond to changes in iron status, each test reflects different aspects of iron metabolism. For this reason, various tests are therefore of different utilities, and results may not always agree between tests.

Serum ferritin is a well-accepted marker of body iron stores and can be determined in venous or capillary bloods or dried blood spots using enzyme-linked immunosorbent assays (ELISA) or two-site immunoradiometric assays [30, 31]. Although still expensive for field-based settings, the ability to measure serum ferritin from dried blood spots is a major contribution. One of the problems with serum ferritin, however, is that infection and inflammation can falsely elevate the levels and is therefore a concern in areas where infections and parasitic diseases are common. The inclusion of a marker of infection such as C-reactive protein and alpha(1)-acid glycoprotein (AGP) to adjust ferritin concentrations or a slightly higher cutoff value (<15 µg/L vs. <12 µg/L) has been recommended to address this concern [32, 33].

Other markers of iron status are based on the transport form namely transferrin which can be measured using chromogenic methods. The measurement of serum transferrin receptors either from venous blood or whole blood using ELISA techniques is also another good indicator of iron status. Elevated expression of serum transferrin receptors is indicative of iron-deficient erythropoiesis which may be common in regions where iron deficiency is common but the prevalence of anemia is not that high. Total body iron can also be calculated by the ratio of serum transferrin receptor to serum ferritin as described by Cook et al. [34]; (total body Fe (mg/kg) = −[log (serum transferrin receptor/serum ferritin) − 2.8229]/0.1207) and is useful to measure iron status. Similarly, elevated levels of free erythrocyte protoporphyrin (FEP) are indicative of impaired heme synthesis due to lack of iron and can be measured in whole blood using hematofluorometry. Although field friendly equipment has been developed, problems remain in the use of these methods for large population-based surveys. It should be noted that a WHO and CDC Technical Consultation on the Assessment of Iron Status at the

Table 10.1 Assessment of iron deficiency and iron deficiency anemia [29, 30, 32, 129, 130]

Indicator	Measure	Cutoffs	Indication	Commonly used methods	Special considerations
Serum ferritin	Total body iron stores	<15 μg/L <12 μg/L	Depleted iron stores in individuals 5 years or older Depleted iron stores in individuals less than 5 years of age	Venous or capillary blood, dried blood spots (DBS) ELISA method	Infection and inflammation may cause inflated ferritin values Use of DBS convenient for field work
Serum transferrin concentration (TIBC)	Concentration of iron transport protein	360 μg/dL	Depleted iron stores	Venous blood Assay in which transferrin is saturated with excess iron; chromogenic methods	Influenced by infection and inflammation More complicated laboratory procedure that requires quality-control sera
Serum transferrin saturation	Iron transport protein	<15%	Iron-deficient erythropoiesis	Venous blood Calculated from TIBC and serum iron values	Influenced by infection and inflammation Diurnal variation
Soluble Serum transferrin receptor (STfR)	Expression of STfR, which bind ferritin for uptake in cells	High (10 mg/L)	Iron-deficient erythropoiesis	Venous blood ELISA method	Possible to quantify STfR using a dried blood spot Not significantly influenced by infection and inflammation Can be influenced by other nutritional deficiencies such as B12 and folate deficiency and specifically by acute malaria infection
Free erythrocyte protoporphyrin (FEP)	Serves as a precursor in heme biosynthesis	>70 mmol FEP/mol heme	Iron-deficient erythropoiesis	Whole blood (drop) Hematofluorometry	Influenced by infection and inflammation Portable hematofluorometer available
Hemoglobin (SCN 2000)	Blood hemoglobin concentration	<11.0 g/dL <12.0 g/dL	Anemia in pregnant women Anemia in nonpregnant women >15 year	Venous or capillary blood Dried blood spot HemoCue or cyanmethemoglobin method	Influenced by certain parasitic infections and other micronutrient deficiencies It is necessary to make adjustments to cutoff values for persons living in high altitudes Less expensive, field friendly equipment available
Hematocrit	Packed red blood cell volume	<0.36 <0.33	Anemia in nonpregnant women >15 year Anemia in pregnant women	Whole blood Centrifugation method	Less expensive, but methods can be difficult to standardize in a field setting
Erythrocyte	Color and shape or erythrocyte	Microcytic or hypochromic	Anemia	Whole blood Microscopy	

Population level recommended the use of hemoglobin and serum ferritin as the most efficient combination for monitoring programs that aim to improve iron status [35]. In addition, new method advances on assessing ferritin, transferrin receptor, CRP, AGP, and retinol-binding protein from a combined sandwich ELISA requiring a small amount of serum that can be obtained by finger prick may allow for infection and nutritional status to be obtained simultaneously and cost-effectively in field settings [36].

Anemia

Anemia as measured by low hemoglobin concentration or low hematocrit is by far the most commonly used indicator for detecting iron deficiency. Common causes of anemia other than iron deficiency include malaria, hereditary hemoglobinopathies or red cell production defects such as thalassemia minor, recent or current infections including human immunodeficiency virus (HIV) infection, and any chronic conditions with an inflammatory response. On an individual basis, anemia cannot be used to detect those with milder forms of iron deficiency (iron deficiency without anemia). Because it is not generally feasible to perform iron biochemistry tests in many settings, hemoglobin response to iron treatment is a common approach in diagnosing iron deficiency. Evidence from randomized control trials of iron supplementation in anemic subjects has demonstrated mean hemoglobin increases of 10.17 g/L for pregnant women, 8.64 g/L for nonpregnant women, and 8.0 g/L for children [27, 37, 38]. These hemoglobin shifts can then be applied to estimate the proportion of all anemia amenable to iron supplementation for global estimates of iron deficiency. One common reason for the misdiagnosis of anemia is inadequate laboratory procedures for hemoglobin determination related to capillary blood sampling or owing to inaccurate laboratory methods or procedures.

Field Testing for Hemoglobin

A portable photometer, the HemoCue system (Anglholm, Sweden), has been used in many different field surveys for the evaluation of anemia [39]. This system consists of a battery-operated photometer and a disposable cuvet, which is coated with the dried reagent (sodium azide) and serves as the blood collection device. This one-step blood collection that does not require handling any wet reagents makes the system uniquely suited for rapid field surveys. Non-laboratory personnel can be quickly and easily trained to operate the device, which is not dependent on electricity. Most importantly, when used by well-trained personnel, the HemoCue system has satisfactory accuracy and precision when compared to laboratory-based methods of measuring hemoglobin [40]. Long-term field experience also demonstrates that the instrument is stable and durable. However, in humid climates, care must be taken in the proper storage of cuvettes to ensure accuracy. These features make the HemoCue system suitable for the inclusion of hemoglobin measurements in nutrition surveys.

Detection of Anemia by Clinical Examination

In resource-poor settings where it is not feasible to detect anemia by measurement of hemoglobin or hematocrit, clinical examination has been widely used to detect those with severe anemia. The extents of pallor of skin, conjunctiva, tongue, and palms are typically evaluated but may be subject to inter-examiner errors. In one study, sensitivity and specificity for the detection of severe anemia (hemoglobin < 70 g/L) was reported to reach the range of 50–60 and 90%, respectively [41].

Use of Frequency Distributions of Hemoglobin in Assessing Iron Status

Hemoglobin measurements have been used traditionally to estimate iron nutrition among women and young children in large surveys, and the prevalence of anemia serves as the index of severity of iron deficiency in the population. This approach is useful in areas where iron deficiency is the predominant cause of anemia, as is generally the case in many low- and middle-income countries (LMICs). In settings where poor iron intake is the main etiologic factor, children and women are disproportionately affected, and the hemoglobin concentration of adult men whose requirements are lower is virtually unaffected. If conditions other than poor dietary iron intake also are present at a significant level, men can also have a high prevalence of anemia. For this reason, inclusion of a sample of men for anemia surveys can be useful in defining the nature of a high prevalence of anemia among children and women. If the prevalence of anemia for men is low, poor dietary iron intake is almost certain to be the cause of anemia in children and women. If men also have a high prevalence of anemia, factors other than poor dietary iron intake are usually present. This can include severe hookworm infection causing iron deficiency owing to blood loss [42].

Prevalence of Iron Deficiency and Anemia

Globally 43% of children under five and 38% of pregnant women are anemic [27]. The prevalence is particularly high in south Asia and west Africa (Table 10.2). Although there is considerable variation by region, young children and women of reproductive age are at greatest risk. Iron deficiency is the most common cause of anemia; recent estimates suggest 50% of anemia in nonpregnant and pregnant women and 42% of anemia in children are amendable to iron supplementation [27]. For severe anemia the proportions amenable to iron supplementation are more than 50% for children and nonpregnant women and over 60% for pregnant women. Other key factors that contribute to anemia include other nutrient deficiencies (folate, vitamin B12, vitamin A), genetic traits (including sickle cell anemia and thalassaemia), malaria, schistosomiasis, hookworm and trichuris infection, and HIV and some non-communicable diseases [27].

The complex etiology of anemia in certain settings may explain the limitation of using hemoglobin as an indicator of response for programs aiming to reduce the burden of iron deficiency. Nevertheless, because the presence of anemia reflects a more severe form of iron deficiency, it is safe to assume that the actual presence of iron deficiency is about two to three times that of the prevalence of iron deficiency anemia. For example, if a survey found that 30% of young children were anemic, and further testing using an iron-specific test found that two out of three of these children had clear evidence of iron deficiency, then 20% of the children would have iron deficiency anemia. The estimated prevalence of iron deficiency for this childhood population would be 40–60%.

Risk Factors/Etiology

The highest risk groups for iron deficiency are preterm and low birth weight infants, infants, and children during periods of rapid growth, infants receiving undiluted cow's milk before one year (see also Chap. 15 on milk), premenopausal women, pregnant women, and individuals with nematode infections in the gastrointestinal tract (Table 10.3). Low consumption of iron-containing foods and consumption of high phytate foods, tannin containing tea, coffee, and other foods that inhibit iron absorption also increase the risk of iron deficiency. These individual risk factors will be discussed throughout the following sections.

Table 10.2 Mean hemoglobin concentration and anemia prevalence by region in 1995 and 2011

	1995			2011		
	Mean hemoglobin (g/L)	Anemia (%)	Severe anemia (%)	Mean hemoglobin (g/L)	Anemia (%)	Severe anemia (%)
Children aged <5 years						
High-income regions	123 (120–124)	11% (7–17)	0.3% (0.0–1.1)	123 (119–125)	11% (6–20)	0.1% (0.0–0.5)
Central and Eastern Europe	116 (109–122)	29% (15–47)	1.4% (0.2–5.1)	117 (111–123)	26% (13–45)	0.2% (0.0–1.1)
East and Southeast Asia	118 (115–120)	29% (22–37)	0.9% (0.5–1.5)	118 (113–123)	25% (16–38)	0.2% (0.1–0.6)
Oceania	111 (102–118)	42% (23–64)	2.0% (0.2–7.7)	112 (105–120)	43% (21–65)	0.5% (0.0–2.6)
South Asia	100 (96–105)	70% (59–78)	5.9% (3.0–9.1)	106 (102–111)	58% (44–69)	2.1% (0.8–4.4)
Central Asia, Middle East, and North Africa	111 (108–114)	43% (35–53)	1.5% (0.6–3.0)	114 (110–118)	38% (25–51)	0.4% (0.1–1.2)
Central and West Africa	95 (92–98)	80% (74–84)	9.7% (7.4–12.1)	100 (99–102)	71% (67–74)	4.9% (3.8–6.2)
East Africa	96 (93–100)	74% (65–81)	10.2% (7.7–12.6)	107 (105–108)	55% (50–59)	2.5% (1.8–3.6)
Southern Africa	116 (111–119)	30% (21–42)	1.1% (0.3–2.3)	110 (105–116)	46% (31–62)	0.9% (0.3–2.4)
Andean and central Latin America and Caribbean	113 (110–116)	38% (30–46)	1.4% (0.8–2.4)	116 (113–118)	33% (28–40)	0.4% (0.2–0.7)
Southern and tropical Latin America	117 (106–124)	28% (11–55)	1.3% (0.0–6.2)	119 (112–124)	23% (10–41)	0.2% (0.0–1.1)
Globe	109 (107–111)	47% (43–51)	3.7% (2.8–4.7)	111 (110–113)	43% (38–47)	1.5% (1.1–2.2)
Nonpregnant women aged 15–49 years						
High-income regions	131 (129–132)	14% (12–18)	0.6% (0.3–1.1)	130 (128–132)	16% (12–22)	0.5% (0.2–1.0)
Central and Eastern Europe	129 (124–134)	23% (13–37)	0.9% (0.3–2.2)	128 (123–132)	22% (13–37)	0.5% (0.2–1.4)
East and Southeast Asia	126 (123–128)	29% (22–39)	1.0% (0.6–1.7)	129 (124–133)	21% (12–36)	0.5% (0.2–1.2)
Oceania	123 (115–130)	37% (21–56)	2.8% (0.8–6.9)	126 (119–132)	28% (14–47)	1.8% (0.4–5.2)
South Asia	117 (113–121)	53% (42–64)	3.8% (2.3–5.8)	119 (115–124)	47% (33–59)	2.4% (1.0–4.6)
Central Asia, Middle East, and North Africa	123 (120–126)	38% (31–45)	2.0% (1.2–3.2)	125 (121–129)	33% (23–43)	1.0% (0.5–2.1)
Central and West Africa	118 (114–123)	52% (39–61)	2.8% (1.8–4.1)	119 (115–123)	48% (37–58)	2.2% (1.4–4.0)
East Africa	123 (120–127)	40% (33–47)	2.7% (1.8–3.8)	128 (126–131)	28% (23–34)	1.4% (1.0–1.9)
Southern Africa	124 (119–130)	33% (21–47)	2.0% (0.7–4.5)	128 (122–134)	28% (16–44)	1.2% (0.5–2.9)
Andean and central Latin America and Caribbean	126 (123–129)	30% (24–37)	1.7% (1.1–2.7)	131 (128–134)	19% (14–26)	0.7% (0.4–1.2)
Southern and tropical Latin America	129 (120–137)	22% (9–46)	1.2% (0.2–3.7)	130 (122–138)	18% (7–41)	0.7% (0.1–2.5)
Globe	125 (123–126)	33% (29–37)	1.8% (1.3–2.3)	126 (124–128)	29% (24–35)	1.1% (0.7–1.7)

(continued)

Table 10.2 (continued)

	1995			2011		
	Mean hemoglobin (g/L)	Anemia (%)	Severe anemia (%)	Mean hemoglobin (g/L)	Anemia (%)	Severe anemia (%)
Pregnant women aged 15–49 years						
High-income regions	119 (116–121)	23% (18–30)	0.5% (0.1–1.1)	119 (117–122)	22% (16–29)	0.2% (0.0–0.4)
Central and Eastern Europe	117 (111–124)	30% (17–47)	0.9% (0.2–2.2)	119 (113–125)	24% (14–40)	0.3% (0.1–0.9)
East and Southeast Asia	115 (112–117)	34% (28–43)	1.3% (0.7–2.0)	119 (114–123)	25% (17–38)	0.4% (0.1–1.0)
Oceania	110 (104–117)	48% (31–63)	2.8% (0.8–5.9)	115 (107–124)	36% (18–59)	1.1% (0.2–3.2)
South Asia	108 (104–111)	53% (43–63)	2.9% (1.8–4.4)	108 (105–113)	52% (40–63)	1.3% (0.7–2.4)
Central Asia, Middle East, and North Africa	114 (111–117)	37% (30–46)	1.1% (0.5–2.0)	117 (113–120)	31% (22–42)	0.4% (0.1–0.8)
Central and West Africa	105 (103–109)	61% (53–66)	3.3% (2.2–4.7)	108 (105–111)	56% (46–62)	1.8% (1.1–3.2)
East Africa	111 (109–114)	46% (41–52)	2.9% (1.9–4.1)	116 (113–118)	36% (30–41)	1.2% (0.8–1.7)
Southern Africa	117 (110–124)	34% (21–51)	1.2% (0.4–2.7)	118 (111–124)	31% (20–48)	0.4% (0.2–0.9)
Andean and Central Latin America and Caribbean	115 (112–118)	37% (30–44)	1.4% (0.8–2.3)	119 (116–122)	27% (21–34)	0.3% (0.2–0.6)
Southern and tropical Latin America	115 (106–125)	37% (18–60)	1.3% (0.2–3.8)	117 (108–127)	31% (13–56)	0.5% (0.1–1.7)
Globe	112 (111–113)	43% (39–47)	2.0% (1.5–2.6)	114 (112–116)	38% (34–43)	0.9% (0.6–1.3)

Reprinted with permission from Elsevier (The Lancet, 2013;1(1):e16–25) [27]

Table 10.3   Risk factors for iron deficiency

Prematurity
Low birth weight
Rapid growth
Menstruation
Pregnancy
Young age at first birth
Short birth spacing
Sensitivity to cow's milk
Low consumption of meat
High consumption of phytates (common in largely plant-source-based diets)
Nematode infection in gastrointestinal tract

Increased Requirement for Iron

In general, the etiology of iron deficiency can be viewed as a negative balance between iron intake and iron need and loss. Whenever there is rapid growth, as occurs during infancy, early childhood, adolescence, and pregnancy, iron requirement is much greater, and hence, a positive iron balance is difficult to maintain. The blood volume expands in parallel with growth, with a corresponding increase in iron requirement [43]. Table 10.4 compares the iron requirement of infants, women, and men. It is clear that infancy and pregnancy are times when requirement is high, increasing the risk for iron deficiency. Iron loss, related to monthly menstrual blood loss as well as iron transfer to the fetus during pregnancy, is a major factor in the increased risk of iron deficiency for women of childbearing age [44]. Risks of iron deficiency during pregnancy are especially high because pregnancy-associated iron losses approximate 480–1150 mg (including losses to the fetus, placenta, and blood loss at delivery) [45]. In a 55-kg woman the total iron requirement during pregnancy is approximately 1040 mg and corresponds to daily absorbed iron needs of roughly 0.8 mg, 4–5 mg, and 6–8 mg/d for each of three trimesters of pregnancy, respectively [46]. Many women struggle to meet the iron demands required for nonpregnant women (1.5 mg/d), so meeting these increased requirements during pregnancy from dietary sources alone is especially difficult. Pregnant adolescents are at an even higher risk of developing iron deficiency compared with pregnant adults because they also face the increased nutrient demands of growth and development. During adolescence, girls have a peak weight gain of 9 kg/year, which requires an additional 280 mg of iron to maintain circulating hemoglobin concentrations [3]. Even otherwise healthy adolescents are at increased risk of developing iron deficiency due to these high iron demands. Finally, closely spaced pregnancies do not provide adequate time to rebuild iron stores and thereby significantly increase the risk of iron deficiency for the next pregnancy. The intergenerational cycle of iron deficiency is further perpetuated as women who are iron deficient are more likely to give birth to infants with insufficient iron stores and at greater risk for developing iron deficiency [47].

Poor Dietary Intake

Worldwide, the majority of iron deficiency is the direct result of low dietary iron content, especially of bioavailable iron. The dietary source of iron strongly influences the efficiency of the absorption. For infants, the iron content of milk consumed is a major determinant of iron status. The iron content of breast milk is low, in comparison to that of cow's milk. However, 50% of the iron in breast milk

Table 10.4 Iron recommended daily allowance[a]

Age (year)	Male	Female
Infants		
0–0.5	0.27[b]	0.27
0.5–1	11	11
Children		
1–3	7	7
4–8	10	10
9–13	8	8
14–18	11	15
Adults		
19–50	8	18[c]
>51	8	8
Pregnant	N/A	27
Lactating	N/A	9

[a]Assuming medium bioavailability (10% iron absorption)
[b]Mean adequate intake to be all by breast-fed infants
[c]Nonpregnant non-lactating. Institute of Medicine, Dietary Reference Intakes. National Academy Press, 2001

can be absorbed, in contrast to less than 10% from cow's milk. The higher absorption efficiency of human breast milk does not entirely make up for the low iron content. Premature and LBW infants in particular may be at risk of developing iron deficiency before 6 months and there is an urgent need to address this issue [48]. After 6 month of age, breast-fed infants require an additional source of iron from the diet to meet their iron requirement. Unfortunately, in most settings, complementary food is low in iron content and bioavailability. The amount of iron absorption from foods ranges from less than 1% to more than 20%. Foods of vegetable origin are at the lower end of the range, dairy products are in the middle, and meat is at the upper end. Meat is a good source of iron, because most iron is in the form of heme iron, which has an absorption efficiency of 10–20%, which is two to three times greater than that for nonheme iron (2–7%). Nonheme iron is not only less well absorbed, but the absorption is strongly influenced by the other foods ingested at the same meal. Ascorbic acid and meat protein are among the most potent enhancers of nonheme iron absorption. Tannin in tea and phytic acid in grain fibers are among the better known inhibitors of nonheme iron absorption.

Abnormal Iron Loss

The normal turnover of intestinal mucosa with some blood loss can be regarded as physiological blood loss, which is accounted for in the daily requirement. Normal menstrual blood loss is also an obligatory or physiological loss. The most common reason for abnormal blood loss in infants and younger children is the sensitivity of some children to the protein in cow's milk, resulting in increased gastrointestinal occult blood loss. In many tropical communities where hygienic conditions are inadequate, hookworm infection is a major cause of gastrointestinal blood loss for older children and adults. Hookworms cause bleeding in the upper intestine, and the severity of blood loss as measured by the hemoglobin content of feces is proportional to the intensity of the hookworm infestation and infecting species. *A. duodenale* causes a greater level of bleeding than *N. americanus*. For example in a study in Tanzania, among children with only *N. americanus* there was a 61% prevalence of anemia and 33% prevalence of iron deficiency. However, among children infected with *A. duodenale* there was nearly a twofold increase in iron deficiency (59% iron deficiency, 81% anemia) [49]. *Trichuris*, found in the colon, has also been shown to contribute to blood loss, but to a lesser extent than hookworm.

Functional Consequences of Iron Deficiency

Hemoglobin contains the majority of functional iron in the body, and in addition, there are a number of other iron-dependent enzymes that can be adversely affected by iron deficiency [50]. The functional consequences of iron deficiency especially maternal and child health outcomes which are of major public health importance are briefly reviewed in this section.

Anemia and Maternal Mortality

Iron deficiency is widely recognized as a substantial risk factor for maternal death [51]. In late pregnancy, a 10 g/L increase in mean hemoglobin is associated with an odds ratio of 0.71 (95% CI 0.60–0.85) for maternal death. Previous WHO estimates have attributed 18% of maternal deaths to anemia [52]. These estimates vary by context. Recently, researchers in India estimated that approximately 40% of maternal mortality is directly or indirectly caused by anemia [53] with severe anemia contributing up to 15% of maternal deaths [54]. Although mild anemia (10–20 g/L below the cutoff) is not accompanied by health impairment, at a moderate level of anemia, reduced oxygen-carrying capacity begins to interfere with aerobic function [55]. In areas where severe anemia (hemoglobin < 80 g/L) is common, iron deficiency is usually one of multiple causes of anemia [56]. Very severe anemia (hemoglobin < 50 g/L) is associated with increased childhood and maternal mortality, and is often regarded as the underlying cause of death [57, 58]. Deaths associated with severe anemia generally occur in time of increased physiological stress, for example, during an acute febrile illness for a young child, or during the peripartum period, when oxygen delivery and cardiovascular function are further compromised by worsening hemoglobin concentrations. In contrast to the known effects of severe anemia, the role of mild to moderate anemia and iron deficiency in reducing mortality remains controversial [59–61]. The causal association between iron deficiency and maternal mortality has been questioned and a major limitation is the dearth of randomized placebo-controlled trials (RCT) which are difficult to conduct in settings where there may be an impact, since prenatal iron–folate (IFA) supplementation is part of routine care [62, 63].

Birth Outcomes and Mortality

Maternal iron deficiency anemia is an important contributor to poor birth outcomes [51]. Iron deficiency and anemia during pregnancy are associated with increased risk of low birth weight and increased perinatal mortality [64–66]. In a recent meta-analysis of controlled trials, routine daily iron supplementation during pregnancy was associated with a 20% reduction in low birth weight [67]. In a study by Mwangi et al. [68], even in malaria-endemic areas in Kenya the benefits of antennal iron supplementation remained high, a 150 g increase in birth weight and a 58% reduction in the prevalence of LBW with no effect on risk of maternal Plasmodium infection. Fewer studies have examined other outcomes but a large study from Indonesia showed that prenatal IFA supplementation was associated with a 34% reduction in death among children under 5 [69]. In China, iron and folic acid compared to folic acid supplementation alone were associated with over a 50% reduction in neonatal mortality [70]. Similarly in Nepal, prenatal IFA compared to vitamin A only was associated by a 31% reduction in death among children under 7 years [71]. However, a recently completed double-blind RCT among Chinese women with no or mild anemia showed that, compared to folic acid only, prenatal IFA and MM supplements containing iron prevented only later pregnancy anemia and had no significant impact on mortality or other infant outcomes [72]. The mechanisms in which iron supplementation may impact child survival are still unclear and require further investigation.

Child Behavior and Development

The relationship between iron nutritional status and the cognitive development of children has been an area of active investigation. The 2013 Lancet series recently reviewed this evidence [51]. Among children 5 years and older, iron supplementation has a positive impact on child development in populations where iron deficiency is common; however, the evidence for children 3 years and younger is less clear. Many studies have shown that iron deficiency anemia in children under 3 negatively impacts development; however, research from iron supplementation trials has only demonstrated consistent relations with improved motor development with no consistent evidence on mental development [51]. As suggested by Black et al., further evidence is needed as it may be that longer duration trials are needed to demonstrate impact on mental development or that the impact of iron deficiency in young children is irreversible. For this reason, control of childhood iron deficiency anemia should be based on primary prevention, rather than relying on the detection of anemia in children after significant iron deficiency has occurred.

In addition to the direct impact of the child's iron status, iron-deficient women may be at increased risk of depression which in turn would impact mother–child interactions and influence child growth and development. Maternal iron supplementation in high-income counties has been associated with improved maternal mental health and reduced fatigue [73]; however, there is limited data from LMICs of the impact on mother's mental health and mother–child interactions [51]. In a study by Perez et al. [74], iron deficiency anemia among South African mothers both negatively altered mother–child interactions and was associated with poorer infant development scores at 10 week and 9 months of age. Furthermore, research by Christian et al. [75] demonstrated that the impact of maternal iron and folic acid supplementation may have lasting positive impacts on child development. Children 7–9 years of age whose mother received iron and folic acid supplementation during pregnancy scored better in several areas of child development (working memory, inhibitory control, and fine motor functioning).

Work Performance and Productivity

It is well established that significant anemia related to iron deficiency will reduce work performance. The classic study by Viteri [76] demonstrated a linear dose–response relationship between hemoglobin concentration and Harvard step-test performance. The adverse effect of iron deficiency on work or energy output appears to be mediated through a combination of decreased oxygen-carrying capacity from anemia and the effect of iron deficiency on muscle function. In animal studies, it has been shown that both aerobic and anaerobic functions are reduced [77].

In low-income countries, where a large proportion of the economic output is based on physical labor, a major reduction in work capacity can be of great economic consequence. Iron supplementation studies among rubber tappers in Indonesia and tea pickers in Sri Lanka have clearly shown that gain in productivity is secondary to treatment of significant anemia [78, 79]. If the average reduction in productivity is 20% for an anemic individual, in a country where 50% of the women and 20% of the men are affected, the impact of iron deficiency anemia equals a total loss of 5–7% of the national economic output. Therefore, the economic consequence of iron deficiency for some poor countries may be substantial [80].

Heavy Metal Absorption

In high-income countries such as the United States and in some situations in LMICs, an important consequence of iron deficiency is an increased risk of lead poisoning [81]. In the United States, young children who have iron deficiency have a three to four times higher prevalence of lead poisoning than children who are not iron deficient [82]. This association is partly socioeconomic: poor children are more likely to have nutritional disorders and are also more likely to live in inadequate housing where risk to lead exposure is greater [82]. However, there is strong evidence of a direct association between iron deficiency and lead toxicity, related to the fact that iron-deficient individuals have increased efficiency of lead absorption [83]. This increased absorptive capacity is not specific for iron, and the absorption of other divalent metals, including toxic heavy metals such as lead and cadmium, is also increased [84]. The microcytic anemia thought in the past to be owing to lead poisoning is in fact iron deficiency anemia, which is frequently observed among children with lead poisoning [85]. Prevention of iron deficiency would reduce the number of children who arc susceptible to lead poisoning through greater lead absorption, and one study suggests that iron treatment of children with lead poisoning may also help reduce their lead burden [86]. In a controlled clinical trial conducted among lead-exposed Mexican schoolchildren showed that daily supplementation with iron and/or zinc reduced blood lead concentrations but had no impact on cognition [87]. The investigators concluded that iron or zinc supplementation could not be recommended as the sole treatment for improving cognition in lead-exposed children. In conjunction with efforts to prevent iron deficiency, contextualized public health efforts are needed to limit child exposure to lead. In a recent review, it was found that US refugee children were nearly twice as likely to have elevated blood lead levels compared to non-refugee US children due to country of origin-specific pre-entry risk exposure and traditional practices (for example use of lead-based cosmetic around the eyes) [88].

Iron and Infection

While the benefits of iron supplementation are clear, in malaria-endemic areas it has been controversial whether these benefits would outweigh potential increased risk of malarial infection. In a classic paper by Sazawal et al. [89], a large community-based controlled clinical trial conducted in a malaria-endemic region in Zanzibar showed that routine supplementation with iron and folic acid increased hospitalizations and mortality. A recent Cochrane review that looked at the collective evidence concluded that iron supplementation is not harmful as long as regular malaria surveillance and treatment services are provided [90]. Currently the WHO recommends intermittent iron supplementation in children in malaria-endemic regions and that these programs be conducted in conjunction with adequate measures to prevent, diagnose, and treat malaria [91]. Additional research is needed to better understand how supplements and malaria interact within specific target groups (e.g., age, sex, pregnant, nonpregnant women) based on prior malaria exposures.

Furthermore, in areas where hookworm prevalence is 20% or greater, it is recommended to also provide anthelminthic treatment with iron supplementation. However, there is limited evidence of the impact of anthelminthic treatment in pregnancy. A recent meta-analysis of randomized trials did not demonstrate any clear benefits in maternal and child health outcomes; however, observation studies have reported associations with reduced maternal anemia, low birth weight, and mortality [92]. Current evidence suggests that it is safe to deworm women after the first trimester of pregnancy, and the decision of deworming all children and women can be based on the local prevalence, because screening and treatment on the individual level may be less feasible.

Another emerging area of research is the impact of iron supplementation on the gut microbiome and intestinal inflammation. In a study by Jaeggi et al. [93], iron fortification among Kenyan infants was associated with increased pathogen abundance and diarrhea. Further research is needed to weigh the cost: benefit ratio of small increases in illness with sometimes large impacts on iron deficiency and anemia, and their consequences, among deficient children and to examine the need of targeted versus population-based programs in areas with a high burden of infectious disease.

Control of Iron Deficiency and Anemia

Given the widespread prevalence and dire consequences of iron deficiency anemia there is an immediate need to implement effective prevention and treatment interventions in women and children. Combining strategies that address both diet quality and quantity with public health interventions such as improved hygiene and sanitation, routine deworming, and increased access to health service are often needed in many settings where the etiology of iron deficiency and anemia is complex. Table 10.5 summarizes some of the key interventions for combating iron deficiency and anemia. Below is a brief summary of some of the key nutritional interventions.

Iron Supplementation

Iron supplementation is the most common approach to combating iron deficiency anemia across the globe. The WHO has recently released guidelines for supplementation for women and children as described in Table 10.6. Beyond the target groups listed in the table, earlier iron supplementation for preterm or LBW infant may be necessary given their low iron stores at birth. However, further work is needed to establish the optimal timing, duration, and long-term effects in this vulnerable population [48].

Table 10.5 Intervention strategies for the prevention and treatment of iron deficiency/anemia

Nutritional	Non-Nutritional
• Supplementation	• Hookworm/parasite treatment
• Fortification/Biofortification	• Malaria treatment
• Home fortification (MNP)	• Increasing birth interval (>2 year)
	• Increasing age at 1st pregnancy

• Other food-based strategies
    – Dietary diversification
    – Balance of enhancers and inhibitors of iron bioavailability
    – Community gardens
    – Animal production
	• Income-generating activities
	• Delayed cord clamping

Table 10.6 WHO Guidelines on iron supplementation [91, 131–134][a]

Target group	Children 6–23 months	Preschool-age children (24–59 months)	School-age children (5–12 years)	All menstruating adolescent girls and adult women	All pregnant adolescents and adult women	Non-anemic pregnant adolescents and adult women	Postpartum women
Supplement composition	2 mg/kg of body weight	25 mg of elemental iron	45 mg of elemental iron	Iron: 60 mg of elemental iron Folic acid: 2800 µg (2.8 mg)	Iron: 30–60 mg of elemental iron[b] Folic acid: 400 µg (0.4 mg)	Iron: 120 mg of elemental iron Folic acid: 2800 µg (2.8 mg)	1 table t = 60-mg, folic acid = 400-µg[c]
Frequency	One supplement daily	One supplement per week		One supplement per week	One supplement daily	One supplement once a week	One supplement daily
Duration		3 months of supplementation followed by 3 months of no supplementation after which the provision of supplements should restart. If feasible, intermittent supplements could be given throughout the school or calendar year			Throughout pregnancy Iron and folic acid supplementation should begin as early as possible		At least three months after delivery
Settings	Prevalence of anemia in children approximately 1 year of age is above 40% or the diet does not include foods fortified with iron	Prevalence of anemia in preschool or school-age children is 20% or higher		Prevalence of anemia among nonpregnant Women of reproductive age is 20% or higher	All settings	Prevalence of anemia among pregnant women is lower than 20%.	All settings

[a]In malaria-endemic areas, provision of iron and folic acid supplements should be implemented in conjunction with measures to prevent, diagnose, and treat malaria

[b]In settings where anemia in pregnant women is a severe public health problem (40% of higher), a daily dose of 60 mg of elemental iron is preferred over a lower dose. If a woman is diagnosed with anemia in a clinical setting, she should be treated with daily iron (120 mg of elemental iron) and folic acid (400 µg or 0.4 mg) supplementation until her hemoglobin concentration rises to normal. She can then switch to the standard antenatal dose to prevent recurrence of anemia. Note, current evidence suggests multiple micronutrient supplements may provide additional advantage in reducing the risk of LBW and SGA compared IFA alone [97]. However, WHO policies have not been modified at this point

[c]If severe anemia (Hb < 7), give double dose of iron (1 tablet 60 mg twice daily for 3 months)

Iron supplementation is a very effective means for combatting iron deficiency anemia. For example, in a recent meta-analysis, daily maternal iron supplementation during pregnancy led to a 69% reduction in the incidence of anemia at term and 66% reduction in IDA [67]. However, despite widespread universal iron supplementation policies anemia remains one of the most prevalent nutrient deficiencies in the world. One key reason for the seeming paradox is poor coverage and implementation of iron supplementation programs. In a review of 2003–2009 DHS data, coverage across the globe is extremely poor, in Sub-Saharan Africa 40% of women do not receive any iron during pregnancy and less than 20% receive the supplement for at least 90 days [94]. Also, few LMICs have effective iron supplementation programs for young children and efforts have been hampered by the lack of low-cost preparation or drops for distribution in developing countries and lack of experience for large-scale supplementation. One major limitation of the iron supplementation strategy is the need to establish a system for supply and distribution of iron tablets through the primary health care system, and such supply and distribution is not always reliable in a resource-constrained setting. As with any system where there are multiple steps in getting supplies to a target population, it is not uncommon to have breakdowns in the supply chain. Poor compliance is another common problem for any medication required over a long period of time by asymptomatic individuals. At higher doses of iron (60 mg or more of elemental iron), the gastrointestinal side effects are common and may contribute to a lack of compliance. To overcome these problems, proper education on the importance of the supplement and awareness and management of potential side effects need to be provided as part of the distribution program. Efforts to improve the effectiveness of the program include assuring the supply and distribution, communication towards primary health care workers and women on the benefits and non-harmful side effects of supplementation [95, 96]. Another potential reason for lack of substantial anemia reduction could be the presence of other limiting factors (i.e., beyond iron deficiency), such as vitamin A deficiency, or infections such as hookworm, malaria, or HIV infection. Thus far, the evidence indicates that greater effort is still needed to improve the effectiveness of such programs. Another approach under investigation is whether to provide multivitamin–mineral supplements instead of iron–folate supplements during pregnancy. Although policy recommendations have not yet been made, several meta-analyses of controlled trials that compared prenatal multiple micronutrients (MM) to iron–folate including the latest Cochrane review [97] have reported small ($\sim 10\%$) but significant reductions in the incidence of LBW and SGA but no differences in the prevalence of maternal anemia [97, 98]. There were also no differences in maternal or neonatal mortality [97, 98] that were raised as potential concerns earlier [98, 99]. It is interesting to note that iron–folate supplements contain 60 mg iron, whereas the multiple micronutrient supplements contain 30 mg, which was apparently equally effective for addressing maternal anemia and is associated with less side effects.

Nevertheless, considerable progress has been made during the past decade in the development and testing of alternative approaches to deliver micronutrients such as iron along with other critical nutrients such as vitamin A, zinc, and multiple micronutrient combinations to young children. These include micronutrient powders (MNP) that can be added to complementary foods, low-cost fortified processed complementary foods, micronutrient foodlets or enriched spreads, etc. In the past decade, there has been increased global uptake of MNPs. MNPs are specially designed to prevent changes in the appearance, texture, or taste of meal, making it more palatable to children [11]. The powders are provided in single-serving sachets which may be sprinkled once daily over the food before consumption. MNPs, highlighted in the 2008 Lancet Series on Maternal and Child Under Nutrition [22], represent an alternative strategy that overcomes many of the barriers of traditional supplementation and are growing in popularity as an increasing evidence base supports their efficacy and effectiveness [100]. According to a recent Cochrane review, home fortification with micronutrient powders reduced anemia in young children by 31% and iron deficiency by 51% [101]. Given the strength of the evidence base for the efficacy of this product the WHO released strong recommendations in support of home fortification of foods with micronutrient powders to improve iron status and reduce anemia among young children [100].

Nutrition Education and Promotion

Among various micronutrients of interest, more is known about the bioavailability of iron in dietary sources than perhaps any other micronutrient. Factors that can either enhance or inhibit iron absorption have been well-studied. To date, there is limited evidence from LMICs that suggest that dietary selection is an effective approach to improving iron status. This might be attributed to the fact that the main iron-rich foods are animal sources, which are relatively expensive. There is some encouraging evidence from HICs that nutrition education can lead to improved feeding patterns and iron status among infants and younger children, because iron-fortified foods such as infant cereal are commonly used. In most LMIC settings, however, complementary foods are mainly locally home prepared with both low iron content and low iron bioavailability, which can also interfere with the absorption of iron in breast milk. Promotion of exclusive breast feeding may help protect the higher absorption of iron from breast milk. Promoting the earlier introduction of meat-based complementary foods may be helpful. In the Middle East and northern Africa, tea is often introduced during infancy. Education efforts to delay the age at which tea is introduced and avoiding tea near meal times can be considered to be part of the education-based approach. The promotion of certain traditional food processing techniques such as fermentation and germination which can reduce phytate levels and thereby increase iron bioavailability has also been shown to be successful in some settings [102]. It is recommended that the phytate:iron molar ratio is <1.0:1.0 given the strong dose-dependent inhibitory effect on iron absorption [103, 104]. Since the inhibitory effect of phytic acid occurs even at rate as low as 0.2:1.0, where possible all phytate should be degraded, which can be associated with a four–fivefold increase in nonheme iron absorption. Special attention to the high phytate content and poor iron bioavailability of complementary foods in particular is needed given the high iron demands of young children. Key strategies to address this issue include pretreatment methods such as fermentation, soaking, germination, and enzymatic treatment of grains with phytase, combined with introduction of animal sources foods and biofortification/fortification [103, 105, 106].

Fortification

Food fortification of commonly consumed foods is one of the most cost-effective options to improve iron status [107]. There is evidence of the efficacy of iron-fortified foods in improving iron status and reducing anemia [108]; however, there is limited and mixed effectiveness data at a national scale. Common problems with programs include the use of poorly absorbed forms of iron (atomized and hydrogen-reduced iron) and inadequate levels of fortification given the average level of consumption of the fortified food [109]. These factors are related to the required stability and cost of the final product. Depending on the level of refinement of flour and total flour consumption, the WHO interim consensus statement on flour fortification recommends specific iron forms and addition rates [110]. One strong example though of the impact of well-implemented food fortification is Costa Rica [111]. By fortifying a variety of foods (wheat flour, maize flour, milk) with iron, iron deficiency and anemia were substantially reduced in children at a national scale. Another example of the effectiveness of fortification in the prevention of iron deficiency anemia was seen in a project to fortify milk powder with iron and vitamin C for low-income families in Chile [112]. Iron fortification of common food items such as wheat flour will affect the iron intake of all segments of the population except for low consumers of wheat, for example, young infants and selected subgroups that rely on other staples like maize or rice. Women of childbearing age may potentially gain the most from this untargeted approach. Experience to date indicates that it is highly feasible to fortify wheat and maize flour with iron and other micronutrients. The additional cost of fortification is approximately 0.5% of the overall cost of the processed flour. This is a small margin that can reasonably be passed on to the consumer without undue burden. One concern with flour fortification is that it is only suitable for areas where the consumption of flour and flour related products is at least 75 g/person/day [110]. There are, however, several settings where this is feasible and other food items such as curry powder, soy sauces, salt and fish sauce, and milk powder have also been shown to be useful for iron fortification [113, 114]. More recently, progress has been made in fortifying rice with iron using an extruded product and small studies have demonstrated the acceptability and bioefficacy of this product in improving iron status. A study of non-anemic Filipino women, consumption of iron-biofortified rice improved iron stores by 20% [115]. Efforts have also been made in examining the feasibility of biofortification as a potential means of improving iron status especially in populations that consume staples such as wheat and maize which have high levels of phytates that inhibit iron absorption [116]. Traditional plant breeding techniques along with more modern techniques are being pursued to develop and promote varieties of staples that have high content of bioavailable iron either by increasing the actual iron content and/or reduce phytate levels. Implementation research, however, is needed to evaluate these approaches on a large scale.

Delayed Cord Clamping

Delayed cord clamping represents a promising simple and cost-effective intervention to prevent iron deficiency among neonates recently highlighted in the Lancet 2013 nutrition series [100]. By delaying the timing of clamping the umbilical cord by only 2–3 min it increases blood flow to the fetus and thus iron endowment at birth. In a 2009 Cochrane review, delayed cord clamping improved infant iron status up to 6 months of age [117]. Infants with early cord clamping compared to delayed cord clamping were over twice as likely to be iron deficient. Although there are no clear cutoffs or established norms to define suboptimal neonatal iron stores, cord serum ferritin values at birth have been associated with cognitive and motor development. For example, in a study by Tamura et al. [118], infants born with cord serum ferritin values <76 µg/L scored significantly worse on language ability, fine motor, and tractability at age 5. Also in a study by Siddappa et al. [119], researchers found that infants born with cord serum ferritin <34 µg/L had impaired infant auditory recognition memory and lower psychomotor development scores after one year, thus emphasizing the critical need for early intervention in improving infant iron status through interventions such as maternal iron supplementation and delayed cord clamping. Further research is needed to examine the feasibility and safety of scaling up this intervention in existing health systems and effectively influencing behavior change among health care personnel [100].

Iron Overload

Concerns have been raised that iron fortification may potentially harm individuals who may be at risk for iron overload owing to various diseases that cause excess iron accumulation, such as hereditary hemochromatosis, a genetic condition in which iron absorption is enhanced, or thalassemia. Hereditary hemochromatosis is an autosomal recessive disorder with a homozygote frequency of 100–500 per 100,000 in North America and Europe [120]. In hereditary hemochromatosis hepcidin levels are inappropriately low given the individual's iron stores due to abnormalities in the genes encoding HFE, hemojuvelin, and transferrin receptor that lead to the dysregulation of hepcidin production or to mutations that affect hepcidin directly [8]. It is possible to screen for affected individuals and treat these individuals with prophylactic phlebotomy in order to prevent clinical disease [121]. This strategy should be combined with dietary counseling on reducing intake of iron-rich foods such as red meat. The potential to use therapeutic hepcidin is under investigation [122]. In developing countries, incidence of hereditary hemochromatosis is lower because it is a genetic disorder that is generally associated with northern European ancestry. In Asia and Africa, rare and severe hereditary anemias such as thalassemia major are more common, and these affected individuals often become iron-overloaded because of repeated transfusion. Individuals with thalassemia have altered iron metabolism, in which iron absorption is not reduced in response to their higher iron status [123]. For the most part, these individuals have been identified, and specific measures can be taken to protect these individuals from iron overload. However, further research is needed to examine the public health significance in regions such as Cambodia where up to 60% of the people are carriers of a mutation of the β–globin gene [124].

Other concerns have been raised regarding the possible contribution of high iron levels to the development of chronic diseases. The evidence for this association is contradictory [125, 126] and it is possible that chronic disease may alter iron metabolism, giving rise to an apparent association that is not causal in nature. However, there is no advantage to higher iron stores as long as the body's iron requirement is met. The association between higher iron status and chronic diseases should be viewed as hypothetical, requiring more refined confirmatory studies. Because chronic diseases are the leading cause of mortality in many countries, these studies have generated a great deal of concern and have affected efforts to improve iron nutrition even in areas with severe iron deficiency.

Conclusions

Considerable progress has been made in our understanding of the causes and consequences of iron deficiency and anemia but there is a lot of work to be done in moving toward the elimination of these conditions in many developing countries [127, 128]. Without doubt, the challenge of reducing iron deficiency and anemia worldwide depends upon the development of sound approaches to intervention but also needs the commitment of the public, private, and civic sectors to work together. Assessing iron status for monitoring program impact does not always require the full compendium of iron laboratory tests. The effective use of hemoglobin in combination with serum ferritin can be implemented easily even in settings with limited resources [110, 112]. The most promising approach is dietary improvement by iron fortification of common staples, using fortificants of good bioavailability, while for selected groups at higher risk such as infants, young children, and pregnant women, iron supplementation may still be needed [113–115]. Prevention of iron deficiency anemia among younger children especially needs to be a high-priority issue, in light of the evidence that links it to impaired cognition. The limited overlap in dietary intakes of young children compared to adults needs special attention and although strategies like increasing the consumption of animal products can be effective, economic and cultural barriers remain. A holistic approach is also required in many resource-poor settings and programmatic approaches to improve iron intakes should be complemented with public health interventions such as improving sanitation and hygiene, improved access to health care and disease control for maximizing impact [116, 117].

Recommendations/Areas of Future Research

Although iron deficiency is one of the best characterized of all nutritional deficiency disorders, there are several areas that need to be characterized further through scientific investigation at various levels that range from basic science to implementation research as summarized below:

- Heme iron absorption, transport, and regulation.
- Evaluate the effect(s) of iron supplementation on immune responses to different infectious diseases.
- The association between chronic diseases and iron status needs further elucidation.
- Development of possible therapeutic applications of hepcidin for combating anemia and iron overload.
- Reexamination of biomarkers and cutoff values to define anemia and iron deficiency among young children.
- Identification of appropriate cutoff values of hemoglobin or hepcidin that would be most efficient for screening young children who will benefit the most from iron-containing supplements or home fortificants.
- Development of strategies to improve the iron status of premature and LBW infants.
- Development and evaluation of tailored nutrition promotion and education-based interventions combined with approaches that increase availability and affordability of iron-rich foods that will improve iron status in various settings in LMICs.
- Identification of appropriate strategies to improve the delivery and effectiveness of programs for the prevention and control of iron deficiency (supply chain management for iron supplements/implementation science).

Discussion Points

- List two and describe in detail one compensatory mechanism for maintaining iron homeostasis under conditions of low iron intake.
- Describe why hemoglobin is described as having low sensitivity and specificity as an iron status indicator.
- A new study is released documenting low serum ferritin levels among newborns born in a rural hospital in India. What may be the implications of low serum ferritin levels in infants? What interventions would you recommend to address this issue? Explain your rationale.
- You are a nutritionist working in a Department of Public Health that is applying for maternal and child health program funds. Provide a convincing brief summary and argument for why **iron** intervention/programs should be a part of this package.

References

1. Yip R. The challenge of improving iron nutrition: limitations and potentials of major intervention approaches. Eur J Clin Nutr. 1997;51(Suppl 4):S16–24.
2. Huebers HA, Finch CA. The physiology of transferrin and transferrin receptors. Physiol Rev. 1987;67(2):520–82.
3. Dallman PR, Siimes MA, Stekel A. Iron deficiency in infancy and childhood. Am J Clin Nutr. 1980;33(1): 86–118.

4. Yip R. Age related changes in iron metabolism. In: Brock JH, Halliday JW, Pippard MJ, Powell LW, editors. Iron metabolism in health and disease. London: W. B. Saunders; 1994. p. 427–48.

5. Hentze MW, Muckenthaler MU, Andrews NC. Balancing acts: molecular control of mammalian iron metabolism. Cell. 2004;117(3):285–97.

6. Green R, Charlton RW, Seffel H, et al. Body iron excretion in man: a collaborative study. Am J Med 1968;45:336–53.

7. Hallberg L, Hogdahl AM, Nilsson L, Rybo G. Menstrual blood loss—a population study. Variation at different ages and attempts to define normality. Acta Obstet Gynecol Scand. 1966;45(3):320–51.

8. Munoz M, Garcia-Erce JA, Remacha AF. Disorders of iron metabolism. Part 1: molecular basis of iron homoeostasis. J Clin Pathol. 2011;64(4):281–6.

9. Andrews NC, Schmidt PJ. Iron homeostasis. Annu Rev Physiol. 2007;69:69–85.

10. Shayeghi M, Latunde-Dada GO, Oakhill JS, Laftah AH, Takeuchi K, Halliday N, et al. Identification of an intestinal heme transporter. Cell. 2005;122(5):789–801.

11. Qiu A, Jansen M, Sakaris A, Min SH, Chattopadhyay S, Tsai E, et al. Identification of an intestinal folate transporter and the molecular basis for hereditary folate malabsorption. Cell. 2006;127(5):917–28.

12. West AR, Oates PS. Mechanisms of heme iron absorption: current questions and controversies. WJG (World Journal of Gastroenterology). 2008;14(26):4101–10.

13. Krishnamurthy P, Ross DD, Nakanishi T, Bailey-Dell K, Zhou S, Mercer KE, et al. The stem cell marker Bcrp/ABCG2 enhances hypoxic cell survival through interactions with heme. J Biol Chem. 2004;279(23): 24218–25.

14. Quigley JG, Yang Z, Worthington MT, Phillips JD, Sabo KM, Sabath DE, et al. Identification of a human heme exporter that is essential for erythropoiesis. Cell. 2004;118(6):757–66.

15. Andrews NC. Understanding heme transport. New Engl J Med. 2005;353(23):2508–9.

16. Hallberg L. Perspectives on nutritional iron deficiency. Annu Rev Nutr. 2001;21:1–21.

17. Cook JD. Adaptation in iron metabolism. Am J Clin Nutr. 1990;51(2):301–8.

18. Hentze M, Muckenthaler M, Galy B, Camaschella C. Two to tango: regulation of Mammalian iron metabolism. Cell. 2010;142(1):24–38.

19. Muckenthaler MU, Galy B, Hentze MW. Systemic iron homeostasis and the iron-responsive element/iron-regulatory protein (IRE/IRP) regulatory network. Annu Rev Nutr. 2008;28:197–213.

20. Han O. Molecular mechanism of intestinal iron absorption. Metallomics (Integrated Biometal Science). 2011;3(2): 103–9.

21. Ganz T. Hepcidin—a regulator of intestinal iron absorption and iron recycling by macrophages. Best Pract Res Clin Haematol. 2005;18(2):171–82.

22. Ganz T. Systemic iron homeostasis. Physiol Rev. 2013;93(4):1721–41.

23. Krause A, Neitz S, Magert HJ, Schulz A, Forssmann WG, Schulz-Knappe P, et al. LEAP-1, a novel highly disulfide-bonded human peptide, exhibits antimicrobial activity. FEBS Lett. 2000;480(2–3):147–50.

24. Park CH, Valore EV, Waring AJ, Ganz T. Hepcidin, a urinary antimicrobial peptide synthesized in the liver. J Biol Chem. 2001;276(11):7806–10.

25. Pigeon C, Ilyin G, Courselaud B, Leroyer P, Turlin B, Brissot P, et al. A new mouse liver-specific gene, encoding a protein homologous to human antimicrobial peptide hepcidin, is overexpressed during iron overload. J Biol Chem. 2001;276(11):7811–9.

26. Nemeth E, Ganz T. Regulation of iron metabolism by hepcidin. Annu Rev Nutr. 2006;26:323–42.

27. Stevens GA, Finucane MM, De-Regil LM, Paciorek CJ, Flaxman SR, Branca F, et al. Global, regional, and national trends in haemoglobin concentration and prevalence of total and severe anaemia in children and pregnant and non-pregnant women for 1995–2011: a systematic analysis of population-representative data. Lancet Glob Health. 2013;1(1):e16–25.

28. Yip RD. Iron. In: Ziegler EE, Filer LJ Jr, editors. Present knowledge in nutrition. 7th ed. Washington, DC: International Life Sciences Institute, ILSI Press; 1996.

29. WHO. Haemoglobin concentrations for the diagnosis of anaemia and assessment of severity. Vitamin and mineral nutrition information system. Geneva: World Health Organization (WHO/NMH/NHD/MNM/11.1); 2011. Available from: http://www.who.int/vmnis/indicators/haemoglobinpdf.

30. Gibson R. Principles of nutritional assessment. 2nd ed. Oxford: Oxford University Press; 2005.

31. Ahluwalia N, Lonnerdal B, Lorenz SG, Allen LH. Spot ferritin assay for serum samples dried on filter paper. Am J Clin Nutr. 1998;67(1):88–92.

32. Lynch S, Green R. Assessment of nutritional anemias. In: Ramakrishnan U, editor. Boca Raton: Nutritional Anemias, CRC Press LLC; 2001. p. 23–42.

33. Thurnham DI, McCabe LD, Haldar S, Wieringa FT, Northrop-Clewes CA, McCabe GP. Adjusting plasma ferritin concentrations to remove the effects of subclinical inflammation in the assessment of iron deficiency: a meta-analysis. Am J Clin Nutr. 2010;92(3):546–55 (Epub 2010/07/09).

34. Cook JD, Flowers CH, Skikne BS. The quantitative assessment of body iron. Blood. 2003;101(9):3359–64 (Epub 2003/01/11).
35. World Health Organization/Centers for Disease Control. Assessing the iron status of populations. A joint report of a World Health Organization and Centers of Disease Control and Prevention Technical Consultation on Assessment of Iron Status of Populations; 2005.
36. Erhardt JG, Estes JE, Pfeiffer CM, Biesalski HK, Craft NE. Combined measurement of ferritin, soluble transferrin receptor, retinol binding protein, and C-reactive protein by an inexpensive, sensitive, and simple sandwich enzyme-linked immunosorbent assay technique. J Nutr. 2004;134(11):3127–32 (Epub 2004/10/30).
37. Fernandez-Gaxiola AC, De-Regil LM. Intermittent iron supplementation for reducing anaemia and its associated impairments in menstruating women. Cochrane Database Syst Rev. 2011(12):CD009218 (Epub 2011/12/14).
38. De-Regil LM, Jefferds ME, Sylvetsky AC, Dowswell T. Intermittent iron supplementation for improving nutrition and development in children under 12 years of age. Cochrane Database Syst Rev. 2011(12):CD009085 (Epub 2011/12/14).
39. Cohen AR, Seidl-Friedman J. HemoCue system for hemoglobin measurement. Evaluation in anemic and nonanemic children. Am J Clin Pathol. 1988;90(3):302–5.
40. Hudson-Thomas M, Bingham KC, Simmons WK. An evaluation of the HemoCue for measuring haemoglobin in field studies in Jamaica. Bull World Health Organ. 1994;72(3):423–6.
41. Gjorup T, Bugge PM, Hendriksen C, Jensen AM. A critical evaluation of the clinical diagnosis of anemia. Am J Epidemiol. 1986;124(4):657–65.
42. Stoltzfus RJ, Albonico M, Chwaya HM, Savioli L, Tielsch J, Schulze K, et al. Hemoquant determination of hookworm-related blood loss and its role in iron deficiency in African children. Am J Trop Med Hyg. 1996;55 (4):399–404 (Epub 1996/10/01).
43. Dallman PR. Changing iron needs from birth through adolescence. In: Fomon SJ, Zlotkin S, editors. Nutritional anemias. New York, NY: Raven Press; 1992. p. 29–38.
44. Bothwell T, Charlton RW, Cook JD, Finch CA. Iron metabolism in man. Oxford: Blackwell Scientific; 1979.
45. Viteri FE. The consequences of iron deficiency and anemia in pregnancy. In: Allen L, King J, Lonnerdahl B, editors. Nutrient regulation during pregnancy, lactation and growth. New York: Plenum Press; 1994.
46. Bothwell TH. Iron requirements in pregnancy and strategies to meet them. Am J Clin Nutr. 2000;72(1 Suppl):257S–64S.
47. Viteri. Iron endowment at birth: maternal iron status and other influences. Nutr Rev. 2011;69:S3–S16.
48. Mills RJ, Davies MW. Enteral iron supplementation in preterm and low birth weight infants. Cochrane Database Syst Rev. 2012;3:CD005095 (Epub 2012/03/16).
49. Albonico M, Stoltzfus RJ, Savioli L, Tielsch JM, Chwaya HM, Ercole E, et al. Epidemiological evidence for a differential effect of hookworm species, Ancylostoma duodenale or Necator americanus, on iron status of children. Int J Epidemiol. 1998;27(3):530–7 (Epub 1998/08/11).
50. Dallman PR. Tissue effects of iron deficiency. In: Jacobs A, Worwood M, editors. Iron in biochemistry and medicine. London: Academic Press; 1974.
51. Black RE, Victora CG, Walker SP, Bhutta ZA, Christian P, de Onis M, et al. Maternal and child undernutrition and overweight in low-income and middle-income countries. Lancet. 2013;382(9890):427–51.
52. WHO. Global health risks: mortality and burden of disease attributable to selected major risk factors. Geneva: WHO; 2009.
53. Kalaivani K. Prevalence & consequences of anaemia in pregnancy. Indian J Med Res. 2009;130(5):627–33.
54. Gupta SD, Khanna A, Gupta R, Sharma NK, Sharma ND. Maternal mortality ratio and predictors of maternal deaths in selected desert districts in rajasthan a community-based survey and case control study. Women's Health Issues (Official Publication of the Jacobs Institute of Women's Health). 2010;20(1):80–5.
55. Varat MA, Adolph RJ, Fowler NO. Cardiovascular effects of anemia. Am Heart J. 1972;83(3):415–26.
56. Brooker S, Peshu N, Warn PA, Mosobo M, Guyatt HL, Marsh K, et al. The epidemiology of hookworm infection and its contribution to anaemia among pre-school children on the Kenyan coast. Trans R Soc Trop Med Hyg. 1999;93(3):240–6.
57. Allen LH. Pregnancy and iron deficiency: unresolved issues. Nutr Rev. 1997;55(4):91–101.
58. Murphy JF, O'Riordan J, Newcombe RG, Coles EC, Pearson JF. Relation of haemoglobin levels in first and second trimesters to outcome of pregnancy. Lancet. 1986;1(8488):992–5.
59. Rush D. Nutrition and maternal mortality in the developing world. Am J Clin Nutr. 2000;72(1 Suppl):212S–40S.
60. Brabin BJ, Hakimi M, Pelletier D. An analysis of anemia and pregnancy-related maternal mortality. J Nutr. 2001;131(2S-2):604S–14S (Discussion 14S–15S).
61. Brabin BJ, Premji Z, Verhoeff F. An analysis of anemia and child mortality. J Nutr. 2001;131(2S-2):636S–45S (Discussion 46S–48S).
62. Rasmussen K. Is there a causal relationship between iron deficiency or iron-deficiency anemia and weight at birth, length of gestation and perinatal mortality? J Nutr. 2001;131(2S-2):590S–601S (Discussion S–3S).

63. Ramakrishnan U. Functional consequences of nutritional anemia during pregnancy and early childhood. In: Ramakrishnan U, editor. Nutritional anemias. Boca Raton, FL: CRC Press; 2001. p. 43–68.
64. Rasmussen KM, Stoltzfus RJ. New evidence that iron supplementation during pregnancy improves birth weight: new scientific questions. Am J Clin Nutr. 2003;78(4):673–4.
65. Allen LH. Biological mechanisms that might underlie iron's effects on fetal growth and preterm birth. J Nutr. 2001;131(2S-2):581S–9S.
66. Christian P. Micronutrients, birth weight, and survival. Annu Rev Nutr. 2010;30:83–104.
67. Imdad A, Bhutta ZA. Routine iron/folate supplementation during pregnancy: effect on maternal anaemia and birth outcomes. Paediatr Perinat Epidemiol. 2012;26(Suppl 1):168–77.
68. Mwangi MN, Roth JM, Smit MR, Trijsburg L, Mwangi AM, Demir AY, et al. Effect of daily antenatal iron supplementation on plasmodium infection in kenyan women: a randomized clinical trial. JAMA. 2015;314(10): 1009–20.
69. Dibley MJ, Titaley CR, d'Este C, Agho K. Iron and folic acid supplements in pregnancy improve child survival in Indonesia. Am J Clin Nutr. 2012;95(1):220–30.
70. Zeng L, Dibley MJ, Cheng Y, Dang S, Chang S, Kong L, et al. Impact of micronutrient supplementation during pregnancy on birth weight, duration of gestation, and perinatal mortality in rural western China: double blind cluster randomised controlled trial. BMJ. 2008;337:a2001.
71. Christian P, Stewart CP, LeClerq SC, Wu L, Katz J, West KP Jr, et al. Antenatal and postnatal iron supplementation and childhood mortality in rural Nepal: a prospective follow-up in a randomized, controlled community trial. Am J Epidemiol. 2009;170(9):1127–36.
72. Liu JM, Mei Z, Ye R, Serdula MK, Ren A, Cogswell ME. Micronutrient supplementation and pregnancy outcomes: double-blind randomized controlled trial in China. JAMA (Internal Medicine). 2013;173(4):276–82.
73. Murray-Kolb LE. Iron status and neuropsychological consequences in women of reproductive age: what do we know and where are we headed? J Nutr. 2011;141(4):747S–55S.
74. Perez EM, Hendricks MK, Beard JL, Murray-Kolb LE, Berg A, Tomlinson M, et al. Mother-infant interactions and infant development are altered by maternal iron deficiency anemia. J Nutr. 2005;135(4):850–5.
75. Christian P, Murray-Kolb LE, Khatry SK, Katz J, Schaefer BA, Cole PM, et al. Prenatal micronutrient supplementation and intellectual and motor function in early school-aged children in Nepal. JAMA. 2010;304(24):2716–23.
76. Viteri F, Torun B. Anemia and physical work capacity. Clin Hematol. 1974;3:609–26.
77. McLane JA, Fell RD, McKay RH, Winder WW, Brown EB, Holloszy JO. Physiological and biochemical effects of iron deficiency on rat skeletal muscle. Am J Physiol. 1981;241(1):C47–54.
78. Basta SS, Soekirman D, Karyadi D, Scrimshaw NS. Iron deficiency anemia and the productivity of adult males in Indonesia. Am J Clin Nutr. 1979;32(4):916–25.
79. Edgerton VR, Gardner GW, Ohira Y, Gunawardena KA, Senewiratne B. Iron-deficiency anaemia and its effect on worker productivity and activity patterns. Br Med J. 1979;2(6204):1546–9.
80. Horton S, Ross J. The economics of iron deficiency. Food Policy. 2003;28:51–75.
81. Kwong WT, Friello P, Semba RD. Interactions between iron deficiency and lead poisoning: epidemiology and pathogenesis. Sci Total Environ. 2004;330(1–3):21–37.
82. Yip R, Norris TN, Anderson AS. Iron status of children with elevated blood lead concentrations. J Pediatr. 1981;98(6):922–5.
83. Yip R. Multiple interactions between childhood iron deficiency and lead poisoning: evidence that childhood lead poisoning is an adverse consequence of iron deficiency. In: Hercberg SGP, Dupin H, editors. Recent knowledge on iron and folate deficiencies in the world. Paris: INSERM1990. p. 523–32.
84. Tandon SK, Khandelwal S, Jain VK, Mathur N. Influence of dietary iron deficiency on acute metal intoxication. Biometals (An International Journal on the Role of Metal Ions in Biology, Biochemistry, and Medicine). 1993;6(2): 133–8.
85. Clark M, Royal J, Seeler R. Interaction of iron deficiency and lead and the hematologic findings in children with severe lead poisoning. Pediatrics. 1988;81(2):247–54.
86. Hammad TA, Sexton M, Langenberg P. Relationship between blood lead and dietary iron intake in preschool children. A cross-sectional study. Ann Epidemiol. 1996;6(1):30–3.
87. Rico JA, Kordas K, Lopez P, Rosado JL, Vargas GG, Ronquillo D, et al. Efficacy of iron and/or zinc supplementation on cognitive performance of lead-exposed Mexican schoolchildren: a randomized, placebo-controlled trial. Pediatrics. 2006;117(3):e518–27.
88. Shrestha R, Taren DL. Lead toxicity: an under appreciated harm for refugee children entering the USA. In: Nutrition information in crises situations. United Nations Standing Committee on Nutrition, Report No. 16, Mar 2008 http://www.who.int/hac/orioo/nioo16.pdf. Accessed 7 July 2015.
89. Sazawal S, Black RE, Ramsan M, Chwaya HM, Stoltzfus RJ, Dutta A, et al. Effects of routine prophylactic supplementation with iron and folic acid on admission to hospital and mortality in preschool children in a high malaria transmission setting: community-based, randomised, placebo-controlled trial. Lancet. 2006;367(9505): 133–43.

90. Okebe JU, Yahav D, Shbita R, Paul M. Oral iron supplements for children in malaria-endemic areas. Cochrane Database Syst Rev. 2011(10):CD006589.
91. WHO. Guideline: intermittent iron supplementation in preschool and school-age children. Geneva: World Health Organization; 2011.
92. Imhoff-Kunsch B, Briggs V. Antihelminthics in pregnancy and maternal, newborn and child health. Paediatr Perinat Epidemiol. 2012;26(Suppl 1):223–38.
93. Jaeggi T, Kortman GA, Moretti D, Chassard C, Holding P, Dostal A, et al. Iron fortification adversely affects the gut microbiome, increases pathogen abundance and induces intestinal inflammation in Kenyan infants. Gut. 2015;64(5):731–42 (Epub 2014/08/22).
94. Lutter CK, Daelmans BM, de Onis M, Kothari MT, Ruel MT, Arimond M, et al. Undernutrition, poor feeding practices, and low coverage of key nutrition interventions. Pediatrics. 2011;128(6):e1418–27.
95. Ekstrom EC. Supplementation for nutritional anemias. In: Ramakrishnan U, editor. Nutritional anemias. Boca Raton, Florida: CRC Press; 2001. p. 129–52.
96. Galloway R. Anemia prevention and control: what works. In: USAID TWB, UNICEF, PAHO, FAO, editors. The Micronutrient Initiative; 2003.
97. Haider BA, Bhutta ZA. Multiple-micronutrient supplementation for women during pregnancy. Cochrane Database Syst Rev. 2015; Issue 11. Art. No.: CD004905. doi:10.1002/14651858.CD004905.pub4.
98. Ramakrishnan U, Grant FK, Goldenberg T, Bui V, Imdad A, Bhutta ZA. Effect of multiple micronutrient supplementation on pregnancy and infant outcomes: a systematic review. Paediatr Perinat Epidemiol. 2012;26 (Suppl 1):153–67.
99. Ronsmans C, Fisher DJ, Osmond C, Margetts BM, Fall CH. Maternal micronutrient supplementation study G. Multiple micronutrient supplementation during pregnancy in low-income countries: a meta-analysis of effects on stillbirths and on early and late neonatal mortality. Food Nutr Bull. 2009;30(4 Suppl):S547–55.
100. Bhutta ZA, Das JK, Rizvi A, Gaffey MF, Walker N, Horton S, et al. Evidence-based interventions for improvement of maternal and child nutrition: what can be done and at what cost? Lancet. 2013;382(9890): 452–77.
101. De-Regil LM, Suchdev PS, Vist GE, Walleser S, Pena-Rosas JP. Home fortification of foods with multiple micronutrient powders for health and nutrition in children under two years of age (Review). Evid-Based Child Health (A Cochrane Review Journal). 2013;8(1):112–201.
102. Gibson RS, Hotz C. Dietary diversification/modification strategies to enhance micronutrient content and bioavailability of diets in developing countries. Br J Nutr. 2001;85(Suppl 2):S159–66.
103. Gibson RS, Bailey KB, Gibbs M, Ferguson EL. A review of phytate, iron, zinc, and calcium concentrations in plant-based complementary foods used in low-income countries and implications for bioavailability. Food Nutr Bull. 2010;31(2 Suppl):S134–46 (Epub 2010/08/19).
104. Hallberg L, Brune M, Rossander L. Iron absorption in man: ascorbic acid and dose-dependent inhibition by phytate. Am J Clin Nutr. 1989;49(1):140–4 (Epub 1989/01/01).
105. Troesch B. How can phytase improve public health nutrition? III World Congress on Public Health Nutrition. Sight Life. 2015;29(1):108–10.
106. Gupta RK, Gangoliya SS, Singh NK. Reduction of phytic acid and enhancement of bioavailable micronutrients in food grains. J Food Sci Technol. 2015;52(2):676–84 (Epub 2015/02/20).
107. Horton S, Alderman H, Rivera J. Hunger and malnutrition. Copenhagen consensus 2008: malnutrition and hunger. In: Lomborg B, editor. Global crises, global solutions. Cambridge: Cambridge University Press; 2009. p. 305–33.
108. Das JK, Salam RA, Kumar R, Bhutta ZA. Micronutrient fortification of food and its impact on woman and child health: a systematic review. Syst Rev. 2013;2:67.
109. Hurrell R, Ranum P, de Pee S, Biebinger R, Hulthen L, Johnson Q, et al. Revised recommendations for iron fortification of wheat flour and an evaluation of the expected impact of current national wheat flour fortification programs. Food Nutr Bull. 2010;31(1 Suppl):S7–21.
110. WHO, FAO, UNICEF, GAIN, MI, & FFI. Recommendations on wheat and maize flour fortification. Meeting Report: Interim Consensus Statement. Geneva: World Health Organization; 2009. http://www.who.int/nutrition/publications/micronutrients/wheat_maize_fort.pdf. Accessed 14 July 2015.
111. Martorell R, Ascencio M, Tacsan L, Alfaro T, Young MF, Addo OY, et al. Effectiveness evaluation of the food fortification program of Costa Rica: impact on anemia prevalence and hemoglobin concentrations in women and children. Am J Clin Nutr. 2015;101(1):210–7 (Epub 2014/12/21).
112. Heresi G, Pizarro F, Olivares M, Cayazzo M, Hertrampf E, Walter T, et al. Effect of supplementation with an iron-fortified milk on incidence of diarrhea and respiratory infection in urban-resident infants. Scand J Infect Dis. 1995;27(4):385–9.
113. Thuy PV, Berger J, Davidsson L, Khan NC, Lam NT, Cook JD, et al. Regular consumption of NaFeEDTA-fortified fish sauce improves iron status and reduces the prevalence of anemia in anemic Vietnamese women. Am J Clin Nutr. 2003;78(2):284–90.

114. Mannar V, Gallego EB. Iron fortification: country level experiences and lessons learned. J Nutr. 2002;132(4 Suppl):856S–8S.
115. Haas JD, Beard JL, Murray-Kolb LE, del Mundo AM, Felix A, Gregorio GB. Iron-biofortified rice improves the iron stores of nonanemic Filipino women. J Nutr. 2005;135(12):2823–30.
116. Bouis HE. Micronutrient fortification of plants through plant breeding: can it improve nutrition in man at low cost? Proc Nutr Soc. 2003;62(2):403–11.
117. McDonald SJ, Middleton P, Dowswell T, Morris PS. Effect of timing of umbilical cord clamping of term infants on maternal and neonatal outcomes. Cochrane Database Syst Rev. 2013;7:CD004074.
118. Tamura T, Goldenberg RL, Hou J, Johnston KE, Cliver SP, Ramey SL, et al. Cord serum ferritin concentrations and mental and psychomotor development of children at five years of age. J Pediatr. 2002;140(2):165–70.
119. Siddappa AM, Georgieff MK, Wewerka S, Worwa C, Nelson CA, Deregnier RA. Iron deficiency alters auditory recognition memory in newborn infants of diabetic mothers. Pediatr Res. 2004;55(6):1034–41.
120. Olynyk JK, Cullen DJ, Aquilia S, Rossi E, Summerville L, Powell LW. A population-based study of the clinical expression of the hemochromatosis gene. New Engl J Med. 1999;341(10):718–24.
121. Felitti VJ, Beutler E. New developments in hereditary hemochromatosis. Am J Med Sci. 1999;318(4):257–68.
122. Pietrangelo A. Hepcidin in human iron disorders: therapeutic implications. J Hepatol. 2011;54(1):173–81.
123. Zimmermann MB, Fucharoen S, Winichagoon P, Sirankapracha P, Zeder C, Gowachirapant S, et al. Iron metabolism in heterozygotes for hemoglobin E (HbE), alpha-thalassemia 1, or beta-thalassemia and in compound heterozygotes for HbE/beta-thalassemia. Am J Clin Nutr. 2008;88(4):1026–31 (Epub 2008/10/10).
124. Angastiniotis M, Modell B. Global epidemiology of hemoglobin disorders. Ann NY Acad Sci. 1998;850:251–69 (Epub 1998/07/21).
125. Giles WH, Anda RF, Williamson DF, Yip R, Marks J. Body iron stores and the risk of coronary heart disease. New Engl J Med. 1994;331(17):1159–60.
126. Sempos CT, Looker AC, Gillum RF, Makuc DM. Body iron stores and the risk of coronary heart disease. New Engl J Med. 1994;330(16):1119–24.
127. Mason J, Lotfi M, Dalmiya N, Sethuraman K, Deitchler M, Geibel S, et al. Progress in controlling micronutrient deficiencies. MI/Tulane University/UNICEF. The Micronutrient Initiative; 2001.
128. Galloway R, Dusch E, Elder L, Achadi E, Grajeda R, Hurtado E, et al. Women's perceptions of iron deficiency and anemia prevention and control in eight developing countries. Soc Sci Med. 2002;55(4):529–44.
129. WHO. Serum ferritin concentrations for the assessment of iron status and iron deficiency in populations. Vitamin and mineral nutrition information system. Geneva: World Health Organization, WHO/NMH/NHD/MNM/11.2;2011. Available from: http://www.who.int/vmnis/indicators/serum_ferritinpdf.
130. WHO. Assessing the iron status of populations: report of a joint World Health Organization/Centers for Disease Control and Prevention technical consultation on the assessment of iron status at the population level. 2nd edn. Geneva: World Health Organization; 2007. Available from: http://www.who.int/nutrition/publications/micronutrients/anaemia_iron_deficiency/9789241596107.pdf.
131. WHO. Guideline: daily iron and folic acid supplementation in pregnant women. Geneva: World Health Organization; 2012.
132. WHO. Guideline: intermittent iron and folic acid supplementation in menstruating women. Geneva: World Health Organization; 2011.
133. WHO. Guideline: intermittent iron and folic acid supplementation in non-anaemic pregnant. Geneva: World Health Organization; 2012.
134. World Health Organization Pregnancy. Childbirth, postpartum and newborn care: a guide for essential practice; 2006. Available from: http://www.who.int/elena/titles/iron_supplementation_children/en/.

Chapter 11
Zinc Deficiency

Sonja Y. Hess

Keywords Zinc · Zinc status · Assessment · Zinc deficiency · Supplementation · Fortification · Dietary diversification and modification · Biofortification · Diarrhea · Growth

Learning Objectives

- Identify the causes of zinc deficiency.
- Describe the health consequences of zinc deficiency.
- Understand the assessment of zinc deficiency.
- Analyze intervention strategies to prevent zinc deficiency.

Introduction

Adequate zinc nutrition is essential for human health because zinc is involved in numerous metabolic processes as a catalyst, regulatory ion, or structural element of proteins. Over 300 zinc metalloenzymes require zinc as a catalyst, and about 2500 transcription factors require zinc for their structural integrity [1, 2]. Zinc is involved in the regulation of gene expression and as a regulator of cell signaling pathways [1]. Because zinc participates in so many metabolic pathways, zinc deficiency affects multiple physiological systems, children's physical growth, the risk and severity of a variety of infections and pregnancy outcomes. Based on available evidence, the number of child deaths attributable to zinc deficiency in 2011 was estimated at 116,000 [3]. In recent years, the recognition of the importance of zinc deficiency worldwide has expanded dramatically [4], and more experience has accumulated on the design and implementation of zinc intervention programs, as described below.

Estimates of Zinc Requirements

The estimated average requirement (EAR), for any micronutrient, is the level at which half of the healthy individuals within a specific population group meet the physiological requirements for that micronutrient. The World Health Organization (WHO) [5], the US Institute of Medicine (IOM) [6],

S.Y. Hess (✉)
Nutrition Department, University of California Davis, One Shields Avenue, Davis, CA 95616, USA
e-mail: syhess@ucdavis.edu

© Springer Science+Business Media New York 2017
S. de Pee et al. (eds.), *Nutrition and Health in a Developing World*,
Nutrition and Health, DOI 10.1007/978-3-319-43739-2_11

Table 11.1 Estimated average requirement (EAR)[a] from the US Institute of Medicine (IOM) [6], the International Zinc Nutrition Consultative Group (IZiNCG) [7], and the European Food Safety Authority (EFSA) [8] for dietary zinc intake according to life stage and diet type

Life stage	Sex	IOM [6] (mg/day)	IZiNCG [7] (mg/day)		EFSA [8][b]	
			Mixed or refined vegetarian diets	Unrefined, cereal-based diets	300 mg phytate intake per day	1200 mg phytate intake per day
6–11 month	All	2.5	3	4	2.4	
1–3 year	All	2.5	2	2	3.6	
4–8 year	All	4	3	4	4.6–6.2[c]	
9–13 year	All	7	5	7	6.2–8.9[c]	
14–18 year	M	8.5	8	11	11.8	
14–18 year	F	7.3	7	9	9.9	
Pregnancy 14–18 year	F	10.0	9	12	+1.3[d]	
Lactation 14–18 year	F	10.9	8	9	+2.4[d]	
Adult > 19 year	M	9.4	10	15	7.5	12.7
Adult > 19 year	F	6.8	6	7	6.2	10.2
Pregnancy > 19 year	F	9.5	8	10	+1.3[4]	+1.3[d]
Lactation > 19 year	F	10.4	7	8	+2.4[4]	+2.4[d]

[a]The estimated average requirements represent the mean dietary requirement at which 50% of individuals would meet their physiological requirement
[b]EFSA estimated the Average Requirements for adults according to the phytate intake of 300, 600, 900 1200 mg/day (only 300 and 1200 shown here), and body weight. Median body weight for women and men were estimated based on body heights measured in 13 European Union Member States and assuming a body mass index of 22 kg/m^2
[c]EFSA estimated the Average Requirements for zinc to be 4.6 mg/day for 4–6 year olds, 6.2 mg/day for 7–10 year, and 8.9 mg/day for 11–14 year old boys and girls combined
[d]EFSA estimated the additional Average Requirements for zinc needed during pregnancy and lactation based on the estimated additional physiological requirements for each life stage

the International Zinc Nutrition Consultative Group (IZiNCG) [7], the European Food Safety Authority (EFSA) [8], and other international expert groups have published estimates of human zinc requirements (Table 11.1). But these estimates lack consistency because they are based on different conceptual frameworks and/or statistical techniques, and they rely on diverse sources of empirical information. It has been recognized that aligning recommended nutrient intakes is important so that they can be used across countries for establishing public and clinical health objectives and food and nutrition policies, such as fortification programs, and for addressing regulatory and trade issues [9].

Causes of Zinc Deficiency

The risk factors for zinc deficiency are similar to those for other minerals and trace elements. In particular, four main factors are responsible for the development of zinc deficiency: (1) inadequate dietary zinc intake, (2) poor zinc absorption from high-phytate, plant-based diets, (3) physiological states that increase zinc requirements, and (4) disease states that either induce excessive losses or impair absorption and utilization of zinc.

Inadequate Dietary Zinc Intake

Inadequate dietary intake of absorbable zinc is likely to be the primary cause of zinc deficiency in most situations [7]. Animal source foods, in particular, shellfish, small whole fish, beef, and organ meats, such as liver and kidney, are rich sources of zinc, and zinc is highly bioavailable from these foods. Plant source foods, such as most fruits and vegetables including green leaves, and starchy roots and tubers, have relatively low zinc content. While whole grains, nuts and legumes have moderate to high-zinc content, these foods also contain large quantities of phytate (phytic acid or myo-inositol hexaphosphate), the most potent identified dietary inhibitor of zinc absorption [10]. Phytate chelates metal ions, especially, zinc, iron, and calcium, forming insoluble complexes in the gastrointestinal tract that cannot be digested or absorbed in humans because of the absence of intestinal phytase enzymes [11]. The inhibitory effect of phytate on zinc absorption appears to follow a dose-dependent response, and the phytate: zinc molar ratio can be used to estimate the proportion of absorbable zinc [12].

The phytate: zinc molar ratio of foods or diets is calculated as follows:

$$\frac{mg\ phytate/660}{mg\ zinc/65.4}$$

where 660 equals the molecular weight of phytate and 65.4 the molecular weight of zinc.

Unrefined cereal and/or legume-based diets generally have phytate: zinc ratios >18, which is associated with relatively low zinc bioavailability and results in zinc absorption of 18% for men and 25% for women [13]. In contrast, mixed diets containing higher amounts of animal source foods and less plant source foods, or refined plant-based diets generally have phytate: zinc ratios between 4 and 18, which are associated with higher zinc bioavailability. Zinc absorption of mixed diets is about 26% for men and 34% for women [13].

Conditions Increasing Physiological Requirements

During growth and pregnancy, the incorporation of zinc into newly synthesized tissue increases zinc requirements [6, 7]. Similarly, the amount of zinc transferred from mother to infant in breast milk must be added to the lactating women's physiological requirement for absorbed zinc [8, 14] (Table 11.1). These increased needs for zinc add to the challenge of consuming adequate amounts of bioavailable zinc from the food supply. Consequently, infants (particularly those born prematurely), young children, children recovering from malnutrition or diarrhea, adolescents and pregnant, and lactating women are at elevated risk of zinc deficiency.

Another population group at potential risk of zinc deficiency is the elderly because of multiple physiological, social, psychological, and economic risk factors [15]. Available information from Europe is inconsistent and little is known about the zinc status of elderly populations in other parts of the world, particularly low-income countries. A high prevalence of zinc deficiency was found in the ZINCAGE Project of five European countries (Italy, Greece, Germany, France and Poland) where 31% of 851 healthy elderly people 60–84 years of age had low plasma zinc concentration [16]. In contrast, the ZENITH study of adults 55–70 years of age living in three European countries (France, Italy, and United Kingdom) found a low prevalence (<5%) of zinc deficiency [17]. Since these studies did not use a representative population sampling scheme, the estimated prevalences are not reflective of the elderly population in these countries, but they highlight that zinc deficiency may be an issue in some of the elderly. Representative surveys of elderly populations are needed to assess the prevalence of zinc deficiency and associated risks both in lower and higher income countries.

Other Causes of Zinc Deficiency

Zinc is absorbed from the small intestine, primarily from the duodenum and jejunum. Under normal physiological conditions, zinc is secreted into the small intestine in large quantities together with digestive juices, but is largely reabsorbed. Given the important role of the small intestine in regulating dietary zinc absorption, and the secretion and reabsorption of endogenous zinc during digestion, conditions that affect its health or integrity could interfere with the adequate maintenance of zinc balance. Diarrhea not only leads to an increased loss of endogenous zinc [18], but may also lead to reduced absorption of dietary zinc during the episode due to decreased intestinal transit time. Environmental enteropathy, a subclinical, chronic disorder of the small intestine, is hypothesized to be a key cause of childhood undernutrition including zinc deficiency [19, 20]. Environmental enteropathy is characterized by changes in the small bowel morphology, including villous atrophy, hyperplasia of crypt cells, infiltration of inflammatory cells, and increased permeability [21]. Although its etiology is unknown, it is very common in young children living in conditions of poor sanitation and hygiene [19]. Lindenmayer et al. [20] recently reviewed the evidence for interactions between zinc deficiency and environmental enteropathy. The authors concluded that environmental enteropathy may impair zinc homeostasis, and zinc deficiency may contribute to environmental enteropathy by impairing intestinal barrier function, increasing the risk of gastrointestinal infections, and inducing intestinal inflammation [20]. The extent to which diarrhea, environmental enteropathy, and similar conditions contributes to the risk of zinc deficiency in lower income countries requires further investigation.

Assessment of Zinc Deficiency

Plasma and Serum Zinc Concentration

Zinc homeostasis in the cell, tissue, and whole blood is tightly controlled to sustain metabolic functions over a wide range of zinc intakes. This strong homeostatic control makes assessing zinc status very challenging. Nevertheless, several expert committees have endorsed plasma or serum zinc concentration as a useful biomarker of zinc status, especially for assessing the risk of zinc deficiency in populations [22, 23]. This recommendation was based on the fact that plasma zinc concentrations consistently respond to zinc supplementation and that the results of dietary depletion/repletion studies indicate that plasma zinc concentrations respond to severe dietary zinc restriction, although there is considerable variation between individuals [24]. It has to be noted that plasma zinc concentration is not a reliable indicator of an individual's zinc status [24], except when very low in that case there is a strong association between low plasma zinc concentration (<50 µg/dL) and clinical signs of deficiency [25]. Plasma zinc concentration is influenced by the time of day and time since last meal [26, 27]. Specific cut-offs have been proposed for women and men separately based on a large sample of the US population, assessed during the second National Health and Nutrition Examination Survey (NHANES II) [28]. These cut-offs have been adopted by IZiNCG and are widely used (Table 11.2) [7, 22]. Because clinical signs of zinc deficiency only occur in severely zinc deficient individuals and little was known about the level of plasma zinc concentration at which clinical signs of zinc deficiency occur, Wessells et al. [25] recently completed an analyses of studies of severe zinc-restricted diets and patients with acrodermatitis enteropathica and proposed a new cut-off of 50 µg/dL to define severe zinc deficiency (Table 11.2).

Several important technical issues have to be considered when collecting blood, analyzing plasma, and interpreting results for plasma zinc concentration. Because only small amounts of the total body

Table 11.2 Cutoffs recommended by IZiNCG for serum and plasma zinc concentration (µg/dL) by age group, sex, time of day, and time since last meal [7, 25]

| | Lower cut-offs for serum zinc concentration (µg/dL)[a] | | |
| | <10 years | ≥ 10 years | |
	Males and females	Nonpregnant females	Males
Morning, fasting[b]	n/a	70	74
Morning, nonfasting	65	66	70
Afternoon, nonfasting	57	59	61
Severe zinc deficiency	n/a	50	50

n/a not available
[a]For conversion to µmol/L, divide by 6.54
[b]Fasting is defined as no food or beverage consumption for at least 8 h

zinc are circulating in blood, any contamination from external sources has to be prevented as they can falsely increase the zinc concentration measured. Ideally, blood samples are collected from fasting participants because the zinc concentration is influenced by the time of day and last meal consumed, as described above. Another challenge, when assessing plasma zinc concentration, is that the concentration is reduced during inflammation and infection. Thus in areas where infections are common, it is recommended to assess acute-phase proteins such as C-reactive protein (CRP) and α1-acid glycoprotein (AGP) and to adjust plasma zinc concentration categorically based on elevated acute-phase proteins (defined as CRP > 5 mg/L, AGP > 1 g/L, or both) [29]. Further details of appropriate blood collection techniques, suitable supplies, and analyses are provided by IZiNCG [30, 31]. Zinc deficiency is considered a public health concern when the prevalence is >20%, and interventions to improve zinc status should be considered [22].

Dietary Zinc Intake

Inadequate dietary intake of absorbable zinc is one of the major causes of zinc deficiency. Therefore, assessment of the adequacy of zinc intakes through the use of 24-h recalls or weighed dietary records is an important component in evaluating the risk of zinc deficiency in a population [32]. To assess the risk of zinc deficiency in a population, WHO, the United Nations Children's Fund (UNICEF), the International Atomic Energy Agency (IAEA), and IZiNCG recommend assessing dietary zinc intake to determine the prevalence of zinc intakes below the EAR [22]. Recommendations for dietary surveys of zinc intake were described by IZiNCG [13]. As described above, the bioavailability of zinc depends on the presence of phytate in the food, which has to be considered in any dietary zinc assessment. Where possible, local food composition data for zinc and phytate should be used, as their content can vary with both local soil conditions and food preparation and processing methods [33]. When zinc and phytate composition of foods cannot be derived from composition tables, direct chemical analyses of food samples should be considered using the strategy of choosing food samples suggested by Gibson and Ferguson [34]. A population is considered at risk of zinc deficiency, where the prevalence of inadequate intakes of zinc is >25% [22].

Stunting

Somatic growth and susceptibility to infection are considered zinc-related functional outcomes because meta-analyses have found a consistent beneficial impact of zinc supplementation as described in more detail below. Of these indicators, growth is the only one recommended to assess the risk of zinc deficiency in a population. For population assessment, the recommended indicator to use is the prevalence of stunting, i.e., the percentage of children under 5 years of age with length-for-age z-score (0–24 months of age) or height-for-age z-score (2–5 years) less than -2.0 SD below the age-specific median of the reference population [35]. The Growth Standards proposed by WHO in 2006 are a useful tool for international assessments, as they reflect early child growth under optimal environmental conditions [36]. A prevalence of stunting >20% of the population indicates a public health concern [22]. Because zinc deficiency is not the only factor affecting children's growth, assessment of dietary zinc intake and plasma zinc concentration is recommended to decide whether zinc intervention strategies should be considered when the prevalence of stunting is elevated.

Other Indicators

Several potential other indicators of zinc status have been identified including hair, nail and urinary zinc levels, concentrations of zinc-dependent proteins, zinc kinetic markers, and other markers. Urinary zinc excretion and hair zinc concentration responded to zinc status overall [23]. However, more research is needed before these indicators can be used to assess the zinc status of individuals or populations because of the lack of reference values. Efforts are also continuing to identify new biomarkers of zinc status.

Prevalence of Zinc Deficiency

In the past two decades, several low- and middle-income countries included the assessment of plasma or serum zinc concentration in their national nutrition surveys, and the number of planned surveys assessing zinc status is increasing. Surveys in four African countries found a prevalence of low plasma zinc concentration ranging from 45 to 83% in children and 52–82% in women of reproductive age [37–40] and similar rates were found in Bangladesh, Vietnam, and Colombia [41–43] (Table 11.3). Although to a lesser extent, zinc deficiency was also highly prevalent in Pakistan, the Republic of Maldives, the Philippines, and Mexico [44–47]. Except in young children in the Republic of Maldives, where 16% were found to be zinc deficient [46], in all of the above mentioned surveys, the prevalence of low serum or plasma zinc concentrations was greater than 20% indicating that the risk of zinc deficiency is of public health concern. In all surveys, regional differences were identified and the authors concluded that large-scale programs to improve zinc intake are needed.

There is less information available from national nutrition surveys in high-income countries. In the United Kingdom, a national nutrition survey of children and adolescents (4–18 years) implemented in 1997 found that only 2% had low plasma zinc concentration [48]. A subsequent national survey of adolescents and adults completed in the United Kingdom from 2008 to 2011 did not present results of low plasma zinc concentration, but mean plasma zinc concentrations were high (102.8 μg/dL for 11–18 years olds and 100.9 μg/dL for 19–64 years old, respectively) [49]. The United States has not included the assessment of zinc status since the second National Health and Nutrition Examination Survey (NHANES II; 1976–1980), which was the basis for the IZiNCG cut-offs (see above section on plasma and serum zinc concentration) [7, 28].

Although more national surveys have included the assessment of plasma zinc concentration in recent years, there is still insufficient data on the global prevalence of zinc deficiency. In an effort to estimate the risk of zinc deficiency globally, Wessells and Brown [50] estimated the prevalence of inadequate zinc intake based on the estimated absorbable zinc content of the national food supplies as

Table 11.3 Prevalence of zinc deficiency from nationally representative surveys

Country, year	Year of survey	Age of population groups (sample size)		Prevalence of low plasma zinc concentration (%)		Plasma zinc concentration adjustments	Cut-offs used	Ref.
		Children	Women	Children	Women			
Africa								
Cameroon	2009	12–59 month (*n* = 845)	15–49 years (*n* = 879)	83	82	Adjusted for presence of inflammation[b] and methodological factors	IZiNCG cut-offs[a]	[37]
Kenya	1999	2–72 month (*n* = 541)	Mothers of participating children (*n* = 1093)	51	52	Controlled for infection[c]	IZiNCG cut-offs[a]	[38]
Senegal	2010	12–59 month (*n* = 1496)	15–49 years (*n* = 1082)	50	58	Adjusted for presence of inflammation[b]	IZiNCG cut-offs[a]	[39]
South Africa	2005	1–9 years (*n* = 400)	–	45	–	Adjusted for presence of inflammation[d]	IZiNCG cut-offs[a]	[40]
Americas								
Colombia	2008–2010	12–59 month (*n* = 4279)	–	43	–	–	IZiNCG cut-offs[a]	[43]
Mexico	2006	1–11 years (*n* = 3964)	12–49 years (*n* = 2421)	26	34	–	IZiNCG cut-offs[a]	[44]
Eastern mediterranean								
Pakistan	2011	0–59 month (*n* ~ 12,000)	15–49 years (*n* ~ 12,000)	38	48		<60 μg/dL	[45]
Europe								
United Kingdom	1997	4–18 years (*n* = 1193)	–	2	–	Not required[e]	fasting <70 μg/dL; nonfasting <65 μg/dL	[48]

(continued)

Table 11.3 (continued)

Country, year	Year of survey	Age of population groups (sample size)		Prevalence of low plasma zinc concentration (%)		Plasma zinc concentration adjustments	Cut-offs used	Ref.
		Children	Women	Children	Women			
South-East Asia								
Bangladesh	2011–12	6–59 month (n = 662)	15–49 years, nonpregnant, nonlactating (n = 1073)	45	57	Adjusted for presence of inflammation[b]	IZINCG cut-offs[a]	[41]
Republic of Maldives	2007	6–59 month (n = 1262)	15–49 years (n = 1304)	16	27	–	<60 µg/dL	[46]
Western Pacific								
Philippines	2008	6–12 years (n = 2905)	20–59 years (n = 2892)	31	31	–	IZINCG cut-offs[a]	[47]
Vietnam		0–59 month (n = 563)	15–49 years, nonpregnant (n = 1522)	52	67	–	IZINCG cut-offs[a]	[42]

[a]Cut-offs suggested by IZiNCG [7]

[b]Plasma zinc concentration adjusted for elevated C-reactive protein and α1-acid-glycoprotein

[c]Controlled for infection, details not provided

[d]Plasma zinc concentration adjusted for elevated C-reactive protein and α1-acid-glycoprotein

[e]Adjustment not required; plasma zinc concentrations not significantly associated with plasma α-1-antichymotrypsin

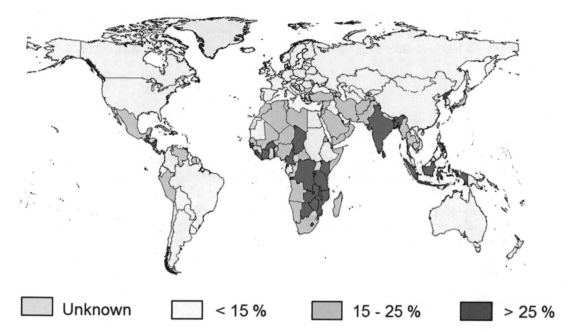

Unknown   < 15 %   15 - 25 %   > 25 %

Fig. 11.1 Estimated country-specific prevalence of inadequate zinc intake based on FAO's food balance sheets [50]. Copyright: © 2012 Wessells, Brown; Open Access

derived from national food balance sheet data obtained from the Food and Agriculture Organization of the United Nations. These analyses suggest that at least 17% of the world's population is at risk of inadequate zinc intake (Fig. 11.1). The estimated prevalence of inadequate dietary zinc intake was particularly high in Sub-Saharan Africa (26%) and South Asia (30%) [50, 51]. To confirm these estimated prevalences of zinc deficiency, it is recommended to assess plasma zinc concentration and/or to assess dietary zinc intake using 24 h dietary recalls in a representative population sample of countries identified with a high prevalence of inadequate dietary zinc intake derived from food balance sheets.

Importance of Zinc for Human Health

Evidence of human zinc deficiency began to emerge from studies in male adolescents in Egypt and Iran during the 1960s. In these individuals, zinc deficiency resulted in delayed sexual maturation, short stature, anemia, enlarged liver and spleen, and abnormalities in skeletal maturation [52, 53]. Zinc supplementation significantly increased height, weight, bone development, and sexual maturation [54].

Studies of patients suffering from acrodermatitis enteropathica provide insight into the functional consequences of zinc deficiency. Acrodermatitis enteropathica is an autosomal recessive disorder caused by a gene mutation which results in defective absorption of dietary zinc causing severe zinc deficiency. Severe zinc deficiency as occurs in acrodermatitis enteropathica is characterized by skin lesions, reduction in growth, alopecia (hair loss), diarrhea, emotional disorders, weight loss, intercurrent infections due to cell-mediated immune dysfunction, hypogonadism in males, and neurosensory disorders [55, 56]. In patients suffering from acrodermatitis enteropathica, only high-dose zinc supplementation can overcome the reduced zinc absorption resulting in rapid resolution of clinical symptoms.

Evidence of the effects of mild to moderate zinc deficiency has been derived from animal studies, observational studies of the association between zinc status and functional outcomes, and clinical or community-based intervention trials assessing the impact of zinc supplementation on functional outcomes [7].

Child Growth

Impaired growth is considered a functional outcome of zinc deficiency. Studies from different regions of the world consistently show an increase in growth and weight gain with preventive zinc supplementation, as reviewed in more detail below. The importance of zinc for normal growth is not surprising, considering zinc's involvement in DNA replication, RNA transcription, endocrine function and metabolic pathways [7]. However, exact factors responsible for the effects of zinc deficiency on growth remain to be defined [1].

Immune Function and Morbidity

Zinc is important for proper immune function, as deficiency can affect both innate and adaptive immunity. Zinc deficiency impairs macrophage functions (phagocytosis, intracellular killing), neutrophil functions (generation of oxidative burst, chemotaxis), NK cell activity, and complement activity [57, 58]. Zinc deficiency also adversely affects the growth and function of T- and B-cells [55]. Moreover, it has become evident that zinc acquisition is a key element of the host–pathogen interaction, similar to iron and other metals such as manganese and copper [59]. During an infection, the host and the pathogen compete over these metals, and the host's metabolism is adjusted in an effort to limit the pathogens' access to these metals [60]. Specifically for zinc, a typical early response to bacterial infection is the rapid fall of plasma zinc concentration accompanied by accumulation of zinc in the liver [59]. Although the mechanism and function of zinc sequestration by the host remain unclear, limiting microbial access to zinc has the potential to disrupt a number of processes that are critical to progression of the infection [60].

There is consistent evidence that preventive zinc supplementation reduces the incidence of diarrhea and that therapeutic zinc supplementation reduces the duration of the current diarrhea episode, as described below. Several mechanisms have been suggested through which zinc reduces diarrhea at the level of the intestine. These include modulation of ion transport, stimulation of enterocyte growth and differentiation, maintenance of normal intestinal permeability, and regulation of oxidative stress and inflammation [61].

Pregnancy Outcome

Findings from studies in animals and in pregnant women suffering from acrodermatitis enteropathica suggest that severe zinc deficiency during pregnancy has devastating effects on pregnancy outcome, such as fetal malformations, embryonic or fetal death, fetal growth restriction and life-threatening complications during pregnancy and birth [62]. However, mild and moderate zinc deficiency is more common, and observational studies have failed to show a consistent association between maternal zinc deficiency and maternal and fetal outcomes [63, 64]. Similarly, there is inconclusive evidence from observational studies investigating associations between maternal zinc status and infant birth weight. Donangelo and King [64] hypothesize that in cases of mild zinc deficiency homeostatic adjustments during pregnancy and lactation improve zinc utilization sufficiently to meet the elevated zinc requirement and consequently prevent immediate adverse effects due to a low zinc intake. In contrast, zinc supplementation trials consistently found an overall significant reduction in prematurity in the zinc supplemented group compared to the placebo group, as described below.

Neurobehavioral Development

Animal studies suggest that zinc deficiency early in life has long-lasting effects on the animals' response to stress, which results in poor learning performance [65]. Moreover, maternal and infant zinc deficiency in animals was linked with deficits in activity, attention, and memory [66]. In a recent review, Prado and Dewey [67] concluded that preventive zinc supplementation during infancy may positively affect motor development and activity levels, but that it does not seem to affect measures of early cognitive ability.

Zinc Intervention Strategies

Preventive Zinc Supplementation in Children

An updated analysis published in the 2013 Lancet series on maternal and child nutrition concluded that preventive zinc supplementation is among the interventions with the largest potential impact on mortality in children under 5 years of age [68]. The other interventions recommended by the Lancet series for reducing child mortality are management of severe-acute malnutrition, optimal breast-feeding practices and vitamin A supplementation. A considerable number of clinical trials investigated the impact of preventive zinc supplementation given in tablet or syrup form with or without other micronutrients on growth, morbidity, and other outcomes during childhood. Most of these trials were implemented in low-income countries. Many investigated the impact of daily supplements, but some provided the zinc supplements several times per week or once weekly. The zinc doses ranged from 1 to 70 mg, resulting in a daily dose equivalent ranging from 0.9 to 21.4 mg/day [69]. The zinc compound in the supplements also varied, with zinc sulfate being most frequently used. Although the trials differed by many of the above described factors, the common objective was the prevention of zinc deficiency and other zinc-related functional outcomes.

Meta-analyses investigating the impact of these trials consistently found that preventive zinc supplementation has a small, but highly significant impact on linear growth and weight gain [69–72]. Although the impact on growth of studies providing different doses was significantly different, there was no clear pattern of increasing or decreasing effect with higher doses [72]. Imdad and Bhutta [71] did a subgroup analysis of studies in children <5 years of age that reported actual increase in length (cm) and showed that a dose of 10 mg zinc/d for a duration of 24 weeks led to a net gain of 0.37 (±0.25) cm in the zinc supplemented group compared to placebo. An earlier meta-analyses found that the beneficial impact of zinc on the change in height was negatively associated with concurrent supplementation of either iron or vitamin A and the change in weight with concurrent supplementation of iron [69]. This was confirmed in the most recent meta-analysis by Mayo-Wilson et al. [72], where concurrent supplementation with iron did not show an impact on growth. Only groups that received zinc supplements without iron showed a beneficial impact on growth.

Four meta-analyses investigated the impact of preventive zinc supplementation during childhood on diarrhea incidence and found a reduction of 12–20% in the zinc group compared to the placebo group [69, 72–74]. The beneficial impact on diarrhea incidence seems to be greater in studies that enrolled children with mean initial age >12 months compared to 6–12 months (reduction of 15% compared to 8%, respectively) [69, 72].

Three of four meta-analyses also concluded that preventive zinc supplementation reduced the incidence of acute lower respiratory infection, and that this reduction was greater in studies where the symptoms were clinically diagnosed rather than just based on caregiver's reports [69, 74, 75]. The challenges of diagnosing acute lower respiratory tract infection accurately may be the reason for the conclusion of the most recent meta-analyses by Mayo-Wilson et al. [72], which found no significant impact of preventive zinc supplementation on the incidence of lower respiratory tract infection. At present, the impact of preventive zinc supplementation on malaria is inconclusive [69, 72]. There is mixed evidence on the impact of preventive zinc supplementation on the incidence of otitis media in healthy children under the age of 5 years living in low- and middle-income countries [76]. The impact of preventive zinc supplementation is borderline significant for all-cause mortality. Depending on the meta-analyses, the mortality reduction ranged from 5% (relative risk (RR) = 0.95; 95% confidence interval (95% CI): 0.86, 1.05 [72]) to 9% (RR = 0.91; 95% CI: 0.82, 1.01 [74]). An analysis by Brown et al. [69] showed a significant 18% reduction in all-cause mortality (RR = 0.82; 95% CI: 0.70, 0.96) in children aged >12 months. Borderline significant effects were identified for diarrhea-specific (RR = 0.82; 95% CI: 0.64, 1.05) and pneumonia-specific mortality (RR = 0.85; 95% CI: 0.65, 1.01) [74].

In summary, the available evidence suggests a beneficial impact of preventive zinc supplementation on selected childhood infections, a significant impact on childhood mortality in children >12 months of age, and a significant increase in children's physical growth. Thus, in populations at high risk of zinc deficiency and a high burden of childhood morbidity and stunting, there is a need for intervention programs to enhance zinc intake through preventive zinc supplementation. There are a number of programmatic delivery platforms available, including bi-annual Child Health Days which often also provide high-dose vitamin A supplements, anthelminthic medication and nutrition counseling, growth monitoring and promotion programs, community-based or community-directed distribution programs, and social marketing through private-sector distribution channels [77]. The most appropriate delivery platform or combination thereof needs to be determined at the country or regional level.

Preventive Zinc Supplementation in Pregnant Women

Two recent meta-analyses compared the effects of prenatal zinc supplementation on maternal, fetal, neonatal, and infant outcomes in healthy pregnant women [78, 79]. Both meta-analyses included 20 independent intervention trials, but due to some differences in the inclusion criteria only 17 of these were included in both analyses. In all cases, zinc was the only factor that differed between the comparison groups, and zinc doses varied from 5 to 50 mg/day. The initiation of the supplementation ranged from preconception to 26 weeks of gestation. Both meta-analyses found a significant reduction of 14% in preterm births in the zinc supplemented group compared to the placebo group (RR 0.86, 95% CI: 0.75, 0.99 [78, 79]). Chaffee and King [78] hypothesized that prenatal zinc supplementation may reduce the incidence or the severity of maternal infections that may lower the risk of preterm birth. There was no evidence that supplemental zinc affected any parameter of fetal growth (risk of low birth weight, birth weight, length at birth or head circumference at birth) or other maternal outcomes.

Interestingly, three randomized controlled trials found decreased incidence of diarrhea during infancy in children whose mother received zinc supplementation during pregnancy (note that this outcome was not included in any of the other prenatal zinc supplementation studies) compared to children of mothers in the placebo group [80–82]. While one study in Peruvian infants found greater weight, calf, and chest circumference beginning at 4 months and continuing through 12 months of age in the prenatal zinc supplemented group compared to the placebo group [82], the other two trials in Bangladesh and Indonesia did not find an impact on postnatal growth by 6 months of age [80, 81]. It may be that maternal prenatal supplementary zinc is prioritized toward the development of immunity rather than growth in the fetus. The impact of maternal zinc intake on infant and child postnatal health needs further investigation. Also, available evidence to date suggests that preventive zinc supplementation during pregnancy does not improve childhood cognitive or motor development [67].

In summary, the evidence of the impact of preventive zinc supplementation during pregnancy is less consistent than for preventive zinc supplementation of children. However, the benefit of prenatal zinc supplementation on reducing the risk of premature birth is important to consider, since prematurity is associated with an increased risk of neonatal and infant mortality and stunting [83, 84]. Thus, in areas at risk of zinc deficiency, maternal zinc supplementation should be considered.

Therapeutic Zinc Supplementation

WHO and UNICEF recommend that zinc supplementation should be included as a component in the treatment of all cases of diarrhea [85], by providing children 20 mg supplemental zinc per day for 10–14 days (10 mg per day for infants under 6 months old) along with oral rehydration salt solution and continued feeding. The aim is that the recommendations become routine practice both in the home and health-care facility and that caretakers will act quickly at the first sign of diarrhea. To distinguish between the preventive use of zinc supplementation and use of supplementary zinc in the treatment of diarrhea, the latter is commonly referred to as therapeutic zinc supplementation.

A recent meta-analysis of the impact of therapeutic zinc supplementation [86], which included 24 trials, confirmed previous meta-analyses of therapeutic zinc supplementation [87–93]. Therapeutic zinc supplementation shortens the duration of diarrhea by around 10 h (mean difference (MD) = −10.44 h; 95% CI: −21.13, 0.25) and probably reduces the number of children whose diarrhea persists until day 7 (RR = 0.73; 95% CI: 0.61, 0.88) [86]. However, the authors judged the evidence quality as low to moderate. The beneficial impact on both diarrhea outcomes mentioned above was limited to children older than 6 months of age. The authors also concluded that therapeutic zinc supplementation probably reduces the duration of persistent diarrhea (diarrhea lasting >14 days) by about 16 h (MD = −15.84 h; 95% CI: −25.43, −6.24), but that there was insufficient evidence from well-conducted trials on the impact of zinc supplementation during acute diarrhea on the risk of death or hospitalization [86].

Since the joint statement by WHO and UNICEF in 2004 [85], efforts are underway to reinforce national diarrhea programs and roll out therapeutic zinc supplementation provided in the form of dispersible tablets in many countries [94]. However, initial experiences encountered a number of challenges. In particular, it became evident that the scale up required a strong communication component to ensure that doctors, health-care workers, and pharmacists are informed about the benefits of zinc in the treatment of diarrhea [95]. Another important programmatic challenge is the low rate of care seeking for childhood diarrhea [96], as caregivers frequently fail to recognize children's diarrhea when illness signs are less severe [97]. Thus, continued efforts are needed to strengthen diarrhea control programs and ensure the inclusion of therapeutic zinc supplementation in the treatment of diarrhea [98].

Food Fortification with Zinc

Fortification is the practice of intentionally increasing the content of an essential micronutrient in a food, with the aim of improving the nutritional quality of the food and providing a public health benefit with minimal risk [99]. Food fortification is increasingly recognized as an effective approach to improve a population's micronutrient status, including zinc. There are different types of food fortification: foods fortified that are widely consumed by the general population (mass fortification); foods fortified for specific population subgroups, such as complementary foods for young children, therapeutic foods used in the treatment of malnutrition such as ready-to-use therapeutic foods (RUTF) and ready-to-use supplementary foods (RUSF), or rations for displaced populations (targeted fortification); and food fortified voluntarily by the manufacturers and available in the market place (market-driven fortification) [99].

The nutritional effect of zinc fortification can be assessed in several ways, namely, by measuring its impact on dietary zinc intake, total absorbed zinc, and biochemical and functional indicators of zinc status, among either individuals or populations who are exposed to zinc fortified foods [100]. Available absorption studies clearly show that zinc fortification can increase dietary zinc intake and total daily zinc absorption [101]. Most studies also indicate that adding zinc to food does not adversely affect the sensory properties of the food or the absorption of other micronutrients, such as iron. The results of available trials of milk products fortified with or without zinc suggest that zinc-fortified milk products appear to boost the zinc status of infants and young children and increase the growth of premature infants and malnourished children [101, 102]. In contrast, the impact of zinc-fortified cereal products on plasma zinc concentration is inconsistent. Several studies compared the provision of zinc in form of a supplement or added to food and found that a zinc dose given as a supplement increased plasma zinc concentration, whereas the same dose added to food did not [103–105]. This may be due to the reduced absorption when zinc is mixed with food or because zinc provided in food is metabolized differently from zinc supplements post-absorption. High-zinc intakes of 100–300 mg zinc/d over a long duration has been found to induce copper deficiency [106]. However, a meta-analysis investigating the effect of zinc fortification on hemoglobin and copper status found no negative effects [102]. There is insufficient information to determine whether zinc fortification of cereal products could enhance growth or reduce morbidity among individuals at risk for zinc deficiency because of the small number of available studies [101]. With regard to large-scale zinc fortification programs, a few rigorous evaluations of ongoing programs have been reported to date.

Although the impact of food fortification with zinc as a public health intervention remains unknown, WHO issued an interim consensus statement on the fortification of wheat and maize flour for national fortification programs with the rational that wheat and maize flour fortification is a preventive food-based approach to improve micronutrient status of populations over time that can be integrated with other interventions in the efforts to reduce vitamin and mineral deficiencies when identified as public health problems [107]. The recommended levels of zinc to consider adding to fortified wheat flour is based on extraction, fortificant compound, and estimated per capita flour consumption (for further details see [100]). In response to the above-mentioned WHO recommendations for wheat flour fortification, the eight-nation West African Economic and Monetary Union (UEMOA) drafted new guidelines and standards that mandate fortification of flour with iron and folic acid and allow voluntary fortification with zinc, vitamin B_{12} and other B vitamins [108]. Thus, the number of countries worldwide with either mandatory or voluntary zinc fortification of wheat flour is increasing [100].

In a recent review, de Pee [109] also proposed nutrients and nutrient levels for rice fortification, which can be achieved by mixing fortified with unfortified rice kernels. In regions where rice consumption is 150–300 g per capita per day, the addition of 6 mg zinc per 100 g rice is recommended in addition to iron, vitamin A, folic acid, niacin, and B vitamins [109].

Food fortification can also be targeted to a specific population group with high nutrient requirements. Various strategies for home fortification, or point-of-use fortification (POUF), have been developed to ensure adequate micronutrient intakes by infants and young children. These types of products include micronutrient powders, crushable tablets, and small-quantity lipid-based nutrient supplements, which are added to the complementary food at the time of consumption. To date, there is only inconsistent evidence that zinc fortified complementary foods or home fortification products can improve zinc status, as measured by biochemical or functional indicators [101, 110, 111]. This is the case even when zinc is added in amounts that are identical to the levels of zinc provided in supplements, as reviewed above. Whether this is due to the low bioavailability of zinc from cereal-based complementary foods (due to the high-phytate concentration) or to other reasons needs further investigation.

In summary, zinc fortification programs either at the national level or targeted toward vulnerable populations groups increases zinc intake as shown in absorption studies. Considering the absence of any adverse effects, and the relatively low cost of adding zinc to food, public health managers should consider including zinc in their planned mass and targeted food fortification programs [77, 101].

Dietary Diversification and Modification

Ensuring access to foods with adequate zinc content and good bioavailability is the most desirable approach to eliminate zinc deficiency. This strategy is typically referred to as dietary diversification and modification, which has the potential to prevent deficiencies of zinc and other micronutrients simultaneously. There are several main dietary strategies that can be used at the household level to enhance both the content and the bioavailability of zinc and other micronutrients. The best strategy for enhancing the zinc content of diets is to promote the consumption of meat, poultry and fish, all good sources of highly bioavailable zinc [112]. Potential approaches include increasing production and consumption of small livestock such as poultry, guinea fowl, rabbits, guinea pigs, and small ruminants. An advantage of this approach is that increased consumption of livestock will also simultaneously enhance intakes of heme iron, riboflavin, vitamin B_6, vitamin B_{12}, and, when liver is consumed, preformed vitamin A [113, 114]. The introduction of aquaculture can be another useful strategy to enhance the consumption of bioavailable zinc [115]. However, any effort of production or promotion of animal source foods through animal husbandry or aquaculture should be combined with behavior change communication to encourage consumption of the foods by those household members most at risk of zinc deficiency, namely young children and pregnant and lactating women [112].

Several household strategies can be used to reduce the phytate content of cereal- and legume-based foods, including soaking, fermentation, and germination. Soaking has been shown to remove about half of the phytate from maize and mung bean flour [115, 116]. Fermentation can induce phytate hydrolysis and germination can increase endogenous phytase activity in some cereals and legumes, both resulting in decreased inhibitory effects of phytate on zinc absorption [112]. Partial dephytinization at the industrial level can be achieved by milling or the addition of exogenous phytase enzymes [117]. In a recent review of phytate, iron, zinc, and calcium concentrations in plant-based complementary foods used in low-income countries, Gibson et al. [118] found that many indigenous and processed complementary foods had phytate: mineral molar ratios associated with poor mineral bioavailability. The authors proposed the use of the above mentioned strategies to reduce the phytate content, but recommended that additional strategies, including fortification of the complementary foods should be considered.

Promotion and support of appropriate breastfeeding practices should also be considered among the recommended dietary strategies to enhance the zinc status of infants and young children, for two reasons: breast milk is an important source of bioavailable zinc [14], and breastfeeding protects against diarrhea [119], which causes excessive zinc losses. As recommended by WHO, public health programs targeting young children should consider the promotion of the three key recommendations: (1) Early initiation of breastfeeding, (2) exclusive breastfeeding to 6 months, and (3) continued breastfeeding to 24 months or beyond [120].

Biofortification

Another promising approach to increase zinc intake through food is biofortification. Biofortification is an intervention strategy with the goal of increasing the content and/or bioavailability of selected micronutrients, including zinc, in the edible portion of staple food crops by selective breeding agronomic, or genetic modification techniques [121]. At present, efforts are ongoing to understand the translocation of zinc from soil to seed [122], and to develop and test different techniques to increase zinc content of some of the most important staple food crops including rice, wheat, pearl millet, and beans [123–125]. Other efforts focus on the reduction of the phytate content in the crops [126].

The absorption of zinc from some biofortified foods has also been assessed. In Bangladeshi preschool children, total zinc absorption, calculated as the product of zinc intake and fractional absorption, did not differ between the biofortified high-zinc rice cultivar and the conventional rice [127] and efforts are ongoing to breed another cultivar with higher zinc and/or lower phytate content. In contrast, a stable isotope study of biofortified pearl millet, which contained almost twice the amount of zinc compared to the conventional pearl millet, resulted in increased amounts of absorbed zinc compared to a conventional variety in preschool children in India [128].

Discussion Points

- What are the causes of zinc deficiency?
- Which population groups are most at risk of zinc deficiency and why?
- Which foods are good sources of zinc?
- How can the risk of zinc deficiency be assessed in a population?
- What intervention strategy(ies) is(are) the most suitable to prevent zinc deficiency among young children?
- What are the consequences of zinc deficiency for human health?

References

1. King J, Cousins R. Zinc. In: Shils MESM, Ross AC, Caballero B, Cousins RJ, editors. Modern nutrition in health and disease. 11th ed. Philadelphia: Lippincott Williams & Wilkins; 2014. p. 189–205.
2. Liuzzi JP, Cousins RJ. Mammalian zinc transporters. Annu Rev Nutr. 2004;24:151–72.
3. Black RE, Victora CG, Walker SP, Bhutta ZA, Christian P, de Onis M, et al. Maternal and child undernutrition and overweight in low-income and middle-income countries. Lancet. 2013;382(9890):427–51 Epub 2013/06/12.
4. Hess SY, Lönnerdal B, Hotz C, Rivera J, Brown KH. Recent advances in knowledge on zinc nutrition and human health. Food Nutr Bull. 2009;30(1):S5–11.
5. World Health Organization, Food and Agriculture Organization. Vitamin and mineral requirements in human nutrition. Report of a joint FAO/WHO expert consultation. Geneva, Switzerland: World Health Organization; 2004.

6. US Institute of Medicine. Dietary reference intakes for vitamin A, vitamin K, arsenic, boron, chromium, iodine, iron, manganese, molybdenum, nickel, silicon, vanadium, and zinc. Washington, DC: National Academy Press; 2001.
7. Brown KH, Rivera JA, Bhutta Z, Gibson RS, King JC, Lönnerdal B, et al. International Zinc Nutrition Consultative Group (IZiNCG) technical document #1. Assessment of the risk of zinc deficiency in populations and options for its control. Food Nutr Bull. 2004;25(1 Suppl 2):S99–203.
8. EFSA NDA Panel (EFSA panel on dietetic Products Nutrition and Allergies (NDA)). Scientific opinion on dietary reference values for zinc. EFSA J. 2014;12(10):3844–920.
9. King JC, Garza C. Harmonization of nutrient intake values. Food Nutr Bull. 2007;28(1 Suppl International):S3–12.
10. Gibson RS, Perlas L, Hotz C. Improving the bioavailability of nutrients in plant foods at the household level. Proc Nutr Soc. 2006;65(2):160–8 Epub 2006/05/05.
11. Iqbal TH, Lewis KO, Cooper BT. Phytase activity in the human and rat small intestine. Gut. 1994;35(9):1233–6 Epub 1994/09/01.
12. Miller LV, Krebs NF, Hambidge KM. A mathematical model of zinc absorption in humans as a function of dietary zinc and phytate. J Nutr. 2007;137(1):135–41.
13. International Zinc Nutrition Consultative Group (IZiNCG). Determining the prevalence of zinc deficiency: assessment of dietary zinc intake. IZiNCG technical brief no. 3. Davis, CA: University of California, 2007. Available at www.izincg.org.
14. Brown KH, Engle-Stone R, Krebs NF, Peerson JM. Dietary intervention strategies to enhance zinc nutrition: promotion and support of breastfeeding for infants and young children. Food Nutr Bull. 2009;30(1 Suppl):S144–71.
15. McClain CJ, McClain M, Barve S, Boosalis MG. Trace metals and the elderly. Clin Geriatr Med. 2002;18(4):801–18, vii–viii. Epub 2003/03/01.
16. Marcellini F, Giuli C, Papa R, Gagliardi C, Dedoussis G, Herbein G, et al. Zinc status, psychological and nutritional assessment in old people recruited in five European countries: zincage study. Biogerontology. 2006;7(5–6):339–45 Epub 2006/09/14.
17. Andriollo-Sanchez M, Hininger-Favier I, Meunier N, Toti E, Zaccaria M, Brandolini-Bunlon M, et al. Zinc intake and status in middle-aged and older European subjects: the ZENITH study. Eur J Clin Nutr. 2005;59(Suppl 2):S37–41 Epub 2005/10/29.
18. Castillo-Duran C, Vial P, Uauy R. Trace mineral balance during acute diarrhea in infants. J Pediatr. 1988;113(3):452–7.
19. Humphrey JH. Child undernutrition, tropical enteropathy, toilets, and handwashing. Lancet. 2009;374(9694):1032–5.
20. Lindenmayer GW, Stoltzfus RJ, Prendergast AJ. Interactions between zinc deficiency and environmental enteropathy in developing countries. Adv Nutr. 2014;5(1):1–6 Epub 2014/01/16.
21. Haghighi P, Wolf PL. Tropical sprue and subclinical enteropathy: a vision for the nineties. Crit Rev Clin Lab Sci. 1997;34(4):313–41.
22. de Benoist B, Darnton-Hill I, Davidsson L, Fontaine O, Hotz C. Conclusions of the joint WHO/UNICEF/IAEA/IZiNCG interagency meeting on zinc status indicators. Food Nutr Bull. 2007;28(3 Suppl):S480–4.
23. Lowe NM, Fekete K, Decsi T. Methods of assessment of zinc status in humans: a systematic review. Am J Clin Nutr. 2009;89(6):2040S–51S Epub 2009/05/08.
24. Hess SY, Peerson JM, King JC, Brown KH. Use of serum zinc concentration as an indicator of population zinc status. Food Nutr Bull. 2007;28(3 Suppl):S403–29.
25. Wessells KR, King JC, Brown KH. Development of a plasma zinc concentration cutoff to identify individuals with severe zinc deficiency based on results from adults undergoing experimental severe dietary zinc restriction and individuals with acrodermatitis enteropathica. J Nutr. 2014. Epub 2014/05/23.
26. Hambidge KM, Goodall MJ, Stall C, Pritts J. Post-prandial and daily changes in plasma zinc. J Trace Elem Electrolytes Health Dis. 1989;3(1):55–7.
27. King JC, Hambidge KM, Westcott JL, Kern DL, Marshall G. Daily variation in plasma zinc concentrations in women fed meals at six-hour intervals. J Nutr. 1994;124(4):508–16.
28. Hotz C, Peerson JM, Brown KH. Suggested lower cutoffs of serum zinc concentrations for assessing zinc status: reanalysis of the second National Health and Nutrition Examination Survey data (1976-1980). Am J Clin Nutr. 2003;78(4):756–64.
29. Thurnham DI, McCabe LD, Haldar S, Wieringa FT, Northrop Clewes CA, McCabe GP. Adjusting plasma ferritin concentrations to remove the effects of subclinical inflammation in the assessment of iron deficiency: a meta-analysis. Am J Clin Nutr. 2010;92(3):546–55 Epub 2010/07/09.

30. International Zinc Nutrition Consultative Group (IZiNCG). Assessing population zinc status with serum zinc concentration. IZiNCG technical brief no. 2. 2nd ed. Davis, CA: University of California, 2012. Available at: www.izincg.org.
31. International Zinc Nutrition Consultative Group (IZiNCG). Practical tips to collect blood in the field for assessment of zinc concentration. Davis, CA, USA: IZiNCG; 2012; Available from: http://izincg.org/publications/practical-tips.
32. Hotz C. Dietary indicators for assessing the adequacy of population zinc intakes. Food Nutr Bull. 2007;28(3 Suppl):S430–53.
33. Gibson RS. Principles of nutritional assessment. 2nd ed. New York: Oxford University Press; 2005.
34. Gibson RS, Ferguson EL. An interactive 24-hour recall for assessing the adequacy of iron and zinc intakes in developing countries. Washington, DC and Cali: International Food and Policy Research Institute (IFPRI) and International Center for Tropical Agriculture, 2008.
35. World Health Organization. Physical status: the use and interpretation of anthropometry. Technical Report Series No. 854. Geneva: World Health Organization, 1995.
36. World Health Organization. WHO growth standards: length/height-for-age, weight-for-age, weight-for-length, weight-for-height and body mass index-for-age: methods and development. Geneva: World Health Organization; 2006.
37. Engle-Stone R, Ndjebayi AO, Nankap M, Killilea DW, Brown KH. Stunting prevalence, plasma zinc concentrations, and dietary zinc intakes in a nationally representative sample suggest a high risk of zinc deficiency among women and young children in Cameroon123. J Nutr. 2014;144(3):382–91 Epub 2014/01/24.
38. Mwaniki DL, Omwega AM, Muniu EM, Mutunga JN, Akelola R, Shako BR, et al. Anaemia and status of iron, vitamin A and zinc in Kenya. The 1999 national survey. Nairobi, Kenya: Ministry of Health, 2002.
39. Wade S, Idohou-Dossou N, Diouf A, Seydi AB, Guiro AT, Sall MG, et al. Adjusting plasma zinc concentrations of ferritin, retinol, and zinc affect the prevalence of micronutrient deficiencies in children but not in women. Ann Nutr Metab. 2013;63(suppl 1):821.
40. Dhansay MA, Marais CD, Labadarios D. Zinc status. The national food consumption survey (NFCS): South Africa, 2005. Pretoria, South Africa: Directorate: Nutrition, Department of Health; 2007.
41. iccdr'b, UNICEF, GAIN, Institute of Public Health and Nutrition. National micronutrients status survey 2011–12. Dhaka, Bangladesh: icddr'b, 2013.
42. Laillou A, Pham TV, Tran NT, Le HT, Wieringa F, Rohner F, et al. Micronutrient deficits are still public health issues among women and young children in Vietnam. PLoS ONE. 2012;7(4):e34906. Epub 2012/04/25.
43. Martinez-Torres J, Ramirez-Velez R. Zinc deficiency and associated factors in colombian children; results from the 2010 national nutrition survey; a cross sectional study. Nutr Hosp. 2014;29(4):832–7 Epub 2014/04/01.
44. Villalpando S, Rivera J, de la Cruz V, A. G. Prevalence of zinc deficiency in Mexican children and women of childbearing age. Ann Nutr Metab. 2013;63(suppl 1):82.
45. Soofi S, Habib A, Bhutta ZA, Hussain I, Alam D. Evaluation of zinc status and community perceptions in Pakistan: the national nutrition survey 2011. Ann Nutr Metab. 2013;63(suppl 1):207.
46. Ministry of Health and Family, UNICEF Maldives, The Agha Khan University P. Project report. National micronutrient survey 2007, Republic of Maldives. Male', Republic of Maldives: Ministry of Health and Family, 2007.
47. Marcos J, Perlas L, Trio P, Ulanday J, Cheong R, Desnacido J, et al. 7th National nutrition survey, Philippines 2008: Serum zinc levels in selected Filipino population groups. Manila, The Philippines: Research and Development; 2008.
48. Thane CW, Bates CJ, Prentice A. Zinc and vitamin A intake and status in a national sample of British young people aged 4–18 y. Eur J Clin Nutr. 2004;58(2):363–75.
49. Bates B, Lennox A, Bates C, Swan G. National diet and nutrition survey. Headline results from years 1 and 2 (combined) of the rolling programme (2008/2009–2009/10). London, UK: Department of Health and Food Standards Agency, 2010.
50. Wessells KR, Brown KH. Estimating the global prevalence of zinc deficiency: results based on zinc availability in national food supplies and the prevalence of stunting. PLoS ONE. 2012;7(11):e50568. doi:10.1371/journal.pone.0050568.
51. Wessells KR, Singh GM, Brown KH. Estimating the global prevalence of inadequate zinc intake from national food balance sheets: effects of methodological assumptions. PLoS ONE. 2012;7(11):e50565. Epub 2012/12/05.
52. Prasad AS, Miale A Jr, Farid Z, Sandstead HH, Schulert AR. Zinc metabolism in patients with the syndrome of iron deficiency anemia, hepatosplenomegaly, dwarfism, and hypognadism. J Lab Clin Med. 1963;61:537–49.
53. Halsted JA, Ronaghy HA, Abadi P, Haghshenass M, Amirhakemi GH, Barakat RM, et al. Zinc deficiency in man. The Shiraz experiment. Am J Med. 1972;53(3):277–84.
54. Prasad AS. Discovery and importance of zinc in human nutrition. Fed Proc. 1984;43(13):2829–34.
55. Prasad AS. Zinc in human health: effect of zinc on immune cells. Mol Med. 2008;14(5–6):353–7 Epub 2008/04/04.

56. Sehgal VN, Jain S. Acrodermatitis enteropathica. Clin Dermatol. 2000;18(6):745–8 Epub 2001/02/15.
57. Wintergerst ES, Maggini S, Hornig DH. Contribution of selected vitamins and trace elements to immune function. Ann Nutr Metab. 2007;51(4):301–23 Epub 2007/08/30.
58. Ibs KH, Rink L. Zinc-altered immune function. J Nutr. 2003;133(5 Suppl 1):1452S–6S Epub 2003/05/06.
59. Cerasi M, Ammendola S, Battistoni A. Competition for zinc binding in the host-pathogen interaction. Front Cell Infect Microbiol. 2013;3:108 Epub 2014/01/09.
60. Kehl-Fie TE, Skaar EP. Nutritional immunity beyond iron: a role for manganese and zinc. Curr Opin Chem Biol. 2010;14(2):218–24 Epub 2009/12/18.
61. Berni Canani R, Buccigrossi V, Passariello A. Mechanisms of action of zinc in acute diarrhea. Curr Opin Gastroenterol. 2011;27(1):8–12. Epub 2010/09/22.
62. King JC. Determinants of maternal zinc status during pregnancy. Am J Clin Nutr. 2000;71(5 Suppl):1334S–43S Epub 2000/05/09.
63. Hess SY, King JC. Effects of maternal zinc supplementation on pregnancy and lactation outcomes. Food Nutr Bull. 2009;30(1 Suppl):S60–78.
64. Donangelo CM, King JC. Maternal zinc intakes and homeostatic adjustments during pregnancy and lactation. Nutrients. 2012;4(7):782–98 Epub 2012/08/02.
65. Black MM. The evidence linking zinc deficiency with children's cognitive and motor functioning. J Nutr. 2003;133(5 Suppl 1):1473S–6S.
66. Golub MS, Keen CL, Gershwin ME, Hendrickx AG. Developmental zinc deficiency and behavior. J Nutr. 1995;125(8 Suppl):2263S–71S Epub 1995/08/01.
67. Prado EL, Dewey KG. Nutrition and brain development in early life. Nutr Rev. 2014;72(4):267–84 Epub 2014/04/02.
68. Bhutta ZA, Das JK, Rizvi A, Gaffey MF, Walker N, Horton S, et al. Evidence-based interventions for improvement of maternal and child nutrition: what can be done and at what cost? Lancet. 2013;382(9890):452–77 Epub 2013/06/12.
69. Brown KH, Peerson JM, Baker SK, Hess SY. Preventive zinc supplementation among infants, preschoolers, and older prepubertal children. Food Nutr Bull. 2009;30(1 Suppl):S12–40.
70. Brown KH, Peerson JM, Rivera J, Allen LH. Effect of supplemental zinc on the growth and serum zinc concentrations of prepubertal children: a meta-analysis of randomized controlled trials. Am J Clin Nutr. 2002;75(6):1062–71.
71. Imdad A, Bhutta ZA. Effect of preventive zinc supplementation on linear growth in children under 5 years of age in developing countries: a meta-analysis of studies for input to the lives saved tool. BMC Public Health. 2011;11 Suppl 3:S22. Epub 2011/04/29.
72. Mayo-Wilson E, Junior JA, Imdad A, Dean S, Chan XH, Chan ES, et al. Zinc supplementation for preventing mortality, morbidity, and growth failure in children aged 6 months to 12 years of age. Cochrane Database Syst Rev. 2014;5:CD009384. Epub 2014/05/16.
73. Aggarwal R, Sentz J, Miller MA. Role of zinc administration in prevention of childhood diarrhea and respiratory illnesses: a meta-analysis. Pediatrics. 2007;119(6):1120–30.
74. Yakoob MY, Theodoratou E, Jabeen A, Imdad A, Eisele TP, Ferguson J, et al. Preventive zinc supplementation in developing countries: impact on mortality and morbidity due to diarrhea, pneumonia and malaria. BMC Public Health. 2011;11 Suppl 3:S23. Epub 2011/04/29.
75. Roth DE, Richard SA, Black RE. Zinc supplementation for the prevention of acute lower respiratory infection in children in developing countries: meta-analysis and meta-regression of randomized trials. Int J Epidemiol. 2010;39(3):795–808 Epub 2010/02/17.
76. Gulani A, Sachdev HS. Zinc supplements for preventing otitis media. Cochrane Database Syst Rev. 2014;6:CD006639. Epub 2014/06/30.
77. Brown KH, Baker SK, IZiNCG Steering Committee. Galvanizing action: conclusions and next steps for mainstreaming zinc interventions in public health programs. Food Nutr Bull. 2009;30(1 Suppl):S179–84.
78. Chaffee BW, King JC. Effect of zinc supplementation on pregnancy and infant outcomes: a systematic review. Paediatr Perinat Epidemiol. 2012;26(Suppl 1):118–37 Epub 2012/07/07.
79. Mori R, Ota E, Middleton P, Tobe-Gai R, Mahomed K, Bhutta ZA. Zinc supplementation for improving pregnancy and infant outcome. Cochrane Database Syst Rev. 2012;7:CD000230. Epub 2012/07/13.
80. Osendarp SJ, van Raaij JM, Darmstadt GL, Baqui AH, Hautvast JG, Fuchs GJ. Zinc supplementation during pregnancy and effects on growth and morbidity in low birthweight infants: a randomised placebo controlled trial. Lancet. 2001;357(9262):1080–5.
81. Wieringa FT, Dijkhuizen MA, Muhilal, Van der Meer JW. Maternal micronutrient supplementation with zinc and beta-carotene affects morbidity and immune function of infants during the first 6 months of life. Eur J Clin Nutr. 2010;64(10):1072–9 Epub 2010/08/05.
82. Iannotti LL, Zavaleta N, Leon Z, Huasquiche C, Shankar AH, Caulfield LE. Maternal zinc supplementation reduces diarrheal morbidity in Peruvian infants. J Pediatr. 2010;156(6):960-4, 4 e1-2. Epub 2010/03/17.

83. Katz J, Lee AC, Kozuki N, Lawn JE, Cousens S, Blencowe H, et al. Mortality risk in preterm and small-for-gestational-age infants in low-income and middle-income countries: a pooled country analysis. Lancet. 2013;382(9890):417–25 Epub 2013/06/12.

84. Christian P, Lee SE, Donahue Angel M, Adair LS, Arifeen SE, Ashorn P, et al. Risk of childhood undernutrition related to small-for-gestational age and preterm birth in low- and middle-income countries. Int J Epidemiol. 2013;42(5):1340–55 Epub 2013/08/08.

85. World Health Organization, UNICEF. Clinical management of acute diarrhoea. Geneva: WHO/Unicef joint statement. WHO/FCH/CAH/04.7, 2004 WHO/FCH/CAH/04.7.

86. Lazzerini M, Ronfani L. Oral zinc for treating diarrhoea in children. Cochrane Database Syst Rev. 2013;1: CD005436. Epub 2013/02/27.

87. The Zinc Investigator's Collaborative Group, Bhutta ZA, Bird SM, Black RE, Brown KH, Gardner JM, et al. Therapeutic effects of oral zinc in acute and persistent diarrhea in children in developing countries: pooled analysis of randomized controlled trials. Am J Clin Nutr. 2000;72(6):1516–22.

88. Lazzerini M, Ronfani L. Oral zinc for treating diarrhoea in children. Cochrane Database Syst Rev. 2008(3): CD005436.

89. Lukacik M, Thomas RL, Aranda JV. A meta-analysis of the effects of oral zinc in the treatment of acute and persistent diarrhea. Pediatrics. 2008;121(2):326–36.

90. Patro B, Golicki D, Szajewska H. Meta-analysis: zinc supplementation for acute gastroenteritis in children. Aliment Pharmacol Ther. 2008.

91. Haider BA, Bhutta ZA. The effect of therapeutic zinc supplementation among young children with selected infections: a review of the evidence. Food Nutr Bull. 2009;30(1 Suppl):S41–59.

92. Patel A, Mamtani M, Dibley MJ, Badhoniya N, Kulkarni H. Therapeutic value of zinc supplementation in acute and persistent diarrhea: a systematic review. PLoS ONE. 2010;5(4):e10386. Epub 2010/05/06.

93. Lamberti LM, Walker CL, Chan KY, Jian WY, Black RE. Oral zinc supplementation for the treatment of acute diarrhea in children: a systematic review and meta-analysis. Nutrients. 2013;5(11):4715–40 Epub 2013/11/29.

94. Santosham M, Chandran A, Fitzwater S, Fischer-Walker C, Baqui AH, Black R. Progress and barriers for the control of diarrhoeal disease. Lancet. 2010;376(9734):63–7 Epub 2010/07/09.

95. Fischer Walker CL, Fontaine O, Young MW, Black RE. Zinc and low osmolarity oral rehydration salts for diarrhoea: a renewed call to action. Bull World Health Organ. 2009;87(10):780–6.

96. Nasrin D, Wu Y, Blackwelder WC, Farag TH, Saha D, Sow SO, et al. Health care seeking for childhood diarrhea in developing countries: evidence from seven sites in Africa and Asia. Am J Trop Med Hyg. 2013;89(1 Suppl):3–12 Epub 2013/05/01.

97. Wilson SE, Ouedraogo CT, Prince L, Ouedraogo A, Hess SY, Rouamba N, et al. Caregiver recognition of childhood diarrhea, care seeking behaviors and home treatment practices in rural Burkina Faso: a cross-sectional survey. PLoS ONE. 2012;7(3):e33273. Epub 2012/03/20.

98. Baker S, Breyne C, Brown KH, Coulibaly-Zerbo F, David P, Diop M, et al. The way forward: repositioning children's right to adequate nutrition in the Sahel. Matern Child Nutr. 2011;7:182–5.

99. World Health Organization, Food and Agriculture Organization. Guidelines on food fortification with micronutrients. Edited by Allen L, Benoist de B, Dary O, Hurrell RF. Geneva: World Health Organization; 2006.

100. Brown KH, Hambidge KM, Ranum P. Zinc fortification of cereal flours: current recommendations and research needs. Food Nutr Bull. 2010;31(1 Suppl):S62–74 Epub 2010/07/16.

101. Hess SY, Brown KH. Impact of zinc fortification on zinc nutrition. Food Nutr Bull. 2009;30(1 Suppl):S79–107.

102. Das JK, Kumar R, Salam RA, Bhutta ZA. Systematic review of zinc fortification trials. Ann Nutr Metab. 2013;62 (Suppl 1):44–56 Epub 2013/05/25.

103. Brown KH, López de Romaña D, Arsenault JE, Peerson JM, Penny ME. Comparison of the effects of zinc delivered in a fortified food or a liquid supplement on the growth, morbidity, and plasma zinc concentrations of young Peruvian children. Am J Clin Nutr. 2007;85(2):538–47.

104. Aaron GJ, Ba Lo N, Hess SY, Guiro AT, Wade S, Brown KH. Plasma zinc concentration increases within 2 weeks in healthy Senegalese men given liquid supplemental zinc, but not zinc-fortified wheat bread. J Nutr. 2011;141:1369–74. Epub 2011/05/13.

105. Ba Lo N, Aaron GJ, Hess SY, Idohou-Dossou N, Guiro AT, Wade S, et al. Plasma zinc concentration responds to short-term zinc supplementation, but not zinc fortification, in young children in Senegal1,2. Am J Clin Nutr. 2011;93(6):1348–55. Epub 2011/04/15.

106. Prasad AS, Brewer GJ, Schoomaker EB, Rabbani P. Hypocupremia induced by zinc therapy in adults. JAMA. 1978;240(20):2166–8.

107. World Health Organization. Recommendations on wheat and maize flour fortification. Meeting report: Interim consensus statement. Geneva, Switzerland: World Health Organization, 2009.

108. Hess SY, Brown KH, Sablah M, Engle-Stone R, Aaron GJ, Baker SK. Results of fortification rapid assessment tool (FRAT) surveys in sub-Saharan Africa and suggestions for future modifications of the survey instrument. Food Nutr Bull. 2013;34(1):21–38 Epub 2013/06/19.

109. de Pee S. Proposing nutrients and nutrient levels for rice fortification. Ann N Y Acad Sci. 2014;1324:55–66.
110. Hess SY, Abbeddou S, Jimenez EY, Some JW, Vosti SA, Ouedraogo ZP, et al. Small-quantity lipid-based nutrient supplements, regardless of their zinc content, increase growth and reduce the prevalence of stunting and wasting in young burkinabe children: a cluster-randomized trial. PLoS ONE. 2015;10(3):e0122242.
111. Salam RA, Macphail C, Das JK, Bhutta ZA. Effectiveness of micronutrient powders (MNP) in women and children. BMC Public Health. 2013;13 Suppl 3:S22. Epub 2014/02/26.
112. Gibson RS, Anderson VP. A review of interventions based on dietary diversification or modification strategies with the potential to enhance intakes of total and absorbable zinc. Food Nutr Bull. 2009;30(1 Suppl):S108–43.
113. International Zinc Nutrition Consultative Group (IZiNCG). Preventing zinc deficiency through diet diversification and modification. IZiNCG technical brief no. 5 Davis, CA: University of California, 2007. Available at www.izincg.org.
114. Allen LH. Global dietary patterns and diets in childhood: implications for health outcomes. Ann Nutr Metab. 2012;61(Suppl 1):29–37 Epub 2013/02/21.
115. Gibson RS, Hotz C. Dietary diversification/modification strategies to enhance micronutrient content and bioavailability of diets in developing countries. Br J Nutr. 2001;85(Suppl 2):S159–66.
116. Perlas LA, Gibson RS. Household dietary strategies to enhance the content and bioavailability of iron, zinc and calcium of selected rice- and maize-based Philippine complementary foods. Matern Child Nutr. 2005;1(4):263–73 Epub 2006/08/03.
117. Troesch B, Egli I, Zeder C, Hurrell RF, de Pee S, Zimmermann MB. Optimization of a phytase-containing micronutrient powder with low amounts of highly bioavailable iron for in-home fortification of complementary foods. Am J Clin Nutr. 2009;89(2):539–44.
118. Gibson RS, Bailey KB, Gibbs M, Ferguson EL. A review of phytate, iron, zinc, and calcium concentrations in plant-based complementary foods used in low-income countries and implications for bioavailability. Food Nutr Bull. 2010;31(2 Suppl):S134–46 Epub 2010/08/19.
119. Horta B, Victora C. Short-term effects of breastfeeding: a systematic review on the benefits of breastfeeding on diarrhoea and pneumonia mortality. Geneva, Switzerland: World Health Organization; 2013.
120. World Health Organization. Optimal duration of breast feeding. Report of an expert consultation. Geneva, Switzerland: World Health Organization, 2002 Contract No.: WHO/ NHD/ 01.09.
121. Hotz C. The potential to improve zinc status through biofortification of staple food crops with zinc. Food Nutr Bull. 2009;30(1 Suppl):S172–8.
122. Olsen LI, Palmgren MG. Many rivers to cross: the journey of zinc from soil to seed. Front Plant Sci. 2014;5:30 Epub 2014/02/28.
123. Blair MW. Mineral biofortification strategies for food staples: the example of common bean. J Agric Food Chem. 2013;61(35):8287–94 Epub 2013/07/16.
124. Cakmak I. Enrichment of fertilizers with zinc: an excellent investment for humanity and crop production in India. J Trace Elem Med Biol. 2009;23(4):281–9 Epub 2009/09/15.
125. Cakmak I, Kalayci M, Kaya Y, Torun AA, Aydin N, Wang Y, et al. Biofortification and localization of zinc in wheat grain. J Agric Food Chem. 2010;58(16):9092–102 Epub 2010/08/25.
126. Aluru MR, Rodermel SR, Reddy MB. Genetic modification of low phytic acid 1-1 maize to enhance iron content and bioavailability. J Agric Food Chem. 2011;59(24):12954–62.
127. Islam MM, Woodhouse LR, Hossain MB, Ahmed T, Huda MN, Ahmed T, et al. Total zinc absorption from a diet containing either conventional rice or higher-zinc rice does not differ among Bangladeshi preschool children. J Nutr. 2013;143(4):519–25 Epub 2013/02/22.
128. Kodkany BS, Bellad RM, Mahantshetti NS, Westcott JE, Krebs NF, Kemp JF, et al. Biofortification of pearl millet with iron and zinc in a randomized controlled trial increases absorption of these minerals above physiologic requirements in young children. J Nutr. 2013;143(9):1489–93 Epub 2013/07/12.

Chapter 12
Iodine

Michael B. Zimmermann

Keywords Iodine · Iodine deficiency · Thyroid · Goiter · Cretinism · Hyperthyroidism · Hypothyroidism · Iodized salt · Iodized oil

Learning Objectives

- Describe the epidemiology of iodine nutrition on the global and regional level.
- Compare the methods that can be used to determine the prevalence of iodine deficiency and how they may be best utilized during different stages of the life cycle.
- Justify a strategy that can be used to prevent and treat childhood iodine deficiency in low-income countries.
- Explain three strategies that can be used to prevent and treat iodine deficiency during pregnancy.

Introduction

Iodine is an essential component of hormones produced by the thyroid gland. Thyroid hormones, and therefore iodine, are essential for mammalian life. Optimal dietary iodine intakes for healthy adults are 150–250 µg/day. In regions where iodine in soils and drinking water is low, humans and animals may become iodine deficient. Iodine deficiency has multiple adverse effects in humans due to inadequate thyroid hormone production that are termed the iodine deficiency disorders (IDD). Iodine deficiency during pregnancy and infancy may impair growth and neurodevelopment of the offspring and increase infant mortality. Deficiency during childhood reduces somatic growth and cognitive and motor function. Mild-to-moderate iodine deficiency in adults results in more toxic nodular goiter and an increase in hyperthyroidism in the population. Correcting iodine deficiency in adult populations may shift thyroid cancer subtypes toward less malignant forms. Overall, iodine deficiency produces subtle but widespread adverse effects in individuals, including decreased educability, apathy, and reduced work productivity. Because in iodine deficient regions most of the population is affected, this results in impaired social and economic development. Assessment of iodine status includes

M.B. Zimmermann (✉)
Department of Health Sciences and Technology, ETH Zurich, Schmelzbergstrasse 7,K LFVD20,
ETH Zentrum, Zurich 8092, Switzerland
e-mail: michael.zimmermann@hest.ethz.ch

© Springer Science+Business Media New York 2017
S. de Pee et al. (eds.), *Nutrition and Health in a Developing World*,
Nutrition and Health, DOI 10.1007/978-3-319-43739-2_12

measurement of urinary iodine concentration, goiter, newborn TSH, and blood thyroglobulin. In most countries, the best strategy to control iodine deficiency in populations is iodization of salt, one of the most cost-effective ways to contribute to economic and social development.

Ecology and Dietary Sources, Absorption, Metabolism, and Excretion

Iodine (as iodide) is widely but unevenly distributed in the earth's environment. In many regions, over millions of years, leaching from glaciation, flooding, and erosion have depleted surface soils of iodide, and most iodide is found in the oceans. The concentration of iodide in sea water is ≈50 µg/L. Iodide ions in seawater are oxidized to elemental iodine, which volatilizes into the atmosphere and is returned to the soil by rain, completing the cycle [1]. However, iodine cycling in many regions is slow and incomplete, leaving soils and drinking water iodine depleted. Crops grown in these soils will be low in iodine, and humans and animals consuming food grown in these soils become iodine deficient. Iodine deficient soils are common in mountainous areas because of glaciation and areas of frequent flooding. Iodine deficiency in populations residing in these areas will persist until iodine enters the food chain through addition of iodine to foods (e.g. iodization of salt) or dietary diversification introduces foods produced outside the iodine deficient area.

The native iodine content of most foods and beverages is low. In general, commonly consumed foods provide 3–80 µg per serving [2, 3]. Foods of marine origin have higher iodine content because marine plants and animals concentrate iodine from seawater. Iodine in organic form occurs in high amounts in certain seaweeds. Major dietary sources of iodine are iodized salt, bread (made with iodized salt), marine fish, and milk and milk products [2, 3]. Although milk and milk products typically contain low amounts of native iodine, iodophors used by the dairy industry for cleaning milk cans and teats and iodine supplements given to cows often increase the iodine content of dairy products. Less frequently, iodine content in foods is also influenced by iodine-containing compounds used in irrigation, fertilizers, and livestock feed.

Iodine is ingested in several chemical forms. Iodine compounds in foods and iodate used in salt iodization are rapidly reduced to iodide in the gut and nearly completely absorbed in the stomach and duodenum. Iodate is widely used in salt iodization because it is more stable than iodide in the presence of moisture and impurities. In healthy adults, the absorption of iodide is >90% [4]. Iodine deficiency is the main cause of endemic goiter (see below), but other dietary substances that interfere with thyroid metabolism can aggravate the effect, and they are termed goitrogens [5]. They are found in cassava, millet, sweet potato, beans, and crucifera vegetables (e.g., cabbage). Most of these substances do not have a major effect on thyroid function unless there is coexisting iodine deficiency. Deficiencies of selenium, iron, and vitamin A can also exacerbate the effects of iodine deficiency [6].

The body of a healthy adult contains 15–20 mg of iodine, of which 70–80% is in the thyroid. In chronic iodine deficiency, the iodine content of the thyroid may fall to <20 µg. In iodine sufficient areas, the adult thyroid traps 50–60 µg of iodine/day to balance losses and maintain thyroid hormone synthesis. A sodium–iodide symporter (NIS) in the basolateral membrane transfers iodide into the thyroid at a concentration gradient 20–50 times that of plasma [7]. Iodine comprises 65 and 59% of the weights of thyroxine (T4) and triiodothyronine (T3), respectively. In target tissues, such as liver, kidney, heart, muscle, pituitary, and the developing brain, T4 is deiodinated to T3. T3 is the main physiologically active form of thyroid hormone. Thyroid hormone regulates a variety of physiologic processes, including reproductive function, growth, and development. More than 90% of ingested iodine is ultimately excreted in the urine, with only small amounts appearing in the feces.

The Effects of Deficiency

Iodine deficiency has multiple adverse effects on growth and development in animals and humans. These are collectively termed the IDD (Table 12.1), and are one of the most important and common human diseases [8]. They result from inadequate thyroid hormone production due to lack of sufficient iodine.

Thyroid enlargement (goiter) is the classic sign of iodine deficiency. It is a physiologic adaptation to chronic iodine deficiency. As iodine intake falls, secretion of thyrotropin (TSH) increases in an effort to maximize uptake of available iodine, and TSH stimulates thyroid hypertrophy and hyperplasia. Initially, goiters are characterized by diffuse, homogeneous enlargement, but over time, thyroid follicles may fuse and become encapsulated, a condition termed nodular goiter. Large goiters may be cosmetically unattractive, can obstruct the trachea and esophagus, and may damage the recurrent laryngeal nerves and cause hoarseness.

Effects on Pregnancy and Infancy

Although goiter is the most visible effect of iodine deficiency, the most serious adverse effect is damage to the developing central nervous system of the fetus if women are iodine deficient during pregnancy. Normal levels of thyroid hormones are required for neuronal migration, glial differentiation, and myelination of the central nervous system [9]. Because ID continues to affect large populations, particularly in Africa and South Asia [8], it is an important preventable cause of cognitive impairment. Two systematic reviews have highlighted the benefits of correcting iodine deficiency. The first looked at 89 studies that provided iodized salt to populations and found a significant 72–76% reduction in risk for low intelligence (defined as IQ < 70) and an 8.2–10.5 point overall increase in IQ [10]. A previous smaller review also found IQ was 10–13 points lower in moderate-to-severely iodine deficient populations compared to iodine sufficient populations [11]. Severe iodine deficiency during pregnancy is associated with a greater incidence of stillbirths, abortions, and congenital abnormalities. Iodine prophylaxis with iodized oil in pregnant women in areas of severe deficiency reduces fetal and perinatal mortality [12]. The most severe form of

Table 12.1 The iodine deficiency disorders, by age group

Age groups	Health consequences of iodine deficiency
All ages	Goiter
	Increased susceptibility of the thyroid gland to nuclear radiation
Fetus	Abortion
	Stillbirth
	Congenital anomalies
	Perinatal mortality
Neonate	Infant mortality
	Endemic cretinism
Child and adolescent	Impaired mental function
	Delayed physical development
Adults	Impaired mental function
	Reduced work productivity
	Toxic nodular goiter; iodine-induced hyperthyroidism
	Hypothyroidism in moderate-to-severe iodine deficiency

neurological damage from fetal hypothyroidism is called cretinism. It is characterized by gross mental retardation along with varying degrees of short stature, deaf mutism, and spasticity [13]. Two distinct types have been described. The more common, neurologic cretinism has specific neurologic deficits that include spastic quadriplegia with sparing of the distal extremities. The myxedematous form is seen most frequently in central Africa, and has the predominant finding of profound hypothyroidism, with thyroid atrophy and fibrosis [13]. Up to 10% of people in populations with severe iodine deficiency may be cretinous.

Effects in Childhood

Whether mild-to-moderate ID in children has adverse effects has long been debated. Several older randomized, controlled trials in school-aged children have tried to measure the effect of iodized oil on cognition; three of the studies found no effect [14–16] and one found cognition improved with treatment [17]. However, two of the studies were confounded by a significant improvement in iodine status in the control group [14, 17], while in the other two, the treated group remained iodine deficient at retesting [15, 16]. Two more recent randomized, placebo controlled, double-blind intervention trials in mild-to-moderately deficient school-aged children have shown clear benefits of iodine on cognitive and motor function [18, 19]. Moderately iodine deficient 10–12-years-old children ($n = 310$) in Albania were randomized to receive either 400 mg of iodine as oral iodized oil or placebo [18]. Compared to placebo, iodine treatment significantly improved performance on tests of information processing, fine motor skills, and visual problem solving. The second placebo-controlled, double-blind trial was conducted in mildly iodine deficient New Zealand school-aged children ($n = 184$) randomly assigned to receive 150 μg iodine daily or placebo for 28 week [19]. The overall cognitive score of the iodine-supplemented group was 0.19 SDs higher than that of the placebo group ($P = 0.011$).

A recent systematic review [20] examined the effects of iodine supplementation and/or status on mental development of children ≤5 years. Organized by study design, average effect sizes were: (a) 0.68 (2 randomized controlled trials with iodine supplementation of mothers); (b) 0.46 (8 non-randomized trials with iodine supplementation of mothers and/or infants); (c) 0.52 (9 prospective cohort studies stratified by mothers' iodine status); and (d) 0.54 (4 cohort stratified by infants' iodine status). Overall, this translated into 6.9–10.2 lower IQ points in iodine deficient children compared with iodine-replete children [20]. Thus, the available data, although limited, suggest ID of mild-to-moderate severity in school-age children and in children ≤5 years has adverse effects on cognitive/motor performance and likely prevents children from attaining their full intellectual potential. The intellectual deficits caused by iodine deficiency during pregnancy and childhood can be entirely prevented by adequate iodine intake.

Effects in Adults

Iodine status is also a key determinant of thyroid disorders in adults [21]. Severe iodine deficiency causes goiter and hypothyroidism because, despite an increase in thyroid activity to maximize iodine uptake and recycling, there is simply not enough iodine to produce thyroid hormone. In mild-to-moderate iodine deficiency, increasing thyroid activity can compensate for deficient intake and maintain euthyroidism in most individuals, but at a price: chronic thyroid stimulation results in more frequent formation of autonomous nodules in goiters that overproduce thyroid hormone (called toxic nodular goiters), and this results in an increase in hyperthyroidism in the population [22]. This high prevalence of nodular autonomy usually results in a further increase in hyperthyroidism if iodine intakes are increased by salt iodisation. But this is transient because iodine sufficiency normalizes thyroid activity and this will, in the long term, reduce nodular autonomy [23]. Variations in population iodine intake do not affect risk for Graves' disease or thyroid cancer, and correcting iodine deficiency may shift thyroid cancer subtypes toward less malignant forms [21].

Requirements and Prevalence of Iodine Deficiency Worldwide

The U.S. Food and Nutrition Board of the National Academy of Sciences has set an Adequate Intake (AI) for iodine in infancy and a Recommended Dietary Allowance (RDA) for children, adults, and pregnant and lactating women [4] (Table 12.2). The WHO has established recommended nutrient intakes for iodine [8] (Table 12.2).

Several methods are available for assessment of iodine nutrition [13]. The most commonly used are measurement of thyroid size and concentration of urinary iodine [8]. Additional indicators include newborn TSH, and blood concentrations of thyroglobulin, T4 or T3. Urinary iodine concentration is a sensitive indicator of recent iodine intake (days) and serum thyroglobulin shows an intermediate response (weeks to months), whereas changes in the goiter rate reflects long-term iodine nutrition (months to years).

Until 1990, only a few countries: Switzerland, some of the Scandinavian countries, Australia, the U.S. and Canada were completely iodine sufficient based on adequate urinary iodine concentrations in their populations. Since then, globally, the number of households using iodized salt has risen from <20% to >70%, dramatically reducing iodine deficiency [8]. This effort has been achieved by a coalition of international organizations, including WHO, the International Council for the Control of Iodine Deficiency Disorders (renamed the Iodine Global Network in 2014), the Global Alliance for Improved Nutrition (GAIN), the Micronutrient Initiative and UNICEF, working closely with national IDD control committees and the salt industry; this informal partnership was established after the World Summit for Children in 1990.

The two most commonly used approaches to assessing iodine nutrition at population level are estimation of the household penetration of adequately iodized salt (HHIS) and measurement of urinary iodine concentrations (UICs) [8]. UIC surveys are usually done in school-aged children, because they are a convenient population, easy to reach through school based surveys, and usually representative of the general population. Therefore, the WHO recommends the use of UICs from 6 to 12 years-old children in nationally representative surveys, expressed as the median in µg/L, to classify a population's iodine status [8] (Table 12.3). More countries are beginning to carry out studies in high-risk population groups, i.e., women of reproductive age, pregnant women and younger children;

Table 12.2 Recommendations for iodine intake (µg/day) by age or population group

Age or population group	U.S. Institute of Medicine [4]		Age or population group	World Health Organization [8]
	EAR	AI or RDA		RNI
Infants 0–12 months	–	110–130	Children 0–5 years	90
Children 1-8 years	65	90	Children 6-12 years	120
Children 9–13 years	73	120		
Adults ≥ 14 years	95	150	Adults > 12 years	150
Pregnancy	160	220	Pregnancy	250
Lactation	200	290	Lactation	250

EAR Estimated Average Requirement; *AI* Adequate Intake; *RDA* Recommended Daily Allowance; *RNI* Recommended Nutrient Intake

Table 12.3 Epidemiological criteria from the World Health Organization for assessment of iodine nutrition in a population based on median or range of urinary iodine concentrations [8]

	Iodine intake	Iodine nutrition
School-aged children		
<20 µg/L	Insufficient	Severe iodine deficiency
20–49 µg/L	Insufficient	Moderate iodine deficiency
50–99 µg/L	Insufficient	Mild iodine deficiency
100–199 µg/L	Adequate	Optimum
200–299 µg/L	More than adequate	Risk of iodine-induced hyperthyroidism in susceptible groups
>300 µg/L	Excessive	Risk of adverse health consequences (iodine-induced hyperthyroidism, autoimmune thyroid disease)
Pregnant women		
<150 µg/L	Insufficient	
150–249 µg/L	Adequate	
250-499 µg/L	More than adequate	
≥500 µg/L[a]	Excessive	
Lactating women[b]		
<100 µg/L	Insufficient	
≥100 µg/L	Adequate	
Children less than 2 years of age		
<100 µg/L	Insufficient	
≥100 µg/L	Adequate	

[a]The term excessive means in excess of the amount needed to prevent and control iodine deficiency
[b]In lactating women, the numbers for median urinary iodine are lower than the iodine requirements, because of the iodine excreted in breast milk

however, data is limited and the majority of countries still conduct routine iodine monitoring in children.

Currently, nationally representative UIC surveys are available for 117 countries, including low-, middle- and high-income countries, and for 33 countries, subnational surveys are available [24]. There are no UIC data available for 43 countries, but the majority of these have small populations. Available UIC data now cover 97.4% of the world's population of SAC. Classified by iodine nutrition according to degree of public health importance based on the median UIC, iodine intake is inadequate in 32 countries, adequate in 71, more than adequate in 36, and excessive in 11. Of the 32 countries with iodine deficiency, nine are classified as moderately deficient, 23 as mildly deficient and none as severely deficient [24]. Based on the current estimates, the iodine intake of 30.0%, or 246.2 million of SAC worldwide is insufficient (Table 12.4). Over one-half of the children with low intakes are in two regions: 78 million children in Southeast Asia and 58 million children in Africa. The smallest proportions with low intakes are in the Americas (13.7%) and the Western Pacific (19.8%), while the greatest proportions of children with inadequate iodine intake are in European (43.9%) and the African (39.5%) regions [24]. Inferring from the proportion of SAC to the general population, 1.92 billion people globally have inadequate iodine intakes.

Although all European countries endorsed the goal of eliminating iodine deficiency at the 1992 World Health Assembly, control of iodine deficiency has received low priority in much of Europe. As mentioned above, over the past decade, compared to other WHO regions, Europe has had the largest percentage of iodine deficient school-age children, as well as the lowest household coverage by iodized salt, despite its relative wealth and high standard of health care [24]. Why? Many European governments still equate iodine deficiency with visible goiter, a historical problem and thus a low priority, and may be unaware of the adverse effects of more subtle iodine deficiency on brain

Table 12.4 Number of countries, proportion of population, and number of individuals with insufficient iodine intake in school-aged children and in the general population, by WHO region, 2012 [24]

WHO region[2]	Insufficient iodine intake (urinary iodine concentration <100 µg/L)				
	Countries (n)	Children 6–12 years-old	Total n (millions)	General population	
		Proportion (%)		Proportion (%)	Total n (millions)
Africa	10	39.5	58.1	40.1	322.2
Americas	2	13.7	14.6	13.7	125.7
Eastern Mediterranean	4	38.6	30.7	37.4	199.2
Europe	11	43.9	30.5	44.2	393.1
Southeast Asia	0	31.9	78.4	31.7	565.3
Western Pacific	5	19.8	33.9	17.9	319.4
Global total	32	29.8	246.2	28.7	1924.9

Based on the 193 WHO Member States, and United Nations population estimates in the year 2010

development. In Europe, an increasingly smaller amount of salt is consumed as discretionary salt added at home: thus, it is crucial that salt in processed foods be iodized, but legislation in most countries does not cover the food industry. Moreover, legislation on use of iodized salt in foods, where enacted, varies from country to country, and these differences limit the marketing of common processed foods containing iodized salt across all countries in Europe.

Data on household coverage with iodized salt is available for 128 out of 196 UNICEF member states, most of which are low-income countries. Adequately iodized household salt is defined as salt that contains at least 15 ppm, measured quantitatively by titration. Out of 128 countries with data, 37 countries have salt iodization coverage that meets the international goal of at least 90% of households consuming adequately iodized salt [24]. Fifty-two countries have coverage rates of between 50 and 89%, and 39 countries have coverage rates of <50%. Overall, approximately 70% of households worldwide have access to adequately iodized salt [24]. Those with the greatest access are living in the WHO regions of the Western Pacific and the Americas, and those with the least access are residing in the Eastern Mediterranean region.

Prophylaxis and Treatment

There are two methods commonly used to correct iodine deficiency in a population: iodized oil and iodized salt. In nearly all regions affected by iodine deficiency, the most effective way to control iodine deficiency is through salt iodization [13]. All salt for human consumption, including salt used in the food industry, should be continuously iodized. In Switzerland, previously affected by endemic goiter and cretinism, a monitored national salt iodization program, in place for over half a century, has effectively eliminated iodine deficiency. Iodine can be added to salt in the form of potassium iodide (KI) or potassium iodate (KIO3). Because KIO3 has higher stability in the presence of salt impurities, humidity, and porous packaging, it is the recommended form [8]. Iodine is usually added at a level of 20–40 mg iodine/kg salt, considering per capita salt intakes of 5–10 g per day in the target population. But in industrialized countries, because ca. 90% of salt consumption is from purchased processed foods, if only household salt is iodized it will not supply adequate iodine. Thus, it is critical that the food industry use iodized salt. The current push to reduce salt consumption to prevent chronic diseases and the policy of salt iodization to eliminate iodine deficiency do not conflict: iodization methods can fortify salt to provide recommended iodine intakes even if per capita salt intakes are reduced to <5 g/day. Worldwide, sustainability of iodized salt programs has become a major focus.

These programs are fragile, and require a long-term commitment from national governments, donors, consumers, and the salt industry.

In some regions, iodization of salt may not be practical for control of iodine deficiency, at least in the short term. This may occur in remote areas where communications are poor or where there are numerous very small-scale salt producers. In these areas, other options for correction of iodine deficiency should be considered, such as iodized oil [13]. Iodized oil is a long-lasting, "depot" form, of iodine supplementation, prepared by esterification of the unsaturated fatty acids in seed or vegetable oils, and addition of iodine to the double bonds. It can be given orally or by intramuscular injection. The intramuscular route has a longer duration of action (up to 2 years), but oral administration is more common because it is simpler and safer. Iodized oil is recommended for populations with moderate-to-severe iodine deficiency that do not have access to iodized salt, and may be targeted to women of child-bearing age, pregnant women, and children. The recommended dose is 400 mg iodine/year for women and 200 mg iodine/year for children 7–24 months of age [8]. Iodine can also be given as potassium iodide or iodate as drops or tablets, and iodine supplements ($\approx$150 µg/day) are often recommended for pregnant and lactating women residing in areas of mild-to-moderate iodine deficiency [12].

Iodine Excess

Most people are remarkably tolerant to high dietary intakes of iodine. In iodine sufficient populations, large excesses of iodine in the mg to g range inhibit thyroid hormone production, leading to increased TSH stimulation, thyroid growth and goiter [21]. A rapid increase in iodine intake of populations with chronic iodine deficiency may precipitate iodine-induced hyperthyroidism [8]. This is more likely to occur if the iodine is given in excess, usually because the iodine content of iodized salt is set too high, and occurs mainly in older people with nodular goiter. The incidence of iodine-induced hyperthyroidism tends to abate after 3–5 years [23]. To reduce risk, the iodine level in salt should be monitored and reduced if too high.

Discussion Points

- Why is it important to use various indicators of Iodine status?
- Is it worthwhile to iodize salt in areas where there is no signs of iodine deficiency?
- What can be the economic impact of iodine deficiency in a community?
- Are there reasons that Iodine deficiency can be considered a global issue or only an issue that affects isolated area of the world?

References

1. Goldschmidt VM. Geochemistry. Oxford: Clarendon Press; 1954.
2. Haldimann M, Alt A, Blanc A, Blondeau K. Iodine content of food groups. J Food Compos Anal. 2005;18(6):461–71.
3. Pearce EN, Pino S, He X, Bazrafshan HR, Lee SL, Braverman LE. Sources of dietary iodine: bread, cows' milk, and infant formula in the Boston area. J Clin Endocrinol Metab. 2004;89(7):3421–4.
4. Institute of Medicine, Academy of Sciences. Iodine. In: Dietary reference intakes for Vitamin A, Vitamin K, Arsenic, Boron, Chromium, Copper, Iodine, Iron, Manganese, Molybdenum, Nickel, Silicon, Vanadium and Zinc. Washington DC, National Academy Press, 2001.
5. Gaitan E. Goitrogens in food and water. Annu Rev Nutr. 1990;10:21–39.

6. Zimmermann MB, Kohrle J. The impact of iron and selenium deficiencies on iodine and thyroid metabolism: biochemistry and relevance to public health. Thyroid. 2002;12(10):867–78.

7. Eskandari S, Loo DD, Dai G, Levy O, Wright EM, Carrasco N. Thyroid Na+/I- symporter. Mechanism, stoichiometry, and specificity. J Biol Chem. 1997;272(43):27230–8.

8. World Health Organization, United Nations Children's Fund, International Council for Control of Iodine Deficiency Disorders. Assessment of iodine deficiency disorders and monitoring their elimination: a guide for programme managers. 3rd edition. Geneva: World Health Organization, 2007.

9. Auso E, Lavado-Autric R, Cuevas E, Del Rey FE, Morreale De Escobar G, Berbel P. A moderate and transient deficiency of maternal thyroid function at the beginning of fetal neocorticogenesis alters neuronal migration. Endocrinology 2004;145(9):4037–47.

10. Aburto N, Abudou M, Candeias V, Wu T. Effect and safety of salt iodization to prevent iodine deficiency disorders: a systematic review with meta-analyses. WHO eLibrary of Evidence for Nutrition Actions (eLENA). Geneva: World Health Organization, 2015.

11. Bleichrodt NR, Shrestha RM, West CE, Hautvast JG, van de Vijver FJ, Born MP. The benefits of adequate iodine intake. Nutr Rev. 1996;54(4):S72–8.

12. Zimmermann MB. Iodine deficiency in pregnancy and the effects of maternal iodine supplementation on the offspring: a review. Am J Clin Nutr. 2009;89(2):668S–72S.

13. Zimmermann MB, Jooste PL, Pandav C. Iodine-deficiency disorders. Lancet. 2008;372(9645):1251–62.

14. Bautista A, Barker PA, Dunn JT, Sanchez M, Kaiser DL. The effects of oral iodized oil on intelligence, thyroid status, and somatic growth in school-age children from an area of endemic goiter. Am J Clin Nutr. 1982;35:127–34.

15. Huda SN, Grantham-McGregor SM, Tomkins A. Cognitive and motor functions of iodine deficient but euthyroid children in Bangladesh do not benefit from iodized poppy seed oil (Lipiodol). J Nutr. 2001;31:72–7.

16. Isa ZM, Alias IZ, Kadir KA, Ali O. Effect of iodized oil supplementation on thyroid hormone levels and mental performance among Orang Asli schoolchildren and pregnant mothers in an endemic goitre area in Peninsular Malaysia. Asia Pac J Clin Nutr. 2000;9:274–81.

17. Shrestha RM. Effect of iodine and iron supplementation on physical, psychomotor and mental development in primary school children in Malawi. Doctoral thesis, Wageningen Agricultural University, Wageningen, The Netherlands, 1994.

18. Zimmermann MB, Connolly K, Bozo M, Bridson J, Rohner F, Grimci L. Iodine supplementation improves cognition in iodine-deficient schoolchildren in Albania: a randomized, controlled, double-blind study. Am J Clin Nutr. 2006;83:108–14.

19. Gordon RC, Rose MC, Skeaff SA, Gray AR, Morgan KM, Ruffman T. Iodine supplementation improves cognition in mildly iodine-deficient children. Am J Clin Nutr. 2009;90(5):1264–71.

20. Bougma K, Aboud FE, Harding KB, Marquis GS. Iodine and mental development of children 5 years old and under: a systematic review and meta-analysis. Nutrients. 2013;5(4):1384–416.

21. Zimmermann MB, Boelaert K. Iodine deficiency and thyroid disorders. Lancet Diabetes Endocrinol. 2015.

22. Carlé A, Pedersen IB, Knudsen N, Perrild H, Ovesen L, Rasmussen LB, Laurberg P. Epidemiology of subtypes of hyperthyroidism in Denmark: a population-based study. Euro J Endocrinol. 2011;164(5):801–9.

23. Burgi H, Kohler M, Morselli B. Thyrotoxicosis incidence in Switzerland and benefit of improved iodine supply. Lancet. 1998;352(9133):1034.

24. http://www.ign.org/cm_data/Scorecard_ICCIDD_website_18_12_2012_updated_MCD.pdf. Accessed 10 Feb 2015.

Chapter 13
Nutritional Rickets and Vitamin D Deficiency

John M. Pettifor and Kebashni Thandrayen

Keywords Nutritional rickets · Vitamin D deficiency · Low dietary calcium intakes · Non-skeletal functions

Learning Objectives

- Explain why rickets remains a major cause of infant and young child morbidity.
- Define what the determinants of rickets are.
- Evaluate why recommendations for vitamin D intake over the lifespan are unique compared with other nutrients.
- Describe the clinical and subclinical effects of vitamin D deficiency.

Introduction

Over the past 20–30 years, nutritional rickets has received considerable attention from public health specialists in a number of high-income countries, as there appears to have been resurgence in the prevalence of the disease over this period, having almost been eradicated by the middle of the last century in many of these countries. In many low-income countries too, attention has been focused on the disease, not only because of its effects on bone growth and mineral homeostasis but also because of its association with increased infant and childhood mortality especially when accompanying lower respiratory tract infections. Further, the long-term sequelae of the bony deformities, which are characteristic of the acute disease, may be associated with considerable morbidity during child birth and have permanent effects on the joints of affected individuals.

As will be discussed later (c.f. Public Health Importance section of this chapter), it is now apparent that nutritional rickets is caused not only by vitamin D deficiency but also by low dietary calcium intakes, and that it is likely that these two factors play synergistic roles in many children who develop the disease.

J.M. Pettifor (✉)
MRC/Wits Developmental Pathways for Health Research Unit, Department of Paediatrics,
Faculty of Health Sciences, University of the Witwatersrand, 7 York Road, Parktown,
Johannesburg 2193, South Africa
e-mail: john.pettifor@wits.ac.za

K. Thandrayen
Department of Paediatrics, Chris Hani Baragwanath Academic Hospital, Faculty of Health Sciences,
University of the Witwatersrand, P O Bertsham, Johannesburg, Gauteng 2013, South Africa

© Springer Science+Business Media New York 2017
S. de Pee et al. (eds.), *Nutrition and Health in a Developing World*,
Nutrition and Health, DOI 10.1007/978-3-319-43739-2_13

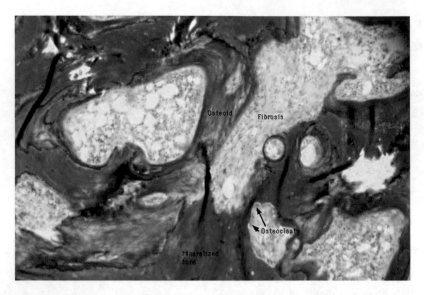

Fig. 13.1 The histological features of osteomalacia on bone biopsy. An iliac crest bone biopsy showing the excessive orange osteoid lining the trabecular surfaces. Mineralized bone is *stained blue*

Definition

Rickets is a disease of growing bones, which results from a failure of or delay in the calcification of newly formed cartilage at the growth plates of long bones, and is associated with a failure of mineralization of newly formed osteoid (this latter feature is termed osteomalacia) at the trabecular bone surfaces and the endosteal and periosteal surfaces of cortical bone (Fig. 13.1). These osseous changes result in the long bones in particular no longer being able to maintain their normal shapes in response to physical forces, such as produced by weight bearing or muscle insertions. The results are the characteristic bony deformities, which are described in the Pathophysiology/Clinical Features section of this chapter.

There are numerous causes of rickets, however, they can be divided broadly into three large categories: those associated with a primary inability to maintain serum calcium concentrations (calciopenic rickets), those associated with a primary inability to maintain normal serum phosphorus concentrations (phosphopenic rickets), and those associated with a primary defect of mineralization. Nutritional rickets is a form of calciopenic rickets and has classically been associated with vitamin D deficiency. Nutritional phosphopenic rickets only occurs in a very specific situation—that of very low birthweight infants being fed predominantly unfortified breast milk—this condition is known as rickets or bone disease of prematurity. Outside of prematurity, dietary phosphate is generally in abundance.

Historical Background

Although there are reported to be references to rickets in Greek and Roman writings nearly 2000 years ago, and a report has been published of skeletal evidence of rickets in an infant skeleton found in South Africa [1], which was radiocarbon dated to nearly 5000 BP, it has been only in the last 400 years that good descriptions of the disease have been recorded [2].

Historically, nutritional rickets is a disease that is associated with urbanisation and the industrial revolution. The first clear descriptions of the disease were published in the middle of the seventeenth century by Francis Glisson (1597–1677) and Daniel Whistler (1619–1684) [3], at which time it became known as the "English disease" because of its high prevalence among urban English children then. Francis Glisson provided a clear description of its peak prevalence in children between the ages of 6 and 30 months. At that time the disease was more common among children of the affluent than of the poor, reflecting the parental protection of affluent infants from sunlight [4]. However with the development of inner city slums with their narrow sunless streets and atmospheric pollution, the disease became much more prevalent among the infants and young children of the poor and destitute. A number of hypotheses was proposed at that time as to its aetiology including digestive disturbances, poor and incorrect feeding, and the breathing of foul air.

A couple of centuries later, Trousseau, the famous French physician (1801–1867), noted that the disease was "unquestionably more common in damp cold countries than elsewhere" and also that cod liver oil and fish oils in general were effective in its management [5], however, it was not until the beginning of the twentieth century that his advice was generally accepted.

In the eighteenth, nineteenth and early twentieth centuries, a number of studies noted the almost universal finding of the features of rickets in infants and young children living in the industrialised cities of Northern Europe and northern North America [6, 7]. It was noted too that children living in rural and farming communities were generally spared [8].

A number of physicians had concluded in the late 1800s that sunlight was beneficial in both preventing and treating the disease [9, 10], however it was not until the early twentieth century that the discovery of vitamin D by McCollum [11] and of the role of UV light in the formation of vitamin D in the 1920s [12] provided a rational and acceptable approach to the prevention and management of vitamin D deficiency rickets. Following the isolation of vitamin D, a number of countries introduced supplementation programmes and food fortification, especially of infant milk formulas almost universally and of cow's milk in USA and Canada. These measures were associated with a rapid reduction in the prevalence of rickets in young children and by the latter half of the twentieth century, infantile rickets had become a relatively uncommon disease in many high-income countries in the more northern latitudes. However, with the relatively recent encouragement of exclusive breast-feeding during the first months of life and the immigration of darker skinned populations into many of these industrialised countries after the Second World War resurgence of the disease in certain communities in these countries has been observed [13–15]. Until recently, little attention has been paid to the prevalence of rickets in other countries, but it is clear that nutritional rickets has been and remains a problem in northern parts of Asian countries, the Indian subcontinent, the Middle East and in a number of countries in Africa (see "Public Health Importance" Section).

Epidemiology

Although humans can obtain their vitamin D supply through two routes, namely through the diet or via skin synthesis under the influence of ultraviolet-B radiation, it is the latter epidermal synthesis which plays the major role in maintaining the vitamin D status of the majority of populations [16] (Fig. 13.2). Few unfortified foods, except for foods such as oily fish and fish oils, contain adequate quantities of vitamin D to ensure vitamin D sufficiency [17].

Ultraviolet-B radiation between the wavelengths of 290 and 315 nm induces the photolysis of 7-dehydrocholesterol in the skin to form previtamin D_3, which then undergoes thermal isomerisation over the next 24–36 h to form vitamin D_3 (cholecalciferol). Once formed in the deeper layers of the epidermis, vitamin D_3 is transported in the blood stream attached to vitamin D binding protein (DBP) to the liver, where it is hydroxylated to 25-hydroxyvitamin D_3 ($25(OH)D_3$). This latter

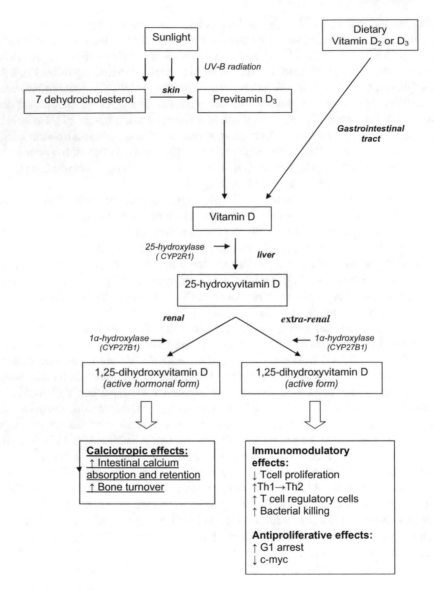

Fig. 13.2 Vitamin D metabolism

compound is the major circulating form of the vitamin and measurement of its serum concentration provides a good index of the vitamin D status of an individual [18]. Ingested and absorbed vitamin D (in the form of either vitamin D_2 or D_3) is also transported to the liver where it is hydroxylated mainly by P450 CYP2R1 to 25(OH)D (the absence of a subscript is used to denote that the vitamin D compound may be derived from either vitamin D_2 or D_3) [19, 20]. Vitamin D_2 (ergocalciferol) is formed by the UV radiation of the plant sterol, ergosterol. Neither vitamin D nor its hydroxylated compound (25(OH)D) is physiologically active at normal concentrations; 25(OH)D must first be converted to 1,25-dihydroxyvitamin D (1,25-$(OH)_2$D) in the proximal tubules of the kidney before becoming a calciotropic hormone. 1 α- hydroxylation is the major rate-limiting step in the synthesis of 1,25-$(OH)_2$D and its synthesis is tightly mediated and regulated by the enzyme 1 α- hydroxylase. *CYP27B1* is the gene encoding 1 α- hydroxylase and *CYP27B1* mRNA is expressed in a number of vitamin D target tissues including bone, kidney, intestine, skin and macrophages [21]. The active form of vitamin D, $1,25\text{-}(OH)_2D$, acts largely through its intracellular vitamin D receptor to influence gene transcription and protein synthesis; its major target organs related to calcium and bone homeostasis being the gastrointestinal tract where it enhances dietary calcium and to a lesser extent phosphorus absorption, and the bone itself where it stimulates bone resorption and the release of calcium and phosphorus into the blood stream (Fig. 13.2). It has minor effects on the kidney where it increases calcium reabsorption and on the parathyroid gland where it influences parathyroid hormone secretion (see reference [22] for a review of vitamin D physiology).

The amount of vitamin D_3 formed in the skin is dependent on a number of factors [23], the most important of these being the amount of solar UV-B radiation that is available at the skin surface. This is dependent to a large extent on the zenith angle of the sun which in turn is dependent on the latitude of the country, the season of the year and the time of day. Studies suggest that areas above a latitude of $35°$ receive insufficient UV radiation during the winter months for cutaneous synthesis of vitamin D [24], thus cities such as Boston ($42°N$) or Calgary ($52°N$) in the north and Ushuaia ($55°S$) in the south receive negligible amounts of UV-B radiation during the winter months [25, 26]. Even in Cape Town at $32°S$ the amount of vitamin D that can be formed during sunlight hours during the winter months is small (Fig. 13.3) [27]. A further factor which influences UV-B radiation is the extent of atmospheric pollution, such that in areas of high atmospheric pollution in an industrialised city UV radiation is reduced compared to that in less polluted areas in the same city [28].

Personal factors also influence the formation of vitamin D in the skin. These include the amount of time spent outside, the extent of skin area exposed to sunlight, the time of day of the sunlight exposure, and the use of sunscreens, which can very effectively prevent UV penetration into the skin. Elderly subjects appear to form less vitamin D_3 than their younger counterparts, as the amount of 7-dehydrocholesterol in the skin is reduced, thus reducing the substrate available for the formation of vitamin D_3. Further, the degree of melanin pigmentation has a major effect on the amount of vitamin D formed in the skin. In numerous studies, in which serum concentrations of 25(OH)D have been compared between black and white subjects, values in black and Asian subjects are significantly lower than those of their white peers living in the same community [29–31].

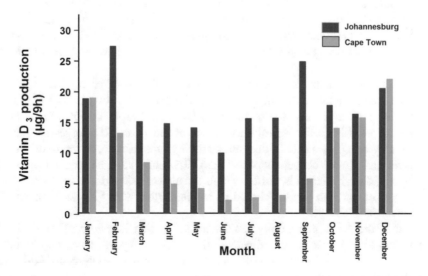

Fig. 13.3 The formation of vitamin D in cities at two different latitudes in South Africa. Johannesburg has a latitude of $26°S$ while Cape Town has a latitude of $32°S$. Vials containing 7-dehydrocholesterol were placed in the sun for 9 h on one day a month throughout the year. The vitamin D formed in the vials was measured. Note the limited vitamin D formation that occurs during the winter months from April to September in Cape Town. Reproduced with permission [27]

Factors Influencing the Formation of Vitamin D in the Skin

The amount of UV-B reaching the earth

- The zenith angle of the sun (the distance from the equator)
- The season of the year
- Time of day
- Atmospheric pollution
- Cloud cover

Human factors

- Amount of skin exposed (clothing coverage)
- Duration of exposure
- Use of sunscreens
- Degree of melanin pigmentation (more pigment, less vitamin D formation)
- Amount of 7-dehydrocholesterol in the skin (aging).

It is clear from the above discussion that vitamin D deficiency rickets is characteristically a disease of infants and young children, as once children start to walk, they will tend to spend more time out of the house in the open air and thus be exposed to sunlight. Furthermore, it is typically a disease of young children living in countries of high latitude. Breastfed infants are further disadvantaged as breast milk normally contains very little vitamin D or its metabolites (estimated to be between 20 and 60 IU/l) [32, 33]. It is estimated that a lactating mother probably requires 4000 IU/d of vitamin D (some 6–7 times the currently recommended intake) to provide sufficient vitamin D in breast milk to maintain vitamin D sufficiency in the nursing baby who has limited access to sunlight [34]. Of all the vitamin D metabolites, 25(OH)D crosses the placenta most readily. The newborn infant has circulating levels of 25(OH)D which are approximately 60–80% of those of the mother, thus the infant is protected for several months from vitamin D deficiency without an additional source of vitamin D, provided the mother is vitamin D replete [35]. However, numerous studies have highlighted that many pregnant mothers have either vitamin D insufficiency or deficiency [36]; this being particularly true of mothers with increased melanin pigmentation living in countries of high latitude (for example, African Americans and the Asian and African communities in the UK and Europe) [37–40]. These low maternal levels predispose the young infant to earlier and more severe vitamin D deficiency and rickets [41].

Over the last 20 years, rickets has been described from all the inhabited continents of the world. In the USA, African American infants are mainly at risk. The age group is typically less than 30 months of age and the vast majority of affected infants is or has been breastfed (96%) [13]. An interesting study by Carpenter and his group from the east coast of the USA [42] suggested that low dietary calcium intakes may also play a role in the pathogenesis of the disease, as many of the infants who developed rickets had normal concentrations of 25(OH)D and had been weaned onto diets low in calcium. In Canada, darker skinned breastfed infants are also at risk and it is suggested that breastfed infants living north of the 55th parallel should be supplemented with Vitamin D at 800 IU/d rather than the customary 400 IU/d [43].

In Europe, it is the Asian community (Pakistani and Indian immigrants) living in the United Kingdom that has been the most investigated, as numerous reports have highlighted the high prevalence of vitamin D deficiency not only in infants but also in adolescents [44] and pregnant mothers [14, 45–47]. Although vitamin D deficiency is central to the pathogenesis of the disease in this community, it is suggested that low dietary calcium intakes associated with the high phytate

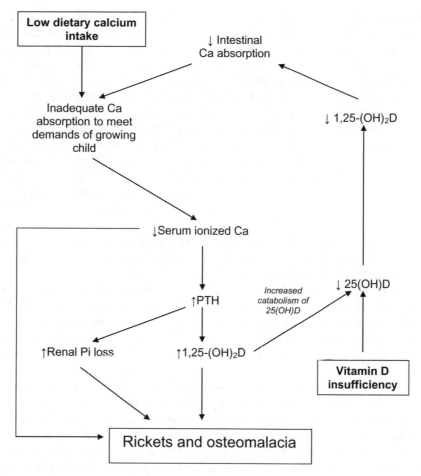

Fig. 13.4 The pathogenesis of rickets. The interrelationship between low dietary calcium intakes and vitamin D insufficiency is shown

content of the typical vegetarian diet increase vitamin D requirements through increased catabolism of 25(OH)D [48] (Fig. 13.4). Besides the increased melanin pigmentation, it appears that greater clothing coverage of the skin and less time spent outside might contribute to the greater prevalence of vitamin D deficiency in the Asian community compared to the indigenous population. In other northern European countries, reports of rickets being more prevalent in dark-skinned immigrants have also appeared [49–52].

Vitamin D deficiency and rickets are common in Middle Eastern countries, where social and religious customs, such as purdah and veiling, which prevent adequate skin exposure to UV-B radiation, are primarily responsible [53–55]. Vitamin D deficiency in young infants is also aggravated by a high prevalence of vitamin D deficiency in pregnant mothers [56]. Low calcium and high phytate intakes have been reported to be responsible for osteomalacia among the Bedouins in Israel [57]. In the Yemen some 50% of children admitted for pneumonia had rickets [58], a finding similar to that was noted in Ethiopia [59].

As Africa straddles the Equator, it might be expected that rickets would be uncommon on that continent, yet the disease has been reported from a number of African countries, including Algeria, Tunisia, Libya, Egypt, Sudan, Ethiopia, Nigeria, Kenya and South Africa. In the majority of these countries, the disease presents in infants and young children [51, 60–62] and is likely to be due to vitamin D deficiency caused by poverty (associated with overcrowding), and social and religious customs preventing sunlight exposure [63]. However, in Nigeria the mean age of presentation is older (46 months) and a number of researchers have noted that affected children have 25(OH)D concentrations above the accepted vitamin D deficient range and have elevated 1,25-(OH)$_2$D levels [64, 65]. Furthermore, the bone disease responds to dietary calcium supplements alone [64, 66, 67]. Calcium intakes in these children are typically low ($\sim$ 200 mg/d) as the diet is almost devoid of milk and dairy products, and the phytate content of the diet is high. However in the Nigerian studies no difference in calcium intakes between control and affected children has been found [65]. Thus although it appears that low dietary calcium intakes play a pivotal role in the pathogenesis of the disease in these children, other unknown factors may predispose susceptible children to the development of the disease.

In South Africa, vitamin D deficiency was frequently seen some 50 years ago in infants in the southern most regions [62], but the prevalence has dropped markedly with the provision of vitamin D supplements to breastfed infants in their first year of life and the fortification of infant milk formulas with vitamin D. More recently, calcium deficiency rickets in association with normal 25(OH)D and elevated 1,25-(OH)$_2$D concentrations has been described in children (aged between 4 and 16 years) living in rural parts of the country. As in the Nigerian children, the calcium intakes were estimated to be very low (150–250 mg/d), however unlike the Nigerian situation, calcium intakes of control children were generally higher than those of affected children [68–71].

Rickets is well described in northern China [72, 73] (including Tibet where the prevalence of clinical rickets has been estimated to be about 66% in one study [74]), and Mongolia [75]. Not only is the disease prevalent during infancy but low vitamin D status and symptomatic hypocalcaemia is reported during the winter months in adolescents as well [76]. Excellent descriptions of the effects of osteomalacia on the skeleton and in particular on the pelvis of women in China were made by Maxwell over 70 years ago [77].

In India, the prevalence of rickets is more common in the Muslim than Hindu communities [78]. Also, although vitamin D deficiency probably plays the dominant role in the pathogenesis of the disease, there is evidence emerging that low dietary calcium intakes may be an important contributor in young children [79]. In urban communities, air pollution and overcrowding probably play a role in the pathogenesis of vitamin D deficiency [28]. Endemic fluorosis is well described in certain parts of India [80], and recent studies suggest that vitamin D deficiency and low dietary calcium intakes might aggravate the clinical picture, through the increased calcium demands associated with endemic fluorosis [81].

Dietary calcium deficiency rickets has also been described in the south-eastern region of Bangladesh [82], where 0.9% of children between the ages of 1–15 years were found to have rickets as detected by radiology [83].

Rickets and vitamin D deficiency in South America are uncommon, because most countries are reasonably close to the equator. However vitamin D deficiency is well described in the southern most regions of Argentina, especially during the winter months [84] and rickets is also described from this region and from urban areas around Buenos Aires, where it is associated with overcrowding and low socio-economic status [85].

In Australia, a growing concern is apparent about the rising prevalence of rickets in the major cities such as Sydney [15]. Over a 10 year period spanning the beginning of this century over 125 cases were diagnosed as having vitamin D deficiency rickets in three large teaching hospitals. As in other high-income countries, the disease is now occurring almost exclusively in children of immigrant families, especially from the Indian subcontinent, Africa and the Middle East [86], although some thirty years ago a study from Melbourne suggested that it was immigrants from the Mediterranean region who were most at risk [87]. Studies also indicate that many of the pregnant women of immigrant families are vitamin D deficient, thus exposing their newborn infants to a greater risk of more severe and earlier rickets [88].

Public Health Importance

The global prevalence of rickets is not known, as many of the community surveys that have been conducted rely on, for the diagnosis of the disease, the finding of bony deformities and clinical findings which are not specific to rickets. Furthermore, these deformities do not necessarily imply the presence of active rickets as deformities which develop during the active stage of the disease may persist for months or years after the disease has been treated. Despite the lack of accurate information, it is clear that rickets and vitamin D deficiency are common in many countries throughout the world [89, 90] as described in the previous section, including Middle Eastern countries [91–93] and a number of low–middle income countries, such as Ethiopia [94], the Yemen [58], and areas of Asia, such as China [74] and Mongolia [75, 95]. Furthermore, the disease is prevalent among immigrant and dark-skinned populations in a number of high-income countries [15].

Besides the classical effects of active rickets on bone growth and development and on calcium homeostasis (cf. Pathophysiology/Clinical Features section), vitamin D deficiency may have adverse effects on a number of other systems. These and the current controversies surrounding the diagnosis of vitamin D status have been recently reviewed [96]. Vitamin D has effects on the immune system [97]. Activated T and B lymphocytes, monocytes, and macrophages express the vitamin D receptor and vitamin D has been shown to modulate B and T lymphocyte function [98, 99]. Innate immunity involving monocytes, macrophages, and mucosal cells causes activation of the toll-like receptors (TLRs) and up-regulates the expression of CYP27B1 [100]. Adaptive immunity (learned mechanisms for fighting invaders) is mediated by T cells producing cytokines and B cells producing immunoglobulins [101]. Vitamin D itself actually suppresses the adaptive immune response by reducing the proliferation and differentiation of B cells, and inhibiting the production of immunoglobulins and proliferation of Th_1 and Th_{17} cells (T cells that encourage destruction of offenders). Interleukins beneficial for Th_2 and T regulatory cells are increased by 1,25-$(OH)_2D$, protecting the body against self-damage or preventing autoimmunity. The TLRs have specific functions for innate immunity and stimulate the production of 1,25-$(OH)_2D$ which plays an autocrine role in the immune response to bacterial, viral, cancerous, proinflammatory and autoimmune diseases. The appropriate concentrations of vitamin D and/or its metabolites required to facilitate the ability of immune cells to defend against bacterial and viral infections need further investigation [102]. However, there is compelling experimental evidence of the importance of vitamin D in stimulating cathelicidin production and controlling Mycobacterium tuberculosis infection in vitro [97]. Further, studies suggest that vitamin D deplete or insufficient states are prevalent among children with viral respiratory tract infections [103] and wheezing [104], although the effect of vitamin D supplementation on the incidence of allergy and wheezing is not consistent [105].

A study from Ethiopia found that children admitted to hospital with pneumonia had a 13 times greater incidence of rickets than children without pneumonia and the combination was associated with a 40% mortality rate [59]. In a study from Jordan 11% of children under 2 years of age admitted for acute illnesses were found to have rickets, and 85% of those with rickets had lower respiratory tract infections compared to only 30% of the children without rickets [106]. There are several possible mechanisms for rachitic children to be predisposed to lower respiratory tract infections; the first is the role that vitamin D has been shown to play in the innate immune system, a second mechanism relates to the muscle weakness and hypotonia which is characteristic of severe vitamin D deficiency, and the third is the effect of rickets and osteomalacia on the rigidity and support provided by the ribs during respiration. The results of vitamin D supplementation studies on the incidence of respiratory infections in children and adults have been inconsistent [107–109]. Despite good laboratory and animal studies suggesting a role for vitamin D in the management and prevention of tuberculosis, a recent randomised controlled trial of vitamin D supplementation did not find any beneficial effects of intermittent bolus therapy on the morbidity and mortality of adults with tuberculosis [110].

The vitamin D status of the subjects was generally good with less than 10% having 25(OH)D concentrations <50 nmol/l, thus it is possible that the results would have been different in a population with a more deplete vitamin D status.

Vitamin D deficiency during pregnancy and early infancy has been associated with poorer maternal weight gain, a higher incidence of neonatal hypocalcaemia, poor neonatal bone mineralization and fractures, and reduced longitudinal growth [29], however these findings are not consistent and a recent review suggests that the quality of the evidence is poor [111].

Further, there is evidence to suggest that vitamin D supplementation in infancy reduces the risk of type 1 diabetes mellitus in later life [112]. Vitamin D deficiency has been shown to be positively associated with type 1 diabetes and other autoimmune diseases such as multiple sclerosis [113] and other studies have shown that vitamin D sufficient states are protective against type 1 diabetes [114] and multiple sclerosis [115]. Children in Finland who received 2000 IU of vitamin D a day from 1 year of age and who were followed for the next 25 years had an 80% decreased risk of developing type 1 diabetes, whereas children who were vitamin D deficient had a 4-fold increased risk of developing this disease later in life [116]. Furthermore, more recent studies worldwide have reported a higher prevalence of low 25(OH) D levels in patients with type 1 diabetes compared to healthy controls [117–119], but it is unclear from these cross-sectional studies whether the lower 25(OH)D levels have a causal relationship with prevalence of diabetes. There is also equivocal evidence on the association between maternal 25(OH)D levels during pregnancy and the risk for type 1 diabetes in the offspring [120, 121]. Furthermore the intake of vitamin D in at-risk children (first degree relatives of subject with type 1 diabetes or with HLA class II typing) showed no correlation with the presence of islet autoimmunity [122] and intervention trials with 25(OH)D and 1,25-(OH)$_2$D in newly diagnosed type 1 diabetes patients showed variable results in the protection of pancreatic beta cell function, which produces insulin [123].

The risk for multiple sclerosis is higher in people living above 35° latitude than in those who live below this latitude [124] and the lower the serum 25(OH)D concentrations the higher the risk for multiple sclerosis [125]. Vitamin D supplementation has also been shown to have protective effects against rheumatoid arthritis [126] and inflammatory bowel disease [127, 128].

It has also been suggested that in addition to multiple sclerosis, other neurological disorders such as schizophrenia and bipolar disorders are associated with vitamin D deficiency during pregnancy or early neonatal life [129]. Many studies have confirmed that schizophrenics are more likely to be born during winter than other seasons. The same winter excess of births has been reported in bipolar affective disorders. These data suggest that vitamin D deficiency and poor sun exposure of pregnant mothers may be associated with a higher risk of schizophrenia and bipolar disorders in their offspring [130]. Low maternal vitamin D levels may have an impact on fetal brain maturation, given that vitamin D is also involved in the development and functioning of the nervous system [131].

Recent epidemiological studies have provided interesting but as yet unproven data which suggest that low vitamin D status during adulthood may increase the risk of colon and prostate cancers among a number of others [132]. The mechanisms through which vitamin D exerts its effects are varied, ranging from altering the calcium concentration in the colonic contents to providing substrate for the local formation of 1,25-(OH)$_2$D which is important in regulating cellular division and differentiation. Currently there are no studies reporting the association between vitamin D deficiency and cancer risk in children. In a study conducted in Israel, nearly half the children who had malignancies had vitamin D insufficiency or deficiency, but there was no control group against which to compare the prevalence of vitamin D deficiency [133]. Further research in the field of childhood cancers and vitamin D needs to be conducted to determine the association of vitamin D status and cancer risk.

In conclusion, although the wide range of possible positive extra-skeletal effects of vitamin D have generated considerable interest among both researchers and the lay public, there are few controlled trials to support the findings of observational and epidemiological studies. Until such time that these findings are supported by clinical trials, the Institute of Medicine (IOM) and others have cautioned against excessive enthusiasm [134]. The IOM suggests that there is no evidence to indicate that serum 25(OH)D levels above 20 ng/ml (50 nmol/l) are beneficial. The committee further suggests that in children the risk of symptomatic vitamin D deficiency increases below 30 nmol/l [135]. In the 2010 recommendations of the IOM, the committee specifically determined the DRIs for vitamin D based on the assumption that there was no skin synthesis of vitamin D, even though in most populations skin synthesis of vitamin D accounts for up to 90% of the circulating 25(OH)D.

Pathophysiology/Clinical Features

Nutritional rickets is primarily a result of disturbed calcium homeostasis consequent on impaired dietary calcium absorption or inadequate dietary calcium intake to meet the demands of the growing skeleton. As discussed earlier, the principal physiological role of vitamin D (or more specifically 1,25-(OH)$_2$D) is the control of intestinal calcium absorption, thus a deficiency of vitamin D results in impaired absorption and hypocalcaemia. The latter stimulates secondary hyperparathyroidism, which results in a reduction in urinary calcium excretion and an increase in urinary phosphate loss. A possible rationale for this reciprocal relationship between calcium and phosphorus excretion is an attempt by the body to protect serum ionised calcium concentrations, which are vital for normal neuromuscular function. Further, increased parathyroid hormone secretion increases bone resorption and bone turnover, resulting in bone loss, which increases the supply of both calcium and phosphorus into the extracellular fluid. Without the increased renal excretion of the resultant surplus phosphate, rising serum phosphorus concentrations would suppress ionised calcium increasing the risk of hypocalcaemic neuromuscular symptoms. The combination of hypocalcaemia and/or hypophosphataemia results in impaired mineralization at the growth plate and the development of the typical pathological features of rickets (see reference [136] for a more detailed discussion).

Clinically, the typical features of rickets are a result of the widening and splaying of the growth plates and resultant deformities of the metaphyses of the long bones. Thus widening of the wrists, knees and ankles, palpable and enlarged costochondral junctions (the rachitic rosary) and deformities of the long bones as a result of weight bearing are the characteristic features [137]. The type of long bone deformity is dependent on the age of the child; in young infants deformities associated with fractures of the forearm are not uncommon and are associated with swaddling, while in the lower limb, anterior bowing of the distal third of the tibia may be found as a result of the infant lying with the legs crossed. In the child who has just started walking bow legs are a common feature, while in the older child, knock knees or a windswept deformity are more common (Fig. 13.5). In the young infant, softening of the skull and a delay in mineralization result in craniotabes (ping pong sign over the petrous temporal bone) and enlargement of and delay in closure of the anterior fontanelle. In young children with severe rickcts, softening of the ribs with narrowing of the lateral diameter of the chest producing the 'violin case deformity' and the development of the Harrison's sulcus along the site of attachment of the diaphragm to the inner surface of the ribs may result in severe respiratory distress and recurrent lower respiratory tract infections. Fractures of ribs and long bones are common manifestations of severe rickets.

Hypotonia and myopathy associated with vitamin D deficiency (possibly in association with bone pain) result in delayed motor milestones and in older children these may present with difficulty in walking up stairs or rising from the sitting position [138].

Hypocalcaemia may manifest clinically without features of bony deformities especially in the early stages of vitamin D deficiency in the young infant less than six months of age [139, 140]. In the neonate hypocalcaemia with apnoeic attacks, convulsions or tremor is more common in infants born to vitamin D deficient mothers [141, 142]. Hypocalcaemic symptoms without bony deformities are also frequently noted in adolescent children [55].

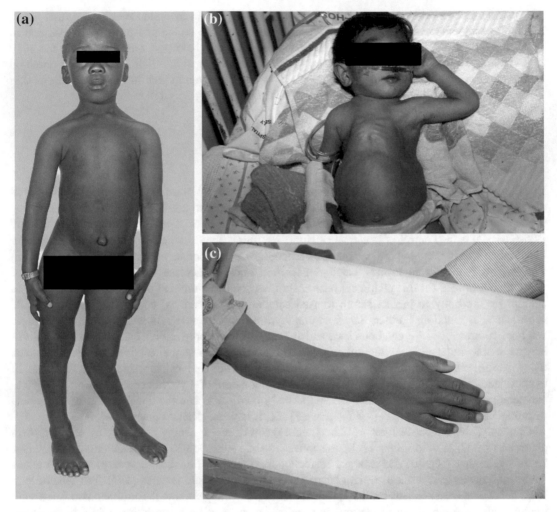

Fig. 13.5 Typical bony deformities associated with rickets. **a** Windswept deformities in a child with dietary calcium deficiency rickets. **b** Chest deformities in a child with severe rickets. The child presented with severe respiratory distress. **c** Enlarged wrist in a child with vitamin D deficiency

Diagnosis

The diagnosis of rickets is suspected clinically by the presence of the typical bony deformities [137], however these do not necessarily indicate active disease as they may persist for months or years following the correction of dietary calcium or vitamin D deficiencies. Craniotabes too may occur in young normal infants, especially in those who were born prematurely [143]. A further difficulty in diagnosing rickets clinically may be created by active rickets being present without clinically apparent bony deformities; this is typically the situation in the early stages of rickets, when the infant only presents with hypocalcaemic symptoms or in the adolescent in whom the growth plates are almost fused.

The presence of active rickets should be confirmed by radiological examination of the growth plates of rapidly growing regions of the skeleton. Radiographs of the wrists and knees are the typical

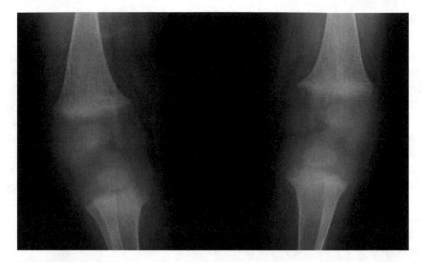

Fig. 13.6 Radiographic changes at the knees of an 18 month old child with severe rickets. Note the loss of the provisional zone of calcification at end of the metaphyses, the widening of the growth plates, and splaying, irregularity and fuzziness of the metaphyses

sites examined. Early features of the disease are a loss of the provisional zone of calcification at the junction of the growth plate and metaphysis and progressive widening of the growth plate [144]. As the growth plates widen, physical forces disrupt the normal cartilage plates and under-mineralized metaphyses result in cupping, fraying and splaying of the metaphyses (Fig. 13.6). The epiphyses are typically underdeveloped and the trabecular pattern of the metaphyses is coarse and sparse. The cortices of the diaphyses are thin and periosteal new bone formation may be seen, especially during the early stages of healing. Fractures of the long bones and ribs are frequently noted in severe rickets. A grading system of the radiographic changes at the knees and wrists has been found to be useful in assessing the severity of rickets and its response to treatment [145].

Biochemically, active rickets manifests classically with hypocalcaemia, hypophosphataemia, and elevated alkaline phosphatase and parathyroid hormone concentrations. In the early stages of vitamin D deficiency, hypocalcaemia may be the only biochemical finding, but as the disease progresses and secondary hyperparathyroidism becomes manifest, hypocalcaemia may partially correct and hypophosphataemia and elevated alkaline phosphatase levels become apparent. In the severe stages of the disease, calcium levels once again fall as the homeostatic mechanisms fail to maintain normocalcaemia.

Confirmation of vitamin D deficiency is dependent on the finding of low 25(OH)D concentrations. It is generally considered that values <10–12 ng/ml (25–30 nmol/l) are indicative of vitamin D deficiency, however, children with vitamin D deficiency rickets typically have values <5 ng/ml (12.5 nmol/l) [146]. The Institute of Medicine (IOM) in its 2011 report [135] has proposed that persons are at increasing risk for vitamin D deficiency and rickets at serum 25(OH)D levels below 12 ng/ml (30 nmol/l). The measurement of 1,25-$(OH)_2$D concentrations is not helpful in the diagnosis of vitamin D deficiency as levels have been found to be low, normal or elevated even in the face of what are considered to be low 25(OH)D levels [146–148].

Rickets due to dietary calcium deficiency presents with very similar biochemical findings to those of vitamin D deficiency, however 25(OH)D levels are characteristically within the normal range and 1,25-$(OH)_2$D concentrations are elevated [65, 66, 69].

Treatment

Vitamin D deficiency rickets responds rapidly to vitamin D supplements or adequate UV radiation. Thus radiographic changes, and hypocalcaemia and elevated alkaline phosphatase levels may normalise during the summer months in children living in countries of high latitude [149]. Vitamin D deficiency rickets is most frequently treated with oral vitamin D_2 or D_3 at doses ranging from 2000 to 10,000 IU/d for 8–12 weeks [150]. Response to therapy may be assessed by an improvement in serum calcium or phosphorus values within 2–3 weeks, while radiographic signs of healing may be seen within a month [146]. Elevated alkaline phosphatase values may persist for several months after the commencement of therapy. Bony deformities as a result of both vitamin D deficiency and dietary calcium deficiency rickets improve in the majority of patients following therapy, although the lower limb deformities of genu valgum and varus tend to respond better in the younger than older child. Improvement in the deformities may take many months to occur, so parents should be advised that patience is required for improvements to be seen. Residual deformities may require orthopaedic corrective surgery.

A single large dose of oral or parenterally administered vitamin D (150,000–600,000 IU) has been found to be useful in situations where patient compliance may be problematic. Healing occurs more rapidly than when smaller daily doses of vitamin D are administered, and no evidence of symptomatic hypercalcaemia has been noted if doses between 150,000 and 300,000 IU are used [151]. Concerns have been expressed about the use of 600,000 IU, especially in young children, and care givers should be cautioned about the dangers of hypervitaminosis D if these large doses are used more frequently than recommended by the health professional [152].

In most low-income countries and in certain situations in industrialised countries, vitamin D deficiency is frequently associated with low dietary calcium intakes, thus it is prudent to provide calcium supplements at the same time as correcting vitamin D deficiency as response to therapy is more rapid [67, 153]. A daily supplement of 50 mg/kg/d of elemental calcium for several months is recommended.

Where dietary calcium deficiency is suspected to be the primary aetiological factor in the pathogenesis of the disease, as in Nigeria or Bangladesh, or in older children in South Africa, children have been shown to respond rapidly to calcium supplements alone (1000 mg/d) [67], however unless the measurement of 25(OH)D concentrations are readily available, it is appropriate to combine the calcium supplements with vitamin D therapy [79]. Vitamin D alone is less effective than either calcium alone or a combination of calcium and vitamin D in these situations [67, 154].

Prevention

Since the discovery of vitamin D over 80 years ago, cheap and effective means of preventing vitamin D deficiency rickets have existed, yet despite this, rickets prevention has not been universally effective as has been highlighted by the resurgence of rickets in certain communities in the USA and Europe and its still common occurrence in many low–middle income countries.

Several different approaches were taken to address the high prevalence of rickets that existed in children living in temperate climates at the turn of the last century. In the USA and Canada, fortification of all dairy milk and infant milk formulas with vitamin D ($\sim$400 IU/litre) has dramatically reduced the prevalence of the disease. However the promotion of exclusive breastfeeding for the first six months of life, the greater use of sunscreens and the advice to avoid direct sunlight in the early months of life are all thought to have increased the risk for developing rickets in young children. In the United Kingdom, vitamin D fortification of a number of foods including milk took place in the middle of the last century, but because of a suspected (but not proven) link to an apparent increase in distal renal tubular acidosis, this practice was discontinued, although margarines and a few cereals remain fortified.

The US Institute of Medicine and Endocrine Society's Clinical Practice guidelines recommend that all infants and children aged 0–1 year receive at least 400 IU/d and children aged 1 year and older have an intake of 600 IU/d to maximise bone health [155, 156], which is higher than generally recommended intakes by other international organisations, such as the FAO/WHO. The increase is as a result of the IOM being conscious of the recommendations for no direct sunlight exposure in young infants and limited sunshine in older children, and to ensure that the recommended serum 25(OH)D levels are achieved. The possible role that vitamin D plays in other physiological actions besides its well-recognised central role in calcium homeostasis [157], has raised concerns that the recommendations of the Institute of Medicine may be insufficient to optimise the many functions that vitamin D might have. However, it is unclear at what levels of 25(OH)D these other functions are optimised [158], and future research needs to focus on the different requirement levels for vitamin D in relation to the non-skeletal actions of vitamin D.

In the United Kingdom, vitamin D supplementation of all infants is recommended, with at-risk older toddlers and children, defined as infants born to mothers who are vitamin D deficient, dark-skinned and who for religious or social customs limit skin exposure to sunlight, receiving supplementation. Many paediatricians believe that vitamin D supplementation should be routine for all infants [159] and for all at-risk children who do not get sufficient sunlight exposure because of clothing, religious or social customs or who have increased skin pigmentation. In areas where at-risk communities are in the majority, routine vitamin D supplementation to pregnant mothers and children under 5 years of age has been shown to be effective in reducing the incidence of rickets [160].

Certainly more attention must be paid to pregnant women in many countries. There is indeed a greater awareness of the role that maternal vitamin D deficiency plays in exacerbating the development of vitamin D deficiency and rickets in infants, but it appears that healthcare professionals pay little attention to the recommendation that dark-skinned mothers should be supplemented during pregnancy [142]. High doses of vitamin D (4000-6400 IU) taken by lactating mothers maintains the vitamin D status of the mother–infant pair, without the need for supplementing the infant [161], however insufficient long-term information on the safety of such high doses is available. Thus, these doses cannot be recommended until further large scale trials have been conducted to assess safety to both the mother and breastfeeding infant.

Education programmes to promote vitamin D supplement consumption targeting at-risk communities have met with some success, but the messages need continual reinforcement and a champion within the health sector to ensure that health professionals comply with the recommendations.

The prevention of rickets in low income countries is even more problematic than in high-income nations. The enormous burden of infectious diseases (including HIV), malnutrition and poverty means that little attention is paid by health authorities to the problem of rickets, especially when health resources are severely curtailed. In these countries too rickets is more likely to be due to a combination of vitamin D deficiency and low dietary calcium intakes, as once breastfeeding ceases the diets are typically devoid of dairy products.

Several studies have reported the effectiveness of intermittent large doses of vitamin D orally or parenterally. In areas where parental compliance or regular vitamin D supplies may be problematic, the use of vitamin D 100,000 IU every three months has been shown to maintain normal serum 25 (OH)D levels [162]. Doses higher than this have resulted in markedly elevated levels of 25(OH)D and occasional episodes of hypercalcaemia. Further studies are required to see if intermittent doses can be linked to the Extended Programme of Immunization or to high dose vitamin A administration in countries where the prevalence of rickets in infants is high (e.g. China, Mongolia, Ethiopia and the Middle East).

Food fortification is a strategy that should be considered in those countries where the majority of the population has or is at risk of low vitamin D status. Careful consideration needs to be given not only to the foods that should be fortified to reach the at-risk communities in a particular country, but also to levels of fortification, and the legislation needed to control and monitor such a fortification policy. Innovative techniques may need to be used in low income countries where subsistence farming may reduce access of the most vulnerable to customary fortified foods. Some examples of targeted fortified foods are the fortification of chapattis in the UK to target the immigrant Asian community, laddoos in a trial in India to target children at school, and milk and margarine in high-income countries to target the general population.

Dairy products are expensive and often not accessible in many low income countries, thus national or community programmes to increase calcium intakes in children who have been introduced to complementary foods may be difficult as there are few cheap and acceptable alternative foods high in calcium. In countries or areas where dried fish is available, this can be ground with the bones and may provide an acceptable condiment to be added to porridge [163]. Powder limestone, added to porridge, has also been shown to be an effective way of treating children with rickets [154]. The addition of limestone to corn in the manufacture of tortillas markedly improves calcium intakes in populations in Central America, and is an accepted part of the diet. Similar food additions to staples should be experimented with in other low income countries, where dietary calcium intakes are low and associated with rickets.

Future Directions

The control of rickets in low income countries is dependent on the control of poverty and over-crowding and the development of effective primary health care facilities and programmes for early treatment and preventive supplementation. Further, dietary diversification is an important aspect of the improvement of calcium intakes. Improvement in vitamin D intakes requires that food fortification becomes a reality, and that the foods are consumed by at-risk groups. In areas where social or religious customs can result in inadequate sunlight exposure for pregnant and lactating mothers and their young infants, attention must be paid to ensuring an adequate vitamin D status of pregnant women through the provision of vitamin D supplements during antenatal care. Health promotion and education programmes should highlight the ease of combating vitamin D deficiency and the prevention of long-term morbidity through ensuring adequate sunlight exposure and/or vitamin D supplementation.

International bodies must highlight the continuing morbidity and mortality associate with nutritional rickets in many low income countries and attention must be paid to placing programmes for the prevention of the disease on the world health agenda.

Although a lot is known about the pathogenesis and treatment of nutritional rickets, there are still a number of unanswered questions concerning the interrelationship between environmental and genetic factors which may predispose individual children to the development of rickets. For instance in Nigeria, dietary calcium intakes of children with and without rickets have been found to be similar [65], yet the disease in affected children is cured by the provision of calcium supplements alone. These findings suggest that other genetic or environmental factors may play a role in the pathogenesis. Some 30 years ago, Greek researchers suggested that there was a genetic component to the predisposition for the development of vitamin D deficiency rickets [164], and more recently work from the USA points to increased catabolism of vitamin D in Asian Indians compared to whites living in the same country [165], possibly indicating genetic differences and a predisposition to develop vitamin D deficiency.

Conclusions

Despite cheap and effective means of both treating and preventing nutritional rickets, the disease remains a major cause of infant and young child morbidity and mortality in several low–middle income countries across the world. Rickets continues as a public health problem in low–middle income countries lying at high latitude in the temperate zones, while in the Middle East and some other countries, religious customs often prevent adequate sunlight exposure not only in young infants but also in adolescent children and pregnant women. In other tropical countries, increasing evidence is accumulating which indicates that low dietary calcium intakes by themselves or in synergy with relative vitamin D deficiency exacerbate and promote the development of the disease.

Effective prevention programmes are not in place in most low-income countries, thus there needs to be a concerted effort from international agencies to ensure that rickets is placed on the health agenda of these countries. Innovative food fortification strategies, for example of vegetable oil, together with vitamin A, should be considered as a sustainable approach to improving the vitamin D status of at-risk populations. Treatment of most patients with rickets can be effectively managed using daily vitamin D supplements for several months; however consideration should be given to the use of single large doses of vitamin D in those situations where compliance might be problematic. In all cases, attention should be paid to ensuring an adequate dietary calcium intake during treatment. A recent global consensus statement by concerned child health professionals has highlighted the need for a global effort to prevent and eradicate nutritional rickets [166].

Future Research Needs

- There are still a number of unanswered questions concerning the interrelationship between environmental and genetic factors which may predispose individual children to the development of rickets as highlighted by those children in Nigeria with rickets who respond to calcium therapy and yet, prior to treatment, had similar dietary calcium intakes and vitamin D status as age matched community controls.
- Further studies are required to assess if intermittent doses of vitamin D can be linked to the Extended Programme of Immunization or to high dose vitamin A distribution in countries where the prevalence of rickets in infants is high. To ensure maternal vitamin D sufficiency, studies need to assess the most appropriate means of vitamin D delivery to pregnant women to optimise compliance.
- There needs to be a concerted effort from international agencies to ensure that rickets is placed on the health agenda of those countries where rickets incidence remains high. Further research is needed to determine how effective prevention programmes for rickets can be established in low–middle income countries where the risk of vitamin D deficiency and dietary calcium deficiency are high.
- Before recommendations can be made about how to ensure appropriate 25(OH)D concentrations to optimise the possible non-skeletal actions of vitamin D, further well-designed studies are required to support the suggested role of vitamin D in the prevention of non-skeletal diseases, such as cancer and diabetes.

Discussion Points

- Why do rickets prevention programs need to understand the biochemical synthesis of vitamin D when planning, implementing and evaluating their impact?
- How do sociocultural factors have to be taken into account when developing nutrition specific and nutrition sensitive approaches to rickets prevention?
- Why may different approaches need to be used to prevent rickets in different parts of the word?
- Why could vitamin D be considered a neglected nutrient deficiency and what would be the reasons for this description?

References

1. Pfeiffer S, Crowder C. An ill child among mid-Holocene foragers of Southern Africa. Am J Phys Anthropol. 2004;123(1):23–9.
2. O'Riordan JL, Bijvoet OL. Rickets before the discovery of vitamin D. Bonekey Rep. 2014;3:478.
3. Dunn PM. Francis Glisson (1597–1677) and the "discovery" of rickets. Arch Dis Child Fetal Neonatal Ed. 1998;78(2):F154–5.
4. Gibbs D. Rickets and the crippled child: an historical perspective. J R Soc Med. 1994;87(12):729–32.
5. Dunn PM. Professor Armand Trousseau (1801–67) and the treatment of rickets. Arch Dis Child Fetal Neonatal Ed. 1999;80(2):F155–7.
6. Chick DH. Study of rickets in Vienna 1919–1922. Med Hist. 1976;20(1):41–51.
7. Larocque R. Deaths at an early age in the city of Quebec, 17th-19th centuries. Can Bull Med Hist. 1999;16 (2):341–61.
8. Snow J. On the adulteration of bread as a cause of rickets. 1857. Int J Epidemiol. 2003;32(3):336–7.
9. Holick MF. Photosynthesis, metabolism, and biologic actions of vitamin D. In: Glorieux FH, editor. Rickets. Nestle Nutriton Workshop Series. 21. New York: Nestec Ltd., Vevey/Raven Press; 1991. P. 1–20.
10. Gibbs D. Rickets and the crippled child: an historical perspective. J R Soc Med. 1994;87:729–32.
11. Rafter GW. Elmer McCollum and the disappearance of rickets. Perspect Biol Med. 1987;30(4):527–34.
12. Rajakumar K, Thomas SB. Reemerging nutritional rickets: a historical perspective. Arch Pediatr Adolesc Med. 2005;159(4):335–41.
13. Weisberg P, Scanlon KS, Li R, Cogswell ME. Nutritional rickets among children in the United States: review of cases reported between 1986 and 2003. Am J Clin Nutr. 2004;80(6):1697S–705S.
14. Iqbal SJ, Kaddam I, Wassif W, Nichol F, Walls J. Continuing clinically severe vitamin D deficiency in Asians in the UK (Leicester). Postgrad Med J. 1994;70(828):708–14.
15. Munns CF, Simm PJ, Rodda CP, Garnett SP, Zacharin MR, Ward LM, et al. Incidence of vitamin D deficiency rickets among Australian children: an Australian Paediatric Surveillance Unit study. Med J Aust. 2012;196 (7):466–8.
16. Norman AW. Sunlight, season, skin pigmentation, vitamin D, and 25-hydroxyvitamin D: integral components of the vitamin D endocrine system. Am J Clin Nutr. 1998;67(6):1108–10.
17. Calvo MS, Whiting SJ, Barton CN. Vitamin D intake: a global perspective of current status. J Nutr. 2005;135 (2):310–6.
18. Zerwekh JE. Blood biomarkers of vitamin D status. Am J Clin Nutr. 2008;87(4):1087S–91S.
19. Wikvall K. Cytochrome P450 enzymes in the bioactivation of vitamin D to its hormonal form. Int J Mol Med. 2001;7(2):201–9.
20. Shinkyo R, Sakaki T, Kamakura M, Ohta M, Inouye K. Metabolism of vitamin D by human microsomal CYP2R1. Biochem Biophys Res Commun. 2004;324(1):451–7.
21. Kim SY. The pleiomorphic actions of vitamin D and its importance for children. Ann Pediatr Endocrinol Metab. 2013;18(2):45–54.
22. Bikle D. Nonclassic actions of vitamin D. J Clin Endocrinol Metab. 2009;94(1):26–34.
23. Holick MF. Environmental factors that influence the cutaneous production of vitamin D. Am J Clin Nutr. 1995;61 (3 Suppl):638S–45S.
24. Holick MF, Chen TC, Lu Z, Sauter E. Vitamin D and skin physiology: a D-lightful story. J Bone Miner Res. 2007;22(Suppl 2):V28–33.

25. Webb AR, Kline L, Holick MF. Influence of season and latitude on the cutaneous synthesis of vitamin D_3: exposure to winter sunlight in Boston and Edmonton will not promote vitamin D_3 synthesis in human skin. J Clin Endocrinol Metab. 1988;67:373–8.

26. Ladizesky M, Lu Z, Oliveri B, San Roman N, Diaz S, Holick MF, et al. Solar ultraviolet B radiation and photoproduction of vitamin D_3 in central and southern areas of Argentina. J Bone Miner Res. 1995;10(4):545–9.

27. Pettifor JM, Moodley GP, Hough FS, Koch H, Chen T, Lu Z, et al. The effect of season and latitude on in vitro vitamin D formation by sunlight in South Africa. S Afr Med J. 1996;86(10):1270–2.

28. Agarwal KS, Mughal MZ, Upadhyay P, Berry JL, Mawer EB, Puliyel JM. The impact of atmospheric pollution on vitamin D status of infants and toddlers in Delhi, India. Arch Dis Child. 2002;87(2):111–3.

29. Pawley N, Bishop NJ. Prenatal and infant predictors of bone health: the influence of vitamin D. Am J Clin Nutr. 2004;80(6 Suppl):1748S–51S.

30. Looker AC, Dawson-Hughes B, Calvo MS, Gunter EW, Sahyoun NR. Serum 25-hydroxyvitamin D status of adolescents and adults in two seasonal subpopulations from NHANES III. Bone. 2002;30(5):771–7.

31. Poopedi MA, Norris SA, Pettifor JM. Factors influencing the vitamin D status of 10-year-old urban South African children. Public Health Nutr. 2011;14(2):334–9.

32. Specker BL, Tsang RC, Hollis BW. Effect of race and diet on human-milk vitamin D and 25-hydroxyvitamin D. Am J Dis Child. 1985;139:1134–7.

33. Hollis BW, Roos BA, Draper HH, Lambert PW. Vitamin D and its metabolites in human and bovine milk. J Nutr. 1981;111:1240–8.

34. Hollis BW, Wagner CL. Vitamin D requirements during lactation: high-dose maternal supplementation as therapy to prevent hypovitaminosis D for both the mother and the nursing infant. Am J Clin Nutr. 2004;80(6):1752S–8.

35. Hillman LS, Haddad JG. Human perinatal vitamin D metabolism 1: 25-hydroxyvitamin D in maternal and cord blood. J Pediatr. 1974;84:742–9.

36. Dawodu A, Wagner CL. Mother-child vitamin D deficiency: an international perspective. Arch Dis Child. 2007;92(9):737–40.

37. Nesby-O'Dell S, Scanlon KS, Cogswell ME, Gillespie C, Hollis BW, Looker AC, et al. Hypovitaminosis D prevalence and determinants among African American and white women of reproductive age: third National Health and Nutrition Examination Survey, 1988–1994. Am J Clin Nutr. 2002;76(1):187–92.

38. Brunvand L, Haug E. Vitamin D deficiency amongst Pakistani women in Oslo. Acta Obstet Gynecol Scand. 1993;72(4):264–8.

39. Grover SR, Morley R. Vitamin D deficiency in veiled or dark-skinned pregnant women. Med J Aust. 2001;175(5):251–2.

40. Mukamel MN, Weisman Y, Somech R, Eisenberg Z, Landman J, Shapira I, et al. Vitamin D deficiency and insufficiency in Orthodox and non-Orthodox Jewish mothers in Israel. Isr Med Assoc J. 2001;3(6):419–21.

41. Dawodu A, Wagner CL. Prevention of vitamin D deficiency in mothers and infants worldwide - a paradigm shift. Paediatr Int Child Health. 2012;32(1):3–13.

42. DeLucia MC, Mitnick ME, Carpenter TO. Nutritional rickets with normal circulating 25-hydroxyvitamin D: a call for reexamining the role of dietary calcium intake in North American infants. J Clin Endocrinol Metab. 2003;88(8):3539–45.

43. Ward LM. Vitamin D deficiency in the 21st century: a persistent problem among Canadian infants and mothers. CMAJ. 2005;172(6):769–70.

44. Das G, Crocombe S, McGrath M, Berry J, Mughal Z. Hypovitaminosis D among healthy adolescent girls attending an inner city school. Arch Dis Child. 2006;91:569–72.

45. Dunnigan MG, Paton JP, Haase S, Mc NG, Gardner MD, Smith CM. Late rickets and osteomalacia in the Pakistani community in Glasgow. Scott Med J. 1962;7:159–67.

46. Datta S, Alfaham M, Davies DP, Dunstan F, Woodhead S, Evans J, et al. Vitamin D deficiency in pregnant women from a non-European ethnic minority population–an interventional study. BJOG. 2002;109(8):905–8.

47. Dunnigan MG, McIntosh WB, Ford JA. Rickets in Asian immigrants. Lancet. 1976;i:1346.

48. Clements MR. The problem of rickets in UK Asians. J Hum Nutr Diet. 1989;2:105–16.

49. Meulmeester JF, van den Berg H, Wedel M, Boshuis PG, Hulshof KF, Luyken R. Vitamin D status, parathyroid hormone and sunlight in Turkish, Moroccan and Caucasian children in The Netherlands. Eur J Clin Nutr. 1990;44(6):461–70.

50. Pedersen P, Michaelsen KF, Molgaard C. Children with nutritional rickets referred to hospitals in Copenhagen during a 10-year period. Acta Paediatr. 2003;92(1):87–90.

51. Markestad T, Elzouki AY. Vitamin D-deficiency rickets in Northern Europe and Libya. In: Glorieux FH, editor. Rickets. New York: Nestec, Vevey; Raven Press; 1991. p. 203 13.

52. Yeste D, Carrascosa A. Nutritional rickets in childhood: analysis of 62 cases. Med Clin (Barc). 2003;121(1):23–7.

53. Gannage-Yared MH, Chemali R, Yaacoub N, Halaby G. Hypovitaminosis D in a sunny country: relation to lifestyle and bone markers. J Bone Miner Res. 2000;15(9):1856–62.

54. Taha SA, Dost SM, Sedrani SH. 25-Hydroxyvitamin D and total calcium: extraordinarily low plasma concentrations in Saudi mothers and their neonates. Pediatr Res. 1984;18(8):739–41.
55. Narchi H, El Jamil M, Kulaylat N. Symptomatic rickets in adolescence. Arch Dis Child. 2001;84(6):501–3.
56. Elidrissy AT, Sedrani SH, Lawson DE. Vitamin D deficiency in mothers of rachitic infants. Calcif Tissue Int. 1984;36(3):266–8.
57. Shany S, Hirsh J, Berlyne GM. 25-Hydroxycholecalciferol levels in bedouins in the Negev. Am J Clin Nutr. 1976;29(10):1104–7.
58. Banajeh SM, al-Sunbali NN, al-Sanahani SH. Clinical characteristics and outcome of children aged under 5 years hospitalized with severe pneumonia in Yemen. Ann Trop Paediatr. 1997;17(4):321–326.
59. Muhe L, Luiseged S, Mason KE, Simoes EAF. Case-control study of the role of nutritional rickets in the risk of developing pneumonia in Ethiopian children. Lancet. 1997;349:1801–4.
60. Lawson DEM, Cole TJ, Salem SI, Galal OM, El-Meligy R, Abdel-Azim S, et al. Aetiology of rickets in Egyptian children. Hum Nutr Clin Nutr. 1987;41C:199–208.
61. el Hag AI, Karrar ZA. Nutritional vitamin D deficiency rickets in Sudanese children. Ann Trop Paediatr. 1995;15(1):69–76.
62. Dancaster CP, Jackson WP. Studies in rickets in the Cape peninsula. II. Aetiology. S Afr Med J. 1961;35:890–4.
63. Belachew T, Nida H, Getaneh T, Woldemariam D, Getinet W. Calcium deficiency and causation of rickets in Ethiopian children. East Afr Med J. 2005;82(3):153–9.
64. Okonofua F, Gill DS, Alabi ZO, Thomas M, Bell JL, Dandona P. Rickets in Nigerian children: a consequence of calcium malnutrition. Metabolism. 1991;40:209–13.
65. Thacher TD, Fischer PR, Pettifor JM, Lawson JO, Isichei CO, Chan GM. Case-control study of factors associated with nutritional rickets in Nigerian children. J Pediatr. 2000;137(3):367–73.
66. Oginni LM, Worsfold M, Oyelami OA, Sharp CA, Powell DE, Davie MW. Etiology of rickets in Nigerian children. J Pediatr. 1996;128(5 Pt 1):692–4.
67. Thacher TD, Fischer PR, Pettifor JM, Lawson JO, Isichei CO, Reading JC, et al. A comparison of calcium, vitamin D, or both for nutritional rickets in Nigerian children. N Engl J Med. 1999;341(8):563–8.
68. Pettifor JM, Ross P, Wang J, Moodley G, Couper-Smith J. Rickets in children of rural origin in South Africa: is low dietary calcium a factor? J Pediatr. 1978;92:320–4.
69. Pettifor JM, Ross FP, Travers R, Glorieux FH, DeLuca HF. Dietary calcium deficiency: a syndrome associated with bone deformities and elevated serum 1,25-dihydroxyvitamin D concentrations. Metab Bone Rel Res. 1981;2:301–5.
70. Marie PJ, Pettifor JM, Ross FP, Glorieux FH. Histological osteomalacia due to dietary calcium deficiency in children. N Engl J Med. 1982;307:584–8.
71. Eyberg C, Pettifor JM, Moodley G. Dietary calcium intake in rural black South African children. The relationship between calcium intake and calcium nutritional status. Hum Nutr Clin Nutr. 1986;40C:69–74.
72. Fraser DR. Vitamin D-deficiency in Asia. J Steroid Biochem Mol Biol. 2004;89–90(1–5):491–5.
73. Strand MA, Peng G, Zhang P, Lee G. Preventing rickets in locally appropriate ways: a case report from north China. Int Q Community Health Educ. 2003;21(4):297–322.
74. Harris NS, Crawford PB, Yangzom Y, Pinzo L, Gyaltsen P, Hudes M. Nutritional and health status of Tibetan children living at high altitudes. N Engl J Med. 2001;344(5):341–7.
75. Tserendolgor U, Mawson JT, Macdonald AC, Oyunbileg M. Prevalence of rickets in Mongolia. Asia Pac J Clin Nutr. 1998;7(3/4):325–8.
76. Du X, Greenfield H, Fraser DR, Ge K, Trube A, Wang Y. Vitamin D deficiency and associated factors in adolescent girls in Beijing. Am J Clin Nutr. 2001;74(4):494–500.
77. Maxwell JP. Further studies in adult rickets (osteomalacia) and foetal rickets. Proc Roy Soc Med. 1934;28:265–300.
78. Bhattacharyya AK. Nutritional rickets in the tropics. In: Simopoulos AP, editor. Nutrtional triggers for health and in disease. World Rev Nutr Diet. 67. Basel: Karger; 1992. P. 140–97.
79. Balasubramanian K, Rajeswari J, Govil YC, Agarwal AK, Kumar A, Bhatia V, et al. Varying role of vitamin D deficiency in the etiology of rickets in young children vs. adolescents in northern India. J Trop Pediatr. 2003;49(4):201–6.
80. Teotia SP, Teotia M. Endemic fluorosis in India: a challenging national health problem. J Assoc Physicians India. 1984;32(4):347–52.
81. Khandare AL, Harikumar R, Sivakumar B. Severe bone deformities in young children from vitamin D deficiency and fluorosis in Bihar-India. Calcif Tissue Int. 2005;76(6):412–8.
82. Fischer PR, Rahman A, Cimma JP, Kyaw-Myint TO, Kabir AR, Talukder K, et al. Nutritional rickets without vitamin D deficiency in Bangladesh. J Trop Pediatr. 1999;45(5):291–3.
83. Kabir ML, Rahman M, Talukder K, Rahman A, Hossain Q, Mostafa G, et al. Rickets among children of a coastal area of Bangladesh. Mymensingh Med J. 2004;13(1):53–8.

84. Olivieri MB, Ladizesky M, Mautalen CA, Alonso A, Martinez L. Seasonal variations of 25 hydroxyvitamin D and parathyroid hormone in Ushuaia (Argentina), the southernmost city of the world. Bone Miner. 1993;20:99–108.
85. Oliveri MB, Ladizesky M, Sotelo A, Griffo S, Ballesteros G, Mautalen CA. Nutritional rickets in Argentina. In: Glorieux FH, editor. Rickets. New York: Nestec, Vevey; Raven Press; 1991. P. 233–45.
86. Robinson PD, Hogler W, Craig ME, Verge CF, Walker JL, Piper AC, et al. The re-emerging burden of rickets: a decade of experience from Sydney. Arch Dis Child. 2006;91:564–8.
87. Mayne V, McCredie D. Rickets in Melbourne. Med J Aust. 1972;2(16):873–5.
88. Nowson CA, Margerison C. Vitamin D intake and vitamin D status of Australians. Med J Aust. 2002;177(3):149–52.
89. Thacher TD, Fischer PR, Strand MA, Pettifor JM. Nutritional rickets around the world: causes and future directions. Ann Trop Paediatr. 2006;26(1):1–16.
90. Prentice A. Nutritional rickets around the world. J Steroid Biochem Mol Biol. 2013;136:201–6.
91. Lubani MM, al-Shab TS, al-Saleh QA, Sharda DC, Quattawi SA, Ahmed SA, et al. Vitamin-D-deficiency rickets in Kuwait: the prevalence of a preventable disease. Ann Trop Paediatr. 1989;9(3):134–9.
92. Fida NM. Assessment of nutritional rickets in Western Saudi Arabia. Saudi Med J. 2003;24(4):337–40.
93. Ozkan B, Doneray H, Karacan M, Vancelik S, Yildirim ZK, Ozkan A, et al. Prevalence of vitamin D deficiency rickets in the eastern part of Turkey. Eur J Pediatr. 2009;168(1):95–100.
94. Lulseged S, Fitwi G. Vitamin D deficiency rickets: socio-demographic and clinical risk factors in children seen at a referral hospital in Addis Ababa. East Afr Med J. 1999;76(8):457–61.
95. Uush T. Prevalence of classic signs and symptoms of rickets and vitamin D deficiency in Mongolian children and women. J Steroid Biochem Mol Biol. 2013;136:207–10.
96. El-Hajj Fuleihan G, Bouillon R, Clarke B, Chakhtoura M, Cooper C, McClung M, et al. Serum 25-Hydroxyvitamin D Levels: Variability, Knowledge Gaps, and the Concept of a Desirable Range. J Bone Miner Res. 2015;30(7):1119–1133.
97. Hewison M. Vitamin D and immune function: an overview. Proc Nutr Soc. 2012;71(1):50–61.
98. Mathieu C, Adorini L. The coming of age of 1,25-dihydroxyvitamin D(3) analogs as immunomodulatory agents. Trends Mol Med. 2002;8(4):174–9.
99. Tsoukas CD, Provvedini DM, Manolagas SC. 1,25-dihydroxyvitamin D3: a novel immunoregulatory hormone. Science. 1984;224(4656):1438–40.
100. Liu PT, Stenger S, Li H, Wenzel L, Tan BH, Krutzik SR, et al. Toll-like receptor triggering of a vitamin D-mediated human antimicrobial response. Science. 2006;311(5768):1770–3.
101. Iyer P, Diamond F. Detecting disorders of vitamin D deficiency in children: an update. Adv Pediatr. 2013;60 (1):89–106.
102. Walker VP, Modlin RL. The vitamin D connection to pediatric infections and immune function. Pediatr Res. 2009;65(5 Pt 2):106R–13R.
103. Cannell JJ, Vieth R, Umhau JC, Holick MF, Grant WB, Madronich S, et al. Epidemic influenza and vitamin D. Epidemiol Infect. 2006;134(6):1129–40.
104. Devereux G, Litonjua AA, Turner SW, Craig LC, McNeill G, Martindale S, et al. Maternal vitamin D intake during pregnancy and early childhood wheezing. Am J Clin Nutr. 2007;85(3):853–9.
105. Goldring ST, Griffiths CJ, Martineau AR, Robinson S, Yu C, Poulton S, et al. Prenatal vitamin d supplementation and child respiratory health: a randomised controlled trial. PLoS ONE. 2013;8(6):e66627.
106. Najada AS, Habashneh MS, Khader M. The frequency of nutritional rickets among hospitalized infants and its relation to respiratory diseases. J Trop Pediatr. 2004;50(6):364–8.
107. Remmelts HH, Spoorenberg SM, Oosterheert JJ, Bos WJ, de Groot MC, van de Garde EM. The role of vitamin D supplementation in the risk of developing pneumonia: three independent case-control studies. Thorax. 2013;68 (11):990–6.
108. Camargo CA Jr, Ganmaa D, Frazier AL, Kirchberg FF, Stuart JJ, Kleinman K, et al. Randomized trial of vitamin D supplementation and risk of acute respiratory infection in Mongolia. Pediatrics. 2012;130(3):e561–7.
109. Manaseki-Holland S, Maroof Z, Bruce J, Mughal MZ, Masher MI, Bhutta ZA, et al. Effect on the incidence of pneumonia of vitamin D supplementation by quarterly bolus dose to infants in Kabul: a randomised controlled superiority trial. Lancet. 2012;379(9824):1419–27.
110. Wejse C, Gomes VF, Rabna P, Gustafson P, Aaby P, Lisse IM, et al. Vitamin D as supplementary treatment for tuberculosis: a double-blind, randomized, placebo-controlled trial. Am J Respir Crit Care Med. 2009;179(9):843–50.
111. Karras SN, Anagnostis P, Bili E, Naughton D, Petroczi A, Papadopoulou F, et al. Maternal vitamin D status in pregnancy and offspring bone development: the unmet needs of vitamin D era. Osteoporos Int. 2014;25(3):795–805.
112. Harris SS. Vitamin D in type 1 diabetes prevention. J Nutr. 2005;135(2):323–5.

113. Grant WB, Cross HS, Garland CF, Gorham ED, Moan J, Peterlik M, et al. Estimated benefit of increased vitamin D status in reducing the economic burden of disease in western Europe. Prog Biophys Mol Biol. 2009;99(2–3):104–13.

114. Willis JA, Scott RS, Darlow BA, Lewy H, Ashkenazi I, Laron Z. Seasonality of birth and onset of clinical disease in children and adolescents (0–19 years) with type 1 diabetes mellitus in Canterbury, New Zealand. J Pediatr Endocrinol Metab. 2002;15(5):645–7.

115. Willer CJ, Dyment DA, Sadovnick AD, Rothwell PM, Murray TJ, Ebers GC. Timing of birth and risk of multiple sclerosis: population based study. BMJ. 2005;330(7483):120–4.

116. Hypponen E, Laara E, Reunanen A, Jarvelin MR, Virtanen SM. Intake of vitamin D and risk of type 1 diabetes: a birth-cohort study. Lancet. 2001;358(9292):1500–3.

117. Bin-Abbas BS, Jabari MA, Issa SD, Al-Fares AH, Al-Muhsen S. Vitamin D levels in Saudi children with type 1 diabetes. Saudi Med J. 2011;32(6):589–92.

118. Greer RM, Portelli SL, Hung BS, Cleghorn GJ, McMahon SK, Batch JA, et al. Serum vitamin D levels are lower in Australian children and adolescents with type 1 diabetes than in children without diabetes. Pediatr Diabetes. 2013;14(1):31–41.

119. Azab SF, Saleh SH, Elsaeed WF, Abdelsalam SM, Ali AA, Esh AM. Vitamin D status in diabetic Egyptian children and adolescents: a case-control study. Ital J Pediatr. 2013;39:73.

120. Sorensen IM, Joner G, Jenum PA, Eskild A, Torjesen PA, Stene LC. Maternal serum levels of 25-hydroxy-vitamin D during pregnancy and risk of type 1 diabetes in the offspring. Diabetes. 2012;61 (1):175–8.

121. Miettinen ME, Reinert L, Kinnunen L, Harjutsalo V, Koskela P, Surcel HM, et al. Serum 25-hydroxyvitamin D level during early pregnancy and type 1 diabetes risk in the offspring. Diabetologia. 2012;55(5):1291–4.

122. Simpson M, Brady H, Yin X, Seifert J, Barriga K, Hoffman M, et al. No association of vitamin D intake or 25-hydroxyvitamin D levels in childhood with risk of islet autoimmunity and type 1 diabetes: the diabetes autoimmunity study in the young (DAISY). Diabetologia. 2011;54(11):2779–88.

123. Gabbay MA, Sato MN, Finazzo C, Duarte AJ, Dib SA. Effect of cholecalciferol as adjunctive therapy with insulin on protective immunologic profile and decline of residual beta-cell function in new-onset type 1 diabetes mellitus. Arch Pediatr Adolesc Med. 2012;166(7):601–7.

124. Hernan MA, Olek MJ, Ascherio A. Geographic variation of MS incidence in two prospective studies of US women. Neurology. 1999;53(8):1711–8.

125. Munger KL, Levin LI, Hollis BW, Howard NS, Ascherio A. Serum 25-hydroxyvitamin D levels and risk of multiple sclerosis. JAMA. 2006;296(23):2832–8.

126. Merlino LA, Curtis J, Mikuls TR, Cerhan JR, Criswell LA, Saag KG. Vitamin D intake is inversely associated with rheumatoid arthritis: results from the Iowa Women's Health Study. Arthritis Rheum. 2004;50(1):72–7.

127. Cantorna MT, Munsick C, Bemiss C, Mahon BD. 1,25-Dihydroxycholecalciferol prevents and ameliorates symptoms of experimental murine inflammatory bowel disease. J Nutr. 2000;130(11):2648–52.

128. Ananthakrishnan AN, Khalili H, Higuchi LM, Bao Y, Korzenik JR, Giovannucci EL, et al. Higher predicted vitamin D status is associated with reduced risk of Crohn's disease. Gastroenterology. 2012;142(3):482–9.

129. Grant WB, Holick MF. Benefits and requirements of vitamin D for optimal health: a review. Altern Med Rev. 2005;10(2):94–111.

130. Boyd JH, Pulver AE, Stewart W. Season of birth: schizophrenia and bipolar disorder. Schizophr Bull. 1986;12 (2):173–86.

131. Garcion E, Wion-Barbot N, Montero-Menei CN, Berger F, Wion D. New clues about vitamin D functions in the nervous system. Trends Endocrinol Metab. 2002;13(3):100–5.

132. Holick MF. Vitamin D: importance in the prevention of cancers, type 1 diabetes, heart disease, and osteoporosis. Am J Clin Nutr. 2004;79(3):362–71.

133. Modan-Moses D, Pinhas-Hamiel O, Munitz-Shenkar D, Temam V, Kanety H, Toren A. Vitamin D status in pediatric patients with a history of malignancy. Pediatr Res. 2012;72(6):620–4.

134. Rosen CJ, Taylor CL. Common misconceptions about vitamin D–implications for clinicians. Nat Rev Endocrinol. 2013;9(7):434–8.

135. Institute of Medicine. Dietary reference intakes for calcium and vitamin D. Washington, DC.: The National Academies Press; 2011.

136. Pettifor JM. Nutritional rickets. In: Glorieux FH, Pettifor JM, Juppner H, editors. Pediatric bone: biology and diseases. 2nd ed. San Diego: Academic Press; 2012. p. 625–54.

137. Thacher TD, Fischer PR, Pettifor JM. The usefulness of clinical features to identify active rickets. Ann Trop Paediatr. 2002;22(3):229–37.

138. Glerup H, Mikkelsen K, Poulsen L, Hass E, Overbeck S, Andersen H, et al. Hypovitaminosis D myopathy without biochemical signs of osteomalacic bone involvement. Calcif Tissue Int. 2000;66(6):419–24.

139. Bonnici F. Functional hypoparathyroidism in infantile hypocalcaemic stage I vitamin D deficiency rickets. S Afr Med J. 1978;54(15):611–2.

140. Fraser D, Kooh SW, Scriver CR. Hyperparathyroidism as the cause of hyperaminoaciduria and phosphaturia in human vitamin D deficiency. Pediatr Res. 1967;1(6):425–35.
141. Zeghoud F, Vervel C, Guillozo H, Walrant-Debray O, Boutignon H, Garabedian M. Subclinical vitamin D deficiency in neonates: definition and response to vitamin D supplements. Am J Clin Nutr. 1997;65(3):771–8.
142. Shenoy SD, Swift P, Cody D, Iqbal J. Maternal vitamin D deficiency, refractory neonatal hypocalcaemia, and nutritional rickets. Arch Dis Child. 2005;90(4):437–8.
143. Pettifor JM, Pentopoulos M, Moodley GP, Isdale JM, Ross FP. Is craniotabes a pathognomonic sign of rickets in 3-month-old infants? S Afr Med J. 1984;65:549–51.
144. Steinbach HL, Noetzli M. Roentgen appearance of the skeleton in osteomalacia and rickets. Am J Roentgen. 1964;91:955–72.
145. Thacher TD, Fischer PR, Pettifor JM, Lawson JO, Manaster BJ, Reading JC. Radiographic scoring method for the assessment of the severity of nutritional rickets. J Trop Pediatr. 2000;46(3):132–9.
146. Kruse K. Pathophysiology of calcium metabolism in children with vitamin D-deficiency rickets. J Pediatr. 1995;126(5 Pt 1):736–41.
147. Markestad T, Halvorsen KS, Aksnes L, Aarskog D. Plasma concentrations of vitamin D metabolites before and during treatment of vitamin D deficiency rickets in children. Acta Paediatr Scand. 1984;73:225–31.
148. Chesney RW, Zimmerman J, Hamstra A, DeLuca HF, Mazees RB. Vitamin D metabolite concentrations in vitamin D deficiency. Are calcitriol levels normal. Am J Dis Child. 1981;135(11):1025–8.
149. Gupta MM, Round JM, Stamp TCB. Spontaneous cure of vitamin-D deficency in Asians during summer in Britain. Lancet. 1974;i:586–8.
150. Shaw NJ, Mughal MZ. Vitamin D and child health part 1 (skeletal aspects). Arch Dis Child. 2013;98(5):363–7.
151. Cesur Y, Caksen H, Gundem A, Kirimi E, Odabas D. Comparison of low and high dose of vitamin D treatment in nutritional vitamin D deficiency rickets. J Pediatr Endocrinol Metab. 2003;16(8):1105–9.
152. Pettifor JM. How should we manage vitamin D deficiency rickets? Indian Pediatr. 2014;51:259–60.
153. Kutluk G, Cetinkaya F, Basak M. Comparisons of oral calcium, high dose vitamin D and a combination of these in the treatment of nutritional rickets in children. J Trop Pediatr. 2002;48(6):351–3.
154. Thacher TD, Fischer PR, Pettifor JM. Vitamin D treatment in calcium-deficiency rickets: a randomised controlled trial. Arch Dis Child. 2014;99(9):807–11.
155. Holick MF, Binkley NC, Bischoff-Ferrari HA, Gordon CM, Hanley DA, Heaney RP, et al. Evaluation, treatment, and prevention of vitamin D deficiency: an Endocrine Society clinical practice guideline. J Clin Endocrinol Metab. 2011;96(7):1911–30.
156. Ross AC, Manson JE, Abrams SA, Aloia JF, Brannon PM, Clinton SK, et al. The 2011 report on dietary reference intakes for calcium and vitamin D from the Institute of Medicine: what clinicians need to know. J Clin Endocrinol Metab. 2011;96(1):53–8.
157. Greer FR. Issues in establishing vitamin D recommendations for infants and children. Am J Clin Nutr. 2004;80(6):1759S–62S.
158. Whiting SJ, Calvo MS. Dietary recommendations to meet both endocrine and autocrine needs of Vitamin D. J Steroid Biochem Mol Biol. 2005;97(1–2):7–12.
159. Wharton B, Bishop NR. Lancet. 2003;362(9393):1389–400.
160. Moy RJ, McGee E, Debelle GD, Mather I, Shaw NJ. Successful public health action to reduce the incidence of symptomatic vitamin D deficiency. Arch Dis Child. 2012;97(11):952–4.
161. Basile LA, Taylor SN, Wagner CL, Horst RL, Hollis BW. The effect of high-dose vitamin D supplementation on serum vitamin D levels and milk calcium concentration in lactating women and their infants. Breastfeed Med. 2006;1(1):27–35.
162. Zeghoud F, Ben-Mekhbi H, Djeghri N, Garabedian M. Vitamin D prophylaxis during infancy: comparison of the long- term effects of three intermittent doses (15, 5, or 2.5 mg) on 25- hydroxyvitamin D concentrations. Am J Clin Nutr. 1994;60:393–6.
163. Thacher TD, Bommersbach TJ, Pettifor JM, Isichei CO, Fischer PR. Comparison of limestone and ground fish for treatment of nutritional rickets in children in Nigeria. J Pediatr. 2015;167(1):148–54 e1.
164. Doxiadis S, Angelis C, Karatzas P, Vrettos C, Lapatsanis P. Genetic aspects of nutritional rickets. Arch Dis Child. 1976;51(2):83–90.
165. Awumey EM, Mitra DA, Hollis BW, Kumar R, Bell NH. Vitamin D metabolism is altered in Asian Indians in the southern United States: a clinical research center study. J Clin Endocrinol Metab. 1998;83(1):169–73.
166. Munns CF, Shaw N, Kiely M, Specker BL, Thacher TD, Ozono K, et al. Global consensus recommendations on prevention and management of nutritional rickets. J Clin Endocrinol Metab. 2016;101(2):394–415.

Chapter 14
Essential Fatty Acids

Esther Granot and Richard J. Deckelbaum

Keywords Essential fatty acids · DHA · EPA · Arachidonic acid (AA) · Alpha-linolenic acid (ALA) · Polyunsaturated fatty acids

Learning Objectives

- Review the role that essential fatty acids should have as part of nutrition interventions for low- and middle-income countries
- Identify the dietary sources for essential fatty acids and their conversion to other n-3 and n-6 fatty acids
- Describe how essential fatty acids are associated with birth outcomes
- Explain the mechanisms for how essential fatty acids are associated with chronic diseases
- Describe how dietary requirements for essential fatty acids can be determined.

Introduction

Essential polyunsaturated fatty acids, of both the n-3 and n-6 series, play a critical role in a myriad of complex biologic and metabolic pathways. They thereby affect various processes relevant to human health and disease throughout the life course, from fetal and infantile neurodevelopment to immune modulation, with an impact on diverse conditions as asthma, rheumatoid arthritis, inflammatory bowel disease, and atherosclerosis.

This review focuses on basic science research and clinical/epidemiological studies relating to essential polyunsaturated fatty acids, with an emphasis on areas of importance to developing countries, specifically those pertaining to mother and child health. Attempts to assess dietary requirements of essential fatty acids and maintain their adequate intake during pregnancy, lactation, and early childhood, in vulnerable middle- and low-income populations, will be addressed.

E. Granot (✉)
Department of Pediatrics, Kaplan Medical Center, Rehovot,
Hebrew University—Hadassah Medical School, Jerusalem, Israel
e-mail: ettie.granot@ekmd.huji.ac.il

R.J. Deckelbaum
Institute of Human Nutrition, Departments of Pediatrics and Epidemiology,
Columbia University Medical Center, New York, USA
e-mail: rjd20@cumc.columbia.edu

© Springer Science+Business Media New York 2017
S. de Pee et al. (eds.), *Nutrition and Health in a Developing World*,
Nutrition and Health, DOI 10.1007/978-3-319-43739-2_14

Essential Fatty Acids and Their Metabolism

Essential polyunsaturated fatty acids (PUFA) cannot be synthesized in the body and must be ingested in food. There are two series of essential fatty acids: omega 3 fatty acids characterized by a double bond at the third carbon from the methyl end of the fatty acid and omega 6 fatty acids which have a double bond at the position of the sixth carbon from the methyl end.

The n-3 fatty acids originate from synthesis in plants and algae. The main n-3 fatty acid consumed is alpha-linolenic acid (ALA)(C 18:3 n-3). The major dietary source of two n-3 fatty acids, eicosapentanoic (EPA) acid and docosahexaenoic acid (DHA), is fish. The proportion of linolenic acid that can be converted to the longer chain n-3 fatty acids EPA (C 20:5 n-3) and DHA (C 22:6 n-3) is very low, estimated at less than 1% [1–4].

The main essential n-6 fatty acid present in diet, from which longer n-6 fatty acids are synthesized, is linoleic acid (LA) (C 18:2 n-6). The longer chain-6 fatty acid arachidonic acid (AA) (20:4,n-6), is also present in diet, but to a lesser degree. Linoleic acid can be metabolized to arachidonic acid (C 20:4 n-6). Arachidonic acid is further metabolized, by chain elongation, via docosatetraenoic acid (C 22:4 n-6) to tetracosapentaenoic acid (C 24:5 n-6). The metabolism of n-3 and n-6 fatty acids is interrelated and uses the same enzymes for elongation and desaturation; high intakes of the n-6 linoleic acid inhibit the metabolism of the n-3 linolenic acid so that the conversion of linolenic acid to DHA is decreased (Fig. 14.1).

In 1999 an NIH sponsored Workshop on the Essentiality of the Recommended Dietary Intakes for n-6 and n-3 Fatty acids [5] emphasized the importance of decreasing n-6 PUFA in face of an increase in dietary n-3 PUFAs, in order to reduce adverse effects of excesses of AA and its eicosanoid products

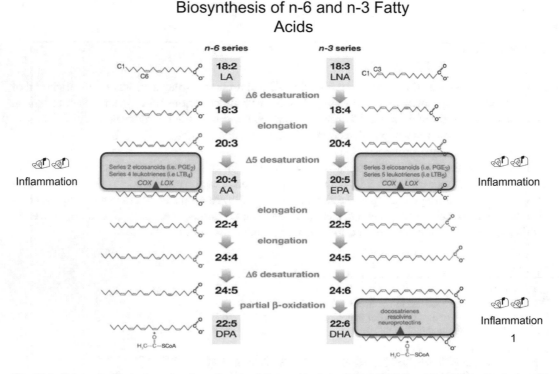

Fig. 14.1 Schematic illustration of major n-3 and n-6 fatty acids derived from linoleic acid and alpha-linolenic acid. Adapted from Marszalek and Lodish [99]

that can occur when too much linoleic acid and AA are present in the diet. Linoleic acid converts to AA via the enzyme Δ-6 desaturase, which is the same enzyme necessary to desaturate alpha-linolenic acid, the parent compound of the n-3 class.

Traditionally human diets contained almost equal amounts (1–2:1) of n-6 and n-3 fatty acids. Over the past 100–150 years there has been a decrease in n-3 FA intakes and an enormous increase in consumption of n-6 FA, due to intake of vegetable oils from corn, sunflower seeds, safflower seeds, and soybeans. In Western diets the n-6/n-3 ratio is estimated at 15:1–16:1 but can reach as high as 20–30:1 [6–8].

Reducing the large amounts of dietary n-6 LA (present in corn, safflower and soybean oils) or increasing dietary ALA will better balance n-6/n-3 ratios. The known competition between the two pathways of essential fatty acids is very difficult to untangle biologically and it is not known in what proportions C20 & C22 unsaturated long-chain fatty acids will be produced from different dietary mixtures of linoleic and alpha-linolenic acids.

Polyunsaturated Fatty Acids and Immunomodulation

Polyunsaturated fatty acids are basic constituents of phospholipid membranes and affect membrane structure and fluidity. They are also precursors of eicosanoids (prostaglandins, prostacyclins, thromboxanes, and leukotrienes) via which they exert an effect on the immune response. PUFA also modulate nuclear receptors and intracellular enzyme activities. Leukotrienes derived from AA via the lipoxygenase pathway stimulate production of proinflammatory cytokines, and the prostanoids derived from AA via the cyclooxygenase pathway promote vasoconstriction and aggregation of thrombocytes. EPA competes for the same initial enzymes in the lipoxygenase and cyclooxygenase pathways leading to inhibition of eicosanoid synthesis from AA. Thus, n-6 FA are expected to shift the physiologic state to one that is proinflammatory and prothrombotic while n-3 FA are expected to result in production of eicosanoids that posses more anti-inflammatory, antithrombotic, and vasodilation properties [9].

PUFA are incorporated into membrane phospholipids, specifically in distinct micro domains of the plasma membrane which are known as lipid rafts. Lipid rafts play a critical role in signal transduction; PUFA regulate gene expression either directly by interaction with nuclear receptors as the peroxisome proliferators-activated receptor (PPAR) and liver X receptor (LXR), or indirectly via pathways initiated at the plasma membrane such as T cell receptors of Toll—like receptors. The effects of PUFAs on various nuclear receptors are receptor-specific and fatty-acid-specific. PUFAs which activate PPARγ inhibit expression of proinflammatory cytokines. Conversely, as LXR agonists exert an anti-inflammatory effect via inhibition of COX2 and IL6, PUFAs that inhibit the LXR, would be expected to have a proinflammatory effect [10, 11]. n-3 fatty acids, in contrast to saturated fatty acids, have been shown to decrease endothelial lipase which is one of the lipases synthesized and secreted by macrophages [12]. In mice, endothelial lipase deficiency is associated with a decrease in atherosclerotic lesions. PPARγ, highly expressed in macrophages—derived foam cells in atherosclerotic plaques is regulated by EPA, leading to a decrease in endothelial lipase and a parallel decrease in proinflammatory markers and increase in anti-inflammatory markers [12].

Recently, novel di- and trihydroxy-containing n-3 fatty acid-derived mediators have been defined. These mediators named resolvins and protectins are of importance in terminating a state of inflammation. The noninflamed state is described not as a passive process but rather as an actively regulated program of resolution [13, 14].

Associations Between N-3 and N-6 PUFA Dietary Intakes and Disease

Various epidemiological studies link a high dietary n-6/n-3 ratio with an increased risk of cardio-vascular diseases, diabetes, asthma, autoimmune disorders, and even cancer suggesting that a Western-type diet based on a high dietary intake of n-6 FA can have detrimental effects [8]. Adopting a Western diet has been shown to be associated with increased morbidity from noncommunicable diseases—some examples are reviewed below.

Noncommunicable Diseases

Raheja et al. [15] reported a sharp increase in the prevalence of non-insulin-dependent diabetes mellitus and coronary artery disease among the upper socioeconomic classes in India after they adopted diets high in total fat and with high n-6/n-3 ratios. Indeed, in Japanese women a low incidence of breast cancer has been observed among those women who conserved their traditional diet which contains fats derived mainly from marine sources rich in n-3 PUFA. Similarly, Greenland Inuits have a very low incidence of breast cancer, cardiovascular diseases, and autoimmune disorders despite their relatively high fat diet, presumably because of its high n-3 FA content [8, 16, 17].

While results are mixed, administering of n-3 PUFA as fish oil or as individual or a combination of n-3 FA, in different ratios and amounts, has been studied in the prevention and control of a multitude of disease states including CHD, hypertension, type II diabetes, rheumatoid arthritis, renal disease, inflammatory bowel disease, asthma, multiple sclerosis, depression, schizophrenia, and Alzheimer's dementia [18, 19].

Increased dietary amounts of n-3 FA have proven beneficial in the secondary prevention of cardiovascular disease; a ratio of 4:1 was associated with a 70% decrease in total mortality [20, 21]. Yet, despite other studies in cardiovascular patients demonstrating beneficial effects of n-3 FA supplementation [22], a systematic review of 48 RCT and 26 cohort studies reached the conclusion that the positive effects of n-3 FA supplementation is nonsignificant [23]. Indeed, more recent, large intervention studies with marine n-3 fatty acids failed to replicate earlier findings of reduced cardiovascular mortality in at-risk patients [24, 25]. Attempts to reconcile these conflicting data emphasize different background intakes of the different n-6 and n-3 fatty acids in the different populations studied, sample size differences, timing of initiation of the n-3 fatty acid supplements, and the relative amounts of EPA versus DHA used [26].

Asthma

Population studies in Australia showed that regular fish intake was associated with a 50% reduction in asthma prevalence and increased airway responsiveness [27] and that children whose parents reported eating oily fish have significantly less asthma [28]. Yet, the effect of n-3 FA is likely complex—in patients with asthma, an n-6/n-3 ratio of 5:1 was linked to a beneficial effect whereas a 10:1 ratio had adverse consequences [29]. In a Japanese study of 6–15-year olds, which compared 1673 asthmatics versus 22,109 healthy children, increased fish intake (1–2/week) was associated with a significantly higher prevalence of asthma [30]. However, a review of 9 RCT (in both children and adults) comparing n-3 FA supplementation for at least 3 weeks versus placebo found no convincing evidence regarding the ability of n-3 FA to improve asthma symptoms [31]. These differences might be related to different baseline n-3 (or n-6) intakes in different populations.

Other Conditions

Studies on the effect of n-3 FA on ADHD, autism, and related disorders similarly yielded conflicting results [32, 33] but given their relative safety and general health benefits n-3 FA are considered as a promising complementary approach to standard treatments [34].

Similarly, when assessing benefit of n-3 PUFA supplementation in rheumatoid arthritis patients (on pain, swollen joints, laboratory parameters of disease activity), in over 19 RCTs, results are inconsistent, but in some studies patients did show a definite improvement in clinical findings and laboratory parameters [35, 36].

In cancer patients there is limited data regarding benefits of n-3 FA. A dietary ratio of n-6/n-3 of 2.5:1 reduced rectal cell proliferation in patients with colorectal cancer but interestingly, no beneficial effect was observed with the same amount of n-3 but when the ratio of n-6/n-3 was maintained at 4:1 [37, 38]. A recent review highlighting controversies relating to dietary fatty acids in disease [39] addressed the contradictory studies relating to the effect of fish oil and fish oil fatty acids on lung cancer and the conflicting data on the association between plasma phospholipids fatty acids and prostate cancer [40, 41]. An association has been reported between higher blood n-3 fatty acids and increased cancer prostate cancer risk [42, 43]. Yet, a meta-analysis of eight prospective studies concluded that intake of marine n-3 fatty acids is not associated with prostate cancer development [44]. Currently, there is insufficient evidence for establishing any relationship of PUFA consumption with cancer.

It is noteworthy that results of different trials are not consistent, likely as amount and type of PUFA used are not uniform and include different dietary fish, fish oils and/or flaxseed oil, rapeseed oil, primrose oil and EPA, DHA and ALA in variable doses and ratios and for different time periods. As the conversion of ALA to EPA and DHA is highly inefficient, the beneficial effect of rapeseed or flaxseed oil may result from the ALA itself. The potential, independent immunomodulatory effects, if any, of ALA are yet to be determined [45]. Furthermore, optimal doses or combinations of n-3 fatty acids, or perhaps optimal n-6/n-3 ratios or absolute amounts of n-6 FA and n-3 FA, may be disease dependent so that in future treatment should be tailored to the specific disease/condition and even to its degree of severity.

Effect of N-6 and N-3 Fatty Acids in Pregnancy, Lactation, and Infancy

DHA is deposited in appreciable amounts in the central nervous system during the perinatal brain growth spurt with fetal DHA accretion during the third trimester of gestation estimated at 45–60 mg/day. It is noteworthy that AA accretion occurs mainly postnatally.

Dietary fat intakes and specifically intakes of AA and DHA are important during pregnancy and early infancy, affecting pregnancy outcome, fetal growth, and infants' neural maturation and retinal function [46–50]. In a study encompassing 11,875 pregnant women, low maternal sea food consumption was found to be associated with offspring achieving lower social scores, decreased fine motor skills, and higher risk of IQ scores at the lowest quartiles [51]. Observation and intervention studies involving pregnant and lactating women and infants-fed DHA-supplemented formulas show that a greater intake of DHA is associated with better scores on tests of visual and neural development in infancy and early childhood [4, 52].

Although the fractional conversion of ALA to n-3 long-chain PUFAs may be greater in women than in men, it is limited and cannot meet the increased demands for DHA which must therefore be met by an increase in dietary DHA intake. The recommended daily allowance of DHA during pregnancy and lactation is 300 mg/day [5] with women urged to aim at an intake of at least

200 mg/day [53]. This desired intake can be reached with the consumption of one to two portions of fish per week, of which tuna, herring, mackerel, salmon, and trout are those richer in EPA and DHA. As for AA, plasma and tissue content is relatively stable and not influenced by the dietary intake of preformed AA. There is no indication that women of childbearing age with an adequate dietary intake of the precursor fatty acid, linoleic acid, need an additional supply of AA [53]. Most pregnant women do not meet the recommended dietary intake of DHA. In a survey of pregnant Canadian women mean DHA intake was only 82 ± 33 mg/day and in 90% of low-income Midwest American women intake was far below 300 mg/day [54, 55].

Levels of maternal DHA decline with multiple pregnancies; levels have been shown to be significantly less in multiparous compared with primiparous mothers and when pregnancies are closely spaced [56]. Low consumption of fish has been linked to a higher percentage of preterm deliveries [57, 58] and the effects of n-3 long-chain PUFA supplementation (150–1200 mg of DHA daily or up to 2.7 gr total n-3 long-chain PUFA), in pregnant women, on length of gestation and birth weight have been evaluated. In a number of trials a slight increase in birth weight, and length of gestation coupled with a reduced risk of preterm delivery, were observed [59–61].

One of us (E.G) recently studied the effect of 400 mg/day of DHA supplementation starting after the 12th week of gestation in multiparous mothers with all of them in at least their third pregnancy (40% in their fifth–seventh pregnancies). Gestational length and infants' birth weight, in the DHA-supplemented group were compared to a non-supplemented control group and were also compared within groups to the mothers' previous pregnancies. DHA supplementation did not have any effect on the infants' birth weight. However, an effect of DHA supplementation on length of gestation was observed in highly multiparous mothers, those with six or more pregnancies [62].

Long-Chain Polyunsaturated Fatty Acids in Human Milk

Maternal dietary intake of DHA affects levels of DHA in breast milk. In a study comparing the composition of long-chain PUFAs in diet and breast milk of Chinese women from a rural area and Swedish women residing in Stockholm the Chinese diet was found to contain more linoleic acid and less AA, EPA, and DHA than that of Swedish mothers [63]. These dietary differences were mirrored in breast milk fatty acid composition; the ratio of AA to DHA was 3.1 in the Chinese women's breast milk and 1.6 in that of Swedish mothers [63]. A comparison of breast milk fatty acid composition of Chinese women residing in five different geographical regions demonstrated a highly variable AA to DHA ratio (g/g) with mean levels of 2.77 in inland areas to 0.42 in coastal/sea areas [64]. In a meta-analysis that considered 65 studies encompassing 2474 women worldwide, breast milk fatty acid composition demonstrated mean DHA concentrations (% of total fatty acids) of 0.32 ± 0.22 (range 0.06–1.4%) and mean AA concentrations of 0.47 ± 0.13(% of total fatty acids) (range 0.24–1.0%). The mean ratio of AA to DHA in breast milk, even within the same geographical region, varies widely. The highest breast milk DHA concentrations were observed primarily in coastal populations and were associated with marine food consumption [65]. Populations with the highest breast milk DHA concentrations, in the range of 0.6–1.4%, included women from Japan, Philippines, Congo, Sweden, Dominican Republic, and Canadian women residing in arctic regions. All of these, with the exception of Congo, are coastal or island populations. In Congo, proximity to lakes and rivers likely results in high dietary fish intake. The lowest DHA levels were noted in breast milk samples from Pakistan, rural South Africa, Canada, the Netherlands, and France with DHA levels in the range of 0.06–0.14% [65]. These populations reside inland or are from developed countries, both of which are usually associated with low marine food consumption. Indeed, in Chinese women residing in the coastal regions of China breast milk mean DHA levels are 2.78% of total fatty acids whereas levels were only 0.68% in breast milk of Chinese women residing in inland rural areas of

China [64]. Notably, the concentration of AA in breast milk samples is much less variable than that of DHA. Based on these studies, the best estimates of worldwide mean breast milk AA and DHA concentrations (% of total fatty acids) are 0.47 for AA and 0.32 for DHA [65].

The amount of AA and DHA in infant formulas is currently based on these mean breast milk levels, with a ratio of AA/DHA of 1–1.5:1, thereby aiming to have infant formulas which simulate the essential fatty acid composition of human milk. The recommended DHA level in infant formulas is 0.2–0.5% of fatty acids with the amount of AA being at least equal to the DHA level. The total fat content in most infant formulas is 4.4–6.0 g/100 kcal, equivalent to ∼40–54% of energy content.

The comparison of levels of AA and DHA in mature and premature human milk is of special interest as both play a pivotal role in brain development and visual function maturation. The critical period of placental transfer of these fatty acids is believed to be in the third trimester of pregnancy. It has been estimated that approximately 45–60 mg of DHA per day accrues in the fetal brain during this time period [47, 49]. Thus, in infants born prematurely depleted DHA stores, coupled with limited ability to synthesize long-chain PUFAs [4] and enhanced needs due to accelerated growth, places them at high risk for ARA and DHA deficiency.

Long-chain PUFAs and especially DHA are preferentially transported across the placenta to the developing fetus and accumulate extensively in the fetal brain during the last trimester of pregnancy. Thus, infants born prematurely are at a disadvantage as their body stores of long-chain PUFAs are limited while at the same time requirements for fatty acid deposition in their rapidly growing tissues are high [66]. After delivery, endogenous long-chain PUFAs synthesis is relatively low and supply of long-chain PUFAs to the breast-fed infant depends on the amount of these fatty acids in breast milk.

Human milk fatty acid composition is influenced by factors such as maternal parity, maternal diet, and stage of lactation. As infants born prematurely have increased requirements for long-chain PUFAs, it is of interest to determine whether human milk fatty acid composition is also influenced by duration of pregnancy. To date, studies on long-chain PUFAs content in milk of mothers who gave birth to preterm infants have yielded conflicting results [67–70].

One of us (E.G) recently compared fatty acid composition in human milk of mothers giving birth to full-term and preterm infants. In the mothers of preterm infants, breast milk fatty acid composition was also studied during the first 2 weeks after delivery [71]. This study did not observe differences in the proportion of either AA or DHA nor did these levels increase, in breast milk of mothers giving birth to preterm infants during the 2 weeks post delivery period studied. Furthermore, even in the "very small" premature infants (26–30 weeks gestation), included in our study, mothers' breast milk AA and DHA levels did not differ from mean levels in breast milk of mothers giving birth to full-term infants. Thus, the results of this study are in accord with the studies by Luukkainen [68] and Kovacs [70] showing that breast milk of mothers of preterm infants does not compensate for the special needs and increased requirements for long-chain PUFAs, which result from prematurity. Optimal daily amount of AA & DHA required by the premature infant should be defined so one can determine if there is a need to add essential fatty acids not only to infant formulas but also to supplement breastfeeding mothers.

Breastfeeding confers protection against infections during infancy. Breast-fed infants have an enhanced local humoral immune response, resulting in a lower prevalence of gastrointestinal and respiratory tract infections than in formula—fed infants [72, 73]. Exclusive breastfeeding for the first few months has also been suggested to be protective against the development of atopic disease [74]. Immunoglobulins, lymphocytes, proteins like lactoferrin and lysozyme, which are present in breast milk, play a specific immunologic role.

Another component, which may be of high importance to maturation and function of the immune system, is the fatty acid pattern of dietary milks. Human milk contains long-chain PUFAs (20–22 carbons) of both n-3 and n-6 class which constitute ∼2% of total fatty acids and which are undetectable in unsupplemented formulas prepared from vegetable oils. The type of dietary milk which infants consume results in changes in the fatty acid pattern of cell membrane phospholipids [75].

As the ratio of arachidonic acid-derived eicosanoids and those derived from n-3 fatty acids has been suggested to play a role in immune modulation [76, 77] we designed a study to assess whether the beneficial effects of breast milk on the immune response might be related to its essential fatty acid composition. We measured RBC membrane fatty acid composition, as a surrogate marker for WBC membrane fatty acid composition, by gas–liquid chromatography in breast-fed and non-supplemented formula-fed, 2–4 month old, infants. Release of the proinflammatory cytokines IL-1 and TNF was measured in whole blood culture in bacterial endotoxin stimulated and nonstimulated cells. Significant differences were observed in cell membrane fatty acid composition between breast-fed and formula-fed infants; breast-fed infants had a significantly greater percentage of n-3 fatty acids and specifically a twofold greater level of DHA than infants fed a non-supplemented formula, with similar membrane levels of AA and % total n-6 fatty acids. Despite differences in cell membrane fatty acid composition, the release of proinflammatory cytokines by immunocompetent cells did not differ between breast-fed and formula-fed infants [78]. Although our study failed to prove our hypothesis that increased mononuclear cell membrane DHA levels would likely reduce cellular production of proinflammatory cytokines, it was credited for providing "a new glimpse into neonatal nutrition and its effects on the immune response" [79].

Various parameters relating to the immune response have been compared in infants-fed human milk, infants-fed non-supplemented formulas, and infants-fed long-chain PUFAs-supplemented formulas. Infants receiving long-chain PUFAs fortified formula showed an increase in the proportion of activated "memory" CD4 and CD8 cells [80], but no changes were observed in older children receiving AA and DHA for a 7-month period [81].

In vitro and in vivo studies in animals and humans have demonstrated that long-chain PUFAs reduce release of the proinflammatory cytokines IL-2 TNFα and IFNγ from mononuclear cells [82–84], although other researchers did not observe any change in IFNγ release following long-chain PUFAs supplementation [81].

As maternal DHA levels decline with multiple, closely spaced pregnancies we questioned whether DHA supplementation during pregnancy and lactation, in a population with a high percentage of multiparous mothers would affect the immune response of their infants, solely breast-fed up to the age of 4 months [85]. DHA supplementation did not exert an effect on the humoral immune response and infants in both groups did not differ in levels of immunoglobulins of IgG, IgM, and IgA classes and the specific antibody response as reflected by measuring the titer of antibodies to HBsAg after two doses of vaccine (at 2 days and at 1 month of age) was similar in both groups.

Infants in the DHA-supplemented group had a similar number of CD4 cells as the non-supplemented group but the number of CD8 cells was significantly reduced (CD4/CD8 ratio 2.6 in DHA-supplemented infants as compared with 1.9 in the non-supplemented group). Of CD4 cells the fraction of CD45RA+ cells, representing naïve helper cells, was significantly higher in the DHA-supplemented group and the proportion of CD8 + CD45RO + activated cells was significantly higher, constituting 35% of CD8 cells as compared with 16% in the non-supplemented group. In both CD4 & CD8 cells the production of IFNγ was found to be markedly lower in lymphocytes of the infants in the DHA-supplemented group [85].

Thus, in our study DHA supplementation during pregnancy and lactation did not result in changes in the infants' humoral immune response, as assessed by levels of antiHBs antibodies and total immunoglobulins, but did affect lymphocyte subset profile and cytokine production. A lymphocyte profile with a higher percentage of CD4 naïve cells and decreased IFNγ production in both CD4 & CD8 cells is likely compatible with attenuation of a proinflammatory response. The clinical implications of the changes observed in cellular immune response are as yet speculative and whether supplementation of DHA to breast feeding mothers confers an advantage to their infants remains to be elucidated.

Essential Fatty Acid Requirements in Healthy Infants, Children, and Adults

The Joint FAO/WHO Expert Consultation on Fats and Fatty Acids, Geneva 2008, recommended that total n-3 FA intake range between 0.5 and 2.0% of total energy with a minimum dietary requirement of alpha linoleic acid being 0.5% energy [86]. For adult males and nonpregnant, nonlactating females 0.25–0.5 g/day of EPA plus DHA, together, is recommended, with insufficient evidence to set a specific minimum intake of either EPA or DHA alone; both should be consumed. For pregnant and lactating mothers the minimum intake, for both their own optimal health and that of the fetus and infant, is 0.3 g/day of EPA&DHA of which at least 0.2 g/day should be DHA [86]. As for n-6 FA there is no sufficient data for establishing a precise quantitative estimate of the LA requirement needed in order to prevent deficiency. An adequate intake of LA of 2–3% of energy is proposed. Arachidonic acid is not essential for a healthy adult whose habitual diet provides LA at an amount that is at least 2.5% of total caloric energy supply. There is as yet no compelling scientific evidence upon which to base recommendations regarding specific ratios of dietary n-6 FA to n-3 FA or ratio of LA to ALAs [86, 87].

The expert panel reiterated the recommendations that the minimum concentration of DHA in infant formulas and baby foods should be 0.2% of total fatty acids and should not exceed 0.5% of total FA. Levels of added AA should, at least, equal that of added DHA. The amount of EPA added should not exceed the amount of DHA. For infants 0–6 months of age AA should be supplied in the diet within the range of 0.2–0.3% E, based on human milk composition. For older infants (6–24 months of age), the LA adequate intake range recommended is 3.0–4.5% of total caloric energy intake. Sources of long-chain PUFAs during the first year of life include breast milk, infant formulas, or follow-on formulas enriched with long-chain PUFAs and complementary foods such as eggs and fatty fish. Highly refined oils from single-cell organisms (algae and fungi), eggs, or fish are appropriate as DHA and AA sources for use in infant formulas and complementary foods [86].

Essential Fatty Acids and Specific Needs in Developing Countries

A special concern is the lack of data regarding dietary intake of PUFA in low and middle income countries (LMICs). A recent review compiled information, from the few studies available, on the content of PUFA in breast milk and in major foods using national food balance sheets from the United Nations' Food and Agriculture Organization Statistical Database (FOASTAT) for 13 LMICs [88]. This review indicated that breast milk DHA content is very low in populations living mainly on a plant-based diet but is higher in fish-eating communities. Per capita supply of fat and n-3 FA increases markedly with increasing gross domestic product (GDP). In most of the 13 countries surveyed, 70–80% of the supply of PUFA comes from cereals and vegetable oils, some of which have very low alpha-linolenic acid content. In the nine countries with the lowest GDP, the total n-3 FA supply was found to be below or close to the lower end of the recommended intake range (0.4% of energy supply) for infants and children and below the minimum recommended level (0.5% of energy) for pregnant and lactating women [88]. As breast milk is one of the best sources of alpha-linolenic acid and DHA, breast-fed infants are less likely to be at risk of insufficient intakes than infants who are not breast-fed. If needed, where maternal diets have insufficient n-3 intakes mothers can be given DHA supplementation during pregnancy and lactation; this may be particularly of benefit when breast feeding is continued for 2 years or more [89].

The issue of optimal infant nutrition, specifically of n-3 FA "fortified" foods is an area of interest, with a special emphasis on the needs of infants and young children from low-income populations, with a high prevalence of malnutrition. The potential for small quantity lipid-based nutrient supplements (LNS), i.e., 20 g/d providing <120 kcal/d to promote growth and development after 6 months of age, is currently being investigated. A recent study showed that infants receiving such supplements do not reduce their intake of breast milk so that the beneficial effects of breast milk are not concomitantly decreased [90, 91]. In infants who are 6 months of age, the introduction of complementary feeding coupled with continued breast feeding is of special interest. Ensuring an adequate intake of micronutrients, (including calcium, iron, zinc, B vitamins), fat-soluble vitamins (vitamins A, D, E, and K), appropriate amounts of protein and fat, and specifically the recommended allowance of EFA, is of major importance [92].

The Food and Agriculture Organization (FAO) reports that adequate intakes of ALA should be 0.4–0.6% of energy intake and that of LA 3.0–4.5% of energy intake, for children aged 6–23 months. For children residing in LMICs, where the prevalence of underweight is high, essential fatty acid recommendations based on percentage of daily energy intake would be expected to result in calculated lower recommended daily amounts of EFA than those of children in well-nourished populations. Furthermore, the lower stores of EFA that these children likely have and the conversion of EFA to longer chain derivatives, which is thought to be defective in malnourished children, should also be considered [94–96]. Daily recommended intakes for EFA in LMICs should be adjusted accordingly and not be based only on the children's body weight as this would likely underestimate their needs and increase the risk of inadequate intake and consequent nutritional deficiency. Yang and Huffman [93] suggested that adequate requirements should therefore be calculated based on the WHO Reference Growth Standards, of median body weights of children of similar age, thereby "correcting" the lower estimated EFA in undernourished children.

Enhancing intake of alpha-linolenic acid through complementary plant food products (soy beans, soy oil, canola oil, lipid-based supplements) is feasible but due to the low conversion rates of ALA to DHA it may be more efficient to enhance DHA status by increasing fish consumption or DHA fortification. An industry that specializes in farmed fish that are fed specific oils, and in the growing of microalgae, on a large scale, can serve as adequate sources of EPA and DHA. Obtaining n-3 fatty acids through genetically selected or modified plants is also being studied [97].

Fortification of foods with n-3 long-chain PUFA, specifically DHA, is of growing interest. Designing products with these long-chain fatty acids for developing countries is especially challenging as they should be designed so as to address the nutritional needs of the target population and to withstand environmental conditions that may affect the fatty acids' stability and cause them to undergo lipid peroxidation. Other concerns include palatability of fortified foods, and preparation of appropriate formulations (powder, capsules, oils) according to the age group (infants, adults) for which they are intended [98].

In order to achieve adequate intake of EFA worldwide recognition of their importance is needed. Effective strategies to address adequate intakes should address the optimal balance of dietary LA and ALA based on the metabolism of these fatty acids, determine the appropriate recommended intake for different periods of life (pregnancy, infancy, early childhood), and allow for differences in requirements based on nutritional status. Still, more information is needed to recommend appropriate EFA intake in populations with undernutrition.

Conclusion

Long-chain polyunsaturated fatty acids act as major mediators of processes relating to health and disease throughout the life course both in developed and LMIC populations. Their role in fetal and early infancy is critical and their intake has also been linked to major causes of morbidity and mortality as cardiovascular diseases, diabetes, asthma, autoimmune disorders, and even cancer.

The optimal intake of essential fatty acids at various milestones in life and whether intake should be modified to account for the differing needs in LMICs and in less economically privileged populations warrants further research.

Discussion Points

- What are the key mechanisms through which essential fatty acids affect health throughout the lifespan?
- Describe the factors that affect the dietary requirements for essential fatty acids.
- How can changing dietary patterns in the world affect the essential fatty acid status of people living in low and middle income countries?
- What role can essential fatty acids have as part of nutritional interventions in low and middle income countries?

References

1. Salem N Jr, Wegher B, Mena P, Uauy R. Arachidonic and docosahexanoic acids are biosynthesized from their 18-carbon chain precursors in human infants. Proc Natl Acad Sci USA. 1996;93:49–54.
2. Hussein N, Ah-Sing E, Wilkinson P, et al. Long-chain conversion of ^{13}C linoleic acid and alpha linolenic acid in response to marked changes in their dietary intake in men. J Lipid Res. 2005;46:269–80.
3. Goyens PL, Spilker ME, Zock PL, et al. Compartmental modeling to quantify alpha linolenic acid conversion after longer term intake of multiple tracer boluses. J Lipid Res. 2005;46:1474–83.
4. Innis SM. Omega3 fatty acids and neural development to 2 years of age: do we know enough for dietary recommendations? J Pediatr Gastroenterol Nutr. 2009;48:S16–24.
5. Simopoulos AP, Leaf A, Salem N Jr. Workshop Statement on the essentiality of and recommended dietary intakes for omega-6 and omega-3 fatty acids. Prostagland Leuk Essent Fat Acid. 2000;63:119–21.
6. Simopoulos AP. Essential fatty acids in health and chronic diseases. Am J Clin Nutr. 1999;70:560S–9S.
7. Simopoulos AP. The importance of the ratio of omega-6/omega-3 essential fatty acids. Biomed Pharmacother. 2002;56:365–79.
8. Yam D, Eliraz A, Berry EM. Diet and disease—the Israeli paradox: possible dangers of a high omega 6 polyunsaturated fatty acid diet. Isr J Med Sci. 1996;32:1134–43.
9. Seo T, Blaner WS, Deckelbaum RJ. Omega 3 fatty acids: molecular approaches to optimal biological outcomes. Curr Opin Lipidol. 2005;16:11–8.
10. Fritsche K. Fatty acids as modulators of the immune response. Ann Rev Nutr. 2006;26:45–73.
11. Calder PC. Polyunsaturated fatty acids and inflammatory processes: new twists in an old tale. Biochimie 2009; 791–795.
12. Jung UJ, Torrejon C, Chang CL, Hamai H, Worgall TS, Deckelbaum RJ. Fatty acids regulate endothelial lipase and inflammatory markers in macrophages and in mouse aorta, a role for PPARγ. Arterioscler Thromb Vasc Biol. 2012;32:2929–37.
13. Weylandt KH, Chui CY, Gomolka B, Waechter SF, Wiedenmann B. Omega-3 fatty acids and their lipid mediators: towards an understanding of resolving and protectin formation. Prostaglandins Other Lipid Mediat. 2012; 97:73–82.
14. Bannenberg GL, Chiang N, Ariel A, Arita M, Tjonahen E, Gotlinger KH, Hong S, Serhan CN. Molecular circuits of resolution: formation and actions of resolvins and protectins. J Immunol. 2005;174:4345–55.
15. Raheja BS, Sadikot SM, Phatak RB, Rao MB. Significance of the w-6/w-3 ratio for insulin action in diabetes. Ann NY Acad Sci. 1993;683:258–71.
16. Horrobin DF, Huang YS. The role of linoleic acid and its metabolites in the lowering of plasma cholesterol and the prevalence of cardiovascular disease. Int J Cardiol. 1987;17:241–55.
17. Kromann N, Green A. Epidemiological studies in the Upernavik district, Greenland. Incidence of some chronic diseases 1950–1974. Acta Med Scand. 1980;208:401–6.

18. Lorente–Cebrian S, Costa AG, Navas–Carretero S, Zabala M, Martinez JA, Moreno-Aliaga MJ. Role of omega-3 fatty acids in obesity, metabolic syndrome and cardiovascular disease: a review of the evidence. J Physiol Biochem 2013; 69:633–651.

19. Cabre E, Manosa M, Gassull MA. Omega-3 fatty acids and inflammatory bowel disease—a systematic review. Br J Nutr. 2012;107(Suppl 2):S240–52.

20. de Lorgenile M, Renaud S, Mamelle N, Salen P, Martin JL, Monjaud I, Guidollet J, Touboul P, Delaye J. Mediterranean alpha linolenic acid-rich diet in secondary prevention of coronary artery disease. Lancet. 1994;343:1454–9.

21. Saravanan P, Davidson NC, Schmidt EB, Calder PC. Cardiovascular effects of marine omega-3 fatty acids. Lancet. 2010;376:540–50.

22. Wang C, Harris WS, Chung M, et al. w-3 fatty acids from fish or fish-oil supplements but not alpha-linolenic acid acid, benefit cardiovascular disease outcomes in primary and secondary prevention studies: a systematic review. Amer J Clin Nutr. 2006;84:5–17.

23. Hooper L, Thompson RL, Harrison RA, Summerbell CD, Ness AR, Moore HJ, Worthington HV, Durrington PN, Higgins JP, Capps NE, Riemersma RA, Ebrahim SB, Smith G. Risks and benefits of omega 3 fats for mortality, cardiovascular disease and cancer: a review. BMJ. 2006;332:752–60.

24. Kromhout D, Giltay EJ, Geleijnse JM. For the Alpha Omega Trial Group. W-3 fatty acids and cardiovascular events after myocardial infarction. N Engl J Med. 2010;363:2015–26.

25. Rauche B, Schiele R. Schneider S et al OMEGA, a randomized placebo controlled trial to test the effect of highly purified omega-3 fatty acids on top of modern guideline adjusted therapy after myocardial infarction. Circulation. 2010;122:2152–9.

26. Deckelbaum RJ, Calder PC. Different outcomes for omega -3 heart trials: why? Curr Opin Clin Nutr Metab Care. 2012;15:97–8.

27. Peat JK, Salome CM, Wollcock AJ. Factors associated with bronchial hyper responsiveness in Australian adults and children. Eur Respir J. 1992;5:921–9.

28. Hodge L, Salome CM, Peat JK, Haby MM, Xuan W, Woolcock AJ. Consumption of oily fish and childhood asthma risk. Med J Aust. 1996;164:137–40.

29. Broughton KS, Johnson CS, Pace BK, Liebman M, Kleppinger KM. Reduced asthma symptoms with w3fatty acid ingestion are related to 5-series leukotriene production. Am J Clin Nutr. 1997;65:1011–7.

30. Takemura Y, Sakurai Y, Honjo S, Tokimatsu A, Gibo M, Hara T, Kusakari A, Kugai N. The relationship between fish intake and the prevalence of asthma. Prev Med. 2002;34:221–5.

31. Woods RK, Thien FC, Abramson MJ. Dietary marine fatty acid (fish oil) for asthma in adults and children. Cochrane Database Syst Rev 2002: CD001283.

32. Richardson AJ, Montgomery P. The Oxford-Durham study: a randomized, controlled trial of dietary supplementation with fatty acids in children with developmental coordination disorder. Pediatrics. 2005;115:1360–6.

33. Amminger GP, Berger GE, Schafer MR, Klier C, Friedrich MH, Feucht M. Omega-3 fatty acids supplementation in children with autism: a double blind, randomized, placebo-controlled pilot study. Biol Psychiatr. 2007;61:551–3.

34. Richardson AJ. Omega-3 fatty acids in ADHD and related neurodevelopmental disorders. Int Rev Psychiatry. 2006;18:155–72.

35. Kremer JM. Omega-3 fatty acid supplements in rheumatoid arthritis. Am J Clin Nutr. 2000;71:349–51.

36. MacLean CH, Mojica WA, Morton SC, Pencharz J, Hasenfeld Garland R et al. Effects of omega-3 fatty acids on lipids and glycemic control in type II diabetes and the metabolic syndrome and on inflammatory bowel disease, rheumatoid arthritis, renal disease, systemic lupus erythematosus and osteoporosis. Evid Rep Technol Assess 2004; No 89, AHRQ Publ No 04-E012-2 Rockville MD: Agency Healthcare Res Qual.

37. Bartram HP, Gostner A, Scheppach W, Reddy BS, Rao CV, Dusel G, Richter F, Richter A, Kasper H. Effects of fish oil on rectal cell proliferation, mucosal fatty acid and prostaglandin E2 release in healthy subjects. Gastroenterology. 1993;105:1317–22.

38. Bartram HP, Gostner A, Scheppach W, Reddy BS, Rao CV, Dusel G, Richter F, Richter A, Kasper H. Missing antiproliferative effect of fish oil on rectal epithelium in healthy volunteers consuming a high fat diet. Potential role of the w3:w6 fatty acid ratio. Eur J Can Prev 1995; 4:231–237.

39. Calder PC, Deckelbaum RJ. Dietary fatty acids in health and disease: greater controversy, greater interest. Curr Opin Clin Nutr Metab Care. 2014;17:111–5.

40. Murphy RA, Mourtzakis M, Chu QS, et al. Supplementation with fish oil increases first line chemotherapy efficacy in patients with advanced non small cell lung cancer. Cancer. 2011;117:3774–80.

41. Roodhart JM, Daenen LG, Stigter EC, et al. Mesenchymal stem cells induce resistance to chemotherapy through the release of platinum-induced fatty acids. Cancer Cell. 2011;20:370–83.

42. Brasky TM, Darke AK, Song X et al Plasma phospholipids fatty acids and prostate cancer risk in the SELECT trial J Natl Cancer Inst 2013; 105:1132–1141.

43. Dahm CC, Gorst-Rasmussen A, Crowe FL, et al. Fatty acid patterns and risk of prostate cancer in a case—control study nested within the European Prospective Investigation into Cancer and Nutrition. Am J Clin Nutr. 2012;96:1354–61.

44. Chua ME, Sio MC, Sorongon MC, Dy JS. Relationship of dietary intake of omega-3 and omega-6 fatty acids with risk of prostate cancer development: a meta-analysis of prospective studies and review of literature. Prostate Cancer. 2012;2012:826254.

45. Anderson BM, Ma DW. Are all n-3 polyunsaturated acids created equal? Lipids Health Dis 2009; 10;8:33. doi:10. 1186/1476-511x-8-33.

46. Carlson SE, Neuringer M. Polyunsaturated fatty acid status and neurodevelopment: a summary and clinical analysis of the literature. Lipids. 1999;34:171–8.

47. Descsi T, Koletzko B. Role of long-chain polyunsaturated fatty acids in early neurodevelopment. Nutr Neurosci. 2000;3:293–306.

48. Uauy R, Hoffman DR. Mena P et al Term infant studies of DHA and ARA supplementation on neurodevelopment: results of randomized controlled trials. J Pediatr. 2003;143:17–25.

49. Innis SM. Dietary omega 3 fatty acids and the developing brain. Brain Res. 2008;1237:35–43.

50. Hanebutt FL, Demmelmair H, Schiessl B, Larque E, Koletzko B. Long-chain polyunsaturated fatty acid transfer across the placenta. Clin Nutr. 2008;27:685–93.

51. Hibbeln JR, Davis JM, Steer C, Emmett P, Rogers I, Williams C, Golding J. Maternal seafood consumption in pregnancy and neurodevelopmental outcomes in childhood (ALSPAC Study): an observational cohort study. Lancet. 2007;369:578–85.

52. Birch EE, Garfield S, Castaneda Y, Hughbanks-Wheaton D, Uauy R, Hoffman D. Visual acuity and cognitive outcomes at 4 years of age in a double-blind, randomized trial of long-chain polyunsaturated fatty acid-supplemented infant formula. Early Human Dev. 2007;83:279–84.

53. Koletzko B, Cetin I, Brenna JT for the Perinatal Lipid Intake Working Group. Dietary fat intakes for pregnant and lactating women: Consensus Statement. Br J Nutr 2007; 98:873–877.

54. Denomme J, Stark KD, Holub BJ. Directly quantitated dietary (n-3) fatty acid intake of pregnant Canadian women are lower than current dietary recommendations. J Nutr. 2005;132:206–11.

55. Lewis NM, Widga AC, Buck JS, Frederick AM. Survey of omega3 fatty acids in diets of Midwest low income pregnant women. J Agromed. 1995;2:49–57.

56. Houwelingen AC, Hornstra G. Relation between birth order and the maternal and neonatal DHA status. Eur J Clin Nutr. 1997;51:548–53.

57. Grandjean P, Bjerve KS, Weihe P, Stnerwald U. Birthweight in a fishing community: significance of essential fatty acids and marine food contaminants. Int J Epidemiol. 2001;30:1272–8.

58. Olsen SF, Secher NJ. Low consumption of seafood in early pregnancy as a risk factor for preterm delivery. BMJ. 2002;324(7335):447.

59. Szajewska H, Horvath A, Koletzko B. Effect of n-3 long-chain polyunsaturated fatty acid supplementation of women with low-risk pregnancies on pregnancy outcomes and growth measures at birth: a meta-analysis of randomized controlled trials. Am J Clin Nutr. 2006;83:1337–44.

60. Makrides M, Duley L, Olsen SF. Marine oil and other prostaglandin precursor supplementation for pregnancy, uncomplicated by pre-eclampsia or intrauterine growth restriction. Cochrane Database Syst Rev 2006; 3: CD003402.

61. Horvath A, Koletzko B, Szajewska H. Effect of n-3 long-chain polyunsaturated fatty acid supplementation of women in high -risk pregnancies on pregnancy outcomes and growth measures at birth: a meta-analysis of randomized controlled trials. Br J Nutr. 2007;98:253–9.

62. Jakobovich E. Granot E. Effect of DHA supplementation during pregnancy on birth weight and gestational length. Presented at the 4th World Congress of Pediatric Gastroenterology, Hepatology and Nutrition, Nov. 2012, Taipei, Taiwan (manuscript in preparation).

63. Xiang M, Harbige LS, Zetterstrom R. Long-chain polyunsaturated fatty acids in Chinese and Swedish mothers: diet, breast milk and infant growth. Acta Paediatr. 2005;94:1543–9.

64. Ruan C, Liu X, Man H, Ma X, Lu G, Duan G, DeFrancesco CA, Connor WE. Milk composition in women from five different regions of China: the great diversity of milk fatty acids. J Nutr. 1995;125:2993–8.

65. Brenna JT, Varamini B, Jensen RG, Diersen-Schade DA, Boettcher JA, Arterburn LM. Docosahexaenoic and arachidonic acid concentrations in human breast milk worldwide. Am J Clin Nutr. 2007;85:1457–64.

66. Larque E, Demmelmair H, Koletzko B. Perinatal supply and metabolism of long-chain polyunsaturated fatty acids: importance for the early development of the nervous system. Ann NY Acad Sci. 2002;967:299–310.

67. Bitman J, Wood L, Hamosh M, Hamosh P, Mehta NR. Comparison of the lipid composition of breast milk from mothers of term and preterm infants. Amer J Clin Nutr. 1983;38:300–12.

68. Luukkainen P, Salo MK, Nikkari T. Changes in the fatty acid composition of preterm and term human milk from 1 week to 6 months of lactation. J Pediatr Gastroenterol Nutr. 1994;18:355–60.

69. Genzel-Boroviczeny O, Wahle J, Koletzko B. Fatty acid composition of human milk during the 1st month after term and preterm delivery. Eur J Pediatr. 1997;156:142–7.
70. Kovacs A, Funke S, Marosvolgyi T, Burus I, Decsi T. Fatty acids in early human milk after preterm and full term delivery. J Pediatr Gastroenterol Nutr. 2005;41:454–9.
71. Granot E, Ishay-Gigi K, Malaach L, Flidel-Rimon O. Human milk fatty acid composition after preterm and full term delivery. J Mater Fetal Neonatal Med 2015; (in press).
72. Koutras AK, Vigorita VJ. Fecal secretory immunoglobulin in breast milk versus formula feeding in early life. J Pediatr Gastroenterol Nutr. 1989;9:58–61.
73. Slade HB, Schwartz SA. Mucosal immunity: the immunology of breast milk. J Allergy Clin Immunol. 1987;80:348–58.
74. Kramer MS. Does breast feeding help protect against atopic disease? J Pediatr. 1988;112:181–90.
75. Pita ML, Fernandez MR. De-Lucchi C et al Changes in the fatty acid pattern of red blood cell phospholipids induced by type of milk, dietary nucleotide supplementation and postnatal age, in preterm infants. J Pediatr Gastroenterol Nutr. 1988;7:740–7.
76. Endres S, Ghorbani R. Kelley VE et al The effect of dietary supplementation with w3 polyunsaturated fatty acids on the synthesis of interleukin -1 and tumor necrosis factor by mononuclear cells. N Engl J Med. 1989;320:265–71.
77. Calder PC. Dietary fatty acids and lymphocyte functions. Proc Nutr Soc. 1998;57:487–502.
78. Granot E, Golan D, Berry EM. Breast–fed and formula-fed infants do not differ in immunocompetent cell cytokine production despite differences in cell membrane fatty acid composition. Am J Clin Nutr. 2000;72:1202–5.
79. Sherman MP. Human milk, fatty acids and the immune response: a new glimpse (Editorial). Am J Clin Nutr. 2000;72:1071–2.
80. Field CJ, Thomson CA, Van Aerde JE, et al. Lower proportion of CD45RO+ cells and deficient interleukin-10 production by formula-fed infants, compared with human-fed, is corrected with supplementation of long-chain polyunsaturated fatty acids. J Pediatr Gastroenterol Nutr. 2000;31:291–9.
81. Mazurak VC, Lien V, Field CJ, Goruk SD, Pramuk K, Clandinin MT. Long-chain polyunsaturated fat supplementation in children with low docosahexanoic acid intakes alters immune phenotypes compared with placebo. J Pediatr Gastroenterol Nutr. 2008;48:570–9.
82. Meydani SN. Effect of (n-3) polyunsaturated fatty acids on cytokine production and their biologic function. Nutrition. 1996;12:S8–14.
83. Saedisomeolia A, Wood LG, Garg ML, Gibson PG, Wark AB. Anti-inflammatory effects of long-chain n-3 PUFA in rhinovirus-infected cultured airway epithelial cells. Br J Nutr. 2009;101:533–40.
84. Vaisman N, Zaruk Y, Shirazi I, Kaysar N, Barak V. The effect of fish oil supplementation on cytokine production in children. Eur Cytokine Netw. 2005;16:194–8.
85. Granot E, Jakobovich E, Rabinowitz R, Levy P, Schlesinger M. DHA supplementation during pregnancy and lactation affects infants' cellular but not humoral immune response. Mediators Inflamm 2011:493925.
86. Burlingame B, Nishida C, Uauy R, Weisell R (eds). Fats and fatty acids in human nutrition (from the joint FAO/WHO expert consultation on fats and fatty acids in human nutrition). In: Annals of Nutrition and Metabolism, 2009; vol: 55, Karger AG, Basel.
87. Koletzko B, Lien E, Agostoni C, Bohles H, Campoy C, Cetin I, Decsi T, et al. The roles of long-chain polyunsaturated fatty acids in pregnancy, lactation and infancy: review of current knowledge and consensus recommendations. J Perinat Med. 2008;36:5–14.
88. Michaelsen KF, Dewey KG, Perez-Exposito AB, Nurhasan M, Lauritzen L, Roos N. Food sources and intake of n-6 and n-3fatty acids in low-income countries with emphasis on infants, young children (6–12 months) and pregnant and lactating women. Mater Child Nutr 2011; Suppl 2:124–140.
89. Huffman SL, Harika RK, Eilander A, Osendarp SJ. Essential fats: how do they affect growth and development of infants and young children in developing countries? A literature review. Mater Child Nutr 2011; Suppl 3:44–65.
90. Kumwenda C, Dewey KG, Hemsworth J, Ashorn P, Maleta K, Haskell MJ. Lipid based nutrient supplements do not decrease breast milk intake of Malawian children. Am J Clin Nutr. 2014;99:617–23.
91. Briend A, Dewey KG. Complementary feeding: keeping the message simple. J Pediatr Gastroenterol Nutr. 2014;58:275.
92. Chaparro CM, Dewey KG. Use of lipid-based nutrient supplements (LNS) to improve the nutrient adequacy of general food distribution rations for vulnerable sub-groups in emergency settings. Matern Child Nutr. 2010;6 (Suppl 1):1–69.
93. Yang Z, Huffman SL. Modeling linoleic acid and alpha linolenic acid requirements for infants and young children in developing countries. Mater Child Nutr. 2013;9:S72–7.
94. Franco VH, Hotta JK, Jorge SM, Dos Santos JE. Plasma fatty acids in children with grade III protein malnutrition in its different forms: marasmus, marasmus kwashiorkor and kwashiorkor. J Trop Pediatr. 1999;45:71–5.
95. Decsi T, Koletzko B. Effects of protein-energy malnutrition and human immunodeficiency virus-1 infection on essential fatty acid metabolism in children. Nutrition. 2000;16:447–53.

96. Marin MC, Rey GE, Pedersoli LC, Rodrigo MA, Alaniz MJ. Dietary long-chain fatty acids and visual response in malnourished nursing infants. Prostagland Leukotrien Essent Fatty Acids. 2000;63:385–90.
97. Racine RA, Deckelbaum RJ. Sources of very- long-chain unsaturated omega-3 fatty acids: eicosapentanoic acid and docosahexanoic acid. Current Opin Clin Nutr Metab Care. 2007;10:123–8.
98. Gotz N, Bulbarello A, Konig-Grillo S, Dusterioh A, Volker M. Long-chain polyunsaturated omega-3 fatty acids in food development. Sight Life. 2013;27:12–7.

Chapter 15
The Role of Human and Other Milks in Preventing and Treating Undernutrition

Benedikte Grenov, Henrik Friis, Christian Mølgaard and Kim Fleischer Michaelsen

Keywords Milk protein · Whey · Lactose · Cow's milk · Breastfeeding · Linear growth · Undernutrition · Malnutrition · MAM · SAM

Learning Objectives

- To describe human milk and how breastfeeding benefits the child and the mother
- To outline the composition and importance of macronutrients and micronutrients of common milk types in relation to undernutrition
- To summarize the influence of milk consumption on linear growth
- To describe the use of cow's milk in prevention and treatment of undernutrition in vulnerable groups (infants below 6 months, children above 6 months, pregnant and lactating women, adults with HIV or tuberculosis)
- To discuss the optimal amount of milk ingredients in products used in treatment of severe and moderate acute malnutrition.

Introduction

Mammals have the unique capacity of producing milk that contains all the nutrients and bioactive compounds that are needed to support growth and development of their offspring during early life. In humans, breastfeeding has been shown to have many beneficial effects, especially in low-income countries with high rates of infections and undernutrition. The use of nonhuman milk for human consumption and feeding of young children dates back to the time of animal domestication and later breeding of animal species to obtain high milk yields. Today millions of people consume milk every day and production and intake of milk is increasing rapidly worldwide especially in low- and middle

B. Grenov · H. Friis · C. Mølgaard · K.F. Michaelsen (✉)
Department of Nutrition, Exercise and Sports, Science, University of Copenhagen,
Rolighedsvej 26, 1958 Frederiksberg, Copenhagen, Denmark
e-mail: kfm@nexs.ku.dk

B. Grenov
e-mail: bgr@nexs.ku.dk

H. Friis
e-mail: htr@nexs.ku.dk

C. Mølgaard
e-mail: cm@nexs.ku.dk

© Springer Science+Business Media New York 2017
S. de Pee et al. (eds.), *Nutrition and Health in a Developing World*,
Nutrition and Health, DOI 10.1007/978-3-319-43739-2_15

income countries. This is facilitated by growing economies and urbanization. As an example, India has increased the production of milk fourfold between 1963 and 2003 and today India is the largest global producer of milk with approximately 16% of the global milk production [1]. The increased milk production in India is mainly driven by small-scale dairy farms and may therefore contribute to poverty reduction. However, the nutritional status of Indian children has not improved during the same period and India still has some of the highest prevalence of underweight, stunting and wasting globally [1]. This may be due to the fact that milk intake per capita is very low and the poorest segments of the population do not have access to milk. Continued growth of dairy production is expected due to economic growth and increasing purchasing power as well as increasing urbanization and general population growth.

Cow's milk is a key ingredient in products used for treating severe acute malnutrition (SAM) and has been shown to be effective in preventing and treating undernutrition. Only a small fraction of the global milk production is needed to prevent and treat moderate and severe acute malnutrition.

The key objectives of this chapter are described in box "28 Key Objectives." Other health and nutrition aspects of milk intake in relation to the healthy general population, such as non-communicable diseases, milk hypersensitivity or allergy, and dental and bone health are not covered. A comprehensive and broad description of the effects of milk and dairy products in human nutrition is given in a recent book published by FAO [2], which also covers the effects in undernourished populations in low-income countries.

Breastfeeding, the Composition of Human Milk and Effects on Infant and Mother

The current WHO recommendations regarding breastfeeding are that newborn infants should start breastfeeding within 1 h after delivery, be exclusively breastfed for about 6 months and thereafter continue to be breastfed together with complementary food until the age of 2 years or beyond [3]. In many high-income countries the recommendation is to continue partial breastfeeding only to about 12 months, as the evidence for beneficial effects during the second year of life is not strong in high-income populations. However, there are large differences between breastfeeding rates in different parts of the world and between different socioeconomic groups. Globally, only half of all children below 1 month and 30% of children aged 1–5 months are exclusively breastfed [4]. The importance of breastfeeding is underlined by recent estimates showing that 800,000 children die every year due to suboptimal breastfeeding practices [4, 5].

Composition

The composition of breast milk is very dynamic. Colostrum, human milk produced during the first few days after delivery, has a very high level of immunoglobulins, lactoferrin, leukocytes, and other immune protecting factors supporting that a main function of colostrum is to protect the child from infections and stimulate gut function [6]. After the first days of colostrum, the milk gradually changes and it is considered mature breast milk after approximately four weeks. The composition of mature breast milk fluctuates diurnally and within the same feed. For example, the last milk of a feed, the hindmilk, contains 2–3 times more fat than foremilk. The nutritional components of breast milk are synthesized in the lactocyte (milk producing cell in the mammary epithelium) or come from the maternal stores and are to some degree influenced by the diet of the mother. The content of energy and macronutrients of mature human milk is described in Table 15.1. In general the macronutrient

Table 15.1 Proximate composition of human, cow's, buffalo's, goat's, and sheep's milk (average per 100 g of milk)[a]

Proximates	Human	Cow	Buffalo	Goat	Sheep
Energy (kJ)	291	262	412	270	420
Energy (kcal)	70	62	99	66	100
Water (g)	87.5	87.8	83.2	87.7	82.1
Protein (g)	1.0	3.3	4.0	3.4	5.6
Fat (g)	4.4	3.3	7.5	3.9	6.4
Lactose (g)	6.9	4.7	4.4	4.4	5.1
Ash (g)	0.2	0.7	0.8	0.8	0.9

[a]Modified after Wijesinha-Bettoni and Burlingame [28]. The table is based on average composition. The composition varies depending on the actual mammal species/breed, feeding efficiency, lactation state of the animal and seasonal variation

content of milk from undernourished mothers seems to be similar to a well-nourished mother [7]. As for micronutrients, the content of some nutrients in human milk is dependent on the status of the mother (e.g., vitamin B-6, B-12, iodine, and selenium), while others are not (e.g., calcium, iron, and folate) [8]. The amount of long-chain polyunsaturated fatty acids is directly depending on the intake of the mother [9]. The content of docosahexaenoic acid (DHA) in breast milk is very low in populations living mainly on a plant-based diet with a low fish intake, and much higher in populations consuming fish [9]. The number and potential functions of bioactive molecules in human milk are numerous and some of them are described below.

Benefits for the Child

The most important benefits of breastfeeding in low-income countries are reductions in child mortality and morbidity, mainly due to protection against infections [10–12]. As shown in Table 15.2, all-cause mortality and mortality due to diarrhea and pneumonia are 10–15 times higher in children below 5 months that are not breastfed in comparison to similar groups of exclusively breastfed children. The table also shows that partial breastfeeding (other liquids or solids in addition to breast milk) has moderately higher relative risks than predominant breastfeeding (only water and tea in

Table 15.2 Relative risk of suboptimum breastfeeding

Outcome	0–5 months—compared to exclusive breastfeeding			6–23 months—compared to any breastfeeding
	Predominant breastfeeding	Partial breastfeeding	Not breastfeeding	Not breastfeeding
All cause mortality	1.48 (1.13–1.92)	2.85 (1.59–5.10)	14.40 (6.09–34.05)	3.68 (1.46–9.29)
Diarrhea mortality	2.28 (0.85–6.11)	4.62 (1.81–11.77)	10.53 (2.80–39.64)	2.83 (0.15–54.82)
Pneumonia mortality	1.75 (0.48–6.43)	2.49 (1.03–6.04)	15.13 (0.61–373.84)	1.52 (0.09–27.06)
Diarrhea incidence	1.26 (0.81–1.95)	3.04 (1.32–7.00)	3.65 (1.69–7.88)	1.20 (1.05–1.38)
Pneumonia incidence	1.79 (1.29–2.48)	2.48 (0.23–27.15)	2.07 (0.19–22.64)	1.17 (0.37–3.65)

Data are point estimate (95% CI). Data are based on meta-analysis of data from Bangladesh, India, Ghana, Peru, and United Arab Emirates, published between 1981 and 2006. After Black et al. [10]

addition to breast milk). A protective effect of breastfeeding during the third year of life has also been shown in a study from Bangladesh [13].

Infants are born with an immature immune system and therefore to some degree depend on maternal antibodies and other immunological factors in breast milk to protect against infections. Secretory IgA is the predominant antibody of breast milk, but also IgM and IgG are present [6]. In addition, the innate immune cells in breast milk such as macrophages and lymphocytes, cytokines, and bioactive peptides like lactoferrin contribute to the protective effect against infections. Other bioactive components may support maturation of the infant intestine (e.g., epidermal growth factor), growth regulation (e.g., insulin-like growth factor), metabolism, and body composition (leptin, adiponectin), and formation of the gut microbiota (oligosaccharides) [6].

In addition to the immediate effects of breastfeeding, there are also long-term effects, which were evaluated in a WHO systematic review [14]. The most consistent finding was that breastfeeding is associated with a small increase in intelligence test performance with an average increase of 2–3 IQ points, depending on the adjustments [14]. The cited studies were mainly performed in high-income countries. Breastfeeding seems to be associated with lower risk of obesity and diabetes later in life, but the effect seems to be small and confounding by socioeconomic factors cannot be ruled out [14, 15]. Breastfeeding also seems to protect against some forms of allergic diseases, sudden infant death syndrome, necrotizing enterocolitis, childhood leukemia, and inflammatory bowel disease, but the evidence is not always strong [16].

Human milk contains chemicals from the environment, e.g., organic pollutants and lead. Although such pollutants might have potential negative effects, there is no evidence that these effects can outweigh the positive effects of breastfeeding [16].

Beside the nutritional and health benefits of breastfeeding the care and close physical contact between the mother and child during breastfeeding may also have both short- and long-term positive consequences for the well-being of children.

Benefits for the Mother

Longer duration of exclusive breastfeeding is prolonging lactational amenorrhea [17] and thus contributes to birth spacing. Longer birth intervals may allow the mother to replete her nutritional status before the subsequent pregnancy and lower the risk of stunting among offspring [17]. Long-term benefits of breastfeeding seem to include reduced risk for the mother of developing breast cancer and ovarian cancer [18]. Beside nutritional, health and developmental benefits associated with breastfeeding, breast milk is free of charge and safe to use.

Breastfeeding Promotion and Support

A review evaluating the effect of counseling and educational interventions on exclusive breastfeeding found that these interventions can considerably improve breastfeeding on the first day of life as well as breastfeeding for up to 5 months. A combination of individual and group counseling seemed to increase breastfeeding practice more than individual or group counseling alone [19]. Studies with both pre- and/or postnatal counseling were included.

Kangaroo mother care is a concept of neonate handling involving early skin-to-skin contact between the mother and newborn baby, early and continued breastfeeding, support by parents and health workers, and early discharge from hospital (for births that took place in the hospital). Review of studies in pre-term [20] and term neonates [21] have shown that the improvement of breastfeeding duration associated with Kangaroo mother care may be extended to community settings and thereby also support breastfeeding.

An important obstacle in promoting good breastfeeding practices, i.e., 6 months exclusive breastfeeding followed by continued breastfeeding until 2 years of age or beyond, is the challenge of working mothers, especially in low-income countries where there may be no or very limited possibilities for maternity leave or breastfeeding during often very long working hours. Chapter 16 provides more information about breastfeeding policies and programs.

HIV and Breastfeeding

HIV can be transmitted via human milk. If no antiretroviral drugs are provided, 20% of HIV-infected mothers will transmit HIV to their babies during pregnancy or delivery [22], and breastfeeding may account for an additional 5–20% [23], depending on breastfeeding practices. A randomized trial in Kenya, found that breastfeeding led to an additional 16% transmission compared to formula feeding, but adherence to the specific feeding regimens was not perfect [24]. However, if both the HIV-infected mother and her HIV-exposed child receive antiretroviral treatment (ARVs), then the transmission rate can be as low as 1–2% [25, 26]. The WHO guidelines from 2013 regarding use of antiretroviral drugs (ARV) for treating and preventing HIV infection [27] recommend that HIV positive pregnant and breastfeeding women should receive lifelong antiretroviral treatment (ART) with a specified triple drug combination. If this is not possible due to limited resources, WHO recommends lifelong ART for pregnant and breastfeeding women with CD4 counts <500 or clinical stage 3 or 4. For women with CD4 counts >500, ART can be stopped 1 week after complete cessation of breastfeeding. HIV-exposed infants should be treated with ARV for 6 weeks if breastfed and 4–6 weeks if formula fed. National guidelines have been developed to reduce and prevent transmission of HIV infection from mother to child. In a number of countries, caregivers who can afford and always have access to infant formula and boiled water are recommended to give infant formula to their children. In all other countries and situations, caregivers are recommended to exclusively breastfeed their children for 6 months followed by complementary feeding and continued breastfeeding.

Composition of Human Milk, Cow's Milk, and Other Milks

Milk composition of different mammal species varies a lot and is adapted to the environment and growth velocity of the newborn animal with more energy dense milk in cold climates and high levels of protein and growth supporting minerals in fast growing animals.

Table 15.1 shows the composition of the most common types of milk used for human consumption and in dairy production. The composition of more seldom used types of milk for human consumption (e.g., camel and reindeer milk) can be found elsewhere [28].

Human milk has a low concentration of protein and minerals (main content of ash in the table above) and a high concentration of lactose compared to milk of dairy animals. The low content of protein and minerals is a reflection of a slower growth of the human infant compared to dairy animals. Due to high content of protein, undiluted milk is poorly tolerated in young infants and undiluted milk should not be used before the age of 12 months.

Buffalo and sheep milk both have a high content of fat, protein, and minerals (ash) compared to cow's milk and are therefore more energy dense. This may be an advantage in settings of low access to energy dense food but should be considered with caution for treatment of young malnourished children, because the protein and mineral content, which is also higher, results in a high renal solute load, which the kidneys may not be able to handle.

Other differences between cow's milk and other milks include differences in milk fat composition, micronutrients and vitamins. Goat's milk contains more short and medium chain fatty acids (6–10 carbon atoms) which are absorbed more easily compared to long chain fatty acids [28]. This is relevant for those suffering from malnutrition as they often have some degree of fat malabsorption. In addition, the fat globule size of goat's milk and sheep's milk is smaller compared to cow's milk which may improve the digestibility of goat's and sheep's milk. All the milks contain high amounts of vitamin B-12 and riboflavin which are often lacking in the diets of malnourished populations. Other important milk vitamins include vitamin A, especially from buffalo's and sheep's milk, and vitamin C which is high in sheep's milk. Together with other sources of vitamin A and C, milk can contribute significantly to the daily recommended intake of these vitamins [28].

In 2012, more than 80% of the global milk production was cow's milk [29] and the remaining part of the chapter is therefore describing cow's milk unless otherwise specified.

Protein

Protein quality is assessed by the ability of a dietary protein to meet human requirements for indispensable amino acids. FAO and WHO currently recommend DIAAS (digestible indispensable amino acid score) for evaluation of protein quality [30]. This method is based on the first indispensable (essential) amino acid that becomes a limiting factor in relation to a reference pattern. Three reference patterns have been defined, but for regulatory purposes only two reference patterns are used: For infant formula, the reference pattern is equivalent to the amino acid composition of breast milk and for all other foods and age groups, the reference pattern is based on the needs of a young child aged 6 months–3 years. In comparison to the PDCAAS method (protein digestibility corrected amino acid score) which was recommended until 2013, the main differences are that DIAAS is based on true ileal protein digestibility and not on fecal crude digestibility as ileal output is considered to better reflect the amount of amino acids absorbed [30]. DIAAS scores may be higher than 100% (i.e., if the lowest amount of indispensable amino acid content multiplied by the ileal digestibility index exceeds the reference pattern) and should only be truncated if calculating the DIAAS score for mixed diets or sole source foods like infant formula. For many foods, the DIAAS score is not yet known as the ileal digestibility has not been assessed. Dairy proteins all have DIAAS scores greater than 100% and whole milk powder has a DIAAS value of 122% [30, 31].

Cow's milk protein contains approx. 80% casein and 20% whey protein. Casein proteins are α_{s1}-, α_{s2}-, γ-, and κ-casein and the major whey proteins include β-lactoglobulin, α-lactalbumin, immunoglobulins, serum albumin and lactoferrin, and all the proteins have different biological activities [32, 33]. Human milk has a casein-whey ratio of 40:60. This is likely to influence digestibility of the proteins as casein and whey protein are categorized as slow and fast proteins, respectively, corresponding to how fast amino acids appear in the blood circulation after ingestion [32, 34].

For further information about the effect of whey protein, please refer to the "Whey Protein" section in this chapter.

Lactose

Human milk contains approx. 6.9% (w/w) of lactose and up to 40% of the energy in human milk comes from lactose compared to approx. 4.7% (w/w) lactose and 30 energy% in cow's milk. The significant amount of lactose may contribute to growth and development in the young child through several mechanisms that are discussed in the "Lactose" section in this chapter. In addition lactose has a sweet taste which increases the preference, especially among young children [35].

Minerals

Milk contains high amounts of minerals supporting growth, so-called type II nutrients, including potassium, magnesium, and phosphorus but only small amounts of zinc. These minerals are characterized by having no body stores and being used in all body tissues for cell division and growth. Depletion in any of these minerals results in growth limitation or stunting [36]. Very often malnourished children have clinically relevant phosphorus deficiency, associated with increased mortality. According to Golden [36], the success of cow's milk in treatment of malnutrition is likely to be partly accounted for by correction of phosphate deficiency.

Milks also contain very high amounts of calcium which is important in bone mineralization. In low-income countries the intake of calcium is often very low and combined with a diet which often contains high amounts of antinutrients this may result in children with demineralized bones which is likely to be due to calcium deficiency and which in some cases results in rickets which in high-income countries most often is due to vitamin D deficiency [36, 37].

Milk, including human milk, contains very little iron. Furthermore, the high content of calcium, phosphorus and casein in cow's milk may impair iron absorption from other sources [28, 38]. This is important as iron deficiency is very common in many low-income countries.

The bioavailability of milk minerals is high compared to plant minerals. Phytate, an antinutritional factor, is present in cereal staples, legumes, and other edible plants and impairs absorption of important minerals like iron, zinc and calcium [39].

Fat

Cow's milk contains approx. 3.5 g fat/100 g milk before processing to varieties with different fat content. Whole milk contains approximately 2.3 g of saturated fatty acids (SFA)/100 g (mainly C12–C18:0), 0.8 g/100 g of mono-unsaturated fatty, mainly oleic acid (C18:1), and 0.1 g/100 g of polyunsaturated fatty acids [40]. Mature human milk contains more fat (4.1 g/100 ml), has less saturated fat (1.8 g/100 g) and considerable higher contents of monounsaturated fatty acids (1.6 g/100 g) and of polyunsaturated fatty acids (0.5 g/100 ml) [40].

Fat is an important energy source for young children. Breast milk contains approx. 50 energy% fat and it has been recommended that complementary food for moderately malnourished children should contain 35–45 energy% from fat [39]. Although the amount of saturated fatty acids in cow's milk compared to human milk is considerably higher and the amount of polyunsaturated fatty acids (PUFA) is considerably lower including zero or negligible amounts of the essential fatty acids eicosapentaoic acid and docosahexaenoic acid, whole milk is considered a good energy and fat source in treatment of malnourished children [9].

Much research has focused on the potential negative role of milk fat on low-density lipoprotein cholesterol and cardiovascular disease. Obesity and cardiovascular diseases are increasing health problems worldwide, where the same population and sometimes even individuals of the same household may suffer from undernutrition and overweight (double burden). Currently, WHO and FAO recommend that intake of SFAs should not exceed 10 energy% and should be replaced by PUFAs in order to reduce the risk of coronary heart disease [41]. But the claimed negative effect of saturated fat on cardiovascular disease has been challenged by a recent large meta-analysis [42].

Milk fat also includes small amounts of conjugated linoleic acid which has been associated with a range of health promoting activities including inhibition of cancer, hypertension, atherosclerosis, diabetes and immune stimulation. Furthermore, cow's milk contains ruminant trans-fatty acids which constitute up to 5% of the total fatty acids. Industrially produced trans-fatty acids have been strongly associated with coronary heart disease, metabolic syndrome and diabetes while the effects of ruminant trans-fatty acids seem to be much more limited [40, 43, 44]. Human milk does not contain any trans-fatty acids.

The Effects of Cow's Milk in Prevention and Treatment of Undernutrition

Milk is the only or main energy and nutrient source of newborn humans and animals and is biologically adapted to support high growth velocity during the first period of life. It is therefore plausible that milk has the potential to support growth and rehabilitation in individuals with acute malnutrition. The growth promoting effect of milk is likely to be caused by a combination of whey protein, casein, specific amino acids and growth promoting milk minerals including phosphorus, magnesium and potassium. The specific effects of the individual components on bone growth and muscle mass accretion are not understood in detail. The effect of cow's milk on linear growth and in prevention and treatment of human undernutrition in different age groups is discussed below.

Of the world's population of children below 5 years, 52 million are wasted (weight for length or height below −2 SD) of which 19 million are severely wasted (weight for length or height below −3 SD) [4]. Acute undernutrition (low weight for length or height or low mid-upper arm circumference) affects especially children below 5 years in low-income countries and is more prevalent in south Asia and sub-Saharan African countries than elsewhere [4]. Chronic malnutrition, or stunting, affects 165 million children under 5-years of age [4]. Every year, approx. 3 million child deaths—or 45% or all child deaths below 5 years—are directly or indirectly attributable to undernutrition, including wasting, stunting, micronutrient deficiencies, and suboptimal breastfeeding practices. Adults are rarely affected by acute malnutrition except in emergency situations, and among adults with chronic diseases, e.g., TB or HIV. In vulnerable groups of adults, e.g., pregnant and lactating women, prevention of undernutrition is important.

Although milk seems to have specific positive effects on growth and rehabilitation of malnourished individuals, other animal source foods (ASF) also have positive effects on growth as well as effects on cognitive development, morbidity, and immune functions. An often cited study in Kenyan school children evaluated the effect of iso-energetic school meals of a plant-based stew plus meat, milk or oil versus a non-supplemented control group over 2 years. All supplemented groups gained more weight than children in the control group and both meat, and milk increased lean body mass measured as mid-upper arm muscle area [45]. The meat group performed significantly better in a range of school tests compared with groups with no animal source foods and the milk group performed better than the non-supplemented group in a few school tests [46]. The study supports findings from other studies with ASF indicating that milk supports linear growth whereas meat has better effect on cognitive performance [38]. In addition to the high protein quality of milk and meat, minerals in ASF have a high bioavailability and micronutrients like iron (meat), zinc (meat and milk) and vitamin B-12 (milk) are thought to contribute to the positive effects of animal source foods.

Cow's Milk and Linear Growth

There is considerable evidence, both from high- and low-income countries, that cow's milk has a stimulating effect on linear growth [47, 48]. The strongest evidence comes from both intervention and observational studies in low-income countries. Additionally, many but not all observational studies from well-nourished populations show an association between milk intake and linear growth. The stimulating effect of cow's milk on linear growth is likely to be mediated via an increased synthesis of Insulin-like Growth Factor 1 (IGF-1). IGF-1 is regulated both by growth hormone but also by nutrition, especially in the first years of life.

Infants being exclusively breastfed have a higher growth velocity during the first 2–3 months of life. Thereafter formula fed infants grow at a faster rate continuing until the age of about 12 months [49]. At 12 months breastfed infants are slightly shorter than formula fed infants and have also a lower weight and body mass index. It is most likely the higher protein content in cow's milk based infant formula compared to human milk, which has a greater effect on linear growth. Protein content in infant formula is only about 1/3 of the content in cow's milk, but still considerably higher than in breast milk. Some studies suggest that breastfed infants have a catch-up in linear growth later in childhood and are taller as adults, which might be mediated via a programming effect on the IGF-I axis (insulin-like growth factor) [50].

The classic Boyd Orr study was conducted in the early 1900s in Scotland among school children of mainly working class families. Their diet was supplemented with whole milk, skimmed milk, or biscuits with an equivalent amount of energy and compared to an unsupplemented control group. The groups receiving milk, irrespective of age, grew 20% more in height compared to the control group during the 7 month intervention period [51].

Later, randomized controlled trials (RCTs) in undernourished or underprivileged preschool children [52] as well as school children in Kenya, New Guinea, and Vietnam [45, 53, 54] demonstrated increased linear growth in most of the groups receiving milk. In one study [45] the weight and lean body mass increased in milk-supplemented compared to control groups, but height only increased in a subgroup of children whose weight-for-height Z-score was below median at baseline.

Following a systematic review including a meta-analysis of 12 randomized and nonrandomized controlled trials performed in undernourished (2 studies) or well-nourished children and adolescents between 3 and 13 years, de Beer concluded that "the most likely effect of dairy products supplementation is 0.4 cm additional growth per annum per ca 245 ml of milk daily" [55].

It has also been suggested that population mean adult height is influenced by milk intake. In Africa, pastoralist, e.g., the masaais, tend to be taller than populations not drinking milk [56] and in Europe, where the Dutch are the tallest, it has been suggested that it could be because of a high intake of milk in the Netherlands [57].

Overall the short-term results of intervention studies with milk or milk products suggest a positive effect of intake of cow's milk on linear growth in both well-nourished and undernourished children. Long-term effects of high intake of cow's milk during childhood may however influence the IGF-level later in life and possibly increase the risk of non-communicable diseases like coronary heart disease, and cancer [58].

Cow's Milk in Prevention and Treatment of SAM and MAM

Severe Acute Malnutrition (SAM) is defined as severe wasting or mid-upper arm circumference (MUAC) <11.5 cm or bipedal pitting edema, and moderate acute malnutrition (MAM) is defined as moderate wasting or MUAC between 11.5 and 12.5 cm. Cow's milk plays a key role in treatment of SAM. Although milk seems effective in treatment of MAM, the use of milk is being debated because of its high price.

Children below 6 Months

Approximately 8.5 million infants below 6 months are wasted [59]. Despite this high number, global guidelines for management of infants below 6 months with MAM or SAM are lacking. If a child is undernourished before the age of 6 months it is often due to suboptimal breast feeding, which in some cases may relate to poor nutritional status or health of the mother. Infants below 6 months with SAM have a very poor prognosis and should be referred to inpatient care with intensive breastfeeding support. If too weak to suckle, human milk can be expressed and given by naso-gastric tube, a cup or the supplementary suckling technique. This technique is used to start or reestablish breastfeeding and involves that the child is suckling at the breast and simultaneously fed with expressed human milk or a human milk substitute from a cup via a tube placed along the nipple. In this way human milk or human milk substitute can slowly drip into the mouth of the infant and ensure adequate intake of energy and nutrients while the breast is stimulated to produce more milk.

In some cases breastfeeding is not considered an option, e.g., for HIV positive mothers who decide not to breastfeed and for infants who do not have a mother or wet nurse. For these children, a human milk substitute, i.e. diluted therapeutic milks (F-75 and F-100) or infant formula, can be provided under medical supervision [60]. F-75 is only given during stabilization of the child and diluted F-100 or commercial infant formula (manufactured according to codex alimentarius) is given during the transition and rehabilitation phase. After discharge the child can receive infant formula or homemade formula based on diluted, heat treated animal milk with sugar, and micronutrients. Reconstituted dried skimmed milk or other low fat milks are also inappropriate for long-term feeding of infants due to their low fat content.

There are many challenges in relation to use of infant formula for children below 6 months in low-income countries. The main concerns are hygiene problems due to lack of access to clean water and inappropriate cleaning of feeding bottles or utensils which may result in infections. In addition, wrong preparation and dosage of infant formula may lead to repeated undernutrition or mineral imbalances and the high price of infant formula is likely to prevent mothers and caregivers with a low and unstable income to feed their children appropriately. Breastfeeding has repeatedly been shown to protect against infections and reduce infant mortality in low-income countries [4]. To support the promotion of breastfeeding, advertising, and promotion of infant formula is not allowed according to the WHO International Code of Marketing of Breast milk Substitutes [61].

Despite the positive effects of dairy protein given to infants with MAM or SAM, undiluted cow's milk should never be given to infants below 12 months. The content of protein and minerals is very high and especially during the first 6 months the kidneys might not be able to excrete the surplus, which might lead to hypernatremic dehydration.

Children above 6 Months

Cow's milk is a key ingredient in products used for treatment of MAM and SAM. According to WHO guidelines [62], children with SAM and medical complications should be treated in inpatient facilities and the recommended food is F-75 during initial stabilization. F-75 has a low content of dried skimmed milk. The protein level is low to protect children from the negative impact protein breakdown may have on liver function in severely malnourished children [36] and the increased renal solute load of urea resulting from breakdown of protein. The lactose level is low to reduce the risk of lactose intolerance and osmotic diarrhea (see "Lactose" section in this chapter). During the initial stabilization phase children do not gain weight. When children improve, they are transferred to ready-to-use-therapeutic-food (RUTF) or—in settings where F-100 is available or considered more appropriate—children are first transferred to F-100 and then RUTF before discharge to outpatient treatment. Compared to F-75, RUTF and F-100 are more energy dense and designed to support

Table 15.3 Milk ingredients in specialized products for treatment of MAM and SAM

	SAM			MAM		
	F-75	F-100	RUTF	RUSF	Super cereal plus (CSB++)[a]	CSB with 3% WPC 80[b]
Energy density at consumption	75 kcal/100 ml	100 kcal/100 ml	520–550 kcal/100 g	520–550 kcal/100 g	410 kcal/100 g powder	NA
Milk component (w/w %)	DSM 2.5%	DSM 8%	20–25% DSM fulfill the requirements, but other sources/mixtures of milk protein are allowed	13–20% protein, with PDCAAS >70%, may be milk protein[c]	8% DSM	3% WPC80
Milk protein % of total protein	5 energy% protein, 100% from milk	16 energy% protein, 100% from milk	10–12 energy% protein, at least 50% from milk protein	No requirements	Min 16%, approx. 25% from milk	NA

[a]Super cereal plus (CSB++): 410 kcal/100 g
[b]"CSB14" [75], currently being tested in studies, but not yet used in feeding programs
[c]If plant protein, it should be processed to mitigate antinutrients

rehabilitation and growth. The milk content is high with milk protein constituting 100% of the protein content in F-100 and about 50–60% in RUTF; see Table 15.3 for further details. The timing of the transitioning from F-75 to RUTF or F-100 and the gradual increase of their intake are important to avoid re-feeding syndrome which may be fatal.

F-75 and F-100 are both liquid products reconstituted from powder. As this poses a high risk of contamination and spoilage, the use of F-75 and F-100 is restricted to inpatient care and requires careful handling and frequent preparation of fresh milk rations. RUTF was developed to mimic the nutrient content of F-100. It is an energy dense lipid-based paste containing ground peanuts, skimmed milk powder, and/or whey protein, maltodextrin or sugar, vegetable oil and micronutrients. Due to its solid paste form, very low water content and packaging in direct-to-use alu-foil sachets the risk of contamination and spoilage is small enough to allow home-based treatment in community settings. This has revolutionized treatment of children with SAM without medical complications [63] and Community-based Management of Acute Malnutrition has grown substantially over the past 20 years and contributed to reduced global childhood mortality.

Several studies have shown that addition of milk protein (usually whey protein) and/or milk powder (usually skimmed milk powder) has a positive effect on growth and rehabilitation of severely malnourished children [64–67]. Some of these studies are further described in "The Use of Cow's Milk Ingredients in Foods for MAM and SAM" section of this chapter. This section also describes the content of milk ingredients in F-75, F-100, and RUTF (Table 15.3).

For children with moderate acute malnutrition (MAM) there are no firm guidelines from WHO regarding treatment. Recommendations for nutrient content and ingredients of diets for children with MAM have been made by Golden [36], Michaelsen et al. [39], de Pee and Bloem [68] and this has resulted in a Technical Note from WHO on the composition of supplementary foods for treatment of MAM [69]. Traditionally, children with MAM have been treated with fortified blended foods without milk ingredients but the trend is to add more high-quality protein, including milk protein to supplementary foods. This has generally resulted in better recoveries [64–67]. While products cost more per kg, treatment costs are not proportionally higher if the treatment is more effective (greater proportion treated successfully and shorter duration).

School Milk Programs for Prevention of Undernutrition

Many countries around the world promote school milk programs. Milk is perceived as healthy and nutritious for school children and the programs, which also increase the demand for dairy produce, are often supported by public funds and/or the dairy industry. A survey conducted by FAO [70] showed that school milk represents from 3 to 25% of the liquid milk market. School milk programs appear to be more widely supported through governments and public funds in the Asia and Pacific regions [71]. School feeding programs are discussed in more detail elsewhere [71].

Two examples of studies embedded in Asian school milk programs are mentioned here. A 2 year milk intervention study in 10 years old school girls from Beijing, China of UHT milk fortified with calcium or calcium plus vitamin D versus a non-supplemented control group showed that girls receiving calcium fortified milk with or without vitamin D had a higher increase in height and weight compared to the control group and increased bone mineralization which was higher in the calcium plus vit D supplemented group. It was concluded that increase in milk consumption, e.g., by means of school milk programs would improve bone growth during adolescence [72].

A study in Vietnam evaluated the impact of 6 months consumption of 500 ml school milk in 7–8 years old children. Both weight for age (WAZ) and height for age (HAZ) improved significantly during the milk intervention and children in the milk consuming groups had significantly better short-term memory scores. However, each of the three study treatments was only tested in one school [54].

Pregnant and Lactating Women

During pregnancy and lactation the nutritional requirements are increased for particularly protein, iron, iodine, zinc, folic acid, vitamin A, vitamin C, and B-vitamins [73]. With potential impact of nutritional deficiencies on the new generation, pregnant, and lactating women (PLW) are a vulnerable group which is targeted in nutritional programs of NGOs and UN-organizations. General food distributions to adults in emergency situations usually include grain (e.g., rice, cornmeal, wheat flour, sorghum, or millet), fortified blended food, pulse, vegetable oil, sugar, and salt. Food rations based on these commodities often fail to meet the nutritional needs of PLW [74]. Thus, new and improved food supplements are needed. Webb et al. [75] suggested adding 3% of whey protein and enhancing the micronutrient profile of fortified blended foods for young children, PLW and wasted adults with HIV/AIDS and to develop lipid-based nutrient supplement (LNS) products for targeted populations and programs. In line with this, Chaparro and Dewey [74] calculated how to compose LNS products with or without milk that would fulfill the needs of both young children below 24 months and PLW when given as a small daily dose in addition to general food distributions. In an intervention study in Bangladesh LNS with a small amount of milk given to pregnant women resulted in slightly higher weight and length at delivery, but the specific effect of milk is not known [76].

The effect of milk and dairy product intake during pregnancy was evaluated in a meta-analysis based on studies from high-income countries. The evidence was limited but suggestive that a moderate milk intake compared to none or a very low intake was positively associated with birthweight [77].

Adults with Malnutrition—Focus on HIV or Tuberculosis

Acute malnutrition in adults is mainly seen in emergency situations or among those with wasting diseases like HIV and tuberculosis (TB). Malnutrition is a major risk factor for active TB disease and may increase susceptibility to HIV infection. Both TB disease and HIV then cause or exacerbate malnutrition due to lack of appetite, poor nutrient absorption and increased catabolism. Organizations and health ministries that are working in low-income countries are increasingly recognizing the importance of nutrition in management of HIV/AIDS and specialized food products in combination with nutritional counseling as important components of HIV care and treatment programs [78, 79]. Consequently, there is a need for development of effective nutritional support to patients with TB disease and HIV patients as part of comprehensive medical and social care packages.

Specific Effects of Whey and Lactose in Undernutrition

Milk powders, especially dried skimmed milk (DSM) and whey derived ingredients are used in products for treatment of undernutrition. Whey is the liquid remaining after coagulation of cheese curd and it mainly contains whey protein, lactose and milk minerals. Thus, it has traditionally been a low cost surplus product. Casein, which constitutes 80% of protein in cow's milk, is not used as a separate ingredient in foods for undernutrition. Whey is either dried or fractionated into whey protein concentrates with different protein content (see Table 15.4). After removal of all whey proteins, whey permeate remains with approx. 85% lactose and 7% milk minerals. Below, the effects of whey protein and lactose/whey permeate on undernutrition are summarized.

Whey Protein

Immune Effect of Whey Protein

Whey protein may have positive immune modulatory effects relevant for people with HIV. It is known that people with HIV infection develop a systemic deficiency of the tripeptide glutathione (GSH) within weeks after the infection [80]. GSH is an important antioxidant that contains free sulfhydryl groups that mainly comes from cysteine, a semi-essential amino acid. Whey protein is rich in cysteine and GSH precursor peptides and controlled studies in adults [80] and children [81] with advanced stages of HIV infection have shown increased plasma glutathione levels after supplementation with whey protein. Adults received 45 g whey protein per day and children received 20–50% of their protein intake from whey protein. By restoring glutathione concentration and oxidative imbalance, immune functions may also improve. In the study on children with advanced stages of HIV infection mentioned above, the CD4/CD8 lymphocyte ratio in the whey protein supplemented group showed a nonsignificant increase and there was a decrease in co-infections. In a different study in weight stable HIV patients with a history of weight loss, supplementation of 40 g of whey protein

Table 15.4 Composition of milk ingredients used for treatment of MAM and SAM (weight percent)

	DSM[a]	WPC34[a]	WPC80[a]	WPI[a]
Protein content	Whey + casein (20:80) 34–37%	Whey 34–36%	Whey 80–82%	Whey 90–92%
Lactose content	49.5–52%	48–52%	4.0–8.0%	0.5–1.0%
Fat	0.6–1.25%	3.0–4.5%	4.0–8.0%	0.5–1.0%
Ash (mainly minerals)	8.2–8.6%	6.5–8.0%	3.0–4.0%	2.0–3.0%
Moisture	3.0–4.0% (non-instant) 3.5–4.5% (instant)	3.0–4.5%	3.5–4.5%	4.5%

[a]Reference [107]

failed to increase total energy intake but CD4 counts increased in the whey protein supplemented group compared to the control group [82].

In a recent larger study of nutritional supplementation of Ethiopian adult HIV patients starting antiretroviral treatment, whey protein improved immune recovery. After 3 months treatment with LNS containing 16 energy% whey protein compared to a group receiving the same energy content of soy protein isolate, CD3 counts improved significantly with borderline significant increase in CD8 and CD4 counts [83].

A systematic review evaluating the effectiveness of macronutrient interventions for reduction of morbidity and mortality in people with HIV concluded that in general macronutrient supplementations, including whey protein (included in one study [81]), did not significantly alter clinical, anthropometric, or immunological outcomes in HIV-infected adults or children [84]. The review evaluated 14 studies with different nutrient interventions and different HIV populations, but mainly smaller studies from high-income countries. The heterogeneity in nutritional supplement composition, HIV patient characteristics and treatment regimens in studies of HIV and nutrition was also commented by de Pee and Semba [85].

Whey Protein and Muscle Accretion

Whey protein is being consumed by sports athletes and body builders to improve muscle mass formation. Reviews and clinical studies in the field of sports medicine indicate that pre-exercise or post-exercise ingestion of whey protein can increase muscle protein synthesis in young as well as elderly populations [86]. Most studies focused on the acute effect of whey protein supplementation but studies evaluating longer term effects suggested that whey protein can also lead to absolute gain in lean body mass and muscle strength [86]. A hypothesis behind this stimulation of muscle protein synthesis is that whey protein contains a favorable amino acid profile including important branch chained amino acids like leucine which is a key regulator in muscle protein synthesis [32, 87, 88]. In addition whey protein is easily digested and results in a very high blood amino acid peak and stimulation of muscle protein synthesis. In comparison to casein, whey protein results in a more prolonged state of anabolism and inhibition of protein degradation and in a study in young athletes undertaking intense training, whey protein resulted in significantly more lean body mass and better gain in strength compared to casein [87].

The relevance of the above in undernourished populations is currently not known. Very limited knowledge about the effect of whey protein on muscle mass formation and the underlying biology in undernourished individuals is available.

Lactose

In young children, lactose is hydrolyzed by the enzyme lactase to glucose and galactose, which are absorbed in the small intestine. If the lactase activity is too low to digest all the lactose, undigested lactose continues to the large intestine where it is degraded by colonic bacteria, e.g., Bifidobacteria. This leads to formation of short chain fatty acids that have important functions in relation to body homeostasis. This is considered a prebiotic effect and it has been estimated that 50–70% of ingested lactose may pass into the colon of preterm infants and in term infants a smaller unspecified fraction of lactose is likely passed into the colon [89]. In many geographical areas of the world especially in South East Asia and Southern Africa, the synthesis of lactase in the small intestine reduces or even stops some time after weaning [90]. The age at which this happens varies. Some children may experience symptoms of lactose intolerance due to reduced lactase activity and excessive amounts of lactose reaching the colon beginning at 2–3 years of age, but the majority of young children do not experience any symptoms [91–93].

Lactase is synthesized by the enterocytes lining the villi of the small intestine and both diarrhea and enteropathy disrupt the intestinal barrier and may in severe cases cause temporary lactase deficiency which may lead to symptoms of lactose intolerance. In addition helminths, especially Ascaris, have been shown to induce secondary lactase deficiency. Among other factors, anthelmintic treatment could therefore be part of treatment of acute malnutrition to obtain the greatest benefits from cow's milk [94, 95]. Concern about lactose intolerance is frequently expressed by health workers but may be overestimated as the majority of young, undernourished children recover from undernutrition when treated with therapeutic food containing milk powder or whey protein with considerable amounts of lactose. Furthermore, human milk has a considerably higher amount of lactose than foods used for treatment of SAM and breastfeeding is always recommended for infants and young children with SAM.

Lactose may also enhance calcium absorption as well as calcium retention in infants [96, 97] and enhanced absorption of other minerals including magnesium and manganese have also been described [97]. The effect of lactose on calcium absorption was not sufficiently substantiated to be accepted as a health claim by an expert panel collected on behalf of the European Food Safety Agency [98].

A large number of animal studies in piglets have shown that piglets grow faster after weaning if they receive lactose in their diet [99–102]. This mainly affects small piglets just after weaning but even in larger piglets, administration of lactose in the feeds had a positive effect on growth [102]. Human intervention studies investigating the effect of lactose compared to other carbohydrates on growth are lacking.

Lactose has a mild sweet dairy taste and if used in food products alone or in combination with milk protein (see Table 15.3) for treatment or prevention of acute malnutrition it may improve palatability as well as energy density of these foods. Furthermore, lactose is less cariogenic than sucrose [103, 104].

The Use of Cow's Milk Ingredients in Foods for MAM and SAM

Milk ingredients in foods used for treatment of MAM and SAM mainly include DSM and whey protein concentrates (WPC34, WPC80 containing 34 and 80% whey protein, respectively) and whey protein isolates (WPI). Whole milk powder may be used in some locally produced versions of RUTF [105] or therapeutic milk [106] but it is not used in large-scale production due to limited shelf life as the milk fat becomes rancid more easily.

The price of the milk ingredients fluctuate considerably and thereby has a strong effect on the price of foods for preventing and treating SAM and MAM [107]. Calculated per kg dairy protein DSM and WPC34 has fluctuated between 2 and 4 USD during the period from 2010 to 2014, while the more refined types of whey (WPC80 and WPI) have been considerably more expensive, about double the price per kg of protein. Table 15.3 shows the amount of milk ingredients in products used by UNICEF, WFP, USAID, MSF, and others for treatment of SAM and MAM.

Recommended Use of Dairy Ingredients

Specialized food products for treatment of SAM are designed to cover the entire nutrient and energy requirements for catch-up growth of children between 6 and 59 months. As shown in Table 15.3, F-75 has a low content of milk ingredients whereas F-100 and RUTF both have higher content of milk components to support catch-up growth and rehabilitation. The amount of milk ingredients in these products are specified in UNICEF and MSF supplier specifications based on current WHO product recommendations. However, the optimal amount of milk ingredients has not been thoroughly investigated in clinical trials.

The products which have been developed for use in children with MAM are intended as food supplements in addition to home food. The energy content of daily rations does not cover the entire daily need but the amount of nutrients in food supplements is elevated to compensate for home food which often has an inadequate amount of high-quality protein and micronutrients. The food supplements which are supplied by WFP and Unicef which contain milk ingredients include: RUSF and Super cereal plus (CSB++).

In the WHO Technical note: "Supplementary foods for the management of moderate acute malnutrition," the recommended level of high-quality protein (PDCAAS > 70%) is 20–43 g/1000 kcal [69] for children between 6 and 59 months. The source of protein is not specified and can be obtained with plant protein as well as milk or other animal source protein. The Technical Note however, recognizes the high quality of milk protein and its stimulatory effect on linear growth. In a review it was suggested that 25–33% of protein for treatment of MAM should come from milk protein to support weight gain and linear growth [39]. Both papers recommend further research on the amount and source of protein to support rehabilitation of children suffering from acute malnutrition. A recent technical report initiated by USAID to provide recommendations for improvement of FBF recommended addition of 3% of WPC80 to FBF [75]. The recommendation was based on the ability of milk protein to enhance linear growth and lean body mass accretion and a high-protein quality score of milk protein. WPC80 was selected as it has a concentrated form, stable price, and good shelf life. The report and its recommendations were strongly criticized by Noriega and Lindshield [108]. They commented that 3% of whey protein was lower than the amount used in clinical studies and the effect of WPC was not tested separately in malnourished populations in well controlled iso-energetic, iso-nitrogenous interventions against nonanimal source foods (plant protein) when the report was written.

Cost-Effectiveness of Milk Content

The price of milk ingredients is high and may constitute 50% of the ingredient cost of RUTF [105]. It is therefore important to find the optimal dose from a cost-effectiveness perspective and to find out if it is possible to substitute milk protein or combine, e.g., whey protein and plant protein to support healthy growth and rehabilitation of undernourished children on short term and long term.

Substitution of milk protein with plant protein has been tested in several studies. In an un-blinded study in Zambia, children received either peanut based RUTF with milk or a milk free soy-maize-sorghum-based RUTF (SMS-RUTF) [64]. The recovery rate was higher in the peanut-based RUTF with milk (60.8%) compared to the milk free SMS-RUTF (53.3%). Subgroup analyses showed a significant higher recovery rate in children below 24 months and no difference of recovery in children above 24 months.

Two other large studies from Malawi were conducted in children with moderate acute malnutrition and tested different supplementary feedings. The first study compared the effect of RUSF with DSM versus RUSF with soy versus corn soy blend (no milk) [109] and the second study compared the effect of RUSF with whey and soy vs. RUSF with soy alone versus corn soy blend with milk (CSB++) [110]. In the first study recovery rates, weight gain, and MUAC gain were improved for both RUSF products compared to corn soy blend. Length gain did not differ between the groups. In the second study, the recovery rates were similar between the three products. For anthropometric outcomes, weight gain was higher in the two groups receiving RUSF, whereas MUAC gain was significantly higher in RUSF with whey + soy compared to RUSF with soy alone and CSB++. Height gain was similar in all three groups.

Partial substitution of dried skimmed milk with soy was tested in a study comparing standard RUTF with 25% DSM and a modified RUTF with 10% DSM + 15% soy [66]. Children receiving standard RUTF with 25% DSM had higher recovery rates and improved more in weight, height, and MUAC compared to children receiving RUTF with 10% DSM and 15% soy. Children with Kwashiorkor benefited more from the higher content of milk powder compared to children with Marasmus. A different group tried to reduce costs of RUTF by substituting 25% DSM with 25% WPC34 [111]. The results showed that RUTF with WPC34 was non inferior to standard RUTF with DSM in relation to weight gain and recovery rates.

As seen from the above and ongoing studies many researchers are working to find optimal cost of milk from a cost-effectiveness point of view and cheaper sources of protein to reduce the cost of products for prevention and treatment of MAM and SAM. Cost-effectiveness studies have so far focused on price per kg of product and number of days to nutritional recovery. More complex models including differences in the percentage of children that recover or deteriorate with interventions, differences in sharing behaviors, etc. should be developed. Until now milk protein and perhaps other milk ingredients seem to favor rehabilitation of undernourished children more than cheaper sources of high-quality protein.

Conclusions

Mammals produce milk that supports growth and development of their offspring and can serve as the only energy and nutrient source during early life when growth is very high. It seems therefore plausible that animal milk has beneficial effects on growth and recovery also in humans and may be useful in prevention and treatment of undernutrition of children and other vulnerable groups.

WHO recommends exclusive breastfeeding for 6 months and continued breastfeeding until the age of 2 years or beyond [3]. Reduction in child mortality and morbidity are the most important benefits of breastfeeding and it has been estimated that 800,000 children die every year due to suboptimal breastfeeding practices [4]. It is therefore essential to promote and support breastfeeding. Milk composition varies a lot between different mammal species. Compared to milk from dairy animals (cow, buffalo, goat, and sheep), human milk has a low content of protein and minerals and a high content of lactose. For this reason, animal milk needs to be modified, or be mixed with other ingredients, before feeding to infants younger than 12 months. The protein quality of nonhuman milk is high with DIAAS scores above 100% and milk contains important minerals with high bioavailability that support growth as well as bone formation.

Milk or milk components are used in most products intended for treatment of SAM and in some products intended for treatment of MAM. For young children with SAM aged 6–59 months the WHO guideline prescribes use of F-75, F-100 and RUTF for stabilization and rehabilitation. All three products contain (cow's) milk ingredients with a low content of milk in F-75 intended for stabilization of hospitalized patients with SAM and higher contents of milk ingredients in F-100 and RUTF intended for rehabilitation of in- and out-patients with SAM. For children with MAM no official guidelines exist but different groups have come up with suggestions for use of approximately 25–50% milk protein in treatment of MAM. Milk or milk ingredients have also been used in school milk programs to support growth and nutritional needs of school children and in products supplied to vulnerable groups like pregnant and lactating women and adults with HIV or TB.

In relation to undernutrition, the effects of milk protein and particularly whey protein, because of the potential positive effects of specific proteins and peptides in whey, have been investigated. Results indicate that whey protein may have positive immune stimulatory effects relevant for people with HIV and some studies suggest improved muscle accretion if taken immediately after exercise. The effect of milk carbohydrate, i.e., lactose, has achieved little attention. Lactose may have a prebiotic effect and may enhance calcium absorption. Studies have furthermore shown that piglets grow faster if their feed is supplemented with lactose. Future studies are needed to investigate if this can be confirmed in humans.

Dairy ingredients are expensive and researchers are therefore conducting cost-effectiveness studies to define the optimal amounts of milk components for different age groups and stages of undernutrition.

Discussion Points

- An estimated 800,000 children are dying annually due to suboptimum breastfeeding. There is a huge demand for new insight and perhaps new methodologies for supporting breastfeeding in low-income countries. What policy initiatives could address the low breastfeeding rates especially among working women?
- Studies in children with acute malnutrition indicate that feeds containing dried skimmed milk or whey result in higher recovery rates and/or improved anthropometric outcomes. What type of studies and cost-effectiveness analyses are needed to find the optimum amount of dairy ingredients that would support recovery of children with MAM and SAM?
- It is recommended to further investigate if and how milk protein can be (partially) replaced by cheaper sources of high quality protein. What other sources of proteins (e.g., plant protein or low cost animal source proteins from insects or small fish) could be used to replace or complement milk protein? What products would they be used into support recovery from MAM and SAM?
- Lactose constitutes up to 40 energy % of human milk and seems to have several beneficial effects, including potential positive effects on . gut microbiota, mineral absorption and perhaps growth. The role of lactose in treatment of undernutrition is not yet well investigated. Which studies are needed to investigate the effect of lactose in undernourished children?

Conflict of Interest We have received unconditional grants for intervention studies including dairy products from US Dairy Export Council and the Danish Dairy Research Foundation.

References

1. Gerosa S, Skoet J. Milk availability: current production and demand and medium-term outlook (Chap. 2). In: Muehlhoff E, Benneth A, McMahon D, editors. Milk and dairy products in human nutrition. Rome: FAO; 2013.
2. Muehlhoff E, Bennett A, McMahon D, editors. Milk and dairy products in human nutrition. Rome: FAO; 2013.
3. Global strategy for infant and young child feeding. The optimal duration of exclusive breastfeeding, World Health Organization fifty-fourth world health assembly. WHO; 2001. http://www.who.int/nutrition/topics/infantfeeding_recommendation/en/.
4. Black RE, Victora CG, Walker SP, Bhutta ZA, Christian P, de Onis M, et al. Maternal and child undernutrition and overweight in low-income and middle-income countries. Lancet. 2013;382(9890):427–51.
5. Bhutta ZA, Das JK, Rizvi A, Gaffey MF, Walker N, Horton S, et al. Evidence-based interventions for improvement of maternal and child nutrition: what can be done and at what cost? Lancet. 2013;382(9890):452–77.
6. Ballard O, Morrow AL. Human milk composition: nutrients and bioactive factors. Pediatr Clin North Am. 2013;60(1):49–74.
7. Prentice A. Regional variations in the composition of human milk. In: Jensen, RG, editor. Handbook of milk composition. San Diego: Academic Press, Inc.; 1995.
8. Allen LH. Maternal micronutrient malnutrition: effects on breast milk and infant nutrition, and priorities for intervention. SCN News U N Adm Comm Coord Subcomm Nutr. 1994;11:21–4.

9. Michaelsen KF, Dewey KG, Perez-Exposito AB, Nurhasan M, Lauritzen L, Roos N. Food sources and intake of n-6 and n-3 fatty acids in low-income countries with emphasis on infants, young children (6–24 months), and pregnant and lactating women. Matern Child Nutr. 2011;7(Suppl 2):124–40.

10. Black RE, Allen LH, Bhutta ZA, Caulfield LE, de Onis M, Ezzati M, et al. Maternal and child undernutrition: global and regional exposures and health consequences. Lancet. 2008;371(9608):243–60.

11. Lamberti LM, Zakarija-Grković I, Fischer Walker CL, Theodoratou E, Nair H, Campbell H, et al. Breastfeeding for reducing the risk of pneumonia morbidity and mortality in children under two: a systematic literature review and meta-analysis. BMC Public Health. 2013;13(Suppl 3):S18.

12. Lamberti LM, Fischer Walker CL, Noiman A, Victora C, Black RE. Breastfeeding and the risk for diarrhea morbidity and mortality. BMC Public Health. 2011;11(Suppl 3):S15.

13. Briend A, Wojtyniak B, Rowland MG. Breast feeding, nutritional state, and child survival in rural Bangladesh. Br Med J Clin Res Ed. 1988;296(6626):879–82.

14. Horta BL, Cesar VG. Long-term effects of breastfeeding, a systematic review. WHO; Report No.: ISBN 978 92 4 150530 7. http://apps.who.int/iris/bitstream/10665/79198/1/9789241505307_eng.pdf.

15. Arenz S, Rückerl R, Koletzko B, von Kries R. Breast-feeding and childhood obesity—a systematic review. Int J Obes Relat Metab Disord J Int Assoc Study Obes. 2004;28(10):1247–56.

16. ESPGHAN Committee on Nutrition, Agostoni C, Braegger C, Decsi T, Kolacek S, Koletzko B, et al. Breast-feeding: a commentary by the ESPGHAN Committee on Nutrition. J Pediatr Gastroenterol Nutr. 2009;49 (1):112–25.

17. Kramer MS, Kakuma R. Optimal duration of exclusive breastfeeding. Cochrane Database Syst Rev. 2012;8: CD003517.

18. Ip S, Chung M, Raman G, Chew P, Magula N, DeVine D, et al. Breastfeeding and maternal and infant health outcomes in developed countries. Evid Rep Technol Assess. 2007;153:1–186.

19. Haroon S, Das JK, Salam RA, Imdad A, Bhutta ZA. Breastfeeding promotion interventions and breastfeeding practices: a systematic review. BMC Public Health. 2013;13(Suppl 3):S20.

20. Conde-Agudelo A, Belizán JM, Diaz-Rossello J. Kangaroo mother care to reduce morbidity and mortality in low birthweight infants. Cochrane Database Syst Rev. 2011;(3):CD002771.

21. Moore ER, Anderson GC, Bergman N, Dowswell T. Early skin-to-skin contact for mothers and their healthy newborn infants. Cochrane Database Syst Rev. 2012;5:CD003519.

22. Coutsoudis A, Pillay K, Spooner E, Kuhn L, Coovadia HM. Influence of infant-feeding patterns on early mother-to-child transmission of HIV-1 in Durban, South Africa: a prospective cohort study. South African Vitamin A Study Group. Lancet. 1999;354(9177):471–6.

23. HIV transmission through breastfeeding a review of available evidence 2007 update. WHO, Unicef, UNAIDS, UNFPA; 2007. Report No.: ISBN 978 92 4 159659 6. http://www.who.int/maternal_child_adolescent/documents/9789241596596/en/. Accessed Dec 2014.

24. Nduati R, John G, Mbori-Ngacha D, Richardson B, Overbaugh J, Mwatha A, et al. Effect of breastfeeding and formula feeding on transmission of HIV-1: a randomized clinical trial. JAMA. 2000;283(9):1167–74.

25. Siegfried N, van der Merwe L, Brocklehurst P, Sint TT. Antiretrovirals for reducing the risk of mother-to-child transmission of HIV infection. Cochrane Database Syst Rev. 2011;(7):CD003510.

26. Guidelines on HIV and infant feeding 2010. Principles and recommendations for infant feeding in the context of HIV and a summary of evidence. Report No.: ISBN 978 92 4 159953 5. http://www.who.int/maternal_child_adolescent/documents/9789241599535/en/. Accessed Dec 2014.

27. WHO. Consolidated guidelines on the use of antiretroviral drugs for treating and preventing HIV infection. Recommendations for a public health approach. June 2013. World Health Organization, Geneva, Switzerland; Report No.: ISBN 978 92 4 150572 7.

28. Wijesinha-Bettoni R, Burlingame B. Chapter 3. In: Muehlhoff E, Benneth A, McMahon D, editors. Milk and dairy products in human nutrition. FAO, Rome, 2013.

29. FAOSTAT. http://faostat.fao.org/. Accessed Dec 2014.

30. Dietary protein quality evaluation in human nutrition. Report of an FAO Expert Consultation. 31 Mar–2 Apr 2011 Auckland, New Zealand; Report No.: ISSN 0254-4725, ISBN 978-92-5-107417-6. http://www.fao.org/ag/humannutrition/35978-02317b979a686a57aa4593304ffc17f06.pdf. Accessed Dec 2014.

31. Interpretation of the protein quality methodology: change to DIAAS. IDF Factsheet, Mar 2014. www.idfdairynutrition.org. Accessed Dec 2014.

32. Hoppe C, Andersen GS, Jacobsen S, Mølgaard C, Friis H, Sangild PT, et al. The use of whey or skimmed milk powder in fortified blended foods for vulnerable groups. J Nutr. 2008;138(1):145S–61S.

33. Mølgaard C, Larnkjær A, Arnberg K, Michaelsen KF. Milk and growth in children: effects of whey and casein. Nestlé Nutr Workshop Ser Paediatr Programme. 2011;67:67–78.

34. Brun AC, Størdal K, Johannesdottir GB, Bentsen BS, Medhus AW. The effect of protein composition in liquid meals on gastric emptying rate in children with cerebral palsy. Clin Nutr Edinb Scotl. 2012;31(1):108–12.

35. Drewnowski A, Mennella JA, Johnson SL, Bellisle F. Sweetness and food preference. J Nutr. 2012;142 (6):1142S–8S.
36. Golden MH. Proposed recommended nutrient densities for moderately malnourished children. Food Nutr Bull. 2009;30(3 Suppl):S267–342.
37. Oginni LM, Sharp CA, Badru OS, Risteli J, Davie MWJ, Worsfold M. Radiological and biochemical resolution of nutritional rickets with calcium. Arch Dis Child. 2003;88(9):812–7; discussion 812–7.
38. Allen LH, Dror DK. Effects of animal source foods, with emphasis on milk, in the diet of children in low-income countries. Nestlé Nutr Workshop Ser Paediatr Programme. 2011;67:113–30.
39. Michaelsen KF, Hoppe C, Roos N, Kaestel P, Stougaard M, Lauritzen L, et al. Choice of foods and ingredients for moderately malnourished children 6 months to 5 years of age. Food Nutr Bull. 2009;30(3 Suppl):S343–404.
40. Danish Food Composition Databank—Search Food Data [Internet]. [cited 2015 Nov 4]. Available from: http://www.foodcomp.dk/v7/fcdb_search.asp.
41. Interim summary of conclusions and dietary recommendations on total fat & fatty acids. From the Joint FAO/WHO Expert Consultation on Fats and Fatty Acids in Human Nutrition, 10–14 Nov 2008, WHO, Geneva. www.who.int/nutrition/topics/FFA_summary_rec_conclusion.pdf. Accessed Dec 2014.
42. Chowdhury R, Warnakula S, Kunutsor S, Crowe F, Ward HA, Johnson L, et al. Association of dietary, circulating, and supplement fatty acids with coronary risk: a systematic review and meta-analysis. Ann Intern Med. 2014;160(6):398–406.
43. Stanton C, McMahon D, Mills S. Dairy components, products and human health (Chap. 5). In: Muehlhoff E, Benneth A, McMahon D, editors. Milk and dairy products in human nutrition. Rome: FAO; 2013.
44. Mozaffarian D, Aro A, Willett WC. Health effects of trans-fatty acids: experimental and observational evidence. Eur J Clin Nutr. 2009;63(Suppl 2):S5–21.
45. Grillenberger M, Neumann CG, Murphy SP, Bwibo NO, van't Veer P, Hautvast JGAJ, et al. Food supplements have a positive impact on weight gain and the addition of animal source foods increases lean body mass of Kenyan schoolchildren. J Nutr. 2003;133(11 Suppl 2):3957S–3964S.
46. Hulett JL, Weiss RE, Bwibo NO, Galal OM, Drorbaugh N, Neumann CG. Animal source foods have a positive impact on the primary school test scores of Kenyan schoolchildren in a cluster-randomised, controlled feeding intervention trial. Br J Nutr. 2014;111(5):875–86.
47. Hoppe C, Mølgaard C, Michaelsen KF. Cow's milk and linear growth in industrialized and developing countries. Annu Rev Nutr. 2006;26:131–73.
48. Michaelsen KF. Effect of protein intake from 6 to 24 months on insulin-like growth factor 1 (IGF-1) levels, body composition, linear growth velocity, and linear growth acceleration: what are the implications for stunting and wasting? Food Nutr Bull. 2013;34(2):268–71.
49. Dewey KG, Peerson JM, Brown KH, Krebs NF, Michaelsen KF, Persson LA, et al. Growth of breast-fed infants deviates from current reference data: a pooled analysis of US, Canadian, and European data sets. World Health Organization Working Group on Infant Growth. Pediatrics. 1995;96(3 Pt 1):495–503.
50. Larnkjaer A, Ingstrup HK, Schack-Nielsen L, Hoppe C, Mølgaard C, Skovgaard IM, et al. Early programming of the IGF-I axis: negative association between IGF-I in infancy and late adolescence in a 17-year longitudinal follow-up study of healthy subjects. Growth Horm IGF Res Off J Growth Horm Res Soc Int IGF Res Soc. 2009;19(1):82–6.
51. Leighton G, Clark ML. Milk consumption and the growth of school children: second preliminary report on tests to the Scottish board of health. Br Med J. 1929;1(3548):23–5.
52. He M, Yang Y-X, Han H, Men J-H, Bian L-H, Wang G-D. Effects of yogurt supplementation on the growth of preschool children in Beijing suburbs. Biomed Environ Sci BES. 2005;18(3):192–7.
53. Lampl M, Johnston FE. The effects of protein supplementation on the growth and skeletal maturation of New Guinean school children. Ann Hum Biol. 1978;5(3):219–27.
54. Lien DTK, Nhung BT, Khan NC, Hop LT, Nga NTQ, Hung NT, et al. Impact of milk consumption on performance and health of primary school children in rural Vietnam. Asia Pac J Clin Nutr. 2009;18(3):326–34.
55. De Beer H. Dairy products and physical stature: a systematic review and meta-analysis of controlled trials. Econ Hum Biol. 2012;10(3):299–309.
56. Christensen DL, Eis J, Hansen AW, Larsson MW, Mwaniki DL, Kilonzo B, et al. Obesity and regional fat distribution in Kenyan populations: impact of ethnicity and urbanization. Ann Hum Biol. 2008;35(2):232–49.
57. Fredriks AM, van Buuren S, Burgmeijer RJ, Meulmeester JF, Beuker RJ, Brugman E, et al. Continuing positive secular growth change in The Netherlands 1955–1997. Pediatr Res. 2000;47(3):316–23.
58. Martin RM, Holly JMP, Gunnell D. Milk and linear growth: programming of the igf-I axis and implication for health in adulthood. Nestlé Nutr Workshop Ser Paediatr Programme. 2011;67:79–97.
59. Kerac M, Blencowe H, Grijalva-Eternod C, McGrath M, Shoham J, Cole TJ, et al. Prevalence of wasting among under 6-month-old infants in developing countries and implications of new case definitions using WHO growth standards: a secondary data analysis. Arch Dis Child. 2011;96(11):1008–13.

60. Infant Feeding in Emergencies Module 2 Version 1.1 For health and nutrition workers in emergency situations for training, practice and reference. ENN, IBFAN-GIFA, Fondation Terre des hommes, CARE USA, Action Contre la Faim, UNICEF, UNHCR, WHO, WFP. November 2014. http://www.who.int/nutrition/publications/emergencies/ife_module2/en/. Accessed Dec 2014.

61. International Code of Marketing of Breast-milk Substitutes. WHO Geneva 1981. Report No.: ISBN 92 4 154160 1. http://www.who.int/nutrition/publications/code_english.pdf. Accessed Dec 2014.

62. Updates on the management of severe acute malnutrition in infants and children. WHO Guideline, Geneva, World Health Organization; 2013. Report No.: ISBN 978 92 4 150632 8. http://www.who.int/nutrition/publications/guidelines/updates_management_SAM_infantandchildren/en/. Accessed Dec 2014.

63. Ready-to-use therapeutic food for children with severe acute malnutrition, position statement. Unicef, Position paper; 2013. http://www.unicef.org/media/files/UNICEF-Position-Paper_Ready-To-Use-Therapeutic-Food_June2013.pdf. Accessed Dec 2014.

64. Irena AH, Bahwere P, Owino VO, Diop EI, Bachmann MO, Mbwili-Muleya C, et al. Comparison of the effectiveness of a milk-free soy-maize-sorghum-based ready-to-use therapeutic food to standard ready-to-use therapeutic food with 25% milk in nutrition management of severely acutely malnourished Zambian children: an equivalence non-blinded cluster randomised controlled trial. Matern Child Nutr. 2013.

65. Lenters LM, Wazny K, Webb P, Ahmed T, Bhutta ZA. Treatment of severe and moderate acute malnutrition in low- and middle-income settings: a systematic review, meta-analysis and Delphi process. BMC Public Health. 2013;13(Suppl 3):S23.

66. Oakley E, Reinking J, Sandige H, Trehan I, Kennedy G, Maleta K, et al. A ready-to-use therapeutic food containing 10% milk is less effective than one with 25% milk in the treatment of severely malnourished children. J Nutr. 2010;140(12):2248–52.

67. Manary MJ, Ndkeha MJ, Ashorn P, Maleta K, Briend A. Home based therapy for severe malnutrition with ready-to-use food. Arch Dis Child. 2004;89(6):557–61.

68. de Pee S, Bloem MW. Current and potential role of specially formulated foods and food supplements for preventing malnutrition among 6- to 23-months-old children and for treating moderate malnutrition among 6- to 59-month-old children. Food Nutr Bull. 2009;30(3 Suppl):S434–63.

69. Technical note: supplementary foods for the management of moderate acute malnutrition in infants and children 6–59 months of age. Geneva, World Health Organization, 2012. http://www.who.int/nutrition/publications/moderate_malnutrition/9789241504423/en/. Accessed Dec 2014.

70. Griffin, M. Issues in the development of school milk. Paper presented at School Milk Workshop, FAO Intergovernmental Group on Meat and Dairy Products, Winnipeg, Canada, 17–19 June 2004. http://www.fao.org/fileadmin/templates/est/COMM_MARKETS_MONITORING/Dairy/Documents/School_Milk_FAO_background.pdf. Accessed Dec 2014.

71. Iannotti LL. Milk and dairy programs affecting nutrition, Chapter 7. In: Muehlhoff E, Benneth A, McMahon D, editors. Milk and dairy products in human nutrition. Rome: FAO; 2013.

72. Du X, Zhu K, Trube A, Zhang Q, Ma G, Hu X, et al. School-milk intervention trial enhances growth and bone mineral accretion in Chinese girls aged 10–12 years in Beijing. Br J Nutr. 2004;92(1):159–68.

73. Picciano MF. Pregnancy and lactation: physiological adjustments, nutritional requirements and the role of dietary supplements. J Nutr. 2003;133(6):1997S–2002S.

74. Chaparro CM, Dewey KG. Use of lipid-based nutrient supplements (LNS) to improve the nutrient adequacy of general food distribution rations for vulnerable sub-groups in emergency settings. Matern Child Nutr. 2010;6 (Suppl 1):1–69.

75. Webb P, Rogers BL, Rosenberg I, Schlossman N, Wanke C, Bagriansky J et al. Improving the nutritional quality of U.S. food aid: recommendations for changes to products and programs. Boston: Tufts University. http://www.nutrition.tufts.edu/documents/ImprovingtheNutritionalQuality.pdf. Accessed Dec 2014.

76. Mridha MK, Matias SL, Chaparro CM, Paul RR, Hussain S, Vosti SA, et al. Lipid-based nutrient supplements for pregnant women reduce newborn stunting in a cluster-randomized controlled effectiveness trial in Bangladesh. Am J Clin Nutr. 2016;103(1):236–49.

77. Brantsæter AL, Olafsdottir AS, Forsum E, Olsen SF, Thorsdottir I. Does milk and dairy consumption during pregnancy influence fetal growth and infant birthweight? A systematic literature review. Food Nutr. Res. 2012; 56(0).

78. Tumilowicz A. Guide to screening for food and nutrition services among adolescents and adults living with HIV. Washington, DC: Food and Nutrition Technical Assistance II Project (FANTA-2), Academy for Educational Development, 2010. http://www.fantaproject.org/sites/default/files/resources/Nutrition_Interventions_Screening_Guide_Final.pdf. Accessed Dec 2014.

79. World Food Programme. https://www.wfp.org/content/nutrition-assessment-counselling-and-support-adolescents-and-adults-living-with-hiv. Accessed Jan 2016.

80. Micke P, Beeh KM, Buhl R. Effects of long-term supplementation with whey proteins on plasma glutathione levels of HIV-infected patients. Eur J Nutr. 2002;41(1):12–8.
81. Moreno YF, Sgarbieri VC, da Silva MN, Toro AADC, Vilela MMS. Features of whey protein concentrate supplementation in children with rapidly progressive HIV infection. J Trop Pediatr. 52(1):34–8.
82. Sattler FR, Rajicic N, Mulligan K, Yarasheski KE, Koletar SL, Zolopa A, et al. Evaluation of high-protein supplementation in weight-stable HIV-positive subjects with a history of weight loss: a randomized, double-blind, multicenter trial. Am J Clin Nutr. 2008;88(5):1313–21.
83. Olsen MF, Abdissa A, Kæstel P, Tesfaye M, Yilma D, Girma T, et al. Effects of nutritional supplementation for HIV patients starting antiretroviral treatment: randomised controlled trial in Ethiopia. BMJ. 2014;348:g3187.
84. Grobler L, Siegfried N, Visser ME, Mahlungulu SSN, Volmink J. Nutritional interventions for reducing morbidity and mortality in people with HIV. Cochrane Database Syst Rev. 2013;2:CD004536.
85. de Pee S, Semba RD. Role of nutrition in HIV infection: review of evidence for more effective programming in resource-limited settings. Food Nutr Bull. 2010;31(4):S313–44.
86. Graf S, Egert S, Heer M. Effects of whey protein supplements on metabolism: evidence from human intervention studies. Curr Opin Clin Nutr Metab Care. 2011;14(6):569–80.
87. Hayes A, Cribb PJ. Effect of whey protein isolate on strength, body composition and muscle hypertrophy during resistance training. Curr Opin Clin Nutr Metab Care. 2008;11(1):40–4.
88. Phillips SM, Tang JE, Moore DR. The role of milk- and soy-based protein in support of muscle protein synthesis and muscle protein accretion in young and elderly persons. J Am Coll Nutr. 2009;28(4):343–54.
89. Klein CJ. Nutrient requirements for preterm infant formulas. J Nutr. 2002;132(6 Suppl 1):1395S–577S.
90. Itan Y, Jones BL, Ingram CJ, Swallow DM, Thomas MG. A worldwide correlation of lactase persistence phenotype and genotypes. BMC Evol Biol. 2010;10:36.
91. Heyman MB. Committee on nutrition. Lactose intolerance in infants, children, and adolescents. Pediatrics. 2006;118(3):1279–86.
92. Vesa TH, Marteau P, Korpela R. Lactose intolerance. J Am Coll Nutr. 2000;19(2 Suppl):165S–75S.
93. Wilt TJ, Shaukat A, Shamliyan T, Taylor BC, MacDonald R, Tacklind J, et al. Lactose intolerance and health. Evid Rep Technol Assess. 2010;192:1–410.
94. Taren DL, Nesheim MC, Crompton DWT, Holland CV, Barbeau I, Rivera G, et al. Contribution of ascariasis to poor nutritional status of children from Chiriqui Province, Republic of Panama. Parasitology. 1987;95:603–13.
95. Taren DL, Crompton DWT. Mechanisms for interactions between parasitism and nutritional status. Clin Nutr. 1990;8:227–38.
96. Abrams SA, Griffin IJ, Davila PM. Calcium and zinc absorption from lactose-containing and lactose-free infant formulas. Am J Clin Nutr. 2002;76(2):442–6.
97. Ziegler EE, Fomon SJ. Lactose enhances mineral absorption in infancy. J Pediatr Gastroenterol Nutr. 1983;2(2):288–94.
98. Scientific Opinion on the substantiation of health claims related to lactose and increase in calcium absorption leading to an increase in calcium retention (ID 668) pursuant to Article 13(1) of Regulation (EC) No. 1924/20061, EFSA Panel on Dietetic Products, Nutrition and Allergies (NDA), European Food Safety Authority (EFSA), Parma, Italy 2011. http://www.efsa.europa.eu/en/efsajournal/doc/2234.pdf. Accessed Dec 2014.
99. Mahan DC, Fastinger ND, Peters JC. Effects of diet complexity and dietary lactose levels during three starter phases on postweaning pig performance. J Anim Sci. 2004;82(9):2790–7.
100. Pierce K, Callan J, McCarthy P, O'Doherty JV. Effects of high dietary concentration of lactose and increased soyabean meal inclusion in starter diets for piglets. Anim Sci. 2004;2004(82):2790–7.
101. O'Connell JM, Callan J, O'Doherty JV. The interaction between cereal type and lactose level on piglet performance and diet digestibility post weaning. Anim Sci. 2005;81:265–9.
102. Cromwell GL, Allee GL, Mahan DC. Assessment of lactose level in the mid- to late-nursery phase on performance of weanling pigs. J Anim Sci. 2008;86(1):127–33.
103. Neff D. Acid production from different carbohydrate sources in human plaque in situ. Caries Res. 1967;1(1):78–87.
104. Bowen WH, Lawrence RA. Comparison of the cariogenicity of cola, honey, cow milk, human milk, and sucrose. Pediatrics. 2005;116(4):921–6.
105. Manary MJ. Local production and provision of ready-to-use therapeutic food (RUTF) spread for the treatment of severe childhood malnutrition. Food Nutr Bull. 2006;27(3 Suppl):S83–9.
106. ICDDR, B, Ahmed T. Nutrition Rehabilitation Unit at ICDDR, B an ideal home for treatment of children with severe malnutrition. Glimpse. 2004;26(3). http://dspace.icddrb.org:8080/jspui/bitstream/123456789/5505/1/ICDDRBGlimpse-Vol26(3)-2004.pdf. Accessed Dec 2014.
107. Dairy for Global Nutrition, U.S. Dairy Export Council. http://dairyglobalnutrition.org. Accessed December 2014.
108. Noriega KE, Lindshield BL. Is the inclusion of animal source foods in fortified blended foods justified? Nutrients. 2014;6(9):3516–35.

109. Matilsky DK, Maleta K, Castleman T, Manary MJ. Supplementary feeding with fortified spreads results in higher recovery rates than with a corn/soy blend in moderately wasted children. J Nutr. 2009;139(4):773–8.
110. LaGrone LN, Trehan I, Meuli GJ, Wang RJ, Thakwalakwa C, Maleta K, et al. A novel fortified blended flour, corn-soy blend «plus-plus,» is not inferior to lipid-based ready-to-use supplementary foods for the treatment of moderate acute malnutrition in Malawian children. Am J Clin Nutr. 2012;95(1):212–9.
111. Bahwere P, Banda T, Sadler K, Nyirenda G, Owino V, Shaba B, et al. Effectiveness of milk whey protein-based ready-to-use therapeutic food in treatment of severe acute malnutrition in Malawian under-5 children: a randomised, double-blind, controlled non-inferiority clinical trial. Matern Child Nutr. 2014;10(3):436–51.

Chapter 16
The Role of Breastfeeding Protection, Promotion and Support in a Developing World

Douglas Taren and Chessa K. Lutter

Keywords Breastfeeding · Breast milk · Breastfeeding support · Kangaroo method · Baby-friendly hospital initiative · Epidemiology

Learning Objectives

- Evaluate the social determinants of infant feeding and how they may differ between low, middle- and high-income countries.
- Identify the health and economic benefits of breastfeeding.
- Describe the importance of early initiation of breastfeeding and exclusive breastfeeding.
- Describe the major healthcare-based interventions that support the initiation and continuation of breastfeeding.
- Describe community-based policies and programs that can increase exclusive breastfeeding rates.

Introduction

Breastfeeding Definitions and Recommendations

In order to address breastfeeding, there is a need to use common terminology regarding infant feeding. The United Nations Children's Fund (UNICEF) and the World Health Organisation (WHO) have identified five key terms that should be used consistently when addressing infant feeding [1, 2]. These are:

1. Exclusive breastfeeding: infant receives only breast milk (including breast milk that has been expressed or from a wet nurse) and nothing else, except for oral rehydration solution (ORS), medicines and vitamins and minerals.
2. Predominant breastfeeding: infant receives breast milk as the predominant source of nourishment. This includes infants who receive certain liquids (water and water-based drinks, fruit juice), ritual fluids or ORS, drops or syrups (vitamins, minerals, medicines) but excludes consumption of non-human milk or food-based fluids.

D. Taren (✉)
Mel and Enid Zuckerman College of Public Health, University of Arizona,
1295 North Martin Avenue, Tucson 85724, AZ, USA
e-mail: taren@email.arizona.edu

C.K. Lutter
Food and Nutrition, Non-Communicable Diseases and Mental Health,
Pan American Health Organization, 525 23rd Street, NW, Washington, DC, USA
e-mail: lutterch@paho.org

© Springer Science+Business Media New York 2017
S. de Pee et al. (eds.), *Nutrition and Health in a Developing World*,
Nutrition and Health, DOI 10.1007/978-3-319-43739-2_16

3. Breastfeeding: child receives breast milk as well as any other food or liquid, including non-human milk and infant formula.
4. Breast milk substitute: any food being marketed or otherwise represented as a partial or total replacement for breast milk, whether or not it is suitable for that purpose. Infant formula: non-human milks for babies made out of a variety of ingredients, including sugar, animal milks, soybean, vegetable oils, vitamins, minerals, and are usually in powder form, to mix with water.
5. Complementary feeding: solid, semisolid or soft foods that are fed to an infant who is also breastfeeding. It is not recommended to provide any solid, semisolid or soft foods to children less than six months of age.

Exclusive breastfeeding for the first six months of life is recommended by the WHO and universally accepted as the preferred method for feeding an infant because of how it benefits the physical health of mothers and children and the cognitive development of children. WHO and UNICEF recommend that exclusive breastfeeding starts within one hour after birth and continues for the first six months of life. Furthermore, an infant should continue to be breastfed for the first two years of life or more with nutritionally adequate and safe complementary foods that are properly fed starting at six months of age [3]. Breastfeeding has also remained the recommended method of feeding infants of HIV-infected mothers when formula is not available and can be safely used and should be combined with antiretroviral treatment of the mother, and of the child for the first weeks after delivery [4].

The termination of exclusive breastfeeding is often considered to occur the first time a child consumes a liquid, including water or food other than breast milk. The transition from exclusive breastfeeding to predominant breastfeeding should include the introduction of complementary feeding with energy and nutrient dense foods that are present in the community or can be provided as supplements for vulnerable infants in low-resource areas [5].

Although exclusive breastfeeding is considered to have stopped when other liquids or foods are consumed, it is not unusual to have a child go from being exclusively breastfed to predominant breastfeeding and back to being exclusively breastfed. This can occur for several reasons including maternal illness, changing childcare situations and the success of breastfeeding counseling. There is obviously a need to have a defined way to identify when exclusive breastfeeding has stopped for various research studies so data can be comparable [6], but healthcare workers must be aware that women can be encouraged to restart exclusive breastfeeding for their infants that are less than six months of age even if the infant already consumed other liquids or foods. Thus, the current recommendation to assess the prevalence of exclusive breastfeeding is based on feeding practices in the past 24 h using a recall method. However, it is recognized that this method provides a greater estimate for exclusive breastfeeding rates and is not an indicator for the percent of infants who had not received any liquid or solid food before six months of age [2, 7].

Nutrient Content of Breast Milk

Colostrum, the first breast milk that is produced immediately after birth, is rich in cellular and humoral immunological substances including leukocytes and secretory IgA to provide early protection against neonatal infections. Colostrum also is a natural laxative and supports the infants first stool, meconium, and at the same time helps with the excretion of bilirubin for the prevention of jaundice [8]. Nonetheless, many women do not provide colostrum to their infants because they believe it is dirty, and unhealthy for their infant. In India, it has been reported that gold ash is provided in lieu of colostrum to support the removal of meconium [9].

Colostrum usually transitions to breast milk within the first few days postpartum, and breast milk is considered fully mature four to six weeks postpartum. Breast milk continues to contain immunological factors, cells and hormones that support development [10]. It is also a rich source of energy and micronutrients for infants that includes carbohydrates, fats and amino acids. The nutrient composition of breast milk varies based on several factors including the nutritional status of the mother, the feeding pattern of her infant and diurnal changes in its composition. It also differs between the start of a feeding session and the end of a feeding session in which the fat content is greater when the breast is less full [11–13]. The composition also differs depending on whether the infant is preterm or term. Preterm milk is richer in protein but may not have a sufficient nutrient composition to support very preterm and low-birth weight infants without fortification [13].

Breast milk is not a rich source of iron, vitamin K or vitamin D. Supplementing infants with vitamin K and D is recommended, but mainly practiced in high-income countries [14, 15]. For vitamin K, some countries give it by injection at birth while others provide drops for the first couple of weeks or months. Vitamin D is generally given in the form of drops. For iron, infants rely on stores laid down toward the end of the pregnancy. Thus, preterm infants have very small iron stores and hence require supplementation from 1 month of age [14]. Vitamin A content of breast milk can also be low but can be increased by providing mothers a diet rich in (pro)vitamin A or supplements resulting in improved vitamin A status of breastfed infants [15–17]. More recently, dietary patterns have also been shown to affect the B vitamin content of breast milk [18]. Antenatal supplementation of vitamin B12 and during the postpartum period has increased the B12 concentration in colostrum and breast milk and decreased the methylmalonic acid concentration in infants up to 3 months of age. The improvement in the B12 status also improved immune responses of mothers and led to less inflammation in infants [19]. A review of the breast milk concentration of specific group 1 micronutrients (thiamin, riboflavin, vitamin B6, vitamin B12 and choline) suggested that deficient mothers also had deficient breast milk concentrations and that breast milk concentrations could be improved by either improving the mother's diet or providing mothers supplements and supports the need for additional research in this area [20]. Furthermore, additional information about the composition of breast milk is presented in Chap. 15.

Breastfeeding and Infant Health

Breast milk and the act of breastfeeding can never be replaced by the use of infant formula and bottles. Breast milk is safer than formula with the risk of either not mixing formula powder correctly and the potential use of unclean water. Breastfeeding can also decrease a woman's fertility, increasing the time between pregnancies. Breast milk provides nutrients and other substances that protect infants from infectious diseases and promotes growth and development. Breastfed infants have a stimulated immune system and improved response to immunizations compared with non-breastfed infants. Emerging data now indicate that breastfed infants have a decreased risk for developing chronic diseases such as obesity and possibly type 2 diabetes later in life [21]. A systematic review of 17 studies suggests that breastfed infants at six months of age may have greater weight and length than non-breastfed infants and at the same time have a lower body mass index [22]. This effect can also continue into later ages decreasing the risk of obesity, type 2 diabetes and even childhood leukemia [23, 24].

Although data indicate that breastfeeding is able to decrease the risk of developing diarrheal and respiratory infections, it may do so in different ways and its effect may be different based on a child's age. For example, the impact of breastfeeding appears to have a greater impact on decreasing the risk for respiratory infections in the first few months of life and has a greater impact on decreasing diarrheal episodes when exposure risk increases because an infant starts crawling which increases exposure to pathogens [25]. Additional benefits to infant and child health include decreasing the risk of otitis media and dental caries [26, 27]. Breastfeeding slightly decreases the risk for asthma, and meta-analyses suggest that breastfeeding may not decrease the risk for eczema or food allergies [28]. Breastfeeding is even associated with greater cognitive development impacting school performance and economic status [29, 30]. Recently, it was estimated that no or low levels of breastfeeding costs about $302 billion annual or 0.49% of world gross national income because of the lower cognitive development of non-breastfed children [31].

Breastfeeding and Maternal Health

Breastfeeding also benefits maternal health. Immediately following birth, breastfeeding supports the involution of the uterus by stimulating oxytocin. This occurs with skin-to-skin contact and with infant suckling [32]. In fact, external administration of oxytocin is the primary uterotonic drug recommended for the prevention of postpartum hemorrhage in cesarean sections [33]. Breastfeeding also promotes the length of postpartum amenorrhea that reduces fertility leading to increased birth intervals and supports the faster rebuilding of iron stores [34]. There is also evidence that metabolic changes are promoted by breastfeeding well beyond the actual period that breastfeeding takes place. Breastfeeding may decrease the risk of cardiovascular disease, high blood pressure and stroke [35]. Breastfeeding also significantly reduces the risk of type 2 diabetes, ovarian cancer and breast cancer [36].

The energy requirements for women during breastfeeding are greater than during pregnancy. While average energy needs for women during pregnancy peaks during the third trimester at about 1.95 Mj/day, the energy requirement for producing an average of 849 g of fullterm breast milk is 2.62 Mj/day [37]. Not meeting this significantly increased energy need can lead to a negative energy balance and weight loss. Repeated pregnancies and lactation in these conditions can lead to maternal depletion syndrome increasing the risk for poor maternal and infant health [38–40]. Although it is often stated that breastfeeding is associated with maternal weight loss after birth, this is difficult to measure over time and past studies are not conclusive. What does seem to be important when measuring the effect of breastfeeding on weight loss is the amount of gestational weight gain, breastfeeding duration beyond the first six months, the intensity of breastfeeding within a specific time frame and the dietary pattern of breastfeeding women [41, 42].

There are strong biological and psychological reasons supporting the concept that breastfeeding increases maternal–infant bonding due to the hormonal responses that are stimulated with nursing [43]. The presence of oxytocin in maternal and infant blood is also associated with decreased cortisol levels that may be the biological mechanism that supports increased social interaction, and decreased anxiety and blood pressure [32]. On the other hand, few rigorous epidemiological studies have been done on the role of breastfeeding and the mental health of mothers to determine the strength of this impact [44]. Future studies need to better account for self-selection, take into account when measures of bonding are collected and the length and intensity of breastfeeding.

Similarly, the role that breastfeeding has on postpartum depression is important to measure. Although it is clear that depression leads to shorter breastfeeding duration, especially exclusive breastfeeding, it has less of an effect on the intention to breastfeed [45, 46]. Additionally, in Goa India, having troubles with breastfeeding was twice as likely to occur in women with postnatal depression compared with those without depression [47]. This is very important to note given that the prevalence of postpartum depression has been reported to be greater in 22 of 28 low- and middle-income countries compared with high-income countries. The prevalence of post-depression was reported to be between 5 and 33% in 12 Asian countries and between 7 and 33% in 10 African countries [48] compared with a prevalence rates between 8.5 and 19% in high-income countries [49, 50]. These studies support the need for early screening and diagnosis of postpartum depression to not only improve the mother's mental health but also to have her continue to exclusively breastfeed her infant. Similarly, women who are having negative breastfeeding experiences may be at greater risk for developing depressive symptomatology [46]. On the other hand, recent studies suggest that breastfeeding has a strong psychoneuroimmunological role by decreasing stress and the release of cytokines that are related to decreasing depression. Specifically, exclusive breastfeeding may decrease depressive symptoms by improving sleep parameters compared with mixed and formula feeding based on measures of total minutes of sleep, minutes to get to sleep, slow-wave sleep, daytime fatigue and perceived physical health [51].

Infant Feeding After 12 Months

When studying the impact of long-term breastfeeding, i.e., into the second year of life, several factors need to be considered. These include the characteristic of lactation itself, physiological factors, bio-cultural factors, the health effects of breast milk on the child after one year of age, effect on the mother's health and environmental factors. As a mother continues to breastfeed into a child's second year of life, it is done with less frequency and duration as complementary foods become more and more a source of the child's nutrition. Nonetheless, breast milk does remain a rich source of nutrients and other immune promoting substances [10, 52]. During this period, breast milk has a greater concentration of immunologically active compounds such as lactoferrin, lysozyme, Immunoglobulin A and oligosaccharides [52, 53]. However, this may not be the case for some minerals, such as zinc and calcium [53].

Breastfeeding in the second year of life has been associated with decreased morbidity and mortality related to diarrhea. Not breastfeeding has been reported to increase the risk of diarrhea prevalence by 39%, and more than doubled the risk for diarrhea mortality and all-cause mortality for children 12–23 months of age [54]. Even when breastfeeding after one year of life was not associated with an increased weight and length, it was shown to significantly decrease mortality between 12 and 35 months of age [55].

Additional research is still needed to determine the effect of breastfeeding into the second year of life on the growth of children after 12 months of age. The primary issue with studies on the relationship between breastfeeding for longer than 12 months and infant growth has been the fact that these were observational studies that were unable to control breastfeeding choices which were hence not independent from women's health and social status. Studies that have found no effect or a negative effect of longer breastfeeding have been conducted among low-income women who also may not have had the knowledge or resources to properly provide adequate complementary food [56]. Additionally, the effect of breastfeeding on growth after one year is also more likely in environments that lack adequate water and sanitation [57]. Similarly, it is essential to understand the reasons why women stop breastfeeding early. Reverse causality in which women continue to breastfeed because their children are growing poorly may be one reason for associating poor growth with extended breastfeeding [58]. However, there are studies that have reported that extended breastfeeding was associated with greater length-for-age measures compared with weight-for-length when food resources are limited and the timing of appropriate complementary food was delayed [59]. The increased growth of breastfed children may be mediated through breast milk adiponectin that supports the regulation of glucose and fat metabolism [60].

Breastfeeding Initiation

Breastfeeding is an innate, learned and social activity that needs to be integrated into local food systems [61]. Although knowledge about the nutritional and maternal and child health benefits of breastfeeding is a major factor that contributes to breastfeeding, there are still reasons why women may not initiate breastfeeding or stop early. The most common breastfeeding problems that lead to maternal discomfort include breast engorgement, mastitis and sore nipples. One cause of these problems is breast thrush, caused by *candida albicans,* a fungal infection. These problems occur most often in primiparous women who have the least experience with breastfeeding and can be prevented and easily treated with early detection, counseling and treatment [62–65]. Additionally, mothers will often stop exclusive breastfeeding when they think their milk supply is not sufficient, which can be resolved by more frequent and longer breastfeeding sessions [66, 67].

Prelacteal feeding practices still exist, and although sugar solutions are the most common, butter, honey and milk are also given [68, 69]. These practices can lead to not initiating breastfeeding and to early cessation. Home delivered births were associated with prelacteal feeding in Ethiopia [69]. Similarly, mother's expectations and socioeconomic status were especially important along with tobacco use in Greece [70]. The information and support physicians, nurses and other healthcare professionals provide to women as well as their attitudes on breastfeeding are important factors to whether women initiate and continue breastfeeding and are able to manage any of the common discomforts such as mastitis and sour nipples [71, 72].

Kangaroo Method

An important method to promote successful breastfeeding and survival in low-birth weight infants is the Kangaroo method of care. The Kangaroo method is when a premature infant is held skin-to-skin with its mother for a long period of time to promote child development by providing thermal regulation and to enhance breastfeeding practices and maternal–infant bonding. Studies have not consistently reported the length of time babies are exposed to skin-to-skin contact with respect to specific outcomes. However, in Bangladesh it was reported that seven hours a day significantly decreased new born deaths for low-birth weight babies who remained hospitalized compared with infants who had minimal skin-to-skin contact [73]. The increased skin-to-skin contact was also associated with greater antenatal interaction between mothers and community health workers. The Kangaroo method is often incorporated into other clinical practices for infants who are low birth weight, including early hospital discharge for non-symptomatic infants, education on positioning infants in an upright position, breastfeeding support after hospital discharge and part of baby-friendly hospitals that are discussed later in this chapter.

The Kangaroo method was developed to support the growth and development of premature infants and initiated at the San Juan de Dios Hospital in Bogota, Colombia [74]. Venancio and de Almeida have provided a good history of its evolution and explained that its initial conception was for resource-poor areas given the many structural and technological limitations to providing neonatal intensive care [75]. Successful implementation of the Kangaroo method requires strong prenatal and postnatal support [73].

The incorporation of the Kangaroo method has also been shown to increase the duration of exclusive breastfeeding and total time a child is breastfed [76]. In a multicenter randomized trial in the USA, premature infants with an APGAR score greater than six who were exposed to the Kangaroo method with an average of four hours of skin-to-skin contact per day were nearly twice as likely to exclusively breastfeed at six weeks of age and five times more likely to exclusively breastfeed at three months of age as compared to infants with the same characteristics that were not exposed to the Kangaroo method [77].

There is good evidence that there is a strong association between the Kangaroo method and improved morbidity and mortality outcomes in low-income countries. The Kangaroo method provides for increased weight gain for premature infants and decreased risk for hospital acquired infections [78, 79]. Cost savings for reduced intermediate care in India has been observed when hospitals implement the Kangaroo method even when there was no difference in the mortality and morbidity for very low birth weight infants (<1500 g) [79]. The Kangaroo method has focused on stable preterm low and very low birth weight infants, and more information is needed about long-term costs and impact on less stable preterm infants [80].

Most studies on the Kangaroo method have focused on infant outcomes, and less information is known about maternal outcomes. An interesting case report suggested that a woman's mental health improved when she was instructed to provide breast milk with an emphasis on skin-to-skin contact [81]. Other studies have also shown improved psychological outcomes of stressed mothers of low-birth weight infants with skin-to-skin contact [78]. The adaptation of the Kangaroo method has also provided an added value to the bonding and health status for mothers and children in higher-income countries and within the confines of higher technology-based infant care units [75]. Additionally, data suggest that the Kangaroo method may help in preventing and managing post-partum depression [82].

An important supplement to the Kangaroo method can be to provide cup feeding to premature infants in lieu of bottle feeding within neonatal intensive care units. One week following discharge, 47% of infants in Egypt who were cup fed were being exclusively breastfed after discharge compared with 33% who had been bottle fed [83]. A greater percentage of preterm infants who were cup fed continued to be exclusively breastfed for six months (57%) compared with infants who were bottle fed (42%) in hospitals [84]. These results may be due to the need for less suckling effort with bottle feeding by the infant, which may reduce the ability to revert back to breastfeeding. Cup feeding also uses a very different technique and may not affect sucking ability.

Breastfeeding and the 2030 Agenda for Sustainable Development

The promotion of breastfeeding is an integral part of the 2030 Agenda for Sustainable Development [85, 86] and directly contributes to 9 of the 17 goals. Breastfeeding is environmentally sound as breast milk is a natural, renewable food that is produced and fed without packaging or waste. It plays a significant role in improving nutrition, education by increasing health and cognitive development, and maternal and child health and survival [28]. It also contributes to reduced inequalities, as it is one of the few positive health-related behaviors in low- and middle-income countries that are less frequent in higher-income people, both between and within countries. Breastfeeding decreases poverty as breastfed children have lower healthcare costs. Workplace policies that support breastfeeding benefit both employers and mothers as mothers miss less work because of child illness, and this outweighs the time that mothers require for breastfeeding or expressing breast milk while at work [23, 25, 63, 87].

Breastfeeding Trends

Global and Regional Trends

The WHO Global Data Bank on Infant and Young Child Feeding is a rich source on breastfeeding trends by country based on the most current countrywide surveys. Continual updates on breastfeeding rates are also available in the annual UNICEF report *The State of the World's Children*. The World Breastfeeding Trends Initiative (WBTi), coordinated by the International Baby Food Action Network (IBFAN), is an important source of data on the implementation of pro-breastfeeding policies and programs. When comparing information about breastfeeding rates, there are differences in the reported estimates mostly due to the number of countries included in the estimates, choice of indicators, method of analysis and the years used for the estimates.

Population measures of breastfeeding practices should focus on three broad domains that encompass the early initiation of breastfeeding, exclusive breastfeeding and the continuation of breastfeeding into the second year of life [2]. Monitoring breastfeeding rates within these domains should include (1) the proportion of infants who were put to the breast within one hour of birth, (2) the proportion of infants less than six months of age who were fed exclusively with breast milk and (3) the proportion of children 12–15 months of age who receive breast milk.

The World Health Assembly (WHA) has endorsed the goal to have at least 50% of infants being exclusively breastfed during their first six months of life by 2025. In 2016, it was estimated that only 37% of children less than six months of age in low- and middle-income countries were being given only breast milk in the previous 24 h (the definition of exclusive breastfeeding used in most surveys, see explanation of indicators above) [28]. This is a slight increase from the 27.9% estimate for 1990 [88]. According to the UNICEF's Infant and Young Child Feeding Database, the exclusive breast-feeding rates for low-income countries were 47% [89]. This translates to having very few countries that are currently meeting the goal set by the WHA (Fig. 16.1).

Global trends suggest that the percent of infants who are ever breastfed and those infants who are breastfed for six months and 12 months of age occurs at high rates in low- and middle-income countries but is lower for upper-middle- and upper-income countries. However, even in countries with high rates of breastfeeding, only about half the women initiate breastfeeding within an hour after birth and a lower percentage breastfeed exclusively until the child is 6 months of age. Breastfeeding into the second year of life is greatest for the low- and middle-income countries and infrequent in high-income countries [28]. In a review of 11 studies, the pooled prevalence for breastfeeding up to two years of age and beyond was 33% with a wide range among countries from 1% to greater than 90% [90].

In low- and middle-income countries, 63% of infants less than six months of age are not being exclusively breastfed, which means that they are receiving other liquids (including water) and/or

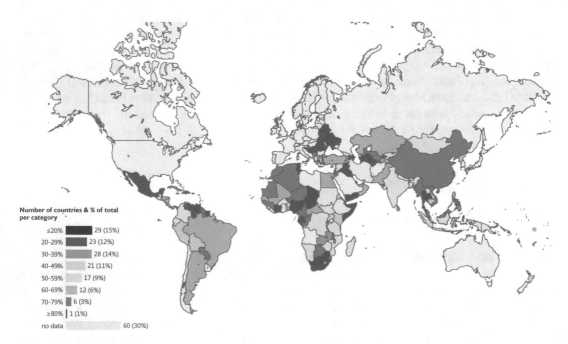

Fig. 16.1 Exclusive breastfeeding rates (<6 months) 2010–2015. Updated November 2015. Values from the data and analytics section; division of data, research and policy, UNICEF. Data Downloaded June 23, 2016 from http://data.unicef.org/nutrition/iycf.html. Map prepared by Ramon Martinez

foods [28]. While water, teas, juices and other liquids and milks are introduced first, semisolid foods follow soon after. Global data are not available on the percentage of children receiving different categories of liquids and foods. However, the Demographic and Health Surveys provide data for some low- and middle-income countries though for most countries recent surveys are not available. Data from surveys conducted since 2010 show varying trends. For example, among infants less than three months of age, formula use ranged from less than 1% in most African countries to more than 20% in Colombia and Peru. The percentages increased only slightly between four and six months. The use of other milks in African countries was more common among infants less than three months and between four and six months compared to Colombia and Peru though the percentages were still less than 10% in most countries. Bottle use was more prevalent in more countries, among infants between four and six months of age reaching more than 15% in Cameroon, Ethiopia, Gabon, Uganda, Armenia, Cambodia, Colombia and Peru. Global data are not available on complementary feeding practices, but the few data that are show that practices are far from optimal. Data from 46 low- and middle-income countries between 2002 and 2008 show that among children less than five years of age only half of children 6–24 months of age met the recommended minimum daily numbers of meals, less than one-third met the minimum criteria for daily dietary diversity and only one in five breastfed children satisfied the criteria for minimum acceptable diet [91].

With the exception of three high-income countries (France, Spain and the USA) where more than 20% of newborns do not initiate breastfeeding, in other countries less than 20% of newborns fall into this category and less than 10% in low-middle-income countries. Robust global data on the prevalence of prelacteal feeds and the use of pacifiers are not available.

Global sales of breast milk substitutes (including milk formula, for infants <6 months of age, follow-on milks and growing-up milks) is large and growing, currently estimated at US$ 44,800 million and projected to increase in 2019 to US$ 70,600 million [31]. Furthermore, growth appears to be recession proof; during the recent global recession sales continued to increase. The increase in milk formula is greatest in middle-income countries as the market is saturated in high-income countries. Indeed, projected growth in two countries, the USA and France is negative. In high-income countries, growth is due to increased sales of follow-on formulas and growing-up milks.

Breastfeeding is one of the few health-related behaviors where practices are better in low- and middle-income countries and among low-income women compared to high-income countries [28]. The most common proximal reason reported by mothers for introducing other liquids and foods is "insufficient milk." Other common reasons include advice from a health professional and employment.

The data in the preceding paragraphs indicate that priority efforts should focus on promoting exclusive breastfeeding and after six months improving the complementary feeding diet by promoting nutrient-dense foods such as eggs and other animal source foods.

Suboptimal breastfeeding practices, including non-exclusive breastfeeding, contribute to the death of children less than 5 years of age [92]. Estimates conducted in 2015 suggest that 823,000 child deaths and 20,000 women deaths from breast cancer could be prevented each year if 95% of all infants younger than 6 months would be exclusively breastfed [28].

There is evidence from Sri Lanka, Cambodia and Malawi that it is possible to increase exclusive breastfeeding rates [93–95]. Knowledge about the importance of exclusive breastfeeding in rural Indonesia was an important determinant for exclusive breastfeeding for 6 months [95]. Early cessation of exclusive breastfeeding occurred more often when formula was provided to infants in hospitals, and when there was a lack of family support [95]. Furthermore, cessation of exclusive breastfeeding before 4 months of age was reported to be due to concerns about inadequate weight gain and after 4 months was associated with returning to work [93]. Greater breastfeeding knowledge was also important but was negated by unsupportive family members [95]. Both the USA and Canada have made significant improvements in breastfeeding promotion by focusing on the healthcare system using baby-friendly hospitals [96]. All countries, including high-income countries, need to improve their exclusive breastfeeding rates [97, 98].

There is also a potential paradox when breastfeeding rates change. Although, breastfeeding rates can increase in a country, a report from Cambodia indicates that even with increasing rates of exclusive breastfeeding, during the same interval the percent of children six to 24 months of age receiving infant formula increased. The greatest increase occurred among children born in private clinics and the urban poor [99]. Also, in Nigeria, a greater initiation of exclusive breastfeeding was associated with supportive hospital practices and higher maternal education. However, while wealth was associated with a higher rate of exclusive breastfeeding, it was also associated with an increased use of infant formula [100]. Similarly, the correlation between the various population-level metrics of exclusive and continued breastfeeding was shown to be of moderate strength and varied by region [28]. Understanding the dynamics of various social, economic, governmental and industrial pressures on these rates is important in order to develop effective breastfeeding promotion programs and to support appropriate infant feeding practices.

Community and Global Issues Affecting Breastfeeding

The direction for how socioeconomic factors are associated with breastfeeding practices is site-specific and based on the economic status and the culture of a population. Additionally, taking a human rights approach to breastfeeding may at times put the right of the mother and the right of a child at odds [101, 102]. Several countries also have criminalized HIV transmission and in high-income countries, a HIV-positive mother's right to breastfeed has been questioned by courts based on having complete access to the conditions required for safely providing formula to her infant [103, 104]. Alternatively, scaling up the implementation of WHO recommendation to prevent mother-to-child HIV transmission, including exclusive breastfeeding, appropriate introduction of complementary foods and the use of ARVs have been shown to consistently reduce new childhood HIV cases [105].

Socioeconomic factors also contribute to breastfeeding rates. In high-income countries, women with higher education, economic status and maternal age are more likely to breastfeed [106]. In contrast, in low-income countries, mothers from households with greater wealth were more likely to delay the initiation of breastfeeding and have a shorter duration of exclusive breastfeeding [107].

Maternal use of pacifiers has also been studied as a factor related to breastfeeding cessation. In a randomized study that reported no effect of prenatal counseling on pacifier use, twice as many women who used a pacifier everyday had stopped breastfeeding by 3 months of age compared with those women who received the education on alternatives to pacifiers [108]. It is possible that pacifier use may have led to less milk production or was a marker for distancing of the mother from her child, an act that is a precursor to the cessation of breastfeeding. Australian breastfed babies also had a greater odds of receiving formula from hospital staff if they perceived that their mother was less likely to continue breastfeeding, including being a primiparous mother, non-English speaking, a mother with a BMI > 30, having a birth by cesarean section, having a child admitted to high-risk unit and being born with a birth weight less than 2500 g [109].

Prior to the advent of the WHO growth charts that are now based on breastfed infants, recommendations on when to introduce complementary feeding may have occurred prematurely by many clinicians. This occurred when breastfed children appeared to fall off the growth curve at around four months of age, decreasing their weight-for-age percentiles because growth curves based on formula-fed infants were used. The WHO growth charts now provide clinicians with information that indicates that the average weight of breastfed infants increases greater in the first few months of life and then more slowly afterward. Thus, the new growth charts allow clinicians and parents to better compare the appropriate growth of breastfed children.

The breastfeeding practices of HIV-positive mothers have also been affected ever since it was known that the HIV virus could pass through breast milk. The primary factors related to mother-to-child transmission of HIV (MTCT) are the health and viral load of the mother and how well her HIV status is being controlled with antiretroviral (ARVs) medication [110]. HIV-positive women who do breastfeed should be provided counseling on breastfeeding methods that decrease the risk of transmission and be able to identify signs of mastitis, breast abscesses and nipple fissures so they may be promptly treated. Exclusive breastfeeding is critical for HIV-positive mothers as this decreases the risk for transmission to her child, especially during the first 2 to 4 months of life [105, 111]. Furthermore, an HIV-positive mother without access to ARVs who decides to breastfeed should be provided information on how to discontinue as soon as possible based on having access to appropriate replacement feedings and local conditions.

Breastfeeding Protection, Promotion and Support

The socioecological model to assess the social determinants of breastfeeding can be used to determine what factors need to be addressed to have a comprehensive approach to breastfeeding promotion (Fig. 16.2). It is increasingly recognized that in addition to providing women with information and counseling, regarding breastfeeding, it is imperative to improve public policies and support systems that are most proximal to their lives. Women live and work within many different organizational structures that can support or provide barriers to breastfeeding infants. Similarly, community norms and public policies can modify the physical and social environment so breastfeeding can be practiced and become a social norm. For example, maternity leave policies can greatly affect breastfeeding rates [112]. In the USA, the length of maternity leave is 12 weeks, if certain conditions are met, but there is no national program to continue a women's salary during this time, while Germany provides 14 months of maternity leave and mothers are able to receive 65% of the wages. Other countries such as Malta, New Zealand, Slovenia, Austria, France, Spain, the Netherlands, Denmark and Russia provide 100% of wages during maternity leave the length of which varies among these countries [113].

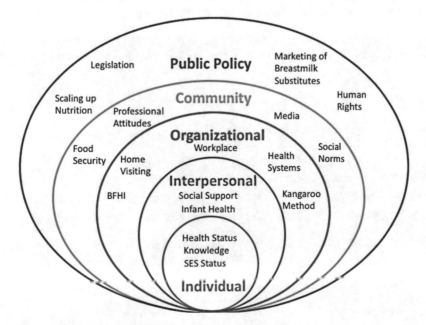

Fig. 16.2 Socioecological model and social determinants of breastfeeding

Policies and Guidelines

The protection, promotion and support of breastfeeding need to occur both within and outside the healthcare systems [11]. WHO and UNICEF support countries to implement the priority actions outlined in the *Global Strategy for Infant and Young Child Feeding* [3]. The focus is on five major areas: national level, health systems level, community level, through communication and advocacy, and during difficult circumstances. The messages and programs that are directed at each of these levels need to be coordinated for the best outcomes [114].

The penetration of breastfeeding promotion tends to be less driven by the socioeconomic status of families in a community compared with other interventions. Data from 54 countries indicated that various efforts to increase the early initiation of breastfeeding appeared to only cover 46% of the target population. This was the third lowest coverage for an intervention among 12 other maternal and child health intervention. Only the number of children who had access to insecticide-treated bed nets (15.4%) and access to oral rehydration therapy (40.1%) had lower coverage [115].

Increases in breastfeeding rates are associated with national policies with the greatest improvements occurring in countries with the lowest initial rates [116]. An analysis from the World Breastfeeding Trends Initiative (WBTi) on national policy and programs to promote breastfeeding supports the concept that there has been a greater impact on increasing the initiation and duration of breastfeeding compared with the duration of exclusive breastfeeding [117]. Implementing the *International Code of Marketing of Breast Milk Substitutes* [1] and providing maternity protection legislation are national policies that have supported an improvement in breastfeeding practices [118, 119]. The Code includes 11 articles starting with the aim, scope and definitions that make up the Code. The next articles provide information about practices that should be maintained by manufacturers and distributors of breast milk substitutes, including what type of information and education should be provided about breast feeding and breast milk substitutes, policies and programs for healthcare systems, professional ethics, and labeling of breast milk substitutes. Additional articles address issues regarding the quality of breast milk substitute products and on requirements regarding the implementation and monitoring of the Code. It is also essential that healthcare systems prevent unscrupulous promotion of breast milk substitutes in any form, including giving out free formula, and formula needs to be properly labeled to state that breast milk is the best source for normal infant feeding [1].

Policies and Practices Regarding the Marketing of Breast Milk Substitutes

Article 4: Information and Education

All information and educational materials should include information on:

(a) Benefits and superiority of breast-feeding.
(b) Maternal nutrition and preparation for breast-feeding.
(c) Negative effect of introducing partial bottle-feeding.
(d) Difficulty of reversing the decision not to breast-feed.
(e) Where needed, proper use of infant formula.

Donations of informational or educational equipment of materials by manufacturers:

(a) Only be given upon request and with written approval by appropriate government authority.
(b) Only distributed through the health system without reference to proprietary products.

Article 5: The General Public and Mothers

(a) No advertising or promotion to the general public of products.
(b) No distribution of product directly or indirectly to pregnant women, or family members.

(c) No point-of-sale advertising or inducements to promote sales of product.

(d) Manufacturers and distributors should not distribute any gifts of articles or utensils to mothers and/or mothers of infants to promote the use of breast milk substitutes or bottle-feeding.

(e) Marketing personnel should not come in direct or indirect contact with pregnant women or mothers of infants and young children.

Article 6: Health Care Systems

(a) Member States should take appropriate measures to encourage and protect breast-feeding.

(b) The healthcare system should not be used to promote infant formula.

(c) Healthcare facilities should not display or promote or distribute materials to promote product.

(d) No healthcare staff should be provided by or paid by manufacturers.

(e) No donations or low-price sales to institutions or organizations of formula should be made except for infants who have to be fed breast milk substitutes.

(f) When donations are made enough needs to be provided to ensure infants have access for as long as needed and should only bear the name of the company but not the product.

Article 7: Health Workers

(a) Health workers should encourage and protect breast-feeding.

(b) Information provided by manufactures to health workers should be restructured to scientific and factual matters.

(c) No financial or material inducements should be given to health workers by manufacturers.

(d) Health workers should not give samples of infant formula to pregnant women, mothers of infants and young children or their family members.

(e) Manufacturers should disclose health workers who have received any benefits from them.

Article 8: Persons Employed by Manufacturers and Distributors

(a) Amount of sales should not be part of bonuses or quotas for distributors.

(b) Employees should not provide any education to pregnant women or mothers of infants and young children.

Article 9: Labelling

(a) Labels should not be designed to discourage breast-feeding.

(b) Label should address the superiority of beast-feeding and instructions on proper use of formula.

(c) No pictures of infants should be on containers or labels.

(d) Other infant feeding products should also meet all the requirements of the code.

Monitoring the marketing of breast milk substitutes can take on many forms, and interventions to stop inappropriate marketing of breast milk substitutes can help meet the global standards for breastfeeding. At the same time, information needs to be given to women who cannot or choose not to breastfeed on when it may be appropriate to use formula, how to properly prepare formula and how to know how much formula to provide an infant based on hunger cues from the child, its age and weight. Situations where this applies include for example when there has been a maternal death, severe illness or when a woman needs to return to work and her employer does not have policies or programs in place that support breastfeeding. Furthermore, as previously stated, it is important to support the infant feeding choice of women based on their rights to care for their children. Supporting women who have difficulty breastfeeding is important to prevent feelings of inadequacy and depression from not breastfeeding that can arise from their own sense of failure and that from society. This positive approach to breastfeeding and infant feeding may actually help improve breastfeeding rates due to decreased stress on women to successfully breastfeed.

Promotion Programs

Hospitals can have a special role as institutions for promoting and supporting the initiation of breastfeeding. Leaving the hospital while exclusively breastfeeding is an important marker as to who will stop breastfeeding early [120]. There are many ways to promote breastfeeding within clinical settings.

The Baby-Friendly Hospital Initiative (BFHI) initiated by the WHO and UNICEF in 1991 following the *Innocenti Declaration* of 1990 [121] is recognized as the foundation for how healthcare systems should support breastfeeding. The BFHI was updated and revised in 2009 and provides curricula, training and support of health workers and health information systems [122]. The BFHI is now being promoted to be a standard component of Integrated Care [123]. An international group from Northern Europe and Canada has recommended an expansion of the BFHI to provide more focus to the neonatal unit [123]. The 10 steps required to fulfill the BFHI are provided below.

Steps for Baby-Friendly Hospital Initiative

1. Have a written breastfeeding policy that is routinely communicated to all healthcare staff.
2. Train all healthcare staff in skills necessary to implement this policy.
3. Inform all pregnant women about the benefits and management of breastfeeding.
4. Help mothers initiate breastfeeding within one half-hour of birth.
5. Show mothers how to breastfeed and maintain lactation, even if they should be separated from their infants.
6. Give newborn infants no food or drink other than breast milk, unless medically indicated.
7. Practice rooming in—that is, allow mothers and infants to remain together 24 h a day.
8. Encourage breastfeeding on demand.
9. Give no artificial teats or pacifiers (also called dummies or soothers) to breastfeeding infants.
10. Foster the establishment of breastfeeding support groups and refer mothers to them on discharge from the hospital or clinic.

Baby-friendly hospitals (BFHs) that have initiated these steps support early production of breast milk and decreases in the initial weight loss of new born infants. In particular, BFHs have obtained these results with policies that support having mothers rooming in with their infants, start breastfeeding within 30 min after birth, feeding on demand, and having more control and comfort with taking care of their infant [124]. BFHs have also been shown to increase rates of exclusive breastfeeding, to reduce the incidence of gastrointestinal disease and atopic eczema during the first year of life, and to improve children's IQ and academic performance [125]. A randomized trial in Brazil indicated that baby-friendly hospital practices increased the duration of exclusive breastfeeding with significant differences occurring as early as one month after birth and continued to be different for infants who were 12 months of age [126]. Additionally, this increase was greater for more underprivileged families compared with families with greater economic status [127, 128]. BFHs increased exclusive breastfeeding by 0.5 months and any breastfeeding by one month after controlling for maternal age, education and occupation [106]. BFHs can continue to impact breastfeeding rates up to 6 months of age [129]. A Russian studied reported that BFHs not only increased exclusive breastfeeding in hospitals but also was associated with an increase in the percent of infants who were breastfed for 6–12 months in the surrounding area [124].

There is evidence that the BFHI supports breastfeeding also for low-birth weight infants [130]. BFHs can even increase breastfeeding metrics when they don't completely sustain implementation of all 10 steps at a high level [131]. BFHs have increased initiation of breastfeeding rates even when formula is provided in-hospital. However, studies that measure the impact of the BFHI must take into account the initial breastfeeding rates. When the rate for the initiation of breastfeeding rates are high (>90%) as in a study from Queensland, possibly due to preexisting cultural norms toward breastfeeding, initiating and promoting new hospital individual practices directly related to breastfeeding such as rooming in, breastfeeding within the first hour after birth and skin-to-skin contact, no hospital supplementation may have little effect in terms of further increasing already high initial breastfeeding rates [132]. However, when women were exposed to all four components they were nearly three times more likely to continue to breastfeed for four months compared with women exposed to fewer support practices.

The BFHI can also provide other clinical support such as additional prenatal visits, daily in-hospital breastfeeding support and postpartum home visits during the first year of life [133]. Interestingly, there is evidence that BFHs have also been associated with decreased cesarean section rates [134].

Although there have been numerous gains in creating BFHs, poor clinical feeding practices still occur that decrease breastfeeding outcomes. Two major factors are cesarean sections and in-hospital feedings of glucose water, which are important barriers to breastfeeding initiation [135, 136]. Thus, even when BFH are started, continual training is needed to keep up with regular staff turnover [137] and a process for recertification every three to five years needs to be established.

Other methods to support breastfeeding and providing breast milk to infants include wet nurses and milk banks. These methods came under scrutiny with the onset of HIV and the knowledge that it could be transmitted through breast milk. However, with new methods for testing multiple compounds in breast milk including hepatitis and HIV, and with the pasteurization of milk, milk banks are once again becoming a reliable source for providing breast milk to infants. In Brasil, there are a total of 336 milk bank centers of which 123 collect human breast milk and 213 store breast milk within the Brazilian Human Milk Banks Network [138]. Pasteurized breast milk from donors has been shown to decrease necrotizing enterocolitis but may not promote increased short-term growth due to its decreasing effect on the activity of growth promoting hormones such as adiponectin and insulin even while nutritional components such as glucose, fatty acids and some vitamins are preserved [139, 140].

How breastfeeding can be supported in the presence of provision of free supplemental formula has been controversial for the United States Special Supplemental Nutrition Program for Women Infants and Children (WIC). Over the 30-year history of the WIC program, various rules and guidelines have increased the use of lactation consultants and food packages for increasing breastfeeding rates and duration. However, the relative results have had a limited impact on increasing breastfeeding rates for these low-income women. The breastfeeding start rate for WIC women was 26.7% in 2010 and only increased to 29.5% in 2013 [141, 142]. These rates remain well below the national estimate of 76.5% breastfeeding start rate for newborn infants in 2013 [143]. These outcomes may not be surprising given a large proportion of women only received one nutrition education session between their first postpartum visit and their six-month follow-up visit and less than half receive two nutrition education contacts during the same six-month period [144]. Furthermore, WIC investment for nutrition education on breastfeeding promotion was less than $350 million compared with $920 million on expenditures for formula in 2010 [145]. Thus, the provision of free formula may outweigh the impact that lactation consultants or an individual breastfeeding promotion program can have on breastfeeding rates for low-income women who are young, lack role models, lack formal and informal supports for breastfeeding or need to return to work [146, 147]. What has appeared to increase breastfeeding rates among WIC participants has been an increase in the amount food and fresh food provided to breastfeeding women [148].

Breastfeeding support also needs to include personalized messages. These messages should be given to the mothers and to her support groups including other family members. Successful breast-feeding includes the presence of support groups that can be developed formally or informally [149]. A home visiting program with community health workers in Nairobi has successfully promoted breastfeeding [150]. Home visits have also been an important method to increase exclusive breast-feeding in high-income countries [151]. Home visiting and the inclusion of peer counselors has also improved the six-month exclusive breastfeeding rate in a randomized multi-country trial that took place in Burkino Faso, Uganda and South Africa [152]. A dose response with the number of home visits also increased exclusive breastfeeding rates in South Africa among women living with HIV [153]. The effect of this program also led to an increased likelihood of participating in additional healthy behaviors such as the use of condoms and growth monitoring. Internet messages have also been successful with increasing breastfeeding rates in high-income countries when they have be been part of a comprehensive approach to breastfeeding promotion [154]. Interestingly, in higher-income countries, phone follow-up may not be very effective for the long-term breastfeeding rates compared with face-to-face programs suggesting the importance of personal approaches to breastfeeding sup-port [155].

Summary

Studies on the social determinants for initiating and continuing breastfeeding have shown com-monalities and differences based on the populations studied. As breastfeeding is related to nine of the 17 goals Sustainable Development Goals (below) for the 2030 Agenda for Sustainable Development, scaling up breastfeeding policies and programs will require increased efforts in advocacy, political will, legislation, research and evaluation [86]. Creating an appropriate policy framework will require reviewing existing national and local breastfeeding policies, and to garner the resources for technical support, program design and strategies to deliver breastfeeding programs [156]. The use of proper communication channels, people and media to develop messages that target specific populations will need to be implemented [157]. The inclusion of training programs for all health professionals, promotion campaigns that are coordinated and the monitoring and evaluation of these programs should use consistent metrics to compare outcomes to better determine how to disseminate best practices.

Nine Sustainable Development Goals Affected by Breastfeeding

1. No Poverty: End Poverty in all its forms everywhere
2. No Hunger: End hunger, achieve food security and improved nutrition and promote sus-tainable agriculture
3. Good Health and Well-Being: Ensure healthy lives and promote well-being for all at all ages.
4. Gender Equity: Achieve gender equality and empower all women and girls.
5. Clean Water and Sanitation: Ensure availability and sustainable management of water and sanitation for all.
6. Decent Work and Economic Growth: Promote sustain, inclusive and sustainable economic growth, full and productive employment and decent work for all.
7. Reduce Inequalities: Reduce inequality within and among countries.

8. Responsible Consumption and Production: Ensure sustainable consumption and production patterns.
9. Partnerships for the Goals: Strengthen the means of implementation and revitalize the global partnerships for sustainable development.

Discussion Points

- What approaches can be taken to increase breastfeeding rates?
- What do you believe are the strengths and weaknesses with the 10 steps that are part of the baby-friendly hospital initiative (BFHI) ? Is there any particular component of the BHFI that you believe would be more difficult to implement and why?
- Compare how different breastfeeding metrics should be used to evaluate breastfeeding promotion policies and programs.
- How have international goals, targets and statements related to breastfeeding practices effected the promotion of breastfeeding?
- What additional information is needed to improve breastfeeding practices in different contexts?

References

1. WHO. International Code of Marketing of Breast-Milk Substitutes. Geneva, Switzerland World Health Organization; 1981.
2. WHO. Indicators for assessing infant and young children feeding practices. Part 1 Definitions. Geneva, Switzerland: World Health Organization; 2010.
3. WHO, UNICEF. Global Strategy for Infant and Young Child Feeding Geneva: 2003.
4. WHO, UNICEF, UNFPA, UNAIDS. Guidelines on HIV and infant feeding. 2010. Principles and recommendations for infant feeding in the context of HIV and a summary of evidence. 2010.
5. UNICEF. Breastfeeding on the worldwide agenda. New York, NY; 2013.
6. Binns CW, Fraser ML, Lee AH, Scott J. Defining exclusive breastfeeding in Australia. J Peadiatr Child Health. 2009;45:174–80.
7. WHO. Indicators for assessing infant and young children feeding practices. Part 2 Indicators. Geneva, Switzerland: World Health Organization; 2010.
8. Joshi SK, Barakoti B, Lamsal S. Colostrum feeding: knowledge, attitude and practice in pregnant women in a teaching hospital in Nepal. WebmedCentral MEDICAL EDUCATION. 2012;3(8).
9. Sabharwal V. Myths and beliefs surrounding complementary feeding practices of infants in India. J Commun Nutr Health. 2014;3(1):34–8.
10. Ballard A, Morrow AL. Human milk consumption. Nutrents and bioactive factors. Pediatr Clin N Am. 2013;60:49–74.
11. Hassiotou F, Filguerira L, Hepworth A, Trengove N, Lai CT, Hartmann P. Coordinated response of the fat and cellular content of breastmilk to the degree of fullness of the breast. FASEB J. 2012;26(390):2.
12. Khan S, Hepworth AR, Prime DK, Lai CT, Trengove NJ, PE H. Variation in fat, lactose, and protein composition in breastmilk over 24 hours: associations with infant feeding patterns. J Human Lactation. 2013;29(1):81–9.
13. Tudehope DI. Human milk and the nutritional needs of preterm infants. J Pediatr. 2013;162(3):S17–25.
14. Baker RD, Greer FR. Nutrition TCo. Clinical report—diagnosis and prevention of iron deficiency and iron-deficiency anemia in infants and young children (0–3 years of age). Pediatrics. 2010;126:1040–50.
15. Taren DL, Kaminsky RG, Alger J, Mourra M, Mhasker R, Canfield LM. Comparing local fruits and vegetables and b-carotene supplements as a vitamin A source for Honduran mothers and infants. In: Bjornson LHAT, editor. Beta Carotene: dietary sources, cancer and cognition. New York: Nova Publishers; 2009.
16. Canfield L, Taren DL, deKaminsky R, Mahel Z. Short-term ß-carotene supplementation of lactating mothers consuming diets low in vitamin A. J Nutr Biochem. 1999;10:532–8.

17. Oliveira-Menegozzo JM, Bergamaschi DP, Middleton P, East CE. Vitamin A supplementation for postpartum women. Cochrane Database of Systematic Reviews. 2010(10).
18. Hampel D, Allen LH. Analyzing B-vitamins in human milk: methodological approaches. Critical Rev Food Sci Nutr. 2015.
19. Siddiqua TJ, Ahmad SM, Ahsan KB, Rashid M, Roy A, Rahman SM, et al. Vitamin B12 supplementation during pregnancy and postpartum improves B12 status of both mothers and infants but vaccine response in mothers only: a randomized clinical trial in Bangladesh. Eur J Nutr. 2016;55(1):281–93.
20. Allen LH. B vitamins in breast milk: relative importance of maternal status and intake, and effects on infant status and function. Adv Nutr. 2012;3:362–9.
21. Horta B, Loret de Mola C, Victora C. Long-term consequences of breastfeeding on cholesterol, obesity, systolic blood pressure and type 2 diabetes: a systematic review and meta-analysis. 2015;14(supplement @467):30–37.
22. Giugliani EJ, Horta BL, de Mola CL, Lisboa BO, Victora CG. Effect of breastfeeding promotion interventions on child growth: a systematic review and meta-analysis. Acta Paediatr. 2015;104:20–9.
23. Horta BL, Victora CG. Long-term effects of breastfeeding. A systematic review. Long-term effects of breastfeeding a systematic review. Geneva, Switzerland: World Health Organization; 2013.
24. Amitay EL, Keinan-Boker L. Breastfeeding and childhood leukemia incidence: a meta-analysis and systematic review. JAMA Pediatr. 2015;169:9.
25. Horta BL, Victora CG. Short-term effects of breastfeeding. A systematic review on the benefits of breastfeeding and diarrhoea and pneumonia mortality. In: Organization WH, editor. Geneva, Switzerland; 2013.
26. Bowatte G, Tham R, Allen KJ, Tan DJ, Lau MXZ, Dai X, et al. Breastfeeding and childhood acute otitis media: a systematic review and meta-analysis. Acta Paediatrica. 2015;104 (85–95).
27. Tham R, Bowatte G, Dharmage SC, Tan DJ, Lau MX, Dai X, et al. Breastfeeding and the risk of dental caries: a systematic review and meta-analysis. Acta Paediatr. 2015;104:62–84.
28. Victora CG, Bahl R, Barros AJD, Franca GVA, Horton S, Krasevec J, et al. Breastfeeding in the 21st century: epidemiology, mechanisms, and lifelong effect. Lancet. 2016;387:475–900.
29. Victora CG, Horta BL, Loret de Mola C, Quevedo L, Pinheiro RT, Gigante DP, et al. Association between breastfeeding and intelligence, educational attainment, and income at 30 years of age: a prospective birth cohort study from Brazil. Lancet Global Health. 2015;3:e199–205.
30. Hanushek EA, Woessmann L. The role of cognitive skills in economic development. J Econ Lit. 2008;46:607–68.
31. Rollins NC, Bhandari N, Hajeebhoy N, Horton S, Lutter CK, Martines JC, et al. Why invest, and what it will take to improve breastfeeding practices? Lancet. 2016;387:491–504.
32. Moberg KU, Prime DK. Oxytocin effects in mothers and infants during breastfeeding Infant. 2013;9(6):201–6.
33. WHO. WHO recommendations for the prevention and treatment of postpartum heamorrhage. Italy: World Health Organization, 2012.
34. Lupton SJ, Shlu CL, Lujic S, Hennessy A, Lind JM. Association between parity and breastfeeding with maternal high blood pressure. American Journal of Obstetrics and Gynecology. 2013;208:454.e1-7.
35. Dieterich CM, Felice JP, O'Sullivan E, Rasmussen KM. Breastfeeding and health outcomes for the mother-infant dyad. Pediatr Clin N Am. 2013;60:31–48.
36. Chowdhury R, Sinha B, Sankar MJ, Taneja S, Bhandari N, Rollins N, et al. Breastfeeding and maternal health outcomes: a systematic review and meta-analysis. Acta Paediatr. 2015;104:96–113.
37. Butte NF, King JC. Energy requirements during pregnancy and lactation. Public Health Nutrition. 2005;8 (7A):1010–27.
38. Kozuki N, Lee ACC, Silveira MF, Victora CG, Adair L, Humphrey J, et al. The associations of birth intervals with small-for-gestational-age, preterm and neonatal and infant mortality: a meta analysis. BMC Public Health. 2013;13((Suppl 3)):9.
39. Winkvist A, Rasmussen KM, Habicht JP. A new definition of maternal depletion syndrome. American Journal Of Public Health. 1992;82(691-694).
40. Wendt A, Gibbs C, Peters S, Hogue CJ. Impact of increasing inter-pregnancy interval on maternal and infant health. Paediatr Perinat Epidemiol. 2012;26(Suppl 1):239–58.
41. Martin RM, Patel R, Kramer MS, Vilchuck K, Bogdanovich N, Sergeichick N, et al. Effects of promoting longer-term and exclusive breastfeeding on cardiometabolic risk factors at age 11.5 years: a cluster-randomized, controlled trial. Circulation. 2014;129(3):321–9.
42. Neville CE, McKinley MC, Holmes VA, Spence D, Woodside JV. The relationship between breastfeeding and postpartum weight change - a systematic review and critical evaluation. International Journal of Obesity. 2014;38:577–90.
43. Kim P, Feldman R, Mayes LC, Eicher V, Thompson N, Leckman JF, et al. Breastfeeding, brain activation to own infant cry, and maternal sensitivity. J Child Psychol Psychiatry. 2011;52(8):907–15.
44. Jansen J, de Weerth C, Riksen-Walraven JM. Breastfeeding and the mother-infant relationship - a review. Dev Rev. 2008;28:503–21.

45. Nishioka E, Haruna M, Ota E, Matsuzaki M, Murayama R, Yoshimura K, et al. A prospective study of the relationship between breastfeeding and postpartum depressive symptoms appearing at 1-5 months after delivery. J Affect Disord. 2011;1330:533–59.

46. Dias CC, Figueiredo B. Breastfeeding and depression: a systematic review of the literature. J Affect Disord. 2015;171:142–54.

47. Patel V, Rodrigues M, DeSouza N. Gender, poverty and postnatal depression: a study of mothers in Goa. India. American Journal of Psychiatry. 2002;159(1):43–7.

48. Parsons CE, Young KS, Rochat TJ, Kringelbach ML, Stein A. Postnatal depression and its effects on child development: a review of evidence from low- and middle-income countries. Br Med Bull. 2012;101:57–79.

49. Lanes A, Kuk JL, Tamim H. Prevalence and characteristics of Postpartum Depression symptomatology among Canadian women: a cross-sectional study. BMC Public Health. 2011;11.

50. Underwood L, Waldie K, D'Souza S, Peterson ER, Morton S. A Review of Longitudinal Studies on Antenatal and Postnatal Depression. Archives of Women's Mental Health. 2016:10.

51. Kendall-Tackett K. The new paradigm for depression in new mothers: current findings on maternal depression, breastfeeding and resiliency across the lifespan. Breastfeed Rev. 2015;23(1):7–10.

52. Perrin MT, Fogleman A, Allen JC. The nutritive and immunoprotective quality of human milk beyond 1 year. Postpartum: Are lactation-duration-based donor exclusions justified. Journal of Human Lactation. 2013;29 (3):341–9.

53. Perrin MT, Fogleman AD, Newburg DS, Allen JC. A longitudinal study of human milk composition in the second year postpartum: implications for human milk banking. Maternal and Child Nutrition. 2016.

54. Lamberti LM, Walker CLF, Noiman A, Victora CG, Black RE. Breastfeeding and the risk for diarrhea morbidity and mortality. BMC Public Health. 2011;11(Suppl 3):15.

55. Briend A, Bari A. Breastfeeding improves survival, but not nutritional status of 12-35 month old children in rural Bangladesh. Eur J Clin Nutr. 1989;43(9):603–8.

56. Kramer MS, Guo T, Platt RW, Shapiro S, Collet JP, Chalmers B, et al. Breastfeeding and infant growth: biology or bias? Pediatrics. 2002;110(2 Pt 1):343–7.

57. Onyango A, Esrey SA, Kramer MS. Continued breastfeeding and child growth in the second year of life: a prospective cohort study in we stern Ke nya. Lancet. 1999;354:2041–5.

58. Marquis GC, Habicht JP, Lanata CF, Black RE, Rasmusen KM. Association of breastfeeding and stunting in Peruvian toddlers: An example of reverse causality. Int J Epidemiol. 1997;26(2):349–56.

59. Taren DL, Chen J. A Positive Association Between Extended Breast-feeding and Growth in Rural Hubei Province. PRC. American Journal of Clinical Nutrition. 1993;58:862–7.

60. Woo JG, Guerrero ML, Guo F, Martin L, Davidson BS, Ortega H, et al. Human milk adiponectin impacts infant weight trajectory during the second year of life. Journal of Pediatric Gastroenterol Nutr. 2012;54(4):532–9.

61. Frank L. Exploring Infant Feeding Practices In Food Insecure Households: What Is The Real Issue? Food and Foodways. 2015;23(3):186–209.

62. Dixon JM, Khan LR. Treatment of breast infection. British Medical Journal. 2011;342.

63. Dyson L, Renfrew MJ, McFadden A, McCormick F, Herbert G, Thomas J. Policy and public health recommendations to promote the initiation and duration of breast-feeding in developed country settings. Public Health Nutrition. 2009;13(1):137–44.

64. Mangesi L, Dowswell T. Treatments for breast engorgement during lactation. Cochrane Database of Systematic Reviews. 2010.

65. Nkala TE, Msuya SE. Prevalence and predictors of exclusive breastfeeding among women in Kigoma region, Western Tanzania: a community based cross-sectional study. International Breastfeeding Journal. 2011;6:7.

66. Lou Z, Zeng G, Huang L, Wang Y, Zhou L, Kavanagh KF. Maternal reported indicators and causes of insufficient milk supply. Journal of Human Lactation. 2014;30(4):466–73.

67. Kent JC, Prime DK, Garbin CP. Principles for Maintaining or Increasing Breast Milk Production. Journal of Obstetric, Gynecology and Neonatal Nursing. 2012;41(1):114–21.

68. Patil CL, Turab A, Ambikapathi R, Nesamvuni C, Chandyo RK, Bose A, et al. Early interruption of exclusive breastfeeding results from the eight-country MAL-ED study. Journal of Health, Population, and Nutrition. 2015;34:10.

69. Legesse M, Demena M, Mesfin F, Haile D. Prelacteal feeding practices and associated factors among mothers of children aged less than 24 months in Raya Kobo district, North Eastern Ethiopia: a cross-sectional study. International Breastfeeding Journal. 2014;9:8.

70. Bouras G, Mexi-Bourna P, Bournas N, Christodoulou C, Daskalaki A, Tasiopoulou I, et al. Mothers' expectations and other factors affecting breastfeeding at six months in Greece. Journal of Child Health Care. 2013;17(4):387–96.

71. Damis E, Gucciardo L, Berrefas L, Goyens P. Breastfeeding: from physiology to practical aspects. Rev Med Brux. 2012;33(4):318–27.

72. Cross-Barnet C. M. A, Gross S, Resnik A, Paige D. Long-term breastfeeding support: failing mothers in need. Matern Child Health J. 2012;16(9):1926–32.
73. Ahmed S, Mitra SN, Chowdhury AM, Camacho LL, Winikoff B, Sloan NL. Community Kangaroo Mother Care: implementation and potential for neonatal survival and health in very low-income settings. J Perinatol. 2011;31 (5):361–7.
74. Whitelaw A, Sleath K. Myth of the marsupial mother: home care of very low birth weight babies in Bogota. Colombia. Lancet. 1985;25:1206–9.
75. Venancio SI, de Almeida H. Kangaroo-Mother Care: scientific evidence and impact on breastfeeding. Jornal de Pediatria. 2004;80(5 Suppl):S173–80.
76. Ahmed AH, Sands LP. Effect of pre- and postdischarge interventions on breastfeeding outcomes and weight gain among premature infants. JOGNN - Journal of Obstetric, Gynecologic, & Neonatal Nursing. 2010;39(1):53–63.
77. Hake-Brooks SJ, Anderson GC. Kangaroo care and breastfeeding of mother-preterm infant dyads 0-18 months: a randomized, controlled trial. Neonatal Network - Journal of Neonatal Nursing. 2008;27(3):151–9.
78. Lizarazo-Medina JP, Ospina-Diaz JM, Ariza-Riano NE. The kangaroo mothers' programme: a simple and cost-effective alternative for protecting the premature newborn or low-birth-weight babies. Revista de Salud Publica. 2012;14(Suppl 2):32–45.
79. Ghavane S, Murki S, Subramanian S, Gaddam P, Kandraju H, Thumalla S. Kangaroo Mother Care in Kangaroo ward for improving the growth and breastfeeding outcomes when reaching term gestational age in very low birth weight infants. Acta Paediatr. 2012;101(12):e545–9.
80. Renfrew MJ, Dyson L, McCormick F, Misso K, Stenhouse E, King SE, et al. Breastfeeding promotion for infants in neonatal units: a systematic review. Child Care Health Dev. 2010;36(2):165–78.
81. Burkhammer MD, Anderson GC, Chiu SH. Grief, anxiety, stillbirth, and perinatal problems: healing with kangaroo care. JOGNN - Journal of Obstetric, Gynecologic, & Neonatal Nursing. 2004;33(6):774–82.
82. Arraes de Alencar AEM. Arraes LC, Cvalcanti de Albuquerque E, Alves JGB. Effect of kangaroo mother care on postpartum depression. J Trop Pediatr. 2009;55(1):36–28.
83. Abouelfettoh AM, Dowling DA, Dabash SA, Elguindy SR, Seoud IA. Cup versus bottle feeding for hospitalized late preterm infants in Egypt: a quasi-experimental study. International Breastfeeding Journal. 2008;3:27.
84. Yilmaz G, Caylan N, Karacan CD, Bodur I, Gokcay G. Effect of cup feeding and bottle feeding on breastfeeding in late preterm infants: a randomized controlled study. Journal of Human Lactation. 2014;30(2):174–9.
85. WHO. Comprehensive Implementation Plan on Maternal, Infant and Young Child Nutrition. Geneva, Switzerland: World Health Organization; 2014.
86. UN. Sustainable Development Goals. Transforming our World : The 2030 Agenda for Sustainable Development: The United Nations; 2016 [Available from: https://sustainabledevelopment.un.org/sdgs.
87. Imdad A, Yakoob MY, Bhutta ZA. Effect of breastfeeding promotion interventions on breastfeeding rates, wtih a special focus on developing countries. BMC Public Health. 2011;11((suppl 3)):S24-S31.
88. Roberts TJ, Carnahan E, Gakidou E. Can breastfeeding promote child health equity? A comprehensive analysis of breastfeeding patterns across the developing world and what we can learn from them. BMC Medicine. 2013;11.
89. UNICEF. Infant and Young Child Feeding Database. Data and Analytics Section; Division of Data, Research and Policy. UNICEF. Data downloaded June 23, 2106 from http://data.unicef.org/nutrition.iycf.html.
90. Delgado C, Matijasevich A. Breastfeeding up to two years of age or beyond and its influence on child growth and development: a systematic review. Cad Saude Publica, Rio de Janeiro. 2013;29(2):243–56.
91. Lutter CK, Lutter RW. Fetal and early childhood undernutrition, mortality and lifelong health. Science. 2012;337:1495–9.
92. Jones G, Steketee RW, Black RE, Bhutta ZA, Morris SS, the Bellagio Child Survival Study Group. How many child deaths can we prevent this year? Lancet. 2003;362:65-71.
93. Perera CR, Fonseca VM, Couto de Oliveira MI, Souza IE, Reis de Mello R. Assessment of factors that interfere on breastfeeding within the first hour of life. Revista Brasileira de Epidemiologia. 2013;16(2):525-34.
94. Prak S, Dahl MI, Oeurn S, Conkle J, Wise A, Laillou A. Breastfeeding trends in cambodia, an the increased use of breast-milk substitute - why is it a danger? Nutrients. 2014;6:2920–30.
95. Susiloretni KA, Hadi H, Prabandari YS, Soenarto YS, Wilopo SA. What works to improve duration of exclusive breastfeeding: lessons from teh exclusive breastfeedign promotion program in rural Indonesia. Matern Child Health J. 2015;19:1515–25.
96. Levitt C, Hanvey L, Kaczorowski J, Chalmers B, Heaman M, Bartholomew S. Breastfeeding policies and practices in Canadian hospitals: comparing 1993 with 2007. Birth. 2011;38(3):228-37.
97. Cattaneo A, Yngve A, Koletzko B, Guzman LR. Promotion of Breastfeeding in Europe Project. Protection, promotion and support of breast-feeding in Europe: current situation.[Erratum appears in Public Health Nutr. 2008 Dec; 11(12):1411]. Public Health Nutrition. 2005;8(1):39–46.
98. CDC. Vital signs: hospital practices to support breastfeeding–United States, 2007 and 2009. MMWR - Morbidity & Mortality Weekly Report. 2011;60(30):1020-5.

99. Prak S, Dahl MI, Oeurn S, Conkle J, Wise A, Laillou A. Breastfeeding trends in Cambodia, and the increase use of breast-milk substitute - why is it a danger? Nutrients. 2014;6:2920–30.
100. Ogbo FA, Agho KE, Page A. Determinants of suboptimal breastfeeding practices in Nigeria: evidence from the 2008 demographic and health survey. BMC Public Health. 2015;15:259–70.
101. UN. Convention on the elimination of all forms of discrimination against women. 1979 December 18, 1979. Report No.
102. UN. Convention on the Rights of the Child. 1989 November 20, 1989. Report No.
103. A Ahmed. HIV and Women: Incongruent Policies, Criminal Consequences. Yale Journal of International Affairs. 2011(Winter):32-42.
104. Tariq S, Elford J, Tookey P, Anderson J, de Ruiter A, O'Connell R, et al. It pains me because as a woman you have to breastfeed your baby": decision-making about infant feeding among African women living with HIV in the UK. Sex Transm Infect. 2016:1-6.
105. Rollins N, Coovadia HM. Breastfeeding and HIV transmission in the developing world: past, present, future. Curr Opin HIV AIDS. 2013;8(5):467–73.
106. Andreassen M, Bale M, Kaaresen PI, Dahl LB. Breast feeding in Tromso before and after the baby-friendly-hospital initiative. Tidsskr Nor Laegeforen. 2001;121(27):3154–8.
107. Titaley C, Loh P, Prasetyo S, Iwan A, Anuraj S. Socio-economic factors and use of maternal health services are associated with delayed initiation and non-exclusive breastfeeding in Indonesia: secondary analysis of Indonesia demographic and health surveys 2002/2003 and 2007. Asia Pacific Journal of Clinical Nutrition. 2014;23(1):91–104.
108. Benis MM. Are pacifiers associated with early weaning from breastfeeding? Advances in Neonatal Care. 2002;2 (5):259–66.
109. Biro MA, Sutherland GA, Yelland JS, Hardy P, Brown SJ. In-hospital formula supplementation of breastfed babies: a population-based survey. Birth. 2011;38(4):302–10.
110. WHO. Antiretroviral drugs for treating pregnant women and preventing HIV infection in infants. Recommendations for a public health approach. Geneva, Switzerland: World Health Organization, 2010.
111. Coovadia HM, Rollins NC, Bland RM, Little K, Coutsoudis A, Bennish ML, et al. Mother-to-child transmission of HIV-1 infection during exclusive breastfeeding in the first 6 months of life: an intervention cohort study. Lancet. 2007;369:1107–16.
112. St Children. Nutrition int eh First 1,000 Days. CT: Westport; 2012.
113. Post Huffington. Maternity leaves around the world: worst and best countries for paid maternity leave. The Huffington Post Canada. 2012;22:2012.
114. Haroon S, Das JK, Salam RA, Imdad A, Bhutta ZA. Breastfeeding promotion interventions and breastfeeding practices: a systematic review. BMC Public Health. 2013;13((Suppl 3)):18.
115. Barros AJ, Ronsmans C, Axelson H, Loaiza E, Bertoldi AD, Franca GVA, et al. Equity in maternal, newborn, and child health interventions in Countdown to 2015: a retrospective review of survey data from 54 countries. Lancet. 2012;379:1225–33.
116. Lutter CK, Morrow AL. Protection, promotion, and support and global trends in breastfeeding. Advances Nutr. 2013;4:213–9.
117. Gupta A, Holla R, Dadhich JP. The State of Breastfeeding in 33 Countries. 2010.
118. ILO. Maternity and paternity at work: law and practice across the world. Geneva, Switzerland; 2014.
119. Soekarjo D, Zehner E. Legislation should support optimal breastfeeding practices and access to low-cost, high-quality complementary foods: Indonesia provides a case study. Maternal Child Nutr. 2011;7(Suppl 3):112–22.
120. Tarrant M, Wu KM, Fong DY, Lee IL, Wong EM, Sham A, et al. Impact of baby-friendly hospital practices on breastfeeding in Hong Kong. Birth. 2011;38(3):238–45.
121. WHO, UNICEF. Innocenti declaration on the protection, promotion and support of breastfeeding. Breastfeeding in the 1990 s: a global initiative; July 30-August 1, 1990; Florene, Italy 1990.
122. WHO, UNICEF. Baby-Friendly hospital initiative, revised, updated and expanded for integrated care. 2009.
123. Nyqvist KH, Haggkvist AP, Hansen MN, Kylberg E, Frandsen AL, Maastrup R, et al. Expansion of the baby-friendly hospital initiative ten steps to successful breastfeeding into neonatal intensive care: expert group recommendations. J Human Lactation. 2013;29(3):300–9.
124. Abolyan LV. The breastfeeding support and promotion in baby-friendly maternity hospitals and not-as-yet baby-friendly hospitals in Russia. Breastfeeding Med Official J Acad Breastfeeding Med. 2006;1(2):71–8.
125. Perez-Escamilla R, Martinez JL, Segura-Perez S. Impact of the baby-friendly hospital initiative on breastfeeding and child health outcomes: a systematic review. Matern Child Nutr. 2016; 16
126. Kramer MS, Chalmers B, Hodnett ED, Sevkovskaya Z, Dzikovich I, Shapiro S, et al. Promotion of Breastfeeding Intervention Trial (PROBIT): a randomized trial in the Republic of Belarus. JAMA. 2001;285(4):413–20.
127. Braun ML, Giugliani ER, Soares ME, Giugliani C, de Oliveira AP, Danelon CM. Evaluation of the impact of the baby-friendly hospital initiative on rates of breastfeeding. Am J Public Health. 2003;93(8):1277–9.

128. Caldeira AP, Goncalves E. Assessment of the impact of implementing the baby-friendly hospital initiative. Jornal de Pediatria. 2007;83(2):127–32.
129. Almeida HD, Venancio SI, Sanches MT, Onuki D. The impact of kangaroo care on exclusive breastfeeding in low birth weight newborns. Jornal de Pediatria. 2010;86(3):250–3.
130. Paes Pedras CT, MA M, da Costa-Pinto EA. Breastfeeding of very low-weight infants before and after implementation of the baby-friendly hospital initiative. J Trop Pediatr. 2012;58(4):324–326.
131. Zakarija-Grkovic I, Segvic O, Bozinovic T, Cuze A, Lozancic T, Vuckovic A, et al. Hospital practices and breastfeeding rates before and after the UNICEF/WHO 20-hour course for maternity staff. J Human Lactation. 2012;28(3):389–99.
132. Brodribb W, Kruske S, Miller YD. Baby-friendly hospital accreditation, in-hospital care practices, and breastfeeding. Pediatrics. 2013;131(4):685–92.
133. Chapman DJ, Morel K, Bermudez-Millan A, Young S, Damio G, Perez-Escamilla R. Breastfeeding education and support trial for overweight and obese women: a randomized trial. Pediatrics. 2013;131(1):e162–70.
134. Di Mario S, Cattaneo A, Gagliotti C, Voci C, Basevi V. Baby-friendly hospitals and cesarean section rate: a survey of Italian hospitals. Breastfeeding Med Official J Acad Breastfeeding Med. 2013;8(4):388–93.
135. Barriuso Lapresa L, Sanchez-Valverde Visus F, Romero Ibarra C, Vitoria Comerzana JC. Hospital guidelines on breastfeeding in the north-center of Spain. Anales Espanoles de Pediatria. 2000;52(3):225–231.
136. Boccolini CS, Carvalho ML, Oliveira MI, Vasconcellos AG. Factors associated with breastfeeding in the first hour of life. Rev Saude Publica. 2011;45(1):69–78.
137. Aryeetey R, Antwi CL. Re-assessment of selected baby-friendly maternity facilities in Accra, Ghana. Int Breastfeeding J. 2013;8(1):15.
138. PR da Silva Maia. Brazilian human milk banks network: numbers in december 2013 and the "Survey of Italian Human Milk Banks. J Human Lactation. 2016;32(1):182.
139. Quigley M, Mcguire W. Formula versus donor breast milk for feeding preterm or low birth weight infants (Review). Cochrane Database Systematic Rev. 2014(4).
140. St-Onge M, Chaudhry S, Koren G. Donated breastmilk stored in banks versus breast milk purchased online. Can Fam Physician. 2015;61(2):143–6.
141. USDA. WIC Breastfeeding data local agency report. Division FSFP; 2012.
142. USDA. WIC Breastfeeding data local agency report. Division FSFP; 2010.
143. CDC. Breastfeeding Report Card 2013. Prevention UCfDCa; 2013.
144. Abt Associates. WIC Nutrition Education Assessment Study. 2013 October 29, 2013. Report No.
145. USDA. WIC Food Cost Report. 2010. Service FaN; 2013.
146. Gross TT, Powell R, Anderson AK, Hall J, Davis M, Hilyard K. WIC peer counselors' perceptions of breastfeeding in African American women with lower incomes. J Human Lactation. 2015;31(1):99–110.
147. Hedberg IC. Barriers to breastfeeding in the WIC population. MCN Am J Matern Child Nurs. 2013;38(4):244–9.
148. Joyce T, Reeder J. Changes in breastfeeding among WIC participants following implementation of the new food package. Matern Child Health J. 2015;19:868–76.
149. Berridge K, McFadden KK, Abayomi J, Topping J. Views of breastfeeding difficulties among drop-in-clinic attendees. Matern Child Nutr. 2005;1(4):250–62.
150. Kimani-Murage EW, Kyobutungi C, Ezeh AC, Wekesah F, Wanjohi M, Muriuki P, et al. Effectiveness of personalised, home-based nutritional counselling on infant feeding practices, morbidity and nutritional outcomes among infants in Nairobi slums: study protocol for a cluster randomised controlled trial. Trials [Electron Resource]. 2013;14:445.
151. Skouteris H, Nagle C, Fowler M, Kent B, Sahota P, Morris H. Interventions designed to promote exclusive breastfeedign in high-income countries: a systematic review. Breastfeeding Med. 2014;9(3):113–27.
152. Tylleskär T, Jackson D, Meda N, IMS E, Chopra M, Diallo AH, et al. Exclusive breastfeeding promotion by peer counsellors in sub-Saharan Africa (PROMISE-EBF): a cluster-randomized trial. Lancet. 2011;378(9789):420–427.
153. Rotheram-Borus MJ, Tomlinson M, le Roux IM, Harwood JM, Comulada S, O'Conner MJ, et al. A cluster randomised controlled effectiveness trial evaluating perinatal home visiting among South African mothers/infants. PLOS One. 2014;9(10).
154. Giglia R, Cox K, Zhao Y, Binns CW. Exclusive breastfeeding increased by an internet intervention. Breastfeeding Med. 2015;10(1):20–5.
155. Tahir NM, Al-Sadat N. Does telephone lactation counselling improve breastfeeding practices? A randomised controlled trial. Int J Nursing Stud. 2013;50(1):16–25.
156. Bhandari N, Kabir AKMI, Salam A. Mainstreaming nutrition into maternal and child health programmes: scaling up exclusive breastfeeding. Matern Child Nutr. 2008;4:5–23.
157. Perez-Escamilla R, Chapman DJ. Breastfeeding protection, promotion, and support in the United States: a time to nudge, a time to measure. J Human Lactation. 2012;28(2):118–21.

Part IV
Tuberculosis, HIV and the Role of Nutrition

Chapter 17
Tuberculosis

Eyal Oren and Joann M. McDermid

Keywords Tuberculosis · *Mycobacterium tuberculosis* · Vulnerable populations · Prevention and control · Epidemiology · Pathogenesis · Treatment

Learning Objectives

- Describe the temporal shifts that have occurred regarding the epidemiology of tuberculosis.
- Analyze why certain population groups are at greater risk of having tuberculosis.
- Evaluate the various stages of tuberculosis infection and disease and factors associated with these stages remaining stable or changing.
- Explain how new diagnostic methods have impacted the identification and treatment of tuberculosis.
- Describe current prevention and management approaches for tuberculosis.

Everything interacts with everything else: each single factor conspires with the others to crush a man, break him physically and mentally, and lay him wide open to disease.... Pack men together like herring in a barrel, deprive 'em of every last ounce of resistance, batten 'em below decks for days at a time, and what do you get? T.B. It's inevitable.

From the novel "HMS Ulysses" by Alistair McLean, Scottish Novelist, 1955

A Global Threat

Although an ancient disease, tuberculosis (TB) has not yet been consigned to the past. Worldwide, TB is the second leading cause of death from an infectious disease, accounting for 1.6–2 million deaths per year, including almost 500 child deaths every day [1]. These figures are shocking since prevention of new infections is possible and drug-susceptible TB is curable with existing drugs costing less than $50 USD for a full course of treatment [1]. Given our extensive medical advances since ancient times, why is TB still haunting humankind?

E. Oren (✉)
Department of Epidemiology and Biostatistics, Mel & Enid Zuckerman College of Public Health, University of Arizona, 1295 N. Martin Ave., PO Box 245211, Tucson, AZ 85724, USA
e-mail: eoren@email.arizona.edu

J.M. McDermid
Department of Medicine, Division of Infectious Diseases and International Health, School of Medicine, University of Virginia, PO Box 801340, Charlottesville, VA 22908, USA
e-mail: joann.mcdermid@virginia.edu

© Springer Science+Business Media New York 2017
S. de Pee et al. (eds.), *Nutrition and Health in a Developing World*,
Nutrition and Health, DOI 10.1007/978-3-319-43739-2_17

Table 17.1 Factors contributing to the global tuberculosis burden

Factors	Mechanism
Human immunodeficiency virus (HIV)	Immunosuppression leading to development of active tuberculosis disease
Drug resistance	Greater treatment failure rates and transmission of drug-resistant *M. tuberculosis*
Political/economic factors	Lack of political will and resources to address poverty, inadequate health care, and inequality
Immigration/air travel	Increasing immigration and air travel from highly endemic countries may introduce tuberculosis into low-incidence communities
Outbreaks in congregate settings	Outbreaks in congregate spaces such as prisons increase infection while incarcerated, as well as transmission in communities after prison release
Drug abuse	Physiologic effects of drug abuse, social environments, behaviors, and barriers to treatment among drug users increase the risk of infection
Global urbanization	Increasing urbanization concentrates groups at high risk for tuberculosis into densely populated cities that increase the risk of *M. tuberculosis* transmission
Diabetes	Diabetes has been shown to increase the risk of progressing to tuberculosis, and the global diabetes burden is increasing
Crowding/poverty	Poverty and household crowding contribute to greater transmission and tuberculosis disease in low-income communities
Malnutrition	Malnutrition has direct biological impact on disease susceptibility through complex mechanisms leading to immunosuppression and is also associated with social factors related to increased transmission

The global TB burden is driven by a complex interplay of factors. These include genetic or biological factors affecting disease susceptibility, bacterial mutations leading to increasing virulence and drug resistance, changes in the physical and ecological environment, and human behavior that is subject to broader political, economic, and social structural factors (Table 17.1). This human–microbe interaction can be summarized by the Institute of Medicine Convergence Model (Fig. 17.1). Of particular relevance to TB are individual-level factors, broader issues of poverty and social inequality, as well as weak healthcare systems and poor access to preventive, diagnostic, and curative care. As a disease that afflicts individuals who breathe "shared air," *M. tuberculosis* is more likely to be transmitted in crowded, congregate environments—which more often than not, correlate with a high degree of poverty [2]. The World Health Organization (WHO) has noted that "circumstances in which we grow, live, work, and age" and the "systems put in place to deal with illness" give rise to unequal, unfair distributions of disease [3].

Emergence of HIV infection has also greatly facilitated the resurgence of TB in regions with previously declining rates, and contributed to an even higher TB burden in regions where TB was already problematic. TB is the leading cause of morbidity and mortality among HIV-infected people worldwide [4]. Incidence and case fatality rates among HIV-positive patients can exceed 50% [5]. The emergence of multidrug-resistant tuberculosis (MDR-TB), and an even deadlier form of TB called extensively drug-resistant TB (XDR-TB), are more recent concerns that require ongoing vigilance and rapid intervention to prevent ongoing transmission (see also *Global Drug Resistance* and *Tuberculosis Therapy* sections of this chapter).

A Brief History

TB has been a disease of humans for over 3000 years, as documented through bone and tissue samples extracted from mummies in Peru [6] and Egypt [7]. Throughout the Middle Ages and well

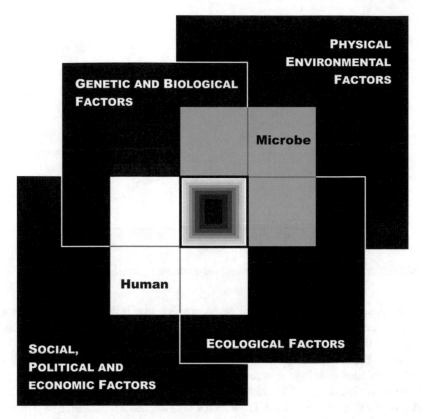

Fig. 17.1 The convergence model. At the center of the model is a box representing the convergence of factors leading to the emergence of an infectious disease. The interior of the box is a gradient flowing from *white* to *black*; the *white outer* edges represent what is known about the factors in emergence, and the *black center* represents the unknown (similar to the theoretical construct of the "black box" with its unknown constituents and means of operation). Interlocking with the center box are the two focal players in a microbial threat to health—the human and the microbe. The microbe–host interaction is influenced by the interlocking domains of the determinants of the emergence of infection: genetic and biological factors; physical and environmental factors; ecological factors; and social, political, and economic factors. From Smolinski, Mark S. et al. Microbial threats to health: Emergence, detection, and response. Reprinted with permission from the National Academies Press, Copyright 2005, National Academy of Sciences

into the industrial age, TB was referred to as phthisis, the "white plague," or consumption—all in reference to the progressive deterioration of health and extensive weight loss experienced. In 1720, Benjamin Marten, an English physician, noted in his publication, *A New Theory of Consumption*, that TB could be caused by "wonderfully minute living creatures...it may be therefore very likely that by an habitual lying in the same bed with a consumptive patient, constantly eating and drinking with him, or by very frequently conversing so nearly as to draw in part of the breath he emits from the lungs, a consumption may be caught by a sound person..." [8]. The disease was also enshrined in the literature as the "captain of death," the slow killer of promise [9]. Prominent European artists who died of TB in the nineteenth century included the English poet John Keats, Polish composer Frédéric Chopin, German author Franz Kafka, and all three Brontë sisters of this English literary family [9].

In 1882, Robert Koch discovered a staining technique that enabled *Mycobacterium tuberculosis*, the causative agent, to be observed by microscopy. In 1921, the Bacillus Calmette–Guerin (BCG) vaccine that confers protection to children from disseminated TB was first administered to a baby. It was not until November 20, 1944, that the antibiotic, streptomycin, was first given to a critically ill TB patient with almost immediate improvement and recovery. This start of the antibiotic era of TB treatment, together with economic improvement, better sanitation, widespread education,

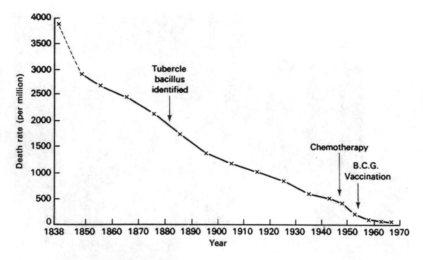

Fig. 17.2 Case fatality rates for tuberculosis, nineteenth and twentieth centuries

and importantly, the establishment of public health practice that included specific measures for TB control, helped to accelerate the dramatic declining trajectory in TB burden within industrialized countries (Fig. 17.2).

In modern times, the global TB epidemic has been fueled by the emergence of the HIV epidemic in the 1980s and insufficient ongoing investment in public health. In many regions where both TB and HIV are endemic, the incidence of TB has doubled. In the early 2000s, as a result of rapid implementation of global efforts to combat the TB and HIV disease, the TB epidemic in Africa slowed and incidence rates stabilized [10]. Complacency is not warranted, however, as many outbreaks, especially in hospitals and other healthcare settings in large cities [11], have been caused by MDR-TB. In South Africa, nearly 10% of all new TB cases are infected with MDR-TB strains, and between 6 and 10% of all MDR-TB cases are found to be infected with XDR-TB strains [12].

Epidemiology

Global Tuberculosis

Roughly one-third of the world's population—over 2 billion people—are thought to be infected with *M. tuberculosis* [5, 13]. Of those infected, 8–12 million will progress to active TB disease each year, resulting in nearly two million deaths [1]. In 2013, the WHO reported that there were 11 million (range 10–13 million) prevalent cases of TB worldwide [1].

While TB disease is widespread throughout the world, over 80% of all new TB cases occur in just 22 high-burden countries—the top six are India, China, Nigeria, Pakistan, Indonesia, and South Africa [1]. In 2013, the global incidence rate of TB was 126 cases per 100,000 population with substantial regional variation [1] (Fig. 17.3). More than half of the reported TB cases occurred in Asia (56%), followed by the African region (29%), where the highest regional- and country-level incidence rates have been reported [1] (see Fig. 17.3). Globally, about 13% of all new TB cases occur among people living with HIV, and this proportion is highest in the African region (37%) where over 75% of the world's HIV-TB-coinfected people reside [1, 14].

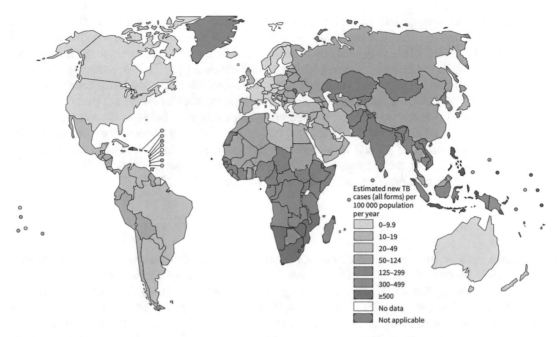

Fig. 17.3 Global incidence of tuberculosis. Estimated TB incidence rates, 2013. Incidence rates of TB remain the highest in sub-Saharan Africa and Asia. Reproduced, with the permission of the publisher, from *Global Tuberculosis Report 2014*. World Health Organization; 2014 (Fig. 2.5, p. 34 http://apps.who.int/iris/bitstream/10665/137094/1/9789241564809_eng.pdf?ua=1, Accessed Nov 27, 2014)

Global Drug Resistance

While the overall incidence and prevalence of TB have declined in recent years, there has been an increase in the incidence of MDR-TB in the past decade [15]. Nearly 4% of all new TB cases and 20% of previously treated TB cases are considered to be MDR-TB. The largest number of MDR-TB cases are in China, India, and the Russian Federation, and in some countries, up to half of all new TB cases are infected with a drug-resistant strain [16]. The proportion of TB cases with MDR-TB in Russian prison populations exceeds 40% in some cases [17]. While less common, over 100 countries have reported cases of XDR-TB, which on average occurs in 8–9% of all MDR-TB cases, with the greatest burden found in former Soviet Union countries [18].

Vulnerable Populations

Race and Ethnicity

In high-income countries, TB is often concentrated among minority populations despite decreasing incidence rates among the overall population [19, 20]. It is unlikely that the concentration of TB in ethnic minorities is driven by biological variation alone, but also includes contributing social factors including disproportionate poverty, crowding, immigration, and asylum seeking from high TB-endemic countries [21, 22]. For instance, in New Zealand, immigrant populations have not been shown to be a significant contributor to TB incidence after controlling for household crowding [22]. In the USA, TB is largely a problem among Hispanic and black populations, with rates eight to nine times those of white populations [23]. Hispanics and blacks disproportionately experience risk factors such as poverty and crowded housing, which may facilitate TB transmission [24, 25]. The burden of pediatric TB in the USA is largely borne by minority populations with heightened transmission from US-born, non-Hispanic black adults to non-Hispanic black children [26]. The disproportionate burden of TB among racial and ethnic groups is largely due to differences in living and social conditions [27]. For example, in the USA, six indicators of socioeconomic status such as crowding, income, poverty, receiving public assistance, unemployment, and education accounted for approximately half of the increased risk for TB among blacks, Hispanics, and Native Americans, when compared to whites [28]. Varying prevalence of TB risk factors such as HIV, substance abuse, lack of health insurance, and homelessness across racial groups also contributes to the disparities seen in both increased exposure and progression from latent infection to active disease [27, 29].

Indigenous Peoples

Indigenous peoples in high-, middle-, and low-income countries continue to bear a high and disproportionate burden of TB [30]. Groups most burdened by TB are located in regions of Latin America (e.g., Peru, Brazil), Southeast Asia (e.g., India, Thailand), Africa (e.g., Chad, Mali), and North America. For example, TB case rates for American (US) Indians are more than five times greater than those for non-Hispanic white people and 13 times as great among Pacific Islanders [31]. High rates of HIV coinfection among indigenous groups in Papua New Guinea and Indonesia may also explain the high risk of TB among these indigenous peoples [32].

Children

An estimated 11% of all TB cases worldwide occur in children younger than 15 years [33]. Pediatric infection is common because of family dynamics: Children in the family of an adult with infectious TB often have frequent and close contact, such that they are at high risk of acquiring infection. If infected, young children are more likely to progress to active disease. While the diagnosis of pediatric TB has unique challenges, if promptly diagnosed and treated, pediatric TB outcomes are favorable [34] (see also Pediatric TB section of this chapter).

Urban and Rural Disparities

In large cities in the USA, TB case fatality rates have been shown to be three times higher in the lowest compared to the highest socioeconomic group among people aged 35 years or younger, increasing to a ratio of six to one among men older than 35 [35]. A Danish study found that TB incidence rates in urban areas were twice as high as rural areas [36], and TB in major cities has been shown to account for more than one-third of all US patients with TB [37]. A cross-sectional study in low-incidence settings across the European Union found the risk of TB to be 2.5 times higher in cities compared to national rates [38]. Social conditions that are observed in high concentrations in urban areas, such as homelessness, HIV, suboptimal access to health care, and migration, are also associated with high TB incidence [39–41]. Living in rural areas may create difficulties in access to health care. Individuals who are more isolated and further removed from services may have a higher risk of developing active TB [42]. Low case finding rates (due to passive case detection) and high rates of transmission and active TB disease have been documented among residents in rural China, Vietnam, and Kenya [43–45]. Disparities in TB rates within countries and across levels of urbanization are often complex and multifactorial, with differences also due to different levels of socioeconomic development and varying financial incentives [46].

The Role of Migration

Migrants are disproportionately affected by TB, often due to high TB incidence in their originating countries (such that they are more likely to have latent TB infection or undiagnosed active TB disease), limited access to health care and infrastructure both during their journey and at their new destination, as well as poverty and social exclusion in their new home [47]. Since persons who were born in countries where TB prevalence is high likely acquire infection before immigrating [48], migrants may progress to TB disease many years after arrival as a result of reactivation of a latent TB infection (LTBI) [20]. In high-income countries, TB is often concentrated among foreign-born minority populations despite decreasing incidence rates among domestic-born populations [19, 20].

Approximately half of new TB cases in the USA occur among foreign-born persons, and TB cases among foreign-born persons were approximately 10–20 times higher than those among persons born in the USA [49, 50]. In Italy, the proportion of TB that occurs among immigrant populations has increased from 19% in 1996 to 53% in 2006 [51]. In Spain, the immigrant population has rates of TB disease three to four times higher than the Spanish population, increasing among the foreign-born population over a 10-year time period from 1994 to 2003. Additionally, the proportion of TB among immigrant populations has also experienced substantial increases in Spain, from 3% in 1997 to over 36% in 1999 [52].

Disparities in Other Settings

Globally, TB rates are substantially higher among incarcerated populations. For instance, in Brazil, TB rates are 100 times higher among incarcerated compared to civilian populations [53, 54]. Transmission risks relevant to correctional institutions include close living quarters among inmates along with poor ventilation and overcrowding [55, 56]. Disparities in TB screening and treatment outcomes are particularly prevalent in this population. Despite being more likely to receive directly observed therapy (see *Tuberculosis Control Strategy* section), inmates are less likely to complete their full course of treatment [55]. In the USA, this is partly due to inmates moving out of institutional jurisdiction before the 6-month treatment is finished or for other reasons associated with the loss of treatment supervision [57]. Further, the high prevalence of HIV coinfection and high-risk behaviors including intravenous drug use (e.g., 12–22% reporting injection drug use [58, 59]) among prisoners may be driving the disease burden in this population [60]. There is also a strong relationship between increases in mass incarceration and relative increase in TB among European and Asian countries, illustrating the hazardous link between TB among incarcerated populations and public health [61]. Mixing of incarcerated and civilian populations upon prisoner release is a contributing factor to TB resurgence [62] because this brings people who have not been fully cured of TB into communities, increasing their risk of now being exposed to infectious TB.

Other High-Risk Populations

Patients in high-risk behavioral groups, including substance abusers (alcohol, injection, and non-injection drug use) and homeless individuals, are more likely to delay seeking timely medical care and if they do, be non-adherent for the 6-month duration of TB treatment. Overall, this leads to a prolonged period of infectivity that increases likelihood of transmission and possible outbreaks [63–65]. Transmission among frequent alcohol or drug users may be due to inability or reluctance of patients to share information about high-risk behavioral patterns that may obstruct screening, diagnosing, and initiating TB treatment [66, 67]. Perceived contagion of TB is also a leading cause of stigmatization [68, 69]. Lack of knowledge regarding routes of TB transmission also contributes to

TB stigma [70]. As a result of this stigma and its social and economic impact, at-risk individuals report that they are less willing to undergo TB screening and to seek medical care after the onset of TB symptoms [71]. TB stigma has also previously been shown to be predictive of decreased TB treatment adherence among certain populations and associated with prolonged patient delay [72, 73]. Other groups at high risk of HIV, such as men who have sex with men, female sex workers, or minority populations (e.g., black populations in the USA), may also be at higher risk for worse TB outcomes given the rate at which HIV hastens progression to active TB [74].

Healthcare workers are also at risk for TB transmission in healthcare settings due to transmission from patients, who may have unrecognized or inappropriately treated TB. In high TB incidence countries, the median estimated annual incidence of TB among healthcare workers is as high as 1180/100,000 persons [75].

Diabetes

Diabetes is a risk factor for disease progression; however, the underlying mechanisms of the association are not well understood [76]. In a cohort of over 17,000 Taiwanese nationals, the risk of TB was over threefold higher among those with two or more diabetic complications. In India, it was estimated that nearly 15% of pulmonary TB (PTB) and 20% of TB smear-positive cases were attributable to diabetes [77]. Further, the risk of failure and death during TB treatment is reportedly higher among diabetic populations [78]. Even after completing treatment, diabetics are up to four times more likely than nondiabetics to have subsequent relapse TB that may be due to either recurrence of previous infection or new infection from a subsequent exposure to infectious TB [78, 79].

How Is Mycobacterium Tuberculosis *Transmitted?*

Following exposure to *M. tuberculosis,* an individual may progress to latent infection and then potentially active TB disease (Fig. 17.4).

The TB pathogen is transmitted through small airborne droplets, called droplet nuclei (1–5 μm in diameter), generated when a person who has disease in their lungs or vocal cords coughs [80–82], sneezes, talks, or sings [83]. Droplets can remain airborne for minutes to hours after expectoration [84]. The number of bacilli in the droplets, the virulence of the bacilli, exposure of the bacilli to ultraviolet light [85, 86], degree of ventilation, and degree of aerosolization all influence transmission likelihood [87]. Transmission occurs when a person inhales the droplet nuclei; introduction of bacteria into the lungs generally leads to infection of the respiratory system or pulmonary TB (PTB); however, bacteria can also spread systemically to other organs, such as the lymphatic system, pleura, bones/joints, or meninges, resulting in extrapulmonary TB (EPTB) [88] (see *Pathogenesis and Clinical Manifestations* section).

While the pathogen is not easily transmissible, and generally requires prolonged exposures to transmit sufficient bacterial doses [89], active disease can develop from a low infectious dose (referred to as the dose of an infectious organism required to produce infection in 50% of the experimental subjects: <10 bacilli). Respiratory transmission is the most common mode of transmission, but less common modes of transmission also include exposure to the bacteria during autopsies [90] and through injury or breaks in skin or mucous membrane [91]. While these bacteria are initially localized, spread to other organs is possible. Congenital transmission of TB, though very rare, has also been documented in case reports [92, 93] (see Pediatric TB section). Bovine TB (*Mycobacterium bovis*) may also be transmitted either through direct exposure to infected cattle or through ingestion of

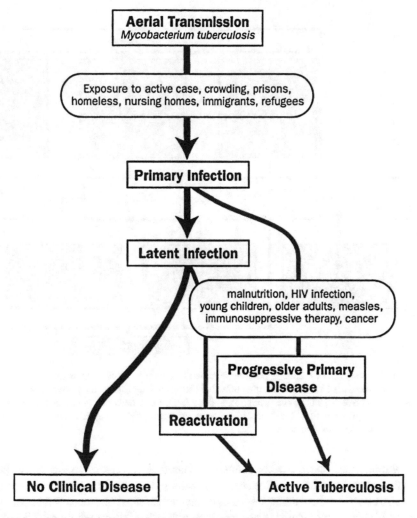

Fig. 17.4 General model for tuberculosis infection and common risk factors

unpasteurized milk and infected meat products, with similar symptoms as those caused by *M. tuberculosis* (see *The Pathogen* section) [94, 95].

It is useful to think of the continuum from exposure through disease, and associated risk factors for each stage of TB pathogenesis (Fig. 17.5). The risk of acquiring TB infection is strongly influenced by environmental risk factors that increase the probability of TB exposure [96]. Environmental factors affect the concentration of *M. tuberculosis* bacilli. For example, if droplet nuclei are more concentrated, there is higher likelihood of transmission, such as in the case of exposure in a small indoor space, where less particle dilution will occur. Adequate ventilation and air circulation serves to dilute or else completely remove droplet nuclei. Ventilation plays a vital role in reducing the transmission of TB, with even intermittent window opening significantly improving ventilation and air quality within a room, as well as overall room volume [97]. If a patient is isolated, rooms are designed such that the positive air pressure in the room will result in the bacilli and other airborne microorganisms flowing outside away from the patient. Ultraviolet (UV) light has also been found to have a significant germicidal effect on *M. tuberculosis*, and UV irradiation has been recommended as a potentially effective TB control strategy in congregate settings with crowded conditions [86, 87].

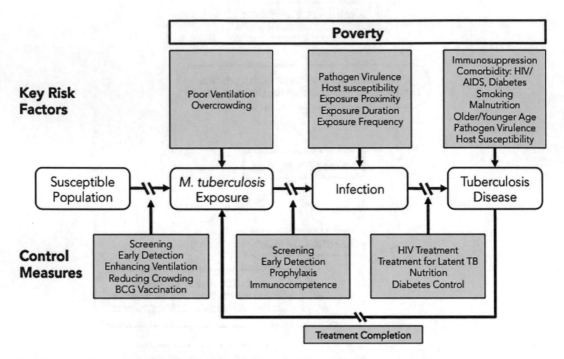

Fig. 17.5 Risk factors and control measures from tuberculosis infection to disease. Overview of key TB risk factors and control measures. The risk of TB exposure, infection, and disease is largely driven by poverty and mediated through social risk factors such as overcrowding, comorbidities, and smoking. Early detection is key in disrupting infection with *M. tuberculosis* and progression to TB disease. Completion of appropriate drug treatment is critical in reducing secondary infections, and drug resistance

Crowding within living spaces, often defined as shared bedrooms or living space, is one of the earliest identified predictors of infection risk. Crowding directly influences risk of infection by increasing the likelihood of close contact exposure between infected and susceptible people that share confined airspace. Many ecological studies have shown the effect of crowding on TB risk on various geographic levels. For instance, Drucker et al. showed that TB risk was over five times higher among children in New York living in neighborhoods with greater household crowding, compared to those neighborhoods with a smaller proportion of crowded households [98]. Other studies in high-income countries have shown the effect on TB risk of crowding at various administrative levels [22]. Studies in prison populations and homeless shelters further demonstrate the effect of crowding on TB risk.

Risk Factors for Infection

There are three factors that influence the risk of becoming infected: (1) the infectivity of the TB source case, (2) the degree of exposure to the index or source case (infectious person), and (3) the degree of susceptibility of the exposed (uninfected person) [99]. The infectiousness (called infectivity) of the source case is largely determined by cough frequency, amount of bacilli present in sputum, degree of pulmonary cavitation, and virulence of the infecting strain type [99]. Infectiousness is largely a function of the number of tubercle bacilli expelled into the air, but also directly related to the duration and appropriateness of TB treatment and whether bacilli are aerosolized through a procedure such as bronchoscopy or sputum induction [100]. Young children are less likely than adults to be infectious TB cases as they generally do not produce sputum with high bacterial loads when they cough [101].

More virulent bacterial strains tend to create greater cavitation and damage to lungs, leading to greater expectoration of bacilli [102]. Indeed, the severity of disease in the index case has been found to be the strongest predictor of secondary infection in household contacts [103]. Degree of exposure is determined by proximity, frequency, and duration of exposure to an infected source case. Longer duration, greater proximity, and higher frequency of exposure are associated with higher transmission risk [87]. Finally, susceptibility to infection is determined by the nutritional status (particularly micronutrient deficiencies, see also Chap. 19 on Tuberculosis Infection and Nutrition), genetics, and general health state of the susceptible person. For example, development of TB disease has been shown to be strongly associated with advanced levels of immunosuppression, while ART initiation is effective in reducing incident TB among HIV-positive children [104]. HIV infection inhibits macrophage bactericidal pathways, leading to increased bacterial survival; the depletion of CD4+ T cells and other aspects of the immune response associated with HIV infection further increase overall susceptibility to TB disease [4].

Risk Factors for Progression from Latent Infection to Disease

A number of risk factors, diseases, and medications can weaken the immune system, such that the body can no longer mount an effective defense against existing TB bacilli. These include deterioration of nutritional status, HIV/AIDS, diabetes, end-stage kidney disease, certain cancers, chemotherapy, heavy or long-term steroid use, organ transplantation, and very young or advanced age [105] (Figs. 17.4 and 17.6). Drug use or alcohol abuse is also immunosuppressive and increases vulnerability to TB, and using tobacco has recently been shown to increase the risk of progressing to active disease [106]. Genetics has been found to play a key role in modulating host susceptibility to the development of active TB [107, 108]. There are a number of candidate genes in humans—one example is the intracellular pathogen resistance 1 gene, which may confer innate immunity to TB by limiting multiplication of *M. tuberculosis* and encouraging apoptosis of *M. tuberculosis*-infected macrophages [107, 109].

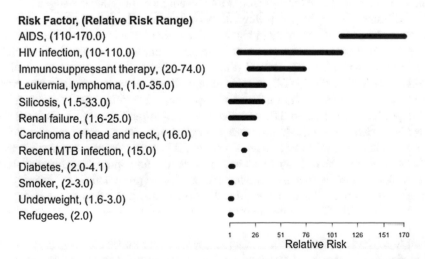

Fig. 17.6 Relative risk of active tuberculosis development by key risk factors. Relative risk of developing active TB disease for various key risk factors

Seasonality

There is evidence of a seasonal dependence of TB; in the USA, the highest incidence of TB occurs in March with over 20% greater reported cases than in November when incidence is lowest [110]. In other regions, notifications are higher in the summer [111, 112]. Globally, vitamin D level variability, indoor activities, seasonal change in immune function, and delays in diagnosis and treatment (e.g., delay in seeking health care in the winter resulting in predominance of tuberculosis notifications in spring and summer) are potential stimuli of seasonal TB disease [111]. However, it is unclear whether these seasonal patterns are largely behavioral, biological, or a combination of both.

Tb $\neq$ Tb $\neq$ Tb

TB is not a uniform disease, but rather a complex infectious disease caused by multiple *Mycobacterium* species, with multiple postinfection outcomes possible (e.g., LTBI vs. active TB disease) and diverse clinical manifestations depending on host factors such as age (e.g., pediatric vs. adult TB) and immune competence (e.g., HIV-negative vs. HIV-positive TB).

The Pathogen

TB is caused by infection with one or more genetically related, slow-growing acid-fast *Mycobacterium* spp. collectively referred to as *M. tuberculosis* complex (MTBC). The most common of these in humans are *M. tuberculosis* and *Mycobacterium africanum*, including *M. africanum* West African-1 (WA-1) and *M. africanum* WA-2, with the latter accounting for up to 50% of PTB cases in some West African regions [113]. *M. bovis* BCG, including *M. bovis* BCG Pasteur and *M. bovis* BCG Tokyo, is a laboratory lineage derived from *M. bovis* (bovine TB). BCG is the only approved TB vaccine at this time; however, this attenuated strain is capable of causing TB disease in immunocompromised individuals [114] (see *Tuberculosis Prevention through Vaccination* section).

Human TB strains were originally thought to have evolved from zoonotic transmissions, specifically bovine-to-human *M. bovis* transmission. More recent genomic analyses suggest that animal TB may actually be human in origin [115]. Regardless of the direction the original species barrier was crossed, understanding MTBC diversity in humans, domestic and wild animals has important clinical and public health implications in terms of monitoring transmission dynamics, maintaining vigilance for emerging strains, and assessing clinical differences. Mammals are known reservoirs for many *Mycobacterium* spp. within the MTBC classification, with *M. bovis* most commonly transmitted to humans [94]. Exposure to *M. bovis* in exhaled air, sputum, urine, feces, pus, unpasteurized dairy or infected meat products can lead to TB. *Mycobacterium pinnipedii* (seals), *Mycobacterium microti* (voles), *Mycobacterium caprae*, *Mycobacterium orygis*, and *Mycobacterium canettii* have been identified in a smaller proportion of human TB cases [116–120]. Despite the importance of understanding MTBC diversity in relation to pathogen virulence and immunogenicity that in turn can impact transmission dynamics, host immune regulation, disease presentation and severity, prioritizing research in this area is a challenge; strain identification is not part of standard clinical laboratory techniques, and the resulting clinical disease has similar presenting signs and symptoms and treatment options.

In addition to *Mycobacterium* species variation, there is variation within *M. tuberculosis*. A small number of clades (e.g., taxonomic grouping according to common ancestor) are responsible for a large proportion of new TB cases in different regions of the world, suggesting that these clades have greater virulence, infectivity, and possibly clinical heterogeneity. Four main phylogenetic *M. tuberculosis* lineages have been identified, namely Indo-Oceanic, East Asian, East African-Indian, and Euro-American [121]. Indo-Oceanic and East Asian strains are predominantly found in East and Southeast Asia, while Euro-American strains are more commonly found in the Americas, Europe, and North Africa. In experimental studies, clinical isolates of Indian strains were less virulent than those of strains from patients in the United Kingdom, while certain clinical strains like East Asian HN878 that have been associated with previous outbreaks in the USA are considered to be "hypervirulent" and characterized by vigorous host immune response, rapid bacterial replication, and significant pathology [121]. Indo-Oceanic and East African lineages are nearly exclusively associated with EPTB, whereas the East Asian lineage is far less likely to manifest in EPTB [122].

The Beijing family of *M. tuberculosis* is the most geographically distributed and appears to rapidly propagate in settings with high TB incidence, especially among children [123]. It is frequently implicated in MDR-TB outbreaks, but the majority of Beijing strains remain drug susceptible. While not drug resistant, there may be variation in virulence, clinical response to treatment, and BCG vaccine efficacy with Beijing strains [124, 125]. The close relationship between geography and strain types may contribute to the observed variability in BCG efficacy by geographic latitude [126]. While strain pathogenicity is a concern for individual disease outcomes, less pathogenic strains are a concern for TB control because they can spread to many people before an outbreak is recognized. For example, strain PG004 was responsible for a large-scale outbreak in Northern California that produced infectious but subclinical cases [127]. Any factor that prolongs the period after which an infection becomes transmissible (e.g., infectious) and before drugs eliminate sufficient bacteria (e.g., treatment sterilization) will lead to new transmissions.

Pathogenesis and Clinical Manifestations

Inhalation of droplet nuclei containing tubercle bacilli leads to various outcomes [128] that depend on a number of factors including the nature of the host immune response and other host (e.g., nutritional status) and pathogen cofactors. Although the exact mechanisms are unclear, some people with known exposure to tubercle bacilli never become infected. In these cases, the mucosal barriers involved in innate immunity may prevent infection or the inoculating dose may have been so low that infection is never established. Others may produce such an effective innate immune response (e.g., involving cells, tissues, and molecules of the innate system) or possess unidentified resistance mechanisms that bacteria are cleared before detectable adaptive immunity is triggered. However, in most people (approximately 90–95%), bacterial exposure leads to an established infection and elicitation of innate and adaptive immune responses. Fortunately, the vast majority remains clinically stable without active TB disease as their immune responses are coordinated and successfully confine bacterial proliferation within a granuloma lesion. This lesion consists of immune cells that form an outer wall ring barrier to restrict escape and dissemination of live bacteria. While bacterial elimination is never achieved in these individuals without active intervention (e.g., TB medication), bacterial containment in well-maintained granulomas halts disease progression and therefore the person remains clinically stable with LTBI throughout their lifetime. In some people (approximately 5%), the early immune response is insufficient to contain recently acquired infection and active TB disease rapidly develops. In others (approximately 5–10% lifetime risk) who develop LTBI but later experience a wane in their immunological control of infection, active TB can develop after years or many decades of successful immunological control. Many factors can affect the likelihood of disease progression including HIV infection and other comorbidities (e.g., diabetes), immunosuppressive medications, advancing age, malnutrition, and others (see Epidemiology section above).

The most common and efficient route of infection is through inhalation of TB-causing *Mycobacterium* spp. contained in aerosolized droplets leading to primary pulmonary infection. Primary extrapulmonary infection results from mucosal membrane exposure in the gastrointestinal and genitourinary systems, or through the conjunctiva or skin lesions. Pulmonary infection requires only a few bacilli to reach terminal airways in order to establish a primary (Ghon) focus, a lesion characterized by granulomatous inflammation [128]. Indeed, *Mycobacterium* has a very low infectious dose, with the human ID_{50} (infectious dose required to cause infection in 50% of experimental participants) estimated to be less than 10 bacilli.

Once bacteria reach an alveolar surface, they encounter alveolar macrophages that ingest them and bacterial replication begins. This process activates infected macrophages, which in turn recruit more macrophages and activated T cells, key immune cells in cell-mediated immunity. A successful immune response includes the development of granulomas, formations containing viable bacilli in the center, with macrophages and other immune cells forming an outer wall [129]. It is essentially the immunological containment of TB-causing bacteria within these granulomas that dictates whether an individual will halt progression after the primary infection, or continue to progress to active TB disease. If progression is halted, an individual is considered to have LTBI. LTBI is asymptomatic; most people are unaware they are infected. LTBI is not infectious as long as there is a sufficient lifelong immune response to keep the living bacteria within granulomas. The challenge from an individual TB disease management or population-level TB control perspective is twofold: difficulty in identifying persons with LTBI who are at high risk for progression to active disease (see *Tuberculosis Diagnosis* section) and difficulty in identifying persons with active disease who are early in the disease course so that curative therapy may be instituted and spread of infection prevented. Lifetime estimated case fatality rates for untreated TB have been estimated to be approximately 70% [130].

When the immune response fails, granulomas weaken and release bacilli that may have remained viable even after decades of quiescence. These bacteria may establish active infection in the lung and may also be transported throughout the lymphatic and circulatory systems to cause disease in any other area of the body. Active disease is classified as PTB or EPTB depending on where the infection is located, and they are not mutually exclusive since both manifestations are possible in the same individual, at the same time. While PTB is the most common manifestation comprising approximately 80% of TB cases, certain subgroups of people including HIV-positive individuals and children and possibly *M. tuberculosis* strain-related factors experience a greater proportion of EPTB cases [34, 131, 132].

Signs and symptoms of active PTB include cough (>3 weeks), hemoptysis (blood in sputum), dyspnea (shortness of breath), and chest pain [133]. Other prominent signs of active TB include chronic (several weeks to months) anorexia, weight loss, low-grade fever, night sweats, chills, and fatigue (Fig. 17.7). Since EPTB can affect any organ system, symptoms are diverse and include cervical lymphadenitis (lymph node inflammation), pleurisy (inflammation of the pleura or lining of the lung), pericarditis (inflammation of the pericardium, the fibrous sac surrounding the heart), synovitis (inflammation of the synovial membrane, the membrane lining joints), meningitis (inflammation of meninges, the membranes covering the brain and spinal cord), and skin or bone infections. Miliary or disseminated TB is characterized by high and sustained fever, night sweats, dry cough, malaise, splenomegaly (enlarged spleen), and skin lesions. TB meningitis is characterized by high fever, cranial nerve deficits, and psychic changes and has a very high mortality rate if untreated. However, individuals with active disease may also be asymptomatic, such as when subclinical disease occurs when bacilli spread from the lungs through the lymphatic system. Tuberculous peritonitis (inflammation of the peritoneum, the lining of the inner wall of the abdomen) is associated with fever, ascites, and increased abdominal girth. Although *M. bovis* causes a disease similar to *M. tuberculosis*, extrapulmonary lesions are more likely if acquired through consumption of *M. bovis*-contaminated milk or meat, while occupations interacting with cattle are prone to pulmonary lesions from exposure to infected aerosol droplets [95, 134].

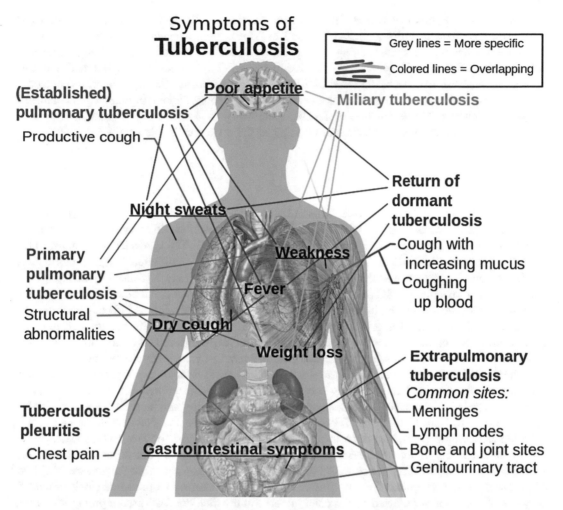

Fig. 17.7 Symptoms and stages of tuberculosis. Main symptoms of different variants and stages of tuberculosis, with many symptoms overlapping with other variants, while others are more (but not entirely) specific for certain variants. Multiple variants may be present simultaneously. From Häggström, Mikael. "Medical gallery of Mikael Häggström 2014." Wikiversity Journal of Medicine 1(2). doi:10.15347/wjm/2014.008. ISSN 20018762

HIV coinfection is the single most potent risk factor for progression from infection to active disease, whether infection is from a new primary infection (e.g., recent exposure to bacteria) and/or reactivation of a latent infection (see **Epidemiology** section above). Since multiple exposures are possible, mixed (or multiple)-strain infections have been described, although the challenges to fully understanding the epidemiology (laboratory detection of mixed strains is difficult leading to gaps in knowledge), clinical (e.g., ability to comprehensively assess individual drug susceptibility/resistance with multiple strain infections), and population (e.g., transmission dynamics of competing strains, vaccine, and preventative therapy effects on circulating strains)-level implications are numerous [135]. Unlike many opportunistic infections that occur only with significant immunosuppression, TB can manifest with any degree of immunosuppression. If TB disease manifests in HIV-positive individuals who are not significantly immunosuppressed, then the disease course is similar to TB in HIV-negative individuals and is dominated by PTB in adults. If TB manifests once advanced HIV-associated immunosuppression has occurred, systemic disease involving multiple organs that lack well-defined granulomas with diffuse lesions is increasingly likely. Notably, all forms of EPTB have been described in HIV-associated TB, and this further complicates the clinical diagnosis of active TB in a resource-restricted setting. The specific nature of the immunological changes caused by HIV infection that drastically increase the likelihood of TB disease is complex and not fully understood [4, 136]. In general, untreated HIV infection leads to an absolute and functional decline in the cell-mediated immune response that is essential for maintaining lifelong immunological control of *Mycobacterium* spp. The destruction of T cells, specifically CD4+ cells in the granuloma by HIV, causes a change in the granuloma structure leading to the escape of viable bacilli.

Pediatric TB

The worldwide prevalence of maternal TB is unknown, but likely mirrors the female population TB burden. In high TB burden regions where TB diagnosis is frequently based on symptoms, diagnosis is challenging since pregnancy weight gain may temporarily mask TB-associated weight loss [137, 138]. Obstetric complications of TB include spontaneous abortion, small fundal height, preterm labor, low birth weight, and increased neonatal mortality. Congenital TB may be caused by hematogenous transmission of maternal MTBC through the umbilical vein to the fetal circulation, forming a primary hepatic complex. Alternatively, it is possible for the fetus to ingest or aspirate infected amniotic fluid or maternal blood during delivery. Congenital TB symptoms are nonspecific and difficult to distinguish from more common neonatal bacterial sepsis or viral infections, thus delaying timely diagnosis and treatment. While transmission via hematogenous spread in utero and/or aspiration of amniotic fluid during delivery is likely a rare occurrence, the true burden is difficult to estimate given the risk of spontaneous abortion and early infancy mortality associated with untreated congenital TB [139]. Indeed, pediatric TB is a major under-recognized cause of morbidity and mortality in young children (<5 years of age) from high-burden TB countries [140]. Newborns and young children can acquire infection in multiple ways, and once infected, they have a high risk of progressing to active TB disease and mortality, if untreated. Most young children who progress to disease do so within the first 12 months following primary infection. A bimodal risk profile is apparent with the greatest likelihood of progression in very young children (<2 years of age), decreasing to the lowest risk around 5–10 years of age. This is followed by a second increase in the likelihood of disease progression at the onset of puberty. Thereafter, TB in adolescents follows a course similar to adult-onset disease with PTB being the dominant phenotype.

Accurate and timely diagnosis and treatment of pediatric TB disease is critical to disease management in this population. Pediatric MDR-TB that is accurately and promptly diagnosed and treated has an excellent prognosis [34]. However, the biggest challenge remains in funneling children into a diagnostic pathway that results in prompt diagnosis and treatment. Diagnosis in resource-restricted regions is frequently based on symptoms, yet pediatric TB symptoms are nonspecific and shared by many other pediatric infections or conditions. Even if laboratory tests are available, obtaining biological specimens (e.g., gastric aspirates, sputum induction, bronchoalveolar lavage, cerebral spinal fluid) from young children is problematic in many settings. If specimens are available, the frequently low pediatric bacterial load may be insufficient for microscopy or culture detection. EPTB is proportionally more common in young children than in adults, and tuberculous meningitis represents the most severe manifestation of childhood TB. TB meningitis mostly affects young children (<3 years of age), and early signs and symptoms include fever, listlessness, failure to thrive, and headache—symptoms that may be misinterpreted as being due to infant malnutrition or other childhood infections. By the time non-TB infections such as pneumonia and non-TB meningitis, food insecurity, and inappropriate infant feeding methods have been ruled out, the prognosis may be grave. Better pediatric diagnostics, drugs, biomarkers and vaccines, improved pediatric TB surveillance that includes intensified tracing of pediatric contacts of active TB cases followed by recommended isoniazid preventive therapy (IPT) and integrated HIV, maternal, and child health services are high priority research and care goals.

Tuberculosis Prevention, Control, and Treatment

Many people still suffer and die from TB each year despite fundamental measures for controlling, treating, and curing TB being available for many decades. Implementation of effective drug treatment strategies resulted in a dramatic reduction in TB prevalence in high-income, low TB prevalence countries, so much so that many people living in these regions are surprised by the magnitude of the global TB burden. While reducing the TB burden remains a shared goal among public health experts, in the past, unintended consequences of declining TB prevalence were shifting healthcare resources needed to maintain TB prevention and control efforts and the abandonment of the drug development pipeline. The worldwide HIV epidemic starting in the 1980s brought TB back to the forefront, with drug-resistant TB demanding further attention, but the fact remains that in low-income countries the TB burden never waned and the high prevalence of LTBI, the ongoing HIV epidemic, emerging drug resistance, and the complex epidemiology and natural history of TB make TB control particularly challenging in LMICs.

Tuberculosis Control Strategy

From the perspective of an individual, TB control implies accurate and prompt diagnosis of persons with infectious TB, timely treatment with potent drugs, and monitoring the course of treatment to ensure disease resolution. Contact tracing of individuals with a known exposure to infectious TB allows implementation of prophylactic treatment to prevent disease progression among individuals at high risk (e.g., the very young) and implementation of TB treatment among individuals with active TB disease that has not yet been diagnosed. From a public health perspective, the goal of effective TB control is to ensure that each infectious TB case is prevented from transmitting the infection to another uninfected individual. Blocking forward transmission at the individual level will reduce the propagation of population-level TB transmission and therefore reduce the global TB burden (see Fig. 17.5).

WHO developed Directly Observed Therapy Short-Course (DOTS) as the cornerstone of global TB control after declaring TB a global emergency in 1994, with subsequent recommendation to reduce TB, summarized in their Stop TB Strategy [141]. The primary goals are to detect at least 70% of (sputum) smear-positive PTB cases and to successfully treat at least 85% of detected cases. Key elements are (1) to encourage government involvement and political will to support and finance TB control; (2) to maintain an accurate surveillance system to monitor the disease burden; (3) to sustain effective case detection through quality-assured diagnostic laboratories; (4) to provide reliable supplies and management of anti-TB drugs; and (5) to offer effective standardized short-course TB treatment for a duration of six months, with direct observation of treatment compliance with the DOTS approach for at least the first two months representing the typical period required to render an infectious case no longer infectious. If successfully implemented, DOTS is effective at reducing infectious TB. However, the program is not without controversy, primarily related to the necessity and efficacy of the direct observation component aimed at improving patient compliance that is linked to a reduction in the risk of treatment failure, relapse, and development of secondary drug resistance [142]. Additionally, since pediatric cases are less likely to be infectious given the paucibacillary nature of pediatric PTB and the higher proportion of EPTB, children have not been recognized as a TB control priority. A heavy reliance on sufficient political will and coordination of many governmental resources and infrastructure needed to fully implement DOTS also remains a barrier in many regions most affected by TB. Nevertheless, by 2013, many countries have made progress implementing DOTS and recent WHO data indicate that on average, 86% of new TB cases complete treatment [1]. Still, further efforts are required to meet targets for active case detection. The current status of 55% for all new and existing cases and the even lower 20% of estimated new MDR-TB cases detected [143] is a long way from the proposed 2020 target of 90% detection. While the proposed 2020 goal that 90% of all people with TB requiring treatment receive appropriate therapy that includes first line, second line as well as preventive therapy, is closer to the current successful treatment estimate of 86% for newly occurring cases, the current estimates of 65% for retreatment cases and 48% for MDR-TB cases indicate that further improvement is needed [143]. New additions to the DOTS strategy, such as integration of HIV, TB, and maternal and child health services, will further improve global control of TB and help lead efforts toward ending rather than only controlling TB.

Tuberculosis Diagnosis

For surveillance, the case definition of TB includes evidence of a positive culture, a positive acid-fast smear using microscopy combined with compatible clinical findings, or a characteristic illness with other evidence suggestive of TB combined with an appropriate response to TB therapy [1]. In many resource-restricted regions, TB diagnosis, and therefore treatment action, is made only on the basis of evidence suggestive of disease (e.g., clinical symptoms). This is problematic as many people are unaware of their MTBC exposure history, TB signs and symptoms are nonspecific, easy to misinterpret or miss altogether, and clinical specimens may be difficult to obtain or have few bacteria. Even if specimens are obtained and sufficient laboratory facilities are available, laboratory diagnostic testing that includes culturing requires a lengthy time between specimen collection and confirmation, from two to six weeks, such that individual patients may be lost to follow-up in the interim. In recent years, there has been considerable research and development of new diagnostic tools, including Xpert MTB/RIF (further described in last paragraph of this section).

The replication of large numbers of bacilli and accompanying inflammatory and tissue damage, usually in the lungs, along with the immune response that is triggered, leads to the signs and symptoms of active TB disease. Epidemiological investigation (e.g., history of MTBC exposure), clinical findings and symptoms (e.g., radiograph, cough, weight loss), skin tests (TST/Mantoux in those without history of BCG vaccination or prior TB disease), appropriate laboratory tests (sputum examination by microscopy and culture), and newer laboratory methods including interferon-gamma release assays (IGRAs) and Xpert MTB/RIF assays are the tools currently available to diagnose infection and active TB. The Mantoux tuberculin skin test (TST or Mantoux test) is a widely used method to detect infection that uses *M. tuberculosis*-derived protein antigen, or purified protein derivative (PPD) [144]. PPD is prepared from cultured tubercle bacilli and injected intracutaneously into the forearm using a standardized dose. After a period of 48–72 h, the size of the induration corresponds to the presence of activated T cells and macrophages. These cells have migrated to the site of PPD injection in order to mount a localized cellular response or delayed-type hypersensitivity reaction among MTBC-infected individuals. False-positive TST results are possible in people with non-tuberculous mycobacteria infection or who have had the BCG vaccination, both of which are common in LMICs. False-negative TST results can occur if a person is very young (e.g., <6 months), elderly, recently infected with *M. tuberculosis* (<8 weeks), recently vaccinated using live vaccines (e.g., measles, smallpox) or if experiencing immunosuppression associated with coexisting malnutrition, HIV or measles infection, leading to an impaired cellular immune response needed for PPD induration. Given the number and frequency of circumstances leading to false-positive and false-negative results, particularly in TB-endemic LMICs, TST can be used to screen for an immune response to infection, but to assess the likelihood of active TB disease, additional investigations (e.g., medical history, physical examination, X-ray, laboratory tests including diagnostic microbiology, culture) may be needed. In addition, some countries are replacing or adding to TST the use of IGRAs (see next paragraph), a decision based on the extent of BCG vaccination coverage, TB endemicity, and national resources. While both TST and IGRAs have advantages and disadvantages, at this time WHO does not recommend replacing TST with IGRAs to diagnose infection in LMICs [145].

IGRAs are whole-blood tests (QuantiFERON®-TB Gold In-Tube test, QFT-GIT; T-SPOT®.*TB* test, T-Spot) that indirectly detect *M. tuberculosis* infection through the measure of immune reactivity to *M. tuberculosis.* These tests have the advantage of providing a result within 24 h, but at a comparably higher cost than TST (e.g., in 2010, the estimated cost of QFT-GIT in Brazil was $48.26 compared to $10.56 for TST [146]). White blood cells in people with exposure to tuberculous bacilli will release interferon-gamma (IFN-γ) when mixed with antigens derived from *M. tuberculosis*, but not from BCG and non-tuberculous mycobacterial antigens. As a result, IGRAs may be particularly useful in people who have been vaccinated with BCG because prior BCG vaccination does not lead to a false-positive result. Given the rapid result, IGRAs are also suitable for people who may be unlikely to return for TST readings. IGRAs are less useful than TST in children <5 years of age because of the limited data available in this age group and high likelihood of false-negative or indeterminate IGRA results related to immune responses of young children. Overall, a positive IGRA result suggests that infection is likely and a negative result suggests that infection is unlikely, while an indeterminate result indicates an uncertain likelihood of infection. Like skin tests, a positive IGRA result should be used as an aid in diagnosing infection but diagnosis of active PTB or EPTB disease requires IGRAs to be considered in combination with a full medical examination to determine the likelihood of active disease [145].

Perhaps the most important recent advance in TB management is the development and rollout of the Xpert MTB/RIF assay [147]. Xpert MTB/RIF is a partially automated, cartridge-based nucleic amplification assay for the simultaneous detection of MTBC, including MDR-TB directly from rifampicin resistance and indirectly from predicted isoniazid resistance (e.g., rifampicin resistance predicts isoniazid resistance since they generally coexist). Key advantages of Xpert MTB/RIF include the ability to detect TB with minimal laboratory capacity (training, biosafety level) even in non-sputum (e.g., EPTB using gastric fluids, urine) and paucibacillary (e.g., HIV, pediatric) samples, and for results to be available in <2 h compared to culture-based methods requiring 2–6 weeks and greater laboratory capacity. Reducing the time to receive an accurate diagnosis ensures that diagnosis and treatment initiation are essentially simultaneous, and this reduces the likelihood TB cases fail to return to clinic to initiate treatment. Rapid diagnosis of rifampicin resistance also leads to appropriate initial treatment that improves individual care and TB control efforts. As with other nucleic acid amplification tests, the Xpert MTB/RIF assay should be interpreted along with clinical, radiographic, and other laboratory findings. In late 2013, WHO expanded its recommendations on the use of Xpert MTB/RIF to include the diagnosis of infection in children and with some forms of EPTB [148].

A current rollout initiative, The TBXpert Project [149] managed by the WHO Global TB Programme and the Stop TB Partnership secretariat and funded by UNITAID, is providing up to US $25.9 million for rollout of the Xpert MTB/RIF technology to 21 recipient countries. As a result of NGO—industry partnerships, PEPFAR, USAID, UNITAID, and the Bill & Melinda Gates Foundation reached an agreement with the manufacturer Cepheid to reduce the price of the Xpert MTB/RIF test to US$9.98 for the public sector in the 145 high TD burden LMICs eligible for concessional pricing [150]. The impact of this concessional pricing structure is notable in that more than 10 million tests have been distributed in four years (as of December 31, 2014).

Tuberculosis Therapy

Isoniazid alone, given for a period of 6 to 9 months, is commonly used for TB prophylaxis. In resource-limited countries, as well as middle-income countries with high TB burdens (>100 incident TB/100,000 population), children younger than five years at risk of infection following close or household contact with a TB case are recommended to receive TB prophylaxis, as are people suspected of having LTBI who are at high risk of disease progression (e.g., people living with HIV) [151]. Although LTBI treatment is unlikely to eradicate all bacilli from the body, if taken as prescribed, LTBI treatment greatly diminishes the chance of progression to active disease. It should be noted that LTBI treatment does not prevent future infections or disease progression from newly acquired infections, and therefore, additional TB treatment may be required, especially in TB-endemic regions where the risk of multiple lifetime transmissions is high.

Despite MTBC differences and the many different clinical manifestations of PTB and EPTB disease, once diagnosed, prophylaxis and treatment options are standardized when drug-resistant bacilli are not detected. Active TB disease is usually effectively treated with a course of four standard or first-line anti-TB drugs: isoniazid, rifampicin, pyrazinamide, and ethambutol. In a basic regimen using a DOTS approach (see *Tuberculosis Control Strategy* section), these four drugs are taken in combination daily during a two-month bacterial sterilizing phase when most of the bacteria are killed, followed by a treatment continuation phase consisting of daily isoniazid and rifampicin for an additional four months to ensure killing of persistent bacteria. Regimen modifications including frequency and drug choices are considered according to the presence of individual drug susceptibility and HIV infection. The comparatively long duration of treatment has an impact on treatment adherence and cure rates, development of side effects, and time to bacterial sterilization (and therefore impact on infection transmission and TB control). Any factor that diminishes the likelihood of a person adhering to the prescribed drug regimen dosage and duration increases the likelihood of developing secondary drug resistance. As a result, current therapeutic research priorities include the development of shorter-duration TB drug regimens.

MDR-TB is resistant to the two most effective first-line TB drugs, isoniazid and rifampicin. Since each of the four TB drugs has different advantages and modes of action, all are required to achieve good treatment outcomes. Drug resistance to isoniazid and rifampicin is associated with an increased risk of treatment failure, disease relapse, additional drug resistance, and death. XDR-TB is disease that is resistant to isoniazid and rifampicin, at least one fluoroquinolone antibiotic (e.g., ciprofloxacin, levofloxacin, ofloxacin), plus at least one of the three injectable second-line drugs (amikacin, kanamycin, or capreomycin) [15]. Primary MDR or XDR-TB occurs when a person is infected with drug-resistant bacilli, while secondary MDR and XDR-TB develop as a result of insufficient treatment efficacy due to poor treatment adherence, drug shortages, inappropriately prescribed medication regimens, drug malabsorption or drug–drug interactions, as well as drug resistance as a result of spontaneous tubercle bacillus mutations [15, 152–154].

Ten new or repurposed anti-TB drugs are currently in the late phases of clinical development, and in the last two years, two new drugs, bedaquiline and delamanid, have been approved for the treatment of MDR-TB under specific conditions [1]. Encouraging news from five of the 27 high MDR-TB burden countries indicates that a treatment success (e.g., cured or completed treatment) rate of ≥ 70% was achieved in Ethiopia, Kazakhstan, Myanmar, Pakistan, and Viet Nam; however, this is offset by the overall treatment success proportion of only 48% in the 126 countries (including all 27 high MDR-TB burden countries) reporting treatment outcomes for people initiating MDR-TB therapy in 2011 due to high mortality and loss to follow-up. While 97,000 patients were started on MDR-TB treatment in 2013, representing a threefold increase compared with 2009, almost 40,000 were on waiting lists. Importantly, the gap between diagnosis and treatment widened between 2012 and 2013 in several countries, with the highest gaps among the high MDR-TB burden countries observed in

Myanmar, Tajikistan, and South Africa [1]. A DOTS-Plus approach has been proposed by the WHO to tackle drug-resistant TB. The DOTS-Plus for MDR-TB management strategy adds components to a well-functioning basic DOTS program and strives for high treatment completion rates and high case detection combined with advocacy for the provision of affordable second-line anti-TB medications. In practice, the high level of financial and governmental capacity required to implement DOTS-Plus is a serious challenge for many of the most affected countries. The drugs for treating an MDR-TB case can cost over $5000 with overall treatment costs exceeding $250,000 in XDR-TB cases [155], and the longer duration of MDR-TB treatment ($\geq$20 months) is burdensome on healthcare systems already under resource constraints.

Additional considerations in the management of HIV-associated TB disease are needed [156]. Intensifying HIV testing efforts, providing isoniazid preventative therapy, and ensuring universal access to antiretroviral therapy soon after HIV diagnosis have been shown to reduce the HIV-associated TB burden as well as the likelihood of immune reconstitution inflammatory syndrome (IRIS) and mortality. In 2013, only 48% of TB cases worldwide had a documented HIV test result, with a greater proportion who knew their status in Africa [1]. While the September 30, 2015, update to WHO guidelines indicating antiretroviral treatment should be initiated as soon as a positive HIV infection diagnosis has been made [157], however, the 2013 estimate of only 70% of TB patients known to have HIV infection who were on antiretroviral treatment falls considerably short of the 100% goal [1]. Estimates of TB prophylaxis in people living with HIV infection lagged far behind with only 21% of countries worldwide, and 14/41 high TB/HIV burden countries, offering recommended prophylaxis in 2013 [1]. WHO strongly recommends that people living with HIV infection who are unlikely to have active TB should receive at least six months of isoniazid preventive therapy as part of a comprehensive package of HIV care [158]. Additionally, there is evidence that giving isoniazid preventive therapy for at least 36 months may be particularly beneficial in setting with a high prevalence of TB and a high likelihood of transmission, i.e., a high risk of new infections, while consensus evidence in support of longer duration or lifelong preventive therapy is unavailable at the present time [158].

Tuberculosis Prevention Through Vaccination

Vaccines remain the single most important tool to prevent infectious diseases. The only currently available TB vaccine, BCG, was developed in 1921 by Léon Charles Albert Calmette (1863–1933) and Camille Guérin (1872–1961). This vaccine was among the first available vaccines and is derived from a live attenuated non-virulent *M. bovis* strain, also known as *M. bovis* BCG. BCG use is widespread, covering over 80% of infants worldwide through its inclusion in the WHO Expanded Programme on Immunization [159]. The vaccine is given to infants at birth or shortly thereafter in a single intradermal or percutaneous injection. Given the increased risk of persistent or disseminated BCG disease in immunocompromised individuals [160], the WHO Global Advisory Committee on Vaccine Safety advises that BCG vaccination is contraindicated if HIV infection is known. Vaccination provides variable protection against disease progression to miliary (disseminated) TB or TB meningitis in uninfected individuals, but does not provide protection against primary TB infection or LTBI [161]. Overall, this means that while vaccinated children may be protected against severe and often fatal forms of early childhood TB, the vaccine does not provide sufficient efficacy to offer longer-term protection against adult TB disease.

Given the significant limitations of BCG, new TB vaccine approaches are needed to reduce the global TB burden and minimize the likelihood of drug-resistant strains [162]. Over the last two decades, considerable progress has been made [163]. Preclinical vaccine candidates and more than a dozen vaccines in clinical trials have been developed either as BCG vaccine boosters or as novel vaccines to replace BCG. Key challenges that new vaccines must meet are the ability to offer protection against infection in people already exposed to non-tuberculous mycobacteria [164] that are ubiquitous in hot climates and may alter vaccine efficacy through unidentified mechanisms (e.g., pre-exposure protection) or those infected with MTBC (e.g., postexposure or postinfection protection against disease progression), against all MTBC strains and forms of TB disease, and among people with HIV infection (e.g., therapeutic protection).

Conclusions

Treatment with multiple antibiotics, ensuring people complete their prescribed treatment course, and actively tracing individuals that may have been infected remain the best measures for containing the spread of TB. However, new tools for early detection and rapid and effective infection control are needed to stem transmission. It is also clear that more "upstream" approaches that take into account the role of poverty, substandard housing, malnutrition, HIV epidemic characteristics, and broader socioeconomic disparities are also needed. Interventions that explore the complex interplay between biological and structural phenomena driving the current TB epidemic may help to change the tide and push back this disease which continues to affect so many people worldwide.

Discussion Points

- How do poverty and tuberculosis interact, before antibiotic treatment became available and now that treatment is available (think of a specific setting)?
- Which factors influence the risk of becoming infected with TB, and which is the risk of progressing from latent infection to disease?
- How does the epidemiology of tuberculosis differ between low-, middle-, and high-income countries? And how should tuberculosis control in high-income countries respond to increased migration from low- and middle-income countries? Think also of higher-risk groups in high-income countries.
- How has the emergence of HIV altered the control of tuberculosis?
- How can tests, such as the Xpert MTB/RIF assay, that give results within <2 h make a substantial difference in TB control?
- For which groups of people is preventive TB therapy indicated and why?

References

1. World Health Organization. Global tuberculosis report 2014. World Health Organization; 2014.
2. Tan de Bibiana J, Rossi C, Rivest P, Zwerling A, Thibert L, McIntosh F, et al. Tuberculosis and homelessness in Montreal: a retrospective cohort study. BMC Public Health. 2011;11:833.
3. Commission on Social Determinants of Health. Closing the gap in a generation: health equity through action on the social determinants of health. Final Report of the Commission on Social Determinants of Health. Geneva: World Health Organization; 2008.
4. Pawlowski A, Jansson M, Skold M, Rottenberg ME, Kallenius G. Tuberculosis and HIV co-infection. PLoS Pathog. 2012;8(2):e1002464.
5. Dye C, Scheele S, Dolin P, Pathania V, Raviglione RC, Project WHOGSM. Global burden of tuberculosis—estimated incidence, prevalence, and mortality by country. JAMA (J Am Med Assoc). 1999;282(7):677–86.

6. Salo WL, Aufderheide AC, Buikstra J, Holcomb TA. Identification of mycobacterium-tuberculosis dna in a pre-columbian peruvian mummy. Proc Natl Acad Sci USA. 1994;91(6):2091–4.
7. Nerlich AG, Haas CJ, Zink A, Sziemles U, Hagedorn HG. Molecular evidence for tuberculosis in an ancient Egyptian mummy. Lancet. 1997;350(9088):1404.
8. Marten B. A new theory of consumptions, more especially of a phthisis or consumption of the lungs. London: Printed for R. Knaplock; A. Bell; J. Hooke, and C. King; 1720.
9. Daniel TM. Captain of death: the story of tuberculosis. Rochester, NY: University of Rochester Press; 1999.
10. Rogers K. Bacterial diseases: leprosy and tuberculosis. In: Rogers K, editor. Infectious diseases (Health and Disease in Society). New York: Rosen Education Service; 2011. p. 35–44.
11. Cantwell MF, Snider DE, Cauthen GM, Onorato IM. Epidemiology of tuberculosis in the United-States, 1985 through 1992. JAMA (J Am Med Assoc). 1994;272(7):535–9.
12. Streicher EM, Muller B, Chihota V, Mlambo C, Tait M, Pillay M, et al. Emergence and treatment of multidrug resistant (MDR) and extensively drug-resistant (XDR) tuberculosis in South Africa. Infect Genet Evol. 2012;12 (4):686–94 (Epub 2011/08/16).
13. World Health Organization. Tuberculosis fact sheet. Geneva, Switzerland: World Health Organization; 2014.
14. Lawn SD, Zumla AI. Tuberculosis. Lancet. 2011;378(9785):57–72.
15. Dheda K, Gumbo T, Gandhi NR, Murray M, Theron G, Udwadia Z, et al. Global control of tuberculosis: from extensively drug-resistant to untreatable tuberculosis. Lancet Respir Med. 2014;2(4):321–38.
16. Glaziou P, Falzon D, Floyd K, Raviglione M. Global epidemiology of tuberculosis. Semin Respir Crit Care Med. 2013;34(1):3–16 (Epub 2013/03/06).
17. Drobniewski F, Balabanova Y, Ruddy M, Weldon L, Jeltkova K, Brown T, et al. Rifampin- and multidrug-resistant tuberculosis in russian civilians and prison inmates: dominance of the beijing strain family. Emerg Infect Dis. 2002;8(11):1320–6.
18. Wright A, Zignol M, Van Deun A, Falzon D, Gerdes SR, Feldman K, et al. Epidemiology of antituberculosis drug resistance 2002–07: an updated analysis of the global project on anti-tuberculosis drug resistance surveillance. Lancet. 2009;373(9678):1861–73.
19. Anderson SR, Maguire H, Carless J. Tuberculosis in London: a decade and a half of no decline. Thorax. 2007;62 (2):162–7.
20. Cain KP, Benoit SR, Winston CA, Mac Kenzie WR. Tuberculosis among foreign-born persons in the United States. JAMA (J Am Med Assoc). 2008;300(4):405–12.
21. de Bruyn G, Adams GJ, Teeter LD, Soini H, Musser JM, Graviss EA. The contribution of ethnicity to *Mycobacterium tuberculosis* strain clustering. Int J Tuberc Lung Dis. 2001;5(7):633–41.
22. Baker M, Das D, Venugopal K, Howden-Chapman P. Tuberculosis associated with household crowding in a developed country. J Epidemiol Comm Health. 2008;62(8):715–21.
23. Centers for Disease Control & Prevention. Trends in tuberculosis—United States, 2011. MMWR (Morb Mortal Wkly Rep). 2012;61(11):181–5.
24. Acevedo-Garcia D. Zip code-level risk factors for tuberculosis: neighborhood environment and residential segregation in New Jersey, 1985–1992. Am J Public Health. 2001;91(5):734–41.
25. Williams G, Applewhite J. Tuberculosis in the Negroes of Georgia: economic, racial and constitutional aspects. Am J Hyg. 1939;29:61–109.
26. Stout JE, Saharia KK, Nageswaran S, Ahmed A, Hamilton CD. Racial and ethnic disparities in pediatric tuberculosis in North Carolina. Arch Pediatr Adolesc Med. 2006;160(6):631–7.
27. AHRQ. National healthcare disparities report. Rockville, MD2010. Available from: http://www.ahrq.gov/research/findings/nhqrdr/nhdr10/Ackno.html.
28. Cantwell MF, McKenna MT, McCray E, Onorato IM. Tuberculosis and race/ethnicity in the United States: impact of socioeconomic status. Am J Respir Crit Care Med. 1998;157(4 Pt 1):1016–20.
29. Serpa JA, Teeter LD, Musser JM, Graviss EA. Tuberculosis disparity between US-born blacks and whites, Houston, Texas, USA. Emerg Infect Dis. 2009;15(6):899–904.
30. Tollefson D, Bloss E, Fanning A, Redd JT, Barker K, McCray E. Burden of tuberculosis in indigenous peoples globally: a systematic review. Int J Tuberc Lung Dis (Official Journal of the International Union against Tuberculosis and Lung Disease). 2013;17(9):1139–50.
31. Bloss E, Holtz TH, Jereb J, Redd JT, Podewils LJ, Cheek JE, et al. TB in Indigenous peoples in the US, 2003–2008; 2011.
32. Pontororing GJ, Kenangalem E, Lolong DB, Waramori G, Sandjaja Tjitra E, et al. The burden and treatment of HIV in tuberculosis patients in Papua Province, Indonesia: a prospective observational study. BMC Infect Dis. 2010;10:9.
33. Nelson LJ, Wells CD. Global epidemiology of childhood tuberculosis. Int J Tuberc Lung Dis (The Official Journal of the International Union against Tuberculosis and Lung Disease). 2004;8(5):636–47.
34. Marais BJ. Tuberculosis in children. J Paediatr Child Health. 2014;50(10):759–67.

35. Rieder H, Cauthen G, Kelly G, Bloch A, Snider DJ. Tuberculosis in the United States. JAMA (J Am Med Assoc). 1989;262(3):385–9.
36. Horwitz O, Knudsen J. A follow-up study of tuberculosis incidence and general mortality in various occupational-social groups of the Danish population. Bull World Health Organ. 1961;24:793–805.
37. Oren E, Winston CA, Pratt R, Robison VA, Narita M. Epidemiology of urban tuberculosis in the United States, 2000–2007. Am J Public Health. 2011;101(7):1256–63.
38. de Vries G, Aldridge RW, Cayla JA, Haas WH, Sandgren A, van Hest NA, et al. Epidemiology of tuberculosis in big cities of the European Union and European Economic Area countries. Eurosurveillance. 2014;19(9):22–9.
39. Chaulk CP, Moore-Rice K, Rizzo R, Chaisson RE. Eleven years of community-based directly observed therapy for tuberculosis. JAMA (J Am Med Assoc). 1995;274(12):945–51.
40. Brudney K, Dobkin J. Resurgent tuberculosis in New York City. Human immunodeficiency virus, homelessness, and the decline of tuberculosis control programs. Am Rev Respir Dis. 1991;144(4):745–9.
41. Rose RC 3rd, McGowan JE Jr. Urban tuberculosis: some modern problems. Am J Med Sci. 1984;287(1):24–6.
42. Clark M, Riben P, Nowgesic E. The association of housing density, isolation and tuberculosis in Canadian First Nations communities. Int J Epidemiol. 2002;31(5):940–5.
43. Chen W, Shu W, Wang M, Hou Y, Xia Y, Xu W, et al. Pulmonary tuberculosis incidence and risk factors in rural areas of China: a cohort study. PLoS ONE. 2013;8(3):e58171.
44. Buu TN, van Soolingen D, Huyen MN, Lan NN, Quy HT, Tiemersma EW, et al. Tuberculosis acquired outside of households, rural Vietnam. Emerg Infect Dis. 2010;16(9):1466–8.
45. Van't Hoog AH, Marston BJ, Ayisi JG, Agaya JA, Muhenje O, Odeny LO, et al. Risk factors for inadequate TB case finding in Rural Western Kenya: a comparison of actively and passively identified TB patients. PLoS ONE. 2013;8(4):e61162.
46. Dowdy DW, Cattamanchi A, Steingart KR, Pai M. Is scale-up worth it? Challenges in economic analysis of diagnostic tests for tuberculosis. PLoS Med. 2011;8(7):e1001063 (Epub 2011/08/05).
47. Hargreaves S, Carballo M, Friedland JS. Screening migrants for tuberculosis: where next? Lancet Infect Dis. 2009;9(3):139–40.
48. Pottie K, Janakiram P, Topp P, McCarthy A. Prevalence of selected preventable and treatable diseases among government-assisted refugees: implications for primary care providers. Can Fam Physician (Medecin de famille canadien). 2007;53(11):1928–34.
49. Centers for Disease Control & Prevention. Trends in tuberculosis–United States, 2012. MMWR (Morb Mortal Wkly Rep). 2013;62(11):201–5.
50. Menzies HJ, Winston CA, Holtz TH, Cain KP, Mac Kenzie WR. Epidemiology of tuberculosis among US- and foreign-born children and adolescents in the United States, 1994–2007. Am J Public Health. 2010;100(9):1724–9.
51. Odone A, Ricco M, Morandi M, Borrini BM, Pasquarella C, Signorelli C. Epidemiology of tuberculosis in a low-incidence Italian region with high immigration rates: differences between not Italy-born and Italy-born TB cases. BMC Public Health. 2011;11:376.
52. Inigo J, Garcia de Viedma D, Arce A, Palenque E, Alonso Rodriguez N, Rodriguez E, et al. Analysis of changes in recent tuberculosis transmission patterns after a sharp increase in immigration. J Clin Microbiol. 2007;45(1):63–9.
53. World Health Organization. Tuberculosis control in prisons: a manual for programme managers. Geneva: WHO; 2000.
54. Kim S, Crittenden KS. Risk factors for tuberculosis among inmates: a retrospective analysis. Public Health Nurs. 2005;22(2):108–18.
55. MacNeil JR, Lobato MN, Moore M. An unanswered health disparity: tuberculosis among correctional inmates, 1993 through 2003. Am J Public Health. 2005;95(10):1800–5.
56. White MC, Tulsky JP, Portillo CJ, Menendez E, Cruz E, Goldenson J. Tuberculosis prevalence in an urban jail: 1994 and 1998. Int J Tuberc Lung Dis (The Official Journal of the International Union against Tuberculosis and Lung Disease). 2001;5(5):400–4.
57. Cummings KC, Mohle-Boetani J, Royce SE, Chin DP. Movement of tuberculosis patients and the failure to complete antituberculosis treatment. Am J Respir Crit Care Med. 1998;157(4 Pt 1):1249–52 (Epub 1998/05/01).
58. Thiede H, Romero M, Bordelon K, Hagan H, Murrill CS. Using a jail-based survey to monitor HIV and risk behaviors among Seattle area injection drug users. J Urban Health (Bulletin of the New York Academy of Medicine). 2001;78(2):264–78 (Epub 2001/06/23).
59. Martin V, Gonzalez P, Cayla JA, Mirabent J, Canellas J, Pina JM, et al. Case-finding of pulmonary tuberculosis on admission to a penitentiary centre. Tubercle Lung Dis (The Official Journal of the International Union Against Tuberculosis and Lung Disease). 1994;75(1):49–53 (Epub 1994/02/01).
60. Drobniewski FA, Balabanova YM, Ruddy MC, Graham C, Kuznetzov SI, Gusarova GI, et al. Tuberculosis, HIV seroprevalence and intravenous drug abuse in prisoners. Eur Resp J. 2005;26(2):298–304.
61. Stuckler D, Basu S, McKee M, King L. Mass incarceration can explain population increases in TB and multidrug-resistant TB in European and central Asian countries. Proc Natl Acad Sci U S A. 2008;105(36):13280–5.

62. Shilova MV, Dye C. The resurgence of tuberculosis in Russia. Philos Trans R Soc Lond Ser B-Biol Sci. 2001;356 (1411):1069–75.
63. Perlman DC, Salomon N, Perkins MP, Yancovitz S, Paone D, Des Jarlais DC. Tuberculosis in drug users. Clin Infect Dis (An Official Publication of the Infectious Diseases Society of America). 1995;21(5):1253–64.
64. Chin DP, Cummings KC, Sciortino S, Snyder DC, Johnson LF, Westenhouse JL, et al. Progress and problems in achieving the United States national target for completion of antituberculosis treatment. Int J Tuberc Lung Dis (The Official Journal of the International Union Against Tuberculosis and Lung Disease). 2000;4(8):744–51.
65. Oeltmann J, Kammerer J, Pevzner E, Moonan P. Tuberculosis and substance abuse in the United States, 1997–2006. Arch Intern Med. 2009;169(2):189–97.
66. Sterling TR. Report from the 38th IDSA: tuberculosis & HIV. Hopkins HIV Rep (A Bimonthly Newsletter for Healthcare Providers/Johns Hopkins University AIDS Service). 2000;12(5):2.
67. Malakmadze N, Gonzalez IM, Oemig T, Isiadinso I, Rembert D, McCauley MM, et al. Unsuspected recent transmission of tuberculosis among high-risk groups: implications of universal tuberculosis genotyping in its detection. Clin Infect Dis (An Official Publication of the Infectious Diseases Society of America). 2005;40 (3):366–73.
68. Macq J, Solis A, Martinez G, Martiny P, Dujardin B. An exploration of the social stigma of tuberculosis in five "municipios" of Nicaragua to reflect on local interventions. Health Policy. 2005;74(2):205–17 (Epub 2005/09/13).
69. Dodor EA, Neal K, Kelly S. An exploration of the causes of tuberculosis stigma in an urban district in Ghana. Int J Tuberc Lung Dis (The Official Journal of the International Union against Tuberculosis and Lung Disease). 2008;12(9):1048–54 (Epub 2008/08/21).
70. Sengupta S, Pungrassami P, Balthip Q, Strauss R, Kasetjaroen Y, Chongsuvivatwong V, et al. Social impact of tuberculosis in southern Thailand: views from patients, care providers and the community. Int J Tuberc Lung Dis (The Official Journal of the International Union against Tuberculosis and Lung Disease). 2006;10(9):1008–12 (Epub 2006/09/13).
71. Coreil J, Lauzardo M, Heurtelou M. Cultural feasibility assessment of tuberculosis prevention among persons of Haitian origin in South Florida. J Immigr Health. 2004;6(2):63–9 (Epub 2004/03/12).
72. Osei E, Akweongo P, Binka F. Factors associated with DELAY in diagnosis among tuberculosis patients in Hohoe Municipality,Ghana. BMC Public Health. 2015;15:721 (Epub 2015/07/30).
73. Kipp AM, Pungrassami P, Stewart PW, Chongsuvivatwong V, Strauss RP, Van Rie A. Study of tuberculosis and AIDS stigma as barriers to tuberculosis treatment adherence using validated stigma scales. Int J Tuberc Lung Dis (The Official Journal of the International Union against Tuberculosis and Lung Disease) 2011;15(11):1540–5, i (Epub 2011/10/20).
74. McShane H. Co-infection with HIV and TB: double trouble. Int J STD & AIDS. 2005;16(2):95–100; quiz 1 (Epub 2005/04/06).
75. Baussano I, Nunn P, Williams B, Pivetta E, Bugiani M, Scano F. Tuberculosis among health care workers. Emerg Infect Dis. 2011;17(3):488–94 (Epub 2011/03/12).
76. Baker MA, Lin HH, Chang HY, Murray MB. The risk of tuberculosis disease among persons with diabetes mellitus: a prospective cohort study. Clin Infect Dis. 2012;54(6):818–25.
77. Stevenson CR, Forouhi NG, Roglic G, Williams BG, Lauer JA, Dye C, et al. Diabetes and tuberculosis: the impact of the diabetes epidemic on tuberculosis incidence. BMC Public Health. 2007;7:8.
78. Baker MA, Harries AD, Jeon CY, Hart JE, Kapur A, Lonnroth K, et al. The impact of diabetes on tuberculosis treatment outcomes: a systematic review. BMC Med. 2011;9:15.
79. Bock NN, Jensen PA, Miller B, Nardell E. Tuberculosis infection control in resource-limited settings in the era of expanding HIV care and treatment. J Infect Dis. 2007;196(Suppl 1):S108–13 (Epub 2007/08/30).
80. Fennelly KP, Martyny JW, Fulton KE, Orme IM, Cave DM, Heifets LB. Cough-generated aerosols of Mycobacterium tuberculosis—a new method to study infectiousness. Am J Respir Crit Care Med. 2004;169 (5):604–9.
81. Loudon RG, Spohn SK. Cough frequency and infectivity in patients with pulmonary tuberculosis. Am Rev Respir Dis. 1969;99(1):109.
82. Jones-Lopez EC, Namugga O, Mumbowa F, Ssebidandi M, Mbabazi O, Moine S, et al. Cough aerosols of Mycobacterium tuberculosis predict new infection: a household contact study. Am J Respir Crit Care Med. 2013;187(9):1007–15 (Epub 2013/01/12).
83. Loudon RG, Roberts RM. Singing and dissemination of tuberculosis. Am Rev Respir Dis. 1968;98(2):297.
84. Riley RL, Mills CC, Nyka W, Weinstock N, Storey PB, Sultan LU, et al. Aerial dissemination of pulmonary tuberculosis—a 2-year study of contagion in a tuberculosis ward (reprinted). Am J Epidemiol. 1995;142(1):3–14
85. Riley RL, Shivpuri DN, Wittstadt F, Ogrady F, Sultan LU, Mills CC. Infectiousness of air from a tuberculosis ward—ultraviolet irradiation of infected air—comparative infectiousness of different patients. Am Rev Respir Dis. 1962;85(4):511.

86. Escombe AR, Moore DAJ, Gilman RH, Navincopa M, Ticona E, Mitchell B, et al. Upper-room ultraviolet light and negative air ionization to prevent tuberculosis transmission. PLoS Med. 2009;6(3):12.
87. Nolan CM, Blumberg HM, Taylor Z, Bernardo J, Brennan PJ, Dunlap NE, et al. American thoracic society/centers for disease control and prevention/infectious diseases society of America: controlling tuberculosis in the United States. Am J Respir Crit Care Med. 2005;172(9):1169–227.
88. Weir MR, Thornton GF. Extrapulmonary tuberculosis—experience of a community-hospital and review of the literature. Am J Med. 1985;79(4):467–78.
89. Comstock GW. Frost revisited—modern epidemiology of tuberculosis. Am J Epidemiol. 1975;101(5):363–82.
90. Lauzardo M, Lee P, Duncan H, Hale Y. Transmission of *Mycobacterium tuberculosis* to a funeral director during routine embalming. Chest. 2001;119(2):640–2 (Epub 2001/02/15).
91. Lauzardo M, Rubin J. Mycobacterial disinfection. In: Block SS, editor. Disinfection, sterilization, and preservation. Philadelphia, PA: Lippincott Williams & Wilkins; 2001. p. 513–28.
92. Espiritu N, Aguirre L, Jave O, Sanchez L, Kirwan DE, Gilman RH. Congenital transmission of multidrug-resistant tuberculosis. Am J Trop Med Hyg. 2014;91(1):92–5 (Epub 2014/05/14).
93. Lee LH, LeVea CM, Graman PS. Congenital tuberculosis in a neonatal intensive care unit: case report, epidemiological investigation, and management of exposures. Clin Infect Dis (An Official Publication of the Infectious Diseases Society of America). 1998;27(3):474–7 (Epub 1998/10/14).
94. Perez-Lago L, Navarro Y, Garcia-de-Viedma D. Current knowledge and pending challenges in zoonosis caused by *Mycobacterium bovis*: a review. Res Vet Sci. 2013;97:S94–100.
95. Torres-Gonzalez P, Soberanis-Ramos O, Martinez-Gamboa A, Chavez-Mazari B, Barrios-Herrera MT, Torres-Rojas M, et al. Prevalence of latent and active tuberculosis among dairy farm workers exposed to cattle infected by *Mycobacterium bovis*. PLoS Neglected Trop Dis. 2013;7(4):e2177.
96. Lienhardt C. From exposure to disease: the role of environmental factors in susceptibility to and development of tuberculosis. Epidemiol Rev. 2001;23(2):288–301.
97. Lygizos M, Shenoi SV, Brooks RP, Bhushan A, Brust JC, Zelterman D, et al. Natural ventilation reduces high TB transmission risk in traditional homes in rural KwaZulu-Natal, South Africa. BMC Infect Dis. 2013;13:300.
98. Drucker E, Alcabes P, Bosworth W, Sckell B. Childhood tuberculosis in the Bronx, New York. Lancet. 1994;343 (8911):1482–5.
99. Lienhardt C, Fielding K, Sillah J, Tunkara A, Donkor S, Manneh K, et al. Risk factors for tuberculosis infection in sub-Saharan Africa: a contact study in The Gambia. Am J Respir Crit Care Med. 2003;168(4):448–55.
100. Dooley SW Jr, Castro KG, Hutton MD, Mullan RJ, Polder JA, Snider DE Jr. Guidelines for preventing the transmission of tuberculosis in health-care settings, with special focus on HIV-related issues. MMWR Recommendations Rep (Morbidity and Mortality Weekly Report Recommendations and Reports/Centers for Disease Control). 1990;39(Rr-17):1–29 (Epub 1990/12/07).
101. Feja K, Saiman L. Tuberculosis in children. Clin Chest Med. 2005;26(2):295–312, vii.
102. Jones-Lopez EC, Kim S, Fregona G, Marques-Rodrigues P, Hadad DJ, Molina LPD, et al. Importance of cough and *M. tuberculosis* strain type as risks for increased transmission within households. PLoS ONE. 2014;9(7):12.
103. Kamat SR, Dawson JJ, Devadatta S, Fox W, Janardhanam B, Radhakrishna S, et al. A controlled study of the influence of segregation of tuberculous patients for one year on the attack rate of tuberculosis in a 5-year period in close family contacts in South India. Bull World Health Organ. 1966;34(4):517–32 (Epub 1966/01/01).
104. Abuogi LL, Mwachari C, Leslie HH, Shade SB, Otieno J, Yienya N, et al. Impact of expanded antiretroviral use on incidence and prevalence of tuberculosis in children with HIV in Kenya. Int J Tuberc Lung Dis. 2013;17 (10):1291–7.
105. Greenaway C, Sandoe A, Vissandjee B, Kitai I, Gruner D, Wobeser W, et al. Tuberculosis: evidence review for newly arriving immigrants and refugees. Can Med Assoc J. 2011;183(12):E939–51.
106. Lonnroth K, Jaramillo E, Williams BG, Dye C, Raviglione M. Drivers of tuberculosis epidemics: the role of risk factors and social determinants. Soc Sci Med. 2009;68(12):2240–6.
107. Möller M, Hoal EG. Current findings, challenges and novel approaches in human genetic susceptibility to tuberculosis. Tuberculosis. 2010;90(2):71–83.
108. Bellamy R. Genetic susceptibility to tuberculosis in human populations. Thorax. 1998;53(7):588–93.
109. Pan H, Yan BS, Rojas M, Shebzukhov YV, Zhou H, Kobzik L, et al. Ipr1 gene mediates innate immunity to tuberculosis. Nature. 2005;434(7034):767–72 (Epub 2005/04/09).
110. Willis MD, Winston CA, Heilig CM, Cain KP, Walter ND, Mac Kenzie WR. Seasonality of tuberculosis in the United States, 1993–2008. Clin Infect Dis (An Official Publication of the Infectious Diseases Society of America). 2012;54(11):1553–60 (Epub 2012/04/05).
111. Fares A. Seasonality of tuberculosis. J Global Infect Dis. 2011;3(1):46–55 (Epub 2011/05/17).
112. Koh GC, Hawthorne G, Turner AM, Kunst H, Dedicoat M. Tuberculosis incidence correlates with sunshine: an ecological 28-year time series study. PLoS ONE. 2013;8(3):e57752 (Epub 2013/03/14).
113. de Jong BC, Antonio M, Gagneux S. Mycobacterium africanum—review of an important cause of human tuberculosis in West Africa. PLoS Neglected Trop Dis. 2010;4(9):e744.

114. Hesseling AC, Cotton MF, Fordham von Reyn C, Graham SM, Gie RP, Hussey GD. Consensus statement on the revised World Health Organization recommendations for BCG vaccination in HIV-infected infants. Int J Tuberc Lung Dis (The Official Journal of the International Union against Tuberculosis and Lung Disease). 2008;12 (12):1376–9.

115. Gagneux S. Host-pathogen coevolution in human tuberculosis. Philos Trans R Soc Lond B Biol Sci. 2012;367 (1590):850–9.

116. Prodinger WM, Indra A, Koksalan OK, Kilicaslan Z, Richter E. Mycobacterium caprae infection in humans. Expert Rev Anti-Infect Ther. 2014;12(12):1501–13.

117. Panteix G, Gutierrez MC, Boschiroli ML, Rouviere M, Plaidy A, Pressac D, et al. Pulmonary tuberculosis due to *Mycobacterium microti*: a study of six recent cases in France. J Med Microbiol. 2010;59(Pt 8):984–9.

118. van Ingen J, Rahim Z, Mulder A, Boeree MJ, Simeone R, Brosch R, et al. Characterization of *Mycobacterium orygis* as *M. tuberculosis* complex subspecies. Emerg Infect Dis. 2012;18(4):653–5.

119. Ueyama M, Chikamatsu K, Aono A, Murase Y, Kuse N, Morimoto K, et al. Sub-speciation of *Mycobacterium tuberculosis* complex from tuberculosis patients in Japan. Tuberculosis (Edinb). 2014;94(1):15–9.

120. Kiers A, Klarenbeek A, Mendelts B, Van Soolingen D, Koeter G. Transmission of *Mycobacterium pinnipedii* to humans in a zoo with marine mammals. Int J Tuberc Lung Dis (The Official Journal of the International Union against Tuberculosis and Lung Dis). 2008;12(12):1469–73.

121. Gagneux S, Small PM. Global phylogeography of *Mycobacterium tuberculosis* and implications for tuberculosis product development. Lancet Infect Dis. 2007;7(5):328–37.

122. Click ES, Moonan PK, Winston CA, Cowan LS, Oeltmann JE. Relationship between *Mycobacterium tuberculosis* phylogenetic lineage and clinical site of tuberculosis. Clin Infect Dis (An Official Publication of the Infectious Diseases Society of America). 2012;54(2):211–9 (Epub 2011/12/27).

123. Cowley D, Govender D, February B, Wolfe M, Steyn L, Evans J, et al. Recent and rapid emergence of W-Beijing strains of *Mycobacterium tuberculosis* in Cape Town, South Africa. Clin Infect Dis (An Official Publication of the Infectious Diseases Society of America). 2008;47(10):1252–9 (Epub 2008/10/07).

124. Parwati I, Alisjahbana B, Apriani L, Soetikno RD, Ottenhoff TH, van der Zanden AG, et al. *Mycobacterium tuberculosis* Beijing genotype is an independent risk factor for tuberculosis treatment failure in Indonesia. J Infect Dis. 2010;201(4):553–7 (Epub 2010/01/13).

125. Grode L, Seiler P, Baumann S, Hess J, Brinkmann V, Nasser Eddine A, et al. Increased vaccine efficacy against tuberculosis of recombinant *Mycobacterium bovis* bacille Calmette-Guerin mutants that secrete listeriolysin. J Clin Investig. 2005;115(9):2472–9 (Epub 2005/08/20).

126. Colditz GA, Brewer TF, Berkey CS, Wilson ME, Burdick E, Fineberg HV, et al. Efficacy of BCG vaccine in the prevention of tuberculosis. Meta-analysis of the published literature. JAMA (J Am Med Assoc). 1994;271 (9):698–702 (Epub 1994/03/02).

127. Cantrell SA, Pascopella L, Flood J, Crane CM, Kendall LV, Riley LW. Community-wide transmission of a strain of *Mycobacterium tuberculosis* that causes reduced lung pathology in mice. J Med Microbiol. 2008;57(Pt 1):21–7 (Epub 2007/12/11).

128. O'Garra A, Redford PS, McNab FW, Bloom CI, Wilkinson RJ, Berry MP. The immune response in tuberculosis. Annu Rev Immunol. 2013;31:475–527.

129. Pagan AJ, Ramakrishnan L. Immunity and immunopathology in the tuberculous granuloma. Cold Spring Harb Perspect Med. 2014.

130. Tiemersma EW, van der Werf MJ, Borgdorff MW, Williams BG, Nagelkerke NJD. Natural history of tuberculosis: duration and fatality of untreated pulmonary tuberculosis in HIV negative patients: a systematic review. PLoS ONE. 2011;6(4):e17601.

131. Naing C, Mak JW, Maung M, Wong SF, Kassim AI. Meta-analysis: the association between HIV infection and extrapulmonary tuberculosis. Lung. 2013;191(1):27–34.

132. Kato-Maeda M, Nahid P. *Mycobacterium tuberculosis* lineage—what's in your lungs? Clin Infect Dis (An Official Publication of the Infectious Diseases Society of America). 2012;54(2):220–4.

133. World Health Organization. Treatment of tuberculosis: guidelines, 4th ed. 2010.

134. Durr S, Muller B, Alonso S, Hattendorf J, Laisse CJ, van Helden PD, et al. Differences in primary sites of infection between zoonotic and human tuberculosis: results from a worldwide systematic review. PLoS Neglected Trop Dis. 2013;7(8):e2399.

135. Cohen T, van Helden PD, Wilson D, Colijn C, McLaughlin MM, Abubakar I, et al. Mixed-strain *Mycobacterium tuberculosis* infections and the implications for tuberculosis treatment and control. Clin Microbiol Rev. 2012;25 (4):708–19.

136. Walker NF, Meintjes G, Wilkinson RJ. HIV-1 and the immune response to TB. Future Virol. 2013;8(1):57–80.

137. Nguyen H, Pandolfini C, Chiodini P, Bonati M. Tuberculosis care for pregnant women: a systematic review. BMC Infect Dis. 2014;14(1):617.

138. Loto OM, Awowole I. Tuberculosis in pregnancy: a review. J Pregnancy. 2012;2012:379271.

139. Mathad JS, Gupta A. Tuberculosis in pregnant and postpartum women: epidemiology, management, and research gaps. Clin Infect Dis (An Official Publication of the Infectious Diseases Society of America). 2012;55 (11):1532–49.
140. Marais BJ. Quantifying the tuberculosis disease burden in children. Lancet. 2014;383(9928):1530–1.
141. World Health Organization. The stop TB strategy: building on and enhancing DOTS to meet the TB-related millennium development goals. 2006.
142. Pasipanodya JG, Gumbo T. A meta-analysis of self-administered vs directly observed therapy effect on microbiologic failure, relapse, and acquired drug resistance in tuberculosis patients. Clin Infect Dis. 2013;57 (1):21–31.
143. World Health Organization. Global tuberculosis report 2014. Geneva; 2014.
144. Prevention CfDCa. Mantoux tuberculin skin testing products. 2012 [cited 2014 11/19/2014]. Available from: http://www.cdc.gov/tb/education/Mantoux/default.htm.
145. World Health Organization. Use of tuberculosis interferon-gamma release assays (IGRAs) in low- and middle-income countries: policy statement. 2011.
146. Steffen RE, Caetano R, Pinto M, Chaves D, Ferrari R, Bastos M, et al. Cost-effectiveness of Quantiferon(R)-TB Gold-in-Tube versus tuberculin skin testing for contact screening and treatment of latent tuberculosis infection in Brazil. PLoS ONE. 2013;8(4):e59546.
147. World Health Organization. Xpert MTB/RIF implementation manual: technical and operational 'how-to'; practical considerations. 2014.
148. World Health Organization. Automated real-time nucleic acid amplification technology for rapid and simultaneous detection of tuberculosis and rifampicin resistance: Xpert MTB/RIF assay for the diagnosis of pulmonary and extrapulmonary TB in adults and children. Policy update. 2013.
149. World Health Organization. TB diagnostics and laboratory strengthening. 2015. Available from: http://www.who.int/tb/laboratory/mtbrifrollout/en/.
150. FIND. Price for Xpert® MTB/RIF and FIND country list. 2015. Available from: http://www.finddiagnostics.org/about/what_we_do/successes/find-negotiated-prices/xpert_mtb_rif.html.
151. World Health Organization. Guidelines on the management of latent tuberculosis infection. 2015.
152. Nechaeva OB, Skachkova EI, Fomina NI. [Drug resistance of Mycobacterium tuberculosis in the Sverdlovsk Region]. Problemy tuberkuleza. 2002(9):8–11 (Epub 2003/01/15). Lekarstvennaia ustoichivost' mikobakterii tuberkuleza v Sverdlovskoi oblasti.
153. Faustini A, Hall AJ, Perucci CA. Risk factors for multidrug resistant tuberculosis in Europe: a systematic review. Thorax. 2006;61(2):158–63.
154. PablosMendez A, Knirsch CA, Barr RG, Lerner BH, Frieden TR. Nonadherence in tuberculosis treatment: predictors and consequences in New York City. Am J Med. 1997;102(2):164–70.
155. Pooran A, Pieterson E, Davids M, Theron G, Dheda K. What is the cost of diagnosis and management of drug resistant tuberculosis in South Africa? PloS ONE. 2013;8(1):e54587 (Epub 2013/01/26).
156. World Health Organization. WHO policy on collaborative TB/HIV activities guidelines for national programmes and other stakeholders. 2012.
157. World Health Organization. Guideline on when to start antiretroviral therapy and on pre-exposure prophylaxis for HIV. 2015.
158. World Health Organization. Guidelines for intensified tuberculosis case-finding and isoniazid preventive therapy for people living with HIV in resource-constrained settings. 2011.
159. World Health Organization. BCG vaccine WHO position paper. Wkly Epidemiol Rec. 2004;4:27–38.
160. Hesseling AC, Schaaf HS, Victor T, Beyers N, Marais BJ, Cotton MF, et al. Resistant Mycobacterium bovis Bacillus Calmette-Guerin disease: implications for management of Bacillus Calmette-Guerin Disease in human immunodeficiency virus-infected children. Pediatr Infect Dis J. 2004;23(5):476–9.
161. Mangtani P, Abubakar I, Ariti C, Beynon R, Pimpin L, Fine PE, et al. Protection by BCG vaccine against tuberculosis: a systematic review of randomized controlled trials. Clin Infect Dis (An Official Publication of the Infectious Diseases Society of America). 2014;58(4):470–80.
162. Groschel MI, Prabowo SA, Cardona PJ, Stanford JL, van der Werf TS. Therapeutic vaccines for tuberculosis—a systematic review. Vaccine. 2014;32(26):3162–8.
163. Andersen P, Kaufmann SH. Novel vaccination strategies against tuberculosis. Cold Spring Harbor Perspect Med. 2014;4(6).
164. Poyntz HC, Stylianou E, Griffiths KL, Marsay L, Checkley AM, McShane H. Non-tuberculous mycobacteria have diverse effects on BCG efficacy against Mycobacterium tuberculosis. Tuberculosis (Edinb). 2014;94 (3):226–37.

Chapter 18
HIV—Medical Perspective

Louise C. Ivers and Daniel Duré

Keywords HIV · AIDS · Antiretroviral therapy · ART · Global health · Equity · Nutrition

Learning Objectives

- To identify major events in the history of, and the global response to the HIV epidemic
- To explain the pathogenesis and clinical features of HIV infection
- To describe the concept of the HIV continuum of care in public health
- To evaluate the many factors associated with HIV risk and access to HIV prevention, treatment and care

Introduction

Human immunodeficiency virus (HIV) infection remains an important public health challenge and a leading cause of death and disability, affecting more than 35 million people worldwide [1]. HIV infection leads to a chronic clinical course of progressive immune dysfunction, susceptibility to a range of opportunistic infections and malignancies, and usually results in death if untreated. More than 39 million people have died of HIV-related diseases since the epidemic began [2]. HIV infection and its associated morbidity, mortality and the social and economic impact of this disease present important challenges for entire populations. Although people from all walks of life are at risk of infection, the global epidemic has illuminated poverty and inequalities. Understanding the history of the epidemic, the activism and mobilization behind access to care and treatment, the social and economic barriers to care and the gaps in access to services are all important in designing successful public health programs going forward. As context for understanding the importance of nutrition and

L.C. Ivers (✉)
Department of Global Health and Social Medicine, Harvard Medical School,
Brigham and Women's Hospital, 15 Francis St., Boston, MA 02115, USA
e-mail: livers@pih.org

D. Duré
Medical Education and Infectious Disease, Mirebalais Teaching Hospital (HUM),
Route Chatulée, Mirebalais, Plateau Central, Haiti
e-mail: ddure@pih.org

© Springer Science+Business Media New York 2017
S. de Pee et al. (eds.), *Nutrition and Health in a Developing World*,
Nutrition and Health, DOI 10.1007/978-3-319-43739-2_18

development as they relate to HIV infection, this chapter highlights key aspects of HIV from a medical perspective—including:

- A brief history of the HIV/AIDS epidemic and access to care
- HIV virology, transmission and pathogenesis
- Clinical history of HIV infection
- Global epidemiology of HIV
- Comprehensive HIV care—the HIV care continuum
- Prevention of HIV
- Overlapping epidemics
- Women and children

Providing medical detail of all aspects of HIV infection and treatment is beyond the scope of the chapter—so medical specifics on antiretroviral therapies, treatment and prevention of opportunistic infections and management of HIV-related complications are not provided. For these kinds of medical detail, the reader is encouraged to review recent guidelines on prevention, treatment and care of HIV (Box 18.1)—these are regularly updated and available free of charge.

Box 18.1 Available Guidelines on the Prevention, Treatment and Care of HIV
Detailed clinical guidelines are provided by a number of sources, including

United States Government Department of Health and Human Service
http://aidsinfo.nih.gov/guidelines/

World Health Organization
http://www.who.int/hiv/pub/guidelines/en/

The European AIDS Clinical Society
http://www.eacsociety.org/Guidelines.aspx

A Brief History of the HIV/AIDS Epidemic and Access to Care

In many ways, the evolution of the HIV pandemic, and the major social and scientific response to it was unprecedented for this generation. Initially charged by fear and discrimination, a global social movement paired with rapid advances in research led to tremendous progress, but much remains to be done. Appreciating the history is important for understanding the ways forward. A number of sources provide detailed and excellent reviews of the history of the HIV epidemic [3, 4], and the following paragraphs note some of the major milestones.

In 1981, the Centers for Disease Control and Prevention (CDC) in Atlanta reported the occurrence of Pneumocystis carinii pneumonia (PCP) in five men in Los Angeles without identifiable cause [5]. Around the same time, at least eight cases of aggressive Kaposi Sarcoma—a rare tumor usually occurring in the elderly—were described in young men who had sex with men (MSM) in New York [6], and speculations began on the possible cause of these diseases which were appearing outside of their typical hosts. Knowledge evolved quickly, and by the end of 1981, cases had also been observed in the UK, and among injection drugs users as well as MSM [5, 7]. Despite the recognition of these clinical cases in the 1980s, later sero-archeological studies documented HIV infection before 1980 and suggest that the pandemic started in the mid- to late 1970s and spread worldwide by 1980 [8, 9].

In July 1982, the acronym AIDS (acquired immune deficiency syndrome) first emerged, and in December of the same year, mother-to-child transmission of the disease was described for the first time

[10, 11]. The following year, researchers from the Institute Pasteur in France reported that they had isolated a new virus that could be the cause of AIDS, initially naming it lymphadenopathy-associated virus [12, 13]. By 1985, at least one case of HIV infection had been reported from each region of the world, and a test was licensed for screening blood supplies [14]. In 1986, early results of a clinical trial showed that zidovudine (AZT), a drug that had been synthesized in 1964 as possible anticancer drug, slowed down HIV infection [15] and it was licensed in 1987 for treating AIDS. By 1994, this drug was shown to substantially reduce the risk of mother-to-child transmission of HIV, and a United States Public Health Service task force recommended that it be provided to HIV-infected pregnant women during pregnancy, in labor, and to their infants for 6 weeks after delivery [16]. Infant HIV infections began to fall in resource-rich countries where access to the drug was available [17].

In 1995, AIDS had become the leading cause of death among all Americans aged 25–44 [18]. In response to the global problem, the Joint United Nations Programme on AIDS (UNAIDS) was established and came into effect on January 1, 1996, bringing together agencies from the UN system to contribute to reducing the impact of the epidemic and harmonizing work at country level. In 1997, according to estimates made later, 22 million people were living with HIV globally [3]. The previous year, studies had demonstrated the effectiveness of combinations of drugs in treating AIDS, and this had led to optimism about the treatment of HIV-infected people [19]. Brazil became the first developing country to provide this combination treatment free of charge to citizens. The combination of antiretroviral drugs (ARVs) used to treat AIDS was often termed "highly active antiretroviral therapy" and initially became known by its acronym HAART. This was later more commonly abbreviated as ART. The introduction of ART revolutionized treatment of HIV infection. However, access to treatment was not universally available, and infections continued to increase globally. Strong grassroots movements evolved, especially of people living with HIV, and battles with multinational pharmaceutical companies attempted to force cuts in drug prices in a push toward access to care [20, 21].

In 2002, the Global Fund for AIDS, Tuberculosis (TB) and Malaria (GFATM) was established to seek and distribute resources to improve the response to those three diseases globally. On World AIDS Day in 2003, the World Health Organization (WHO) announced a new plan called "Three by Five," which aimed to provide 3 million people in resource-poor countries with ART by 2005 [22]. This target was seen as a step toward achieving the ultimate goal of universal access to treatment for those living with HIV infection and AIDS. The campaign did not reach its target, and over 3 million deaths were attributed to AIDS in 2005. However, the campaign contributed importantly to an emphasis on saving the lives of those already living with HIV infection by expanding access to lifesaving therapy. The number of people on ART more than doubled between 2003 and mid-2005, from 400,000 to approximately 1 million [22]. This emphasis on saving the lives of those living with HIV was notable particularly in contrast to the emphasis that some had previously placed on prioritizing HIV prevention as the most important and cost-effective intervention to control the epidemic [23].

Although the movement to begin access to ART in low- and middle-income countries did not begin with GFATM or "Three by five"—for example, Brazil was treating patients through public health programs since 1996, Partners In Health began treating people with AIDS in Haiti in 1998, Médecins Sans Frontières in Cameroon in 2001—these initiatives provided a political commitment and helped to leverage financial resources to scale up services [22, 24, 25].

The US Government Presidents Emergency Fund for AIDS Relief (PEPFAR) with a budget of $15 billion over 5 years was created in 2003, with a goal of increasing access to prevention and treatment in 15 focus countries. Progress in prevention was made scientifically in 2006, when male circumcision was shown to reduce HIV acquisition among heterosexual men [26, 27], and again in 2011 when the HTPN 052 trial showed that early ART initiation reduced HIV transmission by 96% among discordant heterosexual couples [28]. By 2013, 37% of people living with HIV were receiving treatment [29].

Access to Care and Treatment—Antiretroviral Drug Prices and Global Health Initiatives

Governments, communities, people affected by HIV, international organizations and non-governmental organizations together have played a major role in advancing global access to care and treatment for HIV. In May 2000, ART cost US$10,400 per person per year, and so price was a major barrier to treatment for the majority of people living with HIV infection [30]. The work of grassroots activists, people living with HIV, as well as organizations such as Médecins Sans Frontières and the Clinton Health Access Initiative, among others, greatly affected ARV pricing [31]. The introduction of generic antiretroviral medicines (initially produced mostly in India), pressure from activist groups and direct negotiation with manufacturers meant that by 2001, the cost of ARVs per person per year had fallen to US$295, thus paving the way for increased access to treatment for those that needed it [32]. The price of ARVs continues to fall in low- and middle-income countries and in 2013 was US$115 per patient per year [31]. Challenges still remain however, as the cost of second- and third-line ARVs are more expensive, and a number of middle-income countries do not have access to cheaper generic drugs [30, 31].

In 2002, a multi-billion dollar initiative—the aforementioned GFTAM—was established in Geneva, Switzerland, to "[a]ttract and disburse additional resources to prevent and treat HIV and AIDS, tuberculosis and malaria" [33]. Operating as a public–private partnership, by 2012 the organization had authorized US$22.9 billion in funding for over 1000 programs in 151 countries [33]. According to the organization, since its establishment, more than 11.2 million people have benefitted from TB diagnosis and treatment, 360 million insecticide-treated antimalaria nets have been distributed worldwide, and by mid-2013, approximately 6 million people were on lifesaving ART regimes through GFATM-supported programs (of the 12.9 million people on ART in low- and middle-income countries) [33]. Each country receiving funding from GFTAM has their own program coordinating body—the Country Coordinating Mechanism—with representatives from those involved in treating AIDS, TB and malaria, as well as from the communities that are living with these diseases. It is this coordinating committee that applies for the Global Fund grant, and oversees its use in the implementation of their national programs. Actual implementation is carried out by various organizations within the country, such as non-governmental organizations, governmental departments, UN organizations or other faith- or community-based organizations [34].

PEPFAR (President's Emergency Plan for AIDS Relief) was established in 2003 by the US Government and was unprecedented in terms of being such a large, single-health-issue initiative by a single government. It began as a commitment of US$15 billion over 5 years (2003–2008) with specific goals aimed at targeting HIV/AIDS care, treatment and prevention in 15 focus countries: 12 in sub-Saharan Africa, two in Latin America and one in Asia [35]. Its re-authorization in 2008 for an additional 5 years (2009–2013) saw an increase in funding to US$48 billion, with a shift from the initial focus-country approach to a Partnership Framework and with an emphasis on sustainability and long-term strategies for the fight against HIV/AIDS [35]. The primary goal of PEPFAR within this partnership framework was to work with its partner countries that received funding in order to prevent 12 million new infections of HIV globally; to support 12 million people infected with or affected by the disease; to aid partner countries in reaching 80% access to treatment, care and counseling services; and to minimize the spread of HIV, particularly among women, children and mother-to-child transmission [36]. The program continues now in Phase 3 (2013–present) and is focused on sustainable control of the epidemic [37].

Both GFATM and PEPFAR have had challenges and critiques, but together they have been the biggest financial contributors to the scale up of access to prevention, treatment and care worldwide.

Health Systems Strengthening

WHO defines a health system as "all the activities whose primary purpose is to promote, restore or maintain health" [38]. WHO's "Maximizing Positive Synergies" project posed the important question of "How can Global Health Initiatives and national health systems optimize their interactions to capitalize on positive synergies and minimize negative impacts, thereby achieving their common goal of improving health outcomes?" [39]. The WHO Health Systems Framework outlines what it considers to be the fundamental building blocks of a robust health system—service delivery; health workforce; information and research; medical products, vaccines and technologies; healthcare financing; and leadership and governance—and that the interdependence of each of these parts should be recognized when addressing Health System Strengthening [40]. Initially, disease-specific global health initiatives, such as GFTAM and PEPFAR, were more likely to be organized and implemented in a vertical fashion, with a primary focus on the diseases that they aimed to combat, funding programs separately from the rest of the health system, with their own staff, materials and information systems. However, as the initiatives evolved over time, increasing recognition has been given to the role that strong national health systems should play in implementing the disease-specific programs, and how funding might work to strengthen the health systems as a whole, rather than being separate activities that could even detract from primary healthcare if not appropriately integrated and planned. This, in turn, has led to the rethinking of how funding that a country is receiving through such an initiative should be used, not only for disease-specific interventions, but to improve service delivery as a whole and to build a stronger national health system. GFTAM and PEPFAR have increasingly highlighted the importance both of addressing these concerns and of finding new ways to frame both the problems and the solutions of Health System Strengthening. The impact of this is demonstrated by UNAIDS report in 2013 that more than half of countries have either fully integrated HIV and tuberculosis services or strengthened joint service provision, almost two-thirds have integrated services to prevent mother-to-child HIV transmission in antenatal care, and two-thirds have integrated HIV and sexual and reproductive health services. Nearly one in four countries have linked HIV and management of chronic non-communicable diseases, and more than half have integrated HIV testing and counseling and/or antiretroviral therapy in general outpatient care [2].

HIV Virology, Transmission and Pathogenesis

HIV is a retrovirus and member of the Retroviridae family of viruses, genus Lentivirus. There are two types of HIV: HIV-1 and HIV-2, both with similar transmission characteristics. HIV-1 is the predominant virus in the global pandemic of HIV. HIV-2 differs from HIV-1 in that it appears to be somewhat less easily transmitted, the time from infection to clinical illness is longer than for HIV-1, and HIV-2 is mainly present in West Africa. Furthermore, certain antiretroviral drugs are not active against HIV-2. Unless the type is specified, when the term "HIV" is used, it is most often referring to HIV-1 [13, 41–44].

HIV has a high genetic variability that results in part from its rapid replication cycle and its high mutation rate. The different strains of HIV-1 are divided into four groups: M, N, O, P. Group M (for "Major" or "Main") predominates and contributes to more than 90% of HIV/AIDS cases globally. Group N (for "non-M, non-O") and O (for "Outlier") are limited to Gabon and Cameroon, and the Group P is very rare [45]. Group M can be further subdivided into subtypes or clades: A through K. There are also further circulating recombinant forms derived from combinations of viruses of different subtypes. These subtypes do not currently impact antiretroviral treatment choice except that subtype O is resistant to the non-nucleoside reverse transcriptase inhibitor class of drugs [43]. HIV-2 is subdivided into eight groups, from A to H [43].

Biology of HIV

HIV is a cytopathic virus, composed of a central core of RNA surrounded by a spherical lipid envelope. Embedded in the envelope are glycoprotein surface markers. The bullet-shaped viral core contains three enzyme proteins necessary for HIV replication: reverse transcriptase, protease, integrase, and two single strands of RNA. HIV primarily targets CD4+ T cells (also known as CD4 cells, or CD4+ cells, or T cells), dendritic cells and macrophages. To enter CD4 cells and other cells, the HIV attaches to the CD4 protein on the cell surface, but this is not sufficient to enter certain other cells. To enter monocytes and dendritic cells, the HIV virus docks and binds at two separate sites: the CD4 receptor and a 7-transdomain chemokine receptor [46]. The most important of the chemokine receptors are CCR5 and CXCR4 [46]. Once binding has occurred, the viral envelope fuses with the host cell membrane, and the contents of the HIV particle enter the cell. Reverse transcriptase then produces a DNA copy of the viral RNA, the DNA becomes integrated into the host genome using viral integrase, and either one of two things may happen: (i) active viral replication takes place or (ii) a latent stage occurs. The latent stage can persist indefinitely, or be activated and transcribe RNA, thus producing the components of new virions. After assembly, the virions bud from the infected cell and circulate until a new target cell is identified. Each step of the replication process is either a pharmacologic target of, or a site of investigation for ways to disrupt the viral cycle, transmission and development of disease.

HIV Transmission

HIV transmission occurs by three major routes: sexual contact (through semen, cervicovaginal secretions), contaminated blood (through transfusion, blood products or contaminated needles) or vertical transmission from mother to child. Multiple cofactors affect both susceptibility to infection and infectiousness. For example, inflammatory sexually transmitted diseases such as gonorrhea or ulcerative genital lesions increase susceptibility to infection. Male circumcision lowers the risk of HIV acquisition among heterosexual men [47]. Lower blood concentrations of HIV are associated with lower transmission. A study in Uganda noted a dose–response relationship such that increased transmission was associated with increased viral load in HIV serodiscordant couples [48]. Innate and acquired factors in the host may also affect susceptibility to infection—people that are homozygous for a 32-base pair deletion in the CCR5 co-receptor that binds HIV are less likely to become infected than those who do not have it [46]. It is estimated that HIV results in an established systemic infection within 72 h of acquisition, and this contributes to the recommendation that antiretroviral drug therapy be considered to prevent infection after exposure—see below for further discussion of post-exposure prophylaxis (PEP) [49, 50].

Clinical History of HIV Infection

The typical course of HIV infection can be described in characteristic phases:

Early HIV Infection–Acute HIV Infection

"Early HIV infection" is the term frequently used to describe the period of approximately six months after initial acquisition of the virus. "Acute HIV infection" describes the symptomatic illness that may occur during early HIV infection. Although it is difficult to clearly determine, it appears that most early HIV infection is symptomatic, although many patients do not seek medical care during this time. Symptoms of acute HIV infection (also known as "acute seroconversion illness") are typically non-specific, influenza-like or infectious mononucleosis-like. More severe symptoms during acute HIV infection, especially lasting longer than 14 days, have been associated with more rapid progression of disease [51–53]. After acquisition of the virus, HIV viral levels rise rapidly and peak usually at the time when antibodies to HIV are measurable (also known as seroconversion). Initially, there is no HIV-specific immune response and many susceptible CD4 cells are present. Viral levels rise dramatically, and then, with the development of HIV-specific CD8+ cytotoxic T lymphocytes, around six months after infection, plasma viral levels fall to a more steady state known as the individual's "set point." Symptoms usually coincide with rising plasma viral levels and subside with the development of HIV-specific response and the reduction in plasma viremia.

Patients in the early phase of HIV infection have a high risk of transmission of disease because of the high viral loads that occur during this phase. Rare patients maintain a high CD4 cell count and a low or undetectable level of plasma HIV even in the absence of antiretroviral therapy. These so-called elite controllers are characterized by the persistence of an HIV-specific immune response. Research interest in therapeutic intervention in early HIV infection includes trying to recreate a similar immunologic scenario in which HIV-specific immune responses in the host are preserved during early infection, allowing sustained viral control.

Anti-HIV antibodies begin to develop 4–8 weeks after acquisition of the virus. Most patients have seroconverted (i.e., developed antibodies) by 4 weeks after exposure and almost all by 6 months. The pre-seroconversion period of early HIV infection is challenging in terms of epidemic control, as patients are often unaware of their illness, are highly capable of transmission, but are negative on HIV antibody testing [52].

Clinical Latency or Chronic Asymptomatic HIV Infection

After the early infection phase, HIV infection enters an asymptomatic phase that lasts an average of 8–10 years, but can be highly variable. During this time, CD4 counts slowly decline and viral levels of HIV remain relatively stable at the individual's "set point" [54].

Early Symptomatic Infection

After the clinical latency period, HIV infection becomes symptomatic with symptoms that may be more specific than those that may have occurred at the time of initial acute infection. Certain illnesses such as oral thrush, persistent or frequent vaginal candidiasis, oral hairy leukoplakia, peripheral neuropathy or constitutional symptoms such as low-grade fevers and weight loss may occur during this time. For an extensive list of conditions, please see a clinical management guide (Box 18.1). Patients' physical examination during this time may be completely normal, with the exception of lymphadenopathy, which often occurs but may be overlooked by the patient.

Acquired Immune Deficiency Syndrome (AIDS)

AIDS is defined by specific clinical criteria that include a CD4 cell count <200/mm^3, a CD4 cell percentage of total lymphocytes <14%, or by the presence of one or more AIDS-related opportunistic infections or neoplasms, such as Pneumocystis carinii pneumonia, cryptococcal meningitis and central nervous system toxoplasmosis. An extensive list of AIDS-defining conditions is beyond the scope of this chapter, but can be found in clinical management resources. Generally, the term "AIDS" is reserved for those individuals that meet these specific criteria, and otherwise, the terms "HIV infection" or "HIV disease" are used. In addition to depletion of CD4 cells, humoral immunity is also affected during progressive HIV infection, resulting in activation of B cells, and often increased serum immunoglobulins, although these are typically non-specific antibodies, altered in function. Advanced HIV infection results in further decline in CD4 cell count below 50 cells/mm^3, the stage at which most deaths from AIDS occur in the absence of treatment. However, with aggressive management of opportunistic infections and viral control with ART, even patients with advanced AIDS can recover to good health.

Global Epidemiology of HIV

Since the beginning of the epidemic in the 1980s, 78 million people have become infected with HIV, and 39 million have died from AIDS-related illnesses. At the end of 2013, an estimated 35 million people were living with HIV [1]; the annual rate of new infections having decreased by 33% between 2001 and 2012, from 3.4 million to 2.3 million, respectively [2]. Of those 35 million, 31.8 million are 15 years and older, 3.2 million are children under 15 years old, and 16 million are women [56].

One of the Millennium Development Goals, to halve the rate of sexual transmission of HIV infection by 50%, was met by 26 countries. Sub-Saharan Africa is the region most disproportionally affected, with 70% of the total rate of new infections globally. In this region, women account for 58% of the total number of those living with HIV [1]. Worldwide, 15% of women living with HIV aged 15 years and older are young women (15–24 years old), and of these, 80% live in sub-Saharan Africa [29]. Women are physiologically at greater risk of contracting HIV, as during sexual intercourse they risk tissue injury, and have a greater mucosal area exposed to pathogens and infectious fluids. Many other factors also increase women's vulnerability to acquiring HIV, including behavioral, socioeconomic, cultural and structural risks [57].

Often, certain populations are being left behind in the response [29]. People who inject drugs are 28 times more likely to have HIV than the general population. Men who have sex with men are 19 times more likely to be infected, and female sex workers have a prevalence of 13.5 times that found among women aged between 15 and 49 years [29]. Unfortunately, rather than prompt special interventions to address the needs of these key populations, these statistics have often contributed to inappropriate blame, accusation and stigma directed at these groups. This was particularly true at the beginning of the epidemic, but continues in many contexts. Addressing the needs of such key populations including also prisoners and adolescent girls is critical for the response to be successful.

Voluntary HIV testing and counseling is the gateway to accessing treatment; yet, only half of those living with HIV are aware of their status [29]. Only 38% of adults and 24% of children living with HIV, including those who do not know they are HIV positive, have access to treatment globally [29]. At the end of 2013, there were 12.9 million people receiving ART globally, of whom more than 11.7 million were based in low- and middle-income countries [29, 58].

Prevention programs have been shown to be effective in lowering HIV transmission and reinforce the need to invest in preventative measures [29]. Voluntary male circumcision was performed on 2.7 million men in high-priority countries in 2013 [59]. Providing pregnant women living with HIV with access to antiretroviral medicines has averted more than 900,000 new HIV infections among children since 2009 [29]. TB remains the leading cause of death among people living with HIV, although that number has decreased by 36% worldwide between 2004 and the end of 2012 [29]. Of those living with HIV, 2–4 million also have hepatitis B and 4–5 million have hepatitis C; all three are more prevalent among prisoners living with HIV [29].

The HIV Continuum of Care

Comprehensive HIV Care

> Health is a state of complete physical, mental and social well-being – not merely the absence of disease or infirmity [60].

What follows from this quote is that HIV care must address the physical as well as the psychosocial impacts of HIV infection. Providers must also attempt to understand and address the structural and individual barriers to seeking and remaining in care. The "continuum of care" or "cascade of care" for HIV is the name often given to the set of steps that must each be accomplished for a person with HIV infection to reach a healthy state (Fig. 18.1). The continuum includes:

  (i)   HIV diagnosis—counseling and testing for HIV infection
 (ii) Linking to care—once infection has been confirmed, PLHIV must be appropriately linked to care providers that can offer them appropriate treatment and support
(iii) Remaining in care—because treatment is lifelong, PLHIV must stay engaged in care for an indefinite period of time, and this poses challenges that must be addressed
 (iv) Antiretroviral therapy (ART)—the mainstay of treatment for HIV infection
  (v) Viral suppression—regular adherence to effective ART results in viral suppression and immune reconstitution [61].

Viral suppression is not synonymous with complete health of the individual, and those on long-term ART may also have side effects that can impact their health and/or quality of life. So the concept of the "continuum of care" is not really complete and could be further expanded to include stages of physical, mental and social well-being. However, because viral suppression is measurable in the laboratory and is a prerequisite for the reconstitution of physical health, it is a very useful quantitative measure to evaluate the effectiveness of HIV programs—once it is acknowledged that a healthy person is the desired endpoint, rather than a laboratory result. Despite the tremendous advances in science and therapeutics, in 2012 only 30% of people over 18 years of age living with HIV in the USA had achieved viral suppression on their most recent viral load test [62, 63], and substantial racial and age disparities exist such that African-Americans and younger individuals are the least likely to remain in care or to have viral suppression [61, 62]. Detailed information for viral suppression is largely lacking from resource-poor settings because this laboratory test is not widely available. However, using available data UNAIDS estimates that 21–34% of those living with HIV in sub-Saharan Africa are suppressed virologically [29, 64]. This highlights how much remains to be done to identify and address barriers to care and treatment.

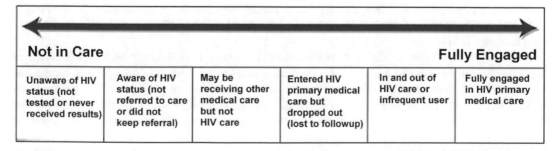

Not in Care					Fully Engaged
Unaware of HIV status (not tested or never received results)	Aware of HIV status (not referred to care or did not keep referral)	May be receiving other medical care but not HIV care	Entered HIV primary medical care but dropped out (lost to followup)	In and out of HIV care or infrequent user	Fully engaged in HIV primary medical care

Fig. 18.1 Continuum of HIV care. Data from *Health Resources and Services Administration, HIV/AIDS Bureau.* Outreach: engaging people in HIV care summary of a HRSA/HAB 2005 consultation on linking PLWH into care. 2006 [online at ftp://ftp.hrsa.gov/hab/HIVoutreach.pdf]

The following section describes stages of the continuum of care of HIV and some potential barriers.

HIV Diagnosis—HIV Counseling and Testing

HIV testing is the process of determining HIV status. Lack of awareness of one's HIV status contributes to significant morbidity and mortality and also contributes to ongoing transmission of the infection. HIV testing policies have been mired in the complex social history of HIV infection and the initial fear and discrimination related to the disease, especially in the pre-ART era. Thankfully, these policies have been changing and this has contributed to increases in (voluntary) testing. In the USA, 16% of those with HIV infection are estimated to be unaware of their status, but globally that may be as high as half of those infected are unaware [65, 66].

Two approaches have evolved for scaling up HIV testing so that individuals know their HIV status as a first step on the continuum of care: voluntary counseling and testing (VCT) and provider-initiated counseling and testing (PICT). In VCT, individuals with the objective of learning their HIV status initiate contact with a health worker. As a strategy for epidemic control, VCT has a number of limitations—for example, there are specific health-seeking barriers to be overcome for an individual to specifically ask for an HIV test, individuals often underestimate their own personal risk of acquiring HIV infection, and the clinical latency of HIV infection means that infected individuals are asymptomatic for a long period of time which may dissuade them from seeking testing. In provider-initiated testing (PICT), the process of offering a test for HIV infection is initiated by a healthcare worker during routine healthcare interactions and is increasingly recommended as a routine part of care (as opposed to just targeting individuals considered to be most at risk and/or showing symptoms). Routine PICT is a sound policy, once the rights of patients to information, treatment and confidentiality are realized. Even in lower burden settings, routine PICT is increasingly recommended and has resulted in increases in HIV testing and diagnosis [66, 67].

Given that transmission of HIV from mother to her infant can almost be eliminated with appropriate preventive methods, an opt-out testing policy is recommended in most settings for pregnant women. This means that HIV counseling and testing are offered as routine to all pregnant women, and women who do not want to be tested must opt-out [66, 68].

Testing involves identifying the presence of HIV antibodies and/or HIV antigen, i.e., a component of the virus. Newer generation tests include combined antibody and p24 antigen detection, the combination of which allows for identification of early HIV infection, which may be missed by protocols that only test for HIV antibodies. In chronic infection, newer generation tests are almost 100% sensitive and specific for HIV infection, but they are less sensitive for early infection, and if this is suspected and a combined test is negative or indeterminate, an additional antigen test such as HIV RNA is required. In the USA, current recommendations are to use a combined HIV p24 antigen and HIV antibody test, followed by confirmation by an HIV-1/HIV-2 antibody differentiation immunoassay [68].

Antibody tests are also available as rapid tests that are easy to administer on blood obtained by finger-prick, can be done in a community or facility setting and have less than 30-min turnaround time, thereby allowing for same-day results. If positive, antibody rapid tests must be confirmed by another test before diagnosis of HIV is confirmed. Many resource-limited settings do not have access to newer generation combined antibody/antigen tests because of cost. In this situation, it is common to use a protocol of sequential rapid antibody testing—a highly sensitive rapid test is used first and followed by a second highly specific rapid test if positive. This may or may not be followed by Western blot for confirmation. Western blot detects IgG antibody to HIV-1 and is usually only available at second- or third-level facilities [69].

HIV testing of infants that have been exposed to HIV in utero is more complex because maternal HIV antibodies that are transplacentally acquired persist in infants for up to 18 months of life. This means that rapid antibody testing is not very specific for HIV infection in the infant during this time period. Furthermore, maternal ART and ART provided to the infant at birth can render the infant's HIV RNA level below detection even if the child is infected. DNA polymerase chain reaction test (DNA PCR) detects HIV proviral DNA in peripheral white blood cells and is the standard test for infants exposed to HIV in utero. It assesses the presence of the proviral DNA that has integrated into the child's white blood cells. Because transmission from mother to child occurs perinatally as well as intrauterine, HIV DNA PCR testing is only 55% sensitive at birth, but this increases to 100% at six months of age [70]. HIV DNA PCR testing is the standard of care diagnostic test for exposed infants where available, but is limited in availability in resource-poor settings.

Linking to Care: Engaging, Retaining and Re-engaging in Care

HIV testing is just the very first step toward engagement in care. When a patient is diagnosed with HIV infection, it is very important to ensure that this contact through testing is continued to encourage them to be linked into ongoing care. Many factors can interfere with the continuum of care, and barriers can occur along the spectrum. For example, many people are tested for HIV infection but never even learn the results of the test, or receive test results but never return to a healthcare provider again. An individual's engagement in care can also fluctuate rather than be static, and it may depend on social, economic, structural or other factors their life. Engaging early in HIV care has many positive benefits on health, and research has shown that people living with HIV who are engaged in care are also less likely to engage in unprotected sex, or injection drug use [71, 72]. The best models of care that ensure linkage and engagement are those that attempt to address the personal, community, cultural and structural barriers to care [23–25, 72, 73].

Antiretroviral Therapy (ART)

Although there are multiple benefits to being engaged in care, ART remains the most powerful weapon in the fight against HIV. When antiretroviral drugs were first licensed, they were used quite aggressively, but side effects of earlier generation treatments, and concern about long-term complications of therapy subsequently resulted in a more measured approach to initiating treatment. Advances in therapeutics are now moving the balance back in the direction of early initiation of ART for treatment as well as for pre- and post-exposure prophylaxis. ART is now recommended for all people with HIV infection in the USA, and European guidelines recommend at least considering ART for all HIV-infected individuals [74, 75]. Some of the factors in favor of early initiation of ART include reduction in HIV RNA (also known as reducing the "viral load"), prevention of immunodeficiency, delay in onset of AIDS and reduction in non-AIDS morbidities such as hepatic, neoplastic and cardiovascular disease, and these are balanced with possible side effects and the need for lifelong therapy [76]. In resource-limited settings, recommendations to wait to start ART until immune suppression had advanced (CD4 cell count of <350 or <500 cells/mm^3) were only changed in 2015 to come into line with what was already being recommended in Europe and the USA—namely that ART should be offered to all those with HIV infection regardless of CD4 count. However, this recommendation has not yet been translated into practice in many resource-limited settings. At least in the USA and Western Europe, studies have demonstrated that individuals with HIV infection on ART have a life expectancy that is similar to those in the general population [77, 78].

People living with HIV infection should be properly assessed for potential barriers to ART adherence, and every effort should be made to address those barriers, in partnership with the individual. This includes evaluation of social and economic challenges, food security, transportation, childcare needs, status of disclosure and a number of other individual challenges. Early after initiation of ART, patients need regular and close medical and psychological monitoring to assess for adherence, tolerance and possible side effects. Monitoring of treatment includes review of clinical status, biological parameters such as blood counts, renal and liver function and viral load. The frequency and type of follow-up required in part depends on the individual's ART regimen. Patients with opportunistic infections because of their degree of immune suppression should be treated appropriately for those infections. Patients should also receive primary and/or secondary prophylaxis to prevent such opportunistic infections when appropriate, based on treatment and prevention guidelines.

Exactly when to start, what ART regimens to start, which prophylaxis is recommended, and the frequency of monitoring and evaluation of patients are all important clinical topics but are beyond the scope of this chapter. Guidelines for clinical management of patients living with HIV infection are updated regularly based on changes in scientific knowledge, so the reader is encouraged to review a recent version of such guidelines—examples are shared in Box 18.1. They also may include local national guidelines, the US Government guidelines [75] or the WHO guidelines [79].

Viral Suppression, CD4 Count Monitoring and Resistance Testing

Historically both CD4 count and HIV viral load monitoring were recommended as part of regular follow-up for patients with HIV infection. As a measure of immune function, CD4 count is a strong predictor of HIV disease progression and survival. It is also an important marker to guide prophylaxis against opportunistic infections. Most opportunistic infections occur in patients with CD4 cell counts <200 cells/mm^3, but some, such as TB, can occur at higher CD4 counts. Access to CD4 monitoring was expanded globally during the first 20 years of the HIV pandemic, but access to viral load monitoring remains limited. Evidence is increasing that if viral load is monitored, routine monitoring of CD4 count for patients on ART may not be necessary, because patients with persistently suppressed viral load tend to have stable or increasing CD4 counts (rather than decreasing). In the USA, almost all individuals with known HIV infection that are engaged in care are on ART (or at least are recommended to be on ART), so CD4 count monitoring is recommended less frequently than in the past, if viral load is measured and suppressed [75].

In addition to high-income countries, some middle-income countries such as Botswana, Brazil, South Africa and Thailand were also early adopters of HIV viral load monitoring [81], and this monitoring is increasingly integrated into the guidelines of national HIV programs. HIV viral load is the most important indicator of initial and sustained response to ART. Ideal viral suppression is considered to be a viral load that is persistently <20–50 copies/mL, or "undetectable" on routine laboratory measures. Viral "blips" are seen to occur in some patients—this is when a patient that is typically suppressed has an isolated viral load in the 20–400 copies/mL range. These blips do not appear to reflect long-term virologic failure [82]. "Virologic failure" is the term used when the virus has become resistant to the individual's antiretroviral therapy regimen, characterized by the individual's viral load increasing despite reliably taking the prescribed drugs. (This is opposed to "immunologic failure," the term given to a fall in CD4 count that occurs at some time after virologic failure, and which precedes "clinical failure," the term given when the individual develops clinical signs and symptoms of HIV progression because of a failing drug regimen). Despite acknowledgement of its importance, and strong recommendation for its use by the WHO [79], viral load monitoring still remains out of reach for many people with HIV infection in resource-poor settings, largely as a result of lack of availability—due to cost and/or lack of laboratory infrastructure. This issue must be addressed to ensure the highest quality of care, and equity in access to services.

Since access to CD4 testing is still limited in some settings (due to cost and lack of laboratory infrastructure), WHO Clinical Staging for HIV infection provides a list of case definitions based on an individual's clinical symptoms, signs and presence of opportunistic infections [55]. Clinical management resources provide more detailed description of WHO stages of HIV disease, but briefly, from asymptomatic through severe symptoms, an individual will be classified as WHO clinical stage 1 through clinical stage 4 [55]. Clinical staging has some correlation with underlying immune status and is a tool for decision making in the absence of access to CD4 testing. However, ideally, all individuals with HIV infection should have access to a care provider that can perform CD4 cell count and HIV viral load testing, and provide them with individualized care.

HIV resistance occurs as a result of viral replication. Billions of new particles of HIV can be made each day in a person that is not on treatment, and because the virus is prone to errors in replication, mutations may occur in the viral genetic material. Those mutations may confer resistance to antiretroviral drugs. If a patient is sub-optimally adherent to ART, and viral replication is occurring in the presence of lower-than-suppressive levels of ART drugs, then there is selective pressure for mutations that are resistant to those drugs.

Drug-resistant virus can be transmitted, and in the USA and Europe, approximately 6–16% [75, 83, 84] of new infections with HIV are with virus that is resistant to at least one antiretroviral drug. HIV resistance can be measured by both genotypic assays—that evaluate the mutations in the reverse transcriptase and protease genes (standard testing) and/or integrase strand transfer inhibitor and co-receptor tropism (supplemental testing), or by phenotypic assays that measure response to antiretroviral drugs in vitro. Phenotypic testing is usually reserved for those with multiple mutations on genotype testing, and a history of multiple treatment regimens. In the USA, HIV drug resistance testing is recommended for all people with HIV infection at the time that they engage in care, and also before ART is initiated (if treatment is deferred after the first measurement). Resistance testing is also recommended to guide ART in patients that are switching regimens as a result of virologic failure, or sub-optimal viral suppression on ART [75]. In resource-limited settings, resistance testing is rarely available to guide patient care.

HIV Prevention

The term "HIV prevention" refers to efforts to prevent transmission of HIV and thus primary prevention of new infections. Universal prevention efforts are centered around the three main routes of transmission: sexual transmission, transmission through blood and mother-to-child transmission. HIV testing, counseling, awareness and risk reduction are mainstays of prevention efforts, but behavioral factors are only one component of vulnerability to HIV infection. There is a complex interaction between behavioral, structural, social, economic and other factors associated with HIV risk, and each of these must be addressed for HIV prevention strategies to be successful.

From a public health perspective, prevention strategies should be country- or region specific and incorporate both generalized prevention and specific prevention for issues that may be driving the epidemic at the regional or national level. For example, a country may have a concentrated epidemic that is driven by the risks associated with injection drug use, whereas other countries have a generalized epidemic, driven by heterosexual transmission. This approach of using multiple aspects of prevention as part of a comprehensive package has come to be known as "combination prevention." This distinguishes it from early initiatives that were highly focused on behavioral aspects of care, such as the "Abstinence, Be faithful, use Condoms" (ABC) approach. UNAIDS defines combination prevention as:

...rights-based, evidence-informed, and community-owned programmes that use a mix of biomedical, behavioural, and structural interventions, prioritised to meet the current HIV prevention needs of particular individuals and communities, so as to have the greatest sustained impact on reducing new infections [85].

Treatment as Prevention

Recently, treatment has been recognized as an important contribution to HIV prevention, and this occurs in one of three ways—pre-exposure prophylaxis (PrEP), post-exposure prophylaxis (PEP) and treatment of infected individuals (secondary prevention) [50, 86]. Some controversy continues to exist with regard to the cost and cost-effectiveness of treatment as prevention (as opposed to treatment for the health of the individual), as well as to its usefulness on a population level for epidemic control of HIV [49]. Antiretroviral drugs are recommended as PEP for people that have potentially been exposed to HIV, especially in occupational settings or after sexual assault. Other non-occupational or consensual sexual exposures could also be considered for PEP, and its use should be determined on a case-by-case basis. ART usually in the form of two- or three-drug combinations is started as soon as possible after the exposure and continued under medical supervision for approximately one month. Regimens may vary, and other treatments may be recommended for other potential harms from the exposure, so consultation with a professional is necessary. The detailed management of potential HIV exposure is beyond the scope of this chapter, but guidelines are regularly updated and made available. Studies on PEP have been largely experimental studies in animals or observational human studies, but given ethical considerations, it is unlikely that a placebo-controlled trial would ever be undertaken [87]. Effectiveness is known to be affected by (i) the timing of ART initiation, with data suggesting that starting less than 72 h after exposure is most effective; (ii) drug resistance, i.e., if the transmitted virus is resistant to the PEP ART, and (iii) the adherence of the recipient to the regimen, which is often low due to side effects—for example, one meta-analysis of sexual assault victims demonstrated only 40% adherence to PEP over one month [88].

Research has demonstrated that pre-exposure prophylaxis with daily oral antiretroviral drugs emtricitabine and tenofovir disoproxil fumarate in a fixed-dose combination decreases HIV acquisition among MSM, serodiscordant couples and heterosexual adults, and tenofovir disoproxil fumarate alone is effective in preventing infection in heterosexual couples and in people who inject drugs [89–93]. Current guidelines suggest the use of the two-drug regimen, although pre-exposure prophylaxis continues to be an active and evolving area of research and practice and guidelines will likely be revised regularly as data emerges from early implementation of pre-exposure strategies.

Other Prevention

Prevention of sexual transmission may be through safer sex practices, condom use, voluntary male circumcision and treatment of those that are infected. There is strong evidence that even brief behavioral counseling delivered to those at risk of HIV infection reduces sexual risk behavior and increases condom use. Identification and treatment of other sexually transmitted infections is also important in prevention, as the presence of cervicitis, vaginitis or other sexually transmitted infections increase the risk of HIV acquisition. Prevention of blood-related transmission includes screening blood products for HIV, eliminating or reducing needle-sharing among injection drug users and reducing or eliminating needle-related occupational accidents [50].

Voluntary male circumcision reduces—HIV acquisition by as much as 60%, and is also protective against transmission of other sexually transmitted infections such as human papilloma virus and herpes simplex virus type 2 [94–97]. UNAIDS recommends voluntary male circumcision as a strategy for HIV prevention in countries with generalized epidemics and low prevalence of male circumcision.

Overlapping Epidemics

In addition to morbidity and mortality directly from HIV, a number of important public health issues overlap with HIV infection. TB, for example, is a leading cause of death globally, and HIV/TB coinfection is a considerable cause of morbidity and mortality. In the earliest days of the HIV epidemic, death was typically due to AIDS-related complications. Now that treatment advances have reduced the risk of HIV-related complications, increasing attention is also being paid to viral coinfections such as hepatitis B and C. This section very briefly highlights the important comorbid issues that are of concern in relation to HIV epidemic control and individual patient care.

TB/HIV Coinfection

TB remains a major global health problem. One-third of the world's population has latent TB infection, and the average lifetime risk of developing TB in those individuals is 5–10%, although the risk is much higher when certain predisposing factors such as malnutrition, or HIV infection are present [98]. TB accelerates replication of HIV, and HIV accelerates the progression of TB. The risk of developing TB is estimated by WHO to be between 12 and 20 times greater in people living with HIV than among those without HIV infection, and 320,000 people died from HIV-associated TB in 2012 [99]. Although that number represented a decrease in deaths compared to 2004, substantial work remains to be done. In people with latent TB infection, HIV is the most important risk factor for progression to active TB disease. Effective responses to either one of the epidemics of TB or HIV require that they each address the other burden. According to WHO guidelines, TB is a criterion for the initiation of ART regardless of CD4 cell count, but only 55% of HIV-infected TB patients were receiving ART in 2013 [99]. A particular medical challenge in the management of coinfection with HIV and TB is that over half of the approved antiretroviral drugs interact adversely with the TB drug rifampin, precluding their concomitant use.

It is recommended to screen all people living with HIV for TB infection and vice versa in areas with high burden of TB. Strategies to improve the control of HIV/TB co-epidemics include: early diagnosis and treatment of HIV infection, treatment of latent TB infection with isoniazid preventive therapy, early diagnosis and treatment of active TB, improvement in diagnostics for TB detection, colocation and joint planning of TB and HIV services.

Hepatitis B

Chronic hepatitis B virus (HBV) coinfection occurs in 5–10% of those with HIV, and progression of HBV is more aggressive in those with HBV/HIV coinfection than in those with HBV alone—HIV increases the risk of cirrhosis and end-stage liver disease in HBV [100–102]. Several antiretroviral drugs (FTC, 3TC and tenofovir) that are used to treat HIV infection also have activity against HBV, and caution must be observed if these drugs are discontinued, as flares in HBV can occur. HBV treatment is recommended for all HIV coinfected patients in whom any HBV replication is present. HBV vaccine is recommended for people with HIV infection who are not coinfected and have close contact with HBV-infected people.

Hepatitis C

All HIV-infected individuals should be screened for hepatitis C virus (HCV) infection as 5–15% of people with HIV also have HCV infection. HIV infection enhances replication of HCV, and the rate of progression to cirrhosis in HIV/HCV coinfected patients is estimated to be three times higher than that in HCV-infected patients alone [20]. Although ART slows the rate of HCV progression in coinfected patients, the rate is still greater than those with HCV alone. For many years, the mainstay of HCV treatment was a combination of peginterferon and ribavirin for 24–48 weeks. This treatment regimen has a number of troublesome side effects, results in a "cure" for between 45 and 70% of mono-infected patients, and has reduced long-term efficacy in HIV/HCV coinfected patients. Recently, successes of so-called direct-acting agents that directly affect HCV are revolutionizing HCV treatment and cure. A study presented at the 2014 International AIDS Society conference found a 94% HCV cure rate for people with HIV and HCV genotype 1 infection using a combination of ribavirin and directly acting agents, and other studies show similarly high rates of cure of HCV with newer agents, depending on viral and patient characteristics [103, 104]. These advances show tremendous promise for both HCV mono-infection and for those with HIV/HCV coinfection, and clinical guidelines are likely to evolve rapidly in the next few years.

Anemia

The prevalence of anemia is higher in people living with HIV infection than in the general population. Risks for HIV-associated anemia are multifactorial, including a direct effect of HIV infection, and drug side effects—of antivirals, antifungals and antineoplastic agents, nutritional deficiencies, blood loss, among others [105]. HIV infection can also magnify the major causes of anemia in the developing world, including iron insufficiency and parasitosis. Although causal relationship has not been established, anemia has been associated with decreased survival and increased disease progression in those with HIV infection [106, 107]. Furthermore, fatigue—a common symptom of anemia—is associated with decreased physical function and impaired quality of life [108]. Special attention must be paid to addressing this comorbidity and its impact.

Food Insecurity and Undernutrition

Food insecurity and HIV infection overlap geographically and have negative additive effects that are bidirectional [109, 110]. In addition to impacting HIV through nutritional pathways (which are discussed in detail in Chap. 20, food insecurity impacts mental health and behavior, contributing to negative outcomes for those with HIV infection, and increasing vulnerability to HIV infection among those that are not yet infected [109].

Schistosomiasis

Schistosomiasis, also known as bilharzia, is an important but neglected tropical disease that has a large public health impact, particularly because it is highly prevalent in individuals of reproductive age in some regions of the world, mostly in sub-Saharan Africa. Evidence suggests that schistosome infection leads to increased susceptibility to HIV-1 infection, more rapid progression of HIV disease and increased transmission of HIV infection. This effect appears to be most important for Schistosoma haematobium infection [111, 112]. The importance of this coinfection has not been sufficiently emphasized to date, but must be addressed.

Women and Children

HIV infection is a leading cause of death of women of reproductive age worldwide and is an important contributor to infant mortality. Transmission of HIV from mother to child occurs in utero, peripartum and postpartum during breastfeeding. Reducing the transmission of HIV from mother to infant has been an important part of the response to the HIV epidemic, with successes beginning in the mid-1990s when research demonstrated that maternal AZT treatment could reduce transmission to infants. Over the subsequent 20 years, advances in research have demonstrated that antiretroviral drugs taken before, during and post-partum can further reduce transmission. Prevention of mother-to-child transmission of HIV (PMTCT) programs have reduced transmission to less than 5% globally for women that are diagnosed with HIV infection and engaged in care. With early intervention and high-quality care, transmission can be even lower—less than 2% [113–115]. Without any intervention, the incidence of mother-to-child transmission is up to 45% [116].

Breastfeeding continues to be an important contributor to HIV transmission to infants. In the USA, replacement feeding is recommended for infants born to HIV-infected mothers. Because of its benefits in protection against diarrheal disease and respiratory illness, its importance in nutrition and overall health of the child, avoidance of breastfeeding is not recommended unless it is safe and affordable to do so, and it is therefore not recommended in many resource-limited settings. The benefits of breastfeeding must be weighed against the risk of transmission of HIV to the infant on the one hand, and the risk of morbidity and death of the infant from unsafe feeding practices on the other. Studies of the use of maternal ART during breastfeeding have demonstrated rates of transmission of HIV to the infant between 1 and 5% [113, 115, 117, 118]. WHO currently recommends that pregnant women with HIV infection are started on ART regardless of their CD4 count and that maternal ART continues at least throughout the period of breastfeeding, to reduce transmission to the child. ART is also recommended for the infant for the first six weeks of life [70, 113, 114]. WHO guidelines then offer the option of either continued ART indefinitely for the mother regardless of her CD4 count (also known as option B+), or stopping ART after the period of breastfeeding if the mother's CD4 count was greater than 500 at the time of initiation (also known as Option B) [81]. Detailed review of PMTCT antiviral protocols is beyond the scope of this chapter, and the reader is referred to the most recently available guidelines to review when and what ART to start, and how long prophylactic ART should continue for the mother and child [79].

Globally, PMTCT strategy involves prevention of HIV infection in women of reproductive age, prevention of undesired pregnancy in women with HIV infection, prevention of mother-to-child transmission of the virus, and provision of ongoing care and treatment to women, their children and their families. Ensuring that women and infants are properly cared for to allow for zero transmission of HIV by definition requires ensuring that women's health is valued, that maternal health services are available to all and that HIV treatment and prevention is integrated with antenatal care services.

Despite the many advances, in 2013, only 54% of pregnant women had an HIV test, only 70% of those that were tested received appropriate treatment for PMTCT [29].

Most young children infected with HIV acquire the virus during pregnancy, childbirth or breastfeeding. Global improvements in PMTCT programs and access to HIV treatment have reduced the number of children newly infected with HIV: From 2002 to 2013, there was a 58% reduction [29]. But infection in children remains an important public health problem, in part because of insufficient investments in diagnostic tools and in treatment formulations for children, and in a lack of sufficient social and economic support for those that are either infected or otherwise affected by HIV. In 2013, 3.2 million children were estimated to be living with HIV [29]. The mortality rate of these children is extremely high during the two first years of life, so it is critical to rapidly diagnose HIV infection and to begin ART in infants (as well as in their caregivers). Children infected with HIV also have special requirements in terms of psychosocial support, not only as it relates to disclosure of their own infection, but also related to the family and life events that they may have experienced, to stigma and loss, as well as the need to address adherence to ART in a way that ensures that they remain healthy. In addition to those infected by HIV, millions of children are indirectly affected by the HIV epidemic. As well as their own pain and suffering, the societal impact of this issue cannot be underestimated.

Conclusion

In 2015, there is cause for optimism as it relates to HIV. Hope exists for the end of deaths due to AIDS, and much progress has been made: Science has been advancing rapidly, many people living with HIV are living decades longer, lives are being saved, and infections are being averted. But nearly half of the people living with HIV infection do not know it, and too few people have access to lifesaving medical care, including ART. Progress in some particular populations has also been very slow—often reflecting societies' preexisting inequities. To ensure that progress continues and expands, a funded, coordinated, integrated HIV approach is critical. Addressing social disparities and structural barriers to care will be essential in the next phase of the response. In the words of UNAIDS Executive Director, Michel Sidibé:

> Ensuring that no one is left behind means closing the gap between people who can get services and people who can't, the people who are protected and the people who are punished… Working together, ending the AIDS epidemic is possible, and it will take leaving no one behind [29].

Discussion Points

- What social factors were important in contributing to access to treatment and care for people living with HIV infection in the first two decades of the HIV epidemic?
- Why were there different guidelines for HIV treatment and care in resource-rich countries compared to resource-poor countries? Is this appropriate?
- What barriers exist to creating an "AIDS-free generation," and how might they be overcome?
- Why does stigma exist around HIV, and how can it be reduced?
- What are "structural" barriers to health care and what social and economic issues are relevant in diagnosing and treating HIV infection?
- How might you design a study to evaluate the effectiveness of post-exposure prophylaxis for HIV? Is such a study ethical?

- Mortality among children with HIV infection is very high in the first two years of life. Why? What strategies could help to reduce this mortality?

Acknowledgments Many thanks to Hannah Hughes and Maeve Montague for contributing to research, summarizing literature reviews, copy editing and other support for the writing of this chapter.

References

1. UNAIDS. Fact Sheet 2014: UNAIDS; 2014. Available from: http://www.unaids.org/en/media/unaids/contentassets/documents/factsheet/2014/20140716_FactSheet_en.pdf. Accessed 31 Aug 2015.
2. UNAIDS. UNAIDS report on the global AIDS epidemic 2013 Geneva, Switzerland: UNAIDS; 2013. Available from: http://www.unaids.org/en/media/unaids/contentassets/documents/epidemiology/2013/gr2013/UNAIDS_Global_Report_2013_en.pdf. Accessed 31 Aug 2015.
3. AVERT. Averting HIV and AIDS; 2014. Available from: http://www.avert.org/. Accessed 31 Aug 2015.
4. AMFAR. 2014. Available from: http://www.amfar.org. Accessed 31 Aug 2015.
5. Masur H, Michelis MA, Greene JB, Onorato I, Stouwe RA, Holzman RS, et al. An outbreak of community-acquired Pneumocystis carinii pneumonia: initial manifestation of cellular immune dysfunction. New Engl J Med. 1981;305(24):1431–8.
6. Hymes KB, Cheung T, Greene JB, Prose NS, Marcus A, Ballard H, et al. Kaposi's sarcoma in homosexual men-a report of eight cases. Lancet. 1981;2(8247):598–600.
7. du Bois RM, Branthwaite MA, Mikhail JR, Batten JC. Primary Pneumocystis carinii and cytomegalovirus infections. Lancet. 1981;2(8259):1339.
8. Mann JM. In: Gottlieb MS, Jeffries DJ, Mildvan D, Pinching AJ, Quinn TC, Weiss RA, editors. Current topics in AIDS, vol 2. Chichester: Wiley; 1989.
9. Quinn TC, Mann JM, Curran JW, Piot P. AIDS in Africa: an epidemiologic paradigm. Science. 1986;234 (4779):955–63.
10. Centers for Disease Control and Prevention. Unexplained immunodeficiency and opportunistic infections in infants–New York, New Jersey, California. MMWR Morbidity and mortality weekly report. 1982;31(49):665–7.
11. Kher U. A Name for the Plague. Time. 30 Mar 2003.
12. Barre-Sinoussi F, Chermann JC, Rey F, Nugeyre MT, Chamaret S, Gruest J, et al. Isolation of a T-lymphotropic retrovirus from a patient at risk for acquired immune deficiency syndrome (AIDS). Science. 1983;220(4599):868–71.
13. Connor S, Kingman S. The search for the virus. London, United Kingdom: Penguin Books Ltd; 1998 35 p.
14. Bureau of Hygiene & Tropical Diseases. AIDS Newsletter. London: Bureau of Hygiene & Tropical Diseases 1986 Contract No.: 1, 30 Jan.
15. Fischl MA, Richman DD, Grieco MH, Gottlieb MS, Volberding PA, Laskin OL, et al. The efficacy of azidothymidine (AZT) in the treatment of patients with AIDS and AIDS-related complex. A double-blind, placebo-controlled trial. New Engl J Med. 1987;317(4):185–91.
16. Public US. Health Service Task Force. Recommendations of the U.S. Public Health Service Task Force on the Use of Zidovudine to Reduce Perinatal Transmission of Human Immunodeficiency Virus. Morb Mortal Wkly Rep. 1994;43(RR11):1–20.
17. AVERT. History of AIDS: 1993–1997. 2015. Available from: http://www.avert.org/history-aids-1993-1997.htm. Accessed 31 Aug 2015.
18. Altman K. AIDS is now the leading killer of Americans from 25–44. New York Times, 1995.
19. Cooper DA, Merigan TC. Clinical treatment. AIDS. 1996;10 Suppl A:S133–4.
20. BBC News. World: Africa AIDS drug trade dispute ends, 1999. 18 Sept 1999.
21. McNeil DG, Jr. Companies to cut cost of AIDS drugs for poor nations. N Y Times Web. 12 May 2000.
22. World Health Organisation. Progress on Global Access to HIV Antiretroviral Therapy: An update on "3 by 5", 2005.
23. Farmer PE. Shattuck lecture. Chronic infectious disease and the future of health care delivery. New Engl J Med. 2013;369(25):2424–36.
24. Farmer P, Leandre F, Mukherjee JS, Claude M, Nevil P, Smith-Fawzi MC, et al. Community-based approaches to HIV treatment in resource-poor settings. Lancet. 2001;358(9279):404–9.
25. Mukherjee JS, Farmer PE, Niyizonkiza D, McCorkle L, Vanderwarker C, Teixeira P, et al. Tackling HIV in resource poor countries. BMJ. 2003;327(7423):1104–6.

26. Bailey RC, Moses S, Parker CB, Agot K, Maclean I, Krieger JN, et al. Male circumcision for HIV prevention in young men in Kisumu, Kenya: a randomised controlled trial. Lancet. 2007;369(9562):643–56.
27. Gray RH, Kigozi G, Serwadda D, Makumbi F, Watya S, Nalugoda F, et al. Male circumcision for HIV prevention in men in Rakai, Uganda: a randomised trial. Lancet. 2007;369(9562):657–66.
28. Cohen MS, Chen YQ, McCauley M, Gamble T, Hosseinipour MC, Kumarasamy N, et al. Prevention of HIV-1 infection with early antiretroviral therapy. New Engl J Med. 2011;365(6):493–505.
29. UNAIDS. The Gap Report, 2014. Available from: http://www.unaids.org/en/media/unaids/contentassets/documents/unaidspublication/2014/UNAIDS_Gap_report_en.pdf. Accessed 31 Aug 2015.
30. Medecins Sans Frontiers. A Matter of Life and Death: The role of patents in access to essential medicines, 2001. Available from: http://www.msf.org/article/matter-life-and-death-role-patents-access-essential-medicines.
31. AVERT. Treatment Access: Antiretroviral drug prices, 2015. Available from: http://www.avert.org/antiretroviral-drug-prices.htm. Accessed 31 Aug 2015.
32. Waning B, Diedrichsen E, Moon S. A lifeline to treatment: the role of Indian generic manufacturers in supplying antiretroviral medicines to developing countries. J Int AIDS Soc. 2010;13:35.
33. The Global Fund to Fight AIDS Tuberculosis and Malaria. Fighting AIDS, Tuberculosis and Malaria, 2014. Available from: http://www.theglobalfund.org/en/about/diseases/. 31 Aug 2015.
34. The Global Fund to Fight AIDS Tuberculosis and Malaria. Structures, 2014. Available from: http://www.theglobalfund.org/en/about/structures/. 18 July 2014.
35. Center for Health and Gender Equity. PEPFAR's Past, 2014. Available from: http://www.pepfarwatch.org/about_pepfar/pepfars_past/. 16 Jul 2014.
36. Congress US. An act: to authorize appropriations for fiscal years 2009 through 2013 to provide assistance to foreign countries to combat HIV/AIDS, tuberculosis, and malaria, and for other purposes. Washington: U.S. Congress; 2008.
37. The Office of the U.S. Global AIDS Coordinator. Controlling the epidemic: delivering on the promise of an AIDS-free generation, 2014. Available from: http://www.pepfar.gov/documents/organization/234744.pdf.
38. World Health Organisation. World Health Report. Health systems: improving performance. Geneva, Switzerland: World Health Organisation; 2000. p. 2000.
39. World Health Organisation. Report on the 3rd expert consultation on maximizing positive synergies between health systems and Global Health Initiatives, WHO, Geneva, 2–3 October 2008. Geneva, Switzerland: World Health Organization; 2008.
40. World Health Organisation. The WHO Health Systems Framework Geneva, Switzerland, 2014. Available from: http://www.wpro.who.int/health_services/health_systems_framework/en/. 21 July 2014.
41. Centers for Disease Control and Prevention. Update: acquired immunodeficiency syndrome–United States. MMWR Morb Mortal Wkly Rep. 1985;34(18):245–8.
42. Reeves JD, Doms RW. Human immunodeficiency virus type 2. J Gen Virol. 2002;83(Pt 6):1253–65.
43. Buonaguro L, Tornesello ML, Buonaguro FM. Human immunodeficiency virus type 1 subtype distribution in the worldwide epidemic: pathogenetic and therapeutic implications. J Virol. 2007;81(19):10209–19.
44. Clavel F, Guetard D, Brun-Vezinet F, Chamaret S, Rey MA, Santos-Ferreira MO, et al. Isolation of a new human retrovirus from West African patients with AIDS. Science. 1986;233(4761):343–6.
45. World Health Organisation. HIV/AIDS Fact Sheet Geneva, Switzerland: World Health Organisation; 2013. Available from: http://www.who.int/mediacentre/factsheets/fs360/en/. 4 Mar 2014.
46. Naif HM. Pathogenesis of HIV Infection. Infect Dis Rep. 2013;5(Suppl 1):e6.
47. Baeten JM, Donnell D, Kapiga SH, Ronald A, John-Stewart G, Inambao M, et al. Male circumcision and risk of male-to-female HIV-1 transmission: a multinational prospective study in African HIV-1-serodiscordant couples. AIDS. 2010;24(5):737–44.
48. Quinn TC, Wawer MJ, Sewankambo N, Serwadda D, Li C, Wabwire-Mangen F, et al. Viral load and heterosexual transmission of human immunodeficiency virus type 1. Rakai Project Study Group. New Engl J Med. 2000;342(13):921–9.
49. Ms C, Ke M, Mk S, Ka P, Ad K. Antiviral agents and HIV prevention: controversies, conflicts, and consensus. AIDS. 2012;26(13):1585–98.
50. Marrazzo JM, del Rio C, Holtgrave DR, et al. HIV prevention in clinical care settings: 2014 recommendations of the international antiviral society–USA panel. JAMA. 2014;312(4):390–409.
51. Tindall B, Barker S, Donovan B, Barnes T, Roberts J, Kronenberg C, et al. Characterization of the acute clinical illness associated with human immunodeficiency virus infection. Arch Intern Med. 1988;148(4):945–9.
52. Schacker T, Collier AC, Hughes J, Shea T, Corey L. Clinical and epidemiologic features of primary HIV infection. Ann Intern Med. 1996;125(4):257–64.
53. Pedersen C, Lindhardt BO, Jensen BL, Lauritzen E, Gerstoft J, Dickmeiss E, et al. Clinical course of primary HIV infection: consequences for subsequent course of infection. BMJ. 1989;299(6692):154–7.
54. Bacchetti P, Moss AR. Incubation period of AIDS in San Francisco. Nature. 1989;338(6212):251–3.

55. World Health Organisation. WHO Case definitions of HIV for surveillance and revised clinical staging and immunological classification of HIV-related disease in adults and children, 2007.
56. World Health Organisation. Global Summary of HIV/AIDS Epidemic 2013. Available from: http://www.who.int/hiv/data/epi_core_dec2014.png?ua=1. 22 July 2014.
57. Ramjee G, Daniels B. Women and HIV in sub-Saharan Africa. AIDS Res Ther. 2013;10(1):30.
58. World Health Organisation. Antiretroviral Drugs in Low- and Middle- Income Countries: technical report July 2014. Melbourne, Australia: World Health Organisation, 2014 July, 2014. Report No.
59. World Health Organisation. WHO Progress Brief - Voluntary medical male circumcision for HIV prevention in priority countries of East and Southern Africa: World Health Organization; 2014. Available from: http://www.who.int/hiv/topics/malecircumcision/male-circumcision-info-2014/en/. July 2014.
60. World Health Organisation. WHO Definition of Health. World Health Organisation, 1948.
61. U.S. Department of Health & Human Services. HIV/AIDS Care Continuum: What is the HIV Care Continuum? 2013. Report No. 18 Dec 2013.
62. Bradley H, Hall HI, Wolitski RJ, Van Handel MM, Stone AE, LaFlam M, et al. Vital Signs: HIV diagnosis, care, and treatment among persons living with HIV–United States, 2011. MMWR Morb Mortal Wkly Rep. 2014;63 (47):1113–7.
63. Signs Vital. HIV Diagnosis, Care, and Treatment Among Persons Living with HIV—United States, 2011. Morb Mortal Wkly Rep. 2014;63(47):1113–7.
64. Barth RE, van der Loeff MF, Schuurman R, Hoepelman AI, Wensing AM. Virological follow-up of adult patients in antiretroviral treatment programmes in sub-Saharan Africa: a systematic review. Lancet Infect Dis. 2010;10 (3):155–66.
65. Kimanga DO, Ogola S, Umuro M, Ng'ang'a A, Kimondo L, Murithi P, et al. Prevalence and incidence of HIV infection, trends, and risk factors among persons aged 15–64 years in Kenya: results from a nationally representative study. J Acquir Immune Defic Syndr. 2014;66(Suppl 1):S13–26.
66. Lin X, Dietz PM, Rodriguez V, Lester D, Hernandez P, Moreno-Walton L, et al. Routine HIV Screening in Two Health-Care Settings—New York City and New Orleans, 2011–2013. MMWR Morb Mortal Wkly Rep. 2014;63 (25):537–41.
67. Ivers LC, Teng JE, Jerome JG, Bonds M, Freedberg KA, Franke MF. A randomized trial of ready-to-use supplementary food versus corn-soy blend plus as food rations for HIV-infected adults on antiretroviral therapy in rural Haiti. Clin Infect Dis (an official publication of the Infectious Diseases Society of America). 2014;58 (8):1176–84.
68. Centers for Disease Control and Prevention. Association of Public Health Laboratories. Laboratory Testing for the Diagnosis of HIV Infection: Updated Recommendations; 2014.
69. Organization Pan American Health. Guidelines for the implementation of reliable and efficient diagnostic HIV testing. Washington, DC: Region of the Americas; 2008.
70. Havens PL, Mofenson LM. Evaluation and management of the infant exposed to HIV-1 in the United States. Pediatrics. 2009;123(1):175–87.
71. Mayer KH. Introduction: linkage, engagement, and retention in HIV care: essential for optimal individual- and community-level outcomes in the era of highly active antiretroviral therapy. Clin Infect Dis (an official publication of the Infectious Diseases Society of America). 2011;52(Suppl 2):S205–7.
72. HIV/AIDS Bureau, Special Projects of National Significance Program. Training manual: innovative approaches to engaging hard-to-reach populations living with HIV/AIDS into care. Rockville, MD: U.S. Department of Health and Human Services, Health Resources and Services Administration, 2013.
73. Fawzi MC, Lambert W, Boehm F, Finkelstein JL, Singler JM, Leandre F, et al. Economic risk factors for HIV infection among women in rural Haiti: implications for HIV prevention policies and programs in resource-poor settings. J Women's Health. 2010;19(5):885–92.
74. European AIDS Clinical Society. Guidelines Version 7.1, November 2014, 2014. Available from: http://www.eacsociety.org/files/guidelines-7.1-english.pdf. 28 Aug 2015.
75. Panel on Antiretroviral Guidelines for Adults and Adolescents. Guidelines for the use of antiretroviral agents in HIV-1-infected adults and adolescents.. In: Services DoHaH, editor. 2014.
76. Sax P, Cohen C, Kuritzkes D. HIV essentials. Burlington, MA: Jones and Bartlett Learning; 2014.
77. Walensky RP, Paltiel AD, Losina E, Mercincavage LM, Schackman BR, Sax PE, et al. The survival benefits of AIDS treatment in the United States. J Infect Dis. 2006;194(1):11–9.
78. Helleberg M, May MT, Ingle SM, Dabis F, Reiss P, Fätkenheuer G, et al. Smoking and life expectancy among HIV-infected individuals on antiretroviral therapy in Europe and North America. AIDS (London, England). 2015;29(2):221–9.
79. World Health Organisation. Guidelines: HIV 2014. Available from: http://www.who.int/hiv/pub/guidelines/en/.
80. World Health Organisation. 2013 Consolidated Guidelines on the Use of Antiretroviral Drugs for Treating and Preventing HIV Infection. Recommendations for a public health approach, 2013.

81. World Health Organisation. March 2014 Supplement to the 2013 Consolidated Guidelines on the Use of Antiretroviral Drugs for Treating and Preventing HIV Infection. Recommendations for a public health approach, 2014.

82. Lee PK, Kieffer TL, Siliciano RF, Nettles RE. HIV-1 viral load blips are of limited clinical significance. J Antimicrob Chemother. 2006;57(5):803–5.

83. Wheeler WH, Ziebell RA, Zabina H, Pieniazek D, Prejean J, Bodnar UR, et al. Prevalence of transmitted drug resistance associated mutations and HIV-1 subtypes in new HIV-1 diagnoses, U.S.-2006. AIDS. 2010;24 (8):1203–12.

84. Ross L, Lim ML, Liao Q, Wine B, Rodriguez AE, Weinberg W, et al. Prevalence of antiretroviral drug resistance and resistance-associated mutations in antiretroviral therapy-naive HIV-infected individuals from 40 United States cities. HIV Clin Trials. 2007;8(1):1–8.

85. UNAIDS. Combination HIV Prevention: Tailoring and Coordinating Biomedical, Behavioural and Structural Strategies to Reduce New HIV Infections. A UNAIDS Discussion Paper, 2010.

86. Mayer K, Gazzard B, Zuniga Jm, Amico Kr, Anderson J, Azad Y, et al. Controlling the HIV epidemic with antiretrovirals: IAPAC consensus statement on treatment as prevention and preexposure prophylaxis, 2013; 2325–9574 (Print).

87. Young TN, Arens Fj Fau - Kennedy GE, Kennedy Ge Fau - Laurie JW, Laurie Jw Fau - Rutherford Gw, Rutherford G. Antiretroviral post-exposure prophylaxis (PEP) for occupational HIV exposure. p. 1469–493X.

88. Chacko L, Ford N Fau - Sbaiti M, Sbaiti M Fau - Siddiqui R, Siddiqui R. Adherence to HIV post-exposure prophylaxis in victims of sexual assault: a systematic review and meta-analysis; 2012:1472–3263.

89. Baeten JM, Donnell D, Ndase P, Mugo NR, Campbell JD, Wangisi J, et al. Antiretroviral prophylaxis for HIV prevention in heterosexual men and women. New Engl J Med. 2012;367(5):399–410.

90. Celum C, Baeten JM. Antiretroviral-based HIV-1 prevention: antiretroviral treatment and pre-exposure prophylaxis. Antiviral Ther. 2012;17(8):1483–93.

91. Celum C, Baeten JM. Tenofovir-based pre-exposure prophylaxis for HIV prevention: evolving evidence. Curr Opin Infect Dis. 2012;25(1):51–7.

92. Thigpen MC, Kebaabetswe PM, Paxton LA, Smith DK, Rose CE, Segolodi TM, et al. Antiretroviral preexposure prophylaxis for heterosexual HIV transmission in Botswana. New Engl J Med. 2012;367(5):423–34.

93. Choopanya K, Martin M, Suntharasamai P, Sangkum U, Mock PA, Leethochawalit M, et al. Antiretroviral prophylaxis for HIV infection in injecting drug users in Bangkok, Thailand (the Bangkok Tenofovir Study): a randomised, double-blind, placebo-controlled phase 3 trial. Lancet. 2013;381(9883):2083–90.

94. Auvert B, Sobngwi-Tambekou J, Cutler E, Nieuwoudt M, Lissouba P, Puren A, et al. Effect of male circumcision on the prevalence of high-risk human papillomavirus in young men: results of a randomized controlled trial conducted in Orange Farm, South Africa. J Infect Dis. 2009;199(1):14–9.

95. Auvert B, Taljaard D, Lagarde E, Sobngwi-Tambekou J, Sitta R, Puren A. Randomized, controlled intervention trial of male circumcision for reduction of HIV infection risk: the ANRS 1265 Trial. PLoS Med. 2005;2(11):e298.

96. Lissouba P, Taljaard D, Rech D, Dermaux-Msimang V, Legeai C, Lewis D, et al. Adult male circumcision as an intervention against HIV: an operational study of uptake in a South African community (ANRS 12126). BMC Infect Dis. 2011;11:253.

97. Mahiane SG, Legeai C, Taljaard D, Latouche A, Puren A, Peillon A, et al. Transmission probabilities of HIV and herpes simplex virus type 2, effect of male circumcision and interaction: a longitudinal study in a township of South Africa. AIDS. 2009;23(3):377–83.

98. World Health Organisation. Latent Tuberculosis Infection (LTBI), 2014. Available from: http://www.who.int/tb/challenges/ltbi/en/.

99. World Health Organisation. Eliminating TB Deaths: Time to Step Up the HIV Response. High level International WHO Consultation. Melbourne, Australia: 2014 Sunday 20 July 2014. Report No.

100. Alter M. Epidemiology of viral hepatitis and HIV co-infection. J Hepatol. 2006;44 (1 Suppl):S6–9.

101. Konopnicki D, Mocroft A, de Wit S, Antunes F, Ledergerber B, Katlama C, et al. Hepatitis B and HIV: prevalence, AIDS progression, response to highly active antiretroviral therapy and increased mortality in the EuroSIDA cohort. AIDS. 2005;19(6):593–601.

102. Thio CL, Seaberg EC, Skolasky R Jr, Phair J, Visscher B, Munoz A, et al. HIV-1, hepatitis B virus, and risk of liver-related mortality in the Multicenter Cohort Study (MACS). Lancet. 2002;360(9349):1921–6.

103. Sulkowski M, Eron J, Wyles D, Trinh R, Lalezari J, Slim J, et al. TURQUOISE-I: safety and efficacy of ABT-450/r/Ombitasvir, Dasabuvir, and Ribavirin in patients co-infected with hepatitis C and HIV-1 [Abstract]. 20th International AIDS Conference Melbourne, Australia, 20–25 July 2014.

104. Sulkowski MS, Naggie S, Lalezari J, et al. Sofosbuvir and ribavirin for hepatitis c in patients with HIV coinfection. JAMA. 2014;312(4):353–61.

105. Volberding PA, Levine AM, Dieterich D, Mildvan D, Mitsuyasu R, Saag M, et al. Anemia in HIV Infection: Clinical Impact and Evidence-Based Management Strategies. Clin Infect Dis. 2004;38(10):1454–63.

106. Sullivan P. Associations of anemia, treatments for anemia, and survival in patients with human immunodeficiency virus infection. J Infect Dis. 2002;185(Suppl 2):S138–42.
107. Sullivan P, Hanson D, Chu S, Jones J, Ward J. Epidemiology of anemia in human immunodeficiency virus (HIV)-infected persons: results from the Multistate Adult and Adolescent Spectrum of HIV Disease Surveillance Project. The Adult/Adolescent Spectrum of Disease Group. Blood. 1998;91:301–8.
108. Breitbart W, McDonald MV, Rosenfeld B, Monkman ND, Passik S. Fatigue in ambulatory AIDS patients. J Pain Symptom Manage. 1998;15(3):159–67.
109. Ivers LC, Cullen KA, Freedberg KA, Block S, Coates J, Webb P. HIV/AIDS, undernutrition, and food insecurity. Clin Infect Dis (an official publication of the Infectious Diseases Society of America). 2009;49(7):1096–102.
110. Weiser SD, Young SL, Cohen CR, Kushel MB, Tsai AC, Tien PC, et al. Conceptual framework for understanding the bidirectional links between food insecurity and HIV/AIDS. Am J Clin Nutr. 2011;94(6):1729S–39S.
111. Secor WE. The effects of schistosomiasis on HIV/AIDS infection, progression and transmission. 1746–6318 (Electronic).
112. Mbabazi PS, Andan O, Fitzgerald DW, Chitsulo L, Engels D, Downs JA. Examining the relationship between urogenital schistosomiasis and HIV infection. PLoS Negl Trop Dis. 2011;5(12):e1396.
113. de Vincenzi I. Triple antiretroviral compared with zidovudine and single-dose nevirapine prophylaxis during pregnancy and breastfeeding for prevention of mother-to-child transmission of HIV-1 (Kesho Bora study): a randomised controlled trial. 1474–4457 (Electronic).
114. Chasela CS, Hudgens Mg Fau - Jamieson DJ, Jamieson Dj Fau - Kayira D, Kayira D Fau - Hosseinipour MC, Hosseinipour Mc Fau - Kourtis AP, Kourtis Ap Fau - Martinson F, et al. Maternal or infant antiretroviral drugs to reduce HIV-1 transmission. p. 1533–4406 (Electronic).
115. Marazzi MC, Nielsen-Saines K, Buonomo E, Scarcella P, Germano P, Majid NA, et al. Increased infant human immunodeficiency virus-type one free survival at one year of age in sub-saharan Africa with maternal use of highly active antiretroviral therapy during breast-feeding. Pediatr Infect Dis J. 2009;28(6):483–7.
116. John G, Kreiss J. Mother-to-child transmission of human immunodeficiency virus type. Epidemiol Rev. 1996;18:149.
117. Shapiro RL, Kitch D, Ogwu A, Hughes MD, Lockman S, Powis K, et al. HIV transmission and 24-month survival in a randomized trial of HAART to prevent MTCT during pregnancy and breastfeeding in Botswana. AIDS. 2013;27(12):1911–20.
118. Shapiro RL, Hughes MD, Ogwu A, Kitch D, Lockman S, Moffat C, et al. Antiretroviral regimens in pregnancy and breast-feeding in Botswana. New Engl J Med. 2010;362(24):2282–94.

Chapter 19
Tuberculosis Infection and Nutrition

Anupama Paranandi and Christine Wanke

Keywords Tuberculosis · HIV and tuberculosis co-infection · Malnutrition · Food security · Macronutrient deficiency · Micronutrient deficiency · Macronutrient intervention · Micronutrient intervention

Learning Objectives

- Explore the relationship between food security, weight loss, wasting and active tuberculosis (TB) in resource limited settings.
- Evaluate the role of macronutrient and micronutrient deficiencies in the risk of developing active TB and their role in TB disease outcomes.
- Explain the nutritional requirements of vulnerable populations suffering from active TB.
- Summarize the nutrition deficiencies and nutrition supplementation recommended for those with HIV and TB co-infection.
- Emphasize the impact of TB and HIV treatment on nutritional status in those suffering from disease in resource limited settings.

Introduction

Tuberculosis (TB) is a globally prevalent disease that affected 8.6 million individuals and killed 1.3 million people in 2012 [1]. HIV and TB are the two most common infectious diseases that cause death; over 95% of deaths related to TB occur in low- and middle-income countries [1]. While sub-Saharan Africa harbors the greatest proportion of TB cases, likely as a result of concurrent HIV disease, Asia, and India in particular, has the greatest absolute number of new cases [1].

TB is caused by the bacteria *Mycobacterium tuberculosis* and is spread via respiratory droplets. The clinical manifestations of TB can be varied, but primary infection involves the lungs and is most commonly called pulmonary TB. TB is transmitted from person-to-person through inhalation of

A. Paranandi (✉)
Department of Medicine, Saint Mary's Hospital, 56 Franklin Street,
Waterbury, CT 06706, USA
e-mail: aparanandi@stmh.org

C. Wanke
Medicine/Infectious Diseases, Tufts Medical Center,
750 Washington Street, Boston, MA 02111, USA
e-mail: Christine.wanke@tufts.edu
© Springer Science+Business Media New York 2017
S. de Pee et al. (eds.), *Nutrition and Health in a Developing World*,
Nutrition and Health, DOI 10.1007/978-3-319-43739-2_19

droplets introduced into the air by infected individuals. Once an individual is exposed to the organism, a number of outcomes are possible. Ninety percent of individuals with intact immune systems will control the disease, whereas 10% will develop a primary pulmonary disease. The 90% of individuals that control the disease enter into a quiescent phase termed latent tuberculosis infection (LTBI), and are asymptomatic. The disease may then remain latent throughout life or may become reactivated in certain conditions, for example, when the immune system is compromised. TB treatment involves multidrug therapy for 6 months or longer, with duration of treatment dependent on the form of active TB. If treated adequately, the mortality from TB falls to 5% globally [2].

There is greater TB morbidity and mortality in the resource limited setting, as compared to resource sufficient countries; these differences can be attributed to a multitude of reasons. Poverty, overcrowding, poor access and development in healthcare, and social stigma represent powerful barriers to efforts to treat TB. An additional factor strongly influencing the outcome of TB is malnutrition. This chapter complements Chap. 17 on TB by Oren and McDermid and reviews the relationship between nutrition and TB, before and after the introduction of anti-tuberculosis therapy (ATT), and the role of food assistance, including nutritional interventions.

History of Nutrition in TB

The most common symptoms of pulmonary TB include fevers, night sweats, weight loss, cough, hemoptysis, and swollen lymph nodes. The weight loss, specifically lean muscle mass, is striking enough that TB was known as consumption in the pre-treatment era, and the resulting malnutrition was severe enough to be linked with high rates of morbidity and mortality [3]. Before ATT, a 10–40% mortality rate was common as treatment was largely symptomatic. While there was recognition of TB as a wasting disease as far back as 81 AD, much of our understanding of the impact of endemic TB comes from the sixteenth to eighteenth centuries. The clinical picture of TB has long been termed phthisis or wasting [4]. Others have used the term "consumption" for the cachexia which develops with untreated TB [3].

Prior to the advent of effective ATT, persons of economic means who were infected with TB would be admitted to a sanitorium in the Swiss Alps for treatment with fresh, clean air, rest and a healthy diet, high in protein and dairy products [5–7]. Cod liver oil, which is rich in omega three fatty acids and vitamins A and D, was widely used in these sanitoria [8–10]. Ultimately the use of cod liver oil spread to France and Germany [9, 11]. A clinical trial using untreated historical controls as a comparator found that cod liver oil was able to decrease mortality from 71 to 10% with one year of follow-up [12]. Another study documented an 8 year rather than a 2 year survival for adults with TB when treated with cod liver oil [13]. Whether cod liver oil's benefit is related to the high concentration of vitamins A and D, or its ability to decrease inflammation, or some other mechanism is not clear. Patients were also recognized to gain weight with the use of cod liver oil. Cod liver oil was widely used throughout the second half of the nineteenth century to the 1920s–1940s when the first ATT began to be used [14]. Another diet that was widely used in TB patients was composed of eggs and milk, both good sources of protein. This diet was recommended from 81 AD to the 1950s [15, 16].

The morbidity and mortality associated with untreated TB was frightening enough that TB captured the imagination of composers: Puccini (La Boheme), (La Traviata), playwrights, Chekhov who died of TB), poets, Elizabeth Barrett Browning (Keats (who died of TB), novelists: (Thomas Man (The Magic Mountain), Victor Hugo (Les Miserables) and even in present day, with effective ATT film-makers: Luhrmann (Moulin Rouge, Vittorio de Sica A Bief Vacation; among many others). In any of these media, the hero or heroine succumbs to the wasting induced by TB. Fortunately, at present there is effective ATT, and like ART, is able to reduce morbidity and mortality related to these infections. Unlike HIV and ART, ATT is able to cure TB. With effective ATT available since the 1940–50s, there has been little nutrition research done since that time [17].

Malnutrition and Risk of TB

Malnutrition is associated with an increased risk of TB disease, likely through its impact on immune function. The risk of developing TB is 37.5 times higher in those with malnutrition than in those with normal nutritional status [18]. Risk for TB is related to body mass index (BMI). A 13.8% reduction in the incidence of TB is observed per unit increase in BMI, within the normal-overweight BMI range of 18.5–30 kg/m^2 [19]. A decrease in incidence of smear positive and smear negative TB can be expected with increasing BMI in all age groups [20]. Infected individuals with BMI, average skin fold thickness, or upper arm muscle area in the lowest decile of these measures in a population, when compared to those in the highest decile, had an increased risk of TB by 6–10-fold [18, 19].

Malnutrition and Outcomes of TB

Malnutrition not only increases the risk for the development of active TB, but can affect outcomes of TB disease, including death. Moderate to severe malnutrition, defined as BMI less than 17 kg/m^2, resulted in twice the risk of early death compared to those with higher BMIs [21]. Malnutrition can also affect severity of disease. BMI and phase angle, calculated from bioelectric impedance analysis, a good predictor and estimator of body fat, were inversely associated with severity of tubercular lung disease as determined by chest X-ray findings [22]. Phase angle is a means of assessing biologic tissue electrical activity and helps gauge cell membrane integrity. The reliability of phase angle is unclear as it is calculated from resistance and reactance of the BIA and their may be multiple factors that influence that calculation. The higher the phase angle is, the healthier the cells, tissues, and ultimately the organism are [23]. Phase angle is an independent predictor of mortality in certain disease states, such as HIV infection [23]. In animal studies, malnutrition was associated with higher bacterial burdens and earlier death from infection [24]. Malnutrition also increases the risk of relapse in treated tubercular disease. Weight less than or equal to 90% of ideal body weight, a BMI less than 18.5 kg/m^2 at the time of diagnosis, or increasing weight by less than 5% by the end of the initial part of treatment (first 2 months), has been shown to be associated with a 2.4-fold increase in relapse [25]. Additionally, those with a weight gain less than or equal to 5% at the end of treatment, usually 6 months, had twice the chance of treatment failure or TB relapse [26]. BMI as a surrogate of nutritional status is strongly predictive of the onset and outcome of TB, but dietary quality is also of importance in looking at outcomes of TB disease.

Food Insecurity and TB

The impact of food insecurity in the cycle of malnutrition and TB is profound and parallels the pathways of food insecurity and HIV. Food insecurity, i.e., inadequate access to the right quantity and quality of food, often caused by poverty, can lead to malnutrition, putting one at increased risk of contracting TB and increased risk of developing active TB (see above). Also, active TB requires increased caloric intake to meet the increased energy demands of active disease [27]. Difficulty in meeting these caloric demands increases weight loss and further malnutrition, which then leads to worsened disease outcomes [27].

Further, TB can affect entire families and worsen food insecurity especially it the person with active TB is also the primary income generator for the family, who is now unable to work due to illness [27]. This can increase the risk of developing TB among family members. Further compounding the issue are the increased expenses while undergoing, often free of charge, TB treatment (i.e. associated health care and medical costs as well as opportunity costs for transport and lost income), leading to the possible diversion of household resources food to disease treatment [27, 28]. Food insecurity is a detriment to maintain nutrition and health and feeds the vicious cycle of malnutrition and TB disease.

Micronutrients and Risk of TB

Increased dietary diversity, as an indicator of dietary quality, particularly greater intake of fruits and vegetables, was associated with a decreased risk of TB [29]. Those with consistently low vitamin C levels were more likely to develop active TB than those with adequate levels [29]. Similarly, vitamin A deficiency has been associated with a higher risk of TB [30–32]. Although not extensively studied, vitamin E deficiency has been found in patients with TB as compared to those without disease [30, 33, 34]. A current topic of interest is vitamin D (one of the components of cod liver oil discussed above). Vitamin D is related to immune function, particularly in macrophages, which help contain TB in its latent, quiescent state [18]. Studies suggest that vitamin D deficiency can predispose an individual to active TB [18]. Deficiencies of zinc, selenium, and iron are more frequent in those with TB infection [35, 36]. These micronutrient deficiencies may have a significant impact on immune function.

Macronutrients and Risk of TB

Protein energy malnutrition (PEM) also affects cell-mediated immunity, and permits the progression of tubercular disease [29]. In animal models, PEM has been found to reduce the inflammatory cytokines that are necessary for the host to control TB. These include IL-2, interferon gamma, and tumor necrosis factor—alpha [24, 37]. There is speculation that PEM can also affect the accuracy of TB skin testing, which may result in false negative results and delay appropriate infection control and treatment [38].

TB and Cachexia

Active TB results in cachexia through several pathways, hence the term "consumption" used to describe TB in the past [29, 39]. Active TB can induce a catabolic or hypermetabolic state, cause nutrient malabsorption and a reduction in appetite. Studies have found that patients with tuberculosis utilized protein for energy production rather than for endogenous protein synthesis, more so than non-infected malnourished or normally nourished subjects [39, 40]. Added to that is the increased energy requirements in pro-inflammatory states due to increased production of cytokines with lipolytic and proteolytic components [39, 40]. Furthermore, dysregulation of enzymes that control appetite induce anorexia and further worsen cachexia. Inflammatory cytokines can increase leptin levels and promote weight loss [41]. Peptide YY and resistin, two of the hormones that decrease appetite were found to be up-regulated in TB infection [42]. Peptide YY was found to be the strongest independent predictor of appetite in cases of tuberculosis [42]. Once treatment was instituted the dysregulated hormone levels slowly normalized to control levels over the 6-month treatment period [42]. ATT, in general, helps reverse many of the processes promoting cachexia and helps in regaining weight lost due to disease.

However, access to treatment and outcome of treatment is not the same among different socio-economic groups and across high, middle or low-income settings. Among the poor in low-resource settings, there is a greater incidence of delayed diagnosis, delayed initiation of treatment, suboptimal adherence and failure to complete treatment [28]. Furthermore, due to high prevalence of food insecurity and malnutrition in low-resource settings, just treating the infection may not be enough to recover nutritional status and health. The emergence of multiple and extremely drug resistant tuberculosis (MRD and XDR) has also revived the interest in nutritional interventions [43]. The impact of nutritional interventions provided in addition to ATT, especially in low-resource settings is reviewed below.

Macronutrient Interventions and TB

To be clear, the truly effective treatment for tuberculosis is antibiotic combination treatment. In fact, without treatment the overall mortality rate can be 50% [2]. However, because malnutrition can have detrimental effects on the progression and outcome of TB, the general recommendation by the WHO and UNAIDS is to improve nutrition as an adjunct to treatment [44, 45]. Providing food assistance in the form of nutritious foods for the TB patient and food or income support for the patient and affected household may not only contribute to reversing malnutrition, but can also encourage infected individuals to remain in care, thereby helping them complete treatment and achieve cure and also protect food security and nutrition of other household members [45, 46].

However, only a few studies objectively assessed the impact of nutritional supplementation on TB disease and treatment related outcomes including retention in care, and showed mixed results. The equivocal benefits of nutritional supplementation found in these studies may be a reflection of study design, variability in populations or treatment, or lack of power to detect a meaningful difference for primary or secondary outcomes rather than a true measure of the intervention itself.

A series of randomized controlled trials done in low- and middle-income countries among adults considered underweight or with low-normal BMIs used a variation of nutritional supplements (cooked meal or high energy supplements with balanced quantities of protein, fat and carbohydrates) with or without nutritional advice, compared to control groups of similar adults being given no intervention and only nutritional advice [2]. The outcomes assessed, which were different trial to trial, were varied and included death, treatment completion, sputum clearance, weight gain, grip strength and quality of life [2]. In terms of death and cure, there was no significant benefit in any of the treatment groups; however the studies were underpowered to effectively demonstrate this [2]. Statistically significant rates of treatment completion and sputum conversion were seen [2]. Additionally, the results also showed increases in weight gain and grip strength, at least within the treatment period [2].

The use of nutritional supplementation in resource limited settings in those who are food insecure to ensure treatment completion is a practical consideration, especially as treatment completion beneficially impacts outcome. Few have rigorously researched the enabling role of food assistance on TB treatment completion. One randomized controlled trial done in Timor-Leste among poor, mostly underweight (80% of study population) men undergoing treatment for newly diagnosed TB, used one nutritionally balanced meal daily and then food packages later in the course of treatment versus nutritional advice alone in the control group, and assessed treatment completion (including cure) in these men [47]. The study found no significant difference in the treatment completion rate among those who were given nutritional supplementation compared to those who only received nutritional advice, which the authors state may be related to the fact that the families were not so much affected by food insecurity [47].

In general, the randomized controlled studies of macronutrient interventions as adjunct to TB treatment have had small sample sizes or flawed study designs and have been unable to demonstrate a consistent benefit on mortality, cure, successful completion of treatment, or clearance of mycobacteria from the sputum [2]. However, there has been some suggestion that there is improvement in weight gain and quality of life with nutrition supplements [2].

However, taking a broader perspective, a recent review that documented substantial costs to the household of TB, distinguished two ways to reduce treatment costs for the patient, either by reducing the direct and indirect costs of seeking a diagnosis and obtaining treatment and/or providing an income transfers to offset some of the incurred costs [28]. In fact, a recent review of studies that provided food assistance in the form of food (e.g. macronutrient supplementation) or as cash or vouchers to people on ART or TB treatment, reported that eight of the ten studies found that the food assistance enabled adherence and/or completion of TB treatment or ART [46]. This indicates that food provision is not only a biological, but also a behavioral intervention, and underscores that unresolved food insecurity can be an impediment to treatment adherence and consequently to good treatment outcomes.

Micronutrient Interventions in TB

Multiple studies have been conducted to elucidate the role and possible benefit of micronutrient supplementation in TB management. Randomized-control trials (RCT), using one, two or multi-micronutrient supplementation in as much as 10 times the recommended dietary intake, showed no evidence of a benefit on TB mortality in HIV negative patients [2]. Various studies have assessed a variety of micronutrient interventions with weight gain as the outcome [48]. However, the general consensus is that micronutrients alone are unlikely to have an impact on weight gain while on TB treatment [2].

Micronutrient supplementation has shown inconsistent effects on sputum clearance [2]. A dual vitamin supplementation of vitamin A plus zinc was studied and in the short term a greater number of patients in the micronutrient group cleared their sputum as compared to the placebo group [35]. Those patients receiving micronutrient intervention showed a greater decrease in the pulmonary lesion size on chest X-ray, and reported increased general well-being [35]. A caveat to these observations is that, in general, vitamin A levels have been found to increase in the plasma of TB-infected patients on treatment independent of supplementation [2]. While this does not provide a clear answer about the role of vitamin A and its supplementation in TB, the benefits of treatment with cod liver oil before the introduction of ATT (see section on history of nutrition in TB above) may have in-part been related to its vitamin A content. Zinc levels are decreased in TB disease, and the supplementation with zinc in this study may have contributed to the benefits seen [35].

Molecular and cellular studies of vitamin D have shown that vitamin D can improve the ability of macrophages to kill TB [29, 49], and vitamin D deficiency has been associated with greater susceptibility to TB [43]. While this would also explain part of the impact observed of treatment with cod liver oil (rich in vitamins A and D and essential fatty acids), the clinical benefits of adding Vitamin D to ATT are not yet clear. In a randomized placebo controlled trial, adult patients with TB starting anti-TB treatment were either given placebo or 100,000 IU vitamin D at inclusion, 5 and 8 months after the start of treatment [50]. No significant difference was observed in the clinical severity of disease, nor 12-month mortality between the two groups [50].

Human and *M. tuberculosis* (MTB) iron metabolism, especially in terms of the onset and mechanism, is incompletely understood. In general, MTB requires iron for many of its enzymatic functions, and flourishes in iron rich environments in experimental models. Furthermore, studies have shown a strong correlation between dietary iron overload and increased risk of developing active TB and mortality from tuberculosis [51]. On the flip side, those afflicted with disease are generally found to have anemia, a state of low hemoglobin. Anemia may result from a number of etiologies, especially due to chronic disease, underlying iron deficiency from baseline malnutrition, the use of host iron stores by the pathogen, or from the body's iron sequestration as a defense against the pathogen [52]. Anemia has been found to be a risk factor for the increased mortality seen in pulmonary TB [53]. Much is still unknown about the sequence and mechanism of iron metabolism and exchange between host and pathogen. Hence, the exact causal relationship between iron stores, disease and mortality has not been established. There are no strong and specific guidelines addressing iron supplementation in terms of TB management.

Not enough data is available in support of any one micronutrient over another in terms of their impact on tuberculosis cure. As a result, the WHO, recognizing micronutrient deficiencies as an indication of overall mal- and under-nutrition, suggest improving overall nutritional status and supplementing micronutrients at the daily recommended nutrient intake level as a potential means to improve disease outcomes [44].

TB Treatment and Nutrition

TB treatment helps normalize nutritional status in those afflicted with disease as noted by an increase in weight throughout and after completing treatment. Much of it has to do with reversing the increased metabolic demands of the disease, as well as improving nutrient absorption and appetite. Weight gain is particularly evident as an increase in fat mass rather than lean muscle mass, though in men, lean mass is regained at faster rate than in women [54]. Treatment also improves levels of micronutrients and trace elements [36], although it is difficult to determine how much of the improvement seen in intervention groups could be attributed to the treatment alone, as opposed to treatment plus improved nutrient intake and absorption. Further confounding the picture, acute changes in several trace elements can be seen during active disease independent of nutritional status. Some examples are decreases in zinc and increases in copper [41]. In some resource limited settings, BMI can be slow to return to normal levels which may be related to poor nutritional intake of those affected by the disease [55]. Important to note is that treatment, while improving weight gain, may not necessarily restore lean muscle [56]. Restoration of lean body mass may take longer than 1 year, especially in those with poor nutritional intake [57] and may also require appropriate physical activity to stimulate growth of muscle tissue.

Vulnerable Populations

Children, Nutrition and TB

TB in children (infants to early adolescence) is much the same as in adults. However, one large difference is that the immune system in young children is immature, with incomplete immune function. It is well known that newborns rely extensively on the innate immune system and maternal antibodies [58]. With the added stress of malnutrition, the impact on immune function is more profound. For example, studies have shown that deficiencies in protein or micronutrients such as vitamin A, D, E, selenium, iron, and zinc may reduce the development and function of the immune system [58]. This may place malnourished children, at any age, at heightened risk of development of TB. It has been suggested that the lower amount of body fat in children contributes to the higher risk of developing active TB [29].

Nutrition is important for any child with acute illness in order to meet the increased metabolic demands of disease. However, few studies have assessed the impact of specific nutritional supplements in children with TB. One randomized trial conducted in Tanzania looked at daily micronutrient supplementation versus placebo on TB outcomes in 255 children aged 6 weeks to 5 years of age [59]. There was no significant effect of multivitamin supplementation on weight gain in the short term [59]. However, supplementation resulted in significant improvements of hemoglobin levels in all age groups [59]. Whether the increased weight or hemoglobin has a clinical impact on mortality, cure, or sputum clearance, remains unknown. As for specific guidelines, the WHO guidelines for nutritional care for patients with TB emphasizes adequate and appropriate nutrition to counter under- and malnutrition in children in general, but given the inconclusive evidence does not recommend any additional nutritional supplementation for children suffering from TB [44]. Adolescents with TB pose additional challenges as rate of weight change and growth need to be monitored carefully. How to position these vulnerable adolescents to provide the maximum opportunity to avoid infection with TB or to be successfully treated for TB is not clear.

Pregnancy, Nutrition and TB

Tuberculosis is one of the top 3 causes of death in women aged 15–45 years [60]. Pregnancy makes women more vulnerable to both malnutrition and to tuberculosis. Additionally, pregnant women infected with TB may have a 20% increase in morbidity, such as disorders of hypertension or pre-eclampsia, when compared to pregnant women not infected with TB. Tuberculosis can also result in obstetrical complications including spontaneous abortion, small-for-gestation age (SGA) fetus, and decreased weight gain in pregnancy [60]. It is also associated with preterm labor, low birth weight and increased neonatal mortality [60]. The average weight for newborn infants of mothers with TB was significantly lower, at 2859 ± 78.5 g, than controls, 3099 ± 484 g, and these infants were more likely to have a low birth weight, on average 2-fold greater likelihood of weighing less than 2500 g [40]. These poor outcomes are related to the difficulty in achieving adequate weight gain [44]. In general, a healthy woman should gain 10–14 kg during pregnancy to ensure a full-term, adequate weight infant [44]. This same recommendation applies to pregnant women with TB [44]. TB treatment is integral to having a safe pregnancy in women suffering from disease, and is also required to enable weight gain, which may need to be further complemented by provision of nutritious foods.

Specific to micronutrients, requirements in any pregnancy can increase by 25–50% compared to non-pregnant state [44]. In pregnant and lactating women with TB, micronutrient supplementation is recommended per the United Nations Multiple Micronutrient Preparation (UNIMMAP), which includes one RDA of Vitamin A, D, E, B1, B2, B6, B12, C, niacin, iron, zinc, copper, iodine and selenium, and 400 micrograms of folic acid [44]. In those with low dietary calcium intake, calcium supplementation at 1.5–2 g of elemental calcium/day, is recommended to prevent complications such as pre-eclampsia [61].

In general, women on appropriate TB treatment for 2 weeks are considered non-contagious and are encouraged to breast feed [60]. However, in resource limited settings breast feeding is recommended from birth despite maternal TB status [60]. While under treatment, anti-TB medications are excreted into breast milk, and detectable levels of anti-TB drugs have been found in infants who are breastfeeding [60]. No toxicity has been reported in infants, which may be related to the small concentrations of anti-TB drugs measured in breast milk [60]. Isoniazid, one of the TB drugs, decreases pyridoxine levels (vitamin B6). Despite the low levels of drug in breast-feeding infants, pyridoxine deficiency may occur and Vitamin B6 need to be supplemented to breastfeeding infants whose mothers are being treated with isoniazid [60].

Conclusion

Malnutrition is common in TB infected individuals and has been found to be associated with severe adverse outcomes. The malnutrition that is seen with TB infections is complex and multifactorial. Medical, socio-economic, cultural and psychological factors all play a role in the development of nutritional compromise in TB infection and vulnerable populations such as children, adolescents, pregnant women and the elderly, as well as the, typically food-insecure, poor in resource-limited settings, are at particular risk. While it is clear that treatment of TB is absolutely critical to improving outcomes, abnormal nutritional status persists despite treatment and continues to contribute to adverse outcomes. In such situations, it becomes important to monitor weight and ensure adequate nutritional intake, which may require provision of food assistance, in the form of nutritious foods and/or income support. According to 2015 WHO guidelines, the goal of nutritional intake of micronutrients should be at the level of one RNI. Balanced macronutrient intake should be such that it restores body weight. In terms of providing supplementation above the WHO recommendations, with the evidence that is currently available, no specific recommendation can be formulated.

Discussion Points

- Discuss the relationship between food insecurity, weight loss, wasting and active tuberculosis (TB) in resource limited settings.
- Discuss the role of macronutrient and micronutrient deficiencies in the risk of developing active TB and their role in TB disease outcomes.
- Discuss the impact of TB treatment on nutritional status in those suffering from disease in resource limited settings.
- Discuss the nutritional requirements of vulnerable populations suffering from active TB.
- Discuss the role of food assistance as additional support to TB patients on treatment and their dependents.

References

1. Tuberculosis Fact Sheet 2014 [internet]. Geneva: World Health Organization; June 2014. Available from http://www.who.int/mediacentre/factsheets/fs104/en/.
2. Sinclair D, Abba K, Grobler L, Sudarsanam TD. Nutritional supplements for people being treated for active tuberculosis. Cochrane Database Syst Rev [internet]. 2011;11:1–76 [cited 2014 June]. Doi:10.1002/14651858. CD006086.pub3/pdf.
3. Morton R. Phthisiologia: or A treatise of consumptions. 2 ed. London: W. and J. Innys; 1720.
4. Cullen W. First lines of the practice of physic, vol. 4. Edinburgh: C. Elliot, and London: T. Cadell; 1786.
5. Bodington G. Essay on the treatment of and cure of pulmonary consumption. London: Longmans and Company; 1840.
6. Bryder L. Below the magic mountain: a social history of tuberculosis in twentieth-century Britain. Oxford: Claredon Press; 1988.
7. Rothman SM. Living in the shadow of death: tuberculosis and the social experience of illness in American history. Baltimore and London: Johns Hopkins University Press; 1994.
8. Bennett JH. Treatise on the Oleum Jecoris Aselli, or Cod Liver Oil, as a therapeutic agent in certain forms of Gout, Rheumatism, and Scrofula, with cases. London: S. Highley; 1841.
9. Schütte D. Beobachtungen über den Nutzen des Berger Leberthrans (Oleum jecoris aselli, von Gadus Asellus L.). Archiv f. med. Erfahrung 1824;79–92 (German).

10. Williams CJB, Williams CT. Pulmonary consumption, its etiology, pathology, and treatment. 2nd ed. London: Longmans, Green, and Co.; 1889.
11. Taufflieb E. De l'huile de foie de morue et de son usage en médecine. Bull Trav Soc Med Prat Paris. 1852;45–135 (French).
12. McConkey M. The treatment of intestinal tuberculosis with codliver oil and tomato juice. Am Rev Tuberc. 1930;21:627–35.
13. Williams CJB, Williams CT. On the nature and treatment of pulmonary consumption. Lancet 1868;i:369–70, 403–4, 431–2, 552–4, 613–5, 711–3, 777–80; ii:3–4, 38–40, 107–9, 211–4.
14. Greenhow EH. On the employment of cod-liver oil in phthisis. With cases. Lancet 1854;ii:502–5, 542–5.
15. Galen. Librorum pars prima [-quinta] (5 volumes). Venetiis, in aedibus Aldi, et Andreae Asulani soceri, 1525.
16. Tui C, Kuo NH, Schmidt L. The protein status in pulmonary tuberculosis. Am J Clin Nutr. 1954;2:252–64.
17. Pottenger FM Jr, Pottenger FM. Adequate diet in tuberculosis. Am. Rev. Tuberc. 1946;54(3):213–8.
18. Nutrition and Tuberculosis: A review of the literature and considerations for TB control programs [internet]. [place unknown]: USAID/Africa's Health in 2010; 2008 [cited 2014 June]. Available from http://digitalcommons.calpoly.edu/cgi/viewcontent.cgi?article=1009&context=fsn_fac.
19. Lonnroth K, Williams BG, Cegielski P, Dye C. A consistent log-linear relationship between tuberculosis incidence and body mass index. Int J Epidemiol. 2010;39(1):149–55.
20. Tverdal A. Body mass index and incidence of tuberculosis. Eur J Res Dis. 1986;69(5):355–62.
21. Zachariah R, Spielmann MP, Harries AD, Salaniponi FM. Moderate to severe malnutrition in patients with tuberculosis is a risk factor associated with early death. Trans R Soc Trop Med Hyg. 2002;96(3):291–4.
22. Van Lettow M, Kumwenda JJ, Harrie AD, Whalen CC, Taha TE, Kumwenda N, et al. Malnutrition and the severity of lung disease in adults with pulmonary tuberculosis in Malawi. Int J Tuberc Lung Dis. 2004;8(2):211–7.
23. Kumar s, Dutt A, Hemraj S, Bhat S, Manipadybhima B. Phase angle measurement in healthy human subjects through bio-impedance analysis. Iran J Basic Med Sci. 2012;15(6):1180–4.
24. Schaible UE, Kaufman SHE. Malnutrition and infection: complex mechanisms and global impacts. PLoS Med [internet]. 2007;4(5):e115 [cited 2014 June]. Available from http://www.ncbi.nlm.nih.gov/pmc/articles/PMC1858706/.
25. Khan A, Sterling TR, Reves R, Vernon A, Horsburgh CR. Lack of weight gain and relapse risk in a large tuberculosis treatment trial. Am J Respir Crit Care Med. 2006;174(3):344–8.
26. Krapp F, Veliz JC, Cornejo E, Gotuzzo E, Seas C. Bodyweight gain to predict treatment outcome in patients with pulmonary tuberculosis in Peru. Int J Tuberc Lung Dis. 2008;12(10):1153–9.
27. Guenther CS, Ivers LC. Food insecurity and tuberculosis. In: Ivers LC, editor. Food insecurity and public health. 1st ed. Boca Raton: CRC Press; 2015. P. 91-112.
28. Grede N, Claros JM, de Pee S, Bloem MW. Is there a need to mitigate the social and financial consequences of tuberculosis at the individual and household level? AIDS Behav. 2014;18:542–53.
29. Cegielski JP, McMurray DN. The relationship between malnutrition and tuberculosis: evidence from studies in humans and experimental animals. Int J Tuberc Lung Dis. 2004;8(3):286–98.
30. Mabedo T, Aukrust P, Berge RK, Lindtjorn B. Circulationg antioxidants and lipid peroxidation products in untreated tuberculosis patients in Ethiopia. Am J Clin Nutr. 2003;78(1):117–22.
31. Mugusi FM, Rusizoka O, Habib N, Fawzi W. Vitamin A status of patients presenting with pulmonary tuberculosis and asymptomatic HIV-infected individuals, Dar es Salaam, Tanzania. Int J Tuberc Lung Dis. 2003;7(8):804–7.
32. Ramachandran G, Santha T, Garg R, Baskaran D, Iliayas SA, Venkatesan P, et al. Vitamin A levels in sputum-positive pulmonary tuberculosis patients in comparison with household contacts and healthy 'normals'. Int J Tuberc Lung Dis. 2004;8(9):1130–3.
33. Ramakrishnan K, Shenbagarathi R, Kavitha K, Uma A, Balasubramaniam R, Thirumalaikolundusubramanian P. Serum zinc and albumin levels in pulmonary tuberculosis patients with and without HIV. Jpn J Infect Dis. 2008;61 (3):202–4.
34. Vijayamalini M, Manoharan S. Lipid peroxidation, vitamins C, E and reduced glutathione levels in patients with pulmonary tuberculosis. Cell Biochem Funct. 2004;22(1):19–22.
35. Karyadi E, Schultink W, Nelwan RH, Gross R, Amin Z, Dolmans WM, et al. Poor micronutrient status of active pulmonary tuberculosis patients in Indonesia. J Nutr. 2000;130(12):2953–8.
36. Kassu A, Yabutani T, Mahmud ZH, Mohammad A, Nguyen N, Huong BTM, et al. Alterations in serum levels of trace elements in tuberculosis and HIV infections. Eur J Clin Nutr. 2006;60(5):580–6.
37. Prezzemolo T, Guggino G, La Manna MP, Di Liberto D, Dieli F, Caccamo N. Functional signatures of humad CD4 and CD8 T cell responses to *Mycobacterium tuberculosis*. Front Immunol [internet]. 2014;5:180 [cited 2014 June]. Available from http://www.ncbi.nlm.nih.gov/pmc/articles/PMC4001014/.
38. Pelly TF, Santillan CF, Gilman RH, Cabrera LZ, Garcia E, Vidal C, et al. Tuberculosis skin testing, anergy and protein malnutrition in Peru. Int J Tuberc Lung Dis. 2005;9(9):977–84.
39. Gupta KB, Gupta R, Atreja A, Verma M, Vishvkarma S. Tuberculosis and nutrition. Lung India. 2009;26(1):9–16.

40. Figueroa-Damian R, Arredondo-Garcia JL. Neonatal outcome of children born to women with tuberculosis. Arch Med Res. 2001;32(1):66–9.
41. Kant S, Gupta H, Ahluwalia S. Significance of nutrition in pulmonary tuberculosis. Crit Rev Food Sci Nutr. 2015;55:955–63.
42. Chang SW, Pan WS, Beltran DL, et al. Gut Hormones, appetite suppression and cachexia in patients with pulmonary TB. PLoS One [internet]. 2013;8(1):e54564 [cited 2014 June]. Available from http://www.ncbi.nlm.nih.gov/pmc/articles/PMC3554726/.
43. Semba RD, Darnton-Hill I, de Pee S. Addressing tuberculosis in the context of malnutrition and HIV coinfection. Food Nutr Bull. 2010;31:S345–64.
44. Nutritional care and support for patients with tuberculosis [internet]. Geneva: World Health Organization; 2013 [cited June 2015]. http://www.who.int/nutrition/publications/guidelines/nutcare_support_patients_with_tb/en/.
45. Nutrition assessment, counselling and support for adolescents and adults living with HIV [internet]. New York: UNAIDS; 2014 [cited July 2015].
46. De Pee S, Grede N, Mehra D, Bloem MW. The enabling effect of food assistance in improving adherence and/or treatment completion for antiretroviral therapy and tuberculosis treatment: a literature review. AIDS Behav. 2014;18:531–41.
47. Martins N, Morris P, Kelly PM. Food incentives to improve completion of tuberculosis treatment: randomized controlled trial in Dili, Timor-Leste. BMJ [internet]. 2009;339:b4248 [cited 2014 June]. Available from http://www.ncbi.nlm.nih.gov/pmc/articles/PMC2767482/pdf/bmj.b4248.pdf.
48. Paton NI, Chua YK, Earnest A, Chee CB. Randomized controlled trial of nutritional supplementation in patients with newly diagnosed tuberculosis and wasting. Am J Clin Nutr. 2004;80(2):460–5.
49. Chacano-Bedoya P, Ronnenberg AG. Vitamin D and tuberculosis. Nutr Rev. 2009;67(5):289–93.
50. Wejse C, Gomes VF, Rabna P, Gustafson P, Aaby P, Lisse IM, et al. Vitamin D as supplementary treatment for tuberculosis—a double-blind randomised placebo-controlled trial. Am J Respir Crit Care Med. 2009;179(9): 843–50.
51. De Voss JJ, Rutter K, Schroeder BG, Barry CE III. Iron acquisition and metabolism by mycobacteria. J Bacteriol. 1999;181(15):4443–51.
52. Boelaert JR, Vandecasteele SJ, Appelberg R, Gordeuk VR. The effect of the host's iron status on tuberculosis. J Infect Dis. 2007;195(12):1745–53.
53. Alavi-Naini R, Moghtaderi A, Metanat M, Mohammadi M, Zabetian M. Factors associated with mortality in tuberculosis patients. J Res Med Sci. 2013;18(1):52–5.
54. Mupere E, Malone L, Zalwango S, Okwera A, Nsereko M, Tisch DJ, et al. Wasting among Uganda men with pulmonary tuberculosis is associated with linear regain in lean tissue mass during and after treatment in contrast to women with wasting who regain fat tissue mass: a prospective cohort study. BMC Infect Dis. 2014;14:24.
55. Kennedy N, Ramsay A, Uiso L, Gutmann J, Ngowi FI, Gillespie SH. Nutritional status and weight gain in patients with pulmonary tuberculosis in Tanzania. Trans R Soc Trop Med Hyg. 1996;90(2):162–6.
56. Schwenk A, Hodgson L, Wright A, Ward LC, Rayner CF, Grubnic S, et al. Nutrient partitioning during treatment of tuberculosis: gain in body fat mass but not in protein mass. Am J Clin Nutr. 2004;79(6):1006–12.
57. Onwubalili JK. Malnutrition among tuberculosis patients in Harrow, England. Eur J Clin Nutr. 1988;42(4):363–6.
58. Jaganath D, Mupere E. Childhood tuberculosis and malnutrition. J Infect Dis. 2012;206(12):1809–15.
59. Mehta S, Mugusi FM, Bosch RJ, Aboud S, Chatterjee A, Finkelstein JL, et al. A randomized trial of multivitamin supplementation in children with tuberculosis in Tanzania. Nutr J [internet]. 2011;10:120 [cited 2014 June]. Available from http://www.ncbi.nlm.nih.gov/pmc/articles/PMC3229564/pdf/1475-2891-10-120.pdf.
60. Loto OM, Awowole I. Tuberculosis in Pregnancy: A Review. J Pregnancy [internet]. 2011; 379271:1–7 [cited 2014 June]. Available from http://www.ncbi.nlm.nih.gov/pmc/articles/PMC3206367/pdf/JP2012-379271.pdf.
61. Guideline: Calcium supplementation in pregnant women [internet]. Geneva: World Health Organization; 2013 [cited July 2015]. Available http://apps.who.int/iris/bitstream/10665/85120/1/9789241505376_eng.pdf.

Chapter 20
HIV and HIV/TB Co-infection in Relation to Nutrition

Anupama Paranandi and Christine Wanke

Keywords HIV · Malnutrition · Food insecurity · Macronutrient deficiency · Micronutrient deficiency · Macronutrient intervention · Micronutrient intervention

Learning Objectives

- Explore the relationship between socioeconomic factors, nutrition status, and HIV in the resource-limited setting.
- Explain the etiology of weight loss in HIV disease and in HIV/TB co-infection.
- Evaluate the role of macro- and micronutrient deficiencies in HIV disease outcomes.
- Explain the nutritional requirements of vulnerable populations suffering from HIV.
- Evaluate the impact of anti-retroviral treatment on nutritional status in PLHIV, in both the short-to-medium term and the long term.
- Understand the dual role of food assistance, distinguishing special nutritious foods and income support, as support to HIV, or HIV and TB, care and treatment.

HIV and Nutrition

Introduction/Background

Many infectious diseases are associated with nutritional compromise. HIV is one of these infections as are tuberculosis, measles, influenza, and diarrhea, among others. The unique characteristic of HIV infection is that while effective treatment is now widely available, the use of effective therapy does not and cannot cure the infection. As the infection is one that will be lifelong, the treatment must also be lifelong. And as the HIV infection is associated with nutritional compromise, the treatment of HIV is also complicated by nutritional issues. The HIV-infected individual or person living with HIV/AIDS (PLWHA) will experience lifelong nutritional issues related to the chronic viral infection, the treatment of the viral infection and by side effects of any opportunistic infections (OI) which

A. Paranandi
Department of Medicine, Saint Mary's Hospital, 56 Franklin Street, Waterbury, CT 06706, USA
e-mail: aparanandi@stmh.org

C. Wanke (✉)
Medicine/Infectious Diseases, Tufts Medical Center, 750 Washington Street, Boston, MA 02111, USA
e-mail: Christine.Wanke@Tufts.edu

© Springer Science+Business Media New York 2017
S. de Pee et al. (eds.), *Nutrition and Health in a Developing World*,
Nutrition and Health, DOI 10.1007/978-3-319-43739-2_20

might develop with immune compromise. Awareness of the full spectrum of possible nutritional compromise and attention to the nutritional status and issues of PLWHA is of great importance.

Malnutrition of any sort is a significant public health concern, especially in the resource-limited setting, and is the most common cause of immune deficiency globally [1]. Eight-hundred and forty-two million people do not have enough to eat and 98% of those live in resource-limited settings [2]. Many people living with HIV (PLWHA) suffer from, or are at risk of suffering from hunger, undernutrition and malnutrition [3]. According to the World Health Organization (WHO), 35.3 million people were living with HIV worldwide in 2012 [4]. In those with HIV infection, the absolute numbers of those with malnutrition are higher in Asia, but the highest prevalence of malnutrition in the HIV-infected population is in sub-Saharan Africa [2]. Such numbers are daunting and bring to light the magnitude of the problem seen with concurrent HIV and malnutrition.

In the resource-limited setting, heterosexual contact has been the most frequent route of HIV transmission, and mother-to-child transmission has been common as well, although hopefully it will decrease if recent WHO recommendations to treat all PLWHA are followed. HIV disease damages the human immune system by methodically targeting and destroying T-lymphocytes. The clinical presentation of HIV disease is diverse and depends on the stage and severity of disease. In acute infection, i.e., within a few weeks of acquisition, HIV presents most typically as a flu-like illness, commonly characterized by fever, chills, night sweats, rash, and swollen lymph nodes. After the initial manifestation, HIV can progress without any specific or associated symptoms. Although slow, progressive weight loss throughout the disease process is not uncommon and may be the only manifestation of disease. Finally, as T-lymphocytes are depleted due to progressive disease, the body's immunity against common infections deteriorates. As a result, PLWHA tend to develop infections that the normal human immune system can suppress. These infections tend to mark the late stage of HIV disease, which is then termed acquired immune deficiency syndrome, or AIDS.

Diagnosis of HIV is made through the detection of HIV antibodies, which are evident after a few weeks of infection. Prior to HIV antibody production, HIV disease can be detected through HIV viral load testing, which is usually very high in the acute phase of infection. However, in infants less than 18 months of age, HIV detection through serology is not accurate as the infant would have maternally acquired HIV antibodies. Instead, HIV DNA PCR (polymerase chain reaction) is the diagnostic test of choice in this situation [5].

After diagnosis, HIV disease can progress through clinical and immunologic stages in those who are untreated, as categorized by the WHO. These criteria have been developed for adults and adolescents as well as for infants and children.

Advanced HIV or AIDS in adults and adolescents is characterized as adult clinical stage 3 or 4 or any clinical stage and CD4 count less than 350 per mm^3 of blood [6]. In children 5 years of age or older, advanced HIV and AIDS is defined as pediatric stage 3 or 4 or any pediatric clinical stage with CD4 count less than 350 per mm^3 of blood [6]. In children less than 5 years of age, advanced HIV or AIDS is defined by clinical stage 3 or 4 or any clinical stage and CD4 <25% in children under 12 months of age, or <20% in children aged 12–59 months [6].

Until the recent WHO recommendation to treat all PLWHA, treatment for HIV has been initiated when an individual presents with stage 3 or 4 of disease, with active TB, severe chronic hepatitis B, pregnancy or breastfeeding, or if the HIV+ individual is in a serodiscordant relationship or if the individual has clinical stage 1 or 2 but the CD4 cell count is ≤ 500 cells/mm^3, whichever comes first [7]. Treatment for HIV/AIDS is based on a combination of drugs and is termed combined anti-retroviral treatment (ART). These medications help control viral replication and disease symptoms but do not cure the disease. Although current recommendations suggest treating all PLWHA, practice varies from country to country. Successful treatment of the virus is indicated by rising CD4 counts and suppression of the viral load below detection.

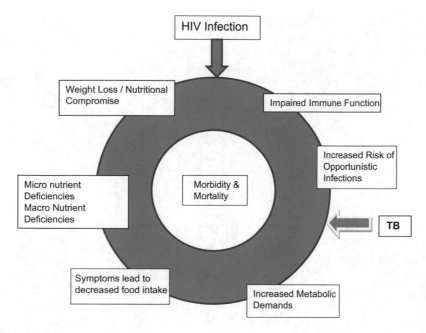

Fig. 20.1 HIV, TB, and nutrition

Mortality and Weight Loss and HIV

In the early days of the HIV epidemic, wasting was so common that HIV was known as "slim disease." Together, malnutrition and HIV infection promote worsened immune function and lead to increased morbidity and mortality (Fig. 20.1).

The CDC definition of HIV wasting is defined as "loss of 10% of total body weight with lack of other detectable cause except HIV" [8], "plus chronic diarrhea (at least two loose stools per day for greater than or equal to 30 days) or chronic weakness and documented fever (for greater than or equal to 30 days, intermittent, or constant) in the absence of a concurrent illness or condition other than HIV infection that could explain the findings" [8]. HIV wasting is considered an AIDS-defining illness by the CDC. Wasting in HIV infection increases the risk of death. A low body mass index (BMI) is an independent prognostic indicator of mortality and morbidity in HIV-infected people [3]. A loss of 5% body weight can increase the risk of death by 2.5 times, particularly in those not on treatment [8].

Etiology of Weight Loss in HIV

The causes of weight loss and malnutrition in HIV-infected individuals fall into two major categories [9].

Etiology of Weight Loss in HIV

Decreased Intake

- Insufficient food
- Anorexia

- Oral/dental lesions
- Gastrointestinal symptoms

  - Nausea
  - Bloating
  - Cramping

- Depression
- Malabsorption/diarrhea

Altered Metabolism/REE

- HIV infection
- Fever
- Opportunistic infection
- Opportunistic malignancy
- Hormonal deficiency

  - Testosterone
  - Adrenal
  - Thyroid

- Cytokine activation

There may be inadequate intake of nutrients and/or there may be inappropriate metabolism of ingested nutrients [9]. Decreased dietary intake may be related simply to the lack of food available to the HIV-infected individual. However, there are other barriers to nutrient intake that may be medical or socioeconomic. HIV can cause symptoms related to dental, oral, or the upper gastrointestinal tract that interfere with ingestion of nutrients (e.g., severe gingivitis, oral ulcers, anorexia, nausea, bloating, pain with swallowing, and abdominal pain) [9]. But many of these symptoms can also be related to side effects of ART or to OI [8]. Psychologically, individuals with HIV may suffer from depression, which can be associated with loss of appetite and decreased nutrient intake, as can significant use of drugs or alcohol. Weight loss in those with HIV may also occur as a result of damaged gut epithelium associated with the virus itself and known as HIV enteropathy which can cause malabsorption of ingested nutrients. Those with advanced HIV disease and low CD4 counts may also be co-infected with intestinal parasites that can cause diarrhea and/or decrease intestinal nutrient absorption [8]. Intestinal bacterial overgrowth or opportunistic enteric infections, such as cryptosporidiosis or mycobacterium avium complex, can also decrease nutrient absorption.

Additionally, replication of the virus itself creates an increased metabolic demand [10]. Fever, OI and malignancies, and hormonal deficiencies (thyroid, adrenal, or gonadal) seen in HIV disease may also increase metabolic demands. When the viral load is fully suppressed on ART, the HIV-infected person who had previously lost weight will regain some weight, particularly if they have access to sufficient food. However, PLWHA are unlikely to return to their premorbid weight. This phenomenon may be due to ongoing cytokine production in the presence of chronic viral infection and may be associated with altered metabolism and ongoing weight loss.

Food Security in HIV

Of particular interest, currently, is the role of food security or insecurity in weight loss in HIV-infected individuals.

HIV and Food Insecurity—Outcomes

Nutritional

- Decreased dietary quality
- Hunger
- Decreased dietary intake
- Decreased weight/BMI

Non-Nutritional

- Increased risk behaviors
- Decreased care seeking
- Decreased willingness to initiate ART
- Decreased ART adherence
- Decreased retention in care

Globally, much of the HIV-infected population is in the lower socioeconomic strata and tends to experience significant food insecurity [11, 12]. Food insecurity is defined as the continual lack of access to adequate quantity or quality of food [11]. Decreased dietary quality, as measured by dietary diversity, has been associated with food insecurity and may result in increased mortality and further immune suppression, particularly in those with CD4 counts lower than 350 cells/mL [13]. While food insecurity may be a significant factor in HIV-associated weight loss and the development of malnutrition, food insecurity may also be a factor in a number of other non-nutritional outcomes in HIV-infected individuals (see above). Many with food insecurity are bound by socioeconomic constraints and have to choose between nutrition and medicine, and/or between nutrition and health care [14]. Those who are food insecure may be at greater risk of infection with HIV as they may need to engage in risky behaviors to acquire food for themselves or their household members. Food insecurity may lead to reluctance to enter care as the time required to attend to health care appointments could distract from time needed to obtain food; similarly, food insecurity has been associated with a reluctance to initiate ART and with lower levels of adherence or greater risk of being lost to follow-up. Supportive of the importance of food insecurity, those with greater food security have reported improved physical and mental health, and better quality of life [15].

Protein Energy Malnutrition in HIV

Whatever the series of events that leads an HIV-infected individual to decreased nutritional intake, which may be predominantly decreased intake of high-quality protein, typically meats and other animal-based foods, as one of the more expensive nutrients, the end result can be protein energy malnutrition (PEM). PEM is also a cause of secondary immune deficiency [16]. PEM causes decreases in immunoglobulin and cytokine production [1]. It is associated with defects in innate and adaptive immunity and is characterized by the loss of lymphoid tissue, decreased T-cell immunity, including CD4 cells, impaired delayed hypersensitivity, and poor antibody responses to vaccinations [8]. PEM can increase the risk of OI and hasten progression to AIDS [1, 15] by 60–170% [8].

Micronutrient Deficiencies in HIV

Micronutrient deficiencies are also common in HIV-infected individuals. Micronutrients are essential factors in antioxidant pathways and are important in human immunity [1, 8]. Particular micronutrients required for this process include zinc, selenium, carotenoids, vitamins A, E, and C, and possibly glutathione and sulfur amino acids such as methionine, taurine, and cysteine [17]. Concurrent PEM and micronutrient deficiencies as described above are present more frequently in the resource-limited setting and may further promote the progression of HIV disease.

Cachexia in HIV

Cachexia is the predominant loss of lean body mass in those who are undergoing involuntary weight loss. Cachexia appears to be driven by the production of TNF-α (tumor necrosis factor) and other inflammatory cytokines. It is seen most commonly in malignancy but can also be seen in hormonal deficiencies, chronic obstructive lung disease, and congestive heart failure. Cachexia is also seen in HIV-infected individuals who have advanced disease and used to be more frequent in the early part of the HIV epidemic. At that time, it was recognized that when true cachexia was present in HIV-infected individuals, the metabolism was so disordered that no amount of oral or parenteral nutrition could successfully improve weight and nutritional status. Fortunately, the number of PLWHA presenting with such advanced metabolic derangements is much lower in the current treatment era.

Resting Energy Expenditure/Metabolic Abnormalities in HIV

Total daily energy expenditure (TDEE) is equivalent to resting energy expenditure (REE) plus physical activity energy expenditure and digestive energy expenditure [16]. In the resource-sufficient world, in chronic illness, REE increases but TDEE generally stays the same as physical activity decreases [16]. Nutritional intake remains the same or increases, so weight is overall maintained [16]. This may not occur in the resource-limited setting. HIV-infected individuals in the resource-limited setting may not have the ability to decrease their physical activity or increase nutritional intake when they are ill. The WHO guidance on nutrient requirements for people living with HIV/AIDS [18] utilized the following: REE in asymptomatic HIV-infected, ART naïve people trying to maintain body weight and baseline activity is considered to be 10% greater than in those without HIV [16] likely due to the metabolic demands of the virus. Those with asymptomatic AIDS were considered to have REEs up to 25% higher than in non-HIV-infected people, and even higher in those with AIDS with concomitant secondary infection [18, 19]. The precise energy requirements for HIV-infected individuals on ART treatment are not clear; it is not known whether all treatment regimens and classes of ART have the same impact on REE and whether the chronic suppression of viral load results in a return to a fully normal REE is also not known. Furthermore, the impact of co-infection with TB or with one of the chronic hepatitis viruses on REE is not clear. The REE of adolescents infected with HIV, who are growing and going through puberty, or the changes that may occur in the population aging with HIV, have not been studied.

Nutritional Assessment in HIV

The precise assessment of nutritional status of HIV-infected individuals is important but complex and difficult. Nutritional assessment of the individual infected with and living with HIV must be comprehensive and incorporate all of the factors that may be pertinent. Nutritional assessment should include nutrient intake, a measure of dietary quality, a measure of food security, and of symptoms that may interfere with nutrient ingestion or metabolism (pain with eating, nausea, vomiting, fever, abdominal pain, bloating, and diarrhea). It should also include brief measures of depression and measures of social and economic support. Availability of clean water for drinking and cooking should be determined. The duration and stage of HIV infection should be determined, and all medications including ART should be recorded. Any other medical issues should also be captured, and any non-HIV medications including herbal or traditional medicines should be recorded. Pregnancy status and breast-feeding status should be determined. Anthropometric measurements, such as height and weight, should be obtained and the body mass index calculated (kg per m^2). Body composition should be evaluated using regional body shape measurements (circumferential measures of chest, waist, hip, mid-upper arm, and mid-thigh) and skinfold thickness measurements (although these are difficult to accurately measure) [20]. Some suggest that the measure of mid-arm circumference should be the preferred screening methodology [20], although this measure has not yet been validated in adults. For a complete assessment, laboratory data including measure of hemoglobin, CD4 count, liver function testing and electrolytes and renal function should be obtained [20]. From these collected data, individuals infected with HIV can be categorized as having normal nutrition status, being nutritionally at risk, or having mild, moderate, or severe malnutrition, and thus be referred for appropriate intervention. After appropriate intervention/treatment is initiated, weight and BMI can then be followed to assess improvement in nutritional status. While weight gain and increase in BMI can be considered a positive outcome of HIV treatment, particularly in HIV-related wasting, it cannot be used as a marker of improved HIV disease, for which one should use increasing CD4 counts or decreasing viral loads. The clinical dilemma in trying to carry out this type of nutrition assessment and intervention in the resource-limited setting is one of time, training, and resources. It is time consuming to obtain the historical data necessary and use the prescribed methods to collect information on dietary intake, dietary diversity, and food security. Often the number of patients presenting at an ART clinic and inadequately trained staff make it challenging to appropriately collect and interpret the suggested nutritional data. And finally, there may be no standardized instruments to measure height and weight, and it may not be possible to collect and analyze the requisite laboratory measures. In the ideal setting, nutritional assessment in some form should occur with each clinic visit.

Macronutrient Interventions in HIV

Increasing caloric intake should increase lean muscle mass and fat mass and hence body weight [16], yet this may not happen in the HIV-infected person. The intervention required to achieve the goal of proportional gain of lean and fat mass is not known. Additionally, the proper indicators to use to assess the success of a nutritional intervention in HIV-infected individuals or as a means to determine the success of study interventions are not clear. On an individual level, simple weight gain is insufficient as there is a need to associate weight gain with improvement in function or quality of life. Changes in mortality, as an outcome, requires a large sample size and a prolonged period of follow-up. Other outcomes such as slowing of HIV progression or decreased risk of OI are also difficult to study. The most appropriate populations and the proper outcomes to study may be complicated by funding or ethical issues and continue to remain a challenge.

The optimal timing or methods of nutritional intervention is also unclear. The evidence generated since the publication of the 2003 WHO guidance on HIV and nutrition is sufficiently scant, or the studies too varied in terms of supplement composition, patient characteristics, or treatments to suggest changes in the recommendations [21]. To summarize, the 2003 WHO guidance on nutritional support in PLWHA stated that "adequate nutrition … best achieved through consumption of a balanced diet, is vital for the health and survival of all individuals regardless of HIV status" [18]. It further acknowledged that energy requirements are increased in asymptomatic HIV-infected adults and children to maintain weight and growth, respectively, and that these requirements increased with the progression of disease [18]. However, data were insufficient to support protein or fat supplementation regardless of age or stage of disease [18]. Similarly, in terms of micronutrients, there was not enough evidence to support supplementation beyond the recommended daily allowances [18, 22].

A Cochrane review [23], in which 14 studies encompassing 1725 HIV-infected, ART-naive adults, that examined the impact of food supplements or no supplement/placebo found there was no difference in the risk of death between the two groups [23]. There was no benefit of supplementation in any clinical, anthropometric, or immunological outcome when compared with no supplementation [23]. However, the studies included in this review had small sample sizes, and the quality of these studies was determined to be of very low-to-moderate quality, with unknown to increased risk of bias [23]. There are some data that suggest that macronutrient supplementation may result in higher CD4 counts and lower viral loads, but these studies were also small, and not otherwise externally validated [24].

Micronutrient Interventions in HIV

As with macronutrients, no new evidence exists to suggest altering the WHO 2003 HIV/AIDS nutrition recommendations related to the intake of micronutrients, which is the intake at recommended dietary allowances (RDA) as in the general population [15, 21, 25]. HIV-infected adults and children are encouraged to consume a healthy diet in order to obtain adequate dietary vitamin levels [18]. However, for those of low socioeconomic status, this may not be feasible. It is important to note that some evidence exists that higher than the recommended nutrient intake of certain micronutrients such as vitamin A, zinc, and iron can result in adverse outcomes in the HIV-infected individual [18]. For example, excess Vitamin A may promote increased viral replication and increased genital secretion of virus [25] with increased risk of HIV transmission, but this has not been replicated in other studies. Furthermore, excess vitamin A can potentially worsen already existent lipid derangements and pre-mature atherosclerosis in PLWHA [21]. Zinc was also found to have some importance in HIV-infected populations in the resource-limited setting. While higher than the required daily allowance of zinc may be harmful, zinc repletion at recommended daily amounts was associated with a decreased risk of diarrhea; higher rates of diarrhea were associated with low serum zinc concentrations [24].

Since the 2003 WHO guidance, studies examining micronutrient supplementation have been heterogeneous in terms of study design, micronutrients provided, dose of micronutrients, study durations, and outcome [21, 22, 25]. There is some evidence that high-dose (multiples of RDA) multi-micronutrient supplementation, specifically thiamine, riboflavin, vitamin B6, vitamin B12, vitamin C, niacin, folic acid, and vitamin E, improved CD4 cell counts, showing HIV progression and increased survival [26]. However, it is not known whether deficiencies of these micronutrients were present at baseline in the HIV-infected, ART-naive subjects in this study. It is not clear whether these PLWHA in resource-limited settings benefitted from meeting the RDA, which is not generally possible with their daily diet, or whether multiples of RDA were necessary and responsible for the benefits seen. Given the limited and wide variability of data available on micronutrient supplementation of PLWHA, the WHO continues to recommend micronutrient intake at the recommended daily allowance either through a healthy diet or if that is inadequate, through additional supplementation.

Nutrition and ART in HIV

Effective combined anti-retroviral therapy (ART) is associated with improved nutritional status in HIV infection. In general, the initiation of ART promotes weight gain in HIV-infected individuals. However, the effects between individual ART components and nutrient metabolism can be varied. Nutrients can alter the metabolism of selected drugs in ART, or ART can affect the metabolism of nutrients [25]. Metabolic pathways can be altered to increase or decrease serum levels of ART [25]. In terms of macronutrients, low protein or fat intake decreases metabolism [25] and may lead to higher serum concentrations of drugs. Excess intake of protein and fats may increase metabolism [25] and results in decreased serum drug concentrations. Conversely, an excess of carbohydrates may also result in decreased drug metabolism [25].

Certain micronutrients can also be associated with alterations in drug metabolism. For example, vitamin C deficiency can lead to a decrease of some hepatic enzymes vital to drug metabolism [25]. In some instances, increasing supplementation can decrease steady-state drug levels in serum [25]. Vitamin D may impact metabolism by altering gene expression and production of enzymes involved in drug metabolism [25]. Finally, vitamin A may increase metabolism and decrease drug levels [25]. It is unclear what level of intake is needed to alter serum drug levels and whether this varies with specific ART agents. Despite these findings and concerns, the data are not necessarily generalizable, and hence recommendations regarding dietary intake in those on ART do not differ from that of the WHO 2003 guidelines.

Much has changed in HIV/AIDS treatment in terms of the discovery and availability of novel anti-retroviral agents in the last decade. Drug development and availability have introduced even more avenues for research in terms of the interaction between nutrition and drug treatment. The focus in HIV and drug research now includes short- and long-term overall health of PLWHA on ART in terms of chronic comorbidities.

Nutrition Programs and HIV

Recognizing that malnutrition significantly worsens morbidity and mortality in PLWHA, the WHO has issued recommendations that emphasize reversal of under- or malnutrition in PLWHA to optimize outcomes and disease treatment. ART is vital to controlling disease and to reversing weight loss and wasting associated with HIV disease. An adjunctive intervention to ART is improvement in nutritional intake. Access to adequate nutrition not only reverses malnutrition, but may also reduce the burdens placed on HIV-infected individuals and their families in terms of access to nutrition and food security. Relieving this burden may help redirect PLWHA to concentrate on treatment rather than access to food and increase their uptake and adherence to treatment and retention in care [27, 28]. Treatment adherence and retention in care can hasten recovery and help infected individuals return to productive lives [27]. Hence, nutrition programs, which provide nutritional assessment, counseling, and support, including nutrient supplementation to meet WHO guidelines to counter under- and malnutrition (which are the same guidelines for malnutrition in non-HIV-infected as well as HIV-infected people given that evidence is insufficient to support nutritional supplementation beyond that required to maintain normal BMI) have been supported [27, 28]. The objectives of nutritional programs are to help PLWHA achieve and maintain normal weight, adequate intake of macro- and micronutrients, decrease the impact of other malnutrition-related illnesses, and improve quality of life [27].

Impact of Fully Suppressed HIV Viral Load on Nutrition/Metabolism

When a PLWHA has a fully suppressed viral load on ART, the nutritional and metabolic issues often begin to evolve. The PLWHA with fully suppressed viral load generally does not continue to lose weight, but as metabolic demand from the virus decreases and inflammation is suppressed, will begin to gain weight. Some with fully suppressed viral load will develop HIV-associated lypodystrophic changes in regional body fat. These include subcutaneous fat atrophy and visceral or intra-abdominal fat accumulation. Fat atrophy is most commonly seen on the face but is also present throughout the body, reducing subcutaneous fat in the trunk and limbs as well. The best predictor of the development of fat atrophy appears to be the use of those nucleoside reverse transcriptase ART agents that are particularly toxic to mitochondria. Visceral fat accumulation has a multifactorial pathogenesis, which includes the use of some protease inhibitor ART agents, pre-HIV amount of body fat, and female gender. Both fat atrophy and visceral fat accumulation can be associated with glucose intolerance and with atherogenic lipid profiles.

HIV infection in ART naïve individuals is associated with high triglyceride levels, low high-density lipoprotein (HDL) levels, low total cholesterol levels, and malnutrition as measured by low BMI [29]. A study done in a resource-limited setting suggests that after being on ART, HDL levels decreased and/or triglyceride levels increased [29]. Other data suggest that triglyceride levels remain high in treated HIV-infected individuals with increased total cholesterol levels and unchanged HDL levels. Other studies also report anti-atherogenic responses to ART, particularly NNRTIs, in which dramatic increases in HDL cholesterol were seen. Some ART agents are also associated with increased rates of insulin resistance and type 2 diabetes.

These atherogenic lipid profiles as well as the inflammation induced by HIV appear to put HIV-infected individuals at higher risk for cardiovascular disease. Obesity has also been reported with increasing frequency in PLWHA with fully suppressed viral load that may be related to continued high dietary intake even as viral metabolic demands decrease. Glucose intolerance and insulin resistance may progress to diabetes mellitus in HIV-infected individuals; and diabetes plays a role in the increased cardiovascular risk.

Vulnerable Populations

Children, Nutrition, and HIV

Current estimates suggest that there are 3.4 million HIV-infected children under the age of 15 globally, with 340,000–450,000 new infections in this population each year [30]. Many of these children also suffer from malnutrition [30]. Mortality from severe malnutrition, defined as weight-for-height less than 3 standard deviations below the reference population's median, or mid-upper arm circumference less than 11.5 cm in children 6 months to 5 years, was three times higher for those with HIV disease than for HIV-negative children [30]. HIV-infected children also have higher rates of infectious comorbidities that may contribute to the high rates of malnutrition [30]. Adolescents may be considered in the same category as children as their continued growth and development must be supported. The precise nutritional needs for adolescents with HIV remain unclear.

From the time of birth, HIV-infected children are at higher risk of malnutrition as they are breast-fed by HIV-infected mothers who are also likely malnourished. Children are particularly vulnerable to gastrointestinal disease that may increase the risk for or worsen pre-existing malnutrition. Children can suffer from chronic diarrhea with viral or parasitic infections [30], or may have repeated acute diarrheal episodes from a series of bacterial infections. Alternatively, they may develop HIV enteropathy that contributes to malabsorption and malnutrition [30].

Children are particularly vulnerable to food insecurity. Many HIV-infected children have one or both parents suffering from HIV, or who have died from HIV. The child's survival depends on their often HIV-infected caretaker, who may or may not be able to provide for them if they have advanced disease and are functionally limited. Children in these households are at higher risk for malnutrition than children in households where neither parent has HIV [30].

The impact of malnutrition in HIV-infected children is generally similar to that in adults, but there are some important differences. Malnutrition can affect a child's thymic development and decrease cellular immunity and antibody production [31]. It also affects innate immune function [31]. The most obvious effect of malnutrition in HIV-infected children is impaired linear growth [31]. The etiology of this stunting appears to be complex. Among the many factors that may contribute to stunting is the suggestion that the pro-inflammatory cytokines that are produced in HIV affect bone remodeling required for linear growth [31].

As in adults, it is unclear whether nutritional supplementation reduces morbidity or mortality in the pediatric HIV-infected population. Certain interventions are clearly beneficial. It is clear that to maintain growth and immune function in asymptomatic pediatric HIV disease, a 10% increase in energy intake is required [18]. For catch-up growth, energy requirements can vary widely between 50 and 100% over the basic requirements [18, 31]. Increased energy demands should be met with caloric intake that includes a balanced mix of protein, fat, and carbohydrates, rather than from only one particular macronutrient. Less is known about nutrient requirements in adolescents with HIV infection. There is speculation that due to growth spurts increased intake of protein may be required [25].

The WHO has made certain recommendations for HIV-infected mothers breast-feeding their infants. In the resource-limited setting, vertical transmission of HIV disease via breast-feeding can be as high as 40% [30] if the mother is not treated with ART. However, this risk decreases dramatically with ART. Pregnant women diagnosed with HIV who met the WHO criteria for clinical stage 3 or 4 disease or have CD4 counts 350 cells/mm^3 or less have been eligible for ART treatment and current WHO recommendations suggest that all infected pregnant women should be treated but it is not clear that this is feasible. A woman must receive ART in order to prevent mother-to-child transmission (PMTCT) [7]. Even in settings where not all PLWHA can receive ART, pregnant and breast-feeding women still require chemoprophylaxis with ART to prevent PMTCT, especially throughout the breast-feeding period and until one week after all breast-feeding has stopped [7]. The infant also requires prophylaxis for four to six weeks after birth.

If ART is available to the mother, then breast-feeding is recommended up to 12 months of age [32]. If ART is unavailable, then formula feeding is recommended, as long as it is acceptable, feasible, affordable, sustainable, and safe [27]. If unable to formula feed, then exclusive breast-feeding is recommended for the first 6 months of life, which can be extended to 12 months as necessary [30]. Exclusive breast-feeding for less than six months can increase the risk of infant mortality, especially due to diarrhea, and exclusive breast-feeding for longer than 12 months can lead to malnutrition [30]. During the first 6 months, mixed feeding, whether breast and formula or breast and food, increases the risk of vertical transmission by 2 and 11 times, respectively [30]. It is hypothesized that mixed feeding damages the integrity of the gut mucosa and thus increases risk of HIV transmission [30]

Regardless of feeding practices, ART reduces the risk of vertical transmission and improves outcomes for both mother and child. In the pediatric population infected with HIV, ART reduces morbidity and mortality. It improves growth patterns and decreases OI, especially diarrheal diseases, which help improve nutrient absorption and metabolism [30].

Pregnancy, Nutrition, and HIV

Nutritional demands during pregnancy are increased for women who are not HIV-infected. TDEE and resting energy expenditure can be heightened by as much as 15–20% by the third trimester, especially in women in resource-sufficient settings [16]. In resource-poor settings, energy requirements only increase slightly, which perhaps indicates that maternal metabolism adapts to ensure that fetal energy requirements are met [16]. In lactating women, energy requirements can increase by 500 kcal/day in resource-sufficient settings [16]. Energy requirements in lactating women in resource-limited settings are not clear.

Whether pregnant or lactating, meeting energy requirements in resource-poor settings, especially for HIV-infected mothers, can be difficult. Pregnant and lactating women are especially susceptible to food insecurity, which affects their nutritional intake. Although pregnant HIV-infected women have greater nutritional demands, they are often less likely to have the physical capability to meet those demands [14]. In addition to concerns about adequacy of caloric intake, there must also be concern over the quality of diet that the pregnant or lactating HIV-infected woman ingests. Poor or inadequate nutrition intake affects maternal weight gain, and less than adequate weight gain in a pregnant woman may increase the risk of pre-term labor and low birth weight [14]. Food insecurity in the pregnant or lactating HIV-infected woman may affect retention in care and decrease ART adherence, which increases the risk of resistant HIV in the mother and of vertical transmission of resistant HIV to the infant [14]. In lactating women, food insecurity can impair breast-feeding activities as mothers may be occupied with employment [14]. Decreased nutritional intake in the HIV-infected woman with food insecurity also results in decreased breast milk production [14]. Review of the evidence produced since the 2003 WHO nutritional guidance suggests that there are no new data that would alter the recommendation that a 10% increase in energy intake is necessary for HIV-infected pregnant or lactating women to meet their increased resting energy expenditure [33]. However, women who have inadequate weight gain during pregnancy, increased weight loss post-partum, other comorbidities, or are also adolescents may need much higher energy intakes [33].

Anemia is a significant concern in pregnant women. However, iron is recommended to be given at the recommended dietary allowance and should only be supplemented at higher levels after confirming iron deficiency anemia, as there are detrimental effects of excessive iron in the HIV-infected population [33, 34].

HIV and HIV–TB Co-infection and Malnutrition

Co-infection with HIV and TB leads to an even greater risk of malnutrition than seen with either infection alone. HIV, TB, and malnutrition either directly or indirectly contribute to immune compromise. Any degree of immune suppression, be it from malnutrition or underlying HIV disease, can increase the risk of developing a concomitant secondary infectious disease, the most common being tuberculosis [35]. In some African countries, the seroprevalence of HIV in those diagnosed with TB can be as high as 75% [35]. In fact, the diagnosis of TB should automatically trigger testing for HIV. As both HIV and TB can precipitate malnutrition, more severe weight loss can be seen in co-infection as compared to either infection alone [35]. However, whether this co-infection promotes an additive or synergistic mechanism in terms of wasting is unclear. Co-infection can heighten energy expenditure, nutrient malabsorption, micronutrient deficiencies, and the production of inflammatory cytokines, inciting weight loss, more so than in either infection alone [35].

Nutritional Status in HIV and HIV–TB Co-infection

Studies conducted in resource-rich as well as resource-limited settings suggest that BMI has been found to be significantly lower in the HIV–TB co-infected population, compared to those with HIV alone [36, 37], even though 24-hour dietary intake was not significantly different between the groups [38]. BMI was significantly lower in those with HIV and TB with CD4 counts less than 200 cells/uL as compared to those with CD4 counts greater than or equal to 200 cells/uL [35, 38], signifying that more severe disease is associated with lower BMI. The studies described above used comparisons between HIV/TB co-infection and HIV alone. Studies comparing nutritional status between co-infected versus only TB-infected patients suggest similar trends [35, 38]. Other measures of body composition such as mid-upper arm circumference were lower in co-infected patients as compared to those with TB alone [35].

Outcomes in HIV and HIV–TB Co-infection

Nutritional status in co-infected patients can contribute to disease outcomes. Individuals infected with HIV and TB with a BMI less than 17 kg/m^2 were at greater risk of early mortality when compared to patients with a BMI greater than or equal to 17 kg/m^2 [35]. Another study showed that in people living with HIV, those with higher BMI had lower rates of development of active TB and associated mortality [39].

Macronutrient Deficiencies in HIV and HIV–TB Co-infection

Malnutrition, as defined by BMI, is associated with macro- and micronutrient deficiencies. Protein–energy malnutrition, as defined by a low serum albumin concentration, is significantly less frequent in those with pulmonary TB alone as opposed to patients with pulmonary TB and HIV [35, 37, 40]. These differences can translate into profound effects on disease outcome as albumin levels are strongly associated with both morbidity and mortality [35, 37, 40]. Appropriate ART and anti-TB treatment would mitigate this effect by decreasing the catabolic processes of disease and improving appetite.

Micronutrient Deficiencies in HIV and HIV–TB Co-infection

The degree of micronutrient deficiencies can be more severe in individuals with HIV and pulmonary TB when compared to those with mono-infection [41]. Vitamin A is important in both HIV and in TB. Vitamin A deficiency can be profound in those presenting with co-infection [42]. Vitamin A plays a vital role in the function of lymphocytes and macrophages, which are important in the control of HIV and TB [35]. Other vitamins, such as vitamin D, vitamin E, and vitamin B complex have not been extensively studied in the HIV/TB co-infected population [35]. Iron deficiency and the resulting anemia are more prevalent in co-infected patients than in HIV-infected patients alone [40]. The trace element selenium also plays a role in immune defense, particularly as an antioxidant [36]. Finally, studies on zinc have shown varied results, but one study did note that levels of zinc were significantly lower in co-infected individuals when compared to those with TB alone or in controls with neither infection [37]. Again, as discussed above, the cornerstone of improving TB and HIV co-infection outcomes rests on anti-TB treatment and ART. Also important, as reflected in the WHO recommendations, is to counter malnutrition and undernutrition to potentially decrease the severity of disease outcomes.

Macronutrient Interventions in HIV and HIV–TB Co-infection

Randomized controlled trials of macronutrient supplementation have only recently been conducted in the TB and HIV co-infected population. A randomized controlled trial conducted in Tanzania sought to determine the effect of energy–protein supplementation in the setting of adequate micronutrient replacement on weight, body composition, and hand grip strength in HIV/TB co-infected patients [43]. Subjects were randomized to receive 1 versus 6 biscuits daily, each biscuit containing 4.5 g of protein and 615 kJ of energy, for 60 days during the first part of TB treatment [43]. About 50% of the subjects had under- or malnutrition, while the other 50% had normal BMIs. Baseline energy intake was not recorded, so the actual supplementation provided by the bars above any particular subject's baseline intake was unclear. However, given the BMIs recorded, it appears that 50% were meeting caloric requirements to maintain their weight within normal margins. Results showed that macronutrient supplementation did not significantly affect weight or body composition, though results were not stratified according to BMI, so it is unclear what the trend was in those with lower than normal BMI. Another small randomized controlled trial in India used macronutrient supplementation (cereal/lentil mixture of 930 kcal) versus nothing and gauged the clinical outcomes of disease in patients with TB with and without HIV [44]. Positive outcomes were defined as cure (cleared sputum), treatment completion, or negative sputum at 2 months after starting treatment (for those without negative sputum recorded at the end of treatment) [44]. Poor outcome was defined as failure, default, death, or relapse [44]. Whether in TB alone or in TB/HIV co-infected patients, macronutrient supplementation did not significantly affect any of the outcomes of either group [44]. It should be noted that this study was conducted prior to the availability of ART (which can substantially alter the course of disease) in India [44].

Micronutrient Interventions in HIV and HIV–TB Co-infection

Studies on micronutrient supplementation have yielded conflicting results with regard to disease outcomes. One study conducted in Tanzania suggested that when zinc, multivitamins, zinc with multivitamins, or placebo was given randomly to HIV/TB co-infected patients, only zinc plus multivitamins had an impact on mortality at 8 months [45]. A second similar study at a different site (Malawi) found no difference in mortality at 24 months [46]. Another trial in a similar population found that in a group randomized to receive micronutrients continuously for the entire duration of follow-up (median of 30 months), there was a significant decrease in TB recurrence at the end of follow-up [47]. While these studies enrolled subjects with similar disease status and BMI, the study designs for these three studies were quite different as were the doses of multivitamins given, with a range from 1 RDA to multiple RDA.

Conclusion

Malnutrition and HIV are inextricably linked, especially in resource-limited settings, and the combination is detrimental to disease outcomes. The malnutrition that is seen with HIV infections is complex and multifactorial, including metabolic derangements, leading to weight loss and wasting, which increases mortality risk, also among people starting anti-retroviral treatment. Malnutrition is even more common in HIV and HIV–TB co-infected individuals and found to be associated with severe adverse outcomes. Medical, socioeconomic, cultural, and psychological factors all play a role in the development of nutritional compromise with HIV or HIV–TB co-infection and vulnerable populations such as children, adolescents, pregnant women, and the elderly, as well as poor and food-insecure people are at particular risk. While it is clear that treatment of the underlying HIV and/or TB is absolutely critical to improving outcomes, abnormal nutritional status persists despite (in case of ARV, lifelong) treatment and continues to contribute to adverse outcomes. Therefore, it is important to monitor nutritional status, including weight, and ensure adequate nutritional intake, which may require specific nutritious foods. According to WHO guidance, micronutrient intake should be at the level of one RNI, as with the evidence that is currently available, it is not possible to recommend other levels for either of these infections. In summary, because of the linkages between malnutrition and HIV and TB infection, as well as the nutrition issues related to long-term ART use and chronic HIV infection, it is important to continue to ensure nutrition assessment and counseling are part of standard care and treatment programs, and that these are augmented where necessary with support in the form of special nutritious foods to support recovery of nutritional status and/or food assistance to support access, adherence, and retention in care and treatment.

Discussion Points

- Discuss the relationship between socioeconomic factors, nutrition status, and HIV in the resource-limited setting.
- Discuss the etiology of weight loss in HIV disease.
- Discuss the role of macro- and micronutrient deficiencies in HIV disease outcomes.
- Discuss the nutritional requirements of vulnerable populations suffering from HIV or HIV–TB co-infection.
- Discuss the impact of anti-retroviral treatment on nutritional status in PLWHA.
- Discuss the impact of TB and HIV treatment on nutritional status in those suffering from disease in resource-limited settings.
- Discuss the possible forms and roles of food assistance in care and treatment of HIV or HIV–TB co-infection.

References

1. Duggal S, Chugh TD, Duggal AK. HIV and malnutrition: effects on immune system. Clin Dev Immunol [internet]. 2012;1–8 [cited 2014 June]. Available from http://www.ncbi.nlm.nih.gov/pmc/articles/PMC3254022/.
2. Hunger Statistics [internet]. [place unknown]: World Food Program; 2014 [cited 2014 June]. Available from http://www.wfp.org/hunger/stats.
3. Koethe JR, Heimburger DC. Nutritional aspects of HIV-associated wasting in sub-Saharan Africa. Am J Clin Nutr. 2010;91(suppl):1138S–42S.
4. HIV/AIDS Global Health Observatory [internet]. Geneva: World Health Organization; 2014 [cited 2014 June]. Available from http://www.who.int/gho/hiv/en/.
5. Havens PL, Mofenson LM. American academy of pediatrics committee on pediatric AIDS. Evaluation and management of the infant exposed to HIV-1 in the United States. Pediatrics. 2009;123:175.
6. WHO case definitions of HIV for surveillance and revised clinical staging and immunological classification of HIV-related disease in adults and children [internet]. Geneva: World Health Organization; 2007 [cited 2015 July]. Available from www.who.int/hiv/pub/guidelines/hivstaging150307.pdf.
7. Consolidated guidelines on the use of antiretroviral drugs for treating and preventing HIV infection [internet]. Geneva: World Health Organization; 2013 [cited 2015 July]. Available from http://www.who.int/hiv/pub/guidelines/arv2013/download/en/.
8. Faintuch J, Soeters PB, Osmo HG. Nutritional and metabolic abnormalities in pre-AIDS HIV infection. Nutriton. 2006;22(6):683–90.
9. Mangili A, Murman DH, Zampini AM, Wanke CA. Nutrition and HIV infection: review of weight loss and wasting in the era of highly active antiretroviral therapy form the nutrition for healthy living cohort. Clin Infect Dis. 2006;15(42):836–42.
10. Mwamburi M, Wilson IB, Jacobson DL, Spiegelman D, Gorbach SL, Knox TA, Wanke CA. Understanding the role of HIV load in determining weight change in the era of highly active antiretroviral therapy. Clin Infect Dis. 2004;15(40):167–73.
11. Ivers LC, Culle KA, Freedberg KA, Block S, Coates J, Webb P. HIV/AIDS, undernutrition, and food insecurity. Clin Infect Dis. 2009;1(49):1096–102.
12. McMahon J, Wanke C, Terrin N, Skinner S, Knox T. Poverty, hunger, education and residential status impact survival in HIV. AIDS Behav. 2011;15(7):1503–11.
13. Rawat R, McCoy SI, Kadiyala S. Poor diet quality is associated with low CD 4 count and anemia and predicts mortality among antiretroviral therapy-naïve HIV-positive adults in Uganda. J Acquir Immune Defic Syndr. 2013;1(62):246–53.
14. Young S, Wheeler AC, McCoy SI, Weiser SD. A review of the role of food insecurity in adherence to care and treatment among adult and pediatric populations living with HIV and AIDS. AIDS Behav [internet]. 2013:12 [cited June 2014]. Available from http://rd.springer.com/article/10.1007%2Fs10461-013-0547-4.pdf.
15. Palermo T, Rawat R, Weiser SD, Kadiyala S. Food access and diet quality are associated with quality of life outcomes among HIV-infected individuals in Uganda. PLoS ONE [internet]. 2013;8(4):e62353 [cited 2014 June]. Available from http://www.ncbi.nlm.nih.gov/pmc/articles/PMC3630150.
16. Kosmiski L. Energy expenditure in HIV infection. Am J Clin Nutr. 2011;94(suppl):1677S–82S.
17. Scrimshaw NS, SanGiovanni JP. Synergism of nutrition, infection, and immunity: an overview. Am J Clin Nutr. 1997;66:464S–77S.
18. Nutrient requirements for people living with HIV/AIDS. Geneva, Switzerland. World Health Organization. 13–15 May 2003.
19. Grunfeld C, Pang M, Shimizu L, Shigenaga JK, Jensen P, Feingold KR. Resting energy expenditure, caloric intake and short-term weight change in human immunodeficiency virus infection and the acquired immunodeficiency syndrome. Am J Clin Nutr. 1992;55:455–60.
20. Gerrior JL, Neff LM. Nutrition assessment in HIV infection. Nutr Clin Care. 2005;8(1):6–15.
21. Forrester JE, Sztam KA. Micronutrients in HIV/AIDS: is there evidence to change the WHO 2003 recommendations? Am J Clin Nutr. 2011;94(suppl):1683S–9S.
22. De Pee S, Semba RD. Role of nutrition in HIV infection: review of evidence for more effective programming in resource-limited settings. Food Nutr Bull. 2010;31:S313–44.
23. Grobler L, Siegfried N, Visser ME, Mahlungulu SSN, Volmink J. Nutritional interventions for reducing morbidity and mortality in people with HIV. Cochrane Database Syst Rev [internet]. 2013;2:1–130 [cited 2014 June]. Available from http://onlinelibrary.wiley.com/doi/10.1002/14651858.CD004536.pub3/abstract;jsessionid=959012C0888CE3A511C8E8F0A730E3D5.f04t02.
24. Chandrasekhar A, Gupta A. Nutrition and disease progression pre-highly active antiretroviral therapy (HAART) and post-HAART: can good nutrition delay time to HAART and affect response to HAART? Am J Clin Nutr. 2011;94(suppl):1703S–15S.

25. Raiten DJ. Nutrition and pharmacology: general principles and implications for HIV. Am J Clin Nutr. 2011;94 (suppl):1697S–702S.
26. Fawzi WW, Msamanga GI, Spiegelman D, Urasse EJN, McGrath N, Mwakagile D, Antelman G, Mbise R, Herrera G, Kapiga S, Willett W, Hunter DJ. Randomised trial of the effects of vitamin supplements on pregnancy outcomes and T cell counts in HIV-1-infected women in Tanzania. Lancet. 1998;16(351):1477–82.
27. World Food Programme (WFP), PEPFAR, USAID, UNAIDS. Nutrition assessment, counselling and support for adolescents and adults living with HIV. New York: UNAIDS; 2014. Available from https://www.wfp.org/content/nutrition-assessment-counselling-and-support-adolescents-and-adults-living-hiv. Accessed 9 May 2016.
28. Mehra, D, De Pee S, Bloem MW. Nutrition, food security, social protection, and health systems strengthening for ending AIDS. In: Ivers LC, editor. Food insecurity and public health. 1st ed. Boca Raton: CRC Press; 2015. p. 69–90.
29. Dillon DG, Gurdasani D, Riha J, Ekoru K, Asiki G, Mayanja BN, et al. Association of HIV and ART with cardiometabolic traits in sub-Saharan Africa: a systematic review and meta-analysis. Int J of Epidemiol. 2013;42:1754–71.
30. Rose AM, Hall CS, Martinez-Alier N. Aetiology and management of malnutrition in HIV-positive children. Arch Dis Child. 2014;99(6):546–51.
31. Schaible UE, Kaufman SHE. Malnutrition and infection: complex mechanisms and global impacts. PLoS Med [internet]. 2007;4(5):e115 [cited 2014 June]. Available from http://www.ncbi.nlm.nih.gov/pmc/articles/PMC1858706/.
32. HIV and infant feeding [internet]. Geneva: World Health Organization; 2010, 2014 [cited 2014 June]. Available from http://www.who.int/maternal_child_adolescent/documents/9789241599535/en/.
33. Raiten DJ, Mulligan K, Papathakis P, Wanke C. Executive summary—nutritional care of HIV-infected adolescents and adults, including pregnant and lactating women: what do we know, what can we do, and where do we go from here? Am J Clin Nutr. 2011;94(suppl):1667S–76S.
34. Rawat R, Humphrey JH, Ntozini R, Mutasa K, Iliff PJ, Stoltzfus RJ. Elevated iron stores are associated with HIV disease severity and mortaliy among postpartum women in Zimbabwe. Pub Health Nutr. 2009;12(9):1321–9.
35. Van Lettow M, Fawzi WW, Semba R. Triple trouble: the role of malnutrition in tuberculosis and human immunodeficiency virus co-infection. Nutr Rev. 2003;61(3):81–90.
36. Shor-Posner G, Miguez MJ, Pineda LM, Rodriguez A, Ruiz P, Castillo G, et al. Impact of selenium status on the pathogenesis of mycobacterial disease in HIV-1—infected drug users during the era of highly active antiretroviral therapy. J Acquir Infect Defic Syndr. 2002;29(2):169–73.
37. Ramakrishnan K, Shenbagarathai R, Kavitha K, Uma A, Balasubramaniam R. Thirumalaikolundusubramanian P. serum zinc and albumin levels in pulmonary tuberculosis patients with and without HIV. Jpn J Infect Dis. 2008;61(3):202–4.
38. Shah S, Whalen C, Kotler DP. Severity of human immunodeficiency virus infection is associated with decreased phase angle, fat mass and body cell mass in adults with pulmonary tuberculosis infection in Uganda. J Nutr. 2001;131(11):2843–7.
39. Hanrahan CF, Golub JE, Mohapi L, Tshabangu N, Modisenyane T, Chaisson RE, et al. Body mass index and risk of tuberculosis and death. AIDS. 2010;24(10):1501–8.
40. Swaminathan S, Padmapriyadarsini C, Sukumar B, Iliayas S, Kumar SR, Triveni C, et al. Nutritional status of persons with HIV infection, persons with HIV infection and tuberculosis, and HIV-negative individuals from Southern India. Clin Infect Dis. 2008;46(6):946–9.
41. Van Lettow M, Harries AD, Kumwenda JJ, Zijlstra EE, Clark TD, Taha TE, et al. Micronutrient malnutrition and wasting in adults with pulmonary tuberculosis with and without HIV co-infection in Malawi. BMC Infect Dis [internet]. 2004;4(1):61 [cited 2014 June]. Available from http://www.ncbi.nlm.nih.gov/pmc/articles/PMC544350/pdf/1471-2334-4-61.pdf.
42. Rwangabwoba JM, Fischman H, Semba RD. Serum vitamin A levels during tuberculosis and human immunodeficiency virus infection. Int J Tuberc Lung Dis. 1998;2(9):771–3.
43. PrayGod G, Range N, Faurholt-Jepson D, Jeremiah K, Faurholt-Jepsen M, Aabye MG, et al. The effect of energy-protein supplementation on weight, body composition and handgrip strength among pulmonary tuberculosis HIV-co-infected patients: randomized controlled trial in Mwanza, Tanzania. Br J Nutr. 2012;107 (2):263–71.
44. Sudarsanam TD, John J, Kang G, Mahendri V, Gerrior J, Franciosa M, et al. Pilot randomized trial of nutritional supplementation in patients with tuberculosis and HIV-tuberculosis co-infection receiving directly observed short-course chemotherapy for tuberculosis. Trop Med Int Health. 2011;16(6):699–706.
45. Range N, Changalucha J, Krarup H, Magnussen P, Andersen AB, Friis H. The effect of multi-vitamin/mineral supplementation on mortality during treatment of pulmonary tuberculosis: a randomised two-by-two factorial trial in Mwanza, Tanzania. Br J Nutr. 2006;95(4):762–70.

46. Semba RD, Kumwenda J, Zijlstra E, Ricks MO, Van Lettow M, Whalen C, et al. Micronutrient supplements and mortality of HIV-infected adults with pulmonary TB: a controlled clinical trial. Int J Tuberc Dis. 2007;11(8): 854–9.

47. Villamor E, Mugusi F, Urassa W, Bosch RJ, Saathoff E, Matsumoto K, et al. A trial of the effect of micronutrient supplementation on treatment outcome, T Cell counts, morbidity, and mortality in adults with pulmonary tuberculosis. J Infect Dis. 2008;197(11):1499–505.

Part V
Nutrition and Health in Different Phases of the Lifecycle

Chapter 21
Reproductive Health and Nutrition

Satvika Chalasani and Nuriye Ortayli

Keywords Reproductive health · Puberty · Menstrual cycle · Pregnancy · Maternal morbidity · Maternal mortality · Sexually transmitted infections · Reproductive organ cancers

Learning Objectives

- Discuss how nutritional status affects reproductive well-being.
- Describe how the major nutrient concerns vary during the reproductive cycle.
- Describe mechanisms through which macronutrients and micronutrients affect reproductive health.
- Evaluate the impact that nutritional interventions have had on reproductive health, especially pregnancy outcomes.

Introduction

In 1994, the International Conference on Population and Development adopted a Programme of Action that represented a remarkable consensus among 179 Governments. The consensus was that individual human rights and dignity, including the equal rights of women and girls and universal access to sexual and reproductive health and rights, are a necessary precondition for sustainable development [1]. The Programme of Action offers the following definition for reproductive health:

> Reproductive health is a state of complete physical, mental and social well-being and not merely the absence of disease or infirmity, in all matters relating to the reproductive system and to its functions and processes. Reproductive health therefore implies that people are able to have a satisfying and safe sex life and that they have the capability to reproduce and the freedom to decide if, when and how often to do so.

Reproductive health thus includes but is not limited to the absence of morbidity and mortality. It includes having a healthy sex life, the capacity to reproduce, a healthy pregnancy and delivery, and a healthy infant as a product of this delivery, and being free of sexually transmitted infections (STIs)

S. Chalasani (✉)
Technical Division, United Nations Population Fund, 605 Third Avenue,
New York, NY 10158, USA
e-mail: satvika.chalasani@gmail.com

N. Ortayli
Technical Division, United Nations Population Fund, 605 Third Avenue,
New York, NY 10158, USA
e-mail: ortayli@unfpa.org

© Springer Science+Business Media New York 2017
S. de Pee et al. (eds.), *Nutrition and Health in a Developing World*,
Nutrition and Health, DOI 10.1007/978-3-319-43739-2_21

and reproductive organ cancers. Nutrition is more closely related to some aspects of reproductive health than others, so this chapter examines those aspects of reproductive health where there are plausible theoretical or empirical links with nutrition.

Reproductive Well-Being

For a long time, medical practice has been interested in the links between nutritional status or diet of women and their ovulation, fertility and childbearing capacities. Plenty of advice was given to treat problems or enhance sexual and reproductive functions using diet, some of which became intertwined with popular culture: Aniseed increases menstrual flow; onion gives "coction to semen"; melon aids sexual intercourse; dates will help women produce sons with ease; garlic dries up semen; on the contrary carrots increase sexual desire and also "provide a good supply of semen"; peas increase both semen and milk are just some of the advices given in the book "Medicine of the Prophet" written by al-Suyuti probably during the second half of fifteenth century [2].

While some remnants of ancient medical advice continue to exist in the thinking and daily practices of several people and communities even today, modern science and medicine has also looked into and tried to better document the linkages between nutritional status and reproductive functions of women and men. A well-known one, the association between polycystic ovaries with accompanying menstrual problems, subfertility and obesity was first described in 1935 by American gynecologists Irving F. Stein, Sr., and Michael L. Leventhal, from whom its original name of Stein-Leventhal syndrome is taken. Some even argue that the written description was made back in 1721, by an Italian named Valisneri: "Young married peasant women, moderately obese and infertile, with larger than normal ovaries" [3]. Another example, the amenorrhea accompanying an eating disorder described and termed as "anorexia nervosa" was described around 1873 by Sir William Gull, one of the personal physicians of Queen Victoria. There are other views saying that French europsychiatrist Ernest Charles Lasègue described it a few weeks earlier than him [4]. Who was first to officially describe the condition is debatable, but in both cases it was observed and documented more than a century ago.

Advances in endocrinology during the second half of the twentieth century, and improvements in our knowledge on the mechanisms by which sex steroid hormones affect the human body, brought new dimensions to our understanding of the interactions between nutrition and reproductive health, and reproductive morbidity. Now we are in an era where we have increasing insight into how our genes are affected by the environment, food we eat, and how they in turn affect our bodies, including our reproductive functions, and thus the future generations we produce. This is still an evolving area where it is not yet possible to show causal relationships, but we actually may not be very far from being able to do so. In this section while we try to give a glimpse of the discussion on the relationship between what we eat and how we reproduce, we will focus on evidence-based, i.e., well-established, well-documented relations between the two.

Onset of Puberty

Reproductive life starts with puberty. Puberty is the process of physical changes by which a child's body matures into an adult body capable of sexual reproduction to enable fertilization. It is initiated by hormonal signals from the brain to the gonads: the ovaries in a girl, the testes in a boy. In response to these signals, the gonads produce hormones that stimulate growth, function and transformation of the brain, bones, muscle, blood, skin, hair, breasts and sex organs. Physical growth, of height and weight, accelerates in the first half of puberty and is completed when the child has developed an adult body.

Puberty is neurochemically initiated by the marked increase in the pulsatile release of gonadotropin-releasing hormone (GnRH) from the preoptic anterior hypothalamus in the brain. The continual GnRH pulse then drives development and maintains the eventual reproductive functioning of gonads which in turn release gonadal sex steroids: testosterone in males and estradiol in females. These hormones enhance development of secondary sex characteristics, breast buds in girls and genital changes in boys. The mean age for starting of secondary sex characteristics are 11.15 years for girls and 11.64 years for boys [5].

Nutritional Problems in Utero and During Early Life

Recent findings indicate that the timing of puberty onset is affected by nutritional deficiencies occurring during certain early critical development windows. Maternal and early-life malnutrition seems to have an impact on the developmental trajectory of a child by leading to early onset of puberty through a number of mechanisms, including modifications in the expression of DNA. The same mechanisms leading to early onset of puberty also increase risks for non-communicable diseases (NCDs) during adulthood. Fetal and neonatal malnutrition causes characteristic disruptions in some of the coordinating mechanisms that regulate onset of puberty, as well as regulation of appetite, and energy balance [6]. Precocious puberty (early onset of puberty) leads to early sexual maturity unmatched with social or emotional maturity. Moreover, owing to a shortened juvenile growth period, and an overall shorter stature, these children are at greater risk of NCDs later in life such as adult obesity, type 2 diabetes, heightened risk of premenopausal breast cancer and cardiovascular disease [7].

Obesity

Several studies from the USA show that girls who have a relatively high body mass index (BMI) are more likely to have their menarche earlier. BMI is also positively associated with other measures of pubertal onset. Studies from other countries like Denmark [8] and Turkey [9] also found a link between BMI and early pubertal development in girls. For boys, however, this link was observed only in a few studies that looked at earlier puberty [10].

Vitamin D Deficiency

According to a case–control study, low level of serum 25OHD may be associated with precocious puberty [11].

Menstrual Cycle: Ovulation and Menstruation

In girls puberty ends with menarche, i.e., the first menstrual bleeding. Menstruation is the cyclic, physiological discharge through the vagina of blood and mucosal tissues from the non-pregnant uterus; it is under hormonal control and normally recurs at approximately four-week intervals, except during pregnancy and lactation, throughout the reproductive period, i.e., from puberty through menopause. Menstruation at regular intervals is the result of ovulatory cycles. In ovulatory cycles, ovaries, under the stimulatory effect of gonadotropic hormones released from the brain, are able to grow and release an ovum (egg). Growth and release of ovum is accompanied by production and release of gonadal steroid hormones, estradiol and progesterone which prepare the uterus for pregnancy (in case fertilization of the ovum happens). In the absence of pregnancy, these hormone levels drop and menstrual bleeding happens.

All the events around menstrual cycle, ovulation, fertilization, implantation of a fertilized egg (i.e., pregnancy) and menstrual bleeding in the absence of fertilization and implantation are the result of intricate interactions between stimulant hormones from the brain, gonadal steroids and reproductive organs. Our current knowledge cannot yet describe very clearly the role of environment, and specifically nutrition, in these complex interactions. However, we know that they play an important role, based on our observations of severe nutritional problems, i.e., nutrition-energy imbalances, such as anorexia nervosa and athletes' triad.

Anorexia Nervosa

Anorexia nervosa is a devastating psychiatric illness marked by extremely low body weight, cognitive distortions related to body shape and weight perception, and either severe restricting of one's food intake or adopting a pattern of binge eating followed by purging. Severe restriction in food intake leads to extreme weight loss (defined as body weight below 85% of expected weight), which in turn leads to the failure to ovulate. Of women presenting with eating disorders, the great majority report the absence of menstruation and a smaller group report other types of menstrual irregularities for at least 3 months during the course of their illness. Low BMI, low caloric intake and excessive exercise are strongly associated with decreased pulsatility of GnRH, and reversion to pubertal pulsatility patterns, which in turn impairs functions of ovaries and disrupts menses [12]. Despite these irregularities in ovulatory function, some women with eating disorders may get pregnant, and they are actually more likely to experience unplanned pregnancies since they (and their healthcare providers) assume they are, temporarily, infertile. The physiological and psychological demands of pregnancy, child delivery and postpartum period present a big challenge to these patients who are already struggling with an eating disorder [13].

Female Athlete Triad

The female athlete triad (also called Triad) is another example where energy deficiency leads to disruption of ovulation and menstruation through weight loss (see point on GnRH above), which in turn causes loss of bone mineral density-hence the triad: eating disorder and/or energy deficiency, amenorrhea and decreased bone mineral density. With proper nutrition, these same relationships promote robust health. However, some female athletes, especially those who are in competitive, demanding sports (i.e., they exercise a lot and need higher energy intake) or in sports where a slim body is needed may suffer from this disorder [14]. Energy availability is defined as dietary energy intake minus exercise energy expenditure. And low energy availability appears to be the factor that impairs reproductive and skeletal health in the Triad, and it may be inadvertent, intentional or psychopathological. Most effects appear to occur below an energy availability of 30 kcal.kg (-1) of fat-free mass per day.

Overnutrition and Obesity

Obesity (BMI more than 30 kg/m^2) is also associated with menstrual dysfunction and decreased fertility. And in men, obesity is associated with abnormal semen parameters and can adversely affect fertility [15]. Fertility rates are lower among overweight and obese women, in spontaneous conception as well as in artificial reproductive techniques [16].

Premenstrual Syndrome

Premenstrual syndrome (PMS), also called premenstrual tension (PMT) is a collection of emotional symptoms, with or without physical symptoms, related to a woman's menstrual cycle. While most women of childbearing age (up to 85%) report having experienced physical symptoms related to normal ovulatory function, such as bloating or breast tenderness, medical definitions of PMS are limited to a consistent pattern of emotional and physical symptoms occurring only during the luteal phase of the menstrual cycle that are of sufficient severity to interfere with some aspects of life. There is evidence of some beneficial effects of calcium and vitamin B6 vis-à-vis PMS, and mixed findings for magnesium and evening primrose oil (which contains omega-6 fatty acids). However, insufficient information about the studies included in the review makes it difficult to assess the reliability of the authors' conclusions [17].

Pregnancy

In nearly every culture around the world, there exist beliefs and traditional wisdom about the links between what a woman eats and her pregnancy, delivery and the health (and even sex) of the infant. In India for example, it is believed that whatever food a woman eats the most of when pregnant, the child will crave and enjoy the same foods in its own lifetime. However, very little of this is actually backed my modern science and standards for evidence. What is backed by such evidence is more linked to the prevention of morbidities and hence mortality, rather than mortality itself. Although it is virtually impossible to link nutrition to maternal mortality in a clinical trial framework (because maternal mortality is a rare event), in examining various possible determinants of maternal mortality in the last 60 years of the twentieth century, including nutrition, the most plausible explanation that emerges for the decline in maternal mortality, at least in the Western world, is the successive improvements in maternal care rather than higher standards of living [18]. Improved maternal care includes safer surgery practices, delivery under aseptic conditions, antibiotics to manage infections, oxytocin to induce labor and safer blood transfusion. A reduction in high-risk pregnancies (at younger ages, and high-parity births) is also a contributing factor.

In this section, we examine the relationship between nutrition and various maternal morbidities, which when health systems are weak, are closely linked to maternal mortality. There is a vast amount of literature examining the impacts of individual (or combined) protein–energy and micronutrient interventions. This section, however, only draws upon large studies or systematic reviews that permit some amount of inference with reasonable confidence (even if not causal).

The World Health Organization has defined reproductive morbidity as consisting of three types: obstetric, gynecologic and contraceptive morbidity [19, 20]. *Obstetric morbidity* refers to morbidity in a woman who has been pregnant (regardless of the site or duration of the pregnancy) from any cause related to or aggravated by the pregnancy or its management, but not from accidental or incidental causes. Obstetric morbidity is the equivalent of maternal morbidity and is further categorized into three types: direct and indirect obstetric morbidity, and psychological obstetric morbidity. Here we focus on the links of nutrition to direct obstetric morbidity which results from obstetric complications of the pregnant state (pregnancy, labor and the puerperium), from interventions, omissions, incorrect treatment, or from a chain of events resulting from any of the above. This can include temporary conditions, mild or severe, which occur during pregnancy or within 42 days of delivery, or permanent/chronic conditions resulting from pregnancy, abortion or childbirth. Some chronic conditions (such as anemia or hypertension) may be caused by pregnancy and delivery, but are equally likely to have other causes.

Maternal death is defined as the death of a woman while pregnant or within 42 days of termination of pregnancy, irrespective of the duration and site of the pregnancy, from any cause related to or aggravated by the pregnancy or its management but not from accidental or incidental causes [19]. Causes of maternal death are classified into direct and indirect causes. Direct maternal deaths are those resulting from obstetric complications of the pregnant state (i.e., pregnancy, delivery and postpartum), interventions, omissions, incorrect treatment or a chain of events resulting from any of the above. Indirect maternal deaths are those resulting from previously existing diseases or from diseases that developed during pregnancy and that were not due to direct obstetric causes but aggravated by physiological effects of pregnancy [21]. Nutrition-related causes would fall under the latter definition.

Energy and Protein

It is well established that nutritional status of women prior to and during pregnancy plays a key role in fetal growth and development. When it comes to the women themselves, malnourished pregnant women may be at increased risk for adverse pregnancy outcomes in terms of maternal morbidity and mortality. One of the better demonstrated relationships is between maternal height, cephalopelvic disproportion (CPD) and obstructed labor, which in turn is one of the major causes of maternal morbidity and mortality. However, height is mostly determined in the first few years of life, even if catch-up growth is possible into adolescence and the start of reproductive years [22]. Better intrapartum care—with better health systems particularly emergency obstetric and neonatal care with C-section capacity—rather than nutrition interventions is thus likely to be the most effective strategies to manage complications resulting from low maternal height and CPD [23]. Over the longer term, however, intergenerational improvements in stature (via better fetal and infant growth) via improvements in maternal nutrition and maternal somatic capital can lead to decreased CPD and a range of other improved outcomes [24].

A recent review examining the impacts of nutritional advice, balanced energy and protein supplementation, high-protein supplementation, and isocaloric protein supplementation on maternal health outcomes of preeclampsia, duration of labor (hours), and mode of birth (cesarean section) concluded that the evidence was generally of low quality (note that this review did not discuss the impacts on birth outcomes such as gestational age, birth weight, head circumference, neonatal mortality). Nutritional advice appears effective in increasing pregnant women's energy and protein intakes. The rather meager data on preeclampsia and duration of labor did not suggest a reduction in risk with balanced energy and protein supplementation, although it results in modest increases in maternal weight gain. High-protein nutritional supplements and isocaloric protein supplementation lack beneficial effects based on available data. And while higher BMI has been shown to be associated with increased risk of preeclampsia [25], among pregnant women who are overweight or exhibit high weight gain, the limited evidence suggests that energy–protein restriction is of no benefit in reducing the risk of preeclampsia or pregnancy-induced hypertension. Studies do not give information on other maternal health outcomes [26, 27].

Vitamin A

Biomedical pathways have been demonstrated from vitamin A to anemia (via its role in red blood cell formation and iron metabolism), obstetric hemorrhage (via its capacity to prevent or decrease the severity of coagulopathy, a cause of hemorrhage), pregnancy-related infections (by promoting wound healing, increasing resistance to infection and immune enhancement if infection occurs) and possibly hypertension (by decreasing endothelial cell damage and promoting vasodilatation, which could decrease the incidence and severity of preeclampsia) [28].

A recent review examines 13 studies comparing vitamin A supplementation with placebo [29]. They concluded that vitamin A supplementation (as well as vitamin A + iron–folic acid) compared with placebo or no treatment had no significant impact on reducing maternal mortality among pregnant and lactating women. No subgroup differences were detected either between general populations of pregnant women and those with HIV nor between pregnant women and those women who had given birth in the past 42 days. Vitamin A supplementation did, however, reduce maternal night blindness by an average 23% in two trials, bacterial vaginosis by 38% in one trial, puerperal fever by 79% in one small trial and increased BMI after birth in one small trial of women with HIV [30].

Vitamins C and E

Antioxidants can inhibit peroxidation and protect enzymes, proteins and cell integrity. They thus contribute to proper cellular function in normal pregnancy [31, 32]. Antioxidants such as vitamins C and E could thus be effective in decreasing oxidative stress, improving vascular endothelial function and thus preventing or ameliorating the pathogenesis of preeclampsia. However, a recent systematic review of nine studies investigating these possible links concluded that there were no significant differences in the risks of preeclampsia between the combined vitamin C and E group compared to the placebo groups, even after restricting the sample to women who were at high risk or low/moderate risk for preeclampsia. In fact, women jointly supplemented with vitamin C (1000 mg per day, far above the 55 mg RNI for pregnant women) and vitamin E (400 IU, also far above the 22.5 IU RNI for pregnant women in some countries) were at increased risk of developing gestational hypertension and premature rupture of membranes, but decreased risk of abruption placentae. There were no significant differences between the vitamin and placebo groups in the risk of other adverse maternal or fetal/perinatal outcomes. The authors conclude that supplementation with vitamins C and E during pregnancy does not prevent preeclampsia [33].

Vitamin D

Vitamin D helps the body maintain normal levels of calcium and phosphate in the blood which in turn contributes to bone mineralization, contraction of muscles, nervous system activities and cellular function [34].

In terms of vitamin D status of pregnant women, hypertensive disorders, especially preeclampsia, are the most studied reproductive health outcomes. Associations have been detected between low concentrations of vitamin D and manifestation of preeclampsia. However, most of the findings in humans are associations, and causality can therefore not be determined. Available scientific data are limited, and well-conducted clinical trials are still lacking. Contradictory results can be explained by methodological differences, as well as genetic, ethnic and racial, and geographic differences. Evidence from observational studies also shows higher rates of preterm birth, bacterial vaginosis and gestational diabetes in women with low vitamin D levels. However, confirmation of experimental observations establishing an association of vitamin D deficiency with adverse reproductive outcomes by high-quality observational and large-scale randomized clinical trials is still lacking [35]. A non-randomized follow-up study of 884 pregnant women with HIV reported that women with low vitamin D status were more likely to develop severe anemia, though no significant differences were seen for anemia overall. Combined death and disease progression (RR 1.23 95% CI 1.04–1.45) were also more likely in women with low vitamin D [36].

Vitamin D supplementation in a single or continued dose during pregnancy increases maternal serum vitamin D concentrations as measured by 25-hydroxy vitamin D at term. However, the clinical significance of this finding for maternal health and whether it should become a part of routine antenatal care for maternal benefit cannot be determined without further high-quality trials [37].

It is important to note that vitamin D, as well as other micronutrients, are part of multiple micronutrient supplements (typically at a dose of 1 RNI) that have been provided to pregnant women to study impact on birth outcomes (see Chaps. 22 and 23).

Calcium

Most studies of the impact of calcium intake on maternal mortality have focused on calcium's links to preeclampsia and eclampsia. A recent review summarizes the various proposed pathways by which calcium influences these major causes of maternal mortality. Low calcium intake may cause high blood pressure by stimulating either parathyroid hormone or renin release, thereby increasing intracellular calcium in vascular smooth muscle (which leads to vasoconstriction) as well as increasing uterine smooth muscle contractility (which can increase risk of preterm labor and delivery). Calcium might also have an indirect effect on smooth muscle function by increasing magnesium levels. It can promote uteroplacental blood flow by lowering the resistance index in uterine and umbilical arteries. And in the second half of pregnancy, it may reduce blood pressure directly rather than preventing the endothelial damage associated with preeclampsia [38].

The same review concluded (based on 13 trials) that calcium supplementation (at least 1 g/day, noting that the World Health Organization recommends calcium 1.5–2 g daily for pregnant women with low dietary calcium intake) is associated with a reduction in the risk of gestational hypertension, preeclampsia and preterm birth. The effects are particularly evident among women with low calcium diets and at high risk of preeclampsia. Calcium also reduces preterm birth and the occurrence of the composite outcome "maternal death or serious morbidity," a result corroborated by another review (11 trials) [29]. However, the authors note that the treatment effect may be overestimated due to small-study effects or publication bias. They also found reduced occurrence of preeclampsia but not of eclampsia. An important conclusion is that in settings of low dietary calcium where high-dose supplementation is not feasible (since calcium is relatively expensive, and the tablets are bulky and heavy to transport and store) the option of lower-dose supplements (500–600 mg/day) might be preferable to no supplementation.

Iron and Vitamin B

Iron as well as folate/folic acid (or vitamin B9) and vitamin B12 are essential to the synthesis of DNA and the production of red blood cells. Fetal growth results in an increase in rapidly dividing cells, which in turns leads to heightened requirements for iron and folate among pregnant women. Combined with the increased deposition or iron in the placenta, this can lead to iron-deficiency anemia and megaloblastic anemia (where cells are abnormally large, and cell contents are incompletely developed) [39, 40]. The pathways by which anemia then increases risk of death among pregnant women need to be better understood. Severe anemia may impair the muscular strength needed for labor (and lead to higher blood loss), or it may decrease resistance to or increase susceptibility to infection. Severely anemic women are more susceptible to death from exsanguinating hemorrhage (extensive internal or external blood loss) [41].

The most recent systematic review concludes that among pregnant and lactating women, iron and folic acid supplement compared to placebo reduced anemia by 36% in pregnant and lactating women [29]. There was no apparent impact on other morbidities and associated outcomes such as postpartum hemorrhage, cesarean section and malarial infection. This confirms the conclusions of an earlier review that found that prenatal supplementation with daily iron was effective in preventing anemia and iron deficiency in pregnancy [42].

Looking at dosage, daily iron or iron and folic acid was significantly more effective than weekly or intermittent supplementation in reducing rates of anemia although adherence was significantly higher in the weekly group compared with the daily group. Iron or iron and folic acid + vitamin A (with or without zinc) were superior to vitamin A alone in regard to anemia control, puerperal infection and endometritis. Universal iron supplementation for pregnant women in Thailand led to significant decreases in anemia in this population [43]. Among women of reproductive age more generally, daily iron and folic acid supplementation, as well as food fortification, both significantly reduced anemia. Large-scale micronutrient and nutrition programs that included iron supplementation were associated with decreased anemia among adolescents [44]. Free weekly iron and folic acid supplement for socioeconomically disadvantaged women of reproductive age, combined with social marketing for those able to purchase low-cost supplements, is also considered practical and effective [45]. However, evidence of associated maternal side effects particularly of high Hb concentrations during pregnancy suggests the need to review and possibly update recommended doses and regimens for supplementation [42].

Despite this important evidence, it is important to note the lack of evidence on the relationship between mild/moderate anemia and maternal mortality [46] as well as the lack of differentiation in the literature on whether iron supplementation can reduce mild/moderate or severe anemia or both. Importantly about 50% of anemia in women is attributable to iron deficiency, with other nutritional and non-nutritional causes explaining the other 50% [47]. This has significant implications for our understanding of the potential impact (or lack thereof) of iron supplementation on maternal mortality. Furthermore, malaria and hookworm infection can inhibit absorption of iron, and contribute to anemia, thus suggesting an important non-nutritional intervention (bed nets and antimalarials, for example) for addressing anemia and its potential consequences for maternal health [48–50].

Zinc

Zinc has been shown to play an important role in protein synthesis, cellular division and nucleic acid metabolism [51]. Among pregnant women, zinc's roles in maintaining immunocompetence, cell membrane integrity, prostaglandin synthesis and function, and estrogen-dependent gene expression are all considered as pathways to its potential impact on pregnancy outcomes [52].

Low serum zinc levels in pregnant women are possibly associated with suboptimal outcomes of pregnancy such as prolonged labor, atonic postpartum hemorrhage, pregnancy-induced hypertension, preterm labor and post-term births, although many of these associations have not yet been established. A 20 trial review concluded that zinc (compared to no zinc) did not make a difference to any maternal outcomes. The conclusions were not altered by subgroup comparisons (low versus normal zinc and nutrition levels, treatment compliant versus non-compliant) [53]. Another recent review of eight trials comparing zinc with placebo among pregnant and lactating women similarly concluded that none of the maternal mortality or morbidity outcomes showed any significant differences [29]. Given this current evidence, efforts to improve overall nutritional status of women of reproductive age in poor areas, rather than focusing exclusively on specific micronutrients (including zinc supplementation in isolation), could be given priority.

Magnesium

Magnesium works with many enzymes to regulate body temperature, synthesize nucleic acids, and protein and maintain electrical potentials in nerves and muscle membranes. Magnesium also has an important role in modulating vasomotor tone and cardiac excitability [54]. Low levels of magnesium could produce vasoconstriction, rise in blood pressure and occurrence and severity of preeclampsia [55].

However, a ten-trial review concludes that magnesium supplementation during pregnancy had no significant effect on preeclampsia [54]. No data were available on maternal mortality. However, a different review of four trials showed that the rate of eclampsia was significantly reduced with magnesium versus no magnesium. Two trials showed no significant difference in maternal mortality with magnesium (versus placebo) [29]. Thus, while there is some evidence that dietary magnesium supplementation during pregnancy can reduce eclampsia, more high-quality evidence is needed and for a wider range of maternal outcomes.

Iodine

Iodine is an essential component of the hormones produced by the thyroid gland. Iodine requirements increase by more than 50% during pregnancy, and iodine deficiency during pregnancy can cause maternal hypothyroidism. The consequences include miscarriages, anemia, preeclampsia, abruptio placenta and postpartum hemorrhage [56] and depend upon the timing and severity of the hypothyroidism. The evidence based on the effects of iodine on maternal pregnancy outcomes is weak. However, in nearly all regions affected by iodine deficiency, salt iodization is the most cost-effective way of delivering iodine and improving maternal health, fetal growth and infant health [57].

Multiple Micronutrients

In many low- and middle-income countries, large proportions of women have poor diets and deficiencies in nutrients and micronutrients that are required for good health, a condition exacerbated by pregnancy when micronutrient needs increase as the fetus grows, and the body's absorption capacities are altered (for better or worse). Multiple micronutrients present advantages in terms of cost-efficiency and possibly interactions effects for greater impact.

Multiple micronutrients (versus two or less) showed no significant effects on maternal anemia, miscarriage, preeclampsia, maternal mortality or risk of delivery via C-section [58]. Note that one review found that multiple micronutrient supplements had the same impact on hemoglobin and iron status indicators as iron with or without folic acid [59].

Overnutrition and Obesity

Obesity (BMI more than 30 kg/m^2) is associated with increased risk of miscarriage and obstetrical and neonatal complications [60]. A recent review concludes that maternal overweight is now a known risk factor that impacts the entire continuum of pregnancy. Overweight women are more susceptible to pregnancy hypertensive disorders, gestational diabetes, respiratory complications and thromboembolic events. As delivery approaches, overweight women have a slower labor progression rate, higher rates of cesarean deliveries and more surgery-related complications such as difficult spinal, epidural or general anesthesia, wound infection and endometritis [61].

Sexually Transmitted Infections (STIs)

Gynecologic morbidity includes any condition, disease or dysfunction of the reproductive system which is not related to pregnancy, abortion or childbirth, but may be related to sexual behavior. It is further categorized into three types: direct and indirect gynecologic morbidity, and psychological morbidity. This section and the next one focus on the links of nutrition to direct gynecologic morbidity which includes bacterial or viral STIs and their sequelae, and reproductive cancers (as well as PMS, discussed in that section).

Very few studies have looked into a possible relationship between nutrition and STIs. A nested case–control study in Pune, India, of individuals attending two sexually transmitted disease (STD) clinics found low serum beta-carotene levels to be independently associated with an increased risk of subsequent HIV seroconversion [62]. One trial reported no impact of vitamin A on the presence of vaginal HIV-1 DNA in 400 women with HIV [63].

Reproductive Organ Cancers

Due to the rarity of cancers and the probable multifactorial mechanisms that lead to their development and their fatality, it is difficult to establish links, particularly causal ones, between nutrition and the prevention and treatment of cancers. Still, in this subsection we try to highlight a number of associations on which we have evidence, focusing on meta-analyses and systematic reviews.

Breast Cancer

Breast cancer is the number one killer of women among all cancers, killing more than half a million women each year [64]. Therefore, its prevention and improvement of treatment is a public health priority.

Obesity

Breast cancer risk among postmenopausal women increases with increasing BMI, but not in premenopausal women [65, 66]. This association has been also observed in cohort studies [67, 68].

Vitamin D

A meta-analysis conducted in 2013, looking at serum 25(OH)D levels showed that there was significant inverse association with breast cancer risk (RR = 0.845, 95% CI = 0.750–0.951). Inversely statistically significant associations were observed in North American studies, postmenopausal women and studies with adjusted and unadjusted RR. No statistically significant associations were observed in European studies and premenopausal women. Dose–response analysis showed that every 10 ng/mL increment in serum 25(OH)D concentration was associated with a significant 3.2% reduction in breast cancer risk [69].

The role of vitamin supplements in preventing breast cancer is still an unclear area. Although there are theoretical pathways which may suggest a benefit, there is no clear evidence for an effect of vitamin supplements on cancer prevention [70].

One analysis of pooled data which included 12,000 breast cancer survivors did not find any relation between post-treatment vitamin supplement use and risk of recurrence or death. Post-treatment use of antioxidant supplements were associated with improved survival, but the associations with individual supplements were difficult to determine [71].

Cervical Cancer

Vitamin A

A meta-analysis of 11 studies showed that pooled odds ratios (ORs) of cervical cancer were 0.59 (95% CI, 0.49–0.72) for total vitamin A intake and 0.60 (95% CI, 0.41–0.89) for blood vitamin A levels. The combined ORs of cervical cancer were 0.80 (95% CI, 0.64–1.00) for retinol, 0.51 (95% CI, 0.35–0.73) for carotene, 0.60 (95% CI, 0.43–0.84) for other carotenoid intake, 1.14 (95% CI, 0.83–1.56) for blood retinol and 0.48 (95% CI, 0.30–0.77) for blood carotene.

Overall, the authors concluded that vitamin A intake and blood vitamin A levels were inversely associated with the risk of cervical cancer in this meta-analysis.

We do not have any evidence yet that we can reduce cancer risk by vitamin A supplementation [72].

Obesity

An association between death from cervical cancer and obesity was observed in a large cohort study conducted in USA [67].

Ovarian Cancer

Obesity

Ovarian cancer is one of the important causes of death due to gynecological malignancy (leading cause in industrialized countries which have controlled cervical cancer prevalence and mortality using effective screening programs). A systematic review and meta-analysis found the pooled effect estimate for female adult obesity was 1.3 (95% CI, 1.1–1.5) with a smaller increased risk for overweight (OR 1.2; 95% CI 1.0–1.3). The pooled OR was stronger among case–control studies than cohort studies (1.5 vs. 1.1). Overweight/obesity in early adulthood was also associated with an increased risk of ovarian cancer [73].

Diets high in glycemic load may actually increase risk of ovarian cancer, especially in overweight/obese women, and diets rich in fibers may provide a modest protection [74].

Various Micronutrients

Australian Ovarian Cancer Study did not observe an overall association between the intake of folate, B vitamins or other methyl donors and ovarian cancer risk [75].

Uterus Cancer

Obesity

Two large cohort studies have found that risk of cancer of the uterus corpus increases in women with obesity [67, 68].

Prostate Cancer

While men face a variety of sexual and reproductive health risks, little is known about links between nutrition and male SRH. One exception is prostate cancer, the most common cancer among men. More than 1.1 million cases of prostate cancer were recorded around the world in 2012, accounting for around 8% of all new cancer cases and 15% in men [76].

Various Micronutrients

No influence on prostate cancer risk was observed for dietary folate or for intake of vitamin C, vitamin E, and beta-carotene [77]. An expert panel on behalf of the World Cancer Research Fund and the American Institute for Cancer Research also concluded that it is unlikely that beta-carotene (whether from foods or supplements) has a substantial effect on the risk of this cancer. SELECT trial, a large randomized control study showed no protective effect of selenium or vitamin E, alone or in combination from prostate cancer, despite encouraging findings from animal models and previous studies [78].

Earlier another large prospective study from USA had found preventative multivitamin use not to be associated with early or localized prostate cancer, but was associated with advanced and fatal prostate cancer, a finding which needs to be further evaluated [79].

However, a recent review on environmental factors in human prostate cancer found that there were protective effects of vitamin E, pulses, soy foods and high plasma 1,25-dihydroxy vitamin D levels. Higher intake of legumes, nuts, shellfish and alpha-tocopherol intake were associated with decreasing prostate cancer risks [80]. Evidence indicates that foods containing lycopene, as well as foods containing selenium, probably protect against prostate cancer. A Danish prospective cohort study of 26,856 men found supplemental folic acid to be inversely associated with prostate cancer risk on a continuous scale [HR 0.88 (95% CI, 0.79–0.98) per 100 mcg increase/day]. However, this inverse association was confined to supplemental folic acid and non-aggressive prostate cancer.

The Mediterranean diet is abundant in foods that may protect against prostate cancer and is associated with longevity and reduced cardiovascular and cancer mortality. Compared with many Western countries, Greece has lower prostate cancer mortality and Greek migrant men in Australia have retained their low risk for prostate cancer. Consumption of a traditional Mediterranean diet, rich in bioactive nutrients, may confer protection to Greek migrant men [80].

Excess consumption of foods or supplements containing calcium is a potential cause of this cancer. A case–control study in 2010 found prostate cancer risk to be associated with an increased intake of dairy products (OR = 2.19; 95% CI, 1.22–3.94). Calcium, the main micronutrient contained in dairy products, showed only a borderline associating with prostate cancer risk (although it has been postulated that it is dairy's phosphate content and not necessarily calcium that is driving this risk) [81]. In another large prospective study in a prostate cancer screening trial, greater dietary intake of calcium and dairy products, particularly low-fat types, was shown to be modestly associated with increased risks for non-aggressive prostate cancer, but was unrelated to aggressive disease [82].

Conclusion

Reproductive health is an important dimension of both women's and men's health. There are strong theoretical underpinnings to the important role that nutrition can play in improving reproductive health. While the evidence of direct causal impacts of specific nutrients on reproductive health outcomes is either weak or sparse, there are numerous studies showing associations between certain nutrients and reproductive health outcomes or intermediate outcomes that we know are linked to reproductive health. For some aspects of nutrition there is stronger evidence of the impact of supplementation, such as calcium and preeclampsia, and iron/folic acid and anemia. Understanding of the precise pathways of impact is still limited and will require further study.

Discussion Points

- How can the definition of reproductive well-being be used to assess the outcome of nutrition interventions?
- What could be the long-term impact of preconceptual and antenatal nutritional interventions on the health of reproductive organs?
- What is the impact of nutritional deficiencies on maternal mortality and why? Are there specific nutrients that lead to specific causes of maternal mortality? If so, describe the pathways for this relationship.
- Nutrition–infection interactions are well described regarding childhood diseases such as diarrhea, measles and respiratory infections. How may this two-way interaction present itself for women of reproductive age?

References

1. UN Economic and Social Council. Framework of actions for the follow-up to the programme of action of the international conference on population and development (ICPD) beyond; 2014.
2. Elgood C. Tibb-ul-Nabi or medicine of prophet. Osiris; 1962:70, 72, 73, 75–7, 82 Accessible at http://isites. harvard.edu/fs/docs/icb.topic1404975.files/Unit%203/Elgood_Tibb-ul-Nabbi%20or%20Medicine%20of%20the%20Prophet%20-%201962.pdf.

3. Farquhar C. Introduction and history of polycystic ovary syndrome. In: Kovacs GT, Norman R, editors. Polycystic ovary syndrome. Cambridge: Cambridge University Press; 22 Feb 2007. p. 4. ISBN 9781139462037. Accessible at http://books.google.com/books?id=bpn1u9hziVgC&pg=PA4#v=onepage&q&f=false.

4. Vandereycken W, van Deth R. A tribute to Lasègue's description of anorexia nervosa (1873), with completion of its English translation. Br J Psychiatry. 1990;157:902–8.

5. Marshall WA, Tanner JM. Variations in pattern of pubertal changes in girls. Arch Dis Child. 1969;44(235): 291–303.

6. Connor N. Impact of fetal and neonatal malnutrition on the onset of puberty and associated noncommunicable disease risks. Adolesc Health Med Ther. 2011;2:15–25. doi:10.2147/AHMT.S10147. Accessed at http://www.ncbi. nlm.nih.gov/pmc/articles/PMC3926776/.

7. Ahmed ML, Ong KK, Dunger DB. Childhood obesity and the timing of puberty. Trends Endocrinol Metab. 2009;20(5):237–42.

8. Juul A, Teilmann G, Scheike T, Hertel NT, Holm K, Laursen EM, Main KM, Skakkebaek NE. Pubertal development in Danish children: comparison of recent European and US data. Int J Androl. 2006;29(1):247–55; discussion 286–90.

9. Semiz S, Kurt F, Kurt DT, Zencir M, Sevinç O. Pubertal development of Turkish children. J Pediatr Endocrinol Metab. 2008;21(10):951–61.

10. Kaplowitz PB. Link between body fat and the timing of puberty. Pediatrics. 2008;121(Suppl 3):S208–17. doi:10. 1542/peds.2007-1813F.

11. Villamor E, Marin C, Mora-Plazas M, Baylin A. Vitamin D deficiency and age at menarche: a prospective study. Am J Clin Nutr. 2011;94:1020–5.

12. Poyastro PA, Thornton LM, Plotonicov KH, et al. Patterns of menstrual disturbance in eating disorders. Int J Eat Disord. 2007;40(5):424–34.

13. Hoffman ER, Zerwas SC, Bulik CM. Reproductive issues in anorexia nervosa. Expert Rev Obstet Gynecol. 2011;6 (4):403–14. doi:10.1586/eog.11.31.

14. Nattiv A, Loucks AB, Manore MM, Sanborn CF, Sundgot-Borgen J, Warren MP. American College of Sports Medicine. American College of Sports Medicine position stand. The female athlete triad. Med Sci Sports Exerc. 2007;39(10):1867–82.

15. Fritz MA, Speroff L. Female infertility. In: Gynecologic Clinical, editor. Endocrinology and infertility. 8th ed. Philadelphia: Lippincott Williams and Wilkins; 2011. p. 1137–90.

16. Yogev Y, Catalano PM. Pregnancy and obesity. Obstet Gynecol Clin North Am. 2009;36(2):285–300.

17. Canning S, Waterman M, Dye L. Dietary supplements and herbal remedies for premenstrual syndrome (PMS): a systematic research review of the evidence for their efficacy. J Reprod Infant Psychol. 2006;24(4):363–78.

18. Loudon I. Maternal mortality in the past and its relevance to developing countries today. Am J Clin Nutr. 2000;72 (1 Suppl.):241s–6s.

19. World Health Organization. International classification of diseases and related health problems, tenth revision, vol. 1. Geneva, Switzerland: World Health Organization; 1992.

20. National Research Council. The consequences of maternal morbidity and maternal mortality: report of a workshop. Washington, DC: The National Academies Press; 2000.

21. World Health Organization. Trends in maternal mortality: 1990 to 2013. Estimates by WHO, UNICEF, UNFPA, The World Bank and the United Nations Population Division; 2014.

22. Rush D. Nutrition and maternal mortality in the developing world. Am J Clin Nutr. 2000;72(suppl):212S–40S.

23. World Health Organization. Balanced energy and protein supplementation during pregnancy; 2014. http://www. who.int/elena/titles/energy_protein_pregnancy/en/.

24. Wells JCK. Maternal capital and the metabolic ghetto: an evolutionary perspective on the transgenerational basis of health inequalities. Am J Hum Biol. 2010;22:1–17. doi:10.1002/ajhb.20994.

25. Duckitt K, Harrington D. Risk factors for pre-eclampsia at antenatal booking: systematic review of controlled studies. BMJ. 2005;330:565.

26. Ota E, Tobe-Gai R, Mori R, Farrar D. Antenatal dietary advice and supplementation to increase energy and protein intake. Cochrane Database Syst Rev. 2012;(9), Art. No.: CD000032. doi:10.1002/14651858.CD000032.pub2.

27. Kramer MS, Kakuma R. Energy and protein intake in pregnancy. Cochrane Database Syst Rev. 2007;(4), Art. No.: CD000032. doi:10.1002/14651858.CD00003.

28. Faisel H, Pitroff R. Vitamin A and causes of maternal mortality: association and biological plausibility. Public Health Nutr. 2000;3:321–7.

29. Middleton PF, Lassi ZS, son Tran T, Bhutta Z, Bubner TK, Flenady V, Crowther CA. Nutrition interventions and programs for reducing mortality and morbidity in pregnant and lactating women and women of reproductive age: a systematic review. ARCH. 2013.

30. Ahmed F, Khan MR, Jackson AA. Concomitant supplemental vitamin A enhances the response to weekly supplemental iron and folic acid in anemic teenagers in urban Bangladesh. Am J Clin Nutr. 2001;74:105–15.

31. Kontic-Vucinic O, Terzic M, Radunovic N. The role of antioxidant vitamins in hypertensive disorders of pregnancy. J Perinat Med. 2008;36:282–90.

32. Al-Gubory KH, Fowler PA, Garrel C. The roles of cellular reactive oxygen species, oxidative stress and antioxidants in pregnancy outcomes. Int J Biochem Cell Biol. 2010;42:1634–50.

33. Conde-Agudelo A, Romero R, Kusanovic JP, Hassan SS. Supplementation with vitamins C and E during pregnancy for the prevention of preeclampsia and other adverse maternal and perinatal outcomes: a systematic review and metaanalysis. Am J Obstet Gynecol. 2011;204:503.e1–12.

34. World Health Organization. Vitamin and mineral requirements in human nutrition, vol 2. Geneva; 2004.

35. Grundman M, von Versen-Höynck F. Vitamin D—roles in women's reproductive health? Reprod Biol Endocrinol. 2011;9:146.

36. Mehta S, Giovannucci E, Mugusi FM, Spiegelman D, Aboud S, Hertzmark E. Vitamin D status of HIV-infected women and its association with HIV disease progression, anemia and mortality. PLoS ONE. 2010;5(1):e8770.

37. De-Regil LM, Palacios C, Ansary A, Kulier R, Peña-Rosas JP. Vitamin D supplementation for women during pregnancy. Cochrane Database Syst. Rev. 2012;(2), Art. No.: CD008873. doi:10.1002/14651858.CD008873.pub2.

38. Hofmeyr GJ, Lawrie TA, Atallah ÁN, Duley L, Torloni MR. Calcium supplementation during pregnancy for preventing hypertensive disorders and related problems. Cochrane Database Syst Rev. 2014;(6), Art. No.: CD001059. doi:10.1002/14651858.CD001059.pub4.

39. Lassi ZS, Salam RA, Haider BA, Bhutta ZA. Folic acid supplementation during pregnancy for maternal health and pregnancy outcomes. Cochrane Database Syst Rev. 2013;(3), Art. No.: CD006896. doi:10.1002/14651858.CD006896.pub2.

40. Charmel R. Cobalamin (Vitamin B12). In: Shils ME, Shike M, Ross AC, Caballero B, Cousins RJ, editors. Modern nutrition in health and disease. 10th ed. USA: Lippincott Williams & Wilkins; 2006. p. 482–97.

41. Rush D. Nutrition and maternal mortality in the developing world. Am J Clin Nutr. 2000;72(suppl):212S–40S.

42. Peña-Rosas JP, De-Regil LM, Dowswell T, Viteri FE. Daily oral iron supplementation during pregnancy. Cochrane Database Syst Rev. 2012;(12), Art. No.: CD004736. doi:10.1002/14651858.CD004736.pub4).

43. World Health Organization. Prevention of iron deficiency anaemia in adolescents: role of weekly iron and folic acid supplementation. Vol. SEA-CAH-02. New Delhi: WHO SEA; 2011.

44. Berti PR, Mildon A, Siekmans K, Main B, MacDonald C. An adequacy evaluation of a 10-year, four-country nutrition and health programme. Int J Epidemiol. 2010;39:613–29.

45. World Health Organization (Western Pacific Region). Weekly iron and folic acid supplementation programmes for women of reproductive age: an analysis of best programme practices. Geneva: WHO; 2011.

46. Pizarro CF, Davidson L. Anemia during pregnancy: influence of mild/moderate/severe anemia on pregnancy outcome. Nutrire: rev. Soc. Bras. Alim Nutr J Brazilian Soc Food Nutr. 2003;25:153–80.

47. World Health Organization. The global prevalence of anaemia in 2011. Geneva: World Health Organization; 2015.

48. Gamble CL, Ekwaru JP, ter Kuile FO. Insecticide-treated nets for preventing malaria in pregnancy. Cochrane Database Syst Rev. 2006;(2), Art. No.: CD003755. doi:10.1002/14651858.CD003755.pub2.

49. McClure EM, Goldenberg RL, Dent AE, Meshnick SR. A systematic review of the impact of malaria prevention in pregnancy on low birth weight and maternal anemia. Int J Gynecol Obstet. 2013;121:103–9. doi:10.1016/j.ijgo.2012.12.014.

50. Brooker S, Hotez PJ, Bundy DAP. Hookworm-related anaemia among pregnant women: a systematic review. PLoS Negl Trop Dis. 2008;2(9):e291. doi:10.1371/journal.pntd.0000291.

51. King JC, Cousins RJ. Zinc. In: Shils ME, Shike M, Ross AC, Caballero B, Cousins RJ, editors. Modern nutrition in health and disease. 10th ed. Philadelphia, PA.

52. Caulfield LE, Zavaleta N, Shankar AH, Merialdi M. Potential contribution of maternal zinc supplementation during pregnancy to maternal and child survival.

53. Mori R, Ota E, Middleton P, Tobe-Gai R, Mahomed K, Bhutta ZA. Zinc supplementation for improving pregnancy and infant outcome. Cochrane Database Syst Rev. 2012;(7), Art. No.: CD000230. doi:10.1002/14651858.CD000230.pub4.

54. Makrides M, Crosby DD, Bain E, Crowther CA. Magnesium supplementation in pregnancy. Cochrane Database Syst Rev. 2014;(4), Art. No.: CD000937. doi:10.1002/14651858.CD000937.pub2.

55. Jain S, Sharma P, Kulshreshtha S, Mohan G, Singh S. The role of calcium, magnesium and zinc in pre-eclampsia. Biol Trace Elem Res. 2010;133:162–70.

56. Obican SG. Jahnke GD. Soldin OP. Scialli AR. Teratology public affairs committee position paper: iodine deficiency in pregnancy. Birth Defects Res (Part A): Clin Mol Teratol. 2012;94:677–82.

57. Zimmermann MB. The effects of iodine deficiency in pregnancy and infancy. Paediatr Perinat Epidemiol. 2012;26:108–17. doi:10.1111/j.1365-3016.2012.01275.x.

58. Haider BA, Bhutta ZA. Multiple-micronutrient supplementation for women during pregnancy. Cochrane Database of Syst Rev. 2015;(11), Art. No.: CD004905. doi:10.1002/14651858.CD004905.pub4.

59. Fall CH, Fisher DJ, Osmond C, Margetts BM. Multiple micronutrient supplementation during pregnancy in low-income countries: a meta-analysis of effects on birth size and length of gestation. Food Nutr Bull. 2009;30(4 Suppl):S533–46.
60. Fritz MA, Speroff L. Female infertility. In: Gynecologic Clinical, editor. Endocrinology and infertility. 8th ed. Philadelphia: Lippincott Williams and Wilkins; 2011. p. 1137–90.
61. Aviram A, Hod M, Yogev Y. Maternal obesity: Implications for pregnancy outcome and longterm risks—a link to maternal nutrition. The impact of obesity and maternal nutrition on short-term pregnancy outcome and long-term child health.
62. Mehendale SM, Shepherd ME, Brookmeyer RS, Semba RD, Divekar AD, Gangakhedar RR, Joshi S, Paranjape RS, Risbud AR, Gadkari DA, Bollinger RD. Low carotenoid concentrations and risk of HIV seroconversion in Pune, India. J Acquir Immune Defic Syndr. 2001;26:352–9.
63. Baeten JM, McClelland RS, Corey L, Overbaugh J, Lavreys L, Richardson BA, Wald A, Mandaliya K, Bwayo JJ, Kreiss JK. Vitamin A supplementation and genital shedding of herpes simplex virus among HIV-1-infected women: a randomized clinical trial. J Infect Dis. 2004;189:1466–71.
64. International Agency for Research on Cancer (IARC). GLOBOCAN 2012: estimated cancer incidence, mortality and prevalence worldwide in 2012. Accessible at http://globocan.iarc.fr/Pages/fact_sheets_population.aspx. 19 Sep 2014.
65. van den Brandt PA, Siegelman D, Yaun SS, et al. Pooled analysis of prospective cohort studies on height, weight, and breast cancer risk. Am J Epidemiol. 2000;152:514–27.
66. International Agency for Research on Cancer (IARC). Weight and weight control: breast cancer. In: IARC handbooks of cancer prevention. Weight control and physical activity. Lyon (France): IARC Press; 2002. p. 95–112.
67. Calle EE, Rodriguez C, Walker-Thurmonnd K, Thun MJ. Overweight, obesity and mortality from cancer in a prospectively studies cohort of U.S. adults. N Engl J Med. 2003;348(17):1625–38.
68. Rapp K, Schroeder J, Klenk J, et al. Obesity and incidence of cancer: a large cohort study of over 145 000 adults in Austria. Br J Cancer. 2005;93:1062–7.
69. Wang D, Vélez de-la-Paz OI, Zhai JX, Liu DW. Serum 25-hydroxy vitamin D and breast cancer risk: a meta-analysis of prospective studies. Tumour Biol. 2013;34(6):3509–17. doi:10.1007/s13277-013-0929-2 (Epub 2013 Jun 27).
70. Misotti AM, Gnagnarella P. Vitamin supplement consumption and breast cancer risk: a review. Ecancermedicalscience. 2013;7:365. doi:10.3332/ecancer.2013.365.
71. Poole EM, Shu X, Chen WY. Post-diagnosis supplement use and breast cancer prognosis in the After Breast Cancer Pooling Project. Breast Cancer Res Treat. 2013;139(2):529–37.
72. Zhang X, Dai B, Zhang B, Vitamin ZW. A and risk of cervical cancer: a meta-analysis. Gynecol Oncol. 2012;124:366–73.
73. Olsen CM, Green AC, Whiteman DC, Sadeghi S, Kolahdooz F, Webb PM. Obesity and the risk of epithelial ovarian cancer: A systematic review and meta-analysis. Eur J Cancer. 2007;43(4):690–709.
74. Nagle CM, Kolandooz F, Ibiebele TI, et al. Carbohydrate intake, glycemic load, glycemic index and risk of ovarian cancer. Ann Oncol. 2011;22(6):1332–8. doi:10.1093/annonc/mdq595.
75. Webb PM, Ibiebele TI, Hughes MC, et al. Folate and related microonutrients, folate-metabolising genes and risk of ovarian cancer. Eur J Clin Nutr. 2011;65(10):1133–40. doi:10.1038/ejcn.2011.99.
76. Ferlay J, Soerjomataram I, Ervik M, Dikshit R, Eser S, Mathers C, Rebelo M, Parkin DM, Forman D, Bray, F. GLOBOCAN 2012 v1.1, Cancer incidence and mortality worldwide: IARC CancerBase No. 11 [Internet]. Lyon, France: International Agency for Research on Cancer; 2014. Available from: http://globocan.iarc.fr. Accessed on 16 Jan 2015.
77. Roswall N, Larrsen SB, Friis S, et al. Micronutrient intake and risk of prostate cancer in a cohort of middle-aged Danish men. Cancer Causes Control. 2013;24(6):1129–35. doi:10.1007/s10552-013-0190-4.
78. Lippman SM, Klein EA, Goodman PJ. Effect of selenium and vitamin E on risk of prostate cancer and other cancers: the selenium and vitamin E Cancer prevention trial (SELECT). JAMA. 2009;301(1):39–51. doi:10.1001/jama.2008.864.
79. Lawson KA, Wright ME, Subar A, et al. Multivitamin use and risk of prostate cancer in the National Institutes of Health-AARP Diet and health Study. J Natl Cancer Inst. 2007;99(10):754–64.
80. Itsiopoulos C, Hodge A, Kaimakamis M. Can the Mediterranean diet prevent prostate cancer? Mol Nutr Food Res. 2009;53:227–39. doi:10.1002/mnfr.200800207.
81. Raimondi S, Mabrouk JB, Shatensteiin B, Maisonneuve P, Ghadirian P. Diet and prostate cancer risk with specific focus on dairy products and dietary calcium: a case-control study. Prostate. 2010;70(10):1054–65. doi:10.1002/pros.21139.
82. Ahn J, Albanes D, Peters U, et al. Dairy products, calcium intake, and risk of prostate cancer in the prostate, lung, colorectal, and ovarian cancer screening trial. Cancer Epidemiol Biomarkers Prev. 2007;16:2623–30.

Chapter 22
Maternal Nutrition and Birth Outcomes

Usha Ramakrishnan, Melissa Fox Young and Reynaldo Martorell

Keywords Maternal nutrition · Birth outcomes · Pregnancy · Preconception · Preterm births · Small for gestational age · Stunting

Learning Objectives

By the end of this chapter, the reader should be able to

- Define maternal nutrition
- Explain the role of nutrition during pregnancy on birth outcomes
  - Preterm birth
  - Birth size
  - Neural tube defects and other congenital anomalies
  - Still birth and perinatal mortality
- Explain the importance of maternal nutrition before and during the periconceptional period.

Introduction

Maternal, newborn and child health (MNCH) outcomes such as anemia, intrauterine growth restriction (IUGR), low birth weight (LBW) and preterm birth (PTB) remain major public health problems that are associated with significant costs to health care and human capital formation [1, 2]. Growing global evidence points to maternal malnutrition and pregnancy at a young age as important determinants of poor fetal growth, LBW, infant morbidity and mortality [2, 3]; but the importance of addressing maternal nutrition both before and during pregnancy has only recently received attention

U. Ramakrishnan · M.F. Young (✉) · R. Martorell
Hubert Department of Global Health, Rollins School of Public Health, Emory University, Atlanta, GA 30322, USA
e-mail: melissa.young@emory.edu

U. Ramakrishnan
e-mail: uramakr@emory.edu

R. Martorell
e-mail: rmart77@emory.edu

U. Ramakrishnan · M.F. Young · R. Martorell
Nutrition & Health Sciences Program, Graduate Division of Biological & Biomedical Sciences, Emory University, Atlanta, GA, USA

© Springer Science+Business Media New York 2017
S. de Pee et al. (eds.), *Nutrition and Health in a Developing World*,
Nutrition and Health, DOI 10.1007/978-3-319-43739-2_22

[4, 5]. This is especially of concern in many low- and middle-income countries (LMIC), where women enter pregnancy while suffering from undernutrition and their nutritional status worsens as pregnancy progresses due to the increasing demand for energy and nutrients [4].

This chapter summarizes the state of current knowledge on the role of maternal nutrition before and during pregnancy in determining birth outcomes especially preterm birth (PTB) and small for gestational age (SGA) that are of considerable public health significance and related to the health, well-being and survival of the next generation with recommendations for action both for programs and future research. Current evidence is presented on the influence of maternal nutrition interventions, especially during pregnancy, on birth outcomes including PTB, SGA and LBW, to help identify what is known and/or needs further research. This is followed by an examination of the importance of maternal nutrition prior to conception including during critical periods such as early childhood and adolescence.

Assessment of Maternal Nutrition

Maternal nutritional status is typically characterized by indicators of body composition and size, adequacy of nutrient intakes before and during pregnancy and to a lesser extent biomarkers of nutritional status. Low body mass index (BMI < 18.5 kg/m^2) is the most widely used indicator of maternal undernutrition, but more recently, mid-upper arm circumference has also been proposed as a useful and simple indicator that is associated with either acute or chronic energy deficits [6, 7]. Maternal short stature (<155 cm) has also been recognized as an independent indicator of adverse pregnancy outcomes such as obstetric complications (pelvic size is related to height), maternal mortality and SGA [8]. This is especially a concern for adolescents who may get pregnant before they have completed growing [9].

Examination of worldwide trends in maternal nutritional status shows reductions in the prevalence of maternal undernutrition (BMI < 18.5) in the past few decades [4], but it remains a significant problem in South Asia where the prevalence exceed 20% as well as parts of Sub-Saharan Africa and Southeast Asia (10–20%). This is further complicated by increases in maternal overweight and obesity in all regions which have also been associated with adverse pregnancy outcomes especially preeclampsia and preterm birth [4, 10, 11]. Data from the nationally representative Demographic and Health Surveys show that more than half of women of reproductive age (20–49 years) are either overweight or obese in countries from the WHO regions of the Americas and the Caribbean, Northern and Southern Africa and Europe (Table 22.1). Maternal short stature remains a concern especially in settings where access to obstetric care is limited and often coexists with thinness in some settings such as South Asia where the burden of undernutrition is very high [8].

Maternal undernutrition (also referred to as thinness and/or underweight characterized as BMI < 18.5 kg/m^2) is typically associated with energy deficits, but poor diet quality remains a problem, including in settings where energy and macronutrient intakes are not limiting. A recent systematic review that examined nutrient intakes and/or patterns of food consumption among women of reproductive age including pregnant women in low- to middle-income countries showed that while overall energy and protein intakes have improved over the past few decades, micronutrient intakes remained problematic with folate and iron intakes being most frequently below the estimated average requirements followed by calcium and zinc [12]. Macronutrient intakes were also relatively higher in women residing in the Caribbean and Central/South America compared to Africa and Asia, and although fat intakes were within the acceptable range of 15–30% of total energy intakes in most settings, data on the types of fat were lacking. Intakes of vitamins A, B complex and C were more variable and may have been influenced by seasonality and access to locally grown fruits and vegetables. Finally, the consumption of micronutrient supplements including antenatal iron–folate which

Table 22.1 Distribution of BMI status of girls and women by MDG region

Regions	Girls 5–20 years			Women 20–49 years			
	BMI < 25 kg/m²	BMI 25–30 kg/m²	BMI 30+ kg/m²	BMI < 18.5 kg/m²	BMI 18.5–25 kg/m²	BMI 25–0 kg/m²	BMI 30+ kg/m²
Asia							
Central	79.4	14.7	5.9	15.3	47.3	23.7	13.7
East	84.3	10.9	2.8	12.7	66.2	15.8	5.3
South	93.8	3.6	2.6	21.3	64.0	10.9	3.8
Southeast	86.3	4.7	9.0	12.2	62.7	17.9	7.2
Africa							
Central	85.4	9.9	4.7	15.7	64.2	14.5	5.6
Eastern	88	9.1	2.9	17.3	65.0	13.3	4.4
Southern	76.9	15.7	7.4	2.0	33.8	30.8	33.4
Western	87.7	9.1	3.2	9.8	63.7	19.1	7.4
Americas and Caribbean							
Caribbean	80.1	13.3	6.6	4.2	45.4	27.8	22.6
Northern	70.9	16.1	13.0	1.3	37.3	32.6	28.8
Central	75.5	18.0	7.5	1.9	34.9	31.7	31.5
South	73.6	17.6	8.8	3.9	48.1	28.5	19.5
Europe							
Eastern	81.2	12.4	6.4	5.1	48.4	26.7	19.8
Western	78.0	15.6	6.4	4.6	59.6	23.8	12.0
Central	79.7	14.0	6.3	4.9	58.6	23.9	12.7
Oceania	77.1	16.5	6.4	2.1	75.5	30.4	22.4

From Ng et al. [11]. Reprinted with permission from Elsevier

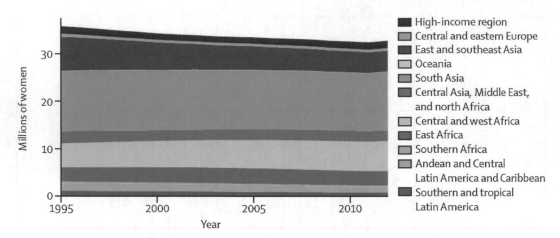

Fig. 22.1 Millions of pregnant women affected by anemia, by region. From Stevens et al. [63] (open access)

is recommended for all pregnant women was also low. These data combined with the rapid changes in food supply and urbanization underscore the need for collecting reliable food consumption data and the need to focus on dietary counseling during pregnancy.

Data based on biomarkers of nutritional status are even more sparse with the exception of anemia which has been measured regularly as part of the Demographic and Health Surveys. Globally, the prevalence of anemia from 1995 to 2011 has modestly declined among non-pregnant (33–29%) and pregnant (43–38%) women [13, 14]. However, the burden of anemia remains unacceptably high especially in regions of South Asia and Central and West Africa (Fig. 22.1). Further, reliable data on the etiology of anemia and relative contribution of nutritional factors (iron, vitamin A, B12, etc.), genetics and infection/disease are lacking. Other common nutrient deficiencies include vitamin A deficiency which is common especially in regions like South Asia based on reports of night blindness during pregnancy [15, 16], as well as riboflavin, vitamin B12 and zinc deficiency.

Nutrition Interventions During Pregnancy

This section is based primarily on several recently published systematic reviews [5, 17–32] that have evaluated the effects of nutrition interventions during pregnancy on key birth outcomes, namely PTB, birth size including SGA and LBW, still birth and perinatal mortality. Many of the reviews include evidence from randomized controlled trials (RCTs) and/or observational studies and have also evaluated the quality of the evidence using criteria recommended by the Cochrane Collaboration and/or the GRADE system [33].

Direct Nutrition Interventions

Several trials and reviews that calculated pooled estimates based on formal meta-analyses of at least 3 or more RCTs have been conducted for single-nutrient interventions such as vitamins A, B, C, D, zinc, calcium, iron and folic acid as well as multi-nutrient interventions that combined two or more micronutrients such as iron and folic acid (IFA), multiple micronutrients (MMN), n-3 polyunsaturated fatty acids (PUFA) or used food-based approaches such as balanced protein–energy (BPE) supplements.

Table 22.2 Effects of direct nutrition interventions during pregnancy on preterm birth as reported by recent meta-analyses

Nutrient [reference]	No. of trials (total n)	Pooled RR (95% CI)
Calcium [19]	11 (15,275)	0.76 (0.60, 0.97)[b]
Iron or IFA [20]	12 (NR)	0.94 (0.84, 1.06)
Iron or IFA [28]	13 (19,286)	0.93 (0.84, 1.03)
Zinc [21]	16 (7637)	0.86 (0.76, 0.97)[b]
Vitamin A [22]	5 (40,137)	0.98 (0.94, 1.01)[a]
Vitamin D [23]	3 (477)	0.36 (0.14, 0.93)[b]
Vitamin C [27]	16 (22,250)	0.99 (0.9, 1.06)[a]
Folic acid [26]	3 (2959)	1.01 (0.73, 1.38)
n-3 PUFA [31]	5 (4343)	0.74 (0.58, 0.94)
MMN [24]	15 (90,892)	0.96 (0.89, 1.03)[a]
Balanced protein–energy [34]	6 (3579)	0.96 (0.80, 1.15)[b]
Balanced protein–energy [25]	5 (3384)	0.96 (0.8, 1.16)[b]

[a]Quality of evidence was high
[b]Quality of evidence was moderate

The amount of nutrients provided was 1–2 times the recommended daily allowance for pregnant women in most supplements (single or multiple) with a few exceptions when higher amounts were used, namely for n-3 PUFA, iron and calcium. For BPE, total energy content ranged from 270 to 1020 kcal and the percentage of energy from protein was between 10 and 25% [34]. In contrast, there are very limited data on prenatal vitamin B12, vitamin B6 or iodine supplementation on their own, i.e., not as part of multi-micronutrient supplements, as well as very few trials on food-based approaches such as lipid-based nutrient supplements (LNS) or home fortification during pregnancy. There are also differences in the nature of the intervention received by the treatment and control group, especially for the trials that evaluated multi-nutrient interventions. For example, for ethical reasons many of the MMN trials used IFA as the control group and the authors defined MMN as 5 or more micronutrients. Thus, the true effect of MMN interventions, which also include iron and folic acid as part of the mix of micronutrients, may be underestimated given the known positive impact of prenatal IFA. A mix of interventions and controls were also used in the BPE trials (e.g., in some trials both groups received micronutrients, and in other trials only the intervention group received micronutrients), and zinc was often provided in addition to other micronutrients (e.g., zinc + MMN versus MMN alone). Vitamins C and E were given concurrently in the included vitamin C trials. The key results on the effect of direct nutrition interventions during pregnancy on selected birth outcomes are summarized in Tables 22.2, 22.3, 22.4 and described in the following sections.

Preterm Birth (PTB)

Several reviews and meta-analyses show that calcium and zinc supplementation significantly decreased the risk of PTB (<37 weeks) [19, 21, 32], while n-3 PUFA supplementation decreased the risk of early preterm birth (<34 weeks) [31]. The quality of evidence for calcium was moderate and was associated with 20–30% reduction in PTB and 50–60% reduction for other related pregnancy complications such as preeclampsia in both developed and developing country settings [19]. In contrast, the quality of evidence was low to moderate for zinc supplementation [21]; in several trials the comparison group received other micronutrient supplements [21, 32]. Evidence from observational studies and several RCTs mostly from high-income countries also supports a role for n-3 polyunsaturated fatty acids (PUFA) in reducing the risk of PTB [31]. Although the differences were not statistically significant for overall PTB, n-3 PUFA supplementation has been shown to decrease

Table 22.3 Effects of direct nutrition interventions during pregnancy on size at birth as reported by recent meta-analyses

Nutrient [reference]	Small for gestational age		Low birth weight		Birthweight	
	No. of trials (total n)	Pooled RR (95% CI)	No. of trials (total n)	Pooled RR (95% CI)	No. of trials (total n)	Mean difference (95% CI)
Calcium [19]	N/A	N/A	6 (14,479)	0.85 (0.72, 1.01)	13 (8574)	86 (38, 134)[d]
Iron or IFA [20]	6	0.94 (0.81, 1.09)	11 (9397)	0.80 (0.71, 0.90)	13 (NR)	42 (9, 75)
Iron or IFA [28]	0	NR	11 (17,613)	0.84 (0.69, 1.03)	15 (18,590)	23.75 (3.0, 50.5)[d]
Zinc [21]	8 (4252)	1.02 (0.94, 1.11)[d]	14 (5643)	0.93 (0.78, 1.12)[d]	17 (6757)	−9 (−22, 24)
Vitamin A [22]	0	NR	4 (14,599)	1.02 (0.89, 1.16)	0	NR
Vitamin D [23]	0	NR	3 (493)	0.40 (0.24, 0.67)[d]	4 (638)	147 (68, 222)
Vitamin C [27]	12 (20,361)	0.98 (0.91, 1.06)	0	NR	13 (17,236)	27 (−19, 73)
Folic acid [26]	0	NR	4 (3113)	0.83 (0.66, 1.04)	4 (625)	136 (48, 224)
n-3 PUFA [31]	0	NR	8 (6511)	0.92 (0.83, 1.02)	9 (6020)	42 (15, 70)
MMN [24][b]	14 (67,036)	0.90 (0.83, 0.97)[d]	15 (70,044)	0.88 (0.85, 0.91)[c]	15 (NR)	53 (43, 62)[d]
Balanced protein–energy [34]	9 (5250)	0.66 (0.49, 0.89)[d]	5 (4196)	0.68 (0.51, 0.92)[d]	16 (6474)	74 (30, 117)[c]
Balanced protein–energy [25]	7 (4408)	0.79 (0.69, 0.9)	0	NR	11 (5385)	41 (4.7, 77.3)[c]

[a]These trials compared iron + folic acid to iron only

[b]the control group received iron or IFA

[c]quality of evidence was high

[d]quality of evidence was moderate

NR not reported

Table 22.4 Effects of direct nutrition interventions during pregnancy on still birth and neonatal mortality as reported by recent meta-analyses

Nutrient [reference]	Still births		Neonatal mortality	
	No. of trials (total n)	Pooled RR (95% CI)	No. of trials (total n)	Pooled RR (95% CI)
Iron or IFA [20]	4 (NR)	0.96 (0.51, 1.83)	4 (NR)	0.82 (0.65, 1.05)
Iron or IFA [28]	NR	NR	4 (16,603)	0.91 (0.71, 1.18)
Zinc[a] [21]	8 (5100)	1.12 (0.86, 1.46)	N/A	N/A
Vitamin A [22]	3 (89,556)	0.97 (0.9, 1.05)	2 (122,850)	1.04 (0.98, 1.1)
Vitamin D [23]	2 (282)	0.27 (0.04, 1.67)	3 (540)	0.35 (0.06, 1.99)
Vitamin C [27]	11 (19,575)	0.79 (0.58, 1.08)	0	NR
Folic acid[a] [26]	3 (3110)	1.33 (0.96, 1.85)	N/A	N/A
MMN [24]	15 (98,808)	0.91 (0.85, 0.98)[b]	11 (83,103)	0.98 (0.90, 1.07)[b]
Balanced protein–energy [34]	4 (3388)	0.62 (0.40, 0.98)	4 (3361)	0.68 (0.59, 0.82)
Balanced protein–energy [25]	5 (3408)	0.60 (0.39, 0.94)	5 (3381)	0.68 (0.43, 1.1)

[a]Still births and/or neonatal deaths
[b]quality of evidence is high

the risk of early preterm birth (<34 weeks) by 26%. The quality of evidence was moderate, but a recent study that was not included in previous reviews also showed significant reductions in early preterm birth (<34 weeks) and longer gestation duration (2.9 d; $P = 0.041$) among women who received 600 mg of algal DHA (docosahexaenoic acid) during the latter half of pregnancy, but no significant differences in overall PTB [35].

Imdad and Bhutta [20] reported a 6% reduced risk of PTB for prenatal IFA supplements, but the differences were not statistically significant and the quality of evidence was moderate. Similar findings were reported in an updated Cochrane review by Pena-Rosas et al. [28]. Several reviews and meta-analysis of controlled trials of dietary interventions including BPE supplements that provided less than 25% energy as protein also found no significant effects on preterm birth [25, 29, 34]. Similarly, the findings from trials of vitamin A [22] as well as vitamin C supplementation [36] which often also included vitamin E have not shown any reductions in PTB; pooled results from 5 trials (17,353 women) actually showed an increased risk of pregnancy-related hypertension in vitamin C group (RR = 1.10, 95% CI = 1.0, 1.2) [27]. Although there is a suggestion of benefit for vitamin D when compared to a placebo, the quality of the evidence was graded as low-moderate [23], and these benefits were not seen when vitamin D was provided with calcium [23] or as part of MMN supplements and compared to IFA which is the recommended standard of care [24, 37]. Finally, the results from two large trials that evaluated the benefits of providing pregnant women with daily lipid-based nutrient supplements (LNS) that contained both the n-6 and n-3 essential fatty acids, linoleic and alpha-linoleic acid, respectively, along with 1–2 times the RDA of several micronutrients, showed no significant differences in mean gestational age or the incidence of PTB when compared to MMN or IFA supplements [38, 39].

Small for Gestational Age and Birth Size

Several RCTs from developed and developing countries have evaluated the benefits of nutrition interventions during the prenatal period on birth size especially birth weight and/or LBW which is defined as birth weight <2.5 kg (Table 22.3). Fewer studies, however, have evaluated the effects on outcomes such as SGA, which is the accepted measure of fetal growth restriction (see Chap. 23 "Small for Gestational Age: Scale and Consequences for Mortality, Morbidity, and Development" for definitions), as well as on measures of linear growth. SGA is more difficult to determine due to the lack of reliable gestational age data (few prospective studies that track last menstrual cycle and/or lack of trained personnel who can assess gestational age at the time of delivery). Supplementation with calcium, balanced protein–energy, MMN, IFA or n-3 PUFA has been shown to increase mean birth weight by 42–86 g ($p < 0.05$) when compared to controls. Although these differences represent a small effect size (~ 0.2 SD), the reductions in those at greatest risk, i.e., LBW, can be substantial depending on the population. For example, babies born to mothers supplemented with IFA, MMN or balanced BPE had a 10–30% lower risk of being born LBW than controls, and the effect sizes are larger among undernourished women (who received BPE) (a limitation of this work is that many of the studies included do not define criteria for "undernourished") [23, 34]. Prenatal supplementation with vitamin A has also been shown to decrease the risk of LBW, but only among HIV + women (RR: 0.79, 95% CI: 0.64, 0.99; data from 3 RCTs), with no significant differences in the total population [40]. Studies of Zn supplementation have also failed to show any overall benefit [21, 32]. In contrast, new evidence suggests a role for vitamin D in reducing the risk of LBW [23, 32]. Supplementation with vitamin B6 has also been associated with higher mean birth weight, but the quality of the evidence is weak [36].

Systematic reviews provide evidence of significant reductions in SGA and LBW for prenatal BPE and MMN interventions [25, 29, 34]. These meta-analyses have shown that interventions that focused on improving macronutrient intakes by including food and/or fortified food products were effective in increasing birth weight and reducing the incidence of LBW (see Tables 22.2, 22.3 and 22.4), and these effects were larger for studies that were conducted in populations with higher prevalence of maternal undernutrition based on body mass index. In contrast, the evidence remains weak and is of poor quality for studies that evaluated the benefits of dietary counseling to improve dietary intakes during pregnancy [29, 41].

Of note are the findings supporting the benefits of MMN interventions when compared to prenatal IFA which has and continues to be the recommended standard of care since the 1960s [42]. Several meta-analyses based on findings from RCTs that were conducted primarily in LMIC have shown that prenatal MMN supplementation significantly reduces the incidence of LBW and SGA by at least 15% when compared to IFA [24, 37]. Mean birth weight was significantly higher by 55 g for MMN with borderline increases in gestational age, but there were no significant differences in the risk of PTB. It should be noted, however, that MMN supplementation was associated with significant decreases in PTB (RR: 0.85, 95% CI: 0.80, 0.90) in the subgroup of four studies that were conducted in settings with more women with undernutrition (mean BMI < 20 kg/m^2), whereas the reductions in the risk of LBW and SGA were seen in the subgroup of trials that were conducted in populations where women were either taller (mean height > 154.9 cm) or with mean BMI > 20 kg/m^2. Greater reductions in SGA and LBW were also seen among studies that used supplements containing 60 mg of iron, but these were not statistically significantly different from those for trials that used 30 mg iron which may have improved compliance in program settings.

Finally, although the meta-analysis by Imhoff-Kunsch et al. [31] did not find any benefits of n-3 PUFA interventions for birth size or LBW, some recent trials show promising findings. In a study of women from the USA, Carlson et al. [35] reported greater birth weight (172 g; $P = 0.004$), length (0.7 cm; $P = 0.022$) and head circumference (0.5 cm; $P = 0.012$) for the DHA group compared to the control group that received a placebo. Large-scale intervention trials in Ghana and Bangladesh using LNS which contained essential fatty acids along with multiple micronutrients have also shown promising findings [38, 39]. Although there were no significant differences in the overall study, babies born to primiparous women in the LNS trial conducted in Ghana were heavier at birth when compared to those who received IFA or MMN. The LNS study from Bangladesh [38] where the rates of SGA are much higher also showed significant increases in birth size among the offspring of women who received LNS compared to IFA, especially among those who were at greatest risk.

Still Birth and Perinatal Mortality

High-quality evidence demonstrates that prenatal iodine supplementation decreased the risk of cretinism (RR: 0.27, 95% CI: 0.12, 0.60; data from 5 RCTs) and improved developmental scores (data from 4 RCTs) in children born to mothers at risk of iodine deficiency [43]. Evidence also suggests that prenatal iodine supplementation decreased the rate of infant mortality (data from 2 RCTs, total $n = 37,400$). BPE supplementation has also been shown to significantly reduce the risk of stillbirths by $\sim 40\%$, but the quality of the evidence was rated as low [17, 23]. The evidence for several other nutrient interventions is also either lacking or of low quality. Although iron-containing supplements have been associated with a lower risk of neonatal mortality or congenital anomalies, the quality of evidence remains low, and the differences were not statistically significant [28]. In contrast, quality of the evidence was ranked as high for MMN supplements, and although concerns of increased risk of perinatal and neonatal mortality have been raised in the past [44], recent reviews found no differences for prenatal MMN supplements when compared to iron or IFA [18, 24]. It should be noted, however, that good obstetric care is needed when these interventions are implemented in settings where maternal malnutrition is common, since larger babies will be born to small women.

Nutrition-Related Factors During Pregnancy

In addition to direct nutrition supplementation interventions, there are also several indirect nutrition-related factors that have the potential to impact birth outcomes that have recently been reviewed [18]. These topics include deworming, nutrition education and counseling during pregnancy and household food production strategies [41, 45, 46]. However, data are limited and most of the evidence is based on observational studies rather than rigorous RCTs. Antihelmintics in pregnancy reduced the risk of very low birth weight; however, the meta-analysis included only 2 trials (1936 women) [45]. Nutrition education and counseling have also shown improvements in anemia, PTB and birth weight [41]. There remains a need to further examine the role of these nutrition-related factors to improve maternal nutrition and birth outcomes.

Role of Maternal Nutrition Before Conception

There is considerable evidence from animal, human, tissue and molecular studies supporting the importance of maternal nutrition in the pre- or periconception period for the subsequent growth and development of the offspring [47]. The maternal environment both in terms of nutrient availability and exposure to environmental toxins has been shown to play a key role in the processes of embryogenesis, implantation and the development of the placenta that occur very early in pregnancy. For example, the availability of selected amino acids, free fatty acids and micronutrients such as folic acid, zinc, vitamin B12 has been shown to influence a wide range of pregnancy outcomes. High-quality evidence supports the importance of folate during the periconceptional period in reducing the risk of neural tube defects (NTD) which has led to widespread efforts to improve folate intakes among women of reproductive age by interventions such as fortification of staples [48, 49]. The most recent estimates attribute a 69% reduction in the risk of NTD based on evidence from well-controlled RCTs that provided folic acid during the periconceptional period [4]. Emerging evidence also suggests reductions for other congenital birth defects [50], although most of this is based on observational studies, since withholding folic acid supplements to a control group in an intervention study would be unethical, and the most recent Cochrane review concluded that there was no clear impact and that the quality of evidence was low [48].

Evidence from observational studies that examined women's nutritional status based on anthropometry (BMI < 18.5 kg/m^2) and/or micronutrient status also suggests a positive relationship with outcomes such as PTB and LBW, but most of the studies were of poor quality and evidence from well-designed trials that evaluate the benefit of interventions that begin before conception is limited [17]. Evidence from observational studies has shown that early age at first childbirth and short interpregnancy interval are associated with significantly increased odds of PTB and LBW [3, 51]. Early age at first childbirth also resulted in increased odds of stillbirth (aOR: 1.35, 95% CI: 1.07, 1.71) and early neonatal death (aOR: 1.29, 95% CI: 1.02, 1.64) [51]. Children born to women under the age of 19 are also more likely to be stunted at two years of age and fail to complete secondary school [3], supporting the need for interventions that delay child bearing especially in settings where many births occur among adolescent girls, i.e., before they have had the opportunity to attain adult stature and body composition.

Two large trials also provide interesting insights on the potential for preconception interventions [52, 53]. The first study was a large food-based intervention study (the Mumbai Maternal Nutrition Project) in which women living in the urban slums of Mumbai, India, received either a nutrient dense snack that contained green leafy vegetables, fruits and milk or a low-nutrient snack from preconception through delivery [46]. There were no differences in birth outcomes in the overall sample, but the intervention increased birth weight for the offspring born to women with a BMI > 18.6 kg/m^2 (birth-weight effect: −23, +34 and +96 g in lowest (<18.6), middle (18.6–21.8) and highest (>21.8) thirds of BMI, respectively), and these effects were also larger among those who received the preconception intervention for at least 90 days (+48 g; 95% CI: 1, 96 g; $P = 0.046$). More recently, a large study evaluated the benefits of weekly micronutrient supplements prior to conception in Vietnam in which women of reproductive age were randomized to receive weekly supplements containing (a) only 2800 µg folic acid (served as the control group), (b) 60 mg of iron and 2800 µg folic acid and (c) multiple micronutrients including IFA and followed up for pregnancies and birth outcomes. All women who conceived, regardless of their preconception supplement group, received daily IFA supplements through delivery. There were no differences in mean birth weight, LBW, SGA or PTB in the intent to treat analysis ($n = 1599$). However, the results of the per-protocol analysis that included only women who consumed the preconception supplements for at least 26 weeks showed that mean birth weight was higher by 67 and 46 g for the MMN and IFA groups compared to FA only [47]. Although nearly a third of the women were underweight, the prevalences of anemia and iron deficiency were much lower compared to the study in India, and no differences were seen in maternal nutritional status at the time of the first prenatal visit by treatment group. However, a secondary analysis of the data from this trial, maternal nutrition before and during pregnancy had similar and independent associations with birth outcomes [54]. A 1 SD higher prepregnancy weight or gestational weight gain was associated with a respective increase in birth weight of 283 and 250 g, indicating that programs aimed at improving birth outcomes will have greatest impact if they target both critical windows, i.e., preconception and pregnancy.

In summary, the evidence on which specific preconceptional interventions best improve birth outcomes remains weak, except for the benefits of folic acid in reducing NTDs. Although we have limited information to design effective and targeted preconception nutrition interventions, ensuring good nutrition for WRA should be a priority in settings where deficiencies are common and access to timely prenatal care remains suboptimal. The findings of several large ongoing trials that are evaluating the benefits of LNS before and during pregnancy in Guatemala, India, Pakistan and the Democratic Republic of Congo [55] and providing animal source foods before and during pregnancy in rural Vietnam [56] will shed more light.

Role of Intergenerational Effects

Strategies to improve nutrition during the first 1000 days can have a profound effect for generations to come. Improving a young girl's nutrition not only improves her health across her lifetime, but also improves birth outcomes for her children as well. As summarized by Martorell et al., the intergenerational influences of maternal nutrition are well established; birth weight is correlated across generations; and maternal short stature (indicator of her poor early nutrition) is linked with delivery complications, offspring low birth weight, stunting and increased child mortality [57]. For example, intergenerational data from the Aberdeen Children of the 1950s study reported that maternal inequalities at birth, her birth weight, early growth and childhood social environment were important determinants for her child's birth weight [58]. In addition, using intergenerational data across four birth cohorts in low- and middle-income counties (COHORTS study), Addo et al. [59] reported that both maternal and paternal early growth (from birth to 2 years) as well as maternal growth from mid-childhood to adulthood was associated with their child's birth weight. The strongest impacts were found on the maternal side (a 1 SD increase in maternal birth weight was associated with a 102 g increase in her child's birth weight), indicating the clear importance of a woman's nutritional status (weight/height) before pregnancy to improve birth outcomes [59]. Overall, the current evidence strongly suggests that improving nutrition prior to and during the first 1000 days is critical for breaking the "intergenerational cycle of growth failure" [60].

Evidence from Programs

While the importance of maternal nutrition for improving birth outcomes is clear, and we have established efficacious interventions, the evidence from maternal nutrition programs at scale, however, is limited and requires further evaluation and prioritizing. In a recent review of global policy and program guidance on maternal nutrition, few countries had maternal nutrition programs beyond anemia control and a clear lack of program guidance to address maternal thinness, gestational weight gain or LBW prevention was noted, citing a lack of priority, financial support and evidence [1, 61].

In order to see similar impacts of maternal nutrition interventions on birth outcomes at scale, there is a critical need to inform and strengthen program implementation strategies. A phenomenon, not unique to maternal nutrition programs, is that we know what do, we know it works, but are failing to effectively implement the program. A key example of this is IFA supplementation during pregnancy, one of the few maternal nutrition programs scaled up across the globe. Although policies and programs are in place to provide IFA to pregnant women, Lutter et al. [62] found that in some regions only 1 in 2 women had ever received IFA and across regions only 17–43% of women reported receiving IFA for at least 90 days during their pregnancy. Thus, it is not surprising that globally we are failing to effectively reduce maternal anemia [63] and the associated preventable poor birth outcomes and maternal and child deaths. There are also major gaps in our understanding of how best to improve dietary intakes among women of reproductive age, especially during pregnancy. Formative research is needed to better understand the underlying factors that limit improvements to nutrient intake during pregnancy in terms of quantity and quality. Based on better insights, strategies and programs can be designed to ensure that macro- and micronutrient intake during pregnancy is in-line with recommendations. This may entail ensuring good coverage and adherence with IFA or MMN supplementation among all pregnant women and increasing access to food in general or to specific fortified foods for women at highest risk of poor birth outcome, e.g., based on young age, poverty or (seasonal) food insecurity. The latter requires coordination between health and food systems and may also involve social protection programs that reach the most vulnerable in the population, for targeting and delivery of interventions to vulnerable pregnant women.

Recently a review of adolescent and women's nutrition programs summarized current program evidence from LMIC [64]. Several programs have reported increased nutrient intake [65–67] and reduced anemia prevalence [68–70], but very few have examined the impact on birth outcomes, as the interventions were not particularly targeted to pregnant women. The Vietnam Folate Supplementation Pilot reported that by providing prepregnancy deworming and weekly IFA supplementation to women the prevalence of LBW infants was significantly reduced [71]. Progesa (Oportunidades) in Mexico reported higher rates of C-sections among overweight participants [72]. The review concludes that too little is known about the most efficacious approaches and there is a critical need for rigorous program research, documentation on lessons learned and impact evaluation. Furthermore, there is need for programs to step beyond the basic services for only pregnant and lactating women to include adolescents/women before pregnancy and WRA in order to maximize impact on health and nutrition [64].

Conclusions

There is increasing recognition of the important role maternal nutrition plays in improving birth outcomes and subsequent growth and development of the next generation. Meta-analyses of intervention trials show that prenatal supplementation with calcium, zinc and n-3 PUFA lowers the risk of PTB, whereas MMN and BPE supplementation resulted in increased birth weight and a lower risk of LBW. Interventions such as iodine and periconceptional folic acid are also important for reducing pregnancy losses and birth defects. Some of these are existing interventions that need to be strengthened with improved program implementation, while others are new interventions that are efficacious but not widely implemented. There also remain some important gaps that need future research to help guide policy and programs to improve birth outcomes.

Key maternal nutrition research priorities
• More rigorous, controlled BPE trials also including micronutrients, fatty acids, etc. (i.e., fortified foods, including lipid-based nutrient supplements and home fortificants such as micronutrient powder) and/or nutrition counseling should be considered along with additional outcomes such as lactation performance, child growth and development during early life
• The relationships between *nutrition and infection during early pregnancy* in predicting subsequent outcomes are unclear
• *The interaction of nutrition and environmental exposures (smoking; air pollution) needs to be explored*
• *Efficacy of balanced protein–energy and/or micronutrient interventions* (IFA; MMN), before and during early pregnancy on MNCH outcomes
• Well-designed observational studies that examine the relationships between *prepregnancy body size and composition* and MNCH outcomes are needed
• Evaluation of integrated approaches that link nutrition with agriculture, water and sanitation and livelihood strategies

In terms of existing interventions, the provision of iodine using iodized salt and/or supplements and fortification of staple foods with folic acid are some of the most successful interventions to date, but constant monitoring and political commitment are still needed especially in resource poor environments. Balanced protein–energy and IFA supplementation during pregnancy is also important *existing interventions* that can significantly improve MNCH outcomes, but face programmatic challenges. Solutions to address barriers related to program delivery, costs and scaling up are needed to improve effectiveness in settings where food insecurity and poor access to care are common.

Furthermore, interventions to improve birth outcomes should be linked with adequate access to obstetric care. Finally, more well-designed studies are needed to estimate the cost effectiveness and barriers to implementation in ongoing programs that promote nutrition education and counseling during pregnancy.

The nutrition interventions that have promise for future implementation are the provision of MMN supplements, calcium and omega-3 fatty acids during pregnancy, but these interventions need more testing in programmatic settings in LMIC. MMN interventions are safe and efficacious, but earlier concerns about possible adverse effects on neonatal mortality and issues related to the dose and composition of these supplements have hampered implementation. In spite of the consistent evidence that supports the benefits of MMN supplements, efforts to change the current guidelines have been slow and are still underway. Calcium supplementation also shows benefit in controlled trials, but additional implementation research is needed to identify the most suitable form(s) of the supplements (multiple large tablets/drinks/other) [73]. Finally, most of the research on n-3 fatty acids has been done primarily in high-income countries, and trials are needed in LMIC where the burden of adverse outcomes is higher. However, cost effective ways of delivering the above interventions are also needed.

In summary, innovative approaches that evaluate targeting and findings solutions to improve effectiveness of existing direct nutrition interventions are needed to improve maternal nutrition. These programs also need to have stronger links with other sectors such as agriculture, water and sanitation, family planning, education and social protection programs to improve birth outcomes. Future research that evaluates the benefits of improving women's nutrition before and during pregnancy as well as postponing age at first marriage/pregnancy is also needed to have better informed strategies that will help reduce the burden of outcomes such LBW, PTB and maternal and neonatal mortality, especially in settings where underlying issues such as poverty, food insecurity and gender discrimination remain.

Discussion Points

- How is maternal nutrition defined?
- Which maternal nutrition interventions are the most effective at improving which specific birth outcomes, and why?
- What are the key limitations of the existing evidence? How can these be addressed?
- What additional evidence is needed to inform maternal nutrition programs to improve birth outcomes?
- In addition to the health sector, which other sectors are important for improving maternal nutrition and birth outcomes and why?

References

1. Victora CG, Adair L, Fall C, Hallal PC, Martorell R, Richter L, et al. Maternal and child undernutrition: consequences for adult health and human capital. Lancet. 2008;371(9609):340–57.
2. Bhutta ZA, Das JK, Rizvi A, Gaffey MF, Walker N, Horton S, et al. Evidence-based interventions for improvement of maternal and child nutrition: what can be done and at what cost? Lancet. 2013;382(9890):452–77.
3. Fall CH, Sachdev HS, Osmond C, Restrepo-Mendez MC, Victora C, Martorell R, et al. Association between maternal age at childbirth and child and adult outcomes in the offspring: a prospective study in five low-income and middle-income countries (COHORTS collaboration). Lancet Glob Health. 2015;3(7):e366–77.

4. Black RE, Victora CG, Walker SP, Bhutta ZA, Christian P, de Onis M, et al. Maternal and child undernutrition and overweight in low-income and middle-income countries. Lancet. 2013;382(9890):427–51.

5. Ramakrishnan U, Imhoff-Kunsch B, Martorell R. Maternal nutrition interventions to improve maternal, newborn, and child health outcomes. Nestle Nutr Inst Workshop Ser. 2014;78:71–80.

6. Ververs MT, Antierens A, Sackl A, Staderini N, Captier V. Which anthropometric indicators identify a pregnant woman as acutely malnourished and predict adverse birth outcomes in the humanitarian context? PLoS Curr. 2013;5.

7. Nguyen P, Ramakrishnan U, Katz B, Gonzalez-Casanova I, Lowe AE, Nguyen H, et al. Mid-upper-arm and calf circumferences are useful predictors of underweight in women of reproductive age in northern Vietnam. Food Nutr Bull. 2014;35(3):301–11.

8. Kozuki N, Katz J, Lee AC, Vogel JP, Silveira MF, Sania A, et al. Short maternal stature increases risk of small-for-gestational-age and preterm births in low- and middle-income countries: individual participant data meta-analysis and population attributable fraction. J Nutr. 2015;145(11):2542–50.

9. Rah JH, Christian P, Shamim AA, Arju UT, Labrique AB, Rashid M. Pregnancy and lactation hinder growth and nutritional status of adolescent girls in rural Bangladesh. J Nutr. 2008;138(8):1505–11.

10. Mission JF, Marshall NE, Caughey AB. Pregnancy risks associated with obesity. Obstet Gynecol Clin North Am. 2015;42(2):335–53.

11. Ng M, Fleming T, Robinson M, Thomson B, Graetz N, Margono C, et al. Global, regional, and national prevalence of overweight and obesity in children and adults during 1980–2013: a systematic analysis for the Global Burden of Disease Study 2013. Lancet. 2014;384(9945):766–81.

12. Lee SE, Talegawkar SA, Merialdi M, Caulfield LE. Dietary intakes of women during pregnancy in low- and middle-income countries. Public Health Nutr. 2013;16(8):1340–53.

13. Taren DL, Duncan B, Shrestha K, Shrestha N, Genaro-Wolf D, Schleicher RL, et al. The night vision threshold test is a better predictor of low serum vitamin A concentration than self-reported night blindness in pregnant urban Nepalese women. J Nutr. 2004;134(10):2573–8.

14. Taren D. Historical and practical uses of assessing night blindness as an indicator for vitamin A deficiency. Panama City, Panama, Geneva: World Health Organization; 2012. 15–17 Sept 2010.

15. Christian P, West KP Jr, Khatry SK, Katz J, LeClerq S, Pradhan EK, et al. Vitamin A or beta-carotene supplementation reduces but does not eliminate maternal night blindness in Nepal. J Nutr. 1998;128(9):1458–63.

16. Katz J, Tielsch JM, Thulasiraj RD, Coles C, Sheeladevi S, Yanik EL, et al. Risk factors for maternal night blindness in rural South India. Ophthalmic Epidemiol. 2009;16(3):193–7.

17. Ramakrishnan U, Grant F, Goldenberg T, Zongrone A, Martorell R. Effect of women's nutrition before and during early pregnancy on maternal and infant outcomes: a systematic review. Paediatr Perinat Epidemiol. 2012;26(Suppl 1):285–301.

18. Ramakrishnan U, Grant FK, Imdad A, Bhutta ZA, Martorell R. Effect of multiple micronutrient versus iron-folate supplementation during pregnancy on intrauterine growth. Nestle Nutr Inst Workshop Ser. 2013;74:53–62.

19. Imdad A, Bhutta ZA. Effects of calcium supplementation during pregnancy on maternal, fetal and birth outcomes. Paediatr Perinat Epidemiol. 2012;26(Suppl 1):138–52.

20. Imdad A, Bhutta ZA. Routine iron/folate supplementation during pregnancy: effect on maternal anaemia and birth outcomes. Paediatr Perinat Epidemiol. 2012;26(Suppl 1):168–77.

21. Ota E, Mori R, Middleton P, Tobe-Gai R, Mahomed K, Miyazaki C, et al. Zinc supplementation for improving pregnancy and infant outcome. Cochrane Database Syst Rev. 2015;2:CD000230.

22. McCauley ME, van den Broek N, Dou L, Othman M. Vitamin A supplementation during pregnancy for maternal and newborn outcomes. Cochrane Database Syst Rev. 2015;10:CD008666.

23. De-Regil LM, Palacios C, Lombardo LK, Pena-Rosas JP. Vitamin D supplementation for women during pregnancy. Cochrane Database Syst Rev. 2016;1:CD008873.

24. Haider BA, Bhutta ZA. Multiple-micronutrient supplementation for women during pregnancy. Cochrane Database Syst Rev. 2015;11:CD004905.

25. Ota E, Hori H, Mori R, Tobe-Gai R, Farrar D. Antenatal dietary education and supplementation to increase energy and protein intake. Cochrane Database Syst Rev. 2015;6:CD000032.

26. Lassi ZS, Salam RA, Haider BA, Bhutta ZA. Folic acid supplementation during pregnancy for maternal health and pregnancy outcomes. Cochrane Database Syst Rev. 2013;3:CD006896.

27. Rumbold A, Ota E, Nagata C, Shahrook S, Crowther CA. Vitamin C supplementation in pregnancy. Cochrane Database Syst Rev. 2015;9:Cd004072.

28. Pena-Rosas JP, De-Regil LM, Garcia-Casal MN, Dowswell T. Daily oral iron supplementation during pregnancy. Cochrane Database Syst Rev. 2015;7:CD004736.

29. Gresham E, Byles JE, Bisquera A, Hure AJ. Effects of dietary interventions on neonatal and infant outcomes: a systematic review and meta-analysis. Am J Clin Nutr. 2014;100(5):1298–321.

30. Taylor PN, Okosieme OE, Dayan CM, Lazarus JH. Therapy of endocrine disease: impact of iodine supplementation in mild-to-moderate iodine deficiency: systematic review and meta-analysis. Eur J Endocrinol. 2014;170(1):R1–15.

31. Imhoff-Kunsch B, Briggs V, Goldenberg T, Ramakrishnan U. Effect of n-3 long-chain polyunsaturated fatty acid intake during pregnancy on maternal, infant, and child health outcomes: a systematic review. Paediatr Perinat Epidemiol. 2012;26(Suppl 1):91–107.

32. Chaffee BW, King JC. Effect of zinc supplementation on pregnancy and infant outcomes: a systematic review. Paediatr Perinat Epidemiol. 2012;26(Suppl 1):118–37.

33. Walker N, Fischer-Walker C, Bryce J, Bahl R, Cousens S, Effects CRGoI. Standards for CHERG reviews of intervention effects on child survival. Int J Epidemiol. 2010;39(Suppl 1):i21–31.

34. Imdad A, Bhutta ZA. Maternal nutrition and birth outcomes: effect of balanced protein-energy supplementation. Paediatr Perinat Epidemiol. 2012;26(Suppl 1):178–90.

35. Carlson SE, Colombo J, Gajewski BJ, Gustafson KM, Mundy D, Yeast J, et al. DHA supplementation and pregnancy outcomes. Am J Clin Nutr. 2013;97(4):808–15.

36. Dror DK, Allen LH. Interventions with vitamins B6, B12 and C in pregnancy. Paediatr Perinat Epidemiol. 2012;26 (Suppl 1):55–74.

37. López-Flores F, Neufeld LM, Sotres-Álvarez D, García-Guerra A, UR. Compliance to micronutrient supplementation in children 3 to 24 months of age from a semi-rural community in Mexico. Salud Publica Mexico. 2012;54:470–8.

38. Mridha MK, Matias SL, Chaparro CM, Paul RR, Hussain S, Vosti SA, et al. Lipid-based nutrient supplements for pregnant women reduce newborn stunting in a cluster-randomized controlled effectiveness trial in Bangladesh. Am J Clin Nutr. 2016;103(1):236–49.

39. Adu-Afarwuah S, Lartey A, Okronipa H, Ashorn P, Zeilani M, Peerson JM, et al. Lipid-based nutrient supplement increases the birth size of infants of primiparous women in Ghana. Am J Clin Nutr. 2015;101(4):835–46.

40. Thorne-Lyman AL, Fawzi WW. Vitamin A and carotenoids during pregnancy and maternal, neonatal and infant health outcomes: a systematic review and meta-analysis. Paediatr Perinat Epidemiol. 2012;26(Suppl 1):36–54.

41. Girard AW, Olude O. Nutrition education and counselling provided during pregnancy: effects on maternal, neonatal and child health outcomes. Paediatr Perinat Epidemiol. 2012;26(Suppl 1):191–204.

42. Bhutta ZA, Imdad A, Ramakrishnan U, Martorell R. Is it time to replace iron folate supplements in pregnancy with multiple micronutrients? Paediatr Perinat Epidemiol. 2012;26(Suppl 1):27–35.

43. Zimmermann MB. The effects of iodine deficiency in pregnancy and infancy. Paediatr Perinat Epidemiol. 2012;26 (Suppl 1):108–17.

44. Ronsmans C, Fisher DJ, Osmond C, Margetts BM, Fall CH. Multiple micronutrient supplementation during pregnancy in low-income countries: a meta-analysis of effects on stillbirths and on early and late neonatal mortality. Food Nutr Bull. 2009;30(4 Suppl):S547–55.

45. Imhoff-Kunsch B, Briggs V. Antihelminthics in pregnancy and maternal, newborn and child health. Paediatr Perinat Epidemiol. 2012;26(Suppl 1):223–38.

46. Girard AW, Self JL, McAuliffe C, Olude O. The effects of household food production strategies on the health and nutrition outcomes of women and young children: a systematic review. Paediatr Perinat Epidemiol. 2012;26(Suppl 1):205–22.

47. King JC. A summary of pathways or mechanisms linking preconception maternal nutrition with birth outcomes. J Nutr 2016;146(7):1437s–44s.

48. De-Regil LM, Pena-Rosas JP, Fernandez-Gaxiola AC, Rayco-Solon P. Effects and safety of periconceptional oral folate supplementation for preventing birth defects. Cochrane Database Syst Rev. 2015;12:CD007950.

49. Hund L, Northrop-Clewes CA, Nazario R, Suleymanova D, Mirzoyan L, Irisova M, et al. A novel approach to evaluating the iron and folate status of women of reproductive age in Uzbekistan after 3 years of flour fortification with micronutrients. PLoS ONE. 2013;8(11):e79726.

50. Dean SV, Lassi ZS, Imam AM, Bhutta ZA. Preconception care: nutritional risks and interventions. Reprod Health. 2014;11(Suppl 3):S3.

51. Gibbs CM, Wendt A, Peters S, Hogue CJ. The impact of early age at first childbirth on maternal and infant health. Paediatr Perinat Epidemiol. 2012;26(Suppl 1):259–84.

52. Potdar RD, Sahariah SA, Gandhi M, Kehoe SH, Brown N, Sane H, et al. Improving women's diet quality preconceptionally and during gestation: effects on birth weight and prevalence of low birth weight—a randomized controlled efficacy trial in India (Mumbai maternal nutrition project). Am J Clin Nutr. 2014;100(5):1257–68.

53. Ramakrishnan U, Nguyen PH, Gonzalez-Casanova I, Pham H, Hao W, et al. Neither preconceptional weekly multiple micronutrient nor iron-folic acid supplements affect birth size and gestational age compared with a folic acid supplement alone in rural vietnamese women: a randomized controlled trial. J Nutr 2016;146(7):1445S–52S.

54. Young MF, Nguyen PH, Addo OY, Hao W, Nguyen H, Pham H, et al. The relative influence of maternal nutritional status before and during pregnancy on birth outcomes in Vietnam. Eur J Obstet Gynecol Reprod Biol. 2015;194:223–7.

55. Hambidge KM, Krebs NF, Westcott JE, Garces A, Goudar SS, Kodkany BS, et al. Preconception maternal nutrition: a multi-site randomized controlled trial. BMC Pregnancy Childbirth. 2014;14:111.

56. Tu N, King JC, Dirren H, Thu HN, Ngoc QP, Diep AN. Effect of animal-source food supplement prior to and during pregnancy on birthweight and prematurity in rural Vietnam: a brief study description. Food Nutr Bull. 2014;35(4 Suppl):S205–8.

57. Martorell R, Zongrone A. Intergenerational influences on child growth and undernutrition. Paediatr Perinat Epidemiol. 2012;26(Suppl 1):302–14.

58. Morton SM, De Stavola BL, Leon DA. Intergenerational determinants of offspring size at birth: a life course and graphical analysis using the Aberdeen children of the 1950s study (ACONF). Int J Epidemiol. 2014;43(3):749–59.

59. Addo OY, Stein AD, Fall CH, Gigante DP, Guntupalli AM, Horta BL, et al. Parental childhood growth and offspring birthweight: pooled analyses from four birth cohorts in low and middle income countries. Am J Hum Biol. 2015;27(1):99–105.

60. Ramakrishnan U, Martorell R, Schroeder DG, Flores R. Role of intergenerational effects on linear growth. J Nutr. 1999;129(2S Suppl):544S–9S.

61. Shrimpton R. Global policy and programme guidance on maternal nutrition: what exists, the mechanisms for providing it, and how to improve them? Paediatr Perinat Epidemiol. 2012;26(Suppl 1):315–25.

62. Lutter CK, Daelmans BM, de Onis M, Kothari MT, Ruel MT, Arimond M, et al. Undernutrition, poor feeding practices, and low coverage of key nutrition interventions. Pediatrics. 2011;128(6):e1418–27.

63. Stevens GA, Finucane MM, De-Regil LM, Paciorek CJ, Flaxman SR, Branca F, et al. Global, regional, and national trends in haemoglobin concentration and prevalence of total and severe anaemia in children and pregnant and non-pregnant women for 1995–2011: a systematic analysis of population-representative data. Lancet Glob Health. 2013;1(1):e16–25.

64. Duffy M, Lamstein S, Lutter C, Koniz-Booher P. Review of programmatic reponses to adolescent and women's nutrition needs in low and middle income countries. Strengthening Partnerships, Results, and Innovations in Nutrition Globally (SPRING) Project. Arlington, VA; 2015.

65. Leroy JL, Gadsden P, Gonzalez de Cossio T, Gertler P. Cash and in-kind transfers lead to excess weight gain in a population of women with a high prevalence of overweight in rural Mexico. J Nutr. 2013;143(3):378–83.

66. Varea A, Malpeli A, Disalvo L, Apezteguia M, Falivene M, Ferrari G, et al. Evaluation of the impact of a food program on the micronutrient nutritional status of Argentinean lactating mothers. Biol Trace Elem Res. 2012;150 (1–3):103–8.

67. Liu J, Jin L, Meng Q, Gao L, Zhang L, Li Z, et al. Changes in folic acid supplementation behaviour among women of reproductive age after the implementation of a massive supplementation programme in China. Public Health Nutr. 2015;18(4):582–8.

68. Kotecha PV, Nirupam S, Karkar PD. Adolescent girls' anaemia control programme, Gujarat, India. Indian J Med Res. 2009;130(5):584–9.

69. Vir SC, Singh N, Nigam AK, Jain R. Weekly iron and folic acid supplementation with counseling reduces anemia in adolescent girls: a large-scale effectiveness study in Uttar Pradesh, India. Food Nutr Bull. 2008;29(3):186–94.

70. Rah JH, de Pee S, Halati S, Parveen M, Mehjabeen SS, Steiger G, et al. Provision of micronutrient powder in response to the cyclone Sidr emergency in Bangladesh: cross-sectional assessment at the end of the intervention. Food Nutr Bull. 2011;32(3):277–85.

71. Passerini L, Casey GJ, Biggs BA, Cong DT, Phu LB, Phuc TQ, et al. Increased birth weight associated with regular pre-pregnancy deworming and weekly iron-folic acid supplementation for Vietnamese women. PLoS Negl Trop Dis. 2012;6(4):e1608.

72. Barber SL. Mexico's conditional cash transfer programme increases cesarean section rates among the rural poor. Eur J Public Health. 2010;20(4):383–8.

73. Baxter JA, Roth DE, Al Mahmud A, Ahmed T, Islam M, Zlotkin SH. Tablets are preferred and more acceptable than powdered prenatal calcium supplements among pregnant women in Dhaka, Bangladesh. J Nutr. 2014;144(7):1106–12.

Chapter 23
Small for Gestational Age: Scale and Consequences for Mortality, Morbidity, and Development

Ines Gonzalez-Casanova, Usha Ramakrishnan and Reynaldo Martorell

Keywords Growth retardation · Birth outcomes · Small for gestational age · Development · Nutrition · Child health · Child mortality · Maternal and child health · Chronic diseases

Learning Objectives

By the end of this chapter, the reader should be able to:

- define small for gestational age (SGA) and enumerate at least three methods of assessment;
- describe the epidemiology and main causes of SGA in developing countries;
- explain the association between SGA and mortality;
- explain and substantiate the association between SGA and morbidity; and
- explain the short- and long-term consequences of SGA on development.

Introduction

Small for gestational age (SGA), which is defined as a birthweight for gestational age below the 10th percentile of the reference, is used frequently as an indicator of inadequate intrauterine growth and also commonly referred to as intrauterine growth restriction (IUGR) or fetal growth restriction (FGR) [1–3]. This is a major public health problem. It is estimated that over 27% of live births are SGA in developing countries, with important short- and long-term repercussions for health and development [4]. This chapter describes the challenges to assess SGA, followed by current knowledge of its epidemiology and determinants especially in developing countries, as well as its main consequences. SGA should not be confused with preterm birth (<37 weeks of gestation) or even with low birthweight (<2500 g), which does not take into account the duration of gestation (Fig. 23.1); these conditions may coexist in certain settings and within individuals and have been described in Chap. 22 as they are also important health concerns.

I. Gonzalez-Casanova (✉) · U. Ramakrishnan
Department of Global Health, Emory University, 1518 Clifton Road, NE, Atlanta, GA 30322, USA
e-mail: igonza2@emory.edu

U. Ramakrishnan
e-mail: uramakr@emory.edu

R. Martorell
Hubert Department of Global Health, Emory University, 1599 Clifton Road, NE, Atlanta, GA 30322, USA
e-mail: rmart77@emory.edu

© Springer Science+Business Media New York 2017
S. de Pee et al. (eds.), *Nutrition and Health in a Developing World*,
Nutrition and Health, DOI 10.1007/978-3-319-43739-2_23

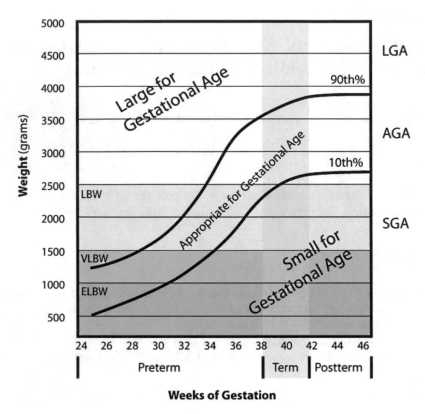

Fig. 23.1 Definition of small gestational age. *LGA* large for gestational age. *AGA* appropriate for gestational age. *SGA* small for gestational age. *LBW* low birthweight. *VLBW* very low birthweight. *ELBW* extremely low birthweight

Assessing Small for Gestational Age

Screening and diagnosis of SGA is challenging, especially in developing countries where access to technological advances may be limited. Different approaches have been used for this purpose [1, 5, 6]. All these methods are prone to error; a key challenge for the assessment of SGA is the accurate estimation of gestational age [6]. Three methods are commonly used to estimate gestational age. Ideally, gestational age should be determined through ultrasound examination, preferably during the first trimester of pregnancy [7, 8]. Although access to ultrasound technology has increased, it is still not available to many women especially those living in resource poor settings and/or it can be less accurate when women do not access prenatal care until the second trimester [9]. Another method to estimate gestational age is through the date of the last menstrual period (LMP), but this often relies on maternal recall, which may be inaccurate. This method is more feasible in low-resource settings and in developing countries, although inaccurate reporting is often more common among less educated and poor women; also, women who are nursing or have irregular menstrual cycles are prone to misreport [7, 10, 11].

Alternatively, physician observation has been used in combination with checklists to approximate gestational age, but this technique performs poorly compared to ultrasound or with recall of LMP as gold standards [11]. A few studies compared the three different methods to estimate gestational age [7, 10–12]. In the USA, Savitz et al. [12] compared the use of LMP to first trimester ultrasound and found gestational age measured by the first method was on average 2.8 days more than that estimated by ultrasound and was less accurate predicting date of birth. The greatest differences were found among younger women, those with low body mass index, and cigarette smokers. In a similar study in the USA, Hoffman et al. [7] compare those two methods and found that LMP estimates were on average 0.8 days longer than those obtained from a first trimester ultrasound. In this case, the differences were greater among young and underweight women, and Hispanics and non-Hispanic Blacks. In developing countries, Rosenberg et al. [11] compared four different methods to estimate gestational age (ultrasound, last menstrual period, and Ballard and Dubowitz physician reported indexes) in Bangladesh. Concordance coefficients were 0.88, 0.91, and 0.88 for LMP, Ballard, and Dubowitz, respectively. Compared to ultrasound, LMP recall and Ballard underestimated gestational age by 2.9 and 1.1 days, respectively, while Dubowitz overestimated it by almost 4 days. In Guatemala, Neufeld et al. [10] compared LMP and physician examination (using Capurro scale) to ultrasound and found that, on average, LMP underestimated gestational age by 0.77 days compared to ultrasound, while physician examination underestimated it by over 3 days. In this study, authors attributed the good performance of the LMP to well-trained village health workers assisting women to recall the dates.

Similarly, anthropometric measurements of the fetus, which are most commonly obtained by measuring uterine height using either calipers, metric tape, or through ultrasound examination, require training and are susceptible to measurement error, complicating the process of screening for SGA [2, 5]. Information obtained from clinical records or at clinical settings might be more susceptible to measurement error, compared to information collected in research settings where training and standardization of measurement techniques minimize potential issues. Another common source of error observed in clinical settings is the practice of rounding birthweights to multiples of 2, 5, 10, 50, and even 100 g [13]. Further, a significant proportion of births may not occur in clinical settings, especially in developing countries, resulting in missing or inaccurate estimates of weight and other anthropometric measurements at birth [14].

Once good quality and reliable information on gestational age and newborn anthropometric measurements is collected, the next challenge in the assessment of SGA is selecting a growth reference to interpret the data. Multiple references are available including international and local, as well as standard or customized by maternal height, parity, ethnicity, etc. For diagnosis and follow-up of pregnancies in clinical settings, local and customized growth charts have been deemed more appropriate. Another challenge is the use of different cutoff values; although the 10th percentile is used most widely, some have used lower values such as below the 3rd and 5th percentile to define SGA [15]. However, to obtain population estimates, standardized and international references are often more convenient and useful for comparisons [5, 16, 17]. An example is the World Health Organization Child Growth Standards, which was released in 2006 and includes children from 0 to 5 years.

After the release of the WHO child growth standards, this and other international and public health organizations identified the development of adequate standards to assess fetal growth in diverse settings as an important research priority. The International Fetal and Newborn Consortium has recently announced the release of "the International Fetal and Growth Standards for the twenty-first century (INTERGROWTH-21st)," which has been developed based on prospective data that were collected from eight geographically diverse populations (Brazil, Italy, Oman, UK, USA, China, India, and Kenya) using a standardized protocol [8]. Each participating country collected data from a sample of healthy pregnant women (non-smokers, healthy weight, no known health problems, etc.) expected to produce full-grown healthy fetuses. This study was implemented from 2008 to 2013 and included repeated ultrasound measurements, as well as measurements of weight and gestational age at birth. The new standards will be adopted by WHO and are complementary to the growth standards published in 2006 for children 0–5 years [18]. The INTERGROWTH-21st website can be accessed at www.intergrowth21.org. The international reference previously supported by WHO was developed in 1970 and was based on data solely from the USA and likely inadequate to assess fetal growth in current populations [19].

It is important to stress that due to the aforementioned complications to produce reliable population-level estimates of SGA, it has been challenging to assess the magnitude of the problem globally and at a country level. Furthermore, it has been anticipated that the use of the new fetal growth standards will not only produce SGA estimates different to those currently available that are based on different references, but also will bring unprecedented opportunity for a comprehensive assessment growth and development [20]. Public health researchers and practitioners interested in maternal and child health need to be aware of these challenges and keep up to date with new developments in this field.

Epidemiology and Determinants of SGA

As a response to the high mortality rates of children under 5 years, the WHO created the Child Health Epidemiology Reference Group (CHERG) in 2001. This group aims to provide reliable epidemiological estimates and technical support for the prevention of mortality and morbidity among children younger than five years in low- and middle-income countries. Many estimates used in this chapter are based on a series of publications, which are a useful resource to complement this reading [2–4, 21–40]. The CHERG Web site can be accessed at www.cherg.org.

As part of this initiative, the CHERG group published the most recent estimates of the extent and magnitude of SGA based on a meta-analysis of several international datasets that include estimates of SGA in 138 low- and middle-income countries (Fig. 23.2).

These estimates were obtained from ultrasound and birthweight information available and in comparison with the 1970 Alexander Ref. [18] that was previously supported by the WHO. Overall, it was estimated that 32.4 million infants (27% of live births) were born SGA in low-to-middle income countries in 2010. The highest prevalence observed was of 41.5% in South Asia, which contrasts with the lowest prevalence of 5.3% observed in East Asia (Fig. 23.3) [4]. The 10 countries with the greatest percent of SGA are presented in Table 23.1, with India, Pakistan, and Nigeria in the top three [41].

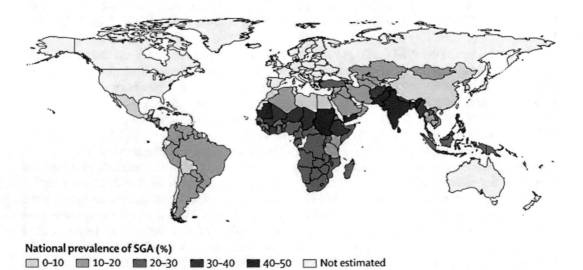

National prevalence of SGA (%)
☐ 0–10   ☐ 10–20   ■ 20–30   ■ 30–40   ■ 40–50   ☐ Not estimated

Fig. 23.2 Estimated prevalence of SGA births in 138 low-income and middle-income countries. From Lee et al. [4] (Open Access)

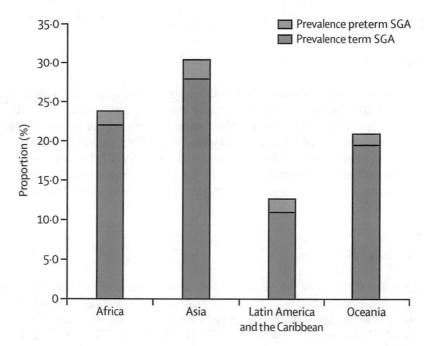

Fig. 23.3 Prevalence of term and preterm SGAs in 4 regions. From Jabeen et al. [39]. *Source* BioMed Central, Open Access

Table 23.1 Top 10 countries in number of small for gestational age (SGA) births per 100 live births in 2010

Rank	Country	Live births 2010	NMR 2010	Term SGA	Preterm SGA	Prevalence of SGA (%)
1	India	27,000,000	33.1	784,626	12,800,000	46.9
2	Pakistan	4,700,000	36.1	166,798	2,228,094	47.0
3	Nigeria	6,300,000	40.2	124,225	1,503,750	23.7
4	Bangladesh	3,000,000	27.5	94,558	1,203,038	39.6
5	China	17,000,000	9.4	261,378	1,072,066	6.5
6	Indonesia	4,400,000	15.9	150,655	1,042,282	23.8
7	Ethiopia	2,600,000	32.4	42,297	838,014	32.1
8	Philippines	2,300,000	12.6	77,791	786,665	33.6
9	Democratic Republic of the Congo	2,900,000	47.4	54,822	629,450	21.9
10	Sudan	1,400,000	31.5	30,237	595,244	41.7

NMR neonatal mortality rate per 1000 live births. From Lee et al. [4]. Reprinted with the permission from Elsevier

This epidemiologic panorama is explained by the multifactorial etiology of SGA. Maternal health and nutrition, placental integrity, and fetal characteristics may be responsible for SGA, but the contribution of these factors may differ among regions and populations. For example, in developed countries, the main cause of SGA is placental dysfunction, while in developing countries, factors associated with malnutrition are primarily responsible [12, 42, 43]. A more detailed description of the main causes of SGA with special emphasis on those associated with nutrition is presented next.

Maternal Factors

Preeclampsia

Severe hypertension is one of the most common complications during pregnancy. Hypertensive disorders are the second cause of maternal mortality worldwide, accounting for 18% of perinatal deaths. During the second half of pregnancy, blood expansion may strain cardiorespiratory capacity and translate into chronic high blood pressure. Hypertension affects placental irrigation and restricts fetal growth. This disorder is associated with maternal micronutrient deficiencies, particularly calcium and vitamin D, as well as with maternal overweight and previous hypertensive disorders. In a study conducted by Rasmussen and Irgens [44], pregnancy hypertension explained 21.9% of preterm cases of SGA and 2.5% of term cases of SGA [44].

Gestational Diabetes (GD)

Gestational Diabetes (GD) is defined as an elevated blood sugar with onset during pregnancy that may or may not be resolved after delivery. It is a result of decreased insulin sensitivity and global inflammation produced by the physiological changes associated with pregnancy. The most common negative effect of this condition is large for gestational age offspring. Nevertheless, GD can also be associated with SGA, since when poorly managed, it can cause vascular and renal complications leading to FGR. Prepregnancy overweight and obesity are the main predictors of gestational diabetes. Other risk factors for this condition include excessive pregnancy weight gain, history of GD, age, and race or ethnicity [45].

Anemia

Anemia is defined as a low level of hemoglobin, which impairs oxygen transportation, and is one of the greatest concerns among women of reproductive age (see Chap. 22). The causes of anemia are diverse, including micronutrient deficiencies (iron, folate, vitamin B12, vitamin A, etc.) as well as blood losses, such as those associated with menstruation and delivery. During pregnancy, anemia is one of the greatest concerns for both maternal and child health. One of the negative consequences of anemia during pregnancy is IUGR and SGA offspring. Potential explanations for this association are the lack of tissue oxygenation that can lead to chronic hypoxia and oxidative stress, as well as an increased production of norepinephrine related to iron deficiency, which, in turn, releases corticosteroids and restricts fetal growth. A recent meta-analysis found that moderate-to-severe maternal anemia (Hemoglobin < 9 or < 8 g/dl) prior to delivery increased the risk of SGA by 53%, whereas mild anemia was not associated with SGA [24].

Undernutrition

Multiple studies have demonstrated the effects of maternal chronic undernutrition on fetal growth. A prepregnancy body mass index under 18.5 kg/m^2 has been demonstrated to increase the risk of SGA by 80% [46]. The biological mechanisms for this effect are not completely understood; however, potential causes are nutritional deficiencies, placental insufficiency, and endothelial damage. It is important to note that many women of reproductive age in developing countries suffer from micro- and macronutrient deficiencies so that when they become pregnant, fetal growth and development and

Table 23.2 Maternal nutritional risk factors for small for gestational age births

OR (95% CI)	Height < 145 cm[a]	BMI < 18.5 kg/m^2 [b]	BMI > 25 kg/m^2 [c]
SGA[c]	2.12 (1.88, 2.39)	1.60 (1.45, 1.77)	0.67 (0.55, 0.83)
Term SGA[d]	2.20 (1.94, 2.50)	1.71 (1.52, 1.92)	0.67 (0.55, 0.83)
Preterm SGA[d]	1.38 (1.15, 1.65)	2.39 (1.69, 3.39)	0.60 (0.38, 0.96)

OR odds ratio; *CI* confidence interval; *AGA* appropriate for gestational age
[a]Relative to ≥155 cm
[b]Relative to 18.5–25 kg/m^2
[c]Relative to AGA
[d]Relative to term AGA
From Jabeen et al. [39]. *Source* BioMed Central, Open Access

maternal health may be impaired due to inability to meet the increased physiological requirements. Insufficient protein intake, inadequate weight gain, and lack of essential micronutrients such as iron, folate, and calcium during pregnancy are some of the examples of undernutrition related to SGA. Nutrition interventions during pregnancy, namely balanced protein energy supplementation in settings where maternal undernutrition is common, are also important and have been shown to reduce the risk of SGA (see Chap. 22); however, preconception interventions and fortification programs (such as flour fortification with folic acid) may be equally necessary to address underlying deficiencies. For example, low maternal height and BMI are associated with increased likelihood of SGA offspring (Table 23.2) [41]. In this sense, low maternal height may be the result of chronic nutritional deficiencies that sometimes go back many generations.

Toxins

Smoking, alcohol, drugs, and other toxins are among the main causes of IUGR and developmental disorders. They impair cell division, may cause hypoxia, and increase oxidative stress. One of the most important factors associated with IUGR is maternal smoking. Rasmussen and Irgens [44] found that maternal smoking explained 12% of SGA among both preterm and term births after controlling for hypertensive disorders [44]. This adds to the body of evidence supporting an association between smoking and growth restriction. Particularly, smoking during the second and third trimester of pregnancy has been shown to significantly decrease fetal growth and increase the likelihood of adverse pregnancy outcomes. This has been attributed to a decrease in the amount of oxygen available for the fetus and, more recently, to epigenetic changes generated by changes in the methylation patterns, which in turn affect the expression of certain genes associated with fetal growth and development [47, 48].

Placental Factors

Malformations or complications related to the placenta are also important causes of SGA. Examples include placenta previa, abnormal thromboblast invasion, and umbilical or placental vascular anomalies. These conditions impair the supply of oxygen and nutrients to the fetus and consequently restrict growth [49].

Fetal Factors

Conditions inherent to the fetus are also related to SGA. For example, genetic abnormalities or malformations, multiple gestation, and intrauterine infections such as malaria or HIV are important causes of SGA worldwide.

Symmetric and Asymmetric SGA

An important consideration is that two different types of SGA have been identified and their etiology can vary significantly [50, 51]. This classification reflects body proportions and time of onset. Symmetric SGA occurs when growth restriction affects weight, length, and head circumference. This type of SGA often occurs during the first trimester and is commonly caused by viral infections, inherited abnormalities, and chemical exposure. The prognosis of symmetric SGA is worse than that of asymmetric SGA [50]. In asymmetric SGA, weight and length are affected, but head circumference remains unaffected; its onset is common during the second or third trimester. The most common cause of asymmetric SGA is nutritional deficiencies during the second trimester and third trimester. Asymmetric SGA is also most prevalent in LMIC [50].

SGA and Mortality

Small for gestational age has been correlated with fetal and perinatal death in several studies from both developing and developed countries [21]. For example, Frøen et al. [52] reported in 2002 that growth restricted fetuses were seven times more likely to suffer from unexplained sudden death compared to AGA. There is a direct association between the severity of growth restriction and the risk of fetal death. Moreover, SGA infants are at higher risk of perinatal death independently of gestational age, prematurity, low birthweight, or type of growth restriction (symmetric or asymmetric). In fact, intrauterine growth retardation is the main risk factor for perinatal mortality and morbidity in developing countries. In terms of infants, SGA is associated with increased risk of complications during the first 24 h of life, such as fetal academia, seizures, sepsis, and neonatal death. In preterm children, the incidence of ventricular hemorrhage and respiratory distress is associated with severe growth restriction (<3% percentile) [53]. Due to these complications and the increase in the risk of being stillbirth, it has been estimated SGA infants have a higher risk of perinatal mortality. In a large meta-analysis which included almost 2 million babies from 20 cohorts in Asia, Africa, and Latin America, Katz et al. (2013) [23] quantified the risk of neonatal mortality among SGA (<10th percentile) and very SGA (<3rd percentile) as two and four times that of AGA infants, respectively (Fig. 23.4). The overall relative risk of neonatal mortality and post-neonatal mortality was 3.12 and 2.85, respectively (Fig. 23.5). Using the above information, Black et al. [41] estimated that the deaths of 817,000 neonates (32.6% of all neonatal deaths and 11.8% of total deaths of children <5 years) could be attributed to SGA in 2011.

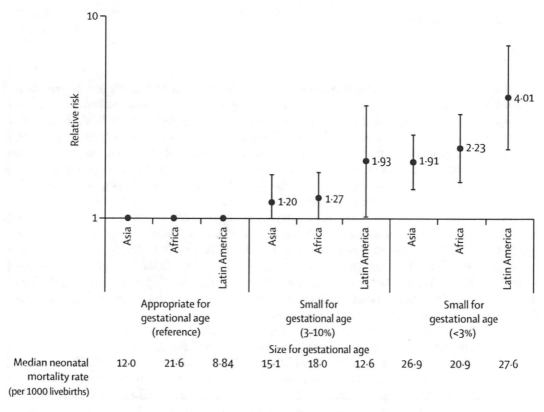

Fig. 23.4 Relative risk of neonatal mortality associated with small for gestational age in developing countries. From Katz et al. [23]. Reprinted with the permission from Elsevier

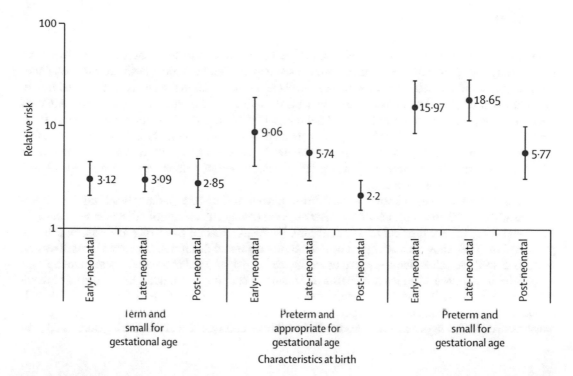

Fig. 23.5 Relative risk of mortality during early neonatal, neonatal, and postnatal periods in developing countries. From Katz et al. [23]. Reprinted with the permission from Elsevier

SGA and Morbidity

Short Term

As mentioned before, SGA increases risk of morbidity during the first 24 h of life in both preterm and term babies; chronic lung disease [54], sepsis, necrotizing enterocolitis, intraventricular hemorrhage, and higher risk of being intubated are a few of the neonatal complications of SGA. Nonetheless, Chauhan et al. [55] followed a cohort of 11,487 births and demonstrated that early detection of FGR by Doppler technique before the 22nd week of gestation may contribute to the prevention of neonatal morbidity, especially in preterm births. This can be achieved through the implementation of early interventions such as those designed to address maternal morbidity (preeclampsia or otherwise), improve maternal nutrition through supplementation or dietary advice, and/or reduce exposure to environmental contaminants or toxins. Among preterm offspring where SGA was detected prenatally, the risk of complications measured by a composite neonatal morbidity score (including thrombocytopenia, respiratory distress syndrome, sepsis, grades III or IV intraventricular hemorrhage, necrotizing enterocolitis, or neonatal seizure) was about 10 times lower compared to prenatally undetected SGA. It is important to note that among the 8% of the offspring born SGA, only 25% were prenatally detected. These results outline the importance of early detection of SGA for timely intervention and prevention of neonatal complications [55].

Finally, being born SGA is also associated with an increased risk of childhood stunting and wasting, which in turn has been associated with increased morbidity and mortality [56]. Using data from 19 large cohorts, Christian et al. [57] estimated a risk attributable to SGA of 20% for stunting and 30% for wasting, and SGA infants were 2–5 times more likely to be wasted, stunted, or underweight at 5 years of age compared to those born AGA. Further, children who were born both preterm and SGA had the greatest risk of these consequences.

Long Term

During the last decade, the focus on SGA has shifted from the treatment of short-term consequences to the study and prevention of its long-term consequences. The biological basis for the association between SGA and its metabolic consequences has been summarized in the theory of the "fetal origins of adult disease" [58]. During early development, the ability of the fetus to adapt to environmental conditions, or plasticity, is most efficient. After this period of developmental plasticity, the functional characteristics become fixed. IUGR appears to alter gene expression through changes in DNA methylation, thus affecting metabolic programming. In other words, gene expression adapts to an adverse and restrictive environment during the plasticity period, which may not correspond with postnatal and long-term exposures.

This phenomenon is also known as the "thrifty phenotype" or "the Barker Hypothesis," as it was first postulated by British physician David Barker, who conducted a study of 5654 men born between 1911 and 1930 in six districts of Hertfordshire, England. Results from this analysis, which was published in 1989, show an association between birthweight and death from ischemic heart disease in adulthood [58]. Another study supporting the increased risk of cardiovascular disease among individuals born SGA was conducted in Helsinki, Finland, a country where adult health records include information on prenatal and birth characteristics. The Helsinki Birth Cohort Study of 1934–1944 included 13,345 individuals born at two hospitals in this city. In this cohort, impaired fetal growth was associated with hypertension, coronary heart disease, and type 2 diabetes during adulthood [59].

More recently, the Consortium of Health-Orientated Research in Transitioning Societies (COHORTS) investigators' initiative [60] was formed with the objective to bring together and analyze all the information available from long-term studies in low- and middle-income countries. Five longitudinal studies met the criteria and were included: the 1982 Pelotas (Brazil) Birth Cohort Study [61], the Institute of Nutrition of Central America and Panama Nutrition Trial Cohort (INTC; Guatemala) [62], the New Delhi Birth Cohort (India) [63], the Cebu Longitudinal Health and Nutrition Survey cohort (CLHNS; Philippines) [64], and the Birth-to-Twenty (Bt20; Soweto-Johannesburg, South Africa) cohort [65]. An analysis of pooled data from these studies showed that in these low- and middle-income settings, being born preterm or SGA was associated with persistent deficits in adult height and schooling but not with increased blood pressure or blood glucose concentration [66].

Three main physiologic adaptations have been reported among SGA newborns to explain the negative long-term consequences: diminished capacity of important organs, for example, the kidney; altered hormonal responses, which may become evident early in life through alterations in the pattern of puberty, which include premature adrenarche and menarche, and polycystic ovarian syndrome; and decreased resilience to adverse outcomes, such as altered response to stress manifested through increased cortisol in blood. These alterations are associated with increased risk of obesity, type 2 diabetes mellitus, dyslipidemias, insulin resistance, and hypertension, which ultimately lead to the onset of cardiovascular disease [67, 68].

SGA and Development

Child Development

The developmental consequences of both preterm birth (before the 37th week of gestation) and low birthweight (<2500 g) have been extensively studied; however, until the last two decades, the impact of being born SGA had barely been explored, especially among infants born to term and heavier than 2500 g. In addition to all the negative physical and metabolic consequences of SGA, deficits in cognition and intellectual development have been reported among children born in the lowest percentiles of weight per gestational age [69]. De Bie et al. [70] reviewed over 25 observational studies reporting on the association between SGA and cognitive outcomes during childhood and adolescence (Table 23.3). Despite a large variability in the definitions, over 90% reported lower intelligence quotient among children classified as SGA compared to the controls. Some of these studies also reported decreased language, spatial and constructive, motor, and learning skills, as well as decreased executive function and attention.

These associations were consistent among both preterm and term SGA infants. An example of a study of the effects of SGA on cognitive development during the preschool years is the one conducted by Sommerfelt et al. [82, 83] in a cohort of Norwegian children. At age 5, children who were born SGA (<15th percentile) scored in the full cognitive scale 4 IQ points less when compared to age-matched controls who were born AGA. A smaller effect of 3 points was found for verbal IQ. Another example, supporting the importance of birthweight for long-term development among schoolchildren from a developing country, is the longitudinal analysis conducted by Torche and Echevarria in Chile [98]. They reported that a 400 g higher birthweight within twin pairs was associated with a 15% higher math score at 9 years of age. The twins participating in this study had an average birthweight of 2500 ± 490 g.

Table 23.3 Intelligence and cognition in children born SGA, compared to children born AGA (matched for gestational age)

Report	Definition of SGA	Sample size (SGA)	Age at assessment (years)	IQ	Cognitive domains				
					Speech and language	Visuospatial and visuoconstructive skills	Manual dexterity and motor skills	Learning and memory	Executive function and attention
Children born at term									
Westwood et al. [71]	P2.3	33	19	▶[a]					
Viggedal et al. [72]	P2.3	17	1.5, 24	▶[a]		▶		▶	
Fitzhardinge and Steven [73]	P3	96	4, 6, 8	▶[a]	▶				
Paz et al. [74]	P3	64	17	▶[a]					
Paz et al. [75]	P3/P10	944	17	▶[a]					
Strauss and Dietz [76]	P5	2719	7	▶[a]	▶				
Strauss [77]	P5	1064	5, 16		▶	▶[a]			▶
O'Keeffe et al. [78]	P10	596	14	—	▶				
Theodore et al. [79]	P10	385	7	—					
Kulseng et al. [80]	P10	60	14	—					—
Harvey et al. [81]	P10	51	5	▶[a] ▶[b]		▶[b]	▶[b]		
Sommerfelt et al. [82, 83]	P15	311	5	▶[a] ▶[c]	—	—	▶	—	
Children born preterm									
McCarton et al. [84]	P3	129	6	▶					
Gutbrod et al. [85]	P10	115	4, 7	▶[a]	—				
Feldman et al. [86]	P10	40	2	▶					
Sung et al. [87]	P10	27	1, 2, 3	▶					

(continued)

Table 23.3 (continued)

Report	Definition of SGA	Sample size (SGA)	Age at assessment (years)	IQ	Cognitive domains				
					Speech and language	Visuospatial and visuoconstructive skills	Manual dexterity and motor skills	Learning and memory	Executive function and attention
Children born at term and preterm (mixed groups)									
Lundgren et al. [88]	P2.3	5890	18	▶					
Frisk et al. [89]	P2.3	71	8	▶	▶e	▶e			▶e
Tideman et al. [90]	P2.3	19	18	▶					▶
Hollo et al. [91]	P2.5	118	10	▶					
Fattal-Valevski et al. [92]	P5	85	3	–					
Leitner et al. [93]	P10	123	9–10	▶a ▶c					
Geva et al. [94–96]d	P10	123–138	9–10	▶a	▶	–	▶	▶	▶
Silva et al. [97]	P10	96	3, 5, 7, 9	▶a					

P2.3 Below the 2.3rd percentile; *P2.5* below the 2.5th percentile; *P3* below the 3rd percentile; *P5* below the 5th percentile; *P10* below the 10th percentile; *P15* below the 15th percentile; ▶ significantly lower than control group; – equal to the control group

aSignificant difference but within the normal range

bIn children born SGA with onset of slow head growth before 26 weeks of gestation

cPerformance IQ only

dWith prematurity as a covariate

eOnly in children with prenatal head growth compromise

Long-Term Performance

The negative impact of SGA on health and development supports the theory that IUGR may impair long-term cognitive performance and educational and economic outcomes. However, few studies have assessed the long-term implications of SGA on human capital and educational attainment in adulthood. A unique example from a developing country was the analysis by Li et al. [99, 100] in Guatemala, where the authors reported no association between size at birth (not necessarily SGA) and women's educational achievement. More recently, Helgertz and Vagero [101] assessed the relative risk of applying for a disability pension in a sample of over 8000 men and women from the Stockholm Birth Cohort, which was established in 1953. For this study, participants who were not on disability pension were enrolled in 1990 and followed prospectively until 2009 when the hazard of disability pension was calculated. Participants who were born with asymmetric SGA had 68% higher risk of starting disability pension during the time of the study compared to those born asymmetric but adequate size for gestational age.

Conclusions

Until recently, the study of SGA and its consequences have been very limited, especially in developing countries. This is partially explained because of the complications to adequately identify children with SGA. Traditionally, studies and interventions have focused on the study and prevention of low birthweight as a marker of IUGR, because it only requires a measurement of weight at birth, not an assessment of gestational age (preferably during the first trimester using ultrasound). However, this leaves out an important proportion of children who are born heavier than 2500 g but still too small for their gestational age. Fortunately, the resources available to assess SGA and the interest of the international community in doing so have significantly increased in the last decade. Technological advances have improved the ultrasound technology, and more affordable and portable devices, which could be used in some low-resource settings, are being developed. This would need to be combined with efforts to promote early prenatal visits and provide adequate health care from the first trimester of pregnancy. The recently released International Fetal Growth Standards are a major advance that will facilitate the screening and estimation of SGA in developing countries. It is imperative to continue the study of the short- and long-term consequences of SGA. For example, a large body of evidence suggests an important link between SGA and cardiometabolic alterations that lead to chronic diseases. These latest findings support the great need of addressing the different factors that lead to SGA as well as integral policies to improve women's health in developing countries. These interventions also have the potential to reduce the numerous child deaths that can be attributed to SGA.

Beyond all the metabolic complications, research supports a detrimental effect of SGA on cognition during infancy and childhood. This impact on development is related to the rapid growth and development of the brain during fetal and first two years of life, which also suffers from the insults that cause SGA, such as poor maternal nutrition and toxic substances. A more in-depth discussion of these issues is presented in Chap. 24: Developmental Disabilities. Intrauterine growth retardation in these children translates into lower IQ and motor skills. In long term, these deficits translate into economic and human capital losses.

Discussion Points

- Discuss potential challenges assessing SGA in developing country settings. What would be the consequences of utilizing inaccurate methodologies and misclassifying newborns with SGA in (a) a clinic in a developing country, (b) a public health intervention trying to prevent SGA, (c) national estimates for comparison across different countries?
- What is the difference among low birthweight, SGA, and preterm birth? Discuss their intersections in term of diagnosis, interventions, and potential complications.
- Select a low- or middle-income country and obtain its WHO country profile. Discuss potential causes of SGA in this particular setting.
- Discuss the potential impact of the increased mortality associated with SGA in low- and middle-income countries. Identify the regions most at risk and describe the factors associated with this problem.
- Elaborate the consequences throughout the life span of being born as an SGA infant in a low- or middle-income country. Discuss the impact of these consequences for the individual, family, community, and country.

References

1. Brodsky D, Christou H. Current concepts in intrauterine growth restriction. J Intensive Care Med. 2004;19 (6):307–19. doi:10.1177/0885066604269663 PubMed PMID: 15523117.
2. Imdad A, Yakoob MY, Siddiqui S, Bhutta ZA. Screening and triage of intrauterine growth restriction (IUGR) in general population and high risk pregnancies: a systematic review with a focus on reduction of IUGR related stillbirths. BMC public health 2011;11(Suppl 3):S1. Doi:10.1186/1471-2458-11-S3-S1 (PubMed PMID: 21501426; PMCID: 3231882).
3. Wu LA, Katz J, Mullany LC, Khatry SK, Darmstadt GL, LeClerq SC, Tielsch JM. The association of preterm birth and small birthweight for gestational age on childhood disability screening using the ten questions plus tool in rural Sarlahi district, Southern Nepal. Child Care Health Dev. 2012;38(3):332–40. doi:10.1111/j.1365-2214. 2011.01221.x PubMed PMID: 21375569.
4. Lee AC, Katz J, Blencowe H, Cousens S, Kozuki N, Vogel JP, Adair L, Baqui AH, Bhutta ZA, Caulfield LE, Christian P, Clarke SE, Ezzati M, Fawzi W, Gonzalez R, Huybregts L, Kariuki S, Kolsteren P, Lusingu J, Marchant T, Merialdi M, Mongkolchati A, Mullany LC, Ndirangu J, Newell ML, Nien JK, Osrin D, Roberfroid D, Rosen HE, Sania A, Silveira MF, Tielsch J, Vaidya A, Willey BA, Lawn JE, Black RE, Group CS-PBW. National and regional estimates of term and preterm babies born small for gestational age in 138 low-income and middle-income countries in 2010. Lancet Glob Health. 2013;1(1):e26–36. Doi:10.1016/S2214-109X(13)70006-8 (PubMed PMID: 25103583; PMCID: 4221634).
5. Chauhan SP, Magann EF. Screening for fetal growth restriction. Clin Obstet Gynecol. 2006;49(2):284–94 PubMed PMID: 16721107.
6. Lynch CD, Zhang J. The research implications of the selection of a gestational age estimation method. Paediatr Perinat Epidemiol. 2007;21(Suppl 2):86–96. doi:10.1111/j.1365-3016.2007.00865.x PubMed PMID: 17803622.
7. Hoffman CS, Messer LC, Mendola P, Savitz DA, Herring AH, Hartmann KE. Comparison of gestational age at birth based on last menstrual period and ultrasound during the first trimester. Paediatr Perinat Epidemiol. 2008;22 (6):587–96. doi:10.1111/j.1365-3016.2008.00965.x PubMed PMID: 19000297.
8. Papageorghiou AT, Ohuma EO, Altman DG, Todros T, Cheikh Ismail L, Lambert A, Jaffer YA, Bertino E, Gravett MG, Purwar M, Noble JA, Pang R, Victora CG, Barros FC, Carvalho M, Salomon LJ, Bhutta ZA, Kennedy SH, Villar J, International F. Newborn growth consortium for the 21st C. International standards for fetal growth based on serial ultrasound measurements: the fetal growth longitudinal study of the INTERGROWTH-21st Project. Lancet. 2014;384(9946):869–79. Doi:10.1016/S0140-6736(14)61490-2 (PubMed PMID: 25209488).
9. McClure EM, Nathan RO, Saleem S, Esamai F, Garces A, Chomba E, Tshefu A, Swanson D, Mabeya H, Figuero L, Mirza W, Muyodi D, Franklin H, Lokangaka A, Bidashimwa D, Pasha O, Mwenechanya M, Bose CL, Carlo WA, Hambidge KM, Liechty EA, Krebs N, Wallace DD, Swanson J, Koso-Thomas M, Widmer R, Goldenberg RL. First look: a cluster-randomized trial of ultrasound to improve pregnancy outcomes in low

income country settings. BMC Pregnancy Childbirth. 2014;14:73. doi:10.1186/1471-2393-14-73 PubMed PMID: 24533878; PMCID: 3996090.

10. Neufeld LM, Haas JD, Grajeda R, Martorell R. Last menstrual period provides the best estimate of gestation length for women in rural Guatemala. Paediatr Perinat Epidemiol. 2006;20(4):290–8. doi:10.1111/j.1365-3016. 2006.00741.x PubMed PMID: 16879501.

11. Rosenberg RE, Ahmed AS, Ahmed S, Saha SK, Chowdhury MA, Black RE, Santosham M, Darmstadt GL. Determining gestational age in a low-resource setting: validity of last menstrual period. J Health Popul Nutr. 2009;27(3):332–8 (PubMed PMID: 19507748; PMCID: 2761790).

12. Savitz DA, Terry JW Jr, Dole N, Thorp JM Jr, Siega-Riz AM, Herring AH. Comparison of pregnancy dating by last menstrual period, ultrasound scanning, and their combination. Am J Obstet Gynecol. 2002;187(6):1660–6 PubMed PMID: 12501080.

13. Emmerson AJ, Roberts SA. Rounding of birth weights in a neonatal intensive care unit over 20 years: an analysis of a large cohort study. BMJ open. 2013;3(12):e003650. doi:10.1136/bmjopen-2013-003650 PubMed PMID: 24319272; PMCID: 3855566.

14. Darmstadt GL, Lee AC, Cousens S, Sibley L, Bhutta ZA, Donnay F, Osrin D, Bang A, Kumar V, Wall SN, Baqui A, Lawn JE. 60 million non-facility births: who can deliver in community settings to reduce intrapartum-related deaths? Int J Gynaecol Obstet. 2009;107(Suppl 1):S89–112. doi:10.1016/j.ijgo.2009.07.010 PubMed PMID: 19815200; PMCID: 3428830.

15. Villar J, Papageorghiou AT, Pang R, Salomon LJ, Langer A, Victora C, Purwar M, Chumlea C, Qingqing W, Scherjon SA, Barros FC, Carvalho M, Altman DG, Giuliani F, Bertino E, Jaffer YA, Cheikh Ismail L, Ohuma EO, Lambert A, Noble JA, Gravett MG, Bhutta ZA, Kennedy SH. Monitoring human growth and development: a continuum from the womb to the classroom. Am J Obstet Gynecol. 2015;213(4):494–9. doi:10. 1016/j.ajog.2015.07.002 PubMed PMID: 26184778.

16. Gelbaya TA, Nardo LG. Customised fetal growth chart: a systematic review. J Obstet Gynaecol. 2005;25(5):445–50. doi:10.1080/01443610500160444 PubMed PMID: 16183577.

17. Unterscheider J, Daly S, Geary MP, Kennelly MM, McAuliffe FM, O'Donoghue K, Hunter A, Morrison JJ, Burke G, Dicker P, Tully EC, Malone FD. Definition and management of fetal growth restriction: a survey of contemporary attitudes. Eur J Obstet Gynecol Reprod Biol. 2014;174:41–5. doi:10.1016/j.ejogrb.2013.11.022 PubMed PMID: 24360357.

18. Borghi E, de Onis M, Garza C, Van den Broeck J, Frongillo EA, Grummer-Strawn L, Van Buuren S, Pan H, Molinari L, Martorell R, Onyango AW, Martines JC, Group WHOMGRS. Construction of the World Health Organization child growth standards: selection of methods for attained growth curves. Stat Med. 2006;25(2):247–65. Doi:10.1002/sim.2227 (PubMed PMID: 16143968).

19. Alexander GR, Himes JH, Kaufman RB, Mor J, Kogan M. A United States national reference for fetal growth. Obstet Gynecol. 1996;87(2):163–8. doi:10.1016/0029-7844(95)00386-X PubMed PMID: 8559516.

20. Garza C. Fetal, neonatal, infant, and child international growth standards: an unprecedented opportunity for an integrated approach to assess growth and development. Adv Nutr. 2015;6(4):383–90. doi:10.3945/an.114.008128 PubMed PMID: 26178022; PMCID: PMC4496737.

21. Liu L, Johnson HL, Cousens S, Perin J, Scott S, Lawn JE, Rudan I, Campbell H, Cibulskis R, Li M, Mathers C, Black RE. Child health epidemiology reference group of WHO, UNICEF. Global, regional, and national causes of child mortality: an updated systematic analysis for 2010 with time trends since 2000. Lancet. 2012;379 (9832):2151–61. doi:10.1016/S0140-6736(12)60560-1 PubMed PMID: 22579125.

22. Liu L, Oza S, Hogan D, Perin J, Rudan I, Lawn JE, Cousens S, Mathers C, Black RE. Global, regional, and national causes of child mortality in 2000–13, with projections to inform post-2015 priorities: an updated systematic analysis. Lancet. 2014;. doi:10.1016/S0140-6736(14)61698-6 PubMed PMID: 25280870.

23. Katz J, Lee AC, Kozuki N, Lawn JE, Cousens S, Blencowe H, Ezzati M, Bhutta ZA, Marchant T, Willey BA, Adair L, Barros F, Baqui AH, Christian P, Fawzi W, Gonzalez R, Humphrey J, Huybregts L, Kolsteren P, Mongkolchati A, Mullany LC, Ndyomugyenyi R, Nien JK, Osrin D, Roberfroid D, Sania A, Schmiegelow C, Silveira MF, Tielsch J, Vaidya A, Velaphi SC, Victora CG, Watson-Jones D, Black RE. Group CS-f-G-A-PBW. Mortality risk in preterm and small-for-gestational-age infants in low-income and middle-income countries: a pooled country analysis. Lancet. 2013;382(9890):417–25. doi:10.1016/S0140-6736(13)60993-9 PubMed PMID: 23746775; PMCID: 3796350.

24. Kozuki N, Lee AC, Katz J. Child health epidemiology reference G. Moderate to severe, but not mild, maternal anemia is associated with increased risk of small-for-gestational-age outcomes. J Nutr. 2012;142(2):358–62. doi:10.3945/jn.111.149237 PubMed PMID: 22190028.

25. Cresswell JA, Ronsmans C, Calvert C, Filippi V. Prevalence of placenta praevia by world region: a systematic review and meta-analysis. Trop Med Int Health TM & IH. 2013;18(6):712–24. doi:10.1111/tmi.12100 PubMed PMID: 23551357.

26. Zhang Y, Chen L, van Velthoven MH, Wang W, Liu L, Du X, Wu Q, Li Y, Car J. mHealth series: measuring maternal newborn and child health coverage by text messaging—a county-level model for China. J Glob Health. 2013;3(2):020402. doi:10.7189/jogh.03.020402 PubMed PMID: 24363920; PMCID: 3868819.

27. Liu L, Li M, Yang L, Ju L, Tan B, Walker N, Bryce J, Campbell H, Black RE, Guo Y. Measuring coverage in MNCH: a validation study linking population survey derived coverage to maternal, newborn, and child health care records in rural China. PLoS ONE. 2013;8(5):e60762. doi:10.1371/journal.pone.0060762 PubMed PMID: 23667429; PMCID: 3646215.

28. Barros AJ, Victora CG. Measuring coverage in MNCH: determining and interpreting inequalities in coverage of maternal, newborn, and child health interventions. PLoS Med. 2013;10(5):e1001390. doi:10.1371/journal.pmed. 1001390 PubMed PMID: 23667332; PMCID: 3646214.

29. Mwaniki MK, Atieno M, Lawn JE, Newton CR. Long-term neurodevelopmental outcomes after intrauterine and neonatal insults: a systematic review. Lancet. 2012;379(9814):445–52. doi:10.1016/S0140-6736(11)61577-8 PubMed PMID: 22244654; PMCID: 3273721.

30. Kalter HD, Salgado R, Babille M, Koffi AK, Black RE. Social autopsy for maternal and child deaths: a comprehensive literature review to examine the concept and the development of the method. Popul Health Metrics. 2011;9:45. doi:10.1186/1478-7954-9-45 PubMed PMID: 21819605; PMCID: 3160938.

31. Acuin CS, Khor GL, Liabsuetrakul T, Achadi EL, Htay TT, Firestone R, Bhutta ZA. Maternal, neonatal, and child health in Southeast Asia: towards greater regional collaboration. Lancet. 2011;377(9764):516–25. doi:10.1016/ S0140-6736(10)62049-1 PubMed PMID: 21269675.

32. Haider BA, Yakoob MY, Bhutta ZA. Effect of multiple micronutrient supplementation during pregnancy on maternal and birth outcomes. BMC Pub Health. 2011;11(Suppl 3):S19. doi:10.1186/1471-2458-11-S3-S19 PubMed PMID: 21501436; PMCID: 3231892.

33. Imdad A, Bhutta ZA. Effect of balanced protein energy supplementation during pregnancy on birth outcomes. BMC Pub Health. 2011;11(Suppl 3):S17. doi:10.1186/1471-2458-11-S3-S17 PubMed PMID: 21501434; PMCID: 3231890.

34. Imdad A, Bhutta ZA. Effect of preventive zinc supplementation on linear growth in children under 5 years of age in developing countries: a meta-analysis of studies for input to the lives saved tool. BMC Pub Health. 2011;11 (Suppl 3):S22. doi:10.1186/1471-2458-11-S3-S22 PubMed PMID: 21501440; PMCID: 3231896.

35. Imdad A, Jabeen A, Bhutta ZA. Role of calcium supplementation during pregnancy in reducing risk of developing gestational hypertensive disorders: a meta-analysis of studies from developing countries. BMC Pub Health. 2011;11(Suppl 3):S18. doi:10.1186/1471-2458-11-S3-S18 PubMed PMID: 21501435; PMCID: 3231891.

36. Imdad A, Yakoob MY, Bhutta ZA. The effect of folic acid, protein energy and multiple micronutrient supplements in pregnancy on stillbirths. BMC Pub Health. 2011;11(Suppl 3):S4. doi:10.1186/1471-2458-11-S3-S4 PubMed PMID: 21501455; PMCID: 3231910.

37. Imdad A, Yakoob MY, Bhutta ZA. Impact of maternal education about complementary feeding and provision of complementary foods on child growth in developing countries. BMC Pub Health. 2011;11(Suppl 3):S25. doi:10. 1186/1471-2458-11-S3-S25 PubMed PMID: 21501443; PMCID: 3231899.

38. Imdad A, Yakoob MY, Bhutta ZA. Effect of breastfeeding promotion interventions on breastfeeding rates, with special focus on developing countries. BMC Pub Health. 2011;11(Suppl 3):S24. doi:10.1186/1471-2458-11-S3-S24 PubMed PMID: 21501442; PMCID: 3231898.

39. Jabeen M, Yakoob MY, Imdad A, Bhutta ZA. Impact of interventions to prevent and manage preeclampsia and eclampsia on stillbirths. BMC Pub Health. 2011;11(Suppl 3):S6. doi:10.1186/1471-2458-11-S3-S6 PubMed PMID: 21501457; PMCID: 3231912.

40. Sapkota A, Chelikowsky A, Nachman K, Cohen A, Ritz B. Exposure to particulate matter and adverse birth outcomes: a comprehensive review and meta-analysis. Air Qual Atmos Health. 2012;5(4):369–81. doi:10.1007/ s11869-010-0106-3.

41. Black RE, Victora CG, Walker SP, Bhutta ZA, Christian P, de Onis M, Ezzati M, Grantham-McGregor S, Katz J, Martorell R, Uauy R, Maternal, Child Nutrition Study G. Maternal and child undernutrition and overweight in low-income and middle-income countries. Lancet. 2013;382(9890):427–51. Doi:10.1016/S0140-6736(13)60937-X (PubMed PMID: 23746772).

42. Maulik D. Fetal growth restriction: the etiology. Clin Obstet Gynecol. 2006;49(2):228–35 PubMed PMID: 16721103.

43. Goldenberg RL, Culhane JF, Iams JD, Romero R. Epidemiology and causes of preterm birth. Lancet. 2008;371 (9606):75–84. Doi:10.1016/S0140-6736(08)60074-4 (PubMed PMID: 18177778).

44. Rasmussen S, Irgens LM. The effects of smoking and hypertensive disorders on fetal growth. BMC Pregnancy Childbirth. 2006;6:16. doi:10.1186/1471-2393-6-16 PubMed PMID: 16630351; PMCID: 1463005.

45. Kanda E, Matsuda Y, Makino Y, Matsui H. Risk factors associated with altered fetal growth in patients with pregestational diabetes mellitus. J Matern-Fetal Neonatal Med. 2012;25(8):1390–4. doi:10.3109/14767058.2011. 636096 PubMed PMID: 22070854.

46. Goetzinger KR, Cahill AG, Macones GA, Odibo AO. The relationship between maternal body mass index and tobacco use on small-for-gestational-age infants. Am J Perinatol. 2012;29(3):153–8. doi:10.1055/s-0031-1284224 PubMed PMID: 21786218; PMCID: 3629943.

47. Suter MA, Anders AM, Aagaard KM. Maternal smoking as a model for environmental epigenetic changes affecting birthweight and fetal programming. Mol Hum Reprod. 2013;19(1):1–6. doi:10.1093/molehr/gas050 PubMed PMID: 23139402; PMCID: 3521486.

48. Suter MA, Aagaard K. What changes in DNA methylation take place in individuals exposed to maternal smoking in utero? Epigenomics. 2012;4(2):115–8. doi:10.2217/epi.12.7 PubMed PMID: 22449181.

49. Jauniaux E, Van Oppenraaij RH, Burton GJ. Obstetric outcome after early placental complications. Curr Opin Obstet Gynecol. 2010;22(6):452–7. doi:10.1097/GCO.0b013e3283404e44 PubMed PMID: 20930630.

50. Vik T, Vatten L, Jacobsen G, Bakketeig LS. Prenatal growth in symmetric and asymmetric small-for-gestational-age infants. Early Human Dev. 1997;48(1–2):167–76 PubMed PMID: 9131317.

51. Maulik D. Fetal growth compromise: definitions, standards, and classification. Clin Obstet Gynecol. 2006;49 (2):214–8 PubMed PMID: 16721101.

52. Frøen JF, Arnestad M, Vege A, Irgens LM, Rognum TO, Saugstad OD, Stray-Pedersen B. Comparative epidemiology of sudden infant death syndrome and sudden intrauterine unexplained death. Arch Dis Child Fetal Neonatal Ed. 2002;87(2):F118–21 (PubMed PMID: 12193518; PMCID: 1721465).

53. McIntire DD, Bloom SL, Casey BM, Leveno KJ. Birth weight in relation to morbidity and mortality among newborn infants. N Engl J Med. 1999;340(16):1234–8. doi:10.1056/NEJM199904223401603 PubMed PMID: 10210706.

54. Gortner L, Reiss I, Hilgendorff A. Bronchopulmonary dysplasia and intrauterine growth restriction. Lancet. 2006;368(9529):28. doi:10.1016/S0140-6736(06)68964-2 PubMed PMID: 16815375.

55. Chauhan SP, Beydoun H, Chang E, Sandlin AT, Dahlke JD, Igwe E, Magann EF, Anderson KR, Abuhamad AZ, Ananth CV. Prenatal detection of fetal growth restriction in newborns classified as small for gestational age: correlates and risk of neonatal morbidity. Am J Perinatol. 2014;31(3):187–94. doi:10.1055/s-0033-1343771 PubMed PMID: 23592315.

56. Pelletier DL. The potentiating effects of malnutrition on child mortality: epidemiologic evidence and policy implications. Nutr Rev. 1994;52(12):409–15 PubMed PMID: 7898782.

57. Christian P, Lee SE, Donahue Angel M, Adair LS, Arifeen SE, Ashorn P, Barros FC, Fall CH, Fawzi WW, Hao W, Hu G, Humphrey JH, Huybregts L, Joglekar CV, Kariuki SK, Kolsteren P, Krishnaveni GV, Liu E, Martorell R, Osrin D, Persson LA, Ramakrishnan U, Richter L, Roberfroid D, Sania A, Ter Kuile FO, Tielsch J, Victora CG, Yajnik CS, Yan H, Zeng L, Black RE. Risk of childhood undernutrition related to small-for-gestational age and preterm birth in low- and middle-income countries. Int J Epidemiol. 2013;42 (5):1340–55. doi:10.1093/ije/dyt109 PubMed PMID: 23920141; PMCID: 3816349.

58. Barker DJ. The fetal and infant origins of adult disease. BMJ. 1990;301(6761):1111 (PubMed PMID: 2252919; PMCID: 1664286).

59. Eriksson JG, Forsen T, Tuomilehto J, Osmond C, Barker DJ. Early growth and coronary heart disease in later life: longitudinal study. BMJ. 2001;322(7292):949–53 (PubMed PMID: 11312225; PMCID: 31033).

60. Richter LM, Victora CG, Hallal PC, Adair LS, Bhargava SK, Fall CH, Lee N, Martorell R, Norris SA, Sachdev HS, Stein AD, Group C. Cohort profile: the consortium of health-orientated research in transitioning societies. Int J Epidemiol. 2012;41(3):621–6. Doi:10.1093/ije/dyq251 (PubMed PMID: 21224276; PMCID: 3378468).

61. Victora CG, Barros FC. Cohort profile: the 1982 Pelotas (Brazil) birth cohort study. Int J Epidemiol. 2006;35 (2):237–42. doi:10.1093/ije/dyi290 PubMed PMID: 16373375.

62. Stein AD, Melgar P, Hoddinott J, Martorell R. Cohort profile: the Institute of Nutrition of Central America and Panama (INCAP) nutrition trial cohort study. Int J Epidemiol. 2008;37(4):716–20. doi:10.1093/ije/dyn028 PubMed PMID: 18285366.

63. Bhargava SK, Sachdev HS, Fall CH, Osmond C, Lakshmy R, Barker DJ, Biswas SK, Ramji S, Prabhakaran D, Reddy KS. Relation of serial changes in childhood body-mass index to impaired glucose tolerance in young adulthood. N Engl J Med. 2004;350(9):865–75. doi:10.1056/NEJMoa035698 PubMed PMID: 14985484; PMCID: 3408694.

64. Adair LS. Size at birth and growth trajectories to young adulthood. Am J Hum Biol. 2007;19(3):327–37. doi:10. 1002/ajhb.20587 PubMed PMID: 17421008.

65. Richter L, Norris S, Pettifor J, Yach D, Cameron N. Cohort profile: Mandela's children: the 1990 birth to twenty study in South Africa. Int J Epidemiol. 2007;36(3):504–11. doi:10.1093/ije/dym016 PubMed PMID: 17355979; PMCID: 2702039.

66. Stein AD, Barros FC, Bhargava SK, Hao W, Horta BL, Lee N, Kuzawa CW, Martorell R, Ramji S, Stein A, Richter L, Consortium of health-orientated research in transitioning societies. Birth status child growth adult outcomes low- middle-income countries. J Pediatr 2013;163(6):1740–6. Doi:10.1016/j.jpeds.2013.08.012 (PubMed PMID: 24064150; PMCID: 3849851).

67. Eriksson J, Forsen T, Tuomilehto J, Osmond C, Barker D. Fetal and childhood growth and hypertension in adult life. Hypertension. 2000;36(5):790–4 PubMed PMID: 11082144.
68. Fall CH. Fetal programming and the risk of noncommunicable disease. Indian J Pediatr. 2013;80(Suppl 1):S13–20. doi:10.1007/s12098-012-0834-5 PubMed PMID: 22829248; PMCID: 3793300.
69. Lee PA, Houk CP. Cognitive and psychosocial development concerns in children born small for gestational age. Pediatr Endocrinol Rev PER. 2012;10(2):209–16 PubMed PMID: 23539832.
70. De Bie HM, Oostrom KJ, Delemarre-van de Waal HA. Brain development, intelligence and cognitive outcome in children born small for gestational age. Hormon Res Paediatr. 2010;73(1):6–14. doi:10.1159/000271911 PubMed PMID: 20190535.
71. Westwood M, Kramer MS, Munz D, Lovett JM, Watters GV. Growth and development of full-term nonasphyxiated small-for-gestational-age newborns: follow-up through adolescence. Pediatrics. 1983;71(3):376–82 PubMed PMID: 6828344.
72. Viggedal G, Lundalv E, Carlsson G, Kjellmer I. Neuropsychological follow-up into young adulthood of term infants born small for gestational age. Med Sci Monit Int Med J Exp Clin Res. 2004;10(1):CR8–16 (PubMed PMID: 14704630).
73. Fitzhardinge PM, Steven EM. The small-for-date infant II. Neurol Intellect Sequelae Pediatr. 1972;50(1):50–7 PubMed PMID: 5038108.
74. Paz I, Gale R, Laor A, Danon YL, Stevenson DK, Seidman DS. The cognitive outcome of full-term small for gestational age infants at late adolescence. Obstet Gynecol. 1995;85(3):452–6 PubMed PMID: 7862391.
75. Paz I, Laor A, Gale R, Harlap S, Stevenson DK, Seidman DS. Term infants with fetal growth restriction are not at increased risk for low intelligence scores at age 17 years. J Pediatr. 2001;138(1):87–91. doi:10.1067/mpd.2001.110131 PubMed PMID: 11148518.
76. Strauss RS, Dietz WH. Growth and development of term children born with low birth weight: effects of genetic and environmental factors. J Pediatr. 1998;133(1):67–72 PubMed PMID: 9672513.
77. Strauss RS. Adult functional outcome of those born small for gestational age: twenty-six-year follow-up of the 1970 British Birth Cohort. JAMA. 2000;283(5):625–32 PubMed PMID: 10665702.
78. O'Keeffe MJ, O'Callaghan M, Williams GM, Najman JM, Bor W. Learning, cognitive, and attentional problems in adolescents born small for gestational age. Pediatrics. 2003;112(2):301–7 PubMed PMID: 12897278.
79. Theodore RF, Thompson JM, Waldie KE, Becroft DM, Robinson E, Wild CJ, Clark PM, Mitchell EA. Determinants of cognitive ability at 7 years: a longitudinal case-control study of children born small-for-gestational age at term. Eur J Pediatr. 2009;168(10):1217–24. doi:10.1007/s00431-008-0913-9 PubMed PMID: 19165501.
80. Kulseng S, Jennekens-Schinkel A, Naess P, Romundstad P, Indredavik M, Vik T, Brubakk AM. Very-low-birthweight and term small-for-gestational-age adolescents: attention revisited. Acta Paediatr. 2006;95(2):224–30. doi:10.1080/08035250500421568 PubMed PMID: 16449031.
81. Harvey D, Prince J, Bunton J, Parkinson C, Campbell S. Abilities of children who were small-for-gestational-age babies. Pediatrics. 1982;69(3):296–300 PubMed PMID: 7199704.
82. Sommerfelt K, Andersson HW, Sonnander K, Ahlsten G, Ellertsen B, Markestad T, Jacobsen G, Hoffman HJ, Bakketeig L. Cognitive development of term small for gestational age children at five years of age. Arch Dis Child. 2000;83(1):25–30 (PubMed PMID: 10868995; PMCID: 1718382).
83. Sommerfelt K, Sonnander K, Skranes J, Andersson HW, Ahlsten G, Ellertsen B, Markestad T, Jacobsen G, Hoffman HJ, Bakketeig LS. Neuropsychologic and motor function in small-for-gestation preschoolers. Pediatr Neurol. 2002;26(3):186–91 PubMed PMID: 11955924.
84. McCarton CM, Wallace IF, Divon M, Vaughan HG Jr. Cognitive and neurologic development of the premature, small for gestational age infant through age 6: comparison by birth weight and gestational age. Pediatrics. 1996;98(6 Pt 1):1167–78 PubMed PMID: 8951271.
85. Gutbrod T, Wolke D, Soehne B, Ohrt B, Riegel K. Effects of gestation and birth weight on the growth and development of very low birthweight small for gestational age infants: a matched group comparison. Arch Dis Child Fetal Neonatal Ed. 2000;82(3):F208–14 (PubMed PMID: 10794788; PMCID: 1721075).
86. Feldman R, Eidelman AI. Neonatal state organization, neuromaturation, mother-infant interaction, and cognitive development in small-for-gestational-age premature infants. Pediatrics. 2006;118(3):e869–78. doi:10.1542/peds.2005-2040 PubMed PMID: 16880249.
87. Sung IK, Vohr B, Oh W. Growth and neurodevelopmental outcome of very low birth weight infants with intrauterine growth retardation: comparison with control subjects matched by birth weight and gestational age. J Pediatr. 1993;123(4):618–24 PubMed PMID: 7692029.
88. Lundgren EM, Cnattingius S, Jonsson B, Tuvemo T. Intellectual and psychological performance in males born small for gestational age with and without catch-up growth. Pediatr Res. 2001;50(1):91–6. doi:10.1203/00006450-200107000-00017 PubMed PMID: 11420424.

89. Frisk V, Amsel R, Whyte HE. The importance of head growth patterns in predicting the cognitive abilities and literacy skills of small-for-gestational-age children. Dev Neuropsychol. 2002;22(3):565–93. doi:10.1207/S15326942DN2203_2 PubMed PMID: 12661971.

90. Tideman E, Marsal K, Ley D. Cognitive function in young adults following intrauterine growth restriction with abnormal fetal aortic blood flow. Ultrasound Obstet Gynecol. 2007;29(6):614–8. doi:10.1002/uog.4042 PubMed PMID: 17523158.

91. Hollo O, Rautava P, Korhonen T, Helenius H, Kero P, Sillanpaa M. Academic achievement of small-for-gestational-age children at age 10 years. Arch Pediatr Adolesc Med. 2002;156(2):179–87 PubMed PMID: 11814381.

92. Fattal-Valevski A, Leitner Y, Kutai M, Tal-Posener E, Tomer A, Lieberman D, Jaffa A, Many A, Harel S. Neurodevelopmental outcome in children with intrauterine growth retardation: a 3-year follow-up. J Child Neurol. 1999;14(11):724–7 PubMed PMID: 10593549.

93. Leitner Y, Fattal-Valevski A, Geva R, Eshel R, Toledano-Alhadef H, Rotstein M, Bassan H, Radianu B, Bitchonsky O, Jaffa AJ, Harel S. Neurodevelopmental outcome of children with intrauterine growth retardation: a longitudinal, 10-year prospective study. J Child Neurol. 2007;22(5):580–7. doi:10.1177/0883073807302605 PubMed PMID: 17690065.

94. Geva R, Eshel R, Leitner Y, Fattal-Valevski A, Harel S. Memory functions of children born with asymmetric intrauterine growth restriction. Brain Res. 2006;1117(1):186–94. doi:10.1016/j.brainres.2006.08.004 PubMed PMID: 16962082.

95. Geva R, Eshel R, Leitner Y, Valevski AF, Harel S. Neuropsychological outcome of children with intrauterine growth restriction: a 9-year prospective study. Pediatrics. 2006;118(1):91–100. doi:10.1542/peds.2005-2343 PubMed PMID: 16818553.

96. Geva R, Eshel R, Leitner Y, Fattal-Valevski A, Harel S. Verbal short-term memory span in children: long-term modality dependent effects of intrauterine growth restriction. J Child Psychol Psychiatry Allied Disciplines. 2008;49(12):1321–30. doi:10.1111/j.1469-7610.2008.01917.x PubMed PMID: 19120711.

97. Silva PA, McGee R, Williams S. A longitudinal study of the intelligence and behavior of preterm and small for gestational age children. J Dev Behav Pediatr JDBP. 1984;5(1):1–5 PubMed PMID: 6699178.

98. Torche F, Echevarria G. The effect of birthweight on childhood cognitive development in a middle-income country. Int J Epidemiol. 2011;40(4):1008–18. doi:10.1093/ije/dyr030 PubMed PMID: 21362701.

99. Li H, Barnhart HX, Stein AD, Martorell R. Effects of early childhood supplementation on the educational achievement of women. Pediatrics. 2003;112(5):1156–62 PubMed PMID: 14595062.

100. Li H, DiGirolamo AM, Barnhart HX, Stein AD, Martorell R. Relative importance of birth size and postnatal growth for women's educational achievement. Early Hum Dev. 2004;76(1):1–16 PubMed PMID: 14729158.

101. Helgertz J, Vagero D. Small for gestational age and adulthood risk of disability pension: the contribution of childhood and adulthood conditions. Soc Sci Med. 2014;119:249–57. doi:10.1016/j.socscimed.2013.11.052 PubMed PMID: 24423878.

Chapter 24
Developmental Disabilities

Burris R. Duncan, Jennifer G. Andrews, Heidi L. Pottinger and F. John Meaney

Keywords Disability · Developmental disability · Prevalence · Genes and environment · Prevention · Social policies · Nutrition and development · Morbidity and mortality · Socioeconomic factors

Learning Objectives

- Define the difference between disabilities and developmental disabilities.
- Identify the etiologic factors that might influence the prevalence of developmental disabilities in low-income and middle-income countries (LMICs).
- Identify some of the genetic and environmental factors that contribute to the occurrence of developmental disabilities in LMICs.
- Describe the nutritional and dietary problems that children with developmental disabilities have and in particular the issues that confront these children in LMICs.
- Compare cultural factors that influence how developmental disabilities are perceived in LMICs and why this is an important consideration for planning and services provision.
- Assess the current status of health, education, employment, and social outcomes among children with developmental disabilities in LMICs.

B.R. Duncan (✉)
Health Promotion Sciences, Mel & Enid Zuckerman College of Public Health,
University of Arizona Health Sciences Center, 1295 N. Martin Ave., Tucson, AZ 85724, USA
e-mail: brduncan@email.arizona.edu

J.G. Andrews · F. John Meaney
Department of Pediatrics, University of Arizona, 1501 N Campbell Avenue, PO Box 245073
85724-5073 Tucson, AZ, USA
e-mail: jandrews@peds.arizona.edu

F. John Meaney
e-mail: fmeaney@email.arizona.edu

H.L. Pottinger
Health Promotion Sciences, Mel & Enid Zuckerman College of Public Health,
1295 N. Martin Ave., 85724 Tucson, AZ, USA
e-mail: heidip@email.arizona.edu

© Springer Science+Business Media New York 2017
S. de Pee et al. (eds.), *Nutrition and Health in a Developing World*,
Nutrition and Health, DOI 10.1007/978-3-319-43739-2_24

Introduction

Overview

This chapter defines developmental disabilities (DDs) as distinct from disabilities. The "Epidemiology" section discusses the epidemiology of DD in LMICs. Although prevalence data for DD in LMICs are still scarcely available, the past two decades have contributed improved estimates of the burden of DD in LMICs. The occurrence of DD in LMICs is likely greater than that in industrialized countries, but cultural perceptions and beliefs that tend to conceal DD and limited resources prevent collection of accurate data. The "Etiology of Developmental Disabilities" section highlights research in genetics and genomics and the dramatic influence of the interplay between genes and the environment. Increasing research on gene-environment interaction has the potential to improve prevention of DD. The "Nutritional Implications for Developmental Disabilities" section discusses nutritional implications for developmental disabilities in LMICs with emphasis on the tremendous influence poverty plays. The "Specific Considerations for Selected Developmental Disabilities" section describes a few selected DDs followed by feeding/nutritional problems particular to that developmental disability and the probable resultant growth deviants. The "Sociopolitical, Policies, and Conventions Adopted by Countries Regulations like Americans with Disabilities Act (ADA)" section discusses two conventions that have been signed by almost every country. Finally, the "Outcomes" section is devoted to morbidity and mortality of children with DD in LMICs, again emphasizing the influence a lack of resources has on their outcomes relative to education and employment.

Definition of Disabilities and Developmental Disabilities

Disability is a very broad term that is defined quite differently by different governmental agencies. Disability includes any impairment in an individual's ability to function; it may be physical, mental, or emotional, or any combination of these. Many types of chronic diseases and/or complications that develop from them may also qualify as a disability. Therefore, disability may be present at birth or may occur any time during a person's lifetime. The prevalence of disability increases with advancing age. Disability may include restriction in participation, and therefore, it not only describes the limitations a person's body may impose but also reflects features of the environment that limit unassisted participation. Thus, disability is a complex term.

The concept of "disability" has changed over time and continues to evolve. In earlier times and even today in some cultures, those who have a disability were shunned, neglected, or estranged from society. In the past several decades, there has been a dramatic shift away from using a medical model in viewing individuals with a disability toward using a functional model, and most recently, individuals with a disability are viewed from a social perspective. From a medical model, the disability is considered the result of a disease, trauma, or health condition that medicine can cure, fix, or at least ameliorate. The focus is on the condition of the individual. The basis of the disability is a derangement of anatomy, physiology, or biochemistry due to disease or damage. Individuals with disabilities are ill or are abnormal and must be treated or "fixed" by a care provider. The disability is viewed in categorical terms (i.e., multiple sclerosis, blindness, or heart disease), and social programs have been established purely based on categorical labels rather than the degree of severity or functional limitations. On the other hand, the functional model of disability focuses not on the particular diagnosis but instead on the individual's limitations or deficits. Regardless of what condition a person has, it is the degree of impairment that is most important; in effect, it is the degree to which function is interrupted or limited. It is the expression of the disability that is addressed, and thus, the approach is to improve functional capacity. This is the model incorporated and clearly stated in Section 223 of the US Social Security Act that defines disability as the "inability to engage in any substantial gainful activity by reason of any medically determinable physical or mental impairment" [1].

The social model diverts the attention from the individual and places the focus on the barriers in the environment that inhibit the ability of people to function without assistance. If the environment is made more accessible, the consequences of the medical condition or functional impairment are lessened. The social model includes social, physical, economic, and political dimensions. Removal of these barriers is difficult and often requires costly environmental modifications, policy changes, governmental financial outlays, employer acceptance, work-site adjustments and, the particularly important, but difficult, shift in public perception and ideally the acceptance and respect of diversity.

The American with Disabilities Act (ADA) is one of only very few pieces of legislation worldwide based on the social model of disabilities [2]. This act provides equal protection for employment, access to state and local governmental programs and services, and access to services of private businesses that are open to the public. The ADA definition of disability emphasizes limitations of function of daily life activities such as seeing, hearing, speaking, walking, breathing, and performing manual tasks, learning, caring for oneself, and working. It encompasses those where the limitation is currently or previously present and includes individuals who do not consider themselves disabled but whom others may regard as having limited functional abilities. This last inclusion addresses the perceptions of others based on a person's outward appearance, not on what functional abilities the individual may actually have.

These three different models of disabilities are germane to how individuals with disabilities are cared for in countries where resources are limited. For example, a child with a categorical diagnosis of cerebral palsy (CP) may have only minimal impairments (awkward skipping or jumping) to severe functional limitations (unable to care for any self-needs and requires around-the-clock total care that may include gastrostomy feedings). The medical "fix it" approach varies tremendously from virtually doing nothing, which may be based on a cultural belief system or limited resources, to extensive surgical interventions where cultural norms are different and where resources are plentiful, either from the family or from the state. The functional approach is to administer physical and occupational therapies and bracing with ankle and/or foot orthotics. The aspects of the social model are addressed through environmental changes such as ramps, toilet stalls sufficient to accommodate a wheelchair, and societal promotion of acceptance and respect of diversity.

Few families can afford the expense of caring for the child with severe CP and hence depend on governmental aid for in-house assistance and environmental alterations. Low- and low-middle-income countries cannot afford to utilize scarce resources on a few when the needs of so many are great. Hence, most of these countries address disabilities using a medical or functional model. The social model will only be incorporated when the political will supports it and economic circumstances allow it.

The concept of developmental disability (DD) is defined more narrowly. In the US Developmental Disabilities Assistance and Bill of Rights Act of 2000, DD is defined as a severe, chronic disability that can be mental or physical or a combination of the two; that manifests itself prior to age 22, is likely to be permanent, and results in a substantial limitation in three or more of the specific areas (self-care, receptive and expressive language, learning, mobility, self-direction, capacity for independent living, and economic self-sufficiency); and that requires a combination of interdisciplinary services for an extended period of time that may be lifelong [3].

Despite the shift in models of disability and the general agreement that both medical and social determinants should be included, the measurement of disabilities continues to be predominately medical with a focus on physical and mental impairments. Just as different agencies in the USA use different definitions of disabilities, so do other countries. The World Health Organization (WHO) developed an International Classification of Functioning Disability and Health (ICF) [4]. This classification views disability based on the body's structure and function in terms of the person's activity and participation in society while also considering the environment in which the person functions. The ICF was originally designed for adults, but then the WHO developed a corollary system for children termed: International Classification of Functioning Disability and Health for Children and Youth (ICF-CY) [5].

Epidemiology

Prevalence of Developmental Disabilities in Low-Income and Middle-Income Countries (LMICs)

Data on the prevalence of DD among children in LMICs are essential for developing prevention policies, allocating resources, and improving the quality of life for individuals with DD [6]. Yet prevalence data are still in scarce supply for LMICs, even almost 15 years since Durkin published a review on the epidemiology of DD in low-income countries that included an evaluation of the state of prevalence studies at that time [7]. We will use Durkin's review as a beginning and then briefly update the progress in obtaining prevalence data of DD in LMICs. All prevalence data are summarized in Table 24.1.

Durkin made a point of stating that prevalence of DD in low-income countries would be expected to be lower than that in other countries since mortality in infants with birth defects and children with DD is high [7]. She then went on to summarize studies in low-income countries reporting overall DD prevalence and condition-specific prevalence of intellectual disabilities (IDs), seizure disabilities, and other disabilities. In one comparative study using the same study design in several countries, a wide range of prevalence for serious non-sensory disabilities (serious cognitive, motor, or seizure disabilities) among children 2–9 years of age was observed, from a low of 0.8% among children in Bangladesh to 1.9% in Jamaica and 3.1% in Pakistan [8]. For serious ID, the estimated prevalence in low-income countries considered by Durkin in 2002 among children ranging from 0 to 15 years was consistently above 0.5% the only exception being the 0.29% reported for Beijing [7]. With respect to seizure disorders, Durkin reported prevalence of epilepsy in children ranging from 0.6 to 1.5% based on the data available from studies at that time [7]. Concerning other disabilities in children, Durkin's evaluation demonstrated there were few data on vision, hearing, and motor disabilities and concluded that prevalence studies on behavior disabilities such as autism and attention deficit/hyperactivity disorder (ADHD) had not been done.

It is fair to say that prevalence data on overall disability among children in LMICs are more readily available now than 15 years ago, but methods of data collection still vary widely and there is a dearth of prevalence data on specific developmental disorders. In the most comprehensive review of childhood disability in LMICs through 2007, the prevalence ranged from 0.4% in Bahrain to 12.7% in India (low-income strata) among 8 cross-sectional studies reporting overall disability in children [9]. Some more recent studies obtained similar prevalence data. For example, the World Report on Disability reported prevalence of combined moderate and severe disability in 0–14-year-olds ranging from 4.2 to 6.4% across World Health Organization regions [10]. Two additional studies in rural Africa and rural Pakistan present prevalence of disability at 6% among children <10 years of age and 0.5% among children 0–5 years of age [11, 12].

Other recent investigations have attempted to apply validated methods of data collection on disabilities in multiple settings [6, 13]. Gottlieb and coinvestigators applied the 3rd round of the Multiple Indicator Cluster Survey, which includes the Ten Questions Screen (TQS) (Table 24.2) for disability, in a study that included over 191,000 children aged 2–9 years living in 18 LMICs and found a median prevalence of 23% for those screening positive for the presence of a disability [13].

Table 24.1 Published prevalence of developmental disabilities (DDs) in low- and middle-income countries (LMICs)

Publication	Case finding method	Source of data	Data collection period	Ages (years)	Surveillance population	Number LMIC	Developmental disability included	Prevalence (%)[a]
Durkin et al. [8]	Population-based household caregiver survey	Survey + clinical evaluation	1987–1989	2–9	22,125	3[b]	Any non-sensory disability	0.8–3.1
Couper [1]	Population-based household caregiver survey	Survey + clinical evaluation	n.d.	0–9	2036	1[b]	Any DD	6
Maulik and Darmstadt [9]	Varied (systematic review)	Varied	1990–2004[c]	Varied 0–19	154,416	8	Any DD	0.4–12.7
Gottlieb et al. [13]	Population-based household caregiver survey	MICS3 – TQ[d]	2005–2006	2–9	191,199	18	Any DD	23 (3–48)
WHO, World Report on Disability [10]	Population-based household caregiver survey	World Health Survey and global burden of diseases	2002–2004	0–14	Not reported	59[e]	GBD composite disability score	4.2–6.4
Ibrahim and Bhutta [12]	Population-based household caregiver survey	Survey + clinical evaluation	2005	0–5	32,204	1[b]	Any DD	0.5
Bornstein and Hendricks [6]	Population-based household caregiver survey	MICS3 – TQ[d]	2005–2006	2–9	101,250	16	Any DD	20.4 (3.1–45.2)
Elsabbagh et al. [16]	Varied (systematic review)	Varied	1992–2009[c]	Varied 0–14	341,283	3	Autism spectrum disorder	0.1–0.2
Elsabbagh et al. [16]	Varied (systematic review)	Varied	2008–2012[c]	Varied 1–12	1,323,017	4	Pervasive developmental disorders	0.1–1.1
Couper [11]	Population-based household caregiver survey	Survey + clinical evaluation	n.d.	0–9	2036	1[b]	Cerebral palsy	1

(continued)

Table 24.1 (continued)

Publication	Case finding method	Source of data	Data collection period	Ages (years)	Surveillance population	Number LMIC	Developmental disability included	Prevalence (%)[a]
Gladstone [14]	Population-based	Clinical evaluation	1997–2004	0–19	405,171	2	Cerebral palsy	0.2–0.3
Ibrahim and Bhutta [12]	Population-based household caregiver survey	Survey + clinical evaluation	2005	0–5	10,464	1[b]	Cerebral palsy	0.1
Mendizabal and Salguero [15]	WHO standard questionnaire and neurological examination	Parent or individual report	n.d.	0–19	1882	1[b]	Epilepsy	0.6
Couper [11]	Population-based household caregiver survey	Survey + clinical evaluation	n.d.	0–9	2036	1[b]	Epilepsy	0.4
Durkin [7]	Varied (systematic review)	Varied	1982–1992[c]	Children	Not reported	>6[b]	Epilepsy	0.6–1.5
Durkin [7]	Varied (systematic review)	Varied	1981–1998[c]	Varied 0–15	Not reported	5[b]	Intellectual disability	0.3–2.4

[a]The prevalence is indicated or the median prevalence if data are from >1 study; otherwise, the range among studies is indicated. We chose to report the prevalence as percentage for ease of interpretation. For reference, 0.1% is 1 in 1000 children studied

[b]Data are from low-income countries only

[c]Dates of published articles in lieu of data collection periods for systematic reviews

[d]Refers to Multiple Indicator Cluster Survey third round (2005–2006), a household survey program developed by UNICEF, and Ten Questions disability module, developed as part of the International Pilot Study of Severe Childhood Disability

[e]Includes high-income countries in count but not in estimate

Table 24.2 The Ten Questions Screen (TQS) for childhood disabilities in children aged 2–9 years[a]

The Ten Questions Screen for childhood disabilities
1. Compared with other children, did the child have any serious delay in sitting, standing, or walking?
2. Compared with other children, does the child have difficulty seeing, either in the daytime or at night?
3. Does the child appear to have difficulty hearing?
4. When you tell the child to do something, does he/she seem to understand what you are saying?
5. Does the child have difficulty in walking or moving his/her arms or does he/she have weakness and/or stiffness in the arms or legs?
6. Does the child sometimes have fits, become rigid, or lose consciousness?
7. Does the child learn to do things like other children his/her age?
8. Does the child speak at all (can he/she make himself/herself understood in words; can he/she say any recognizable words)?
9. For 3–9-year-olds ask:
Is the child's speech in any way different from normal (not clear enough to be understood by people other than his/her immediate family)?
9. For 2-year-olds ask:
Can he/she name at least one object (e.g., an animal, a toy, a cup, and a spoon)?
10. Compared with other children of his/her age, does the child appear in any way mentally backward, dull, or slow?

[a]Stein et al. [131]

The questionnaire screened for functional limitations in the domains of speech, cognition, hearing, vision, seizures, and motor disorders. The indicator for disability was based on the household screening of the parents' perceptions of their child using the TQS, which was adapted for use in resource-poor settings.

Utilizing the same TQS, Bornstein and Hendricks reported data on more than 101,000 children aged 2–9 years living in 16 developing countries [6]. The percentage of children who screened positive for at least one disability was 20.4% across all countries, with a range of 3.1% for Uzbekistan to 45.2% for the Central African Republic.

With respect to individual developmental disorders, we chose to focus first on CP and epilepsy since there are a reasonable number of studies across various ages that report prevalence for these disorders. With respect to CP, the reported prevalence ranged among three studies in LMICs from 0.1 to 1.0% [11, 12, 14]. The low of 0.1% was reported for 0–5-year-olds in a rural area of Pakistan [12] and the high of 1.0% among children <10 years of age in rural KwaZulu-Natal, South Africa [11]. A review of data on CP from resource-poor settings worldwide included a prevalence of 0.3% among over 388,000 children 0–7 years of age in China during 1997 and 0.2% among almost 17,000 children aged 0–19 years in India during 2003–2004 [14].

The prevalence of epilepsy has been reported at similar levels to CP in three studies [7, 11, 15]. The prevalence estimates are related to the ages reported in these studies. They range from 0.4% for seizure disorders in children <10 years of age in KwaZulu-Natal [11] through 0.6% for active epilepsy among children 0–19 years of age in a rural community of Guatemala [15] to 1.5% as the upper range of prevalence reported by Durkin in 2002 for low-income countries [7].

Interest in autism has risen in recent years as data indicate that the prevalence is higher than it was thought to be in the past. But what data exist for LMICs concerning the prevalence of autism? The most recent review of prevalence data worldwide indicates there are no data yet available for any low-income countries [16]. However, the same report indicates that several studies exist for middle-income countries. Estimates are reported for pervasive developmental disorders (PDDs) in 4 middle-income countries and for autistic disorder in 3 middle-income countries. For PDD, estimates ranged from a low of <0.1% in a country-wide study of children age 5 years conducted in Iran and published in 2012 to a high of 1.1% for children 1.5–2.0 years of age in a semiurban area of Sri Lanka published in 2009 [16]. Interestingly, the estimate from Sri Lanka is somewhat higher than that reported in the same year by the Centers for Disease Control and Prevention (CDC) for 11 surveillance sites in the USA, which was 0.9% [16]. The data for autistic disorder do not show as much variance as those for PDD. Prevalence estimates for autistic disorder include 0.1% in a 1992 study that included 5120 children ages 4–7 years in Indonesia and 0.2% in a study published in 2008 including almost 255,000 children ages 3–9 years living in Venezuela [16]. The study by Elsabbagh and colleagues also reported data for 9 studies in China published from 2000 to 2009. The Chinese studies were consistent with each other despite the different diagnostic criteria that were utilized, reporting prevalence of autistic disorder at 0.1–0.2% [16].

Why the Discrepancies

Data on the prevalence of disabilities are scanty in low- and low-middle-income countries, and the results are dependent on the questions asked, who they are asked of, and the way they are asked by the interviewer and interpreted by the respondent. In some societies, children with disabilities are kept at home and parents do not disclose their conditions, and hence, they may not be reported. Surveys that are done through the schools miss many of the children with DD as many do not attend school. But if they do, the staff may not recognize the disability and do not report anything. These factors are potential contributors to underestimation of prevalence in LMICs.

The TQS was originally designed to improve data collection on disabilities worldwide and be applied across cultures and national boundaries. It has been used widely and validated in multiple studies as a method of screening for serious childhood disabilities [13]. What is clear in recent studies that have applied the TQS methodology is that the percent of children screening positive for a disability varies widely among participating countries [6, 13]. We still do not understand how much of this variation represents real population differences and how much reflects the influence of factors such as those described above. It must be emphasized again that the TQS is a screening tool and, therefore, not diagnostic, i.e., children who screen positive have an increased risk of having a disability [6]. Thus, the prevalence data using the TQS provide estimates of the potential needs in LMICs for resources and services to assist these children and their families.

Cultural Perceptions on Developmental Disability

Cultural perceptions on disability vary among and within societies and can contribute to variability in outcomes for individuals with disabilities. Higher income countries have changed their approach to disability in the last 50 years, and the World Health Organization (WHO) actively pursues an agenda to make all nations recognize and value the human rights and societal contributions of individuals with disabilities [10]. The goal is to change the existing cultural perceptions on disability that inform policy and interventional approaches.

The societal values propagated by cultural perceptions are rooted in the primary guiding principles that are fundamental to all aspects of any culture. These guiding principles can be classified into one of the three "Big Ethics" that emphasize the importance of autonomy, community, or divinity within that culture [17, 18]. These Big Three Ethics guide the development of concepts of justice, morality, and causality [17]. Embracing one ethic rather than another will drive individuals in that culture to value life differently and change their approach to issues such as children born with DD. These cultural values affect the types of prevention programs and early interventions that are implemented to change the developmental trajectories and outcomes for children with DD in LMICs [19]. These ethics are grounded in a societal value and belief system that propagates into multiple aspects of life, including health-related concerns. Understanding how to approach and initiate change within a culture requires an understanding of its central belief structure; the most salient approach to management of disease is to understand the cultural perceptions of justice, diversity, human value, and etiology.

Etiology

Cultural perceptions and the beliefs of disease etiology and health management have a direct impact on the types of policies and intervention programs that are or can be implemented in LMICs. Human beings will often rationalize negative events in their life by attempting to determine the cause or the source of blame to provide perspective or a reason for the "suffering" [18]. The manner in which disease etiology is rationalized is based on a cultural causal ontology drawn from the ethic driving that society's value and structure. One can summarize the health-related causal ontologies applied to the etiology of disease into four overarching groups: biomedical, personalistic, naturalistic, and moral source of suffering [18]. Western societies and medicine are heavily rooted in the biomedical ontology of disease etiology, rationalizing that there is a biological process or other material explanation for the incidence of the illness. Personalistic approaches intimate an identifiable and intentional source for the infliction, which could be the result of attacks on the individual performed by witches, ancestors, spirits, or deities. Naturalistic approaches relate to an "equilibrium" model wherein an action or element has caused an imbalance, which either needs to be corrected or has opened a path for the illness to enter [20]. Lastly, moral ontologies are rooted in the belief that illness is punishment or penance for behaviors of the individual affected. Many cultures operate with some combination of the four approaches. How a culture views the reason for developmental disability will substantially affect how that society will manage the diagnosis, prevention, and treatment of the condition, since cultural beliefs and societal values have been shown to affect adherence [21, 22] and the sustainability [23] of Western-based approaches to health care.

Interestingly, individuals are likely to seek biomedical intervention regardless of the perceived causal ontology applied to explain etiology in conjunction with other therapies [18]. Recognition, acceptance, and incorporation of cultural beliefs on disease etiology and disease management, including the involvement of traditional healers, in any approach to prevention and management of DD are critical to ensuring the success of any program or policy. Paying homage to cultural approaches into care management plans will increase adherence, enhance communication, and improve sustainability of prevention and intervention programs [24, 25].

Etiology of Developmental Disabilities

Genetics and Genomics

A decade ago, one textbook on the genetics of DD led to chapters introducing concepts, subfields, programs, and animal models in medical genetics followed by chapters on classical examples of various syndromes with DD and related topics, including ADHD and CP (see definitions in the "Specific Considerations for Selected Developmental Disabilities" section) [26]. It could be easily argued that every topic covered in that textbook has been dramatically influenced, if not changed, as the pace of discovery in genetics has been unprecedented since the completion of the Human Genome Project some dozen years ago. Some of the rapid development has been the result of innovations in technology, but the application of the technology in new ways to discover the genetic causes of DD has been equally impressive. We will only be able to offer a summary to highlight what this research has contributed to the field of DD.

According to one review, three major technical advances in molecular genetics and their application to identifying genes and genotyping individuals for these newly identified genes have contributed significantly to child development research since the late 1990s [27]. These include genome-wide association (GWA) studies, now the dominant method for "finding genes," as Plomin puts it, and for genotyping the use of microarrays and the relatively new technology of whole-genome sequencing. These same techniques have impacted research on the genetics of DD, exemplified by two recent reviews [28, 29]. Coe et al. [28] suggest there has been a convergence regarding the genetics of the multiple conditions that comprise neurodevelopmental disorders. According to Coe et al. [28], many of these conditions, such as autism, epilepsy, and intellectual disability, have evidence of high heritability (i.e., high estimated genetic variance), yet few specific gene variants are associated with them. So, as a consequence of this missing heritability problem, research has shifted to rarer forms of genetic variation like copy number variants (CNVs), to fill the gap. These CNVs occur when an individual has variable copy numbers of a genetic variant, even a small segment of DNA, compared to the reference number in the human genome. Some do not contribute to phenotypic variation, but others have been linked to human diseases, including DD. There is now ample evidence that large CNVs, although rare individually, but considered together relatively common, are shared across many neurodevelopmental disorders, some found in specific conditions and others shared among several conditions and other phenotypic conditions [28]. The sharing of specific genetic causes such as CNVs among conditions that have always been considered separate clinical entities, as well as the extensive co-occurrence of neurodevelopmental disorders, has led some to propose the concept of developmental brain dysfunction to describe the underlying basis of these conditions [29].

What are the implications of the current research in genetics and genomics for low- and middle-income countries (LMICs)? Since the causes of DD are quite heterogeneous, some have assumed in the past that environmental factors such as infectious diseases and suboptimal nutrition might outweigh the importance of genetic factors in low-income countries; however, as Durkin [7] states, the evidence suggests otherwise. If it is true that genetic factors in the etiology of DD are more common in LMICs than in other locations, it may very well have an environmental basis after all, as environmental exposures certainly have been implicated in de novo mutations and could interact with genetic causes such as CNVs during development.

Environmental Exposures

Almost fifteen years ago, a comprehensive review of the epidemiology of DD in low-income countries listed the especially relevant environmental risk factors under five categories: nutritional deficiencies, infectious diseases, environmental toxins, perinatal and neonatal factors, poverty and trauma, or combinations of those factors [7]. The global food crisis continues to be a major concern as a contributor to the occurrence of DD in LMICs [30]. Malnutrition is indicated by Durkin and Gottlieb [30] as both a causal and risk factor for DD, as we describe elsewhere in this chapter and as presented by other investigators [7, 9]. More recent reviews have emphasized the same environmental factors, but have stressed the effects on development associated with intrauterine growth restriction and stunting as well as psychosocial risk factors such as inadequate cognitive stimulation, maternal depression, and exposure to violence [31]. Others have emphasized the effects of maternal stress [19] and of poor hygiene and sanitation [32]. Studies have documented thoroughly the effects of environmental toxins such as lead, mercury, and polychlorinated biphenols on development and less so the effects of other heavy metals, solvents, and pesticides [32]. Their effects may be exacerbated in LMICs where there are fewer environmental regulations. For example, many pesticides that are banned in high-income countries are still being used in many LMICs [33].

Evidence for Gene-Environment Interactions

The concept of gene-environment interaction (GxE) has existed in genetics and been studied in plants and animals for many years, but only recently has it been investigated in human diseases. In terms of disease, a GxE is the contribution to variation in the risk of disease or some outcome of the disease in which the combination of an environmental factor, such as exposure to cigarette smoking, with a specific genetic factor, such as a disease-predisposing mutation or gene variant, results in significantly increased risk or severity for the disease in question. It has been proposed that there are historically two concepts of GxE, the first being the statistical measure of an interaction effect and the other being a concept that reflects the developmental process during which there is interplay between genes and environmental exposures [34]. Both concepts are important, as ultimately any demonstration of GxE statistically has to be studied more thoroughly in terms of development. There is ample evidence of what we will call "developmental thinking" in recent assessments of genetic and environmental factors in DD [35].

Ten years ago, one of us (FJM) predicted that research into gene-environment interaction and intellectual disability would be an area of major expansion during the next two decades [36]. Although we are just at the halfway point of the two decades, recent literature searches suggest the expansion has begun, albeit not at the fast pace of studies of gene-environment interaction in general. Figure 24.1 shows the dramatic increase by decade in the number of publications addressing GxE in contrast to the numbers for GxE combined with DD.

We are beginning to observe more attention to the hypothetical importance of GxE in specific DD, notably autism, as well as research studies demonstrating interactions [37]. A few recent studies have reported GxE interactions for autistic traits or risk of autism. One study reported GxE effects as a significant source of variation in autism spectrum disorder (ASD) symptoms among children with ADHD [38]. In this report, two specific genotypes, one for the catechol-*O*-methyltransferase gene and the other for the serotonin transporter gene, each interacted with maternal smoking during pregnancy to increase stereotyped behavior and increase problems in social interaction, respectively. Another study in northern California has reported evidence of gene x diet interactions with respect to autism risk [39]. Women who had not taken prenatal vitamins were found to have a greater chance of having a child with autism if the mothers had a specific genotype of the 5,10-methylenetetrahydrofolate reductase (MTHFR) gene which is involved in folate metabolism. In the same study, children with a specific genotype of a different gene, the catechol-*O*-methyltransferase gene, had a greater chance of developing autism if their mothers had not taken vitamins during pregnancy. The gene x diet interaction is shown in Fig. 24.2. Since there is evidence that the frequency of these mutations in the

Fig. 24.1 Increase in the number of publications on gene-environment interaction (GxE) for searches excluding neurodevelopmental disorders (NDDs) and searches including NDD only (blue line) by decade: 1950 through 2014

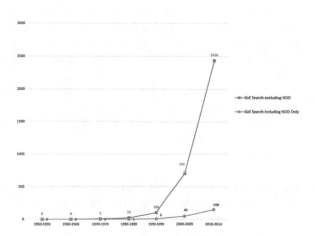

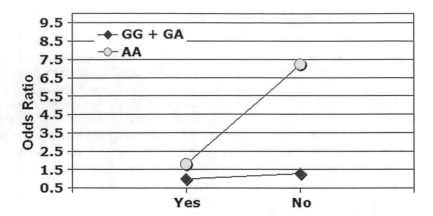

Fig. 24.2 Child genotypes for catechol-*O*-methyltransferase (COMT) 472 gene variants by maternal periconceptional prenatal vitamin intake and odds ratios for autism. *Source* Schmidt [39]. *Note* Children with genotype AA possess two copies of the catechol-*O*-methyltransferase (COMT) 472G>A variant that reduces the activity of this enzyme, which is involved in the metabolism of folate and associated metabolic processes. Children with GG and GA genotypes possess no copy or one copy of the gene variant, respectively, and comprise the reference group. "Yes" indicates mothers who had any reported vitamin intake for three months before pregnancy and first month of pregnancy, and "No" indicates those reporting no vitamin use

general population is high [39], some have hypothesized that the prevalence of autism could be increased in countries such as LMICs where there are problems with inadequate diets during pregnancy [40].

It is widely held that a phenotypic response of individuals with a particular genetic variant given specified environmental exposures does not predict with certitude what the response will be under different environmental conditions. This has important implications for LMICs, which might have populations with frequencies of genetic variants which confer susceptibility to disease and ranges of environmental exposures that dramatically vary from those in higher income countries. For this reason, studies of GxE for diseases might be even more important to conduct in populations of LMICs to provide new insights into the possible causal factors for many DD.

Evidence from Epigenetics/Epigenomics

Although we agree that being able to identify a statistical gene-environment interaction does lay the groundwork for investigations of the "causal-mechanical, biological interaction" that might underlie the statistical result [34], the field of epigenetics, and more recently epigenomics, developed independently to address some of the developmental aspects of interaction among genes and environmental exposures. The NIH "Roadmap Epigenomics Project" defines epigenetics and epigenomics as follows:

Epigenetics is an emerging frontier of science that involves the study of changes in the regulation of gene activity and expression that are not dependent on gene sequence. While epigenetics refers to the study of single genes or sets of genes, epigenomics refers to more global analyses of epigenetic changes across the entire genome [41].

Epigenetics relates to the previously mentioned developmental concept of gene-environment interaction because the sequence of environmental exposures during an individual's development has the potential to change DNA chemically as well as the proteins that are bound to the DNA, which can modify the expression of the gene. The role of epigenetics has been emphasized both in terms of complex disease, which encompasses most if not all DD, and in terms of neurodevelopmental disorders per se, as it involves mechanisms at the molecular level linking the effects of environmental exposures with how genes function [42].

The importance of epigenetics for understanding the basics of human development has been stressed [43], so it is expected that it will strongly impact research concerning DD. There is already increasing research concerning the involvement of epigenetics as a causal factor in neurodevelopmental disorders such as ASD and many syndromes involving ID [42]. Epilepsy is another DD for which epigenetic mechanisms have been implicated [44]. Ongoing research of epigenetic mechanisms involved in neurodevelopmental disorders should ultimately lead to the identification of therapeutic treatments for many of these conditions [42].

The Potential to Prevent Developmental Disabilities

One rationale for investigating GxE interactions is to increase our understanding of what kinds of prevention programs and interventions might work. Identification of GxE interaction can in turn specify the populations that are at higher risk of a disease as a result of having high frequencies of some gene conferring susceptibility to the disease. It also provides information on the environmental risk factors that could be modified through the reduction of specific environmental exposures. The ultimate aim is prevention of the disease in question or reduction in the severity of disease outcomes. A similar argument could be applied to epigenetic research.

One of the lessons of the GxE concept is that "one size might not fit all." We should always be wary that all children might not react favorable to some environmental interventions; the concept of GxE tells us that they will not. With respect to prevention, GxE findings can never offer a complete guide toward the prevention of DD in LMICs, but they do provide important insights. In light of the recent GxE results for autism [39], dietary strategies to ensure adequate intake of folate might be especially important in those LMICs where frequencies of the specific MTHFR gene variant are high.

There is a continuing optimism that a more complete understanding of genetic and environmental effects on human diseases and their interaction will lead to improved disease outcomes and prevention [36]. However, we obviously cannot wait for all the answers, especially given the complexities of DD and the great need for improved interventions. This is especially true in LMICs where resources are limited.

It is well recognized that implementation of programs in LMICs to prevent DD and provide interventions for those children identified with DD is one of immense proportions [45]. Some evaluations of the circumstances in LMICs have stressed that programs addressing early child development need to be systematically implemented across multiple systems in these countries, including the health and education systems as well as community-based organizations [19]. Perhaps the most comprehensive review on childhood disability in LMICs for children <5 years of age included 80 publications, equally divided between low- and middle-income countries [9]. Only a quarter of these publications provided information on prevention and promotion activities concerning disabilities, again about equally divided between low- and middle-income countries. The strategies identified in these studies covered the full range from primary to tertiary prevention and most used methods that could be applied in early childhood when the opportunities for successful intervention are optimal. The activities addressed most of the environmental risk factors addressed above, particularly diet and nutrition and infectious disease prevention. Among the primary prevention strategies identified were increased coverage for immunizations, national programs for dietary supplementation, and development of school meal programs, including preschool. Secondary prevention included increasing community awareness of DD and tertiary strategies focused on activities to improve mother-child interaction and improved education and training of children in need. However, this review in 2007 concluded there remained a tremendous gap in our knowledge about interventions in LMICs for childhood disability.

On a positive note, a team of investigators recently updated a previous review of interventions that assist in preventing adverse outcomes during early child development in LMICs [46]. The coauthors concluded that LMICs should invest in early childhood interventions to reduce loss of developmental potential that is perpetuated by the social and economic circumstances in LMICs. The most effective interventions were those involving support of parenting to promote parent-child interactions and enrollment in early child development or preschool programs. Unfortunately, the team found very few evaluations of interventions for children with DD in LMICs.

Nutritional Implications for Developmental Disabilities in LMICs

Undernutrition in Terms of Macronutrients

The nutritional status of a woman prior to and during pregnancy is of paramount importance for her to give birth to a full-term healthy neonate with a normal birth weight (greater than or equal to 2.5 kg) and without the risk of DD. For instance, poor weight gain during pregnancy doubles the odds of having a preterm birth (delivery prior to 37 weeks' gestation) and almost triples the odds of delivering a neonate with a low birth weight (LBW) (less than 2.5 kg) [47]. Malnutrition during pregnancy as defined by a mid-upper-arm circumference less than 23 cm is associated with adverse neonatal outcomes including preterm birth, small for gestational age (SGA), and intrauterine growth retardation (IUGR) [48, 49].

Malnutrition and poverty are coupled. Undernutrition during pregnancy results in a small neonate, and many of the micronutrient deficiencies also adversely affect the growing fetus and the newborn child. This is particularly detrimental to the brain as it undergoes a rapid rate of growth during the third trimester of gestation and in the early postnatal period. It is during this time that an adequate diet is essential for ensuring appropriate allocation of macro- and micronutrients to the developing brain. Insufficient nutrition during breast-feeding will compound the problem.

Both poverty and malnutrition are most prevalent in Africa and South Asia, regions that produce 52% of all live births and 60% of premature births, and it is in these regions where 75% of neonatal deaths occur. The number of premature births is 22% in East–Southeast Asia-Pacific, 28% in South Asia, and 24% in sub-Sahara Africa. In comparison, only 9% of births are premature in high-income countries. Of the 15 million premature births worldwide, an estimated 13 million survive the first month of life. Those who do survive are at a cognitive risk. The developing brain of the prematurely born infant is vulnerable to many potential insults including respiratory distress syndrome and hypoxia, hypoglycemia, hyper bilirubinemia, and infections. Prenatal malnutrition and its related insults place the premature newborn at an increased risk for developmental impairments. Of those who survive the neonatal period, 7% (900,000) will suffer long-term neurodevelopmental impairment and 2.6% (269,000–420,000) will suffer moderate or severe impairments [50]. The percent of worldwide survivors of prematurity diagnosed with severe neurodevelopmental impairments reaches 12% in high-income countries but is as high as 24% in East–Southeast Asia-Pacific, 25% in South Asia, and 19% in sub-Sahara Africa. The percent with mild impairments are 11, 23, 27, and 20% respectively [50]. Many of the studies Blencowe and colleagues reported demonstrate an association between preterm birth and specific learning and executive function impairments as well as adverse mental health outcomes [51]. The burden is great in LMICs, as an infant born prior to 37-week gestation has a 25% chance of having a severe neurological developmental impairment in SE Asia and a 19% chance in sub-Sahara Africa compared with a 12% chance if born in a high-income country [50].

As reported previously, Gottlieb and colleagues used the Ten Questions Screen in a study of almost 200,000 children aged 2–9 years living in 18 LMICs for their risk of a developmental disability [13]. The results were assessed according to four nutritional variables: breast-feeding, vitamin A supplementation, underweight (weight for age), and stunting (height for age). In all countries, children aged 2–4 who were ever breast-fed screened positive for a disability less frequently than those who were never breast-fed (26 and 36%, respectively). These values were significant in 8 of the 18 LMICs. In the ten countries that were included in the vitamin A analysis, supplementation of vitamin A was associated with a lower prevalence of disabilities among children who had ever received the supplementation versus those that had not (29% vs. 36%, respectively). The difference was significant in 5 of the 10 countries. The percentage of children with risk for a disability was greater for children who were underweight compared to those who were not (36 vs. 26%). These values were significant in 7 of the 15 LMICs. In 12 of 15 LMICs, children who were stunted had a slightly greater percentage of disability risk than those who were not stunted (26 vs. 25%). However, the range was large, and values were significant in only 5 of the 15 LMICs [13].

Food security in low-income households is an outward observable problem, but an underlying hidden condition is that of maternal depression and its impact on DD. Depression during pregnancy is detrimental to both the mother and the fetus, is associated with LBW and SGA, and predicts poorer growth in infants from 2 to 12 months of age [52, 53]. While prevalence rates of postnatal maternal depression (PMD) in high-income countries range from 7 to 13%, in some LMICs the range is between 20 and 30% (South Africa, Lebanon, Bangladesh, Turkey, Brazil, India, and Iran) and is even greater than 30% in some other LMICs. In Malawi, Pakistan, Zimbabwe, Vietnam, Chile, Burkina Faso, and Guyana, half of the women were found to be affected by PMD [54]. Risk factors for PMD include socioeconomic hardships such as food insecurity, overcrowding, lack of potable running water and electricity, and poor sanitation. A depressed mother has poor concentration, lethargy, sleep disturbance, and low mood. These symptoms play an important role in how the child is fed and affect both the quality and quantity of stimulation the child receives. A depressed mother is less likely to provide her child with adequate and appropriate nutrition resulting in poor growth. And mothers living in periurban informal settlements (slums) are more prone to depression, resulting in lack of stimulating play and, too often, inadequate nutritional intake for the newborn infant and young child at a time that is most critical for the rapidly growing brain [55]. Poor nutrition, poor growth, and inadequate stimulation in early childhood are associated with impairment of cognition as well as deficits in school performance and intellectual achievement [56, 57].

Risk factors for developmental delay are particularly prominent in people living in the rapidly growing urban slums as low birth weight is the single most important biological risk for developmental delay. In the slums of Dhaka, Bangladesh, 46% of the newborns are of low birth weight and 70% are small for gestational age. This is the direct influence of poor maternal nutrition and is compounded by a lack of prenatal care and maternal depression. The risk for DD is increased due to home deliveries by inadequately trained traditional birth attendants, who have little to no backup if problems arise. This situation puts the newborn at risk for asphyxia, hypothermia, hypoglycemia, and infections [58]. The Instituto de Nutrición de Centroamérica y Panamá (INCAP) studies in Guatemala demonstrate the impact that supplemental feeding programs have on pregnant women and young children by preventing the ravishes of malnutrition [59]. If malnutrition continues throughout childhood, thereby becoming a chronic condition, the result is stunting. This is particularly detrimental for females as a woman's height is directly proportional to the width of her pelvis [60] A narrow pelvis results in difficult labor and often a small or damaged newborn.

Undernutrition with Respect to Micronutrients

Many poor households do not have the financial resources to consume sufficient quantities of meat and dairy products and instead select less expensive plant source-based foods that are often high in phytate and fiber content that decrease the bioavailability of minerals, such as iron and zinc, increasing the risk of micronutrient deficiency for these essential elements. Over 2 billion people are at risk for deficiencies of vitamin A, iron, and/or iodine [56]. The highest prevalence of micronutrient deficiencies is in sub-Saharan Africa and Southeast Asia. All of these nutritional factors can result in either physical or cognitive developmental defects for their children. These poor health outcomes for women and children do not have to continue. Politicians and health professionals can do something about it, and it is imperative that we do so.

A lack of micronutrients in the maternal diet is detrimental to the growing fetus and also affects the quality of a mother's breast milk. Moreover, if the child's diet continues to be deficient, serious consequences result; often, the outcomes involve DD (Table 24.3).

Iron is not only important in hemoglobin synthesis and production of red blood cells carrying oxygen to the brain, but it is also involved in neurogenesis. Another micronutrient, iodine, is also essential for healthy fetal development. While a severe lack of iodine during pregnancy results in cretinism, a less severe deficiency results in hypothyroidism. Regardless, both types of iodine deficiencies result in irreparable damage to the brain and subsequent intellectual impairment that will persist into adulthood. Calcium is also important, not just for skeletal development and maintaining the integrity of cell membranes but is also necessary for transmission of nerve impulses and mediating muscle function. A lack of calcium is associated with pre-eclampsia and low birth weight infants. A deficiency in magnesium also interferes with fetal growth and hence is associated with intrauterine growth retardation (IUGR). Zinc activates over 100 enzymes, supports the immune system, and is

Table 24.3 Micronutrients, their biological function, and abnormalities leading to a disability when maternal deficiencies occur

Mineral	Function	Maternal deficiency results in
Iodine	Key component of thyroid hormone	Irreversible brain damage
Iron	Hemoglobin synthesis Neurogenesis Thyroid, dopamine	Poor fetal growth Cognitive and behavior problems that persist into adulthood despite treatment
Calcium	Development of skeleton Mediating muscle function Nerve impulse transmission Blood coagulation Cell membrane function Secretion of hormones	Associated with pre-eclampsia and low birth weight May induce intrauterine growth retardation (IUGR)
Copper[a]	Angiogenesis-impaired collagen and elastin cross-linking and therefore responsible for vessel integrity	Brain dysmorphology Vascular hemorrhage
Magnesium	Enzyme cofactor and activator	Interferes with fetal growth Hyperparathyroidism
Zinc	Activation of 100 enzymes Important for embryogenesis and fetal growth Supports immune system	Limits fetal growth If severe → teratogenesis
Selenium	Supports immune system	Associated with abortions, pre-eclampsia, and IUGR

(continued)

Table 24.3 (continued)

Vitamins	Function	Maternal deficiency results in
Vitamins A[b]	Maintenance of mucosal surfaces Cell differentiation and growth Immune system	Low birth weight in HIV-positive women Avoid high doses → teratogenicity—anomalies include [CV (aortic arch), CNS (microcephalia, microphthalmia), cleft palate, thymic hypoplasia, limb reduction]
B1	Coenzyme—lipid and nucleotide synthesis enzymes especially in developing brain	Impairs brain development Impairs fetal growth
B2 riboflavin[c]	Precursor for 2 flavin coenzymes (flavin mononucleotide and flavin adenine dinucleotide	Deficiency in pure form probably does not exist In animal studies, maternal deficiency results in shortened extremities, cleft palate, and hydrocephalus
B6	Coenzyme in protein metabolism especially in CNS	Associated with pre-eclampsia, gastrointestinal carbohydrate intolerance, and neurological diseases of infants
Folate[c]	Enzymatic role in carbon metabolism and synthesis of DNA	Pre-eclampsia, abortions, IUGR Congenital malformation as neural tube defects and congenital heart defects
B12[c]	Support for erythropoiesis	Reduced fetal growth
C and E	Powerful antioxidants	Oxidative stress, important factor for pre-eclampsia
D	Bone growth Immune function and reduction of inflammation	Associated with poor fetal skeletal growth

[a]Keen et al. [132]
[b]Simpson et al. [133]
[c]Rosenthal [134]

important for embryogenesis and fetal growth. A deficiency of selenium is associated with spontaneous abortions, pre-eclampsia, and IUGR.

Vitamins are also vital in fetal and postnatal development (Table 24.3). Vitamin A is important in cell differentiation and growth and maintains mucosal surfaces, whereas high doses are teratogenic. Vitamin B1 is a coenzyme and important in lipid and nucleotide synthesis enzymes, especially in the developing brain. A deficiency of vitamin B1 will impair fetal growth and brain development. Vitamin B6 is a coenzyme in protein metabolism especially in neurons in the central nervous system. A deficiency of vitamin B6 is associated with pre-eclampsia, gastrointestinal carbohydrate intolerance, and neurological deficits in infants. Folate plays an enzymatic role in carbon metabolism and synthesis of DNA, and a deficiency is associated with pre-eclampsia, abortions, IUGR, and congenital malformation such as neural tube defects and congenital heart defects. Vitamin B12 supports erythropoiesis and fetal growth. Vitamins C and E are powerful antioxidants and combat oxidative stress, an important factor in pre-eclampsia, and vitamin D is important in skeletal growth and immune function.

Micronutrient deficiencies can affect cognitive function in young children. A study from North India on children aged 12–18 months correlated plasma levels of several micronutrients with scores on the Bayley III Scales of Infant Development [61]. An increase in folate concentration was associated with a 1.3 times increase in their scores for mental development. The change was even more pronounced when cognitive scores were correlated with concentrations of homocysteine or methylmalonic acid [61]. Below follows a discussion of the effect of specific micronutrient deficiencies on fetal development. For further information on these micronutrients, the reader is encouraged to refer to the respective chapters in this volume.

Iron

Iron deficiency affects nearly 2 billion people or almost one-third of the world's population. The groups most affected by iron deficiency are pubescent women, pregnant women, infants, and children of preschool age. Iron deficiency is most prevalent in low-middle-income countries. In the WHO region of Africa, it affects 32% of children 6–59 months of age, 41% of non-pregnant women 15–49 years of age, and 44% of pregnant women 15–49 years of age. In SE Asia, the percentages are 41, 45, and 47 respectively [62]. Iron deficiency is a risk factor for preterm birth, low birth weight (LBW), and SGA neonates [63]. Since almost two-thirds of the total body iron of a neonate is acquired during the third trimester, all premature births are at risk for iron deficiency [64]. On the other hand, full-term infants developing in an environment where the maternal stores are adequate are born with sufficient iron. However, infants younger than 6 months cannot regulate iron absorption well, and although breast milk is low in iron, the lactoferrin in breast milk promotes iron absorption. During the third trimester extending into the second year of life is a time when iron is vitally important as that is when the brain is most rapidly developing. Even if the fetus receives sufficient iron in utero, if the infant's and toddler's diet is iron insufficient, the result is a deficit in neurocognitive development, particularly in learning and memory. Unfortunately, these problems are not reversible. In fact, five-year-old children who were born iron deficient scored lower on language ability tests and skills of fine motor ability [65].

Iron is essential for neurogenesis, synaptogenesis, dendritogenesis, synthesis of neurotransmitters, and myelination. Myelination is important for rapid impulse transmission along axons and begins in the third trimester of pregnancy and progresses rapidly throughout infancy. Compared to those who received sufficient iron, young adults who were iron deficient in infancy have been shown to perform poorer on tasks involving inhibitory control, set-shifting, and planning, all executive type functions [66]. Fretham and colleagues note that iron deficiency affects at least three major neurobehavioral domains: speed of processing, affect, and learning and memory. The latter is a result of impairment of the hippocampus, the region of the brain responsible for declarative learning and memory [67]. Declarative learning refers to the ability to consciously recall specific facts and events, whereas non-declarative memory refers to memory for cognitive and motor tasks and skills that can be recalled without conscious effort [67]. A meta-analysis of nearly 12,000 children from 6 African countries indicated that iron deficiency anemia is associated with an increased risk of mortality in children from 1 month to 12 years of age. The risk decreases by 24% with each g/dl increase in hemoglobin [68].

Folic Acid

Folic acid is the synthetic stable form of naturally occurring folate, an essential B vitamin and water-soluble compound that occurs naturally in fruits and vegetables. Folates are important in nucleotide synthesis. Early in embryogenesis, the rapidly dividing cells of the neural tube require a large amount of nucleotides to facilitate replication of DNA. Without a sufficient quantity of folate within the first month of embryonic life, the developing embryo may not be able to close the neural tube. Although maternal levels of folate may be "normal," a neural tube defect (NTD) can still develop as the quantity of folate is apparently insufficient. Other factors may also contribute to the development of a NTD, including genetic and environmental influences, maternal obesity, and diabetes [69]. Reports in the early 1980s showed a protective effect of folic acid for the prevention of neural tube defects [70]. This observation was confirmed by the UK Medical Research Council with a double-blind randomized trial. This trial demonstrated that when supplemented daily with 4 mg of folic acid, a woman's rate of a recurrence for birthing a child with a NTD was reduced by 72% [71]. Subsequently, in 1992, the US Public Health Service recommended that all women supplement their daily diet with 4 mg of folic acid at least one month prior to pregnancy and continue throughout the first trimester. And for women who had previously given birth to a child with a NTD, the recommendation extended throughout the entire pregnancy [72]. In 1998, the FDA mandated that flour be enriched with folic acid. Other countries have followed suit, resulting in a rather dramatic decrease in the incidence of NTD. The largest reduction (61%) was in Costa Rica and may have been the result of fortifying not only wheat flour but also corn flour, cow's milk, and rice with folic acid [73]. Of note, not only supplemental folic acid decreased the incidence of NTD by approximately 90%, but it has also been shown to reduce the incidence of congenital heart disease by approximately 40% [74].

Iodine

Iodine deficiency disorder (IDD) affects 13% of the world's population, and greater than 2 billion additional people are at risk [75]. IDD remains a public health problem in 130 countries despite the fact that iodized salt is available to 68% of the population in those countries. Iodine is a key component of the thyroid hormone, and during the first trimester, the fetus is entirely dependent on the adequacy of maternal thyroid levels [76]. Thyroid hormones are critical for brain and neurological development, particularly during gestation. It is well known that severe iodine deficiency in a pregnant woman results in irreversible and devastating impairment to the fetal brain. Unfortunately, no amount of supplemental iodine after birth will negate the cognitive disabilities caused by severe iodine deficiency during pregnancy. However, until recently, little was known about mild or moderate iodine deficiencies in pregnant women. Bath and colleagues analyzed data from the Avon Longitudinal Study of Parents and Children (ALSPAC) in the UK [77]. They reported on the cognitive outcome of children born to mothers who were mildly (urinary iodine-to-creatinine ratio <150 μg/g) and moderately (50 μg/g to 150 μg/g) iodine deficient. Even after adjusting for multiple confounders, when compared to children born to mothers whose ratio was >150 μg/g, their verbal and performance IQs were significantly lower at 8 years of age and at age 9, and children with iodine deficiency scored lower on reading accuracy and comprehension. These authors found a lineal correlation; as the ratio decreased, the same parameters of cognition decreased. The UK study tells us that the problem is not limited to the non-industrialized world. Iodine deficiency is truly a major public health problem worldwide. WHO considers iodine deficiency "the single most important preventable cause of brain damage worldwide" [78].

Vitamin A

Vitamin A deficiency is an endemic problem in the developing world but is most prevalent in sub-Saharan Africa and South Asia. In these regions, poverty rates are high and few households can afford animal source foods that are rich in vitamin A. Beta-carotene, the precursor for vitamin A, is available in plant source foods, but these foods are often not eaten in sufficient quantities to give the individual the amounts needed for conversion into adequate levels of vitamin A. Rice, a staple food in many parts of the world, has virtually no beta-carotene, and corn, another staple food, is also very low in beta-carotene.

The first clinical sign of vitamin A deficiency is "night blindness" or inability to adapt to darkness, and it is estimated that globally 6 million pregnant women suffer from this condition. Furthermore, the fetus of a woman with vitamin A deficiency will also be deficient in vitamin A and the milk she produces will be deficient as well. It is estimated that night blindness affects 5.2 million children under 5 years of age and 190 million children under 5 years of age have low serum retinol concentrations [79]. When vitamin A deficiency is more severe, the outer covering of the eye becomes dry resulting in dry eye or xerophthalmia. In the severe situation, the cornea ulcerates and the lens is extruded leaving the child blind. Vitamin A deficiency is the leading cause of preventable blindness in children and an important cause of death.

Specific Considerations for Selected Developmental Disabilities

Attention Deficit/Hyperactivity Disorder (ADHD)

This is a syndrome complex characterized by lack of attention or focus or concentration together with impulsivity and hyperactivity severe enough to interfere with a child's learning or an adult's employment productivity. If the attention disorder is associated with only a mild degree of hyperactivity or no hyperactivity, the syndrome is referred to as attention deficit disorder (ADD). The number of children diagnosed with this disorder in the USA has mushroomed from 150 thousand in 1970 to 6.4 million (11% of children 4–17 years of age) in 2011 with a male-to-female ratio of 4 to 1 [80]. In comparison, the estimated prevalence is 6% in the Democratic Republic of the Congo [81]. The reasons for this marked increase in the USA are not well understood but may partially be attributed to a perception or overdiagnosis or a greater recognition of the diagnosis plus an expansion of the diagnostic criteria. However, there may also be a true increase in the prevalence of this syndrome. Suggested reasons for the increase include maternal dietary factors and exposure to an increased number of toxins such as lead, mercury, and organic pollutants which, with stricter regulations, is less of a problem in industrialized than in non-industrialized countries. Some have suggested that some children may be more sensitive to certain food additives, including synthetic colorings and a greater array of preservatives. In addition, a child's brain is exposed to an ever-increasing number and degree of stimulants from television and other electronic devices that tend to alter the ability of a child to focus. Most of these suggestions are speculative and have not been proven scientifically.

Feeding/Nutritional Problems

Galler and colleagues published a very interesting but disturbing paper from the Barbados Nutrition Study that linked ADHD in middle adulthood with infant malnutrition [82]. The study participants were of normal birth weight but experienced an episode of moderate-to-severe malnutrition in the first year of life. Following hospital discharge, they were enrolled in a government intervention program that ensured ongoing nutritional support. The control group consisted of healthy classmates without a history of malnutrition. Social and socioeconomic information was collected and considered in the group comparisons. Those children who had experienced malnutrition had lower IQs, poorer academic achievement, and impaired fine motor skills, and the teachers reported a fourfold increase in attention problems that was not the result of a childhood environmental disadvantage or cognitive impairment [83].

Boys with ADHD have a tendency not to adhere to a traditional schedule for meals with a higher frequency of irregular and more frequent eating times. They also have a diminished preference for and hence ingestion of fruits and vegetables and an increased consumption of sweetened beverages [84]. In the early 1970s, Benjamin Feingold presented a paper at the American Medical Association Annual Meeting proposing that many of the behavior and learning problems seen in elementary school children were due to their ingestion of certain foods and food additives [85]. He proposed a diet free of all foods that contained natural salicylates and all artificial food colors and flavors, the Kaiser–Permanente (K-P) diet. However, this diet also provided less calcium, riboflavin, and vitamin C. Feingold's paper and subsequent restricted diets resulted in a number of scientific investigations and reports flourished. This literature of 35 years has been nicely summarized by Stevens and colleagues with a detailed account of dietary sensitivities and artificial food color (AFC) additives on ADHD symptoms [86]. Their review of the literature concluded that whereas AFC additives have not been found to have a link with ADHD, there appears to be a subgroup of children (11–33% of those with ADHD) whose symptoms decreased enough on the K-P diet to improve their functioning at home and at school. And some children with ADHD when challenged with AFC had an increase in their hyperactivity, while other children had exhibited other symptoms after ingesting AFC including irritability, restlessness, and sleep disturbance. Preschool-aged children appeared to be most affected.

Growth Deviants

The side effects of medical stimulants used in the therapy of ADHD include loss of appetite, decreased growth, insomnia, mood disturbance, and headaches. Indeed, there have been reports of decrease in linear growth of children on methylphenidate one of the most commonly used medications for ADHD. To assess this relationship, Durá-Travé and colleagues followed the growth of 187 children over 4 years [87]. At the time of diagnosis, the children had a mean age of 8.1 years and their mean weight and height were lower than the mean of the same-aged cohort of control children, a deficit of 0.70 kg and 0.42 cm, respectively. Thirty months after treatment was started, the weight difference increased to 4.27 kg and the height difference increased to 2.69 cm. After 48 months, the deficits lessened to 1.58 kg in weight and 0.83 cm in height. They concluded that the effect of methylphenidate was transitory and that the relative short stature in children with ADHD was more related to the condition than to the medication [87].

Autism Spectrum Disorders (ASDs)

The spectrum of autistic disorders consists of classic autism, Asperger syndrome, pervasive developmental disorder not otherwise specified (PDD-NOS), childhood disintegrative disorder, and Rett syndrome. These lifelong neurodevelopmental disorders are characterized by severe impairments in social interaction and communication along with behavioral inflexibility and restrictive interests. Prevalence data for ASD in LMICs are presented in Table 24.1.

Feeding/Nutritional Problems

Feeding problems are major issues and include food preferences, food selectivity with limited repertoires of food, food refusal, and excessive intake of certain food categories such as carbohydrates. Whiteley and colleagues reported that 83% of parents reported that their child with ASD had a very restrictive diet and that consistency of food was a major factor [88]. Williams and colleagues surveyed 100 parents of children with ASD aged 22 months to 10 years. Of the 100 parents, 69% reported that their child was reluctant to try new foods; 60% ate very few different foods; 56% of the children were "mouthing" foods; and 46% had rituals surrounding eating. Factors influencing food selection were texture (69%), appearance (58%), taste (45%), smell (36%), and temperature (22%) [89]. Children with ASD have a preference for carbohydrates, snacks, and/or processed foods and a rejection of fruits and vegetables. In addition, food presentation including different foods touching other foods or the use of certain utensils often results in food refusal. Sharp et al. estimated a fivefold increase in the odds that children with ASD will have a feeding problem [90]. Dietary manipulation is becoming more common, and some care providers and parents are using this as treatment for ASD. Particularly prevalent is a diet free of gluten and/or casein. Eliminating casein would mean eliminating milk and all milk-containing foods, which could lead to dietary deficiencies such as calcium and vitamin D. There is no research that supports this practice [91].

Growth Deviants

Cermak and colleagues performed a systematic review of articles on ASD published in English over the past 25 years but uncovered only a few studies that assessed growth parameters [92]. Despite very significant food selectivity and limited intake of certain food categories, weight and linear growth in children with ASD were not found to be adversely affected [92]. From a large longitudinal study of parents and children, Emond et al. compared the feeding patterns and dietary intake of 79 children with ASD with 12,901 controls. The authors found that at 38 months, the intakes of energy, total fat, carbohydrate, and protein were similar, but the ASD group consumed less vitamin C. They found no differences in weight, height, or BMI at 18 months and 7 years [93]. In their extensive review of the literature on this subject, Sharp et al. [90] found specific dietary deficits in children with ASD, specifically a lower intake of calcium and protein. This was consistent with the Hediger et al.'s report a few years earlier that a group of 75 boys with ASD had decreased bone cortical thickness compared with their peers without ASD [94]. Zimmer et al. [95] compared ASD selective eaters with ASD non-selective eaters none of whom were on elimination diets and found lower intake of protein, calcium, and vitamins A, D, and B12 when the combined groups were compared with peers and selective eaters were at greater risk than non-selective eaters.

Cerebral Palsy

Cerebral palsy (CP) is a descriptive term for a group of disorders of movement and posture causing limitations or dysfunction of activity. The etiology is a non-progressive insult or injury to the central nervous system (CNS) when the brain is undergoing its most rapid development [96]. CP is the most frequent cause of childhood disability with overall prevalence rates in the USA of 3.1 per 1000 live births [97]. It is estimated that approximately 70–80% of the insults to the CNS occur prenatally. Perinatal etiologies include hypoxia during the perinatal period, postnatal CNS infections, exposure to toxic drugs, genetic abnormalities, and head injuries. The majority, however, are the result of unknown or undetected mechanisms. Prematurity is the most frequent antecedent of CP, as it predisposes the infant to hypoxic-ischemic encephalopathy, periventricular leukomalacia (PVL) and intraventricular hemorrhage. Despite the intensiveness and multiple advances in neonatal care, there has not been a significant decrease in the prevalence of CP. This is partially explained by the improved survival rate of the very low birth weight preterm newborns. Such is not the case in many LMICs.

There are different types of CP, each of which corresponds to an insult in a different area of the CNS. Spastic CP accounts for about 75% of all individuals with CP and occurs when the neurological insult involves the pyramidal area of the brain and may involve one or all four limbs. The other types are dyskinetic CP (uncontrolled purposeless movements) where the injury is in the extrapyramidal regions and ataxic CP (gait imbalance) where the insult involves the cerebellum. The severity of CP is based on the ability of the child to ambulate with Level 1 being the mildest and Level 5 being the most severe, requiring total care [98]. The degree of disability is closely related to comorbidities and to survival [99, 100].

Whereas the CNS insult is non-progressive, the effects from the motor deficit and muscle imbalance often worsen over time and may result in fixed contractures of major joints, progressive scoliosis, hip dislocation, and body distortion. In addition, many affected children have other comorbidities, such as varying degrees of intellectual disability, seizures, visual and hearing impairments, gastrointestinal problems, drooling, and recurrent aspirations. Treatment of children with the more severe forms of CP and the comorbidities is problematic in LMICs.

Feeding/Nutritional Problems

Motion and colleagues suggest that early, persistent, and severe feeding difficulties can be a marker for CP [101]. Weak sucking at 4 weeks of age was present in 48% (11 of 23) of children diagnosed with CP as compared with 18% (2206 of 12,299) of children not diagnosed with CP. Furthermore, great difficulties with feeding were reported in 10% (2 of 21) of children with CP as compared with 3.3% (373 of 10,941) of control children. In addition, feeding difficulty at 4 weeks was associated with undernutrition at 8 years of age [101]. Reilly and colleagues surveyed 49 children with CP between 12 and 72 months of age and found that 90% had clinically significant oral motor dysfunction [102]. Consistent with Motion et al., they found that in the first 12 months of life, sucking problems were present in 57% and swallowing difficulties in 38%. In 60%, severe feeding problems preceded the diagnosis of CP [102]. In order to identify the presence of feeding and gastrointestinal problems in children with CP, Erkin and colleagues enrolled 120 children consecutively with an age range of 2–12 years [103]. Approximately one-fourth had feeding dysfunction and an equal number had constipation. A lack of appetite was present in 31, and 19% had difficulty in swallowing. The frequency of dysfunction was highest in the children with the greatest levels of severity. Furthermore, as expected, the duration of time required to feed these children was longer [103]. Due to the fact that children with swallowing dysfunction often reject solid foods, spill a lot, choke, cough, and have significant gastroesophageal reflux and aspiration, pneumonia is not uncommon. Those with generalized motor dysfunction are at greater risk for swallowing dysfunction and aspiration. Meal times are often quite stressful for both child and parents [104]. The amount of care involved with these children is particularly difficult when time and resources are limited.

Growth Deviants or Nutritional Deficits

The frequency and degree of growth deviation depend on the extent of the injury to the central nervous system (CNS) and the severity of the CP. Dahlseng and colleagues obtained data on 661 children from the Norwegian CP Register with a mean age of 6 years and 7 months to assess their nutritional status [105]. Only 63% had a normal BMI for age, 20% had mean z-score for weight and/or height <-2 standard deviations (SDs) from the mean, and 16% were overweight or obese. Twenty-one percent were completely dependent on assistance during feeding and 14% were fed through a gastrostomy tube and these were the ones with higher weight and BMI [105]. As might be expected, the greater the degree of severity of feeding dysfunction, the worse the nutritional status unless feedings are done through the gastrostomy tube and then overweight is common. Fung and colleagues used the Child Health Questionnaire to evaluate feeding dysfunction and the nutritional status among 230 children with CP from six centers in the USA and Canada [106]. The mean z-scores for weight were -1.7, -2.5, and -3.3 for those with no, mild, and moderate feeding dysfunctions, respectively. Those who were tube-fed had a mean z-score for weight of -1.8. The findings were similar for height. Children with no feeding problems had mean triceps z-score of -0.3 compared to

−0.9 for those with mild feeding problems [106]. It is quite unusual for children to be tube-fed in LMICs.

Down Syndrome (DS) or Trisomy 21

This is a chromosomal condition observed when an individual possesses a complete or part of an extra copy of chromosome 21. Trisomy 21 due to nondisjunction of chromosome 21, in which a contributed sperm or egg has an extra copy of chromosome 21, occurs in 95% of cases. In remaining cases, the extra chromosomal material is due to a translocation with some part of chromosome 21 breaking off and attaching to another chromosome, usually chromosome 14, or there is mosaicism whereby some cells have extra chromosome 21 material and some do not. In the USA, this is the most common chromosomal condition, occurring once in every 700 live births, with an increasing risk as the maternal age passes age 35. Prenatal screening and diagnostic testing are available, and in some societies, it has resulted in a very high percentage of pregnancy termination. In Western Australia between 1980 and 2013, 93% of women whose tests were positive for trisomy 21 elected termination. If these pregnancies had gone to term, the occurrence would have increased from 1.1 per 1000 to 2.17 per 1000 [107]. The additional chromosomal material results in some degree of cognitive impairment, and the characteristic features that distinguish the DS disorder include low muscle tone, an upward slant to the eyes, a relatively large tongue, a single deep crease across the center of the palm, and short stature. Many with DS have congenital heart disease, and if uncorrected, this results in increased energy expenditure due to an increase in cardiac workload and resultant poor growth. Chromosomal disorders usually also result in disruption of cell proliferation causing a reduction in the number of embryonic cells adding to further growth restriction. In addition, repeated and/or chronic illnesses in those with DS are frequent and can also adversely affect growth.

Growth Deviants

By age 3, 75% of children with DS show some delay in bone maturation and 90% are smaller than their peers. By adolescence, bone maturation is typically delayed by 1–2 years and the adolescent growth spurt is also delayed. Adult height is usually 2–3 SD below the general population. Individuals with DS are less active and have lower physical fitness values with body composition and higher BMIs secondary to obesity accentuated by short stature [108]. Growth problems are so universal in children with DS that special growth charts have been developed for this population.

Spina Bifida

This disorder is the result of failure of closure of the neural tube resulting in either occult (hidden from view) spina bifida, meningocele (a sac lined by the meninges and uncovered by vertebrae, muscle or soft tissue but not containing nerve roots), or myelomeningocele (the sac does contain nerve roots) which is the most severe situation. Worldwide, the incidence of neural tube defects range from 1.0 to 10.0 per 1000 births [109]. The most common lesion is in the lower thoracic or lumbar areas. The height of the motor defect depends on which vertebrae are involved. Bladder and bowel are almost always affected resulting in repeated urinary tract infections (cystitis and pyelonephritis) that may lead to poor growth and eventually to renal failure.

Growth Deviants

Individuals with very low lesions where ambulation is not inhibited attain normal height. However, lesions that affect the ability to ambulate result in short stature. Rosenblum et al. reported that 43% of individuals with mid lesions and 80% of those with high lesions were below the 3rd percentile for height [110]. Adults with spina bifida tend to have an inactive lifestyle, lower aerobic capacity, decreased level of daily physical activity, higher prevalence of obesity, and lower health-related quality of life as compared with a reference group [111].

The caloric needs of individuals with spina bifida who are non-ambulatory are considerably less than those for a very active person. This is particularly important for the adolescent who wants to fit in with peers and hence in social settings finds it difficult to restrict his or her intake of foods. Obesity is not uncommon in this situation. It is therefore important to institute a program of appropriate foods with the recommended caloric amount, self-regulation, and weight control plus an exercise program. Also, constipation is invariably a constant problem and is secondary to weak abdominal muscle, poor dietary fiber intake, neurogenic bowel, inactivity, and anticholinergic drugs used to treat the neurogenic bladder. Dietary management consists of establishing eating habits early with emphasis on foods that have high fiber content, juices, and plenty of water to avoid constipation and facilitate weight control. Children should select their own physical activity, but unfortunately, those in a wheelchair tend to be less active, and if their diets are not restricted to compensate for fewer calories expended, their weights may increase rather rapidly. Also, due to non-weight bearing on their lower extremities, they tend to be shorter than their peers. Hence, dietary restrictions should be instituted when the child is above the 25th percentile on the weight for age chart or above the 10th percentile on the weight for height chart.

Sociopolitical, Policies, and Conventions Adopted by Countries' Regulations like the Americans with Disabilities Act (ADA)

During the past several decades, there have been numerous country-specific as well as "universal" policies and conventions that lay out recommendations that, if enacted, would serve to initiate the lengthy process of eliminating discrimination against individuals with disabilities. Unfortunately, there are many barriers preventing the implementation of well-intended policies such as societal beliefs and perceptions of DD; financial obstacles; lack of resources, both material and adequately trained personnel; and infrastructural issues that require alterations in building construction, sidewalks, and public transportation to allow universal access. Perhaps the most difficult barrier to circumvent is that of effecting a genuine change in people's attitude towards people with disabilities. Unfortunately, individuals with disabilities are often stigmatized, marginalized, and discriminated against. Cultural and attitudinal prejudices are deeply engrained and much harder to change than are physical structures. What is also disturbing is that the prevalence of disabilities in many countries is not even known; therefore, designating appropriate resources is quite imprecise. Moving the rhetoric from paper to practice is difficult. Despite these barriers, the recommendations are explicit in two universal conventions that have been adopted by a majority of countries.

The Convention on the Rights of the Child (CRC) was introduced at the UNICEF-sponsored World Summit for Children held in New York in 1990 [112]. It was one of the most rapidly signed and ratified universal conventions, and to date, only three countries have not ratified this convention (Somalia, the Republic of South Sudan, and the USA). Among other obligations, the CRC guarantees that the rights of all children shall be respected without discrimination and each child will be protected against all forms of discrimination or punishment based on the status or beliefs. Important points include the following:

- Every child should enjoy a full and decent life;
- The disabled child has a right to special care and access to available appropriate resources including social services, training, and opportunities for recreation and employment, and wherever possible, schooling shall be provided free of charge; and
- "in the spirit of international cooperation, the exchange of appropriate information in the field of preventive health care and of medical, psychological and functional treatment of disabled children, including dissemination of and access to information concerning methods of rehabilitation, education and vocational services, with the aim of enabling States Parties to improve their capabilities and skills and to widen their experience in these areas. In this regard, particular account shall be taken of the needs of developing countries" [112].

The Convention on the Rights of Persons with Disabilities (CRPD) is a more recent document that specifically addressed issues of disabilities and was adopted at the United Nations Headquarters in New York in December of 2006 [112, 113]. By March of 2013, the CRPD had been ratified or accepted by 129 countries [114]. The CRPD is of critical importance to children with disabilities. Children who are members of this vulnerable population are more likely to live in poverty, are oftentimes denied education, and are disproportionately at risk for physical and sexual abuse. According to estimates from international agencies, >90% of children with disabilities do not attend school; 500,000 children every year lose some part of their vision due to vitamin A deficiency; 41 million babies are born each year at risk for mental impairment due to lack of maternal iodine; 10,400 children are killed or permanently disabled due to land mines; and over 10 million are psychologically traumatized by armed conflict [115].

The CRPD views individuals with disabilities not as objects of charity who need medical treatment and social protection but rather as capable individuals who have rights and can make decisions for themselves as active members of society. This antiquates the medical model and puts emphasis on the social model for disabilities. It identifies the areas where society needs to both change and adapt the existing environment in order to better fit the needs of individuals with disabilities. The CRPD clarifies and outlines the civil, cultural, political, social, and economic rights of individuals with disabilities as no different from the rights of all human beings. It also identifies areas where adaptations should be made for persons with disabilities, indicates where those rights have been violated, and suggests how those rights should be protected.

Outcomes

Morbidities and Mortalities

Worldwide, child mortality (under age 5) decreased by almost 50% between 1990 and 2013, from 90 deaths per 1000 live births in 1990 to 46 per 1000 in 2013, while neonatal mortality fell by 40% during the same period [116]. Thus, the proportion of the under five mortality due to neonatal mortality rose from 37 to 44%. Child mortality and neonatal mortality are also decreasing dramatically in many LMICs. However, of the 2.8 million neonatal deaths that occurred in 2013, ten LMICs account for about two-thirds of the total, with India accounting for over 25% and Nigeria about 10%. In addition, the ten countries with the highest neonatal mortality rates overall are all LMICs.

The leading causes of neonatal mortality worldwide are preterm birth complications; labor and delivery complications such as birth asphyxia; and infections, particularly sepsis, meningitis, and neonatal tetanus [116–118]. The order changes when we restrict this to low- and low-middle-income countries, i.e., the poorest countries with respect to resources. In these countries, the leading specific cause is birth asphyxia [119].

In LMICs, a decrease in mortality among children under five has also occurred, by 22% [120]. According to UNICEF, in 2013, 12 countries had underfive mortality rates of 100 deaths or more per 1000 live births, all of which are LMICs. Of the worldwide total of deaths in the underfive age group, five countries (India, Nigeria, Pakistan, Democratic Republic of the Congo, and China), all of which are LMICs, account for 50%.

UNICEF reports that child deaths from infectious diseases such as pneumonia, diarrhea, malaria, measles, and AIDS have seen a dramatic decline from 2000 to 2013 [116]. The leading causes of child mortality worldwide now are preterm birth complications, which account for 17% of deaths, pneumonia (15%), complications during labor and delivery (11%), diarrhea (9%), and malaria (7%). Undernutrition contributes to an estimated 45% of the deaths in children under five worldwide [49]. Preterm births continue to rise in importance as one of the leading causes of child mortality [51]. Given this trend, an international review team has stressed the immediate need for improvements in newborn care, particularly in low-income countries [50].

Also within LMICs, lower socioeconomic (SES) circumstances are associated with a higher risk of infant death. A recent analysis of infant mortality among 53 LMICs showed that these deaths are concentrated in households with lower SES [121]. Mortality from specific causes also affects more children in lower socioeconomic circumstances. For example, in low- and low-middle-income countries, i.e., the poorest countries with respect to resources, the leading specific cause is birth asphyxia [119].

Unfortunately, with the decreasing mortality comes increased morbidity among the survivors. Increasing attention to the needs of these surviving children has been observed in recent years. Almost a decade ago, Olusanya described the survivor issues created by mortality reduction in developing countries [122]. By 2008, UNICEF had introduced a report that included data on children with disabilities which prompted the hope that the emphasis on reduction in child mortality would eventually be followed by evaluations of the linkage among survival, disability, and well-being in low-income and many middle-income countries [123].

The same factors that cause neonatal mortality also contribute to child morbidity. For example, birth asphyxia is a main cause of neonatal morbidity, as well as long-term morbidity, including intellectual disability, CP, and other neurodevelopmental disabilities, particularly among children in LMICs [119]. Globally, preterm birth is becoming an increasingly important contributor to morbidity among underfives, and the trend is expected to continue according to Sutton and Darmstadt [124]. These investigators also make the point that adequate data are not available from low-income countries, where the majority of neonatal morbidity occurs, partly the result of the lack of standardized measurement tools in these countries.

While it is established that the same intrauterine and neonatal insults that cause neonatal mortality contribute to morbidity in those infants who do survive, data remain scarce concerning the prevalence of these insults and long-term outcomes in the survivors, especially in resource-poor countries [117]. In an attempt to address this need, Mwaniki et al. [117] completed an extensive literature search to identify publications on a worldwide basis that included data on long-term outcomes after exposure to the intrauterine and neonatal insults that contribute to neonatal mortality, including complications of preterm birth, birth asphyxia, exposure to infections, and conditions such as jaundice and congenital infections. Among 22,161 survivors documented in the 153 studies included in the analyses, the median risk overall of having at least one impairment in any of the outcome domains they included was almost 40%. The most frequent outcomes were learning difficulties, cognitive impairment, or developmental delay (59%), CP (21%), hearing impairments (20%), and visual impairments (18%). These data have serious implications for LMICs since all of them must deal with populations of infants who survive the same intrauterine and neonatal insults.

Just as has been observed for infant mortality, the lowest SES groups in LMICs are the most affected with respect to morbidity from birth asphyxia. There is greater risk both for neonatal morbidity from birth asphyxia and for conditions such as ID, CP, and other neurodevelopmental disorders among children in the lowest SES groups of LMICs [119]. This is not surprising when one considers that malnutrition and undernutrition, as well as exposure to other environmental risk factors, are associated with lower SES.

The reduction of both short- and long-term morbidities among children in LMICs must include both primary and secondary prevention strategies. Recently, Sutton and Darmstadt have stressed preconception health care that focuses on pregnancy prevention in adolescents, prevention of unintended pregnancies, nutritional interventions such as folic acid supplementation, vaccination for rubella and tetanus, and screening for sexually transmitted diseases, as the preferential means for reducing both the mortality and morbidity that result from both full-term and premature births [124]. These investigators and others have also emphasized that improvements in the care of preterm infants could reduce morbidity, particularly in middle-income circumstances [50]. Finally, Scherzer et al. [120] have focused on the need for early evaluation and recognition of conditions and support for families of these children in order to prevent the worst outcomes and move toward improving the quality of their lives.

School

Education, Inclusion, or Exclusion

School administrators have approached the education of children with disabilities in two very different ways, including them with children who do not have disabilities or excluding them from the other children. Unfortunately, the term inclusion is not interpreted in the same way by every country. For some, it only means that those with a disability should be under the responsibility of the ministry of education. Hence, schooling can take place in a variety of settings: centers, special schools, special classes in integrated schools, or regular classes in mainstream schools. For others, inclusion means that students with disabilities should be educated in regular classrooms with age-appropriate peers. For this stricter definition, the whole school system may need to be changed. Physical barriers must be removed, and reasonable accommodations must be made for all students. This of course requires changes in legislation and policies as well as appropriate allocation of sufficient funds.

In the past, children with disabilities were excluded from mainstream education and special schools were established to teach children with specific disabilities, such as schools for the deaf and schools for the blind, which segregated children from their peers. These schools were usually located in urban areas where there were a sufficient number of children to justify the special school. The children living at a distance from these schools were often housed in residential settings at or close to the school grounds, thus separating them from their families and the communities with which they were familiar. Furthermore, many children who might benefit from such schooling were not reached. Placement of children with disabilities in special schools tends to underestimate their abilities, promoting further exclusion and, on graduation, narrows their opportunities to enter the wider community. Myths or cultural beliefs are other factors that foster exclusion. For example, a study published in 2012 found that 48% of the presidents of parent associations in Madagascar believed that disability is contagious [125].

It was initially thought that relegating children with particular disabilities to special schools was good for the student and was cost-effective. However, it is now believed that including children with disabilities with children who do not have disabilities provides a better education for the student with the disability and, at the same time, introduces non-disabled students to diversity. Exclusion has also been found not to be cost-effective. When countries ratified the CRPD, they endorsed Article 24 which promotes inclusion as a goal requiring that: "Effective individualized support measures are provided in environments that maximize academic and social development, consistent with the goal of full inclusion."

Inclusion of children with disabilities in the regular school setting is just beginning in many developing countries. However, it often requires revision of grounds; classrooms and toilet facilities that allow access of wheelchairs or other medical devices; special seating arrangements; adaptive equipment for the hard of hearing or visually impaired; paid aids to assist some who are severely disabled or disruptive if not attended to; and specially trained teachers. All of this is quite expensive and often beyond the reach of schools where resources are limited. However, keeping students with a disability in the mainstream encourages the acceptance in the community following graduation. It increases familiarity with and reduces prejudice against individuals with disabilities. Parents who see other children with disabilities enrolled in school are more apt to also enroll their child with a disability. Inclusion exposes children without disabilities to those with disabilities and encourages them to work together while in school. Inclusion should also become the norm in environments outside the classroom. Without inclusion, countries cannot achieve "Education for All." Unfortunately, children with disabilities are less likely to start school, less likely to be promoted, and less likely to complete the primary grades (Table 24.4). In Malawi, Namibia, Zambia, and Zimbabwe, between 9% and 18% of children without a disability had never attended school as compared to 24% to 39% of children with a disability [10]. Only 300 (3%) of the estimated 10,000 deaf children in Rwanda were enrolled in primary or secondary school [126].

Barriers faced by parents with children who have a disability include hesitancy to send their child to school as they may be the only child with a disability in the school, stigma, myths, harassment, accessibility to classrooms and appropriate desks, toilet facilities that do not accommodate some children with disabilities, and a lack of adequately trained teachers in special education. Other issues include the following:

- Lack of assistive technology: WHO estimates that in many low-income countries, only 5–10% of those who need assistive technology actually have access to it. Devices listed as assistive technology include those for mobility (crutches, wheelchairs, braces, special toilet seats); vision (eyeglasses, white cane, Braille for reading); hearing (hearing aids); communication (cards with text, communication board); and cognition (picture-based instruction, adaptive toys, and games).

Table 24.4 A comparison of educational levels obtained by individuals with disabilities to those without disabilities in LMIC[a]

Individuals	Low-income countries		High-income countries		All countries	
	Not disabled (%)	Disabled (%)	Not disabled	Disabled (%)	Not disabled	Disabled
Male Primary school completed	55.6	45.6	72.3	61.7	61.3	50.6
Female Primary school completed	42.0	32.9	72.0	59.3	52.9	41.7
18–49 years of age Primary school completed	60.3	47.8	83.1	69.0	67.4	53.2
50–59 years of age Primary school completed	44.3	30.8	68.1	52.0	52.7	37.6
Over 60 years of age Primary school completed	30.7	21.2	53.6	46.5	40.6	32.3

[a]*Source* WHO. World Report on Disability 2011. Table 7.1, page 207. [10]

- School problems: accessibility, harassment, poorly trained and underpaid teachers, inappropriate curriculum, grouping of students, labeling of students and either underestimating capabilities, or setting unattainable goals.

In 2008, Snider and Takeda presented a paper to the World Bank outlining the components and benefits of cost-effective, flexible, and inclusive universal design that removes physical barriers, as they are major obstacles to social inclusion for those with limited capacities. The focus of the report was not just on education but included transportation, urban development, water and sanitation, health, as well as postconflict and natural disaster situations [127].

Employment

Data on employment rates in low- and middle-income countries (LMICs) are sparse. However, where there are data, employment rates are universally lower for the population with disabilities than for the overall population. In the USA, the ratio of employment of individuals with disabilities and those without disabilities is around 52%, whereas in South Africa, it is 30% [10]. However, the ratio is quite variable as detailed in the list of countries in Table 24.5.

It is hard to interpret or reconcile such figures as disabilities may be defined differently in the various countries. The World Health Survey of 51 countries gives employment rates for men with disabilities of 52.8% versus 64.9% without disabilities [10]. For women with disabilities, the employment rate is 19.6% versus 29.9% for those without disabilities. However, most of these estimates are not very accurate as statistics are not kept, many individuals with disabilities are not looking for jobs and hence are not counted as part of the workforce, and a significant number of individuals with disabilities work in the informal economy and therefore do not appear in the labor statistics [10]. The type of disability an individual has also influences their employability. Those with physical impairments often need more time to get to work or to maneuver in the workplace and/or need special accommodations to be as productive as those who are not disabled. They have more medical problems and hence require more time off for medical visits. Those who have intellectual impairments have a different disadvantage, and it is estimated that they are 3–4 times less likely to be employed than those without cognitive disabilities [128].

Table 24.5 A comparison of rates of employment of individuals with disabilities to those without disabilities in selected countries[a]

Country	Employment rate (%) of people with disabilities	Employment rate (%) of overall population	Employment ratio
Canada	56.3	74.9	0.75
Netherlands	39.9	61.9	0.64
Australia	41.9	72.1	0.58
USA	38.1	73.2	0.52
Japan	22.7	59.4	0.38
Malawi	42.3	46.2	0.92
Zambia	45.5	56.5	0.81
Mexico	47.2	60.1	0.79
Peru	23.8	64.1	0.37
Poland	20.8	63.9	0.33
South Africa	12.4	41.1	0.30

[a]*Source* WHO. World Report on Disability 2011. Table 8.1, page 238. [10]

The cost of disability is high for the individual, their family, and their community. The impact of disability on poverty for all three levels is great. For instance, the lack of schooling and employment for disabled individuals and their care providers in Bangladesh results in an annual loss of income estimated at $1.2 billion US dollars or nearly 1.7% of the gross national product [129]. A study by the International Labour Organization of LMICs estimated that the economic cost of disability equals 3–5% of the gross domestic product [130].

Conclusions

The major conclusions for this chapter on DD in LMICs are as follows:

- DDs differ from disabilities in general in that DDs are physical or mental conditions (or combinations of these) that impair an individual's ability to function prior to age 22 (US definition), while disabilities can occur throughout life and have increasing prevalence with advancing age.
- Data on the prevalence of DD in low-income and middle-income countries (LMICs) remain limited, but improvements in data collection methods in the last 15 years have provided a better understanding of the underlying burden of disability.
- Knowledge about genetic factors underlying DD has increased at a remarkable pace with the advent of genomics and new technologies in molecular genetics, and all the while, investigators have continued to identify environmental exposures associated with the occurrence of DD.
- The identification of interactions between specific genes (or gene variants) and environmental exposures has increased dramatically in the past few decades; in contrast, the search for gene-environment interactions with respect to DD is just beginning.
- Evaluation of early childhood development programs in LMICs suggests that parenting education and support and enrollment of children in preschools provide the most effective means of improving developmental outcomes in these countries.
- Poverty and malnutrition go hand in hand and are particularly prevalent and severe in LMICs; the coupling of these two maladies results in undernutrition and micronutrient deficiencies in the pregnant women with devastating effects on the brain of the fetus and results in an alarming number of infants born with a DD.
- Children with DD are destined to live with compromised abilities and opportunities and have problems that continue into adolescence and adulthood; the cycle may be repeated.
- Some fairly common DDs such as attention deficit/hyperactivity disorder, autism spectrum disorders, CP, trisomy 21, and spina bifida are associated with feeding and/or nutritional problems that often result in growth deviations.
- Childhood and neonatal mortality have dramatically decreased worldwide and in LMICs since 1990, but children in LMICs are at high risk for many adverse health conditions, including DD.
- Two very important treaties that have strong positive implications for individuals with disabilities, the Convention on the Rights of the Child and the Convention on the Rights of Persons with Disabilities, have been signed by most of the countries in the world, but are worth little without the will of governments to enact the policies they contain and unless societal views change to embrace diversity and respect all people despite their limitations.
- Both these conventions address the right for all children to have an appropriate education in an inclusive environment that will prepare them for life after school and guarantee non-discrimination for employment, but the world awaits their full implementation.

Discussion Points

- What is the role of poverty in the generational cycle of developmental disabilities?
- Which micronutrient(s) if added as a supplement to foods do you think would have the greatest impact on decreasing the prevalence of developmental disabilities and why?
- Why might we expect to find in LMICs' interactions involving gene variants and environmental exposures that have not been previously identified?
- How might the development of new technologies in genetics and genomics affect the frequency with which developmental disabilities are identified in LMICs?
- How might you use the two important conventions (the Rights of the Child and the Rights of Persons with Disabilities) to push governments to enact national policies to improve the lives of those with disabilities?

References

1. Social Security Administration. Section 223 social security laws. 1935.
2. Americans with Disabilities Act of 1990. 1990.
3. Congress 106th. Disabilities assistance and bill of rights act of 2000. 2000.
4. World Health Organization. Towards a common language for functioning, disability and health: ICF The International Classification of Functioning. Geneva: Disability and Health; 2002.
5. UNICEF. The state of the world's children. 2013.
6. Bornstein MH, Hendricks C. Screening for developmental disabilities in developing countries. Soc Sci Med. 2013;97:307–15. Doi:10.1016/j.socscimed.2012.09.049.
7. Durkin M. The epidemiology of developmental disabilities in low-income countries. Ment Retard Dev Disabil Res Rev. 2002;8:206–11. Doi:10.1002/mrdd.10039.
8. Durkin MS, Davidson LL, Desai P, et al. Validity of the ten questions screen for childhood disability : results from population-based studies in Bangladesh, Jamaica, and Pakistan. Epidemiology. 1994;5:283–9.
9. Maulik PK, Darmstadt GL. Childhood disability in low- and middle-income countries: overview of screening, prevention, services, legislation, and epidemiology. Pediatrics. 2007;120 Suppl:S1–55. Doi:10.1542/peds.2007-0043B.
10. World Health Organization. World report on disability. 2011.
11. Couper J. Prevalence of childhood disability in rural Kwazulu-Natal. South African Med J. 2002;92:549–52.
12. Ibrahim SH, Bhutta ZA. Prevalence of early childhood disability in a rural district of Sind, Pakistan. Dev Med Child Neurol. 2013;55:357–63. Doi:10.1111/dmcn.12103.
13. Gottlieb CA, Maenner MJ, Cappa C, Durkin MS. Child disability screening, nutrition, and early learning in 18 countries with low and middle incomes: data from the third round of UNICEF's Multiple Indicator Cluster Survey (2005–06). Lancet. 2009;374:1831–9. Doi:10.1016/S0140-6736(09)61871-7.
14. Gladstone M. A review of the incidence and prevalence, types and aetiology of childhood cerebral palsy in resource-poor settings. Ann Trop Paediatr. 2010;30:181–96. Doi:10.1179/146532810X12786388978481.
15. Mendizabal JE, Salguero LF. Prevalence of epilepsy in a rural community of Guatemala. Epilepsia. 1996;37:373–376. Doi:10.1111/j.1528-1157.1996.tb00574.x.
16. Elsabbagh M, Divan G, Koh Y-J, et al. (2012) Global prevalence of autism and other pervasive developmental disorders. Autism Res 5:160–79. Doi:10.1002/aur.239.
17. Bruce JR. Uniting theories of morality, religion, and social interaction : grid—group cultural theory, the " Big Three " ethics, and moral foundations theory. Psychol Soc. 2013;5:37–50.
18. Schweder RA, Much NC, Mahapatra M, Park L. The "Big Three" of morality (autonomy, community, divinity) and the "Big Three" explanations of suffering. In: Brandt A, Rozin P, editors. Morality and culture. New York: Routeledge; 1997. p. 119–69.
19. Engle PL, Black MM, Behrman JR, et al. Child development in developing countries 3: strategies to avoid the loss of developmental potential in more than 200 million children in the developing world. Lancet. 2007;369:229–42.
20. Foster GM. Disease etiologies in non-western medical systems. Am Anthropol. 1976;78:772–82.
21. McQuaid EL, Everhart RS, Seifer R, et al. Medication adherence among Latino and non-Latino white children with asthma. Pediatrics. 2012;129:e1404–10. Doi:10.1542/peds.2011-1391.

22. DiMatteo MR, Haskard-Zolnierek KB, Martin LR. Improving patient adherence: a three-factor model to guide practice. Health Psychol Rev. 2012;6:74–91. Doi:10.1080/17437199.2010.537592.
23. Ager A. The importance of sustainability in the design of culturally appropriate programmes of early intervention. Int Disabil Stud. 1990;12:89–92.
24. Berlin EA, Fowkes WCJ. A teaching framework for cross-cultural health care: application in family practice. West J Med. 1983;139:934–8.
25. Levin K. I am what I am because of who we all are: international perspectives on rehabilitation: South Africa. Pediatr Rehabil. 2006;9:285–92. Doi:10.1080/13638490500293358.
26. Butler M, Meaney F. Genetics of developmental disabilities. Boca Raton, FL: Taylor and Francis Group; 2005.
27. Plomin R. Child development and molecular genetics: 14 years later. Child Dev. 2013;84:104–20. Doi:10.1111/j.1467-8624.2012.01757.x.
28. Coe BP, Girirajan S, Eichler EE. The genetic variability and commonality of neurodevelopmental disease. Am J Med Genet C Semin Med Genet. 2012;160C:118–29. Doi:10.1002/ajmg.c.31327.
29. Moreno-De-Luca A, Myers SM, Challman TD, et al. Developmental brain dysfunction: revival and expansion of old concepts based on new genetic evidence. Lancet Neurol. 2013;12:406–14. Doi:10.1016/S1474-4422(13)70011-5.
30. Durkin MS, Gottlieb C. Prevention versus protection: reconciling global public health and human rights perspectives on childhood disability. Disabil Health. 2009;J 2:7–8. Doi:10.1016/j.dhjo.2008.08.002.
31. Walker SP, Wachs TD, Gardner JM, et al. Child development in developing countries 2 Child development : risk factors for adverse outcomes in developing countries. Lancet. 2007;369:145–57.
32. Ngure FM, Reid BM, Humphrey JH, et al. Water, sanitation, and hygiene (WASH), environmental enteropathy, nutrition, and early child development: making the links. Ann N Y Acad Sci. 2014;1308:118–28. Doi:10.1111/nyas.12330.
33. Grandjean P, Landrigan PJ. Neurobehavioural effects of developmental toxicity. Lancet Neurol. 2014;13:330–8. Doi:10.1016/S1474-4422(13)70278-3.
34. Tabery J. Biometric and developmental gene-environment interactions: looking back, moving forward. Dev Psychopathol. 2007;19:961–76. Doi:10.1017/S0954579407000478.
35. Karmiloff-Smith A, D'Souza D, Dekker TM, et al. Genetic and environmental vulnerabilities in children with neurodevelopmental disorders. Proc Natl Acad Sci. 2012;109 Suppl:17261–5. Doi:10.1073/pnas.1121087109.
36. Meaney FJ. Mental retardation. In: Ember C, Ember M, editors. Encyclopedia of medical anthropology: health and illness in the world's culture. New York, NY: Kluwer/Plenum; 2004; P. 493–505.
37. Chaste P, Leboyer M. Autism risk factors: genes, environment, and gene-environment interactions. Dialogues Clin Neurosci. 2012;14:281–92.
38. Nijmeijer JS, Hartman CA, Rommelse NNJ, et al. Perinatal risk factors interacting with catechol O-methyltransferase and the serotonin transporter gene predict ASD symptoms in children with ADHD. J Child Psychol Psychiatry. 2010;51:1242–50. Doi:10.1111/j.1469-7610.2010.02277.x.
39. Schmidt RJ, Hansen RL, Hartiala J, et al. Prenatal vitamins, one-carbon metabolism gene variants, and risk for autism. Epidemiology. 2011;22(4):476–85. Doi:10.1097/EDE.0b013e31821d0e30.
40. Schaevitz LR, Berger-Sweeney JE. Gene-environment interactions and epigenetic pathways in autism: the importance of one-carbon metabolism. ILAR J. 2012;53:322–40. Doi:10.1093/ilar.53.3-4.322.
41. NIH Roadmap Epigenomics Mapping Consortium. Overview of the roadmap epigenomics project. http://www.roadmapepigenomics.org/overview. Accessed 28 Sep 2014.
42. Zahir FR, Brown CJ. Epigenetic impacts on neurodevelopment: pathophysiological mechanisms and genetic modes of action. Pediatr Res. 2011;69:92R–100R. Doi:10.1203/PDR.0b013e318213565e.
43. Rivera CM, Ren B; Mapping human epigenomes. Cell. 2013;155:39–55. Doi:10.1016/j.cell.2013.09.011.
44. Roopra A, Dingledine R, Hsieh J. Epigenetics and epilepsy. Epilepsia. 2012;53 Suppl 9:2–10. Doi:10.1111/epi.12030.
45. Msall ME, Hogan DP. Counting children with disability in low-income countries: enhancing prevention, promoting child development, and investing in economic well-being. Pediatrics. 2007;120:182–5. Doi:10.1542/peds.2007-1059.
46. Engle PL, Fernald LCH, Alderman H, et al. Strategies for reducing inequalities and improving developmental outcomes for young children in low-income and middle-income countries. Lancet. 2011;378:1339–53. Doi:10.1016/S0140-6736(11)60889-1.
47. Jariyapitaksakul C, Tannirandorn Y. The occurrence of small for gestational age infants and perinatal and maternal outcomes in normal and poor maternal weight gain singleton pregnancies. J Med Assoc Thai. 2013;96:259–65.
48. Ververs M-T, Anderens A, Sackl A, et al. Which anthropometric indicators identify a pregnant woman as acutely malnourished and predict adverse birth outcomes in the humanitarian context? PLoS Curr. 2013;5.
49. Black RE, Victora CG, Walker SP, et al. Maternal and child undernutrition and overweight in low-income and middle-income countries. Lancet. 2013;382:427–51.

50. Blencowe H, Lee ACC, Cousens S, et al. Preterm birth-associated neurodevelopmental impairment estimates at regional and global levels for 2010. Pediatr Res. 2013;74 Suppl 1:17–34. Doi:10.1038/pr.2013.204.
51. Blencowe H, Cousens S, Oestergaard M, et al. National, regional, and worldwide estimates of preterm birth rates in the year 2010 with time trends since 1990 for selected countries: a systematic analysis and implications. Lancet. 2012;379:2162–72.
52. Rahman A, Iqbal Z, Bunn J, et al. Impact of maternal depression on infant nutritional status and illness: a cohort study. Arch Gen Psychiatry. 2004;61:946–52.
53. Rahman A, Bunn J, Lovel H, Creed F. Association between antenatal depression and low birthweight in a developing country. Acta Psychiatr Scand. 2007;115:481–6.
54. Parsons CE, Young KS, Rochat TJ, et al. Postnatal depression and its effects on child development: a review of evidence from low-and middle-income countries. Br Med Bull. 2012;101:57–79.
55. Nair MKC, Radhakrishnan SR. Early childhood development in deprived urban settlements. Indian Pediatr. 2004;41:227–37.
56. Grantham-McGregor S, Cheung YB, Cueto S, et al. Developmental potential in the first 5 years for children in developing countries. Lancet. 2007;369:60–70.
57. Berkman DS, Lescano AG, Gilman RH, et al. Effects of stunting, diarrhoeal disease, and parasitic infection during infancy on cognition in late childhood: A follow-up study. Lancet. 2002;359:564–571. Doi:10.1016/S0140-6736 (02)07744-9.
58. Ernst KC, Phillips BS, Duncan BD. Slums are not places for children to live: Vulnerabilities, health outcomes, and possible interventions. Adv Pediatr. 2013;60:53–87. Doi:10.1016/j.yapd.2013.04.005.
59. Habicht JP, Martorell R, Rivera JA. Nutritional impact of supplementation in the incap longitudinal study : analytic strategies and inferences. J Nutr. 1995;124:1042S–50S.
60. Ridgeway B, Arias BE, Barber MD. The relationship between anthropometric measurements and the bony pelvis in African American and European American women. Int Urogynecol J. 2011;22:1019–24. Doi:10.1007/s00192-011-1416-1.
61. Strand TA, Taneja S, Ueland PM, et al. Cobalamin and folate status predicts mental development scores in north Indian children 12–18 month of age. Am J Clin Nutr. 2013;97:310–7. Doi:10.3945/ajcn.111.032268.
62. World Health Organization. The Global Prevalence of Anaemia in 2011. WHO Rep. 2011;48. Doi:10.1017/S1368980008002401.
63. Milman N. Iron in pregnancy: how do we secure an appropriate iron status in the mother and child? Ann Nutr Metab. 2011;59:50–4.
64. Allen LH. Anemia and iron deficiency: effects on pregnancy outcome. Am J Clin Nutr. 2000;71:1280S–4S.
65. Tamura T, Goldenberg RL, Hou J, et al. Cord serum ferritin concentrations and mental and psychomotor development of children at five years of age. J Pediatr. 2002;140:165–70. Doi:10.1067/mpd.2002.120688.
66. Lukowski AF, Koss M, Burden MJ, et al. Iron deficiency in infancy and neurocognitive functioning at 19 years: evidence of long-term deficits in executive function and recognition memory. Nutr Neurosci. 2010;13:54–70.
67. Fretham SJB, Carlson ES, Georgieff MK. The role of iron in learning and memory. Adv Nutr An Int Rev J. 2011;2:112–21. Doi:10.3945/an.110.000190.
68. Scott S, Chen-Edinboro L, Caulfield L, Murray-Kolb L. The impact of anemia on child mortality: an updated review. Nutrients. 2014;6:5915–32. Doi:10.3390/nu6125915.
69. Imbard A, Benoist J-F, Blom HJ. Neural tube defects, folic acid and methylation. Int J Environ Res Public Health. 2013;10:4352–89.
70. Smithells RW, Sheppard S, Schorah CJ, et al. Apparent prevention of neural tube defects by periconceptional vitamin supplementation. Arch Dis Child. 2013;56:911–8.
71. Prevention of neural tube defects: results of the medical research council vitamin study. MRC vitamin study research group. Lancet. 1991;338:131–7.
72. Recommendations for the use of folic acid to reduce the number of cases of spina bifida and other neural tube defects. MMWR Recomm Rep. 1992;41:1–7.
73. Barboza Argüello M de la P, Umaña Solís LM. [Impact of the fortification of food with folic acid on neural tube defects in Costa Rica]. Rev Panam Salud Publica. 2011;30:1–6.
74. Czeizel AE, Dudás I, Vereczkey A, Bánhidy F. Folate deficiency and folic acid supplementation: the prevention of neural-tube defects and congenital heart defects. Nutrients. 2013;5:4760–75. Doi:10.3390/nu5114760.
75. Vir SC. Current status of iodine deficiency disorders (IDD) and strategy for its control in India. Indian J Pediatr. 2002;69:589–96.
76. Zimmermann MB. Iodine deficiency. Endocr Rev. 2009;30:376–408. Doi:10.1210/er.2009-0011.
77. Bath SC, Steer CD, Golding J, et al. Effect of inadequate iodine status in UK pregnant women on cognitive outcomes in their children: results from the avon longitudinal study of parents and children (ALSPAC). Lancet. 2013;382:331–7. Doi:10.1016/S0140-6736(13)60436-5.
78. World Health Organization. Assessment of iodine deficiency disorders and monitoring their elimination: a guide for programme management. 2007.

79. World Health Organization. Global prevalence of vitamin A deficiency in populations at risk 1995–2005 : WHO global database on vitamin A deficiency. WHO Iris. 2009;55. Doi:978 92 4 159801 9.
80. Centers for Disease Control and Prevention. Attention-deficit/hyperactivity disorder (ADHD). In: ADHD Data Stat. 2014. http://www.cdc.gov/ncbddd/adhd/data.html.
81. Kashala E, Tylleskar T, Elgen I, et al. Attention deficit and hyperactivity disorder among school children in Kinshasa, Democratic Republic of Congo. Afr Health Sci. 2007;5:172–81. Doi:10.5555/afhs.2005.5.3.172.
82. Galler JR, Bryce CP, Zichlin ML, et al. Infant malnutrition is associated with persisting attention deficits in middle adulthood. J Nutr. 2012;142:788–94. Doi:10.3945/jn.111.145441.
83. Galler JR, Ramsey F. A follow-up study of the influence of early malnutrition on development: behavior at home and at school. J Am Acad Child Adolesc Psychiatry. 1989;28:254–61. Doi:10.1097/00004583-198903000-00018.
84. Ptacek R, Kuzelova H, Stefano GB, et al. Disruptive patterns of eating behaviors and associated lifestyles in males with ADHD. Med Sci Monit. 2014;20:608–13. Doi:10.12659/MSM.890495.
85. Feingold B. Adverse reactions to food additive. Chicago, IL. 1973.
86. Stevens LJ, Kuczek T, Burgess JR, et al. Dietary sensitivities and ADHD symptoms: thirty-five years of research. Clin Pediatr (Phila). 2011;50:279–93.
87. Durá-Travé T, Yoldi-Petri ME, Gallinas-Victoriano F, Zardoya-Santos P. Effects of osmotic-release methylphenidate on height and weight in children with attention-deficit hyperactivity disorder (ADHD) following up to four years of treatment. J Child Neurol. 2012;27:604–9. Doi:10.1177/0883073811422752.
88. Whiteley P, Rodgers J, Shattock P. Feeding patterns in autism. Autism, Whiteley. 2000;P:207–211.
89. Williams PG, Dalrymple N, Neal J. Eating habits of children with autism. Pediatr Nurs. 1999;26:259–64.
90. Sharp WG, Berry RC, McCracken C, et al. Feeding problems and nutrient intake in children with autism spectrum disorders: a meta-analysis and comprehensive review of the literature. J Autism Dev Disord. 2013;43:2159–73. Doi:10.1007/s10803-013-1771-5.
91. Dosman C, Adams D, Wudel B, et al. Complementary, holistic, and integrative medicine: autism spectrum disorder and gluten- and casein-free diet. Pediatr Rev. 2013;34:e36–41. Doi:10.1542/pir.34-10-e36.
92. Cermak SA, Curtin C, Bandini LG. Food selectivity and sensory sensitivity in children with autism spectrum disorders. J Am Diet Assoc. 2010;110:238–46. Doi:10.1016/j.jada.2009.10.032.
93. Emond A, Emmett P, Steer C, Golding J. Feeding symptoms, dietary patterns, and growth in young children with autism spectrum disorders. Pediatrics. 2010;126:e337–42. Doi:10.1542/peds.2009-2391.
94. Hediger ML, England LJ, Molloy CA, et al. Reduced bone cortical thickness in boys with autism or autism spectrum disorder. J Autism Dev Disord. 2008;38:848–56. Doi:10.1007/s10803-007-0453-6.
95. Zimmer MH, Hart LC, Manning-Courtney P, et al. Food variety as a predictor of nutritional status among children with autism. J Autism Dev Disord. 2008;42:549–56. Doi:10.1007/s10803-011-1268-z.
96. Bax M, Goldstein M, Rosenbaum P, et al. Proposed definition and classification of cerebral palsy. Dev Med Child Neurol. 2005;47:571–6.
97. Yeargin-Allsopp M, Van Naarden Braun K, Doernberg NS, et al. Prevalence of cerebral palsy in 8-year-old children in three areas of the United States in 2002: a multisite collaboration. Pediatrics. 2008;121:547–54. Doi:10.1542/peds.2007-1270.
98. Palisano R, Rosenbaum P, Walter S, et al. Development and reliability of a system to classify gross motor function in children with cerebral palsy. Dev Med Child Neurol. 1997;39:214–23.
99. Crichton J, MacKinnon M, White C. The life-expectancy of persons with cerebral palsy. Dev Med Child Neurol. 1995;37:567–76.
100. Strauss DJ, Shavelle RM, Anderson TW. Life expectancy of children with cerebral palsy. Pediatr Neurol. 1998;18:143–149. Doi:10.1016/S0887-8994(97)00172-0.
101. Motion S, Northstone K, Emond A, et al. Early feeding problems in children with cerebral palsy: weight and neurodevelopmental outcomes. Dev Med Child Neurol. 2002;44:40–3.
102. Reilly S, Skuse D, Poblete X. Prevalence of feeding problems and oral motor dysfunction in children with cerebral palsy: a community survey. J Pediatr. 1996;129:877–82.
103. Erkin G, Culha C, Ozel S, Kirbiyik EG. Feeding and gastrointestinal problems in children with cerebral palsy. Int J Rehabil Res. 2010;33:218–24. Doi:10.1097/MRR.0b013e3283375e10.
104. Arvedson JC. Feeding children with cerebral palsy and swallowing difficulties. Eur J Clin Nutr. 2013;67 Suppl 2: S9–12. Doi:10.1038/ejcn.2013.224.
105. Dahlseng MO, Finbråten A-K, Júlíusson PB, et al. Feeding problems, growth and nutritional status in children with cerebral palsy. Acta Paediatr. 2012;101:92–8. Doi:10.1111/j.1651-2227.2011.02412.x.
106. Fung EB, Samson-Fang L, Stallings VA, et al. Feeding dysfunction is associated with poor growth and health status in children with cerebral palsy. J Am Diet Assoc. 2002;102:361–73.
107. Maxwell S, Bower C, O'Leary P. Impact of prenatal screening and diagnostic testing on trends in Down syndrome births and terminations in Western Australia 1980 to 2013. Prenat Diagn. 2015; Doi:10.1002/pd.4698.

108. González-Agüero A, Vicente-Rodríguez G, Moreno LA, et al. Health-related physical fitness in children and adolescents with down syndrome and response to training. Scand J Med Sci Sports. 2010;20:716–24. Doi:10.1111/j.1600-0838.2010.01120.x.

109. Au KS, Ashley-Koch A, Northrup H. Epidemiologic and genetic aspects of spina bifida and other neural tube defects. Dev Disabil Res Rev. 2010;16:6–15. Doi:10.1002/ddrr.93.

110. Rosenblum MF, Finegold DN, Charney EB. Assessment of stature of children with myelomeningocele, and usefulness of arm-span measurement. Dev Med Child Neurol. 1983;25:338–42.

111. Crytzer TM, Dicianno BE, Kapoor R. Physical activity, exercise, and health-related measures of fitness in adults with spina bifida: a review of the literature. PM&R. 2013;5:1051–62. Doi:10.1016/j.pmrj.2013.06.010.

112. UNICEF. Convention of the Rights of the Child. 2013; http://www.unicef.org/crc.

113. United Nations Convention on the rights of persons with disabilities. http://www.un.org/disabilities/convention/conventionfull.shtml.

114. Blanchfield, L., Brougher, C., DeBergh JV. The united nations convention on the rights of persons with disabilities: issues in the U.S. Ratification Debate.

115. Unesco. The right to education for persons with disabilities: towards inclusion. http://www.unesco.org/education/efa/know_sharing/flagship_initiatives/persons_disabilities.shtml. Accessed 8 Jun 2015.

116. UNICEF. Neonatal mortality rates are declining in all regions, but more slowly in sub-Saharan Africa. In: UNICEF Data. 2013; http://data.unicef.org/child-mortality/neonatal.

117. Mwaniki MK, Atieno M, Lawn JE, Newton CRJC. Long-term neurodevelopmental outcomes after intrauterine and neonatal insults: a systematic review. Lancet. 2012;379:445–52. Doi:10.1016/S0140-6736(11)61577-8.

118. Liu L, Johnson HL, Cousens S, et al. Global, regional, and national causes of child mortality: an updated systematic analysis for 2010 with time trends since 2000. Lancet. 2012;379:2151–61. Doi:10.1016/S0140-6736(12)60560-1.

119. Wallander J, McClure E, Biasini F, et al. Brain research to ameliorate impaired neurodevelopment-home-based intervention trial (BRAIN-HIT). BMC Pediatr. 2010;10:27. Doi:10.1186/1471-2431-10-27.

120. Scherzer AL, Chhagan M, Kauchali S, Susser E. Global perspective on early diagnosis and intervention for children with developmental delays and disabilities. Dev Med Child Neurol. 2012;54:1079–84. doi:10.1111/j.1469-8749.2012.04348.x.

121. Hajizadeh M, Nandi A, Heymann J. Social inequality in infant mortality: what explains variation across low and middle income countries? Soc Sci Med. 2014;101:36–46. Doi:10.1016/j.socscimed.2013.11.019.

122. Olusanya BO. State of the world's children: life beyond survival. Arch Dis Child. 2005;90:317–8. Doi:10.1136/adc.2004.062240.

123. Olusanya BO, Renner J, Okolo A. State of the world's children and progress towards the Alma Ata Declaration. Arch Dis Child. 2008;93:451.

124. Sutton PS, Darmstadt GL. Preterm birth and neurodevelopment: a review of outcomes and recommendations for early identification and cost-effective interventions. J Trop Pediatr. 2013;59:258–65. Doi:10.1093/tropej/fmt012.

125. D'Aiglepierre R. Focus development association and united nations children's fund, "Exclusion Scolaire et Moyens D"Inclusion au Cycle Primaire a Madagascar'. 2012.

126. Karangwa, E., Kobusingye M. Consultation report on education of the Deaf in Rwanda. 2007.

127. Snider H, Takeda N. Design for all: implications for bank operations. 2008.

128. Verdonschot MML, de Witte LP, Reichrath E, et al. Community participation of people with an intellectual disability: a review of empirical findings. J Intellect Disabil Res. 2009;53:303–18. Doi:10.1111/j.1365-2788.2008.01144.x.

129. World Bank. Project appraisal document on a proposed credit to the People's Republic of Bangladesh for a disability and children-at-risk project. Washington, DC. 2008.

130. Buckup S. The price of exclusion: The economic consequences of excluding people with disabilities from the world of work. 2009.

131. Stein ZA, Durkin MS, Davidson LL, Hasan ZM, Thorburn MJ, Zaman SS. Guidelines for identifying children with mental retardation in community settings. In: World Health Organization. Assessment of people with mental retardation Geneva: World Health Organization; 1992. P. 12–41.

132. Keen CL, Uriu-Hare JY, Hawk SN, Jankowski MA, Daston GP, Kwik-Uribe CL, Rucker RB. Effect of copper deficiency on prenatal development and pregnancy outcome. Am J Clin Nutr. 1998;67(suppl):1003S–11S.

133. Simpson LJ, Bailey LB, Pietrzik K, Shane B, Holzgreve W. Micronutrients and women of reproductive potential: required dietary intake and consequences of dietary deficiency or excess. Part II - Vitamin D, Vitamin A, Iron, Zinc, Iodine, Essential Fatty Acids. J Matern Fetal Neonatal Med. 2011;24:1–24.

134. Rosenthal DR. Malnutrition and developing fetus: an investigation of the effects of riboflavin, B-12, and folate deficiencies during pregnancy both on mother and fetus. Mt Sinai J Med. 1978;45:581–90.

Chapter 25
Adolescent Health and Nutrition

Jee Hyun Rah, Satvika Chalasani, Vanessa M. Oddo and Vani Sethi

Keywords Adolescents · Adolescent girls · Teenage pregnancy · Child marriage · Platforms for reaching adolescents · Adolescent nutrition

Learning Objectives

- Explain why adolescence is a critical period for improving nutritional status.
- Summarize the major factors that can lead to malnutrition during adolescence.
- Compare the short-term and long-term impacts of social and physiological determinants of nutritional status during adolescences.
- Identify direct and indirect nutritional interventions that are directed toward adolescence.
- List delivery platforms used to reach adolescents with nutrition interventions.

Introduction

The 2012 Lancet Series on Adolescent Health opens by stating that "Adolescence is a life phase in which the opportunities for health are great and future patterns of adult health are established." This is especially important in light of the fact that, of the 7.3 billion people in the world in the year 2015, 42% or more than three billion were under the age of 24, and 16% or an estimated 1.2 billion were adolescents (between the ages of 10–19) [1].

J.H. Rah · V. Sethi
Child Development and Nutrition, UNICEF India Country Office, 73 Lodi Estate, New Delhi 110003, India
e-mail: jhrah@unicef.org

V. Sethi
e-mail: vsethi@unicef.org

S. Chalasani (✉)
Sexual and Reproductive Health Branch, Technical Division, United Nations Population Fund, 605 Third Avenue, New York, NY 10158, USA
e-mail: satvika.chalasani@gmail.com

V.M. Oddo
International Health, Johns Hopkins Bloomberg School of Public Health, 615 N. Wolfe Street, Room W2501, Baltimore, MD 21201, USA
e-mail: voddo1@jhu.edu

© Springer Science+Business Media New York 2017
S. de Pee et al. (eds.), *Nutrition and Health in a Developing World*,
Nutrition and Health, DOI 10.1007/978-3-319-43739-2_25

Although the definition of adolescence varies between geographic and cultural contexts, the UN System generally defines this second decade of life as the period of adolescence [2]. The sheer size of this demographic compels our attention today, as societies across the world grapple with the challenge of how best to respect, protect, and fulfill the rights of individuals in this age group. Adolescents not only have unique needs that must be addressed so they can experience an adolescence befitting their capabilities, but what happens in this period of life often determines their own future outcomes as adults, as well as those of the next generation.

Nutritional status during adolescence and eating behaviors acquired during this period have implications for their current health, their health as adults, as well as the health of their infants and children. This chapter discusses these linkages, and presents various policy and programmatic options that can positively influence these linkages.

Adolescence and Youth—A Window of Opportunity

There is increasing recognition today of the opportunities and challenges a young world presents. While older populations (60 and above) are the fastest growing demographic in many parts of the world, the poorest countries of the world remain young, and over the next 15 years, it will be their large young populations who begin to enter the workforce. Preparing several generations of young people for healthy, safe, and productive lives poses a significant challenge in these countries especially if they are to capitalize on the demographic dividend that now high-income countries like South Korea have benefited from.

The demographic dividend refers to the accelerated economic growth that countries can experience as a result of specific population changes. Countries with large young populations, if they experience reductions in fertility rates, will have a window during which larger shares of the population are of working age than before. The ratio of young and old dependents to working-age adults declines, which can raise output and savings per capita, and lead to improvements in human capital and economic growth. However, the right social and economic policies and investments are needed early on for the window to open, and for the dividend to be realized. Firstly, investments in family health are needed to initiate, accelerate, and sustain a decline in fertility. These include voluntary family planning, maternal health, and child health. Secondly, investments in human capital are needed to create the environment where young people are prepared for absorption into dynamic sectors which will translate into economic growth. The environment can be created with policies that improve access to education and relevant skills, especially for girls, trade portfolio diversity, infrastructure quality, job creation, and labor flexibility [3].

As Fig. 25.1 shows, among all the major regions, sub-Saharan Africa is the youngest, with more than 60% of the population under the age of 24, and the adolescent population as high as 25% of the total population in some countries.

The Unique Lives and Needs of Adolescents

We understand more about adolescence today than we ever did in the past, including exciting new developments in understanding brain development during puberty [4]. Why examine the lives of adolescents as an important demographic in their own right? It is precisely because adolescence is a time distinct from childhood and adulthood. It is a time dense with transitions—physiological, psychological, and social.

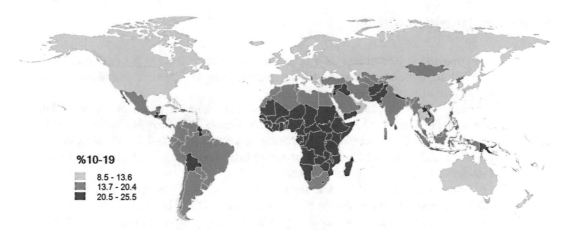

Fig. 25.1 Percentage of each country's total population aged 10–19 years. *Source* Author's calculations using data from World Population Prospects 2015. Map made using DevInfo. *Note* The boundaries and names shown, and the designations used on these maps do not imply official endorsement or acceptance by the United Nations

Focusing briefly on the latter, there are several critical life events that occur during adolescence, social transitions that are widely considered to be markers of adulthood. These events include the transition to citizenship, to work, to marriage, and to parenthood. When young people are physically and psychologically ready for these transitions, and when they have been adequately prepared, these transitions are often considered successful. However, when these transitions are premature, they constitute severe violations of the rights of young people, and they become rights costly to recover, or rights irremediably lost.

The difference in the onset of female and male puberty, the difference in the reproductive roles of males and females, as well as the deeply inegalitarian gender norms that prevail in most contexts, mean that girls are at much higher risk of unsafe transitions to adulthood that impact their health and nutritional status. Therefore, this chapter focuses primarily on adolescent girls, not to the exclusion of adolescent boys but somewhat more proportionate to the gender-specific elevated risks that girls face.

Child Marriage and Adolescent Pregnancy

Two of the most significant unsafe transitions to adulthood among adolescent girls, with important implications for adolescent nutrition, are child marriage and adolescent pregnancy. Child marriage, the accompanying (often non-consensual) sexual initiation, early/unsafe/unwanted pregnancy, school dropout that either precedes or follows both of these events—all of these constitute gross violations of the rights of girls, and also severely impede their preparation for adulthood. Despite repeated international commitments setting the minimum age of marriage at 18, approximately 13.5 million girls are still married under the age of 18 each year in developing countries. Of these, nearly one-third is married before the age of 15 [5]. Further, each year, 7.3 million girls in developing countries will give birth before the age of 18 and 90% of them will give birth within marriage or union [6].

The numerous individual and social costs of early marriage and pregnancy are undeniable. One specific example is their direct effect on the maternal health of adolescents. Complications from pregnancy and childbirth are the second leading cause of death among girls aged 15–19 years in many low- and middle-income countries [7]. Adolescent girls aged 15–19 have a slightly elevated risk of maternal mortality compared to young women aged 20–24. Girls under 15 are thought to be at an even higher risk (although this has been documented only on occasion) [8, 9]. All of these factors impact nutritional status of adolescents as detailed below.

Adolescent Nutrition Globally

Complete and comparable global data on adolescent nutritional status are not currently available. However, the available evidence on undernutrition, overnutrition, and micronutrient deficiency paints a challenging picture of nutrition among adolescents.

Iron deficiency has been identified as one of the main risk factors contributing to disability-adjusted life years in 10–24-year-olds [10]. Figure 25.2 provides some estimates of prevalence of mild, moderate, or severe anemia among adolescent girls aged 15–19, derived from the most recent Demographic and Health Survey (conducted in 2005 or later). Estimates range from a low of 13% in Honduras, to a high of 68% in Yemen.

In terms of undernutrition, a 2014 report shows that among the 47 countries that measure body mass index (BMI) of younger adolescents in the GSHS, at least 10% of boys in 13 countries and 10% of girls in 10 countries are underweight (according to BMI for age). Most of the countries with a high prevalence of underweight are in the Africa or Southeast Asian regions. There are no low- or middle-income countries in the Americas with more than 10% of younger adolescents underweight [11]. Figure 25.3 shows evidence from the most recent Demographic and Health Surveys (2005 and later). Bangladesh, Ethiopia, India, Niger, Senegal, Timor Leste, and Yemen all show very high levels of underweight (as measured by the percentage of adolescents with a body mass index [BMI] of less than 18.5) with 30% or more of adolescents 15–19 being underweight. In all countries, underweight among adolescents was higher than among all women of reproductive age. Note that while the DHS

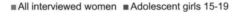

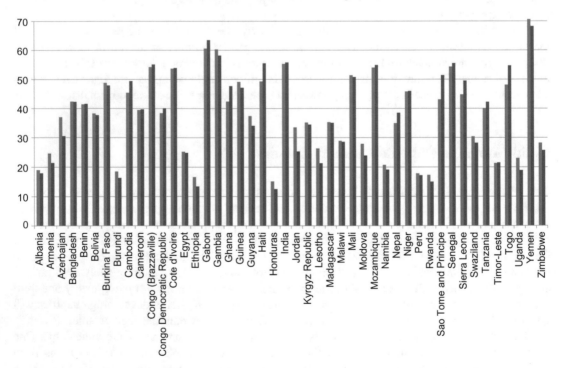

Fig. 25.2 Percentage of women of reproductive age, and adolescent girls 15–19, with mild, moderate, or severe anemia. Graph created with StatCompiler using most recent Demographic and Health Survey conducted in 2005 or later

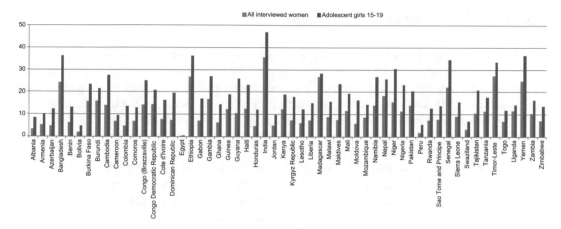

Fig. 25.3 Percentage of women of reproductive age, and adolescent girls 15–19, with a BMI less than 18.5. Graph created with StatCompiler using most recent Demographic and Health Survey conducted in 2005 or later

uses the standard cutoff of BMI of 18.5 for all women of reproductive age 15–49, WHO also has a growth reference chart specifically for school-aged children and adolescents, which includes females 15–19. Use of the BMI-for-age chart classifies a smaller proportion as underweight as compared to applying the cutoff of 18.5.

Undeniably, risks for later life non-communicable diseases are spreading rapidly worldwide, with greater rates of tobacco use and overweight, and lower rates of physical activity, predominantly occurring among adolescents living in low-income and middle-income countries [12]. It must be noted that stunting and overweight coexist in many developing countries, and stunting increases the risk of subsequent obesity and non-communicable diseases.

A 2014 report clearly described regional differences in the prevalence of obesity. African and South and Southeast Asian countries have the lowest levels of obesity among both younger and older adolescents, but there is wide variation within regions. Among the 56 countries where younger adolescents' heights and weights are measured, in 14 countries more than 10% of boys are obese, as is the case for girls in 9 countries. High rates of obesity are reported in some Western Pacific and Eastern Mediterranean countries. In most of the 21 countries with STEPS data (STEPwise approach to non-communicable disease risk factor surveillance) for older adolescents, young women had higher rates of obesity than young men. Again, the highest levels were in the Western Pacific Region. In 6 of the 21 countries, obesity rates were 10% or higher among older adolescents. Rates of overweight and obesity in Europe and North America were measured in the Health Behavior in School-aged Children study, with self-reported height and weight data. Only one country, the USA, reported obesity prevalence of 10% or higher [13].

Trends in most middle- and high-income countries in Europe and North America show no change, but 8 of 32 countries report increases in the proportion of boys or girls who are obese [13]. The limited available data on obesity incidence in Africa suggest that obesity is increasing among adolescents. In South Africa, only 0.2% of children aged 8–11 were overweight or obese in 1994 but by 2004, this had increased to 2.2% of boys and 4.4% of girls [14]. In China, over the past 20 years, there has been a dramatic rise in obesity among children and adolescents. Between 1985 and 2005, overweight and obesity among those aged 8–18 increased from 2% among boys and 1% among girls to 14% of boys and 9% of girls—a total of 21 million children [15].

Growth and Development of Adolescents

Puberty is defined as "a process of physically developing from a child to an adult" which is characterized by acceleration of the growth rate, a growth spurt, and maturation of the reproductive system [16]. Marked alterations in secondary sexual characteristics occur during this period, along with changes in body size, shape, and composition [17]. Whereas a substantial variation exists in the timing and tempo of pubertal growth and maturation, the sequence of events at puberty is relatively consistent [16, 18]. The physical changes and development characteristic of adolescence are secondary to the pubertal hormonal changes.

Due to the acceleration of pubertal height gain, approximately 15% of final adult height is attained during this stage in life. In the course of the pubertal growth period, a total of about 25 cm of height is gained; 7.5–12.5 cm of this gain occurs during the period of peak height velocity [17]. Although most girls grow 5–7.6 cm after menarche, a greater amount of stature may be gained among those with early menarche [16, 17]. Puberty is a time of substantial weight gain during which approximately 50% of final adult weight is gained [16, 17]. Peak weight gain velocity often occurs about six months after peak height gain velocity and reaches 8.3 kg per year [17].

Remarkable changes in body composition take place in adolescence. Before reaching puberty, boys and girls tend to have similar proportions of muscle and fat and lean body mass [16]. However, during puberty, girls accumulate relatively more fat than muscle tissue and major deposition of adipose tissue occurs around the breasts, hips, and gluteal region [16, 18]. An increase in lean body mass, which occurs uniformly in both sexes up until the age of 12–13 years, terminates at around 15 years of age in girls while extending until late puberty in boys [18]. In adults, the percentage of body fat is about 23% in females and 15% in males and lean body mass is 1.5 times greater in males than in females [17, 18].

Adolescence is also a period of rapid bone accumulation. Nearly one-third of total bone mineral is deposited within the first 3–4 years of puberty,[1] and more than 90% of peak bone mass is accumulated by 18 years of age [17, 18]. Impaired skeletal mineral accretion during adolescence in association with delayed puberty may lead to reduced peak bone mass in adulthood, increasing the potential for fractures [17, 18]. Growth in pelvic birth canal is slow and continues through late adolescence, as a large percentage of it is achieved after menarche [19]. The time of pelvic birth canal growth is different from the growth in stature, which is largely completed by the onset of menarche [19].

Determinants of Adolescent Growth

Physical growth and maturation during adolescence are influenced by a number of factors that may be broadly classified as hormonal, genetic, and environmental factors which continuously interact to modify an individual's growth [17, 18]. Environmental conditions such as low socioeconomic status (SES) and poor nutrition may be the major cause of suboptimal growth of teenagers in less-developed countries.

SES has been widely accepted as a determinant of somatic growth and development during adolescence as illustrated by cross-sectional and longitudinal research [20, 21]. In most developing countries, chronic mild to moderate undernutrition influences growth and development at every stage of life including adolescence. In a state of undernutrition, two important concerns regarding adolescent growth emerge. The first concern being whether the pubertal growth spurt is impaired, which

---

[1]Puberty is defined as "a process of physically developing from a child to an adult" which is characterized by acceleration of the growth rate, a growth spurt, and maturation of the reproductive system [16].

may negatively affect final adult size, and the second concern being if catch-up growth takes place during adolescence, which would make up for suboptimal growth during childhood.

The impact of chronic malnutrition on the timing of pubertal growth and sexual development has been well established. There is good evidence to suggest that the onset of puberty, menstruation, and peak height velocity is delayed, and the duration of puberty prolonged in a population that suffered undernutrition [22–26]. Yet, the effect of malnutrition on other physical dimensions of growth, including weight or body composition, has been less well defined as most studies have focused on statural growth. In a state of nutritional stress, pubertal changes represented by other anthropometric indices are likely to be compromised, as reflected by a longitudinal study of rural Indian boys which reported a smaller total weight gain during adolescence compared to that of a well-nourished British population [27].

It is unclear whether catch-up growth takes place in malnourished adolescents who remain in deprived circumstances without nutritional intervention. In situations where malnutrition is pervasive without nutritional interventions, a wide variation exists in compensatory growth during adolescence. Whereas prospective studies of Guatemalan children and rural Indian boys implied an absence of catch-up growth during puberty [23, 27, 28], varying degrees of recovery of early childhood growth retardation occurred in some adolescent populations [29–31]. Adoption and immigration studies consistently show the potential for catch-up growth under improved circumstances [32–36]. However, the specific environmental factors that induce compensatory growth are unknown. It is plausible that improved nutritional intake of macronutrients and micronutrients from late childhood through adolescence will stimulate compensatory growth. Yet, this assumption requires further research as the supplementation may trigger an earlier onset of menarche that would lead to a shorter pubertal growth period. Moreover, further research is also needed to determine whether specific dietary components contribute to accelerated pubertal growth.

Residential factors including rural environment, high altitude, intensive child labor and sports training, and the presence of sickle cell anemia have each been shown to be associated with slow pubertal growth. Teenagers residing in urban areas are known to exhibit better indicators of growth and accelerated sexual maturation compared to those residing in rural areas. High altitude, due to the effect of hypoxia, is generally found to delay pubertal growth and sexual maturation and to decrease the magnitude of growth. This association remains significant after controlling for the influence of confounding factors such as SES and genetic background, although the effect becomes smaller. Growth retardation in combination with delayed sexual and skeletal maturation is commonly observed in children and adolescents with sickle cell disease.

In addition, increasing evidence suggests that iron deficiency and helminthiasis causes slow physical growth during adolescence. It has been postulated that loss of appetite, one of the symptoms of anemia, might be responsible for growth retardation among anemic children, and thus, treating anemia, for example by iron supplementation, might improve growth by correcting anorexia. Based on the existing evidence, it is likely that the provision of iron to anemic adolescents produces accelerated growth in weight, height, and other anthropometric measurements. The determination of whether the acceleration in growth induced by iron supplementation can be extended over a long enough portion of puberty to compensate for earlier growth deficits need further study.

Adolescent Growth and Nutritional Status in Relation to Pregnancy

In low- and middle-income countries, chronic undernutrition may substantially delay physical maturation and extend the adolescent growth period beyond 20 years of age, potentially overlapping with the age of first pregnancy. In general, the increased nutritional needs of the mother and the fetus are delicately fulfilled through physiological and metabolic adaptations that occur during pregnancy.

However, in certain situations of inadequate nutrient supply, a balance between the maternal and fetal demands lies beyond the control of physiological adjustments, and thus, a biological competition for nutrients between the mother and her fetus becomes inevitable.

Pregnancy in adolescence, when active growth is occurring in both the young mother and the fetus, is likely to face limited nutrient availability relative to both maternal and fetal requirements. To date, most studies of nutrient partitioning during adolescent pregnancy have focused on well-nourished populations living in high-income countries [37–42]. Studies conducted in developed countries have suggested that nutrients are favorably partitioned to promote rapid maternal growth at the expense of the fetus in pregnant adolescents [37–42].

In poor rural populations in low-income countries, a large proportion of adolescents enter pregnancy with poor nutritional status and are likely to have suboptimal intake of nutrients during pregnancy and lactation. In this case, both adolescents who undergo pregnancy followed by a long period of lactation and their baby are likely to have less than optimal growth and nutritional status. It has been proposed that normal fetal growth is maintained only when adequate nutrient supply is available to support maternal growth or weight gain [43]. Thus, in conditions of limited nutrient availability, fetal growth is likely to be compromised in order to maintain maternal growth. However, with more severe nutrient restriction, it has been suggested that maternal nutritional depletion and impaired growth of the fetus are likely to occur concurrently due to the competition and inadequate availability of nutrients for both the growing teenage mother and the fetus.

Previously, it was believed that growth was largely completed by the time adolescent girls become pregnant, and thus, the majority of pregnant teenagers did not grow anymore or did so only marginally during pregnancy. This was based on the notion that pregnancy occurs subsequent to menarche, when growth rate drops to nadir [42]. However, in a revolutionary study conducted in Camden, NJ, which measured changes in knee height during adolescent pregnancy, it was demonstrated that a large proportion of adolescents were still growing in stature during pregnancy [44, 45]. Scholl et al. refuted previous studies as being influenced by a "downward bias" due to the tendency of most gravidas to measure slightly less in stature during pregnancy as a result of vertebral compression or weight gain [44, 45]. Using a knee height measurement, which is less susceptible to the "shrinkage" effects of pregnancy on the spine, the study found a significant increase in height [44, 45].

Recent evidence from low- and middle-income countries suggests the negative impact of teenage pregnancy on linear growth of young mothers. In a study of Brazilian adolescents, the attained height at age 19 was inversely associated with having a history of pregnancy during adolescence and each pregnancy was associated with a 0.46 cm reduction in height changes between age 15 and 19 years [46]. A study done in Mexico City showed that pregnant adolescents <18 years of age did not grow in height between the second trimester of pregnancy and 1-month postpartum, whereas never-pregnant adolescents matched on age, menarche age, BMI, and SES continued to grow during a 5-month period [47]. In particular, a study was conducted in rural Bangladesh, where 49% of adolescent girls were stunted and 40% underweight, and where ~25% of pregnancies occur among adolescents [48]. Childbearing during adolescence was found to hamper post-menarcheal linear growth, and it was concluded that the cessation of linear growth in adolescents due to an early pregnancy might result in an overall loss of between 0.6 and 2.7 cm in attained height in rural Bangladeshi women, which may contribute to stunting [48].

The potential negative impact of pregnancy during adolescence on maternal linear growth may be explained by the inadequate nutrient supply to support maternal growth due to the competition for nutrients between the teenage mother and the fetus [43]. Another potential mechanism, which remains to be examined, is the acceleration of epiphyseal closure due to the increased estrogen concentration during pregnancy [49]. Epiphyseal closure is normally induced by an increased secretion of estrogen during puberty [49]. In adolescents, pregnancy may cause an earlier cessation in bone growth and thus a decrease in their final height and increased cephalopelvic disproportion (an unborn child's head being too large to enter or pass through the birth canal) due to the effect of elevated estrogen on stimulating epiphyseal closure [49].

Available information from low- and middle-income countries has also shown that pregnant girls lose weight, body mass index, and mid-upper arm circumference by six months postpartum [48]. The depletion of maternal fat stores and lean body mass during pregnancy and early stages of lactation, especially among adolescents who become pregnant at an earlier gynecological age (defined as time between menarche and first pregnancy), may affect the outcome of future pregnancies and increase the risk of maternal morbidity and mortality [48].

Micronutrient Deficiencies and Anemia in Adolescents in Low- and Middle-Income Countries

Rapid growth and development during puberty markedly elevates the physiological demands for energy and micronutrients in adolescents. Suboptimal food and nutrient intake during this period place adolescents at an increased risk of nutritional deficiencies, which compromise teenagers functionally and developmentally. Specifically, adolescents in developing countries may be challenged to meet their nutritional requirements due to limited food availability in association with poverty, poor quality diets, and lack of nutritional knowledge. Inability to meet nutrition requirements in adolescence may lead to poor growth and nutritional status.

Cross-sectional data on dietary intake of teenagers in low- and middle-income countries revealed that intakes of various nutrients were below the recommended amount, and findings were worse in relation to micronutrients compared to energy and macronutrients [50, 51]. For instance, the percentage of adolescents consuming below 70% of the Recommended Dietary Allowances (RDA) in selected states in India was more than 80% for vitamin A, 70% for riboflavin, 80% for calcium, 75% for iron, and 50% for vitamin C among adolescent girls 16–17 years of age [51].

Anemia is a serious health problem in developing countries affecting 32–97% of teenagers [52]. Among Bangladeshi adolescent girls of low SES aged 12–19 years working in garment factories, 44% were found to be anemic (hemoglobin < 120 g/L) and about 56% had suboptimal serum retinol concentration (<1.05 µmol/l) [53]. In general, about 50% of anemia is assumed to be due to iron deficiency, while in malaria-endemic areas, the proportion can be slightly less at 40% [54].

A few studies that assessed the food consumption of pregnant adolescent women in low- and middle-income countries reported that their overall nutrient intake was insufficient [55]. Evidence of poor nutritional status of adolescents during pregnancy has been reported in some low- and middle-income countries. Among pregnant rural Indian adolescents with a mean age of 17.8 years, 46% were found to be mild to moderately anemic (hemoglobin 70–110 g/L), and 16 and 57% to be vitamin A- and iodine-deficient [56]. Also, in a study of Mexican pregnant adolescents aged 11–17 years who visited a prenatal care clinic, about 80% were found to be anemic due to iron deficiency [57].

Intervention Strategies and Delivery Platforms

Improving the nutritional status of adolescent girls is important for their own health, growth, and development, as well as for addressing intergenerational effects, because women's pre- and periconceptional nutritional status is strongly associated with birth outcomes [58]. Acceleration of pro gress in improving adolescent nutrition will require a range of effective, large-scale, complementary nutrition-specific and nutrition-sensitive interventions. Intervention coverage and the platforms through which these interventions are delivered vary widely by country, but largely include school-, community-, and health-based platforms, as well as social safety nets. Despite increasing evidence of effective intervention strategies and delivery platforms, program implementation gaps persist. This section provides an overview of relevant nutrition-specific interventions addressing the immediate causes of undernutrition (i.e., dietary intake and micronutrient deficiencies in particular), and nutrition-sensitive interventions addressing the underlying and basic causes of undernutrition (i.e., delaying age at marriage and first pregnancy).

Nutrition-Specific Interventions

Overall, nutrition-specific programs targeting adolescents are relatively new, and the coverage is still low in many countries. Nevertheless, international consensus suggests a multi-intervention approach [59]. Primarily, two nutrition-specific interventions have been implemented in order to reduce undernutrition among adolescent girls, including iron or iron and folic acid (IFA) supplementation and improving dietary intake through dietary diversification or fortification.

Improving Iron and Folic Acid Status

Recent reviews demonstrate that iron supplementation may be an effective means of increasing iron stores [60] and more generally, in reducing anemia, in adolescent girls [61]. Improving iron status among adolescent girls preconception is critical as preconception anemia increases the risk of iron deficiency anemia during pregnancy [62] and poor fetal and neonatal outcomes, including low birthweight and fetal growth restriction [63]. Additionally, periconceptional folic acid supplementation among women of reproductive age effectively prevents neural tube defects (NTD) [64]. Globally, two major public health interventions are recommended to improve IFA status including (1) food-based intervention strategies such as dietary diversification and food fortification with iron, folic acid, and other essential vitamins and minerals, and (2) oral iron supplementation and periconception folic acid supplementation.

Among the food-based approaches, *dietary diversification* is the most sustainable approach, but it is difficult to implement given both the actual quantity of iron intake and bioavailability of dietary iron consumed are largely low [58, 65], particularly in low- and middle-income countries where animal source foods, and thus heme iron which has good bioavailability, are less widely available and consumed. *Food fortification* can be an effective way to reduce prevalence of iron deficiency anemia and NTDs [66]. Food fortification can be universal, targeted, or occur at the household level. Universal fortification is the most cost-effective way to reach the population; however, successful universal fortification relies on various factors such as identifying a processed food that most people consume. Therefore, coverage of universal fortified commodities such as wheat or maize flour is often limited in rural areas. Targeted fortification is particularly important in resource-poor areas and for subgroups (e.g., displaced populations). Household- or institutional-level fortification (also called home fortification or point-of-use fortification) typically involves the distribution and utilization of micronutrient powders or small-quantity lipid-based nutrient supplements. However, there is yet very limited experience with the use of home fortification among adolescents. Although an effective and feasible strategy in low- and middle-income countries, levels of fortification, fortificants, and staple foods (wheat, rice, maize) must be tailored to the context of the country and community [67].

Iron supplementation is often recommended given that the iron requirement of adolescent girls is difficult to satisfy even with good-quality, iron-fortified diets [68]. Additionally, periconception *folic acid supplementation* reduces incidence of megaloblastic anemia and improves red cell folate concentrations to levels associated with a reduced risk of NTDs [69–71]. A recent review of intervention strategies targeting adolescents (in both low- and middle- and high-income countries) indicated moderate quality evidence of an overall substantial and significant reduction in anemia with IFA supplementation [61]. Community-based studies did not impact anemia or hemoglobin levels, while school-based delivery of interventions significantly reduced anemia and low ferritin levels, and improved hemoglobin concentration and iron status among adolescents.

The World Health Organization (WHO) recommends preventive iron and folic acid supplementation (60 mg/day iron with 400 mcg folic acid) for 3 consecutive months per year throughout adolescence among populations where anemia prevalence in pubertal girls is severe (>40%) [72]. If anemia is diagnosed in an individual, daily iron (120 mg) and folic acid (400 mcg) supplementation is recommended. However, early trials exploring the effectiveness of IFA among adolescent girls in India found weekly IFA supplementation to be a practical and effective strategy to prevent anemia in school-going adolescent girls [73]. Trials indicated that the differences in hemoglobin concentration among daily and weekly treatment groups were small and that under supervised conditions, weekly IFA would impact on the prevalence of anemia in adolescent girls and be more effective than daily supplementation. As there is limited evidence for the effective dose of folic acid in intermittent supplementation, the recommendation for the folic acid dosage is based on the rationale of providing once a week seven times the daily recommended supplemental dose to prevent neural tube defects (0.4 mg daily or 2.8 mg of folic acid and 60 mg of elemental iron weekly) [74].

Adolescent IFA supplementation has been implemented in several contexts, including India, Mozambique, Cambodia, Egypt, Laos, the Philippines, and Vietnam. In particular, India has implemented a successful IFA supplementation program which was first scaled-up in 2006 utilizing the Integrated Child Development Services (ICDS) channel for school-going adolescent girls and Anganwadi centers. In addition to IFA supplementation, the program introduced biannual deworming, a hot cooked meal or a take-home ration, and counseling and support to adolescent girls on how to improve their diets, prevent anemia, and minimize the potential side effects of IFA supplementation and deworming. By 2011, the Adolescent Girls' Anaemia Control Programme had increased its reach and coverage to 13 states (reaching 27.6 million adolescent girls) [75]; subsequently, the National Weekly Iron and Folic Acid Supplementation Programme was launched in 2012 to expand benefits to all adolescent girls in India.

Despite success in India and other contexts, non-compliance may limit effectiveness of IFA [76], and in malaria-endemic areas, iron and folic acid supplementation should accompany measures to prevent, diagnose, and treat malaria, given the coexistence of anemia of malaria and iron deficiency anemia. Further, because folic acid is needed around the time of conception, when adolescent girls may not be reached by the platform that distributes IFA, and they may not plan to become or know that they are pregnant, fortification of foods may be a more effective way to ensure adequate folic acid status around conception.

Improving Dietary Intake

Balanced energy and protein (BEP) supplementation is one way to improve dietary intake among adolescents; however, BEP is not implemented at scale and there is no evidence that BEP at the time of puberty affects linear growth [77]. However, there are other potential benefits of increasing energy and protein intake and dietary diversity, including weight gain among thin adolescents, and improved micronutrient status. Additionally, BEP may benefit the nutritional status of adolescent girls during future pregnancies given that maternal undernutrition is a risk factor for fetal growth restriction and adverse perinatal outcomes [78]. Among women of reproductive age, providing a total energy supplement, which is comprised of up to 25% protein, effectively reduces SGA and increases birth weight [79, 80].

In India, where 56% of adolescent girls are anemic and 47% have low body mass index [81], several programs aim to improve the dietary intake of adolescent girls, including the National Food Security Act (2013) and the Rajiv Gandhi Scheme for the Empowerment of Adolescent Girls, known as SABLA. Under the provisions of the National Food Security Act, adolescent girls are provided balanced protein/energy supplementation using fortified grains (rice) or flour (wheat or millet) with nine essential micronutrients as a midday meal if they are in school [82]. Additionally, SABLA ensures that over 11 million out-of-school adolescent girls enrolled in the program receive daily supplementary foods either as a hot cooked meal or as a take-home ration [83].

Nutrition of Pregnant Adolescents

Salam et al. [84] systematically analyzed 17 interventions aimed at improving the nutritional status of pregnant adolescents. Interventions included the provision of micronutrient supplements such as calcium and zinc, in addition to the routine IFA supplementation to adolescent mothers or engaging them in nutritional education sessions. The package of interventions provided to adolescents differed across studies; however, data pooled across those interventions suggested an improvement in mean birth weight (standardized mean difference: 0.25, 95% CI: 0.08–0.41, which is estimated to be equivalent to >100 g) and decreased low birth weight prevalence (RR: 0.70, 95% CI: 0.57–0.84), and preterm (RR: 0.73, 95% CI: 0.57, 0.95). Despite evidence that these interventions may be effective at reducing adverse birth outcomes among pregnant adolescent, few low- and middle-income countries have implemented such programs at the national level.

Nutrition-Sensitive Interventions

Anthelmintic Treatment

Hookworm and Schistosoma play a role in the etiology of anemia by causing chronic blood loss [85]. Deworming decreases parasitic load where hookworm anemia is endemic, thereby providing some benefits in improving hemoglobin level. Deworming programs for adolescents have been implemented in several low- and middle-income countries, including India, Indonesia, and Tanzania and often accompany other complementary intervention strategies. For example, in India, biannual deworming was integrated into the scale-up of weekly IFA supplementation program for adolescent girls in 2006, which expanded its reach to all adolescent girls in India in 2012.

Postponing Age at Marriage and First Pregnancy

Postponing age at marriage, and thus first pregnancy, is arguably the most important nutrition intervention among this vulnerable age group. Early age at marriage is common in low- and middle-income countries as indicated by estimates that in South Asia, East and Southern Africa, and West and Central Africa, more than one-third of women are married before the age of 18 [86]. The WHO guidelines on adolescents in developing countries recommend preventing early pregnancy by (1) preventing marriage before 18 years of age; (2) increasing knowledge and understanding of the importance of pregnancy prevention during adolescence; and (3) increasing the use of contraception among adolescents. Age at conception influences the availability of nutrients during pregnancy [87], and teenagers are at increased risk of labor complications [88] and adverse birth outcomes [88, 89].

Optimizing Interval Between Pregnancies

Optimizing duration of inter-pregnancy interval is also critical [88]. Infants conceived 18–23 months after a previous birth have the lowest risks of adverse perinatal outcomes. Both shorter and longer inter-pregnancy intervals are associated with higher risks suggesting a J-shaped relationship; infants conceived less than 6 months after a life birth had 1.4 greater odds (95% CI: 1.3, 1.6) of low birth weight, 1.4 greater odds (95% CI: 1.3,1.5) for preterm birth, and 1.3 greater odds (95 CI%: 1.2, 1.4) for SGA as compared to infants conceived 18–23 months after the previous life birth [90].

Delaying age at marriage and subsequently first pregnancy is difficult to implement in practice because marriage customs are engrained in many cultures. Programs that are able to increase enrollment and retention of girls in schools through cash transfers or reducing access barriers, as well as programs that empower girls with information and skills, have shown potential in delaying age of marriage [91, 92]. In particular, a review of 10 trials showed cash transfers linked with schooling significantly decreased early marriage among adolescents [93]. Additionally, opportunities that increase adolescent girls' labor force participation, such as those in the garment manufacturing industry, often empower girls by providing income, as well as delay marriage.

Delivery Platforms

Improving the nutritional status of adolescent girls in low- and middle-income countries requires a package of services. Intervention strategies should combine complementary nutrition-specific and nutrition-sensitive approaches and incorporate various delivery platforms, as appropriate. Broadly, four types of platforms are used to deliver nutrition interventions to adolescents, which includes school-, community-, and health-based programs, as well as social safety nets. Perhaps most common, school-based platforms are often used to deliver energy-dense meals. These programs are thought to be advantageous in terms of enabling continued school enrollment among adolescent girls (which may delay age at first marriage) and ability to reach a large segment of the population. However, estimates suggest that approximately 58 million children of primary school age are not enrolled in school (and could hence not be enabled to stay in school when they reach adolescence), 31% of who are girls [93]. There is also stark variation in school enrollment by region. In West Africa, 18.8 million children (27%) are not in school, as compared to Eastern and Southern Africa (11.0 million or 15%), South Asia (9.8 million or 6%), East Asia (6.9 million or 5%), or Latin America (3.8 million or 6%) [93]. Rates persist as high as 65% in some contexts (Burkina Faso) and are above average in several countries in Southern Africa including Zambia and Mozambique [94]. Many countries now include several years of secondary school in their national targets; however, in sub-Saharan Africa (40%) and South Asia (26%), more than one-quarter of lower secondary-school-age children are out of school [93]. Therefore, a wide range of non-school-based programs are needed to target out-of-school adolescent girls.

School-based platforms offer an opportunity to promote health and nutrition for adolescents. In particular, school food supplementation programs targeting young adolescents facilitate school enrollment by providing meals, and in some cases, nutrition supplements. These programs are implemented worldwide [95] as they are a relatively simple way to reach this vulnerable population.

School meals make important contributions to children's recommended nutrient intake and also help establish appropriate eating habits. Major effects on height are not expected with school-feeding programs; however, when multiple micronutrient fortified foods are provided, school-based platforms are an effective way to affect micronutrient status among adolescent girls. A review of randomized evaluations of iron-rich school meals (fortified or providing animal source foods) reports that iron status improved in three of four studies [96]. Similarly, evaluations of the World Food Programme's school-based program in Uganda demonstrated positive effects on nutrition outcomes as a result of in-school meals and take-home multiple micronutrient fortified foods [97]. Specifically, the school meals and take-home rations reduced the prevalence of anemia among school-aged girls and adult women [98]. A nutrition-friendly school initiative in Burkina Faso has also shown potential in terms of school and community mobilization toward improved nutrition [59].

Community- and health-based delivery platforms are often utilized for providing preconception care and counseling which aims to educate women of reproductive age about pregnancy and childcare [99–102] as well as for health and nutrition service delivery. Community-based nutrition that targets adolescents often focuses on empowerment and is promoted through peer support groups and info-tainment media (e.g., television), and services are delivered through health care personnel or community health workers. One such example in India includes expanded health days in order to provide health, nutritional, and family planning services to adolescent boys and girls with the launch of the Rashtriya Kishor Swasthya Karyakram [103]. India's package for adolescents includes tetanus toxoid immunization, quarterly monitoring of nutritional status, balanced fortified dry food ration providing 25% of recommended energy and proteins, IFA supplements, deworming and counseling on diet, family and life skills [103].

Adolescent-friendly clinics have been promoted to target this vulnerable group and in order to provide adolescents with an environment where they can share concerns regarding sexual and reproductive health, gain access to medical care, and improve access to and provision of a range of contraceptive methods. While noting the unique needs of and the varied challenges that the poorest adolescent girls face relative to other young people in accessing such services, there is some evidence for the potential effectiveness of this approach. A systematic review of the effectiveness of interventions to improve the use of health services by adolescents in developing countries identified 12 initiatives, including one randomized controlled trial (Nigeria), six quasi-experimental studies (Bangladesh, China, Madagascar, Mongolia, Uganda, and Zimbabwe), two national programs (Mozambique and South Africa), and three projects (Ghana, Rwanda, and Zimbabwe), which demonstrated that actions to make health services adolescent user friendly and appealing had led to increases—sometimes substantial—in the use of health services by adolescents [104]. Adolescent-friendly clinics have also been shown to significantly improve knowledge and demand for contraception [84]. Health-based platforms have been successful at delivering multiple micronutrient supplements to adolescent girls in various contexts including Guatemala [105], Bolivia [106], and throughout Asia [107]. These interventions are inexpensive when added to existing delivery platforms, can have high coverage, and are well accepted [108].

Additionally, mobile technology and text messaging are also potential avenues for intervention, since texting has become the preferred channel of communication between adolescents and their peers. There is emerging rigorous evidence that interactive SMS systems can improve reproductive health knowledge and reduce adolescent pregnancy [109]. However, there is limited data on the impact of community-based delivery on nutrition outcomes.

Social safety nets or social protection programs protect vulnerable individuals and households against risk, and mitigate the impacts of economic shocks. In particular, conditional cash transfer (CCT) programs assign households to receive money, conditional on, for example, children's continued school attendance and being brought in for preventative health and nutrition services [110, 111]. Most

CCTs target transfers to women, as increasing women's control over resources will lead to greater investments in nutrition for the household. For example, [110], Baird et al. [112] found that a cash transfer of $10 per month conditional on school attendance for adolescent girls in Malawi led to significant declines in early marriage and teenage pregnancy, by keeping girls in school, which ultimately could impact nutritional status, also of the next generation. Similarly, a review of 10 trials (1 study in the USA, 8 studies in southeast Africa, and 1 study in Cambodia) showed cash transfers linked with schooling (e.g., secondary education, scholarships, school fee waivers) significantly decreased school dropout rate [RR: 0.48, 95% CI: 0.36, 0.65] and early marriage among adolescents [RR: 0.57, 95% CI: 0.44, 0.74] [113]. Similarly, in 2008, the World Bank launched a public–private partnership to promote continued education and the transition of adolescent girls to productive employment in eight LMIC including Afghanistan, Jordan, Lao PDR, Liberia, Haiti, Nepal, Rwanda, and South Sudan [114].

Conclusion

Adolescence is a critical period marking phenomenal changes in individuals including rapid physical, psychosocial, sexual, and cognitive maturation, and presents a window of opportunity to ensure successful transition to adulthood. Nutritional status and eating behaviors acquired during this life stage have important implications for the health and well-being of adolescents themselves, as well as intergenerational health outcomes. Available evidence suggests that the prevalence of undernutrition, overweight, and micronutrient deficiencies is considerable among adolescents. Rapid growth and development during puberty elevates physiological demands for energy and micronutrients, which is coupled with suboptimal food and nutrient intake. Their inability to meet nutrition requirements due to physiological changes is further complicated by two significant transitions to adulthood among girls that may occur: child/early marriage and adolescent pregnancy. In low-income countries, many adolescents enter pregnancy with poor nutritional status and have a limited intake of nutrients during pregnancy and lactation. In this case, both pregnant and lactating adolescents and their babies are likely to have suboptimal growth and nutritional status. Acceleration of progress in improving adolescent nutrition will require a range of effective, large-scale, complementary nutrition-specific and nutrition-sensitive interventions. Despite evidence of effective strategies and delivery platforms, such as school-, community-, and health-based platforms, program implementation gaps persist.

Discussion Points

- Compare the impact that social factors and physiological changes can have on adolescent nutritional status.
- What are the opportunities and challenges that adolescence presents in the life cycle from a nutrition standpoint?
- What types of nutrition interventions are best provided by the various delivery platforms?
- What makes the nutrition requirements for adolescent pregnancies especially different from pregnancies in older women?
- How will the outcomes of direct and indirect interventions differ in how they affect the nutritional status of adolescents?

References

1. World Population Prospects, the 2015 Revision.
2. UNICEF. The state of the world's children—adolescence: an age of opportunity. New York; 2011. p. 16.
3. United Nations Economic Commission for Africa, African Union Commission. Creating and capitalizing on the demographic dividend for Africa. Issue paper. Abidjan: ECA and UAC; 2013.
4. Sawyer SM, Afifi RA, Bearinger LH, et al. Adolescence: a foundation for future health. Lancet 2012; published online April 25.
5. UNFPA Global Open Database 2015.
6. UNFPA, Motherhood in childhood, state of the world's population. 2013.
7. WHO. Adolescent pregnancy. Fact sheet N°364. 2014.
8. Blanc AK, Winfrey W, Ross JR. New findings for maternal mortality age patterns: aggregated results for 38 countries. PloS One 2013;8(4).
9. Nove A, Matthews Z, Neal S, Camacho AV. Maternal mortality in adolescents compared with women of other ages: evidence from 144 countries. Lancet Glob Health 2014;2:e155–164.0.
10. Gore FM, Bloem PJN, Patton GC, et al. Global burden of disease in young people aged 10–24 years: a systematic analysis. Lancet 2011;377:2093–102.
11. WHO. Health for the world's adolescents: a second chance in the second decade. 2014. http://apps.who.int/adolescent/second-decade/section4/page4/Nutrition.html.
12. Patton GC, Coffey C, Cappa C, et al. Health of the world's adolescents: a synthesis of internationally comparable data. Lancet. 2012;379:1665–75.
13. WHO. Health for the world's adolescents: a second chance in the second decade. 2014. http://apps.who.int/adolescent/second-decade/section4/page5/Obesity-&-physical-activity.html.
14. Armstrong ME, Lambert MI, Lambert EV. Secular trends in the prevalence of stunting, overweight and obesity among South African children (1994–2004). Eur J Clin Nutr. 2011;65:835–40.
15. Ji CY, Cheng TO. Epidemic increase in overweight and obesity in Chinese children from 1985 to 2005. Int J Cardiol. 2009;132:1–10.
16. Spear BA. Adolescent growth and development. J Am Diet Assoc. 2002;102:S23–9.
17. Rogol AD, Clark PA, Roemmich JN. Growth and pubertal development in children and adolescents: effects of diet and physical activity. Am J Clin Nutr. 2000;72:S521–8.
18. Tanner JM. Growth at adolescence. Great Britain, London: Blackwell Scientific Publications; 1990.
19. Moreman ML. Growth of the birth canal in adolescent girls. Am J Obstet and Gynecol. 1982;143:528–32.
20. Malina RM, Little BB, Buschang PH, Demoss J, Selby HA. Socioeconomic variation in the growth status of children in a subsistence agricultural community. Am J Phys Anthropol. 1985;68:385–91.
21. Shi Z, Phil M, Lien N, Kumar BN, Dalen I, Holmboe-Ottesen G. The sociodemographic correlates of nutritional status of school adolescents in Giangsu Province. China J Adol Health. 2005;38:313–22.
22. Kulin HE, Bwibo N, Mutie D, Saniner SJ. The effect of chronic childhood malnutrition on pubertal growth and development. Am J Clin Nutr. 1982;36:527–36.
23. Satyanarayana K, Radhaiah G, MuraliMohan KR, Thimmayamma BVS, Pralhad Rao N, Narasinga Rao BS. The adolescent growth spurt of height among rural Indian boys in relation to childhood nutritional background: an 18 years longitudinal study. Ann Hum Biol. 1989;16:289–300.
24. Kanade AN, Joshi SB, Rao S. Undernutrition and adolescent growth among rural Indian boys. Indian Pediatr. 1999;36:145–56.
25. Cameron N, Mitchell J, Meyer D, Moodie A, Bowie MD, Mann MD, Hansen JDL. Secondary sexual development of 'Cape Coloured' girls following kwashiorkor. Ann Hum Biol. 1988;15:65–76.
26. Satyanarayana K, Nadamuni Naidu A, Swaminathan MC, Narasinga Rao BS. Effect of nutritional deprivation in early childhood on later growth—a community study without intervention. Am J Clin Nutr. 1981;34:1636–37.
27. Satyanarayana K, Nadumuni Naidu A, Narasinga Rao BS. Adolescent growth spurt among rural Indian boys in relation to their nutritional status in early childhood. Ann Hum Biol. 1980;7:359–65.
28. Martorell R, Schroeder DG, Rivera JA, Kaplowitz JH. Patterns of linear growth in rural Guatemalan adolescents and children. J Nutr. 1995;125:1060S–7S.
29. Little MA, Galvin K, Mugambi M. Cross-sectional growth of nomadic Turkana pastoralists. Hum Biol. 1983;55:811–30.
30. Steckel RH. Growth depression and recovery: the remarkable case of American slaves. Ann Hum Biol. 1987;14:111–32.
31. Cameron N, Gordon-Larsen P, Wrchota EM. Longitudinal analysis of adolescent growth in height, fatness and fat patterning in rural South African black children. Am J Phys Anthropol. 1994;93:307–21.
32. Winick M, Meyer KK, Harris RC. Malnutrition an environmental enrichment by early adoption. Science. 1975;190:1173–5.

33. My Lien N, Meyer KK, Winick M. Early malnutrition and late adoption: a study of their effects on the development of Korean orphans adopted into American families. Am J Clin Nutr 1977;30:1734–39.

34. Proos LA, Hofvander Y, Tuvemo T. Menarcheal age and growth pattern of Indian girls adopted in Swedden. II. Catch-up growth and final height. Indian J Pediatr. 1991;58:105–14.

35. Proos LA, Hofvander Y, Tuvemo T. Menarcheal age and growth pattern of Indian girls adopted in Sweden. Acta Peadiatr Scand. 1991;80:852–8.

36. Proos LA, Karlber J, Hofvander Y, Tuveno T. Pubertal linear growth of Indian girls adopted in Sweden. Acta Paediatr. 1993;82:641–4.

37. Wallace JM, Milne JH, Aitken RP. The effect of overnourishing singleton-bearing adult ewes on nutrient partitioning to the gravid uterus. Br J Nutr. 2005;95:533–9.

38. Wallace JM. Nutrient partitioning during pregnancy: adverse gestational outcome in overnourished adolescent dams. Proc Nutr Soc. 2000;59:107–17.

39. Wallace JM, Aitken RP, Cheyne MA. Nutrient partitioning and fetal growth in rapidly growing adolescent ewes. J Reprod Fertil. 1996;107:183–90.

40. Wallace J, Bourke D, Da Silva P, Aitken R. Nutrient partitioning during adolescent pregnancy. Reproduction. 2001;122:347–57.

41. Wallace JM, Da Saliva P, Aitken RP, Cruickshank MA. Maternal endocrine status in relation to pregnancy outcome in rapidly growing adolescent sheep. J Endorinol. 1997;155:359–68.

42. Scholl TO, Hediger ML, Schall JI, Khoo CS, Fischer RL. Maternal growth during pregnancy and the competition for nutrient. Am J Clin Nutr. 1994;60:183–8.

43. King JC. The risk of maternal nutritional depletion and poor outcomes increases in early and closely spaced pregnancies. J Nutr. 2003;133:1732S–6S.

44. Scholl TO, Hediger ML, Cronk CE, Schall JI. Maternal growth during pregnancy and lactation. Horm Res. 1993;39:59S–67S.

45. Hediger ML, Scholl TO, Schall JI. Implications of the Camden study of adolescent pregnancy: interactions among maternal growth, nutritional status, and body composition. Ann N Y Acad Sci. 1997;817(1):281–91.

46. Gigante D, Rasmussen KM, Victora CG. Pregnancy increases BMI in adolescents of a population-based birth cohort. J Nutr. 2005;135:74–80.

47. Casaneuva E, Rosello-Soberon ME, Da-Regil LM, Arguelles M, Cespedes MI. Adolescents with adequate birth weight newborns diminish energy expenditure and cease growth. J Nutr. 2006;136:2498–501.

48. Rah JH, Christian P, Shamim AA, Arju UT, Labrique AB, Rashid M. Pregnancy and lactation hinder growth and nutritional status of adolescent girls in rural Bangladesh. J Nutr. 2008;138:1505–11.

49. Vander A, Sherman J, Luciano D. Human physiology. The mechanisms of body function. 7th ed. Boston, Massachusetts: WCB McGrawHill; 1998.

50. Venkaiah K, Damayanti K, Nayak U, Vijayaraghavan K. Diet and nutritional status of rural adolescents in India. Eur J Clin Nutr. 2002;56:1119–25.

51. National Nutrition Monitoring Bureau (NNMB). Diet and nutritional status of rural population, prevalence of hypertension and diabetes among adults and infant and young child feeding practices. Hyderabad, India: National Institute of Nutrition, Indian Council of Medical Research. Report No 26; 2012.

52. Kurz KM. Adolescent nutritional status in developing countries. Proc Nutr Soc. 1996;55:321–31.

53. Ahmed F, Hasan N, Kabir Y. Vitamin A deficiency among adolescent female garment factory workers in Bangladesh. Eur J Clin Nutr. 1997;51:698–702.

54. Black RE, Allen LH, Bhutta ZA, Caulfield LE, de Onis M, Ezzati M, Materhs C, Rivera J. Maternal and child undernutrition: global and regional exposures and health consequences. Lancet. 2008;371:243–60.

55. Oguntona CRB, Akinyele OI. Food and nutrient intakes by pregnant Nigerian adolescents during the third trimester. Nutrition. 2002;18:673–9.

56. Pathak P, Singh P, Kapil U, Raghuvanshi RS. Prevalence of iron, vitamin A and iodine deficiencies amongst adolescent pregnant mothers. Indian J Pediatr. 2003;70:299–301.

57. Casaneuva E, Jinenez J, Meza-Camacho C, Mares M, Simon L. Prevalence of nutritional deficiencies in Mexican adolescent women with early and late prenatal care. Arch Latinoam Nutr. 2003;53:35–8.

58. Bhutta ZA, Das JK, Rizvi A, Gaffey MF, Walker N, Horton S, Webb P, Lartey A, Black RE. Evidence-based interventions for improvement of maternal and child nutrition: what can be done and at what cost? Lancet. 2013;382(9890):452–77.

59. Delisle H, Receveur O, Agueh V, Nishida C. Pilot project of the Nutrition-Friendly School Initiative (NFSI) in Ouagadougou, Burkina Faso and Cotonou, Benin, in West Africa. Glob Health Promot. 2013;20(1):39–49.

60. Beasley NMR, Tomkins AM, Hall A, Lorri W, Kihamia CM, Bundy D. The impact of weekly iron supplementation on the iron status and growth of adolescent girls in Tanzania. Trop Med Int Health. 2000;5 (11):794–99.

61. Salam RA, Wazny K, Lassi ZS, Das JK, Bhutta ZA. Adolescent health and wellbeing: A review of intervention strategies[Unpublished] Report submitted to Bill and Melinda Gates Foundation. 2014.

62. Brabin L, Brabin BJ. The cost of successful adolescent growth and development in girls in relation to iron and vitamin A status. Am J Clin Nutr. 1992;55(5):955–8.
63. Ronnenberg AG, Wood RJ, Wang X, Xing H, Chen C, Chen D, Guang W, Huang A, Wang L, Xu X. Preconception hemoglobin and ferritin concentrations are associated with pregnancy outcome in a prospective cohort of Chinese women. J Nutr. 2004;134(10):2586–91.
64. Lumley J, Watson L, Watson M, Bower C. Periconceptional supplementation with folate and/or multivitamins for preventing neural tube defects (Review). Cochrane Database Syst Rev. 2002(2).
65. World Health Organization. Iron deficiency anemia: assessment, prevention and control: a guide for programme managers. 2001. http://apps.who.int/iris/bitstream/10665/66914/1/WHO_NHD_01.3.pdf.
66. Ramakrishnan U, Grant F, Goldenberg T, Zongrone A, Martorell R. Effect of women's nutrition before and during early pregnancy on maternal and infant outcomes: a systematic review. Paediatr Perinat Epidemiol. 2012;26(Supplement 1):285–301.
67. Vir SC. Iron deficiency and iron deficiency anemia in adolescent girls. In: Public health nutrition in developing countries. Part 2. New Delhi: Wood head publishing India; 2011. pp. 713–32.
68. Viteri FE. The consequences of iron deficiency and anaemia in pregnancy on maternal health, the foetus and the infant. SCN News. 1994;11:14–7.
69. World Health Organization. Weekly iron folic acid supplementation in women of reproductive age group: its role in promoting optimal maternal and child health. Position statement. Geneva: World Health Organization; 2009.
70. Nguyen P, Grajeda R, Melgar P, Marcinkevage J, Flores R, Martorell R. Weekly may be as efficacious as daily folic acid supplementation in improving folate status and lowering serum homocysteine concentrations in Guatemalan women. J Nutr. 2008;138(8):1491–8.
71. De-Regil LM, Fernandez-Gaxiola AC, Dowswell T, Pena-Rosas JP. Effects and safety of peri-conception folate supplementation for preventing birth defects. Cochrane Database Syst Rev. 2010;10:CD007950.
72. WHO. Guideline: intermittent iron and folic acid supplementation in menstruating women. Geneva, World Health Organization; 2011.
73. Aguayo VM, Paintal K, Singh G. The adolescent girls' anaemia control programme: a decade of programming experience to break the inter-generational cycle of malnutrition in India. Public Health Nutr. 2013;16(09):1667–76.
74. Berry RJ, Li Z, Erickson JD, Li S, Moore CA, Wang H, Mulinare J, Zhao P, Wong LY, Gindler J, Hong SX, Correa A. Prevention of neural-tube defects with folic acid in China. N Engl J Med. 1999;341:1485–90.
75. Aguayo VM, Paintal K, Singh G. The adolescent girls' anaemia control programme: a decade of programming experience to break the inter-generational cycle of malnutrition in India. Public Health Nutr. 2013;16(9):1667–76.
76. WHO. Weekly iron and folic acid supplementation programmes for women of reproductive age: an analysis of best programme practices. WHO Regional Office for the Western Pacific. http://www.wpro.who.int/publications/docs/FORwebPDFFullVersionWIFS.pdf?ua=1.
77. Golden MHN. Is complete catch-up possible for stunted malnourished children. Eur J Clin Nutr. 1994;48(suppl): S58–71.
78. Black RE, Victora CG, Walker SP. Maternal and child nutrition study group. Maternal and child undernutrition and overweight in low-income and middle-income countries. Lancet. 2013;382(9890):427–51.
79. Imdad A, Bhutta ZA. Maternal nutrition and birth outcomes: effect of balanced protein-energy supplementation. Paediatr Perinat Epidemiol. 2012;26(suppl 1):178–90.
80. de Onis M, Villar J, Gulmezoglu M. Nutritional interventions to prevent intrauterine growth retardation: evidence from randomized controlled trials. Eur J Clin Nutr. 1998;52(suppl 1):S83–93.
81. International Institute for Population Sciences (IIPS) and Macro International. National family health survey (NFHS-3) India, 2005–06. Volume II. Mumbai: IIPS; 2007.
82. Ministry of Law and Justice. National food security act. 2013. http://egazette.nic.in/WriteReadData/2013/E_29_2013_429.pdf.
83. United Nations Children's Fund (UNICEF). Nutrition wins: how nutrition makes progress in india. New Delhi, India: UNICEF; 2013.
84. Salam R, Wazny K, Lassi Z, Das J, Bhutta Z. Adolescent health and wellbeing. A review of intervention strategies. Report submitted to Bill and Melinda Gates Foundation; 2014 (Unpublished).
85. World Health Organization. Preventing and controlling iron deficiency anaemia through primary health care: a guide for health administrators and programme managers. Geneva: WHO; 1989.
86. United Nations Population Fund. Marrying too young. End child marriage. 2012. Available at: http://www.unfpa.org/end-child-marriage.
87. Mehra S, Agrawal D. Adolescent health determinants for pregnancy and child health outcomes among the urban poor. Indian Pediatr. 2004;41:137.
88. WHO. Adolescent pregnancy: unmet needs and undone deeds. Geneva: World Health Organization; 2007.
89. Paranjothy S, Broughton H, Adappa R, Fone D. Teenage pregnancy: who suffers? Arch Dis Child. 2009;94 (239):11.

90. Zhu B, Rolfs RT, Nangle BE, Horan JM. Effect of the interval between pregnancies on perinatal outcomes. N Engl J Med. 1999;340(8):589–94.
91. Malhotra A, Warner A, McGonagle A, Lee-Rife S. Solutions to end child marriage: what the evidence shows. International Center for Research on Women [ICRW]; 2011.
92. Amin S, Diamond I, Naved RT, Newby M. Transition to adulthood of female garment-factory workers in Bangladesh. Stud Fam Plann. 1998;29:185–200.
93. UNICEF. Rapid acceleration of progress is needed to achieve universal primary education. 2015. Available: http://data.unicef.org/education/primary#sthash.zdg3pRvl.dpuf. July 2015.
94. Huisman J, Smits J. Effects of household-and district-level factors on primary school enrollment in 30 developing countries. World Dev. 2009;37(1):179–93.
95. Bundy DA, Drake LJ, Burbano C. School food, politics and child health. Public Health Nutr. 2013;16(06):1012–9.
96. Alderman S, Gilligan D, Lehrer K. How effective are food for education programs?: a critical assessment of the evidence from developing countries. Intl Food Policy Res Inst. 2008.
97. Kazianga H, De Walque D, Alderman H. Educational and health impacts of two school feeding schemes: Evidence from a randomized trial in rural Burkina Faso. World Bank Policy Research Working Paper, no. 4976. 2009.
98. Olney DK, Rawat R, Ruel MT. Identifying potential programs and platforms to deliver multiple micronutrient interventions. J Nutr. 2012;142(1):178S–85S.
99. Azad K, Barnett S, Banerjee B, Shaha S, Khan K, Rego AR, et al. Effect of scaling up women's groups on birth outcomes in three rural districts in Bangladesh: a cluster-randomised controlled trial. Lancet. 2010;375 (9721):1193–202.
100. Tripathy P, Nair N, Barnett S, Mahapatra R, Borghi J, Rath S, et al. Effect of a participatory intervention with women's groups on birth outcomes and maternal depression in Jharkhand and Orissa, India: a cluster-randomised controlled trial. Lancet. 2010;375(9721):1182–92.
101. Manandhar DS, Osrin D, Shrestha BP, Mesko N, Morrison J, Tumbahangphe KM, et al. Effect of a participatory intervention with women's groups on birth outcomes in Nepal: cluster-randomised controlled trial. Lancet. 2004;364(9438):970–9.
102. Bhutta ZA, Soofi S, Cousens S, Mohammad S, Memon ZA, Ali I, Feroze A, Raza F, Khan A, Wall S, Martines J. Improvement of perinatal and newborn care in rural Pakistan through community-based strategies: a cluster-randomised effectiveness trial. Lancet. 2011;377(9763):403–12.
103. Rashtriya Kishor Swasthya Karyakram. http://rksklaunch.in/index.html.
104. Dick B, Ferguson J, Chandra-Mouli V, Brabin L et al. A review of the evidence for interventions to increase young people's use of health services in developing countries. In: Ross D, Dick B, Ferguson J, editors. Preventing HIV/AIDS in young people: a systematic review of the evidence from developing countries. Geneva: World Health Organization; 2006.
105. Dhingra U, MacLean A, Boy E. Monitoring adherence and coverage of Sprinkles: the case of Guatemala. Beijing: Micronutrient Initiative; 2009.
106. Micronutrient Initiative. Reducing anemia in Bolivian children using "Chispitas" multiple micronutrient sachets. Ottawa: Micronutrient Initiative; 2008.
107. UNICEF. Workshop report on scaling up the use of micronutrient powders to improve the quality of complementary foods for young children in Asia. Bangkok, Thailand: UNICEF Headquarters, UNICEF Asia Pacific Shared Center and the US CDC; 2009.
108. Loechl CU, Menon P, Arimond M, Ruel MT, Pelto G, Habicht J, Michaud L. Using programme theory to assess the feasibility of delivering micronutrient Sprinkles through a food-assisted maternal and child health and nutrition programme in rural Haiti. Matern Child Nutr. 2009;5(1):33–48.
109. Rokicki S, Cohen J, Salomon J, Fink G. Impact of an interactive mobile phone reproductive health program on knowledge and behavior among adolescent girls: a cluster-randomized trial. 2015. Retrieved on Jan 13, 2016 from https://editorialexpress.com/cgi-bin/conference/download.cgi?db_name=NEUDC2015&paper_id=425.
110. Akresh R, de Walque D, Kazianga H. Alternative cash transfer delivery mechanisms: impacts on routine preventative health clinic visits in Burkina Faso. Washington, D.C.; 2012.
111. Arif S, Syukri M, Isdijoso W, Rosfadhila M, Soelaksono B. Are conditions pro-women?. London, UK: A case study of a conditional cash transfer in Indonesia; 2011.
112. Baird SJ, Garfein RS, McIntosh CT, Ozler B. Effect of a cash transfer programme for schooling on prevalence of HIV and herpes simplex type 2 in Malawi: a cluster randomised trial. Lancet 2012; 379:1320–1329
113. Salam RA, Wazny K, Lassi ZS, Das JK, Bhutta ZA. Adolescent health and wellbeing: a review of intervention strategies. Report submitted to Bill and Melinda Gates Foundation; 2014 (Unpublished).
114. World Bank Group. Adolescent girls initiative, the economic empowerment of adolescent girls and young women: status of pilot implementation. 2014;90767.

Chapter 26
Nutrition in the Elderly from Low- and Middle-Income Countries

Noel W. Solomons and Odilia I. Bermudez

Keywords Aging · Chronic diseases · Senescence · Frailty · Sarcopenia · Anthropometry · Malnutrition · Nutrient requirements · Dietary intake · Food security

Learning Objectives

- Describe the evolutionary approach to how nutrition is associated with aging.
- Identify aging processes that affect nutritional status.
- Compare conditions between low- and high-income countries that affect the nutritional status of elderly.
- Analyze factors that affect the assessment and interpretation of indicators of nutritional status for the elderly.

Introduction

Through the millennia of human evolution, nutrient and physical activity requirements evolved to satisfy the hunter-gatherer lifestyle, survival to reproductive age occurred for a select few, and almost no one survived to advanced age. Yet, there is an underlying chronobiology of *Homo sapiens,* which produces senescent changes from the cellular to the whole body level and limits total lifespan to ∼120 years. Currently, median lifespan is extending throughout the world with the majority of older individuals living in low- and middle-income countries and with increasing numbers of older subjects living well beyond one hundred years. Worldwide, about 8% of the total population are 65 years and older. However, that proportion is expected to grow to 12% by 2030 and to 16% by the year 2050 [1] with the majority of older individuals living in low–middle-income countries.

In low-income societies, the current challenges to medical and nutritional care and services and to public health policy and programs are significant. However, the future is promising as improvements

N.W. Solomons (✉)
Center for Studies of Sensory Impairment, Aging and Metabolism (CeSSIAM),
17th Avenida #16-89, Zona 11, Guatemala City 01011, Guatemala
e-mail: cessiam@cessiam.org.gt

O.I. Bermudez
Public Health and Community Medicine, Tufts University, 136 Harrison Avenue,
Boston, MA 02130, USA
e-mail: Odilia.bermudez@tufts.edu

© Springer Science+Business Media New York 2017
S. de Pee et al. (eds.), *Nutrition and Health in a Developing World,*
Nutrition and Health, DOI 10.1007/978-3-319-43739-2_26

in the medical and nutrition fields, better understanding of the aging process and the support from new discoveries and technologies are facilitating the world's securing successful aging for the elderly.

Finally, aging can be defined in practical terms, as commented by Busuttil and coworkers [2], as a series of time–related processes that ultimately bring life to a close.

The Biology of Human Aging and Survival: An Evolutionary Perspective

For every species, there is a maximal longevity span; that is, there is an age beyond which no member will survive. For humans, this span is judged to be ~ 120 years [3]. Beyond that age, the human organism cannot persist. In the wilds of nature, the risks of infections, the vagaries of food supplies and a food-chain based on a hierarchy of predation assure that most organisms born or hatched do not even survive to reproduce and even fewer survive beyond the reproductive period. As such, for most species, the members do not come close to approaching the maximal, biological lifespan.

For over 90% of the up to 400,000 years of the evolution of the genus *Homo*, our ancestors were part of the community of animal and plant species in a natural wilderness. Humans were just one wild species more. Our way of life was that of migratory hunter-gather clans and tribes. Although a few individuals probably survived to advanced age throughout all epochs of prehistory, the majority of individuals succumbed early in life. As a historical anecdote, the multicenter, international survey research protocol, *Food Habits in Later Life*, called for the enrollment of a cohort of individuals aged 70 years or beyond [4]. When, late in the 1980s, investigators tried to apply it among aboriginal peoples in the north of Australia, the effort was quickly abandoned, as the researchers found no potential subject older than 47 years of age. Such a truncated age pyramid was probably the order of the day among hunter-gather tribes and pastoralist nomadic groups throughout our history. With this evolutionary context, therefore, we might conclude that nature never intended there to be aging societies nor large numbers of older persons in the human populations.

The Evolutionary Paradoxes

Human evolution has been considered to be adaptive [5]. Darwinian theory, correctly interpreted, alludes to "survival of the fittest" in the sense of demographic dominations by the bearers of those genes that provide reproductive superiority. That is, the bearers have a higher propensity to survival to adult life, better chances for procreation and greater fecundity. The strength and agility that made for a better hunter could be generalized over generations, as those men with better skills would both survive the rigors of the hunt and dominate the procreation within the tribe in polygamous societies.

Because the internal and external challenges to the aging organism occur *after* the peak reproductive years, anatomic and functional outcomes in human aging do not obey the conventional norms of natural selection. As a consequence, there is no way for a process of differential fecundity to select for traits that express themselves or become beneficial only *later* in life. In fact, in *Homo sapiens'* natural selection process, we may have accumulated genetic traits directed toward survival within a hunter-gather way of life; these traits could actually affect health detrimentally into the middle and later years of a much longer lifespan.

We also use the word "evolution" in the connotation of *cultural* adaptation [6]. Besides successful reproduction, adequate nutrition is the other fundamental pillar for the basic survival of a species. Until the advent of domestication of animals and the emergence of pastoralist lifestyles some 40,000 years ago [7], tribal hunter-gatherers dominated humanity. Paleonutritionists' opinions vary on the exact composition of "typical" stone-age fare [8–11], but successful hunting societies could have derived over 50% of their calories from the flesh and visceral organs of the available fauna. Animal protein, in the form of dairy foods and meat, has been the dietary fare of pastoralists throughout their history. With respect to aging, one could argue that the cultural (diet and lifestyle) attributes that made for success as a young and vigorous hunter or herder could sow the seeds of poorer health and function if one had the fortune to survive beyond the peak reproductive years. This is explained by the risks associated with such lifestyle, which exposed hunters and herders to arduous and dangerous practices related to killing aggressive wild animals and to eating poorly conserved animal foods high in proteins, fats and probably environmental contaminants.

In summary, when the basic issues of survival confront the individuals of a society on a minute-to-minute and day-to-day basis, genetic biology and cultural adaptation must focus on getting enough individuals to survive up to the age of reproduction in order to assure the mere maintenance of the population. Making provision for **long-term** survival was among the lowest priorities of the evolutionary imperative for any species in the wild, including for us humans.

The Biology of Aging

When the conditions for surviving early and middle life are assured, as with captive wild animals, domesticated pets and livestock, and humans, it becomes evident that underlying senescent processes are operating from conception and throughout life. Since the evolutionary purpose for individuals is reproduction for the maintenance of their species, more redundancy of capacity was focused onto procreative functions; this came about at the expense of capacity for infinite repair of the cells of the host. Molecular gerontology is currently revealing cellular senescence as the basis of the aging process for the whole organism. These changes involve altered remodeling of the chromatin in the nuclear apparatus (telomeres) [12], leakage of free radicals from the energy generation in increasingly porous mitochondria [13], or mutations in their single-stranded DNA [14] and alteration of apoptosis (programmed cell death) [15].

The late Dr. Nathan Shock, a pioneering gerontological physiologist working in Baltimore, Maryland, USA, generalized to the aging process the differential—but inevitable—decline in physiological capacity of almost all human organ systems [16]. Shock and his group were working with white North American men in the mid-twentieth century; the degree to which the genetic constitution of other ethnic groups across the globe might vary in their projected rates of diminished physiological function is still a matter for prospective evaluation. Furthermore, with respect to the low-to-middle-income country perspective and its general social, lifestyle and environmental features, we must take what is currently known about physiological senescence in two speculative directions. What would be the *theoretical* effects of lifestyle and environmental exposures for preservation or deterioration of organ system functions? What would the *projected* effect of physiological decline on day-to-day living demands for older individuals in lower-income societies? The specific physiological and pathophysiological issues of the alimentary tract, and its relation to diet and nutrition, will be discussed in a later section of this chapter. For the general biological aging of humans, a brief profile of physiological senescence of the other systems is illustrative.

Senescence of Tissue and Organ Function with Aging

For the integumentary system (hair, skin, nails), which provides the external protective barrier, greater sun exposure might accelerate the loss of elasticity and the development of wrinkles. Darker skin pigmentation in certain African, Pacific Islander and Amerindian populations, however, might counteract the aging of skin. To the extent that cuts and bruise injuries might be more common among elders in low–middle-income countries, delayed wound healing represents a greater risk to cutaneous infection.

The pulmonary respiratory system function declines due to diaphragmatic weakening and reduction in the compliance of the chest wall. Obviously, lifelong indoor exposure to open hearth-cooking fires damages the alveolar soft tissues of the lungs, themselves. To the extent that relatively strenuous exertion may still be required of older men and women in pre-industrialized settings, greater limitation on desired activities may be imposed by dwindling lung capacity. A similar restriction may be the consequence of cardiovascular and circulatory aging [17]. For the latter systems, however, the fitness conditioning derived from strenuous daily demands may delay various aspects of physiological decline.

An intact musculoskeletal system to maintain agility of movement and weight-bearing capacity is as important for rigorous work capacity in later life as are the roles of breathing and circulation. With respect to joints, bones and muscles, the lifestyle demands of typical manual labor have differential effects. For cartilaginous tissue (joints), wear and tear of running, climbing and lifting accelerates their decline. For bones, the opposite effect is true, with weight-bearing serving to strengthen the vertebral and long bones and retard demineralization [18].

Physiological capacity of the hematological, renal, urogenital and gonadal and reproductive systems declines with age. These systems are relatively less differentiated in their sensitivity to the behavioral and environmental features superimposed on basic aging changes. Endocrine responses dependent upon the pituitary gland (thyroid, adrenal, somatotropic) also decline in capacity with age. Decreased growth hormone secretion and tissue responsiveness of aging (somatopause) have implications for body composition and muscle strength [19]. Lower muscle mass affects the gait of older persons, making them more prone to falls and therefore to bone fractures [20]. In this same metabolic domain, aging is generally associated with a decline in lean body mass and an increase in adiposity, even without overall changes in body weight, in a process termed sarcopenia. Sarcopenia is defined as an age-associated alteration in muscle structure and function with loss of muscle fibers and tensile strength and infiltration of muscle bundles with fat [21, 22].

The function of the immune system and its adequate regulation has important health implication for the aging individual. Given its dependency on the continuous turning over of immune cells, diet and nutrition play a determinant role in immune regulation. Host defenses against microbial pathogens may decline, thus exposing the older person to infections. The inflammatory response becomes dysregulated, and excess production of inflammatory cytokines, such as interleukin-6, advances with age. Tumor vigilance is an aspect of immune protection that takes on increasing importance with aging; the variation in its function represents one of the factors of differential risk of cancer among aging individuals. Autoimmune dysregulation increases with advancing age, increasing an individual's risk to diseases of autoimmunity.

The function of the nervous system declines with age in both the sensory and motor domains of peripheral nerves and at the central level with the special senses and mental cognition. The changes include altered pain sensation and loss of fine motor functions. The special senses, which include sight, hearing, taste, smell and touch, all become less acute with age. Studies have shown that older individuals in all populations around the world suffer a loss of memory and a decline in cognitive functions.

Function of the Alimentary and Digestive Tract in Aging

Aging affects the structure and function of the digestive system beginning in the oral cavity with loosening or loss of dentition and decreasing salivary flow and extending to slowing of propulsive (peristaltic) motility throughout the entire length of the tract. Fecal evacuations become less frequent and more difficult (constipation); the more fiber-rich traditional diets of rural cultures in developing societies, however, would tend to counteract the constipating features of neural and intestinal aging.

The secretory capacity of bile and pancreatic juice in young adulthood is rarely challenged by aging. However, gastric *Helicobacter pylori* infection is more common under the poor sanitation conditions of low-income countries [23]. The parietal cells lining the stomach of older persons, however, often suffer exhaustion. The nutritional consequences are reduced iron solubility and insufficient intrinsic factor secretion for vitamin B_{12} absorption. Assimilation of most other micronutrients, as well as of the macronutrients, is generally adequate to meet nutritional needs throughout the lifespan, if food energy intake is maintained at adequate levels. The background sanitation in low-income countries challenges inhabitants of all ages with the risks of intestinal helminthic and protozoan infestations and recurrent diarrheal episodes.

Successful Aging, Normative Aging and Frail Aging of Individuals Within a Population

One of the hallmark characteristics of an older population is the heterogeneity in functional status that one finds looking across individuals of the same age, that is to say persons of a birth cohort during the same year 60, 70 or 80 years ago. This "splaying" of variation increases with advancing age [24]. One way to conceptualize this heterogeneity is as a dissociation within individuals between *biological* aging and *chronological* aging [4, 25]. The same cumulative numbers of years may have elapsed, but the advance in changes in the anatomic structure, metabolism and physiological function (biological aging) is very non-uniform across a population, even of persons of the same ethnicity and culture, living in the same habitat. The interplay of at least three factors contributes to this dissociation: (1) genetic constitution; (2) environmental exposure; and (3) the burden of disease experience [26, 27].

The eminent gerontologist, Dr. John Rowe [28], advanced the term "successful aging," to characterize the process of growing older while retaining satisfactory health, function and independence. This is contrasted to two other conditions: "normative aging" and "frailty." Normative aging is the experience that covers most of the advanced years of most older persons in which multiple chronic diseases appear and function is compromised to some degree. Frailty is at the other end of the spectrum, in which persons have severe decline in cognitive and physical function, losing independence in activities of daily living [29], often becoming wheelchair bound or bed ridden and requiring assistance and care.

Demography of Aging of Populations in Low- and Middle-Income Countries

The aging of individuals within a population and the aging of a population are not exactly the same phenomenon. Both, however, are increasingly relevant to developing societies [30]. An individual's growing older is a product of surviving the hazards to health and physical safety in the society and environment. The aging of a population is seen in the distribution of a society among different age strata. The typical broad-based pyramidal form of the age pyramid of a young society transforms into a more columnar shape with extension of longer life and reduced falling birth rates. Today, across the world, the most prominent feature of human demography is the aging of individuals and the aging of populations.

The fastest growing subpopulation in the world, in terms of rate of increase, are persons surviving to 100 years of age. A tendency toward longer lives in general, however, can be seen throughout developing and transitional societies across all of the southern continents. Whereas once children had

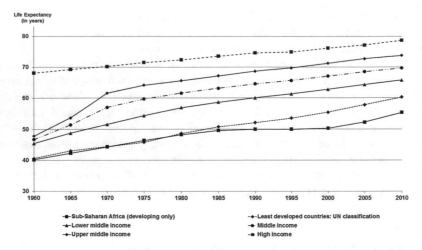

Fig. 26.1 Life expectancy at birth of world countries by levels of development. 1960–2010. *Data source* The World Bank [32]

only a slight chance of ever knowing their grandfather in high-income countries, some 50% of those born currently will come to know their great grandparents [31]. By the year 2020, there will be 7.6 billion inhabitants on earth, with over 1 billion or 13.3% over the age of 60 years; this is up from 8.5% in 1990. Three quarters of these elderly will be living in low- and middle-income countries. By region, 17% of East Asians, 12% of Latin Americans and 10% of Southeast Asians will be over 60 years. China with 231 million estimated elderly for that year, and India with 145 million will be the two most populous nations in terms of elderly citizens [30]. Even more, life expectancy still lags in low-income countries. For the year 2012, the life expectancy at birth in Sierra Leone of only 45 years, mainly due to high mortality of its under-five population, is about half of that for Japan, the most long-lived nation with the highest life expectancy of 84 years in the same year (2012), as can be observed in Fig. 26.1 [32]. Another demographic feature of aging of interest, at least in the USA, is the maintenance of an equitable sex ratio out to age 70 years, followed by a progressive divergence in survival, with women out-surviving their male counterparts Fig. 26.2 [32].

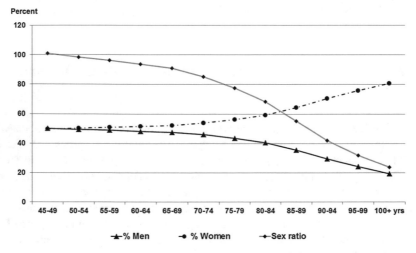

Fig. 26.2 Proportion of older adults by sex categories and sex ratio in the worldwide population for 2014. *Data source* US Census Bureau [1]

The Burden of Chronic Diseases in the Aging

It was conventional wisdom and epidemiological experience in low-income societies that acute infectious diseases, often life threatening, were common, but chronic, degenerative diseases were rare. The aforementioned extension of longevity in developing countries has been termed the "demographic transition" [33], which leads in turn to a change in disease patterns, the so-called "epidemiological transition" [34].

Non-transmissible Disease Epidemiology in Low-Income Country Populations

The epidemiology of non-communicable diseases (NCD) is not well documented in low-income countries, although it is accepted that this situation derives in part from the emergence of the so-called "double burden" of diseases [35–37]. The classical diseases of poverty, related to infections and nutritional deficiency, have not gone away—but they have been *joined* by a growing incidence of degenerative illness. Even more complicated, currently, close to 80% of NCD deaths occur in low- and middle-income countries, with about one-fourth of NCD-related deaths occurring before the age of 60 [38]. Undernutrition early in life, unhealthy diets, insufficient physical activity, tobacco use and alcohol use are five of the main risk factors for NCDs. And those factors are associated with the economic transition, rapid urbanization and changes in lifestyles that occurring at very fast rates in those low- and middle-income countries [38].

Relationship of Chronic Disease to Diet and Nutrition in Low- and Middle-Income Countries

The last three decades have seen the emergence of interest in the nutritional science community with the relationships of diet and nutrition to the risk of chronic diseases [39, 40]. And the international community initiated and mobilized expertise and resources to address the causes, social–economic determinants and the need for the development of policies and regulations needed to address the global burden of NCDs, including obesity and type 2 diabetes [35]. However, those efforts are still insufficient. To date, most nutritional epidemiology inquiry has been focused on dietary patterns in relation to the incidence of overweight and obesity, metabolic syndrome, cardiovascular disease and neoplasms in affluent populations of *high-income*, industrialized nations.

The question of policy and program relevance for low-income countries of accumulated nutritional epidemiological understanding is important to older persons in all low-income societies. Until recently, for instance, the patterns of cancers were sharply distinct between low-income countries in the tropics and high-income countries in temperate zones. Whereas sites in lung and large bowel and the family of hormonal cancers (breast, ovarian, prostatic) were predominant in industrialized population, the uterine cervix, oropharyngeal area, the upper digestive tract and the liver were the most common sites across the developing world. Dietary factors, including nutrient deficiencies, food and beverage constituents, and temperature and charring of foods are clearly implicated in esophageal and gastric malignancy [41]. Overgrowth of staple grains and ground nuts with mycotoxins (e.g., aflatoxins and fumonisins) is a dietary risk factor for liver cancer [42]. By contrast, daily consumption of coffee, more widespread in high-income countries, has been identified as a protective dietary factor against hepatic carcinoma [43]. Many of the putative risk factors for cardiac and circulatory diseases relate to dietary practices including high sodium, high calcium with low vitamin D intakes, hyper-triglyceridemia, hypercholesterolemia, elevated homocysteinemia, systemic inflammation and glycemic load [35]. By contrast, specific diets can provide certain putative protective factors for these diseases such as diets including fruit and vegetables, cocoa, red wine, fish rich in omega-3 fatty acids and calcium-rich sources [44–47]. Within the basic generalization of a traditional diet of low-income populations based on a major grain or tuber and low amounts of animal protein, few of the afore-mentioned or protective dietary components would be expected to be consumed widely. Protection, however, could come from the fiber and phytochemicals in these largely vegetarian fares, plus the absence of the noxious components (e.g., *trans* and saturated fatty acids) in animal sources.

The projection of epidemiological transition reviewed in the previous section portends a rising incidence of chronic diseases across the low- and middle-income countries. To the degree that endemic chronic illness can be prevented, it will improve quality of life of the populace and the budget perspectives of national health authorities. It is important to determine whether the same principles of protective diets and lifestyle are operative in populations experiencing economic development as have been shown in societies of established affluence.

Nutritional Requirements, Nutrient Intake Recommendations and Guidelines for Healthful Eating for the Elderly

Since survival into later life has been infrequent until recent decades, there is also a paucity of information on nutritional requirements of the elderly. Until the mid-1990s, there was insufficiently detailed scientific evidence to differentiate nutrient recommendations for adults over 50 years into any more refined age groupings based on advancing age. This was true for both the US Recommended Dietary Allowances (RDA) and the Recommended Nutrient Intakes (RNI) of the UN System. Until 1997, a uniform requirement level was assigned for everyone over 51 years of age. It has only been recently that official bodies have ventured to specify age-specific recommendations for the oldest segments of populations, based on accumulation of new, age-specific experimental data. For the *Dietary Reference Intakes* (DRI) for the USA and Canada [48–55] and for the Recommended Nutrient Intakes (RNI) of 2004, which come from the UN System [56], and apply across the developing world, new specificity is given to the elderly. The UN System defines 65 year as older, whereas USA–Canada uses two categories for older adults: 51–70 years and above 70 year of age. A series of conceptual definitions govern the expression for normative intakes of macro- and micronutrients.

Definitions Related To Nutrient Intake Recommendations

For the UN System (FAO/WHO/IAEA/UNU):
Recommended Nutrient Intake (RNI): The daily intake, set at the EAR plus 2 standard deviations (SD), which meets the nutrient requirements of almost all apparently healthy individuals in an age- and sex-specific population group.
For the Dietary Reference Intakes (referent to the USA and Canada):
Estimated Average Requirement (EAR): The average daily nutrient intake level estimated to meet the requirement of half the healthy individuals in a particular life stage and gender group.
　　Recommended Dietary Allowance (RDA): The average daily nutrient intake level sufficient to meet the nutrient requirement of nearly all (97–98%) healthy individuals in a particular life stage and gender group.

Adequate Intake (AI): A recommended average daily nutrient intake level based on observed or experimentally determined approximation or estimates of nutrient intake by a group (or groups) of apparently healthy people that are assumed to be adequate—used when an RDA cannot be determined.

Tolerable Upper Intake Level: The highest average daily nutrient intake level likely to pose no risk of adverse health effects to almost all individuals in the general population. As intake increases above the UL, the potential risk of adverse effects increases.

Acceptable Range of Macronutrient Distribution (ARMD): A range of intakes for a particular energy source that is associated with a reduced risk of chronic disease while providing Adequate Intakes of essential nutrients.

Estimated Energy Requirement (EER): The average dietary energy intake that is predicted to maintain energy balance in a healthy adult of a defined age, gender, weight, height and level of physical activity consistent with good health.

The intake recommendations related to specific categories of risk for low or excessive intakes are provided in Tables 26.1 and 26.2 for older men and women, respectively. With respect to nutrient recommendations for older persons, they remain unchanged from the levels recommended from age 19 onward, without any modifications for age. This is true for protein and water requirements. Iron requirement has a unique pattern, as the recommendations **decline** in the latter stages of the lifespan. Based on the 2011 revisions of the DRIs for calcium and vitamin D, both were increased for the older group (70+ years). The upper tolerable level for phosphorus is modified by age. The energy requirement, calculated as the Estimated Energy Requirement (EER), is adjusted by age. There is no Recommended Dietary Allowance (RDA) for energy to prevent the expected weight gain that might occur with energy intakes above the EER [53]. The Adequate Intake (AI) for fiber is also adjusted for age.

The expressions in Tables 26.1 and 26.2 should only be considered first approximations for the purposes of setting them for the elderly in developing countries. To advance to greater certainty and applicability, continuing research efforts are needed, however. With the exception of few nutrients, notably riboflavin [57], the studies on requirements were conducted in subjects living in industrialized country settings. Moreover, the disclaimer in all systems of nutrient recommendations states that they apply only to *healthy* individuals. One can reasonably argue that a diminishingly small number of individuals fit the descriptive term of "healthy" with increasing age. Thus, the recommendations in the tables would strictly speaking apply to only a minority of elderly persons in any population.

Aside from the aging aspect, there is a dimension of the environmental features within human habitats of low-income, tropical—often rural—societies. It has been argued that issues from humidity and high ambient temperatures to the intense concentrations of ecto- and endoparasites and microbes in the environment produce stress [58]. Nutrient requirements may not be a simple linear function of body mass, but rather may have a relation with the underlying composition of tissues. Individuals with short stature, due to early chronic undernutrition, may present this type of metabolic variance. Similarly, the intensive daily physical efforts demanded by non-mechanized agriculture may provoke increased requirements for certain nutrients.

The newer concepts embodied in the DRI include a provision for setting a recommendation considering "health benefits" of a nutrient, above and beyond the basic needs for the nutrients. The recent doubling of folic acid recommendations was motivated by the protective function this can have against neural tube defects in preconceptional women [50, 56]. An additional favorable effect on cardiovascular disease due to suppression of homocysteine levels provided additional support to this public health measure [59]. Generally, however, recommendation panels have been timid in invoking the health benefits criterion, citing the paucity of generalizable evidence and widespread confirmation for findings demonstrating health benefits from supra-requirement intakes of nutrients.

Table 26.1 Nutrient intake recommendations for older men

| | WHO/FAO/IAEA | IoM for USA/Canada | | | |
| | 65+ years | 51–70 years | | >70 years | |
	RNI[a]	RDA/AI/AMDR[b]	UL[b]	RDA/AI/AMDR[b]	UL[b]
Vitamins					
Vitamin A, µg RAE	600 (µg RE)	900	3000	900	3000
Vitamin D, mg	**15**	15	100	20	100
Vitamin E, mg α-toc	10 (mg α-TE)	15	1000	15	1000
Vitamin K, µg	65	120[c]	ND	**120[c]**	ND
Vitamin C, mg	45	90	2000	90	2000
Thiamin, mg	1.2	1.2	ND	1.2	ND
Riboflavin, mg	1.3	1.3	ND	1.3	ND
Niacin, mg	16	16	35	16	35
Vitamin B6, mg	1.7	1.7	100	1.7	100
Biotin, mg	–	30[c]	ND	30[c]	ND
Pantothenic acid, mg	5	5[c]	ND	5[c]	ND
Folate, µg	400	400	1000	400	1000
Vitamin B12, µg	2.4	2.4	ND	2.4	ND
Choline, mg	–	550[c]	3500	550[c]	3500
Boron, mg	–	ND	20	ND	20
Elements					
Sodium, mg	–	1.3[c]	2.3	1.2[c]	2.3
Potassium, mg	–	4.7[c]	–	4.7[c]	–
Chloride, mg	–	2.0[c]	3.6	1.8[c]	3.6
Calcium, mg	**1300**	**1000**	2000	**1200**	2000
Phosphorus, mg	–	700	4000	700	3000
Magnesium, mg	**230**	420	(350)[f]	420	(350)[f]
Iron, mg	14[d]	8	45	8	45
Zinc, mg	7.0[e]	11	40	11	40
Iodine, µg	130	150	1100	150	1100
Copper, µg	–	900	10,000	900	10,000
Fluoride, mg	–	4[c]	10	4[c]	10
Manganese, mg	–	2.3[c]	11	2.3[c]	11
Chromium, µg	–	30[c]	–	30[c]	–
Selenium, µg	**34**	55	400	55	400
Molybdenum, µg	**–**	45	2000	45	2000
Macronutrients					
Energy, EER[b] kcal	–	**2204**	–	**2054**	–
Water, L	–	**3.7[c]**	–	**2.1[c]**	–
Carbohydrate, AMDR	–	45–65%	–	45–65%	–
Protein, AMDR	–	10–35%	–	10–35%	–
Total fat, AMDR	–	20–35%	–	20–35%	–
n-6 PUFA, AMDR	–	5–10%	–	5–10%	–
n-3 PUFA, AMDR	–	0.6–1.2%	–	0.6–1.2%	–
Dietary fiber, g	–	**30[c]**	–	**30[c]**	–

The figures in **bold** denote recommendations specifically modified for aging

ND Values not determined

[a]Recommended Nutrient Intakes from the UN System (WHO/FAO/IAEA). Older adults: ≥65 years

[b]Dietary Reference Intakes from USA/Canada System. *RDA* Recommended Dietary Allowances; *AI* Adequate Intakes; *AMDR* adequate macronutrient distribution range; *EER* Estimated Energy Requirements; *UL* Tolerable Upper Intake Levels

[c]Recommendation in the form of AIs

[d]Based on a 10% bioavailability of iron from the diet

[e]Based on the assumption of a moderate bioavailability of zinc

[f]Based on supplemental intake only

Table 26.2 Nutrient intake recommendations for older women

| | WHO/FAO/IAEA | IoM for USA/Canada | | | |
| | 65+ years | 51–70 years | | >70 years | |
	RNI[a]	RDA/AI/AMDR[b]	UL[b]	RDA/AI/AMDR[b]	UL[b]
Vitamins					
Vitamin A, μg RAE	600 (μg RE)	700	3000	700	3000
Vitamin D, mg	**15**	15	100	20	100
Vitamin E, mg α-toc	7.5 (mg α-TE)	15	1000	15	1000
Vitamin K, μg	55	90[c]	ND	**90**[c]	ND
Vitamin C, mg	45	75	2000	75	2000
Thiamin, mg	1.1	1.1	ND	1.1	ND
Riboflavin, mg	1.1	1.1	ND	1.1	ND
Niacin, mg	14	14	35	14	35
Vitamin B6, mg	1.5	1.5	100	1.5	100
Biotin, mg	–	30[c]	ND	30[c]	ND
Pantothenic acid, mg	5	5[c]	ND	5[c]	ND
Folate, μg	400	400	1000	400	1000
Vitamin B12, μg	2.4	2.4	ND	2.4	ND
Choline, mg	–	425[c]	3500	425[c]	3500
Boron, mg	–	ND	20	ND	20
Elements					
Sodium, mg	–	1.3[c]	2.3	1.2[c]	2.3
Potassium, mg	–	4.7[c]	–	4.7[c]	–
Chloride, mg	–	2.0[c]	3.6	1.8[c]	3.6
Calcium, mg	**1300**	**1200**	2000	**1200**	2000
Phosphorus, mg	–	700	4000	700	3000
Magnesium, mg	**190**	320	(350)[f]	320	(350)[f]
Iron, mg	11[d]	8	45	8	45
Zinc, mg	4.9[e]	8	40	8	40
Iodine, μg	110	150	1100	150	1100
Copper, μg	–	900	10,000	900	10,000
Fluoride, mg	–	3[c]	10	3[c]	10
Manganese, mg	–	1.8[c]	11	1.8[c]	11
Chromium, μg	–	**20**[c]	–	**20**[c]	–
Selenium, μg	**26**	55	400	55	400
Molybdenum, μg	–	45	2000	45	2000
Macronutrients					
Energy, EER[b] kcal	–	**1978**	–	**1873**	–
Water, L	–	**2.7**[c]	–	**2.1**[c]	–
Carbohydrate, AMDR	–	45–65%	–	45–65%	–
Protein, AMDR	–	10–35%	–	10–35%	–
Total fat, AMDR	–	20–35%	–	20–35%	–
n-6 PUFA, AMDR	–	5–10%	–	5–10%	–
n-3 PUFA, AMDR	–	0.6–1.2%	–	0.6–1.2%	–
Dietary fiber, g	–	**21**[c]	–	**21**[c]	–

The figures in **bold** denote recommendations specifically modified for aging

ND Values not determined

[a]Recommended Nutrient Intakes from the UN System (WHO/FAO/IAEA). Older adults: ≥65 years

[b]Dietary Reference Intakes from USA/Canada System. *RDA* Recommended Dietary Allowances; *AI* Adequate Intakes; *AMDR* adequate macronutrient distribution range; *EER* Estimated Energy Requirements; *UL* Tolerable Upper Intake Levels

[c]Recommendation in the form of AIs

[d]Based on a 10% bioavailability of iron from the diet

[e]Based on the assumption of a moderate bioavailability of zinc

[f]Based on supplemental intake only

Supplementation with amounts of nutrients not easily obtained with foods has demonstrated biological effects in humans, including older subjects. Doses of vitamin E in the range of 200–800 mg enhance in vitro indicators of immune function [60]. Daily zinc supplements of 100 mg daily for a month enhanced in vitro lymphocyte responses [61], but such levels are impractical over the long term. The oxo-carotenes, zeaxanthin and lutein, found in certain corn, and certain dark-green leafy vegetables seem to play a protective role in the fovea of the ocular retina, and enhanced intakes are suggested to be preventive against macular degeneration associated with age [62].

Dietary Intake and Eating Behavior by Elderly in Low-Income Countries

Assessing Dietary Intakes in Older Subjects: Caveats for Low-Income Countries

Among the consequences of the global demographic and epidemiological transitions, one could include the increasing numbers of older adults that require nutritional services adequate to their emotional, cultural, social and economic status and health needs; hence, appropriate contextual assessment of their dietary intakes is needed. Dietary data, interpreted in the context of these various needs, would help to identify those dietary factors associated with declining health and the development of chronic conditions. Those linkages between diet and health or diet and disease are only perceived in events followed during periods of time, as the effects of specific dietary practice might take months or even years to influence health.

Several methodologies are regularly applied for the assessment of dietary intakes and food patterns of older adults in high-income countries, with the addition of sophisticated memory enhancing tools that improve situations of short-term memory among elders with compromised cognitive function or with declining physical health. Two of the most commonly used methodologies for dietary assessment are: (1) the 24-h recall and (2) food intake history collected with food frequency questionnaires. Diet history collected in food records (or food diaries) is another methodology used with older adults in high-income countries. However, this methodology requires literate and highly motivated subjects, which could limit its application in some elderly groups. The basic premise when using the 24-h recall is the accurate recalling one could get as it only requests information from the previous 24 h before the information is collected. In addition, the systematization of the 5-step technique developed by the USDA expert group [63] has also improved greatly the application of this technique, particularly in the elderly.

However, there is a shortage of information about which dietary assessment instruments are practical and reliable for extracting the information in older adults from low-income countries. In addition, prior to the adoption of instruments developed in other latitudes, food lists (for food frequency questionnaires) and probing prompts (24-h recalls) need to be developed, as type of foods and eating patterns differ from country to country.

On the one hand, among the elderly in low-income countries, it is presumed that their ability for recalling food consumption and other related dietary facts could be modified not only by their cognitive status and declining health, but also by their level of schooling and their lack of experience as informants. On the other hand, obtaining dietary information from older adults in low-income countries could be facilitated by the monotonous diets that are traditionally associated with these population groups. Moreover, among those groups, there are usually a limited number of staple foods that are consumed frequently and with small variations in portion sizes. It has been observed that in countries like Guatemala, families are very consistent in the dimensions of their homemade tortillas and different members usually consume the same amount of them, making it relatively easy to collect information about amounts and frequencies of use of this food product. Another example pertains to rice, which is the main staple food for older Puerto Ricans living in the US mainland, independent of their length of residency [64], and it is also the main component in diets of older Panamanians [65].

To estimate nutrient and energy composition of foods consumed by older adults, reliable and accurate nutrient databases or food composition tables are needed. However, these reference instruments are scarce in low-income countries, and in many cases, those that are available are outdated and limited in the number of nutrients for analysis and exploring correlations with health outcomes. To correct for these limitations, the International Network of Food Data Systems (INFOODS) has renewed efforts worldwide to collect, systematize and enhance international collaborations around food and nutrient databases [66].

Standards and reference patterns such as nutrient recommendations (discussed in the previous section) as well as dietary guidelines and graphic representations of food groups are used in the interpretation and application of dietary data. After the promulgation of the WHO/FAO guidelines for the development of food-based dietary guidelines [67], countries around the world have produced their own guidelines and used them to guide their efforts in policy making, program planning and evaluation. FAO, through its Nutrition Information, Communication and Education Department, makes efforts to divulgate those dietary guidelines from its online site [66]. Despite all the efforts in improving tools for dietary assessment, few of them have been designed specifically for the elderly, particularly those in low-income countries.

Patterns of Dietary Consumption in Later Life

Traditionally, elderly people had developed lifelong eating patterns partly modulated by sociodemographic and psychosocial determinants of their food-related behaviors, as well as by the environmental circumstances associated with access and availability of their food supply [68]. The attachment of the elderly to their traditional eating practices represents a challenge for interventions to modify intake for the correction of nutritional imbalances, poor health and disease prevention. One could think that food intake of elders from low-income countries, especially those residing in economically deprived areas, could be less than optimal because of food availability issues. All this is in addition to the increased requirements for several nutrients due to physiological changes associated with aging and to pathological effects of some chronic conditions, at the same time that energy intakes are decreasing. However, there is evidence that, whereas for some elder groups, their traditional diets are more health protective than more "modern" ones, for other groups their diets improve with the incorporation of new foods. Earlier studies among Greek elderly in Greece and in Australia revealed that those with traditional eating patterns had lower overall mortality and longer survival [69–71]; that those patterns may be protective for obesity [72]. Among Mexican women in the USA, those of more recent arrival had higher protein, calcium, vitamins A, C and folate intakes and greater overall mean adequacy ratios (constructed with 8 nutrients) than their counterparts that had been in the country for more than a generation [73]. By contrast, older Puerto Ricans in the USA attached to their traditional food patterns with rice as their main source of energy had a higher risk of obesity than those that had incorporated more variety into their eating patterns [74].

The evidence about changes in food accessibility and intake in several countries around the globe, is suggestive of the risk of obesity and the malnutrition-related non-communicable diseases. In Latin America, for example, it was observed that although nutrient availability differs in magnitude across countries, the overall patterns were remarkably consistent. Availability of total fat, animal products and sugars was all increasing, at the same time that rapid declines in the availability of cereals, fruit and vegetables were occurring [75], most likely as responses to consumer and economic changes motivated by increasing purchasing power, urbanization and new dietary profiles.

Although worldwide corrections of poor dietary habits and inadequate food intakes in the elderly are a challenge and could overwhelm governments, societies, households and individuals of low–middle-income countries, the acceleration and magnitude of the changes already occurring in most of those countries are giving little option, but to confront and look for viable solutions for the potential risks of having their elderly populations with the *triple* burden of being old, poor and malnourished.

Nutritional Deficiency and Excess and Its Assessment in the Elderly of Developing Countries

The elderly of developing countries are most likely to suffer in their care and assessment by confusion of the blanket application of the norms and standards of the population at large to this more unique and heterogeneous population in later life. Nutritional status has three domains: The first is global, constitutional nutrition (formerly discussed in terms of "protein-energy" status), related to body composition; the second is status with respect to the body's reserves or availability of micronutrients (vitamins, minerals); and the third relates to hydration and fluid and electrolyte balance. Finally, for evaluating these tiers of status, the aging process, itself, conditions changes that make nutritional assessment more difficult.

Deficiency and Undernutrition States in Low-Income Country Elderly

The most commonly considered imbalance in nutritional status is undernutrition. Chronic energy deficiency is a concern in older persons in all societies. In high-income countries, however, recent weight loss is often secondary, a consequence of a chronic degenerative disease. Although poverty creates the risk of primary dietary deficiencies, a differential diagnosis for underweight representing a secondary consequence of occult illness should be maintained in the elderly of low-income societies as well.

Across all age groups, including the elderly segments, primary vitamin and mineral deficiencies, can arise from consuming diets with low micronutrient density, with nutrients of poor bioavailability or both. The primarily plant-based fare of traditional agrarian societies, combined with environmental stress including parasitosis and recurrent infections, is an established conditioning scenario for undernutrition with respect to a subset of vitamins and minerals. Among the vitamin deficiencies recorded as commonly endemic in low-income settings are vitamin A, riboflavin and vitamin B_{12}. Folate deficiency occurs in certain populations largely dependent on boiled maize. Iodine deficiency is widespread across the globe due to environmental depletion and very low bioavailability of this element from a plant source-based diet. Iron deficiency, and its associated iron deficiency anemia, is reputed to be the most widespread deficiency disorder of humankind. A widespread vulnerability to subadequate zinc deficiency has recently been appreciated [76]. Selenium deficiency occurs when soils are particularly depleted of this mineral.

Specific micronutrient surveys focusing on elderly subpopulations in low-income countries are scarce. Early in the 1990s, in Guatemala, Boisvert et al. [57] found a majority of older persons screened had inadequate riboflavin status. It is widely regarded that gastric hyposecretion adversely influences vitamin B_{12} status with increasing age. Vitamin D deficiency was previously considered to be of a lesser concern in tropical countries, which experience year-round direct penetration of the UV spectrum of sunlight. In fact, little survey experience on vitamin D status in low-income country elderly is available. However, in the absence of general consumption of dairy items or marine fish, tropical populations are virtually totally dependent on solar-dependent vitamin D production. The dermal capacity decreases with aging, and outdoor activities may be curtailed with advancing age. In the context of degenerative diseases, greater amounts of vitamin D than have been considered normative may be protective [77]. Better across the board vitamin D nutriture may emerge as a public health necessity among elderly in the north and south, as epidemiological and intervention trial data continue to emerge, including some evidence from Mayan older adults from Guatemala [78].

Since iron is of slow turnover, reserves of this element actual tend to build with the passage of time. With menopause, the monthly menstrual blood losses cease. For these reasons, the elderly should be considered the most resistant to iron deficiency anemia in any society, and its occurrence raises the specter of some abnormal blood loss conditions. Where hookworm or schistosomiasis is common, bleeding from parasitic lesions may produce anemia in any age group, including adult men and the elderly [77]. Gastric atrophy interferes with the solubility for its intestinal absorption. However, iron deficiency or anemia in an older individual in a tropical country can have the same ominous clinical significance that it has in a developed country setting, i.e., signifying a malignancy at some level of the gastrointestinal tract.

As individuals age several processes occur that make issues of hydration and water and electrolyte balance more precarious. With aging, there is a blunting in thirst sensation, renal function declines and the vascular response to altered blood volume diminishes. In particular, in hot humid climates, this would increase the susceptibility to hypovolemia and dehydration.

Diagnosing Undernutrition

The principles of any diagnosis are: (1) clinical history; (2) physical examination; and (3) laboratory testing. The human aging process itself confounds the assessment of nutritional status both of the older individual in the clinical setting and at the population level in epidemiological screening. Nutritional assessment as applied to the elderly must take into consideration physiological and social changes that occur with advancing age. Cognitive decline distorts the accuracy of answers to clinical history questions, and low levels of schooling and linguistic issues complicate the interview in developing societies. Keys to successful and reliable diagnostic evaluation for undernutrition of the elderly in general—and developing country elders, in particular—are: (1) knowledge of the most common deficiency states, as discussed above, and (2) understanding of the nuances, caveats and pitfalls of assessment techniques with advancing age.

Reflection of undernutrition (underweight) by anthropometric measurements, specifically the body mass index (kg/m^2), is confounded by short stature. The international standards define a BMI <18.5 kg/m^2 as chronic energy deficiency, but up to 40% of free-living elderly in South Asia can have values in that range. Adults lose stature due to settling and curvature of the spine with aging, and arm-span [79] and knee-heel height [79] have been proposed as surrogate measures. Short stature, however, is not an index of ongoing undernutrition in individuals beyond adolescence, such that "stunting" is not applicable in older adults. The laxness of the skin and redistribution of body fat confound the use of skinfolds thickness for representative measurement of subcutaneous fat. Similarly, to the extent that skin turgor is to be used clinically to assess the hydration state, dermal changes with aging can confound assessment. Moisture of mucosal surfaces is a more reliable indicator of hydration of the elderly [79].

Aging has minimal effects on hematological parameters, such that universal standards for hemoglobin, hematocrit and blood cell indices and counts are also applicable in later life. Aging, per se, is associated with elevation of the binding protein of copper (ceruloplasmin) and a slight reduction in albumin concentration [18]. When urinary excretion of nutrient metabolites is employed in nutritional assessment, especially as ambient concentrations or timed excretion, the age-related changes in renal physiology must be considered to avoid diagnostic errors.

Some biochemical and laboratory measures of nutritional status are distorted by some fundamental conditions prevailing in low-income countries, such as inflammatory stimulation by microbes and parasites. This produces redistribution of circulating nutrients (e.g., iron, zinc, vitamin A and copper) and distortion of nutrient indicators (e.g., plasma ferritin). Dehydration in hot climates would tend to produce hemoconcentration, decreasing the acuity of circulating biomarkers to detect deficiency states.

Excess and Overnutrition States in Low- and Middle-Income Country Elderly

The popular image of low-income countries is of populations living in rural poverty. It was also widely regarded that poverty was a restraint on obesity. Contemporary realities debunk both of these generalizations to the status of obsolete myths [80], showing that a lack of social power, choice and a safe environment are more likely to produce weight excess, especially among poor elderly in urban settings.

In real-world experience, the micronutrients most likely to produce adverse effects for older individuals when intake is on the *high* side of exposure are vitamin A, folate, iron, calcium, phosphorus and sodium. Preformed vitamin A has interesting implications in later life, as a postprandial load is cleared more slowly with advancing age [81], and bone demineralization has been related to vitamin A from animal sources [82]. As discussed above, however, culinary customs and economic constraints generally act to produce lower intakes of this form of vitamin A, as well as that of the other aforementioned nutrients, in diets of low-income societies.

The interaction of folate and vitamin B12 has long been topical for the nutritional health of the elderly. In some developed countries, general folic acid fortification has raised some concerns about negative consequences in the face of vitamin B12 scarcity [83]. Folic acid fortification lags behind in most developing countries, but when Chile instituted its national program, fortification levels doubled those in most nations [84], with potential deleterious consequences for vitamin B12 status. Hemochromatosis is rare among the ethnic groups native to low-income countries; a poorly understood syndrome of iron accumulation found in Southern Africa (Bantu siderosis) produces damaging iron overload when soluble forms of iron are available in the diet [85].

Diagnosing Overnutrition

Aging and living in low–middle-income countries impose certain recognized challenges to diagnostic assessment of overnutrition. The BMI increases through the sixth decade and then decreases in the survivors beyond this age. The value of the BMI for any given body weight is influenced by short stature, decreasing the value of the denominator term. Moreover, age-related height loss distorts the accurate assessment of an appropriate stature value for an older individual [79]. Beyond mere body weight are changing proportions of lean and fat mass, with increased visceral deposition of lipids and fatty infiltration of skeletal muscles [20]. All of these aging features are reflected on the widely documented observation that individuals with identical BMIs can have vastly different percentage of body weights as fat or lean mass across ethnic groups [86, 87]. The "Indian paradox" derives from the development of cardiovascular and metabolic risk in South Asians at much lower BMIs [88, 89], leading to a suggested adjustment for a lower cutoff for "overweight" for the populations of Southern and Southeastern Asia of 23 instead of 25 [35]. Finally, the health consequences of a given excessive body mass differ markedly across races [90].

Diagnosis of overload and toxicity states for micronutrients is difficult under any circumstances and in all age groups, requiring interpretive assessment of blood levels of nutrients and metabolites or tissue biopsy findings. No systematic understanding of how aging distorts these challenging diagnoses of vitamin and mineral excess has yet been developed.

Addressing Good Nutritional Status of the Elderly from Low- and Middle-Income Countries

Older adults from low- and middle-income countries are living longer. Therefore, addressing non-communicable diseases, including type 2 diabetes, hypertension, CVD, obesity and other prevalent health conditions, has become an urgent action, particularly in low–middle-income countries. The expectations are that aging groups from those countries do so in good health and as capable of practicing healthy lifestyles, including acceptable dietary cardioprotective behaviors.

In order to maximize country investments in addressing nutritional status of the aging population, it is prudent to investigate and document the mechanisms and potential solutions for those problems that already have proven effectiveness and that offers high potential for translating them to different geographical areas and cultures. It is also important to keep in mind that many of the interventions designed to improve nutritional status of the elderly must be initiated at early ages. For example, working with the under-five population (e.g., to guaranty adequate growth and development) and with adolescents to guaranty acceptable bone health will extend the benefits to the aged. Therefore, addressing nutritional problems of the elderly does not compete with already established proven interventions to improve nutritional status of children. What is expected is that complementary nutrition strategies for the elderly are designed and implemented in order to guaranty good health and nutritional status across the lifespan.

Conclusions

The fact that the populations of low- and middle-income countries are aging and more older persons are surviving is a virtual *Brave New World* for public health for low-income societies. The consequences for diet and nutrition of the older members of all societies have been little explored and are poorly understood. The nutrition transition is bringing forth a dual burden of malnutrition, with problems of under- and overweight. Epidemiological transition is emerging for the populations of low- and middle-income countries with increasing prevalence of the components of the metabolic syndrome and malignant disease.

In the absence of a strong and prolific tradition of "tropical gerontology," the prudent course is to synthesize the substantial knowledge about the unique conditions and challenges in low-income societies and the accumulated understanding of aging biology and senescent changes from affluent societies and prepare an active agenda for inquiry. One would expect a series of interactions between the two domains in which the prevailing conditions of life in low–middle-income nations exacerbate processes of structural and functional senescence as well as those in which the traditional diet and rigorous physical activity will prove protective. This chapter bears testimony to the demographic transition and the prudence of recognizing and acting upon the realities that old age and chronic diseases are important current elements across the panorama of low–middle-income country health and nutrition.

Discussion Points

- How does survival relate to diet along the lifespan and eventually affect the elderly?
- What factors need to be considered when evaluating a nutrition intervention for elderly?
- How do the differing socioeconomic and environmental factors in low- and high-income countries affect the nutritional status of elderly differently?
- What biological and behavioral attributes of elderly contribute to preserving or deteriorating nutritional status?

References

1. U.S. Census Bureau, International Programs Center, and International Data Base. The composition of global population. 2004. URL: https://www.census.gov/population/international/files/wp02/wp-02004.pdf.
2. Busuttil RA, et al. Genomic instability, aging, and cellular senescence. Ann N Y Acad Sci. 2004;1019:245–55.
3. Ruiz-Torres A, Beier W. On maximum human life span: interdisciplinary approach about its limits. Adv Gerontol. 2005;16:14–20.
4. Wahlqvist ML, et al. Food habits in later life: a cross-cultural approach. Melbourne: United Nations University Press/Asia Pacific Journal of Clinical Nutrition; 1996.
5. Bonsall MB. Longevity and ageing: appraising the evolutionary consequences of growing old. Philos Trans R Soc Lond B Biol Sci. 2006;361(1465):119–35.
6. Frisancho AR, ed. Human adaptation and accommodation. Ann Arbor: University of Michigan Press; 1996.
7. Simoons FD. Primary adult lactose intolerance and the milking habit: A problem in biological and cultural interrelations II. A culture history perspective. Am J Dig Dis. 1970;23:963–80.
8. Eaton SB, Konner M. Paleolithic nutrition: a consideration of its nature and current implication. N Engl J Med. 1985;312:283–9.
9. Nestle M. Paleolithic diets: A skeptical view. Nutr Bull. 2000;25:43–7.
10. Cordain L, et al. The paradoxical nature of hunter-gatherer diets: meat-based, yet non-atherogenic. Eur J Clin Nutr. 2002;56(Suppl 1):S42–52.
11. Eaton SB, Konner MJ, Cordain L. Diet-dependent acid load, paleolithic [corrected] nutrition, and evolutionary health promotion. Am J Clin Nutr. 2010;91(2):295–7.
12. Ahmed A, Tollefsbol TO. Telomerase, telomerase inhibition, and cancer. J Anti Aging Med. 2003;6:315–25.
13. Huang H, Manton KG. The role of oxidative damage in mitochondria during aging: a review. Front Biosci. 2004;9:1100–17.
14. Khrapko K, Ebralidse K, Kraytsberg Y. Where and when do somatic mtDNA mutations occur? Ann N Y Acad Sci. 2004;1019:240–4.
15. Fraker PJ, Lill Elghanian DA. The many roles of apoptosis in immunity as modified by aging and nutritional status. J Nutr Health Aging. 2004;8:56–63.
16. Shock NR. Physiological aspects of aging. J Am Diet Assoc. 1970;56:491–6.
17. Sussman MA, Anversa P. Myocardial aging and senescence: where have the stem cells gone? Annu Rev Physiol. 2004;66:29–48.
18. Solomons NW, Older Persons. Physiological changes, in encyclopedia of human nutrition (Caballero B, Allen LH, Prentice AM, editors). 2nd ed. London: Elsevier; 2004. p. 431–436.
19. Lanfranco F, et al. Ageing, growth hormone and physical performance. J Endocrinol Invest. 2003;26: 861–72.
20. Kinney JM. Nutritional frailty, sarcopenia and falls in the elderly. Curr Opin Clin Nutr Metab Care. 2004;7(1):15–20.
21. Mishra SK, Misra V. Muscle sarcopenia: an overview. Acta Myol. 2003;22:43–7.
22. Dufour AB, et al. Sarcopenia definitions considering body size and fat mass are associated with mobility limitations: the Framingham Study. J Gerontol A Biol Sci Med Sci. 2013;68(2):168–74.
23. Perez-Perez GI, Rothenbacher D, Brenner H. Epidemiology of helicobacter pylori infection. Helicobacter. 2004;9 (Suppl 1):1–6.
24. Henry CJK, et al. Impact of human aging on energy and protein metabolism and requirements. Working Group 4 (Schurch B, Scrimshaw NS, editors). Eur J Clin Nutr. 2000;S157–59.
25. Levine ME, Crimmins EM. Evidence of accelerated aging among African Americans and its implications for mortality. Soc Sci Med. 2014;118:27–32.
26. Christiansen MT, et al. Genome-wide high-throughput screening to investigate essential genes involved in methicillin-resistant Staphylococcus aureus Sequence Type 398 survival. PLoS ONE. 2014;9(2):e89018.

27. vB Hjelmborg J, et al. Genetic influence on human lifespan and longevity. Hum Genet. 2006;119(3):312–21.
28. Rowe JW, Kahn RL. Human aging: usual and successful. Science. 1987;237:143–9.
29. Boyle PA, et al. Physical frailty is associated with incident mild cognitive impairment in community-based older persons. J Am Geriatr Soc. 2010;58(2):248–55.
30. Solomons NW. Demographic and nutritional trends among the elderly in developed and developing regions. Eur J Clin Nutr. 2000;54(Suppl 3):S2–14.
31. Laslett P. Interpreting the demographic changes. Phil Trans R Soc Lond Bio Sci. 1998;352:1805–1810 (In: Grimley-Evans J, Holliday R, Kirkwood TBL, Laslett P, Tyler L, editors. Ageing: science, medicine, and society).
32. The World Bank. Life expectancy at birth. 2014. URL: http://data.worldbank.org/indicator/SP.DYN.LE00.FE.IN/countries/1W?display=graph. 28 July 2014.
33. Manton KG. The dynamics of population aging: demography and policy analysis. Milbank Q. 1991;69:309–38.
34. Manton KG. The global impact of noncommunicable diseases: estimates and projections. World Health Stat Q. 1988;41:255–66.
35. World Health Organization, Diet, Nutrition and the Prevention of Chronic Diseases. WHO Technical Report Series 916. Geneva: WHO; 2001.
36. Uauy, R, Solomons N. Role of the international community in addressing the dual burden of malnutrition with a common agenda. SCN News;2006. 32.
37. Moran AE, et al. The global burden of ischemic heart disease in 1990 and 2010: the Global Burden of Disease 2010 study. Circulation. 2014;129(14):1493–501.
38. World Health Organization. Global status report on noncommunicable diseases. 2010. URL: http://whqlibdoc.who.int/publications/2011/9789240686458_eng.pdf?ua=1. ISBN: 978 92 4 156422 9.
39. Willett W. Nutritional epidemiology. 2nd ed. New York: Oxford University Press; 1999.
40. Margetts BM, Nelson M, editors. Design concepts in nutritional epidemiology. 1991, Oxford: Oxford University Press.
41. World Cancer Research Fund, Diet, Nutrition and Prevention of Cancer: A global perspective. London: WCRF; 1997.
42. Liu Y, et al. Population attributable risk of aflatoxin-related liver cancer: systematic review and meta-analysis. Eur J Cancer. 2012;48(14):2125–36.
43. Kurozawa Y, et al. Coffee and risk of death from hepatocellular carcinoma in a large cohort study in Japan. Br J Cancer. 2005;93:607–10.
44. Hendriks HF, van Tol A. Alcohol. Handb Exp Pharmacol. 2005;170:339–61.
45. Keen CL, et al. Cocoa antioxidants and cardiovascular health. Am J Clin Nutr. 2005;81(1 Suppl):298S–303S.
46. Siddiqui RA, et al. Omega 3-fatty acids: health benefits and cellular mechanisms of action. Mini Rev Med Chem. 2004;4:859–71.
47. Peterlik M, Cross HS. Vitamin D and calcium deficits predispose for multiple chronic diseases. Eur J Clin Invest. 2005;35:290–304.
48. Food and Nutrition Board and Standing Committee of the Scientific Evaluation of Dietary Reference Intakes, Dietary reference intakes for calcium, phosphorus, magnesium, vitamin D, and fluoride. Washington, D.C.: Institute of Medicine, National Academy Press; 1999.
49. Food and Nutrition Board and Standing Committee of the Scientific Evaluation of Dietary Reference Intakes, Dietary reference intakes for vitamin C, vitamin E, selenium, and carotenoids. Washington, D.C.: Institute of Medicine, National Academy Press; 2000.
50. Food and Nutrition Board and Standing Committee of the Scientific Evaluation of Dietary Reference Intakes, Dietary reference intakes for thiamin, riboflavin, niacin, vitamin B6, folate, vitamin B12, pantothenic acid, biotin, and choline. Washington, D.C.: Institute of Medicine, National Academy Press; 2000.
51. Food and Nutrition Board and Standing Committee of the Scientific Evaluation of Dietary Reference Intakes, Dietary reference intakes for vitamin A, vitamin K, arsenic, boron, chromium, copper, iodine, iron, manganese, molybdenum, nickel, silicon, vanadium, and zinc. Washington, D.C.: Institute of Medicine, National Academy Press; 2001.
52. Food and Nutrition Board and Standing Committee of the Scientific Evaluation of Dietary Reference Intakes, Dietary reference intakes: Applications in dietary assessment. A report of the Subcommittees on interpretation and uses of dietary reference intakes and upper reference levels of nutrients, and the Standing committee on the scientific evaluation of dietary reference intakes. Washington, D.C.: Institute of Medicine, National Academy Press; 2001.
53. Food and Nutrition Board and Standing Committee of the Scientific Evaluation of Dietary Reference Intakes, Dietary reference intakes for energy, carbohydrates, fiber, fat, protein and amino acids (macronutrients). Washington, D.C.: Institute of Medicine, National Academy Press; 2002.
54. Food and Nutrition Board and Standing Committee of the Scientific Evaluation of Dietary Reference Intakes, Dietary reference intakes for water, potassium, sodium, chloride and sulfate. Washington, D.C.: Institute of Medicine, National Academy Press; 2004.

55. Food and Nutrition Board and Institute of Medicine, Dietary reference intakes for calcium and vitamin D (Ross AC, editors). Washington, D.C.: The National Academy Press; 2011.

56. World Health Organization and Food and Agricultural Organization. Human vitamin and mineral requirements. Geneva: WHO; 2004.

57. Boisvert WA, et al. Riboflavin requirements of the healthy elderly and its relationship to macronutrient composition of the diet. J Nutr. 1993;123:915–25.

58. Solomons NW, Kaufer-Horwitz M, Bermudez OI. Harmonization for mesoamerican nutrient-based recommendations: regional unification or national specification? Arch Latinoam Nutr. 2004;54:363–73.

59. Malinow MR, et al. Reduction of plasma homocyst(e)ine levels by breakfast cereal fortified with folic acid in patients with coronary heart disease. N Engl J Med. 1998;338:1009–15.

60. Meydani SN, Han SN, Nutrient regulation of the immune response: the case of vitamin E. In: Bowman BA, Russell RM, editors. Present knowledge in nutrition. Washington, D.C.: ILSI Press; 2001. p. 449–62.

61. Duchateau J, et al. Beneficial effect of oral zinc supplementation on the immune response of old people. Am J Med. 1981;70:1001–4.

62. Mozaffarieh M, Sacu S, Wedrich A. The role of the carotenoids, lutein and zeaxanthin, in protecting against age-related macular degeneration: a review based on controversial evidence. J Nutr. 2003;2:20.

63. Conway JM, et al. Effectiveness of the US Department of Agriculture 5-step multiple-pass method in assessing food intake in obese and nonobese women. Am J Clin Nutr. 2003;77(5):1171–8.

64. Bermudez OI, Falcon L, Tucker K. Intake and food sources of macronutrients among older Hispanic adults: association with ethnicity, acculturation and length of residence in the United States. J Am Diet Assoc. 2000;100:665–73.

65. Ministry of Health of Panama, Nutritional status and quality of life among older adults attending health centers in Panama City Metropolitan area (Valdes VE, Bermudez O, DeMas M, editors). Panama City: Ministry of Health and Social Security Institute of Panama; 2003.

66. FAO. Food Guidelines by Country. 2005. Available at: http://www.fao.org/ag/agn/nutrition/education_guidelines_country_en.stm. FAO—Nutrition Information, Communication and Education Department. Accessed 18 Dec 2005.

67. World Health Organization and Food and Agriculture Organization of the United Nations, Preparation and use of food-based dietary guidelines. Nicosia. Cyprus: WHO, FAO; 1996.

68. Bermudez OI, Tucker KL. Cultural aspects of food choices in various communities of elders. Generations (Am Society of Aging). 2004;28:22–7.

69. Trichopoulou A, et al. Diet and overall survival in elderly people. Br Med J. 1995;311(7018):1457–60.

70. Trichopoulou A, Lagiou P, Trichopoulos D. Traditional Greek diet and coronary heart disease. J Cardiovasc Risk. 1994;1:9–15.

71. Kouris-Blazos A, et al. Are the advantages of the Mediterranean diet transferable to other populations? A cohort study in Melbourne, Australia. Br J Nutr. 1999;82(1):57–61.

72. Wahlqvist ML, Kouris-blazos A, Wattanapenpaiboon N. The significance of eating patterns: an elderly Greek case study. Appetite. 1999;32(1):23–32.

73. Guendelman S, Abrams B. Dietary intake among Mexican-American women: generational differences and a comparison with White Non-Hispanic women. Am J Public Health. 1995;85(1):20–5.

74. Lin H, Bermudez OI, Tucker KL. Dietary patterns of Hispanic elders are associated with acculturation and obesity. J Nutr. 2003;133(11):3651–7.

75. Bermudez OI, Tucker KL. Trends in dietary patterns of Latin American populations. Cad Saude Publica. 2003;19 (Suppl 1):S87–99.

76. Wuehler SE, Peerson JM, Brown KH. Use of national food balance data to estimate the adequacy of zinc in national food supplies: methodology and regional estimates. Public Health Nutr. 2005;8:812–9.

77. Holick MF, Vitamin D. importance in the prevention of cancers, type 1 diabetes, heart disease, and osteoporosis. Am J Clin Nutr. 2004;79:362–71.

78. Sud SR, et al. Older Mayan residents of the western highlands of Guatemala lack sufficient levels of vitamin D. Nutr Res. 2010;30(11):739–46.

79. Rabe B, et al. Body mass index of the elderly derived from height and arm span. Asia Pac J Clin Nutr. 1996;5:79–83.

80. Monteiro CA, et al. Shifting obesity trends in Brazil. Eur J Clin Nutr. 2000;54:342–6.

81. Solomons NW, Vitamin A, Carotenoids. In: Bowman BA, Russell RM, editors. Present knowledge in nutrition. 8th ed. Washington, D.C.: ILSI Press; 2001. p. 127–45.

82. Crandall C. Vitamin A intake and osteoporosis: a clinical review. J Women's Health (Larchmt). 2004;13:939–53.

83. Flood VM, et al. Folate fortification: potential impact on folate intake in an older population. Eur J Clin Nutr. 2001;55:793–800.

84. Hertrampf E, et al. Consumption of folic acid-fortified bread improves folate status in women of reproductive age in Chile. J Nutr. 2003;133:3166–9.

85. Gordeuk V, et al. Iron overload in Africa: interaction between a gene and dietary iron content. N Engl J Med. 1992;326:95–100.
86. Deurenberg-Yap M, Chew SK, Deurenberg P. Elevated body fat percentage and cardiovascular risks at low body mass index levels among Singaporean Chinese, Malays and Indians. Obes Rev. 2002;3:209–15.
87. Fernandez JR, et al. Is percentage body fat differentially related to body mass index in Hispanic Americans, African Americans, and European Americans? Am J Clin Nutr. 2003;77:71–5.
88. Singh RB, et al. Association of central obesity and insulin resistance with high prevalence of diabetes and cardiovascular disease in an elderly population with low fat intake and lower than normal prevalence of obesity: the Indian paradox. Coron Artery Dis. 1998;9:559–65.
89. Ghosh A, Bala SK. Anthropometric, body composition, and blood pressure measures among rural elderly adults of Asian Indian origin: the Santiniketan aging study. J Nutr Gerontol Geriatr. 2011;30(3):305–13.
90. Stevens J, et al. The effect of decision rules on the choice of a body mass index cutoff for obesity: examples from African American and white women. Am J Clin Nutr. 2002;75:986–92.

Part VI
Tackling Health and Nutrition Issues in an Integrated Way in the Era of the SDGs

Chapter 27
Evaluation of Nutrition-sensitive Programs

Deanna K. Olney, Jef L. Leroy and Marie T. Ruel

Keywords Nutrition sensitive · Evidence of impact · Program evaluation · Plausibility · Probability

Learning Objectives

- Explain the key challenges in evaluating nutrition-sensitive programs and ways to address them.
- Identify three components of a comprehensive evaluation (impact, process, and cost), describe the primary uses of each of these components, and explain how to design these three components to evaluate a nutrition-sensitive program.
- Illustrate how to use a program theory framework and associated program impact pathways in the design and evaluation of nutrition-sensitive programs.
- Analyze the types of challenges that program evaluators and implementers face when working together and explain how to address them in designing and carrying out the evaluation of complex nutrition-sensitive programs.

Introduction

The Lancet Series on Maternal and Child Nutrition called for greater investments in large-scale nutrition-sensitive programs to accelerate progress in improving the nutrition of vulnerable mothers and young children during the first 1000 days (conception to the child's 2nd birthday) [1]. Nutrition-sensitive programs are defined as development programs that address the underlying causes of undernutrition—including poverty, food insecurity, poor maternal health, education, social status and/or empowerment, and limited access to water, sanitation, hygiene, and health services—and also incorporate specific nutrition goals and actions. Nutrition-*specific* interventions and programs, on the other hand, are those that address the immediate determinants of undernutrition such as inadequate food and nutrient intake, sub-optimal care and feeding practices, and poor health [1]. One of the key recommendations from the 2013 Lancet Series was to use nutrition-sensitive programs from sectors

D.K. Olney (✉) · J.L. Leroy · M.T. Ruel
Poverty, Health and Nutrition Division, International Food Policy Research Institute (IFPRI),
2033 K Street, NW, Washington, DC 20006, USA
e-mail: d.olney@cgiar.org

J.L. Leroy
e-mail: j.leroy@cgiar.org

M.T. Ruel
e-mail: m.ruel@cgiar.org

© Springer Science+Business Media New York 2017
S. de Pee et al. (eds.), *Nutrition and Health in a Developing World*,
Nutrition and Health, DOI 10.1007/978-3-319-43739-2_27

such as agriculture, social protection, education, and early child development as platforms to improve the delivery, coverage, and scale of nutrition-specific interventions. For example, agriculture development programs, which target women and promote the production and consumption of nutrient-rich foods, could also be used to deliver specially formulated micronutrient supplements for pregnant/lactating women or young children who have requirements that are difficult to meet with diet alone due to rapid growth and development. These types of integrated agriculture and nutrition programs have been shown to improve the diets of household members, mothers, and children, and using them as delivery platforms for additional nutrition-specific interventions may amplify these positive effects and result in positive changes in the nutritional status of women and children, which to date have been limited [1, 2].

In addition to the recognized importance of nutrition-sensitive programs to improve the nutritional status of at-risk populations, the demand for evidence-based programming has increased in recent years. Recent reviews of the effectiveness of development programs focused on agriculture or social protection highlight the dearth of rigorous evidence of the impact of these programs on nutrition measures, and attribute this lack of evidence to weaknesses in program design and implementation, but even more importantly to poor evaluation designs and methods [3, 4]. A consistent and strong recommendation provided in these reviews is the need for rigorous, theory-based impact evaluations that will generate credible evidence on what works and what does not work to improve nutrition; what are the pathways of impact; what other development measures are improved with different nutrition-sensitive program models; and what is the cost and cost-effectiveness of achieving these improvements.

Key Challenges in Evaluating Nutrition-Sensitive Programs

While the need for rigorous, comprehensive program evaluations is recognized, carrying out such evaluations of complex nutrition-sensitive programs with multiple inputs, goals, pathways of impacts, outcomes, and impacts is challenging. These challenges revolve around five factors. First, nutrition-sensitive programs are, by definition, generally complex in design and implementation because they aim to address both underlying causes of undernutrition (often several of them, such as poverty, food insecurity, and low women's status to name a few) and to incorporate nutrition-specific interventions; second, they require a longer time frame than simpler, more narrowly focused programs, because the pathways of impact are long and often complex (e.g., it takes some time for reductions in poverty and food insecurity to translate into better food and nutrient intake for young children, and for these changes, in turn, to improve their nutritional status); third, programmatic, logistical, or political issues can make the use of randomization and the inclusion of an adequate control group to whom program inputs are withheld unacceptable, thereby possibly reducing the evaluation's rigor; fourth, evaluation of complex nutrition-sensitive programs requires close collaboration between program implementers and evaluators and often requires efforts to overcome potential differences in priorities, expectations, incentives, time frames, and demand for information; and finally, nutrition-sensitive programs are often aimed at improving multiple outcomes among program beneficiaries, but they may also provide benefits for people (or communities) beyond the intended beneficiaries. This complicates the evaluation of the program's overall public health impacts and may also "contaminate" the control group (if non-targeted beneficiaries are part of the control group). These five challenges are discussed below.

Complexity

The complexity of nutrition-sensitive programs stems from their basic design, which relies on the integration of multiple interventions and components, often from different sectors. Within each program intervention, there is potential for variability in the delivery of the intervention by program implementers (both in terms of quantity and quality), utilization by the program beneficiaries, and adherence to the specific protocol for each program intervention (e.g., frequency of participation in program-related activities and dose of nutrition supplement consumed). This makes the evaluation of the overall program impacts more complex and attribution of impact to the different program components particularly difficult unless multiple study arms (which increase cost) are used to disentangle their relative contribution.

Long Impact Pathways and Time Frames

The pathways from program inputs to biological effects on nutritional status for nutrition-sensitive programs are usually long. For example, a homestead food production program that includes home gardens and a behavior change communications (BCC) strategy requires a number of steps before impact on nutritional status could be expected, such as installing garden beds, preparing the soil, sowing, planting, and harvesting; setting up and implementing the BCC strategy, and improving maternal knowledge through repeated BCC sessions; achieving changes in practices and the adoption of the recommendations from the BCC strategy, including preparing dishes using ingredients from the home garden, and adopting optimal child feeding and hygiene practices to improve the diets and nutrient intakes of young children and prevent infections [1–3]. The development and smooth implementation of program components, and the adoption and optimal use of program inputs and services may take several months and up to 1–1.5 years to occur even with experienced program implementers and motivated program beneficiaries. The implementation time frame has critical implications for evaluations: evaluators should carefully plan the baseline, process evaluation, and follow-up surveys based on a realistic timeline for program implementation and complete roll out, and the optimal duration of exposure needed to achieve expected impacts on both intermediary outcomes and final impacts.

Trade-Offs Between Implementation Constraints and Evaluation Rigor

Programmatic, logistical, and political factors that affect how programs are targeted, where they are implemented, and how they are rolled out add to the complexity of rigorously evaluating nutrition-sensitive programs. These factors often compromise the ability to establish a suitable, randomly assigned control group, which is desirable for establishing a proper counterfactual in assessing program impacts. To address this issue, program implementers and evaluators need to work together to identify options, such as using cluster randomization (e.g., randomizing villages or other administrative units) instead of households or individuals, and holding a public lottery to assign clusters to intervention versus control groups to show transparency and obtain endorsement from community leaders and members. If a randomized design is not feasible, the strongest possible non randomized designs need to be considered and discussed with program implementers.

Another trade-off relates to the number of treatment groups that are needed in order to answer specific research questions. If we take the example of a food assistance and BCC program, a typical research question might be what is the contribution of food versus BCC in reducing stunting? In order to properly answer this question, the research design would need to include at least 3 treatment groups (a group that receives only food assistance, one that receives only BCC, and one that receives both interventions) and a control group. The 3 treatment groups would require implementing 3 different program packages across a large number of areas (clusters) and maintaining a control group across these different areas, which clearly have implications for program implementation, logistics, and cost. Any additional research question, such as whether adding a water, sanitation, and hygiene intervention would enhance the impact on stunting, would add yet another treatment group and further complexity for program implementers. For these reasons, researchers and program staff need to spend a significant amount of time discussing key research questions, to come to an agreement on the priority questions, and to identify the ideal research design and set of treatment groups needed to best answer them.

Differing Priorities, Expectations, Incentives, Time Frames, and Demand for Information Among Program Implementers and Evaluators

As noted above, close collaboration between program implementers and evaluators is essential for the successful evaluation of nutrition-sensitive programs, and needs to start as early as possible in the program design phase. Program implementers, however, are often pressured to start rolling out their program as soon as funding is received in order to reach their program targets. Evaluators, on the other hand, typically require a few months before the program is rolled out in order to prepare and conduct a rigorous baseline evaluation. This ensures that the baseline measures adequately represent the status of the beneficiaries before the program started. To achieve an optimal alignment in the priorities, expectations, and time frames of program implementers and evaluators, the two groups need to work jointly and closely as early and often as possible throughout the program and evaluation process [5]. These meetings, especially early on, often require high-level coordination, negotiation, and endorsement.

Assessing Benefits Beyond Targeted Beneficiaries

Lastly, nutrition-sensitive programs are generally aimed at improving multiple outcomes and have the potential to benefit people beyond those directly targeted beneficiaries (pregnant and lactating women and young children), such as other household members, future cohorts of children, and even other households or the community as a whole depending on the types of interventions [1, 3, 6]. This potential "spillover" of benefits beyond the targeted beneficiaries is clearly a positive aspect of such programs and of their potential sustainability, but it adds even more complexity to evaluating and capturing *all* impacts of nutrition-sensitive programs. Evaluations thus need to anticipate the full range of potential benefits and "spillover effects" of the programs and include relevant measures and samples of non-targeted beneficiaries in the evaluation. Related to this is the complexity of measuring the cost-effectiveness of these types of programs that have multiple goals and benefits on multiple measures. To avoid overestimating the cost relative to the program's effectiveness, the multitude of benefits that these types of programs have both in the short and long term must be taken into account.

An additional potential consequence of the spillover of benefits is that some of the non-targeted beneficiaries (or communities) may actually be part of the control group used to assess the program's impact. In that case, the spillover of benefits, although beneficial to households and communities in the control group, may result in a dilution of the program impacts (or cause an underestimation of true impact because both targeted beneficiaries and non-targeted beneficiaries in the control group have received the benefits).

The remainder of this chapter is structured as follows. First, we describe the general sequence of research steps required to document the effects of programs (e.g., efficacy and program effectiveness trials). We then outline a comprehensive evaluation framework for nutrition-sensitive programs and the different components within that framework, including impact evaluation, process evaluation, and cost study. For each component, we highlight how to address the key challenges described above in evaluating nutrition-sensitive programs. We describe ways in which the information generated from comprehensive evaluations of nutrition-sensitive programs can and should be used and disseminated.

Efficacy Trials and Program Effectiveness

In the traditional sequence of determining whether or not an intervention can work to improve a biological outcome at the population level, the effect of a new intervention is first tested in an efficacy trial that evaluates the intervention under ideal and strictly controlled circumstances. Once an intervention is found to be efficacious (i.e., it has a meaningful impact under ideal conditions), the effectiveness of the intervention needs to be evaluated under real-life conditions. This sequence works well with nutrition-specific interventions that generally examine the efficacy and effectiveness of a specific type of intervention such as twice-yearly distribution of high-dose vitamin A capsules or distribution of multiple micronutrient powder (MNP) for home fortification of complementary foods. However, the evaluation of nutrition-sensitive programs does not neatly follow this sequence of steps as they generally combine multiple interventions that may have been shown to be efficacious as individual interventions, but whose combined efficacy may not have been tested.

Efficacy Trials

Efficacy research is used to determine whether nutrition-specific interventions have an impact on biological outcomes. Efficacy research usually starts with lab-based experiments and then moves to human clinical trials. Once efficacy of a given intervention has been proven with clinical trials, it should be tested in a field setting to assess its potential for public health impact [7]. The ideal evaluation design for a field-based efficacy trial is a double-blind randomized controlled trial, which involves the use of a "placebo" (non-intervention) and a treatment group (intervention) and the blinding of both researchers and participants as to who is receiving either the intervention or the placebo. Even though the intervention is implemented under ideal and strictly controlled conditions, it is important in field-based efficacy trials to measure the delivery of the intervention, use of the intervention by the intended recipient, and adherence to the intervention protocol (e.g., dose and frequency of use) [8]. Measurement of delivery, use, and adherence makes it possible to trace the pathway from delivery to intended biological impact, thereby allowing for identification of any potential barriers or facilitators that may limit or improve the potential of the intervention to have the desired impact on the measured outcome [8].[1] Finally, in this type of study, contextual factors (e.g., participant exposure to other interventions that could also impact the biological outcomes that are being measured) are controlled for to minimize potential sources of statistical noise and possibly bias

---

[1]The extent to which adherence can be reliably measured varies. For instance, adherence to vitamin A supplementation, which is provided twice a year under strict supervision, is considerably easier than for micronutrient powders which are consumed at home on daily basis.

and allows for clear attribution of impact to the specific intervention. Once an intervention is shown to be efficacious in a field-based trial, the effectiveness of the intervention at a population level can be tested in a less controlled setting or a more "real-life" situation.

Program Effectiveness Trials

Program effectiveness trials evaluate the impact of a program, or different sets of interventions within a program, under normal as compared to controlled conditions. The complexities of evaluating nutrition-sensitive programs depend on the extent to which each of the five challenges outlined in the introduction come into play.

Historically, program effectiveness has been measured using *adequacy* designs, which are limited to describing whether or not the expected changes and/or targets were achieved. This type of design does not allow the attribution of impact to the specific program being evaluated (or to infer a causal relationship between the program and the outcomes). Measurements are limited to the program recipients or target population. In recent years, however, the increased demand for evidence-based programming [9] has led to the search for more rigorous, yet feasible, evaluations using *plausibility* or *probability* designs. These types of designs do allow for attribution of impact to program interventions when implemented with appropriate rigor. A plausibility design uses a non-experimental control group to minimize the possibility that the observed changes are due to non-intervention related factors. Probability designs use experimental designs with random allocation of program inputs to treatment and control individuals, households, or clusters (e.g., villages or other administrative units). As a result, the (small) probability that the effect is due to confounding can be quantified [9].

Using a Program Theory Framework and Program Impact Pathways Analysis as the Foundation for Understanding and Evaluating Nutrition-Sensitive Programs

This section describes a program theory-based evaluation framework for nutrition-sensitive programs. The program theory framework is used to identify the key program components for each type of intervention included in a program, the factors that may affect optimal delivery or utilization of each of these components, the underlying assumptions associated with each of the key components, and how the components are expected to be linked in order to achieve impact [10]. Depending on the complexity of the program, a program theory framework includes one or more program impact pathways. A clearly documented program theory framework and associated program impact pathways are indispensable to unravel the complexity of nutrition-sensitive programs. In turn, these tools can be used to help identify which measures to assess along the program impact pathways, and when and how to assess them (e.g., who the respondent should be and what method(s) should be used to measure the different inputs, processes, outputs, and outcomes). A clearly documented program theory framework and associated program impact pathways are particularly useful to identify lack of fidelity in implementation or potential bottlenecks in the delivery or utilization of the different components of the program. This information can be fed back to program implementers in a timely fashion, hereby helping them to strengthen program implementation and operation. Similarly, impact pathway analysis results can be used to strengthen the design and implementation of future programs. It is assumed that if the program theory is correct, primary program inputs are provided and utilized as planned, and the processes work as expected, the program should achieve its desired outputs, outcomes,[2,3] and impacts[4] (see Box 27.1) [10]. Conversely, if a program does not achieve its desired impacts, the program theory framework will help identify the inputs and/or processes that may have limited the potential of the program to attain its expected outputs and outcomes and ultimately to achieve its targeted impacts.

Box 27.1 Definitions of Program Inputs, Processes, Outputs, Outcomes, and Impacts [10]

1. Inputs: Resources and constraints applicable to the program (e.g., village health support group identified and trained).
2. Processes (or activities): The services the program is expected to provide (e.g., provision of health, hygiene, and nutrition education).
3. Outputs: Receipt of program services or service utilization (e.g., health, hygiene, and nutrition education received by beneficiaries).
4. Outcomes: The state of the target population or the social conditions that a program is expected to change (e.g., child care and feeding practices).
5. Impacts: The portion of changes in the final measures along the hypothesized program impact pathways that can be attributed uniquely to a program, with the influence of other sources controlled or removed (e.g., maternal and child health and nutritional status).

How to Design a Program Theory Framework and Associated Program Impact Pathways?

Ideally, program theory frameworks should be designed by a group of key stakeholders including program implementers, evaluators, beneficiaries of the program (if the program is already being implemented), and other key stakeholders knowledgeable of the type of program being designed. Program theory frameworks are living documents as programs inevitably change over time and the framework needs to be easily modifiable to reflect these changes. An example of this collaborative effort is in the design of the program theory framework and associated program impact pathways for Helen Keller International's (HKI) homestead food production (HFP) program in Cambodia (Fig. 27.1). This program theory framework was developed at a workshop held in Cambodia which included HKI program staff, evaluation staff from the International Food Policy Research Institute (IFPRI), and a number of key stakeholders, including representatives from the Ministries of Health and Agriculture, other NGOs, and program participants. It was used as the basis to design and conduct a process evaluation of HKI's HFP program in Cambodia to assess which program inputs and processes were working as designed and planned and which ones were not [11]. This basic framework has since served as the basis for some of HKI's HFP programming efforts and associated evaluations in other countries (e.g., Nepal and Burkina Faso).

---

[2]Outcomes may be attributed to the program if a probability design is used to assess them.

[3]Outcomes may be impacts in different studies, depending on the study design, objectives, and selected measures of success.

[4]Impacts can only be assessed if a probability study design is used and a valid counterfactual has been established.

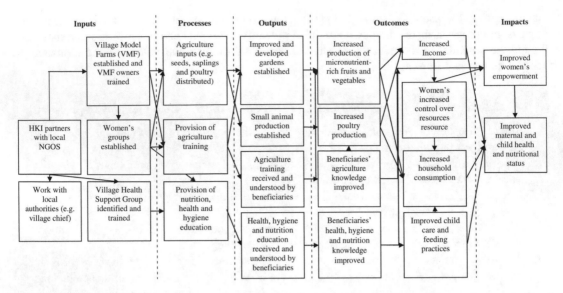

Fig. 27.1 Hypothesized pathways through which homestead food production (HFP) programs may improve maternal and child health and nutrition. Adapted from: Olney DK et al. [11]

How to Use a Program Theory Framework and Associated Program Impact Pathways in Designing the Evaluation of a Nutrition-Sensitive Program?

Once the program theory framework has been clearly outlined and understood by all stakeholders, it should be used to help guide program implementation as well as the monitoring and evaluation activities. By understanding what needs to be delivered by program implementers, what the expected content and quality of each of these intervention components are, what the time frame is for implementation and for utilization by program beneficiaries, and how program impacts are expected to be achieved, evaluators can determine what to evaluate, and when and how to evaluate it. In the case of HKI's HFP program in Cambodia, the program theory framework was used to design the process evaluation related to that program and included both quantitative and qualitative components (Table 27.1). The program theory framework is also an invaluable tool for designing both the impact evaluation and the cost study of a program. Ideally, these different evaluations are included together in a comprehensive evaluation framework to understand what impacts a program has, how it achieves these impacts, and at what cost.

A Comprehensive Evaluation Framework to Assess Program Impacts, Impact Pathways, and the Cost of Nutrition-Sensitive Programs

Understanding the pathways to impact is critical for improving program delivery and effectiveness (i.e., to keep and strengthen components that work and modify or discard components that do not). In addition, when combined with cost information, evidence of fidelity (i.e., the program is implemented as was planned), and confirmation of quality of implementation, this information helps program managers to decide whether the program can be adapted to other settings or scaled up, and at what cost [12]. In the following three subsections, we describe how to assess *what* impact a nutrition-sensitive program has (impact evaluation), *how* this impact is achieved (impact evaluation

Table 27.1 Methods used to assess the implementation and utilization of the primary components of Helen Keller International's homestead food production program[a,b]

Program inputs, processes, outputs, or outcomes identified in the program theory framework	Data collection methods used	Study population or program service delivery point
*Input*s		
HKI partners with local NGO	Semi-structured interview	HKI staff Local NGO staff
VHVs identified and trained (e.g., previous experience, training received through program, motivation, and knowledge)	Semi-structured interview	HKI staff Local NGO staff VHVs
Processes		
Health and nutrition trainings conducted for beneficiaries (e.g., provision, quality, and how these could be improved)	Semi-structured interview	HKI staff Local NGO staff VHVs Beneficiaries
	Focus group discussion	Beneficiaries
	Observation	Health and nutrition training sessions
Outputs		
Beneficiaries received and understood the health and nutrition trainings (e.g., participation, barriers and facilitators to participation and learning)	Semi-structured interview	Beneficiaries HKI staff Local NGO staff VHVs
Outcomes		
Improved agriculture knowledge among beneficiaries	Semi-structured interview	Beneficiaries Non-beneficiaries
Improved health, hygiene, and nutrition knowledge among beneficiaries	Semi-structured interview	Beneficiaries Non-beneficiaries
Increased vegetable production (e.g., types of vegetables produced, perceived barriers, and facilitators to increase production)	Semi-structured interview	Beneficiaries Non-beneficiaries
Increased fruit production (e.g., types of fruit produced, perceived barriers, and facilitators to increase production)	Semi-structured interview	Beneficiaries Non-beneficiaries
Increased poultry production (e.g., perceived barriers and facilitators to increase production)	Semi-structured interview	Beneficiaries Non-beneficiaries
Increased household consumption (e.g., perceived changes in household consumption and perceptions about how consumption has changed due to program participation)	Semi-structured interview Focus group discussion	Beneficiaries Non-beneficiaries Beneficiaries

[a]Adapted from: Olney DK et al. [11]
[b]*HFP* Homestead food production; *HKI* Helen Keller International; *NGO* nongovernmental organization; *VHV* village health volunteer

and process evaluation), and *at what cost* (cost study). In addition, we highlight common challenges within the different evaluation methods that are used to answer these questions.

What Is the Impact of the Program?

A rigorous impact evaluation allows attribution of changes in outcome and impact measures to the program and requires a probability design [9]. Several factors need to be taken into consideration when designing rigorous impact evaluations of nutrition-sensitive programs. These include aspects related to the selection of a valid comparison group (counterfactual), the trade-offs between experimental and non-experimental designs, issues of timing and duration of the evaluation, sample sizes, and choice of impact measures.

The Challenge of Finding a Valid Counterfactual

We consider a program aimed at improving women's nutritional status. Our objective is to estimate the impact of the program on women's nutritional status (N), i.e., we want to know to what extent the program *caused* a change in women's nutritional status. The impact of the program can be calculated as follows:

$$\text{impact} = (N \mid \text{with program}) - (N \mid \text{without program}),$$

that is, the impact of the program is the difference between the nutritional status of a woman receiving the program and the nutritional status of the same woman at the same point in time had she not received the program. By comparing the same woman at the same point, we rule out the possibility that the difference is due to non-program-related differences between women or to changes over time. The problem with this approach is obvious: ($N \mid$ with program) and ($N \mid$ without program) are never both "observable," i.e., no woman can be in the program and not in the program at the same time. For a woman in the program, ($N \mid$ without program) is unknown; conversely, for a woman who is not in the program, we do not know what her nutritional status would have been had she been receiving the program. The key challenge to impact evaluation is thus to determine what would have happened in the absence of the program, which is referred to as the "counterfactual." The counterfactual is constructed by finding a comparison group that is similar to the group receiving the program on all relevant characteristics, except for receiving the program [13–15]. The following subsection describes how different evaluation designs are used to generate valid counterfactuals.

Selecting an Evaluation Design

Experimental (or randomized) designs in which the eligible population is randomly assigned to either a treatment or a control group are considered the gold standard for impact evaluations. Randomization can be done at the individual or group (cluster) level. If the randomization is done well (and the group to be randomized is sufficiently large), one can (reasonably) assume that both groups are comparable and that the only difference between the groups is the program. The control group thus provides a valid counterfactual for the intervention group exposed to the program. As a consequence, differences found in the outcome and impact measures of interest between groups can be attributed to the program.

Experimental designs, even though attractive from a design point of view, are often difficult to implement for practical, logistical, or political reasons. For example, it may be politically unacceptable to withhold a cash transfer program known to have had impacts on poverty in some contexts from households or communities that are equally poor as those receiving the program. Some may even challenge the rationale for conducting an impact evaluation if the program has been previously shown to be efficacious or effective. There are many reasons why new impact evaluations may be justified, such as to assess impacts on other measures (e.g., nutrition, women's empowerment, domestic violence, in addition to poverty) and in other contexts (e.g., testing a successful model implemented in a middle-income country from Latin America in a low-income country in Africa), or to test different modalities or packages of interventions. An important consideration when discussing the creation of a control group is that, given the usually limited resources programs available, only a certain percentage of the poor can be covered by the program. As such, the fairest way to select those included and those excluded is done by random allocation, giving all potential beneficiaries (either individuals or groups) the same probability of getting the program (as opposed to other less fair approaches). Alternatively, a stepped wedge design can be used: Program enrollment (group or individual) is staggered over time, allowing those scheduled to start receiving benefits later to serve as a control until the time they become beneficiaries themselves.

Nonetheless, experimental approaches are often not feasible in programmatic contexts, and quasi-experimental designs are the next best alternative. Short of randomization, quasi-experimental designs use statistical techniques to create a valid comparison group or to address the differences between the treatment and the comparison group. A commonly used method is propensity score matching (PSM), in which (groups of) program beneficiaries are statistically *matched* ex-post to non-beneficiaries on characteristics known to influence the outcome of interest. PSM allows matching on a large number of characteristics. An important limitation is the assumption that all relevant differences between the treatment and comparison group (i.e., all characteristics that could influence the outcome and impact measures and thus potentially bias the impact estimates if not taken into account) can be observed. A second approach is the double difference or difference-in-difference approach.[5] This method compares the difference between the treatment and comparison groups at baseline ($\Delta N_{t=1}$ in Fig. 27.2) and follow-up ($\Delta N_{t=2}$) (hence the term double difference). This method eliminates bias due to unobserved differences between the treatment and the control group provided they are constant over time, i.e., they do not change between baseline and follow-up [16]. Other approaches such as regression discontinuity and instrumental variable regression are beyond the scope of this chapter. Details on these methods can be found elsewhere [13, 14].

It is important to note two widely used evaluation designs that are likely to produce biased impact estimates because of inadequate counterfactuals. These are designs that compare with and without intervention at follow-up only (no baseline), and those that compare program beneficiaries before and after the intervention (intervention group only, no "control" or comparison group). In the first method, individuals who received the program are compared to (non-randomly chosen) individuals who did not receive the program. Any difference between these two groups of individuals can thus be due either to the program or to preexisting differences between the two groups. This is a particularly severe problem when individuals or households self-select into a program (i.e., are eligible to receive program benefits, but can choose to participate or not). In this case, it is likely that those who choose to participate are different from those who choose not to in key aspects such as poverty, employment, education, and other factors that are difficult to measure (e.g., autonomy, and commitment to improve the well-being of their children) that affect both the uptake and the impacts of the program. In the hypothetical example in Fig. 27.2, the comparison group selected at follow-up actually had a higher nutritional status (N) at baseline than the treatment group. But because baseline information is not available, the "with and without estimate" of the program impact at follow-up underestimates the "true impact" of the program.

With the before and after intervention group only method, which compares the outcomes in program beneficiaries before and after program participation, the problem is that no information is available on the potential influence of other factors—shocks (positive or negative) or other programs implemented in the study areas—that may also affect the key outcomes and impacts of interest in the evaluation. Figure 27.2 shows a situation where this approach overestimates the program's impact, simply because it does not consider the improvement in nutritional status that occurred in the area due to factors unrelated to the program (see improvements between baseline and follow-up in hypothetical "valid counterfactual" group). In this case, because information on a valid (counterfactual) comparison group is unavailable, the impact attributed to the program ("before and after estimate") is larger than its real impact (true impact).

---

[5]Note that difference-in-difference estimation is also used to estimate impact on experimental studies.

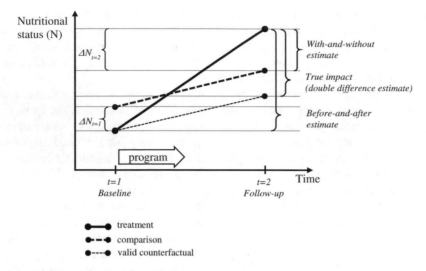

Fig. 27.2 Estimating program impact using the double difference, "follow-up with and without intervention" and the "before and after intervention group only" approaches

The Importance of Time, Duration, and Timing

The proper timing of the impact evaluation and the ideal length of time between baseline and follow-up depend on four different lag times (the first three lag times draw from Habicht et al. [8]) plus seasonality, which are relevant for most nutritional assessments. The first lag time is the time it takes for the program to be fully rolled out, and for program components to reach full coverage at the level of quality of implementation expected. The length of this lag time affects the time it will take after the baseline survey for the program to achieve detectable impacts and thus determines the timing of the follow-up survey (Fig. 27.2). The second lag time relates to the (biological) response time, which depends on the measure of interest. For example, it takes only a few days for vitamin A supplements to improve vitamin A status in deficient populations, but improving children's linear growth takes much longer. In order to improve children's height, it is important to consider not only the duration of the intervention, but also its timing. It is now well recognized that the best time to improve children's height is during the critical first 1000 days (from conception to the child's second birthday), which is considered the period of greatest potential for response to nutritional interventions targeted to mothers and children [17, 18]. To achieve full impact, children should therefore be exposed to the program for almost 3 years (in utero during pregnancy and for at least their first 24 months of life). Since the effect on linear growth is cumulative, the impact should be evaluated after 24 months when the largest effect is expected to be observed. The impact on the behaviors leading to this impact (e.g., nutrition and health practices), on the other hand, should be assessed when they are most important, i.e., before 24 months of age. The third lag time is the time it takes in cohort studies to enroll a sufficiently large number of study subjects in the required age group. Say, for example, that a program aims to enroll mothers during pregnancy and follow them until their child reaches 2 years of age, it will require several months to enroll the target sample of pregnant women, adding to the total time needed for full follow-up of each child until 24 months of age. The fourth lag time relates to the often long pathways from program inputs to the biological effects on nutrition measures (e.g., from installing garden beds to harvesting and feeding the crops to the child; or for mothers receiving BCC to actually adopting recommended feeding practices and for these improvements to translate into improvements in nutritional status measures).

The final time-related factor, seasonality, needs to be taken into account when measuring outcomes such as food availability, dietary intake, or child morbidity or wasting, which are known to vary by season [19]. The potential to benefit from interventions may also vary by season. For instance, the impact of an intervention aimed at alleviating acute malnutrition should be assessed during the lean season when its prevalence is highest. Seasonality is particularly challenging when evaluating the nutrition impact of agricultural interventions, as both the intervention and the impact measures may be sensitive to seasonal variations. To reduce the effect of seasonality, it is generally recommended to conduct the baseline and follow-up surveys at the same time (month) of the year.

Ensuring Appropriate Sample Size

Sample size calculations are conducted to determine the minimal number of observations needed to detect a meaningful effect of the intervention on the impact measures of interest. Calculating the necessary sample size requires information on the hypothesized impact of the intervention, the natural variability in the impact measure of interest, the study design (including whether randomization is done at individual or cluster level), and the level of type I and type II errors the evaluators are comfortable with. The first type of error reflects the possibility of concluding that there is an impact while the program had no effect. One minus the type II error equals the study's statistical power, i.e., the probability of finding the impact if it was truly there [13]. Once the required sample size has been calculated, additional provisions need to be made for missing data, loss to follow-up, and other problems that might reduce the number of observations that can be analyzed.

Choosing Indicators

Selecting appropriate indicators for the evaluation of complex nutrition-sensitive programs with multiple inputs, impact pathways, outcomes, and impacts is challenging. Since these programs integrate interventions from different sectors that often aim to address several underlying determinants of undernutrition (e.g., poverty, food insecurity, and women's empowerment), choosing the right indicators requires consulting with experts from a variety of fields. Indicators need to be selected carefully to ensure that they accurately reflect the phenomenon that is being measured. Other challenges relate to different levels at which measures need to be taken (community, household, and individual) and to the fact that the validity of many indicators depends on the degree or the level at which it will be assessed. For instance, the different stages in the development of iron deficiency require the use of different indicators [19].

Standardized approaches are available for the measurement of a wide variety of outcomes, such as household food security [20], women's dietary diversity [21], women's empowerment [22], and infant and young child feeding practices [23]. The valid measurement of other outcomes, such as agricultural practices, and health and nutrition knowledge require the careful development of data collection tools and analytic approaches that accurately capture the main outcomes and impacts of interest of a given evaluation.

How and Why Did the Program Have (Did Not Have) an Impact?

Understanding the Pathways to Impact

Understanding the pathways to impact is critical to improving program delivery and effectiveness (i.e., to keep and strengthen components that work and modify or discard components that do not), and to identify what is needed to scale up and to adapt the program for implementation in other settings. Information on *how* impact is achieved is typically collected in two different ways. First, data on intermediary measures (outcomes) along the impact pathway are collected in the baseline and follow-up surveys. For example, the evaluation of HKI's HFP program in Burkina Faso assessed a set of intermediary outcomes including changes in agriculture production, women's health and nutrition-related knowledge, and household, women's and children's dietary diversity, all outcomes that lie along the hypothesized program impact pathways for HKI's HFP program (Fig. 27.1) [24]. If no changes are observed in these intermediary outcomes, it is unlikely that improvements will be found in the final impact measures. Conversely, if positive changes, attributable to the program, are seen in both these intermediary outcomes and the final impact measures, the plausibility that the final impacts are due to the program is increased.

Second, a process evaluation study conducted while the program is being implemented will help identify what is working and what might be working less well in terms of fidelity of implementation and delivery and use of program services at different points along the program impact pathway. Process evaluations can help identify bottlenecks or facilitators to optimal program delivery and utilization. This information can be used to improve both ongoing programs and future programs. Note that process evaluation findings that are used to strengthen ongoing programs do not compromise the program evaluation as long as the changes are made uniformly across all program areas. In addition to identifying implementation bottlenecks and providing an opportunity for programs to readjust implementation, process evaluation data are critically important to help understand why a program has (or has not) achieved its desired impacts.

Designing the Process Evaluation

The design of a rigorous process evaluation requires a solid understanding of the overall program theory framework and the associated program impact pathways. Ideally, a process evaluation is designed to examine the primary inputs, processes, outputs, and outcomes along each of the primary program impact pathways (see Fig. 27.1 and Table 27.1) to obtain in-depth information to address five key questions: (1) Are program services being implemented and provided as planned and according to the program design (inputs and processes)? (2) Are program services being utilized as intended (outputs)? (3) What is the quality of the program inputs and services (inputs, processes, and outputs)? (4) What are the barriers and facilitators to optimal service delivery and utilization (inputs and processes)? and (5) Is the program on track to have the desired effect on improving intermediary outputs and outcomes, such as improvements in knowledge (in the example from HKI's HFP program)?

By answering these questions, one can assess the fidelity of the program to its intended design; the adherence to intervention protocols and barriers and facilitators to optimal program delivery; the quality of the services being delivered by program implementers; and the level of utilization of program services by the intended participants and their adoption of recommended practices. In addition, process evaluation results can also provide information related to whether or not the program is likely to have its desired impacts by examining early impacts on intermediary outcomes [5, 25].

The Importance of Timing and Time Frames

Ideally, a process evaluation is conducted once the program is fully up and running in order to give the fairest assessment of what is working well and which processes and services could be improved. With most nutrition-sensitive programs that typically run from 2–3 years, the first process evaluation round should be carried out about one year after the program has started implementing its different intervention components. Depending on the duration of the program, it can be useful to conduct a second round of process evaluation. The purpose of a second round can include documenting whether or not corrective measures implemented by the program team (if applicable) have improved implementation fidelity or successfully addressed previously identified bottlenecks, or furthering the study of specific issues identified during the first round of the process evaluation (e.g., potential time constraints related to beneficiary participation in the program; utilization/sharing of donated commodities or products; and observation of potentially negative impacts of program on household dynamics such as domestic violence).

While program monitoring is usually expected to be designed and implemented by program implementers, linking the process evaluation to well-designed and documented program monitoring activities can provide additional insights into what is working well and what is not with regard to program implementation and utilization. Monitoring data are usually collected starting early in the program life cycle and on a more regular basis than process evaluation data, and thus, combining the two sources of data can provide rich complementary information on program implementation and operations issues. Additionally, linking these two activities can reduce data collection redundancies. Program monitoring, for example, can be used to collect continuous detailed information on program service delivery that a process evaluation (which is conducted at discrete time points) would not be able to assess. However, in order to be useful, program implementers and evaluators need to work together to determine what types of information should be collected, by whom, how, and at what frequency. Lastly, in order to merge the data, common identifiers need to be used.

One of the biggest challenges with conducting a rigorous process evaluation is ensuring that the information collected is both useful and timely. It is relatively straightforward to collect accounting-type data that inform program managers about whether or not services have been delivered as planned and what the uptake by beneficiaries is. This type of information can be collected through either program monitoring or a process evaluation and fed back to program managers within a relatively short time frame and can be used to identify and implement solutions to the problems encountered. However, collecting and analyzing the types of qualitative data that are useful for understanding how and why interventions are or are not working is much more time-consuming. As a consequence, it can be difficult to feed relevant information obtained from these data back to a program within a time frame that is useful for the ongoing program (especially in the case of a 2-year program). Thus, some things to consider when deciding on the overall design of the process evaluation in regard to time and timing are as follows: (1) What is the total duration of the program? (2) When will the program be fully up and running? (3) Is it feasible to evaluate all of the primary intervention inputs, processes, outputs, and outcomes within the program theory framework? (4) If not, which critical inputs, processes, outputs, and outcomes or pathways should be prioritized in the process evaluation? (5) Can the data be collected and analyzed within a time frame that will allow timely feedback to program implementers and give them sufficient time to implement solutions to the problems encountered? and (6) Can the data be used to inform similar programs in the future or help interpret the results from the impact evaluation?

Selecting Data Collection Methods and Tools

Once the overall goals and the key questions to be answered by the process evaluation are determined, the next step is to select appropriate measures and identify the types of service delivery points and respondents (program implementers, program beneficiaries, and other household or community members) to include in the study. Lastly, the choice of methods needs to take into account the program components to be evaluated, the measures to be used, the respondents to be interviewed, and the points of service delivery to be observed. Commonly used approaches in process evaluations include semi-structured interviews, structured/semi-structured observations, and focus group discussions, among others (Table 27.1). As noted above, ideally all program inputs, processes, outputs, and outcomes along the hypothesized program impact pathways are evaluated in a rigorous process evaluation. If there are time and/or resource constraints, however, implementers and evaluators should jointly prioritize which inputs, processes, outputs, and outcomes the research should focus on.

To assess whether or not program inputs, processes, outputs, and outcomes are working as expected requires the collection of data that is subsequently compared to the intended design of the program (e.g., beneficiaries should receive five different types of seeds and attend two trainings per month). In addition, measures of quality of service delivery should be included because it is critically important for uptake and impact. Quality can be assessed using direct (structured or semi-structured) observations at program delivery points and through interviews with program implementers and beneficiaries. Lastly, barriers and facilitators to optimal program delivery and/or utilization should be assessed through the use of observations, interviews, and focus group discussions.

Drawing the Sample

The goal of process evaluation is different from that of an impact evaluation and therefore requires a different sampling approach. Generally, program implementers at various levels and program beneficiaries are the primary respondents. Program implementers are selected using a purposive sampling method whereby the implementers provide a list of staff and the program evaluators select some or all of them. If only a portion of the program implementers is selected, this is done using a random sample or by selecting implementers that meet certain criteria (e.g., gender, age, and skill level). Beneficiaries are either purposively or randomly selected with or without the use of stratification on a few key variables (e.g., poverty, household size, and location) to ensure that a range of respondents is included in the sample.

Summarizing the Results from the Process Evaluation

Given the mix of qualitative and quantitative data collected from a variety of key stakeholders in a process evaluation, it is useful to have a general framework of analysis to determine whether or not program inputs, processes, outputs, and outcomes are working as expected or not, and which aspects of implementation might need strengthening. This is not meant to be an exact science, but rather a general framework that can be used to identify areas that may need attention. One way to do this is to consider the quantitative data related to the primary measure (or set of measures) for a given program input, process, output, or outcome (e.g., beneficiaries established home gardens or attended training) and determine if each of those inputs, processes, outputs, and outcomes are working as expected, and if not, why not, and what could be done to improve them. For example, components with a positive response in more than 75% of the cases could be classified as "working well," those with a positive response in 25–75% as "needs improvement," and those with a positive response in less than 25% as "not working." After this initial classification, the perceptions and opinions of the program implementers and beneficiaries are used for triangulation and the categorization of that component changed as necessary. The final classification needs to consider the frequency with which problems were reported and/or the severity of the respective problems.

Sharing and Feeding the Results Back to Program Implementers

In order for program implementers to fully utilize the results from a process evaluation to improve ongoing and future programs and to identify what was working in the program that should be replicated in similar programs and scaled up if appropriate, the results need to be fed back to them in a timely fashion. This feedback should occur in the context of a workshop where the results are presented and program implementers, evaluators, and other key stakeholders, knowledgeable about the type of program, discuss the implications of the results. In order to make improvements in ongoing and future programs these discussions should focus on what program inputs, processes, or outputs are feasible to improve and how these improvements could take place. The process evaluation of HKI's HFP program in Cambodia, for instance, found that the village health volunteers responsible for conducting nutrition education sessions for program beneficiaries had limited motivation to conduct these sessions which often meant that the sessions were either not conducted or conducted with the help of HKI or supporting staff from HKI's partner NGO, which was not in line with the original program design and may have limited the quality and impact of this part of the program. Participants at the process evaluation workshop identified this as something that could be addressed in the ongoing program and suggested providing the volunteers with small incentives such as chickens to increase their motivation [11]. In relation to replicating and scaling up similar programs, discussions should also include a reflection on what worked well in the program and how optimal program delivery and utilization can be maintained, which can be challenging especially during scale-up processes.

What Is the Cost of the Program?

The objective of the cost study is to estimate the overall cost of the program, the cost of the main program components, and the program's cost-effectiveness. A well-conducted cost study allows for estimation of the savings or cost associated with adding, changing, or dropping program components, adding beneficiaries, or scaling up the program. A preferred method for detailed cost analysis in the context of a theory-driven impact evaluation is the activity-based costing ingredients (ABC-I) approach [26]. Using the program impact pathways, the first step of the ABC-I approach is to conduct a detailed description of all program activities. The description is used to identify the program's main activities. The next step is to define the unit cost algorithms, i.e., the different types, quantities, and costs of the "ingredients" necessary for each activity. Once the unit cost for each ingredient is determined, the total cost for each program activity and for the full program can be determined. This method has been used in several contexts and with a variety of programs, including social transfer programs [26, 27].

Working Together: Evaluation and Program Implementation Teams Working Together Toward a Common Goal

Evaluations of complex nutrition-sensitive programs using a comprehensive evaluation framework require close and continuous collaboration between program implementers and the external evaluation team [5]. This collaboration should be established at the program design phase and maintained throughout. The objective is to align potentially differing priorities, expectations, incentives, and time frames, and to ensure that on the one hand the program implementers share updates and challenges on program roll out and service delivery, and on the other hand, that the evaluators provide regular updates on goals, methods, and findings from their evaluation activities. This collaboration can also be useful for aligning program monitoring and evaluation activities in cases where this would be useful (e.g., collection of detailed program participation information). Some of the key challenges of successful collaboration often relate to differences in (institutional and personal) priorities, expectations, and incentives; conflicting goals, targets, and time frames; and the degree of independence of the evaluators.

Differences in Priorities, Expectations, and Incentives

Program implementers and evaluators often have very different mandates and reporting requirements that are reflected in their differing priorities, expectations, and incentives. Implementers on the one hand are charged with delivering a high-quality program that meets the targets set out in their original proposed plan within the specified budget and time frame. Program evaluators, on the other hand, are responsible for rigorously evaluating the program and producing evidence of program impact (or lack thereof), and are tasked with answering key questions related to why that impact was achieved (or not) and at what cost. A common challenge relates to deciding on the evaluation design. For the evaluator, the most informative design often involves multiple treatment arms receiving different program packages and a control group not receiving any program benefits. Ideally, assignment to these arms is random at the lowest possible level of aggregation (i.e., households rather than villages) to increase statistical power. For the program implementer, this ideal design makes implementation challenging (if not impossible) and increases costs substantially. Agreeing on a workable evaluation design that meets both the evaluators' commitment to rigor and the implementers' mandate to deliver a high-quality program and achieve target coverage numbers within the budgetary limits requires in-depth and regular discussions starting at the inception of the program and evaluation process and continuing until the final evaluation is completed.

A second problem is that evaluators are often wrongly perceived as evaluating the performance of the program implementers themselves, rather than generating evidence on the effectiveness of the program or approach. Likewise, collecting cost data frequently leads to the perception that the evaluators are auditing the program's finances. To build the trust necessary for effective collaboration, it is important for the evaluator to clearly explain the objectives of the different components of the evaluation (impact, process, and cost), present examples of the types of information that will be generated, and discuss how this information can be used to strengthen, replicate, or scale up successful program models.

Differences in Time Constraints and Time Frames

A common constraint in the evaluation of nutrition-sensitive programs is the short time frame imposed by many donors (e.g., 2–3 years). As noted above, nutrition-sensitive programs are by definition complex because they integrate interventions from different sectors that often aim to address several underlying determinants of undernutrition. As can be expected, the more complex the program, the longer it takes to get it fully functional and well implemented, and the more complex (and time- and resource-intensive) is the evaluation process. Moreover, evaluating impacts on biological outcomes such as child anthropometry may require as long as 1000 days of program exposure and must take into account other aspects such as enrollment time to achieve desired sample size and seasonality. The time frame for such evaluations should be at least 4–5 years. By contrast, program implementers are often under high pressure to get their program up and running and may roll out different program components as soon as they are ready. Other components that require extensive training and adaptation of materials, such as BCC and other nutrition interventions, which are important components of nutrition-sensitive programs, however, may take several months of planning and development. For example, a program that involves a community-level BCC strategy requires the BCC strategy to be developed (or adapted), a number of program implementers and frontline workers to be trained (e.g., NGO staff, master-level educators, and community-based educators), and the logistics of delivering the BCC to program beneficiaries needs to be carefully designed and tested. Meanwhile, it also takes time to design a rigorous impact evaluation once the research questions are agreed upon. Preparations include building the program theory framework, developing the evaluation and sampling design, designing and pretesting the data collection tools, training and standardizing enumerators, and planning the logistics of the field work. Ideally, program implementation and evaluation time frames would align so that full program implementation would be ready to go as soon as the baseline survey is completed. If program implementers and evaluators work closely together from the design phase, it is possible to optimize the alignment of the time frames for program and evaluation activities. This type of alignment is illustrated in Fig. 27.3, which shows a program implementation and evaluation time frame for HKI's HFP program in Tanzania. This was designed by program implementers and evaluators working together to understand the different steps and key considerations for both sets of activities. Although it is possible to optimize the alignment of program and evaluation activities, there are cases where program implementation falls behind schedule and in those cases it may be important to conduct a midterm evaluation that in some sense can also serve as a new baseline.

Independence of Evaluators

A final challenge is determining the right degree of independence between the program implementers and the evaluators. To ensure the objectivity and credibility of the evaluation, it is recommended to have an evaluation team that is independent of the institution implementing the program under evaluation. Complete separation, however, is not possible, nor desirable. As explained above, for an evaluation to be successful and relevant, evaluators and implementers must work closely together [13]. The use of an external team is also recommended to ensure the highest possible quality. Rigorous program evaluations require experts with specialized skills which the implementing organization is unlikely to have among its staff. A number of recent capacity building initiatives targeted to development practitioners and policy makers have focused on making communication between implementers and expert evaluators easier. These include books (see for instance Gertler et al. [13]),

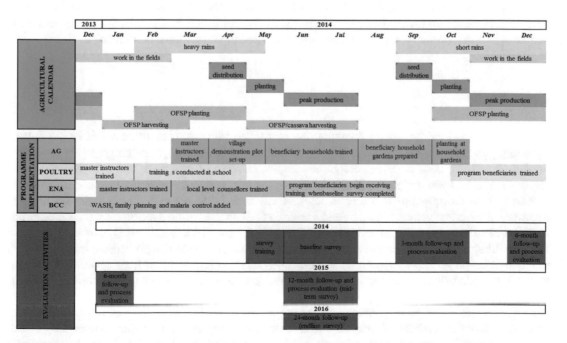

Fig. 27.3 Alignment of program and evaluation activities for HKI's HFP program in Tanzania

and initiatives such as MEASURE Evaluation (www.cpc.unc.edu/measure) and the International Initiative for Impact Evaluation (www.3ieimpact.org). These efforts are likely to be much more valuable than trying to build the capacity of program implementers in conducting rigorous evaluations, just as it would make little sense to train evaluators in designing and implementing programs. Of utmost importance is that program implementers and evaluators learn how to communicate better and work together efficiently.

Using the Results from Evaluation Research

In order to be useful, evaluation results need to be shared widely, in the appropriate fora, and using the most effective and tailored communication approaches for different audiences. For example, program implementers need to know whether they are meeting their targets as agreed with the donors and need information on which program components are working or need improvement. They generally need this information quickly so that they can use it to report back to donors and/or to improve ongoing program delivery and utilization. This information is usually provided by evaluators in the form of reports, and presentation and extensive discussions with implementers of the results and their implications. Lessons learned from synthesis of methods and of results from different studies can also be particularly useful for the wider community of program implementers. Evaluators should use this rich data and work jointly with program implementers to prepare guidance documents on best practices for designing, implementing and evaluating successful nutrition-sensitive programs. Like program implementers, donors need to know if targets are being met, but they also want to know what overall impact the programs they fund have and at what cost. Donors usually have specific reporting requirements that generally include measurement of a given set of performance indicators as well as program and evaluation reports. Widespread dissemination of evaluation results and lessons learned among the donor community is also critically important to inform future investments in nutrition-sensitive programs. Lastly, in order to contribute effectively to building the evidence base and to promote uptake of research methods and findings by the research and development community, results from comprehensive evaluations should be published in the scientific, peer-reviewed literature and disseminated widely at international, regional, and national conferences.

Conclusions

The current global evidence base regarding the nutritional impacts of nutrition-sensitive programs, including popular ones such as social safety nets and agriculture development programs, is generally limited because of poor targeting, design and implementation of programs, and equally important, sub-optimal evaluation designs [1, 3, 6]. Although there is a consensus regarding the need to invest in nutrition-sensitive programs in order to address the underlying causes of undernutrition and to improve the effectiveness, reach, and scale of both nutrition-specific interventions and nutrition-sensitive programs, the evidence of what works, how and at what cost is extremely limited. Thus, building a strong body of evidence from rigorous, theory-based comprehensive evaluations of different nutrition-sensitive program models that bring together interventions from a variety of sectors (e.g., health, education, agriculture, social protection, women's empowerment, water, and sanitation) is essential to provide the needed guidance for future investments for improving nutrition. This chapter provides this type of guidance, focusing on how to design and carry out rigorous process, cost, and impact evaluations of complex nutrition-sensitive programs; and it aims to demystify some of the perceived insurmountable challenges that have prevented investments in rigorous evaluations of such programs in the past. By doing so, we hope that the evidence gap in nutrition-sensitive programming, which has characterized the past decades of development, will quickly be filled and that future investments will benefit from a strong body of evidence on what works to improve nutrition, how it works, and at what cost.

Discussion Points

- What are the five key challenges in evaluating nutrition-sensitive programs? Are there other challenges associated with evaluating nutrition-sensitive programs? How might some of these challenges affect one's ability to rigorously evaluate a nutrition-sensitive program?
- How can some of the key challenges in designing an impact evaluation of a nutrition-sensitive program be addressed?
- What are the three main components of a comprehensive evaluation and what are the primary uses of each of these three components? How can the data collected through each of these components be integrated to enhance one's understanding of the effectiveness of a nutrition-sensitive program?
- How can a program theory framework and the associated program impact pathways analysis be used in the design and evaluation of a nutrition-sensitive program? How else can a program theory framework and the associated impact pathways be used to enhance one's understanding of the impact of a nutrition-sensitive program?

References

1. Ruel MT, Alderman H. Nutrition-sensitive interventions and programmes: how can they help to accelerate progress in improving maternal and child nutrition? Lancet. 2013;382. doi:10.1016/S0140-6736(13)60843-0.
2. Olney DK, Rawat R, Ruel MT. Identifying potential programs and platforms to deliver multiple micronutrient interventions. J Nutr. 2012;142(1):178S–85S. doi:10.3945/jn.110.137182.
3. Webb-Girard A, Cherobon A, Mbugua S, Kamau-Mbuthia E, Amin A, Sellen DW. Food insecurity is associated with attitudes towards exclusive breastfeeding among women in urban Kenya. Matern Child Nutr. 2012;8(2):199–214. doi:10.1111/j.1740-8709.2010.00272.x.
4. Leroy JL, Frongillo EA. Can interventions to promote animal production ameliorate undernutrition? J Nutr. 2007;137(10):2311–6.
5. Rawat R, Nguyen PH, Ali D, Saha K, Alayon S, Kim SS, Ruel M, Menon P. Learning how programs achieve their impact: embedding theory-driven process evaluation and other program learning mechanisms in alive and thrive. Food Nutr Bull. 2013;34(3 Suppl):S212–25.
6. Leroy JL, Ruel MT, Verhofstadt E. The impact of conditional cash transfer programmes on child nutrition: a review of evidence using a programme theory framework. J Dev Effectiveness. 2009;1(2):103–29. doi:10.1080/19439340902924043.
7. Rabin BA, Brownson RC, Haire-Joshu D, Kreuter MW, Weaver NL. A glossary for dissemination and implementation research in health. J Public Health Manag Pract. 2009;14(2):117–23. doi:10.1097/01.PHH.0000311888.06252.bb.
8. Habicht JP, Gretel P, Lapp J. Methodologies to evaluate the impact of large-scale nutrition programs. Washington DC. 2009.
9. Habicht JP, Victora CG, Vaughan JP. Evaluation designs for adequacy, plausibility and probability of public health programme performance and impact. Int J Epidemiol. 1999;28(1):10–8. USA: Division of Nutritional Sciences, Cornell University.
10. Rossi PH, Lipsey MW, Freeman HE. Evaluation: a systematic approach, vol. 7th. Thousand Oaks, CA: Sage Publications; 2004.

11. Olney DK, Vicheka S, Kro M, Chakriya C, Kroeun H, Sok L, Talukder A, Quinn V, Iannotti L, Becker E. Using program impact pathways to understand and improve program delivery, utilization, and potential for impact of Helen Keller International's Homestead Food Production Program in Cambodia. Food Nutr Bull. 2013;34(2): 169–84.

12. White H. Theory-based impact evaluation: principles and practice. J Dev Effectiveness. 2009;1(3):271–84. doi:10. 1080/19439340903114628.

13. Gertler PJ, Martinez M, Premand P, Rawlings LB, Vermeersch CMJ. Impact evaluation in practice. World Bank Publications. 2010.

14. Khandker SR, Koolwal GB, Samad HA. Handbook on impact evaluation: quantitative methods and practices. Washington DC: World Bank Publications; 2010.

15. White H. An introduction to the use of randomised control trials to evaluate development interventions. J Dev Effectiveness. 2013;5(1):30–49. doi:10.1080/19439342.2013.764652.

16. Baker JL. Evaluating the impact of development projects on poverty: a handbook for practitioners. World Bank Publications. 2000.

17. Black RE, Allen LH, Bhutta ZA, Caulfield LE, de Onis M, Ezzati M, Mathers C, Rivera J. Maternal and child undernutrition: global and regional exposures and health consequences. Lancet. 2008;371(9608):243–60. doi:10. 1016/S0140-6736(07)61690-0.

18. Black RE, Victora CG, Walker SP, Bhutta ZA, Christian P, de Onis M, Ezzati M, et al. Maternal and child undernutrition and overweight in low-income and middle-income countries. Lancet. 2013;382(9890):427–51. doi:10.1016/S0140-6736(13)60937-X.

19. Gibson RS. Principles of nutritional assessment. Oxford University Press. 2005.

20. Coates J, Swindale A, Bilinsky P. Household food insecurity access scale (HFIAS) for measurement of food access: indicator guide (v.3). Washington D.C.: Food and Nutrition Technical Assistance Project (FANTA)/ Academy for Educational Development; 2007.

21. FAO (Food and Agriculture Organization of the United Nations), and IRD (Institut de Recherche pour le Développement). Defining a standard operational indicator of women's dietary diversity: the women's dietary diversity follow-up project. Contributors: Martin-Prével Y, Allemand P, Wiesmann D, Arimond M, Ballard TJ, Deitchler M, Dop MC, Kennedy G, Lee WTK. Rome; Montpellier. 2014.

22. Alkire S, Meinzen-Dick R, Peterman A, Quisumbing A, Seymour G, Vaz A. The women's empowerment in agriculture index. World Dev. 2013;52:71–91. doi:10.1016/j.worlddev.2013.06.007.

23. WHO. Indicators for assessing infant and young child feeding practices part 2: measurement. Geneva: World Health Organization; 2010.

24. Olney DK, Dillon A, Pedehombga A, Ouédraogo M, Ruel MT. Using an agricultural platform in burkina faso to improve nutrition during the first 1,000 days. In: International Food Policy Research Institute (IFPRI), editors. Global nutrition report 2014: actions and accountability to accelerate the world's progress on nutrition. Washington D.C: International Food Policy Research Institute; 2014. doi:10.2499/9780896295643.

25. Nguyen PH, Menon P, Keithly SC, Kim SS, Hajeebhoy N, Tran LM, Ruel MT, Rawat R. Program impact pathway analysis of a social franchise model shows potential to improve infant and young child feeding practices in Vietnam. J Nutr. 2014;144(10):1627–36. doi:10.3945/jn.114.194464.

26. Fiedler JL, Villalobos CA, De Mattos AC. An activity-based cost analysis of the honduras community-based, integrated child care (AIN-C) programme. Health Policy Plann. 2008;23(6):408–27. doi:10.1093/heapol/czn018.

27. Margolies A, Hoddinott J. Costing alternative transfer modalities. J Dev Effectiveness. 2015;7(1):1–16. doi:10. 1080/19439342.2014.984745.

Chapter 28
Integrated Approaches to Health and Nutrition: Role of Communities

Olivia Lange, Divya Mehra, Saskia de Pee and Martin W. Bloem

Keywords Communities · Virtual networks · Global trends · Community and health systems linkages · Multi-sectorality · SDG3 · Health enablers · Health system · Community health workers · Task shifting

Learning Objectives

- Understand the different roles of communities in directly or indirectly impacting health.
- Gain insights on key global trends in public health delivery and their influence on development in LMICs.
- Evaluate challenges and opportunities of virtual communities.
- Begin to identify platforms that can be used as entry points for cross-sectoral interventions.
- Distinguish between the different stages of evolution of a society and what this means for communities and individuals.

Introduction

Communities have historically played a significant role in influencing the health outcomes of their populations. Community health workers have existed for half a century to bridge under-served communities and formal health systems. This cadre of lay health workers has enjoyed a prominent place in global health policy discourse, beginning with the Alma-Ata declaration in 1978, which formally recognized the important role of community actors in scaling up primary care. Communities have played an equally important role in generating demand for health by addressing various cultural,

O. Lange · D. Mehra (✉) · S. de Pee · M.W. Bloem
Nutrition Division, World Food Programme, Rome, Italy
e-mail: divya.mehra@wfp.org

O. Lange
e-mail: olivia.h.lange@gmail.com

S. de Pee
e-mail: Saskia.depee@wfp.org

S. de Pee · M.W. Bloem (✉)
Friedman School of Nutrition Science and Policy, Tufts University, Boston, MA, USA
e-mail: martin.bloem@wfp.org

M.W. Bloem
Department of International Health, Bloomberg School of Public Health,
Johns Hopkins University, Baltimore, MD, USA

© Springer Science+Business Media New York 2017
S. de Pee et al. (eds.), *Nutrition and Health in a Developing World*,
Nutrition and Health, DOI 10.1007/978-3-319-43739-2_28

social, informational, and cost barriers to health-promoting lifestyles and care seeking, sometimes at the peril of their own safety.

Community engagement in health may take many forms and embody spectrums from passive to active and informal to formal. While individuals may receive interventions in community settings or participate in externally determined development projects, this chapter focuses primarily on community empowerment, a process by which communities actively work to identify and solve their own health and development problems [1, 2]. The level of formalization with respect to community engagement may also vary. For example, in South Africa, community participation around HIV/AIDS ranges from less formal—for example, members of social networks volunteering to be TB or ART "treatment buddies"—to more formal—for example, community health workers delivering ART and providing adherence support [3]. While this chapter acknowledges that some external mobilization may be needed to facilitate community participation and empowerment, it does not examine the role of external actors such as governments, NGOs or UN agencies [1]. Many proponents of the empowerment approach to participation would like to ignore the uncomfortable fact that participation may require outside prompting; they would rather see spontaneous, self-generating conscientious and participatory action on the part of poor community members. Increasingly, however, they are willing to acknowledge that marginalized or disenfranchised communities are powerless to effect participation precisely because they have no power and that outsiders might succeed in fostering community mobilization as they may act with greater sensitivity and humility.

The role of communities in health continues to evolve as demographic, health, policy and technology trends shift. In the future, geographical communities may play a more limited role in some areas of health—such as delivering specific health information—and a greater role in others—such as educating on how to best navigate the increasingly pluralistic arenas of health, social protection and other social services. The importance of virtual communities, which to date have had a limited application for health, is likely to grow.

This chapter begins by discussing the role—both positive and negative—of geographically bounded communities in health. It then examines changing global dynamics with respect to population demographics, health trends, urbanization, global health policy and technology and analyses the implications of these shifting dynamics on the role of communities in health. In this section, the concept of virtual communities is discussed within the health context. Finally, it proposes an integrated supply and demand-oriented framework for the future role of communities in advancing health and nutrition outcomes.

Historical Perspectives: Communities and Health

Role of Communities in Health

Discourse around communities and health most commonly refers to geographical communities. In this section, we discuss geographical communities, defined as "a group of people with diverse characteristics who are linked by social ties, share common perspectives, and engage in joint action in geographical locations or settings" [4]. In contrast, virtual communities as defined by Demiris are a social unit/group of people who interact with each other using communication technologies to overcome geographical boundaries: "People with mutual interests coming together virtually to ensure mutual support and self-help, share experience and ask questions" [5]. It follows that a virtual community for health care would come together for the purposes of health-related activities and education [6]. We discuss virtual communities further in next section **Shifting Dynamics**.

Communities have a role to play in overcoming both supply and demand barriers to good health and utilization of health services. On the supply side, communities may play a role advocating for

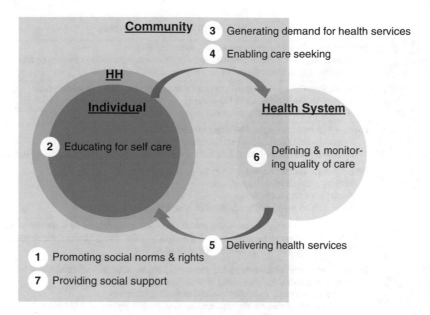

Fig. 28.1 Historical perspective—role of traditional (geographical) communities in health. See Fig. 28.2 for further explanation of numbers

services when lacking, in increasing coverage of health services through community health workers and improving quality and acceptability of health services through engagement with the health system. On the demand side, communities may play a role in addressing various cultural, social, informational, and cost barriers to health-promoting lifestyles and care seeking. Figures 28.1 and 28.2 present various capacities in which communities influence—both positively and negatively—the health outcomes of their populations.

The following section outlines roles that communities have historically played in influencing health outcomes and efforts undertaken in LMICs to harness the power of communities to promote better health outcomes.

Promoting Social Norms and Rights

Attitudes and practices surrounding health and health seeking are strongly embedded in religious, cultural and social norms and values. Female circumcision, early pregnancy, various birthing practices and dietary taboos during pregnancy provide examples of harmful traditional practices [7]. Socio-cultural customs and beliefs can also prove detrimental when they subvert an individual's right to health, including "timely, acceptable, and affordable health care of appropriate quality" [8]. Because of their low status, marginalized groups such as adolescent girls, women and people living with HIV (PLHIV) may face greater economic and social barriers to accessing care. For women, lack of decision-making authority, including decisions around resource allocation for health, may preclude them from seeking care for themselves and their children. A woman's agency tends to be lowest when she lacks education and does not contribute to household income [9, 10]. Women may also face cultural taboos that discourage health seeking, such as resistance to birth control, norms against women leaving home for long periods, and the association of unattended births with strength and good moral character [9, 11].

Global experiences with the HIV and Ebola virus disease (EVD) epidemics highlight that social stigma represents a major obstacle to care seeking. Not only are these diseases themselves devastating

Description and examples

1 Promoting social norms & rights	**Establishing cultural/social norms and rights around health** • Empowering men, women and families to improve and increase control over health • Recognizing right to health and safe motherhood and birth as human rights
2 Educating for self care	**Spreading knowledge about behaviors and practices to treat and prevent disease** • Developing health literacy and knowledge • Behavior interventions to protect and promote health
3 Generating demand for health services	**Encouraging care-seeking and referring individuals to skilled care** • Encouraging care seeking for routine care • Increasing awareness of potential health complications and referring individuals to skilled care
4 Enabling care seeking	**Reduce cost and other barriers to reaching and using services** • Mobilizing health financing resources • Developing transport schemes • Other support e.g. reducing workload of individual, providing childcare
5 Delivering health services	**Filling health system gaps by providing health care services to remote or underserved populations** • Preventative interventions: e.g., malaria prevention, vaccination, nutrition supplements • Disease management: e.g., treating minor illnesses
6 Defining & monitoring quality of care	**Defining and monitoring acceptability and quality based on social and cultural norms** • Identifying needs (e.g., community epidemiological surveillance) • Prioritizing, planning, implementing, and evaluating activities • Ensuring services are culturally appropriate and account for client preferences
7 Providing social support	**Providing social support and encouraging healthy coping mechanisms** • Promoting social integration and affiliation, positive reinforcement and empowerment • Supporting adherence to treatment regimens

Fig. 28.2 Description of traditional (geographical) roles of communities in health

for communities in general, but also for the associated social stigma, including the impact of stigma on disease outcomes. People affected by HIV/AIDS and Ebola and other diseases that carry strong stigma like the plague, cholera and leprosy have been subjected to isolation, violence and ostracism from their communities [12]. For HIV, evidence has shown that stigma has resulted in barriers to prevention, access to treatment and retention in care. It has also lead to an increase in mental health problems. The HIV/AIDS response very early recognized that unless issues of stigma and discrimination are holistically and systemically addressed, achieving the "ends of AIDS" will not be possible. The response aims to address structural issues such as poverty, racism, gender inequality, punitive policy and legal environments for addressing stigma among key populations such as men who have sex with men, injecting drug users and sex workers. During the recent Ebola epidemic in West Africa, communities impacted by EVD stigmatized people in any contact with EVD [13]. For example, children orphaned by EVD and disease free were not cared for by communities and extended families due to fear of disease transmission [12].

Some evidence indicates that community mobilization and empowerment of marginalized groups may create a more positive enabling environment for health; however, accounts are generally descriptive and a more robust evidence base is needed to confirm the effectiveness of these approaches [14]. Strategies such as women's groups and community representative outreach have focused on increasing community awareness of women's rights to reproductive and maternal health and on empowering women to enhance their participation in health-related household decisions [9, 10, 15]. Women's groups may be primarily health-focused, or they may aim to empower women more broadly, which can serve to indirectly impact health outcomes. For example, the Mahila Samkaya programme in India supports a variety of activities—including skills education, literacy training, leadership and negotiating capacity building—and facilitates opportunities to earn modest incomes [10]. Through participation in women's groups, women attest to gaining a more equal status in the household and a greater voice in household decisions, including decisions around health [9, 10].

Educating for Home Care and Care Seeking

Over half of child deaths and most maternal deaths are due to conditions that could be prevented or treated with simple, affordable interventions [16]. The knowledge of health promotion and disease prevention strategies as well as an understanding of when, where and how to seek skilled care is critical to reducing the number of preventable deaths. Relatively simple home-based strategies can address many of the major causes of neonatal and child mortality; however, lack of knowledge represents a major bottleneck. These strategies include:

- **Neonatal care**: 44% of all under-five deaths occur in the neonatal period, or the first 28 days of life [16]. Simple essential newborn care strategies—including skin to skin care, umbilical cord care and early initiation of breastfeeding—can considerably reduce the burden of mortality among this age group when understood and practiced correctly [17, 18].
- **Diarrhoea prevention and treatment**: Diarrhoea causes 15% of under-five deaths, making it the second leading cause of death among this age group [19]. It is estimated that hand washing alone, if practiced appropriately, could reduce the deaths of one million children each year [19]. Other simple, home-based strategies for preventing diarrhoea include environmental sanitation, safe food preparation practices, exclusive breastfeeding in the first six months of life, and good nutrition [18, 19].
- **Malnutrition prevention and treatment**: Malnutrition is an underlying cause of 45% of deaths among children under five. Furthermore, one out of every four children worldwide is stunted, a condition that has livelong and intergenerational consequences, including reduced cognitive and physical potential and increased risk of poor health. Good nutrition during the first 1000 days from conception to a child's second birthday is necessary to prevent stunting. Exclusive breastfeeding in the first six months of life and consumption of nutrient-dense complementary foods in addition to breastfeeding from age 6–23 months is critical [20]. High-dose vitamin A supplementation among children 6–59 months reduces mortality by 25% [21]. However, in many areas, access to nutritious and safe complementary foods represents a bottleneck for prevention of stunting even when appropriate infant and young child feeding practices are well understood.
- **Malaria prevention and treatment**: 216 million cases of malaria and 655,000 malaria deaths occurred in 2010, mostly among African children [19]. Controlled trials have affirmed that sleeping under an insecticide-treated net can substantially reduce mortality among children under five in endemic areas [19, 22]. Furthermore, rapid initiation of malaria treatment reduces mortality, and possibly morbidity, by preventing neurologic complications and severe anaemia [22]. The World Health Organization has advocated for home-based management of malaria (HMM) in Africa, which involves treating children with pre-packaged antimalarial drugs distributed by community members [23].

Furthermore, an understanding of when skilled care is needed, and where and how to seek it is critical to preventing morbidity and mortality. This entails literacy on various health conditions, awareness of associated danger signs, and knowledge of available health services. Poor, vulnerable and remote groups are less likely to benefit from access to health-related information, challenging their ability to make informed decisions around health.

Evidence indicates that communities can play an important role in conveying information about health to improve home-based care practices and generate demand for facility-based health services. Community "agents of change" have historically included community health workers (CHWs), traditional birth attendants (TBAs), women's groups and volunteers. These community representatives have taken on a range of tasks including delivering basic health education and demonstrating essential family practices; identifying sick and malnourished children and encouraging parents to seek care; encouraging attendance at routine prenatal and antenatal care and use of skilled care for delivery; educating on danger signs, particularly for obstetric and neonatal emergencies; and providing information about available services [15, 24]. These outreach services have been demonstrated to positively impact a range of health outcomes, including the prevalence and severity of diseases and adverse health conditions (diarrhoea, malaria, malnutrition); uptake of routine antenatal and postnatal care, use of skilled delivery services, and referrals in obstetric and neonatal emergencies; and under-five and neonatal mortality [9, 14, 15, 18, 24, 25].

CHWs may serve as spokespeople for and intermediaries between excluded, marginalized populations and outside entities [26, 27]. As community leaders with links to various social and health systems, CHWs are well placed to promote structural changes that reduce health iniquities [26, 28]. As policy advocates, CHW can help address the social determinants of health—such as living and working conditions, income inequality and job security, and social exclusion—based on an intimate knowledge of the communities they serve [29].

CHWs have also played a role in building social capital as a means to improve community health. This approach seeks to enhance social connection to increase a community's capacity to achieve mutual goals and respond to emergencies. In several examples, CHWs have mobilized community members to identify pressing health issues and to design community-driven solutions [28, 29]. By promoting civic engagement, CHWs may also empower communities to work with outside entities to lobby for funds, programmes and policies [28].

Overcoming Access Barriers

The cost of seeking care—including direct medical costs, direct nonmedical costs (e.g. transportation) and indirect costs (e.g. the opportunity costs of forgoing paid employment)—may negatively impact demand for health services, particularly for poor and vulnerable populations [9, 30, 31]. Studies in geographies as diverse as Burkina Faso, northeast Brazil and the UK, indicate that transportation represented 25% or more of the total patient costs (including facility costs not incurred by the user) [9, 30]. The opportunity cost of seeking care can be significant, particularly in periods of heavy economic activity, such as the harvest [9]. Furthermore, other household obligations, such as the need to care for children or other household members, may represent barriers to seeking care [32].

Community-driven approaches to social protection have been shown to alleviate consumer cost barriers and increase utilization of health services. A range of local health financing schemes have been observed, including microinsurance, rural health insurance, mutual health insurance, revolving drug funds and community involvement in user-fee management [17]. Community-based strategies for improving transportation for health-related emergencies have included mobilization of vehicles; agreements with local transport unions, private drivers and bus companies; funds for emergency transportation; and communication systems for referrals [9, 17]. Community-based funding and transport mechanisms have been shown to increase utilization of health services and decrease adverse birth outcomes [25].

In remote areas where skilled birth attendants are unavailable or geographically inaccessible, maternity waiting homes (MWHs) can serve as a link between communities and the health system. MWHs are located near health centres and provide facilities where women can stay in the final weeks of pregnancy. While some studies have indicated that MWHs have led to improvements in birth outcomes, others have reported low utilization and poor reception due to factors such as remote locations, poor facilities and no provision of food [9, 25, 33].

Delivering Health Services

Lack of health system capacity, shortage of trained health workers and inequalities in healthcare access and utilization represent enduring concerns for the global health community. Community health workers (CHWs)—a cadre of individuals with basic health training living and working in their communities—have existed for over half a century to reach remote and under-served populations with essential health care (see Box 28.1). By task shifting basic tasks to lesser-trained workers, CHW programmes also free up capacity of overburdened health systems [25, 34].

CHWs play a range of roles, from generalist to specialist, and deliver a diverse set of promotive, preventative and curative interventions. Substantial evidence supports the effectiveness of CHWs in the following areas. Note that these interventions are in addition to health education interventions discussed in section *Educating for Home Care and Care Seeking*, which CHWs may also deliver.

- **Reproductive and maternal health**: CHWs have been effective in increasing the uptake of family planning and delivering contraceptive injections in developing regions [35, 36]. In addition, CHWs have been relied upon to deliver health education for maternal and child health, including breastfeeding promotion and infant and young child feeding counselling [18].
- **Child health and nutrition**: A strong evidence base documents the effectiveness of CHWs in diagnosing and treating serious childhood illnesses. Pneumonia, diarrhoea and malaria are of particular interest, as they cause 41% of deaths among children under five [19]. CHWs also play an important role in delivering routine services such as vaccinations. Child health days, used to deliver multiple maternal and child health interventions during a few days per year, represent an effective setting for routine services such as vaccinations, high-dose vitamin A capsule distribution, growth monitoring and nutrition education, and have demonstrated improvement in under-five mortality [19].
- **Malaria control**: As per latest WHO estimates (December 2015), there were 214 million cases of malaria in 2015 and over 400,000 deaths. Malaria incidence and mortality rates among at risk populations have considerably reduced in recent years—37% reduction in incidence and 60% decrease in mortality. CHW roles have included educating community members on malaria prevention and diagnosis, distributing insecticide-treated bed nets, and providing home-based management and preventative treatment of malaria [19].
- **Tuberculosis care**: Behind HIV, tuberculosis is the second leading cause of death worldwide from a single infectious agent. Patients living with HIV face increased risk of developing tuberculosis, which causes 25% of deaths among PLHIV [37]. CHWs have provided integral support to TB programmes, particularly in community-based directly observed therapy, short-course (DOTS). CHW roles have included detecting symptomatic patients, facilitating testing and ensuring treatment compliance, among other activities [19].
- **HIV prevention and care**: The fastest growing use of CHWs lies in the field of HIV [16]. Treatment is "the cornerstone of an effective response", and under new WHO guidelines,[1] more people are on treatment than ever before [38, 39]. As of 2013, however, only 36% of those eligible for ART treatment were receiving it [40]. Health systems are overburdened and under-equipped to handle the growing caseload, and long distances, costly travel and long wait times at stretched health facilities represent barriers to treatment retention [34]. In 2006, WHO proposed "task shifting" and the training of CHW to decrease the burden on the formal health system and improve coverage among hard-to reach populations [3, 34, 41]. Programmes have engaged CHW to deliver ART at home, provide adherence support, detect side effects and opportunistic infections, and refer sick patients to clinics [34].
- **Treatment of acute malnutrition**: In 2014, 50 million children under five were wasted, with a third severely wasted. While initially treated through in-patient settings, with the advent of ready to use therapeutic foods (RUTFs), the treatment of severe wasting (without complications) can be done in outpatient settings. Community-based management of acute malnutrition (CMAM) started

---

[1]The 2015 WHO guidelines recommend that ART should be initiated in everyone living with HIV at any CD4 cell count.

in 2000, which as the name suggests consists of an integral community component for outpatient treatment of MAM and SAM as well as inpatient management of SAM with complications. The community aspect in CMAM specifically entails case finding, referrals, service delivery and management [42]. Community sensitization through outreach, education and counselling is equally essential components of CMAM [42].

- **Non-communicable Diseases**: To date, the role of CHW for managing NCDs has not been explored in the LMIC context; however, this may change as NCDs have become the leading cause of death in many LMICs, and 85% of NCDs deaths occur in the poorest countries in the world [43]. Evidence from the USA indicates that CHWs can make positive contributions to the management of hypertension, the reduction in cardiovascular risk factors, diabetes control and cancer screening [19].

Defining and Monitoring Quality of Care

Clinic-based services, even when available, accessible and affordable, may fail to adapt to community preferences and expectations, leading to low utilization. Section *Promoting Social Norms and Rights* has described demand barriers related to socio-cultural factors. This section examines the issue from the supply side, specifically how services respond to "consumer" perception of quality.

A range of supply-side factors influence uptake of health services, from staff mix to adequacy of equipment and medicine. In many countries, women may be reluctant to seek clinic-based treatment due to discomfort with male caregivers [11]. Research has highlighted that a respectful provider attitude represents an important factor influencing women's decisions on where to give birth [44]. Women who fear shame and judgement from providers, particularly when the pregnancy is considered illegitimate, are less likely to seek skilled care [11].

Community involvement in the design, planning, implementation and evaluation also increases the likelihood that health services are culturally appropriate and acceptable and account for the "consumer" perception of quality [17]. Community involvement can also improve service uptake by ensuring that health services respond to the specific needs of the population and are culturally appropriate. Communities represent a valuable partner to health systems in gathering and analysing information on health to inform the development and implementation of health strategies. This may entail conducting community epidemiological surveillance, community-based death reviews and verbal autopsies [17]. Different methods have been developed to support ongoing community engagement, also referred to as "community-driven quality". These may include seeking community input through group meetings or household surveys, and establishing community advisory or management boards.

Providing Social Support

Chronic diseases such as HIV and tuberculosis, as well as many types of cancers, require prolonged, physically demanding treatments and demand lifestyle changes that may prevent a patient from working. Feelings of isolation, depression, loneliness and concern for future are common and may be compounded by negative stigma surrounding HIV/TB infections as described under "promoting social norms and rights".

Social support from family, friends and the broader community has been shown to influence health-seeking behaviours, treatment compliance and health outcomes [45]. Social support, defined as the set of relationships and interactions that "lead the subject to believe that he is cared for, loved, esteemed and a member of a network of mutual obligations", can take a variety of forms, including encouragement, financial support and other forms of psychosocial support [46]. For example, members of social networks can support adherence to treatment regimens by reminding or accompanying the patient to the clinic. Contributions of families, friends and communities can also offset the indirect costs of the disease by providing childcare, transportation and food (discussed in detail in section *Overcoming Access Barriers*) [45]. More structured groups such as HIV support groups or "TB clubs" can help patients expand social networks, improve psychosocial well-being, promote a greater understanding of the disease and decrease negative stigma [45].

Box 28.1 History of Community Health Workers (CHWs)

In context of persistent inequality in access to health care and the global shortage of skilled health workers, community health workers (CHWs) have emerged to fill health system gaps and improve coverage of basic health services. CHWs represent a diverse cadre of health workers that perform a wide range of activities in communities outside clinic-based facilities. They generally have some degree of formal health training but do not obtain a professional certificate or educational degree [16, 19, 47].

The concept of the lay health worker operating outside the formal health system has existed for a half-century or more. Chinese "barefoot doctors" in the 1950s and 1960s were peasants and farmers who received limited health training and provided basic care at the brigade (production unit) level [16, 19, 47]. During this period, other countries were struggling with the inability of existing health systems to address the health needs of poor and remote populations. A number of countries looked to the barefoot doctors as an alternate model, and CHW programmes emerged countries such as Indonesia, India, Tanzania, Venezuela, Honduras and Guatemala [19]. In these early programmes, community workers played a range of technical and social roles, which prompted tension over whether they should be considered an extension of the health system or broader agents of social change [3].

The Alma-Ata Declaration in 1978, which called for primary health care to achieve Health For All by 2000, reaffirmed the importance of CHWs; nevertheless, CHW programmes began to lose momentum in the 1980s [19, 47, 48]. Common problems included inadequate training, insufficient remuneration or incentives, and poor supervision and logistical support for supplies and medicines. Poor integration with the health system and lack of acceptance by health professionals hampered CHW programmes [3, 19]. Furthermore, the global economic recession of the 1980s and health sector reforms undermined support and financing for community-level initiatives [17, 19, 47–49].

More recently, however, CHW programmes have regained recognition as a critical link between health systems and hard-to-reach populations, particularly in the light of insufficient and uneven progress towards health-related Millennium Development Goals [19, 50]. CHWs build and stabilize the healthcare system to deliver large-scale programmes. In an eight paper series about Alma-Ata: rebirth and revision, the Lancet highlighted funding, training and supervision for CHWs as a priority action to implement primary health care at scale [50]. As of 2011, the World Health Organization estimated that there were 1.3 million CHWs operating around the world. Large-scale CHW programmes currently exist in many countries including Brazil, Bangladesh, Nepal, Ethiopia, India, Pakistan and South Africa. Brazil's Angentes Comunitarios de Saude (previously Visitadoras) programme is the largest in the world. It engages 240,000 CHWs to provide home visits and services to 110 million people and has driven marked improvements in population health status [19]. The number CHWs per beneficiary may widely vary among programmes. For example, there was 1 CHW for every 100 people in Thailand and 1 CHW for every 300 people in Bangladesh Integrated Nutrition Programme [51]. In CHW models, it is also common to have one supervisor for every 10–30

CHWs [51]. Optimal supervision and number of CHW should be important considerations in programme design.

Extensive global experience with CHWs offers compelling evidence that CHWs can effectively play a range of promotive, preventative and curative roles; however, several critical enablers must be in place to support the success of programmes. Appropriate selection and adequate training for CHWs, including follow-up training, are pre-requisites for success. It is widely acknowledged that strong supervision and support is one of the most important, and often the most overlooked, condition for a well-functioning CHW programme. Governance and accountability, including the role of the communities, and relationships with formal health systems and government structures, must be clearly established at the outset. While many CHWs have relied on volunteers, there is no evidence that this represents a sustainable long-term model, and most reviews of CHW programmes highlight targeted incentives and remuneration as critical success factors [17, 19, 24, 47–49].

Shifting Dynamics

Sustainable Development Goals (SDGs)

The 17 SDGs, adopted by 193 member states in September 2015, pave the way for a new way of addressing global issues. Unlike the MDGs, the SDGs are global, applicable to all countries, owned by member states and are to be implemented through partnerships by leveraging the expertise of all stakeholders. The strong human rights and social inclusion and justice-based agenda emphasize sustainability and linkages between the goals.

In 2000, the MDGs provided the world leaders with 8 goals to meet the needs of the world's poorest.[2] They were revolutionary in providing a clear message and galvanizing efforts around measurable targets by the set date of 2015. While MDGs were "improvement" goals, with perhaps the incentive to "do the easiest first", the SDGs are "zero goals", requiring a strong emphasis on reaching the most vulnerable and hardest to reach. The SDGs address the complexity of the global agenda in a way the MDGs did not. For example, hunger and poverty together formed the first MDGs goal, not distinguishing between the two, particularly with regard to nutrition. The siloed goals of HIV, child mortality and maternal health likely incentivized siloed funding and therefore siloed approaches to these issues. Building on the MDGs, the SDGs, with its 17 goals and 169 targets provide a comprehensive forward-looking framework. Recognizing the trends of climate change, urbanization, increasing conflicts/migration, the SDGs fill several gaps not previously addressed.

Achieving the results of the SDGs by 2030 will require significant shifts and changes from the current way of addressing global challenges. Working across sectors and stakeholders and understanding the inter-connectedness of the goals will be necessary in order to see impact at the individual level, particularly for the most vulnerable. Therefore, it follows that national structures and funding flows will also have to change. In addition, national spending (both public and private) will have to

---

[2]Including goals concerning hunger (Goal 1, Target 1.C); under-five mortality (Goal 4, Target 4.A); maternal mortality (Goal 5, Target 5.A); access to reproductive health (Goal 5, Target 5.B); spread of HIV/AIDS (Goal 6, Target 6.A); access to treatment for HIV/AIDS (Goal 6, Target 6.A); incidence of malaria and other major diseases (Goal 6, Target 6.C); access to safe drinking water and basic sanitation (Goal 7, Target 7.C); and access to affordable essential drugs (Goal 8, Target 8.E).

dramatically increase and reliance on external donor assistance will not only be insufficient but also unreasonable.

Changing Dynamics of Physical Communities (Population Demographics and Urbanization)

Population growth, associated shifts in demographic trends, and growing urbanization will have increasing demands on existing resources and systems. The global population is projected to grow and reach 9 billion by 2050 (from 7 billion in 2011). However, it is expected that the pace of this growth will be slower than it has been in the past. Population growth velocity reached its peak between 1965 and 1970 and has been slowing down ever since. By 2050, it is projected to stagnate in high-income countries and slow down to 0.5% annually and only grow by 1.42% in LMICs [52].

As a country develops, its mortality rate tends to decline as a result of improvements in health, nutrition and social development. Concurrently, fertility rates also decline with improvements in education, delayed age at marriage, empowerment of women and access to contraception. Since this development occurs with great heterogeneity, a couple noteworthy trends with significant impact on health are important to review.

In general, people are living longer and the world population is ageing rapidly. Life expectancy will likely increase to 75.6 years in 2045–2050 from 68 at present [52]. In parallel, the global burden of disease is shifting. NCDs are now causing 60% of deaths and almost 50% actual and effective life years lost due to disability [53]. As compared to 2004, by 2030, diseases such as diarrhoea, neonatal infections and birth trauma as the top ten leading causes of the burden of disease worldwide will be replaced by diabetes and chronic obstructive pulmonary disease (COPD), and ischaemic heart disease will continue to be one of the top leading causes [53]. This growth and changes mean that not only will the burden on health systems increase overall, but it would also necessitate a different system and skill set to prevent and manage non-communicable diseases.

Population growth is expected to be highly concentrated in a few countries and double in the least developed countries, since birth rates still tend to be quite high in LMICs. An increasing number of young people in these countries would require more resources from the national system for health and education, as well opportunities for economic growth. Both these trends are taking place within the context of persistent global inequalities (income and social) and continued environmental degradation.

Another major global shift is urbanization. Already more than half of the world's population lives in urban areas, and this proportion will continue to increase. The rate of urbanization is faster in Asia and Africa as compared to other regions, while simultaneously they still account for more than 90% of the world's rural population. Urbanization itself is characterized by diversity: half of the urban population resides in settlements of less than 500,000 people and a substantial population in "mega-cities" with 10 million or more inhabitants [54]. Urban settings can have both a positive and a negative impact on health. Urban populations have better access to health, education, employment and social services. But, urbanization is also associated with unplanned expansion, people living in slums (one-third of urban residents in LMICs or 860 million people) with suboptimal water and sanitation, overcrowding, increased pollution and other harmful impacts on the environment due to unsustainable production and consumption by a large population. In general, urban areas tend to fare better than rural areas for mortality and morbidity indicators; however, the poorest urban children have the highest risk of mortality [54]. The disparities among urban rich and poor households are stark. For example, in Cambodia and Rwanda, under-five mortality among the poorest fifth of the households was found to be 5 times higher than the richest fifth of the population [54]. In Nigeria, research has shown that urban child mortality increased with urban population growth associated with increasing number of people living in slum-like conditions [54]. Addressing this increasing urbanization trend requires well-resourced systems and services that are equitably distributed, while simultaneously minimizing environmental impact. For further discussion on urban development and implications for food security and nutrition, see Chaps. 31 and 32 by Bloem and S de Pee and by Ruel et al.

Virtual Communities

Similar to traditional communities, virtual communities impact the demand and supply side of good health and utilization of health services. On the demand side, off the roles that traditional or geographical communities have played (as described in **Historical Perspectives: Communities and Health** section above), virtual communities are particularly instrumental for educating for self-care, generating demand for health services and providing psycho/social support. On the supply side, virtual professional communities serving as a cost-effective method for disease management are receiving greater attention. The mix of community members in the virtual community, i.e. general public, patients and/or healthcare providers, depends on the purpose of the engagement. For example, a peer-to-peer disease-specific support group may be limited to patients, whereas a disease management virtual community will also include healthcare providers and care givers.

In an era where technology is enabling communication that is not bound by geography or physical space, there has been a shift in the healthcare field, from "institution-centric" to "patient or consumer centric" systems [6]. At an individual level, virtual communities serve three purposes: (1) a resource for information, (2) access to other community members for support and empowerment, and (3) direct access to certain types of health services. Over the past decades, there has been an increase in online health-related portals and platforms, where people can gather specific information regarding particular conditions, or exchange ideas on a discussion board or through social networking [55]. Patient empowerment through access to health information and the resultant increase in choices is helping individuals in their own disease management.

The evidence for impact of virtual communities on health and social outcomes is sparse and mixed. While it has been found that virtual communities can be effective in providing some of the services from physical groups [6, 56], a recent study suggests that consumer-driven peer-to-peer communities do not show impact on health and social outcomes [57]. However, given that the literature on this topic is very limited, does not include unmoderated virtual groups, and does not distinguish the conditions or people for whom the support is effective, it is difficult and too soon to draw conclusions about the circumstances or conditions under which there may be positive, negative or no impact.

From a systems perspective, the use of virtual communities and the internet are alleviating several challenges faced by healthcare systems (related to capacity and quality) such as barriers to accessing basic health information, connecting with specialists through telemedicine [58], and general disease management. One of the most common non-financial barriers to health access is geographical distance to services, resulting in poor health outcomes in rural or under-served urban populations, which can to an extent be addressed by the use of technology. This could be through support or information available through virtual communities or information available on the internet. Another barrier to accessing or continuing care is stigma associated with certain diseases. Here virtual communities can provide a substitute for physical interaction.

However, given the fact that these fora are almost entirely unregulated, some negative aspects need to be highlighted. First, there is no system of controlling the quality of the information available virtually, unless regulated by a healthcare provider or moderated on certain platforms. The burden of sifting through the information and deciphering its credibility rests with the users. Virtual communities also provide the space and environment for negative health communities, i.e. not in line with good health advice [59]. For example, pro-anorexia networks encourage users to skip meals or fast.

Yet, evidence also shows that in social network portals, users understand that the information may not come from experts and often false information does get corrected through network members, as was the experience in a breast cancer discussion list [59]. Some of the other negative aspects of virtual communities relate to lack of protection against privacy, confidentiality (this is also a positive when people can seek the support they need anonymously) or deception if exposed to someone who falsely joins a community.

Focus Shifting from Communities to Individuals

The shifting focus from communities to individuals is being driven from both the supply and demand sides and also through a natural process as societies evolve from being pre-modern, to modern and post-modern. Therefore, envisioning the role of communities within the context of the macro-trends of changing population dynamics and urbanization must take into account the ability of the community to address the needs of individuals.

Pre-modern societies, typically before industrialization, i.e. predominantly agrarian, consist of communities where people in the same physical space engage in similar activities and have similar beliefs/values, often deeply rooted in religion (whether agrarian, hunter-gatherer, pastoral, etc.). Group identity rather than individual identity is the norm. Modernism, rooted in reason and science, lessens the hold of religion and spiritual beliefs in societies. As technology advances, faster and more efficient methods of production usher in industrialization. Societies tend to move from being largely agrarian to urban. This is also a time when societies start to become more economically diverse and governments guarantee individual rights and establish penal codes. In contrast, post-modernism embraces pluralistic and complex approaches, including science and reason, but it is also not limited to it. Urbanization in turn spurs modernism and post-modernism when populations from different communities interact with each other to exchange and develop individual ideas and beliefs. Even though there is reference/agreement to time and place with regard to the three periods (generally pre-modern, up to the seventeenth century, modern until mid-twentieth century and post-modern from the 1950s and Western societies more modern/post-modern), ethos of the three simultaneously exist at present, including within one country and one physical community, and through increased migration, groups of people at different stages of development live and work alongside each other, often without realizing these differences.

In the context of development, we are now increasingly seeing social transfers being made directly to individuals (either external donor assistance or national social protection), particularly in the form of cash. While this may be a newer phenomenon for LMICs, it has existed as a welfare tool in Western Europe for over a century with most of the increase in public welfare from the mid-twentieth century. In fact, public spending increases as percentage of GDP with increasing per capita income [60]. In high-income countries, sophisticated institutional arrangements including insurance, taxation, good national capacity, accountability and governance protect individual citizens and provide certain rights as contained in the Universal Declaration of Human Rights [61]. These pre-requisites for robust social protection systems are of course limited in LMICs, due to lack of taxation capacity, low employment and inadequate institutional resources and capacities [60].

Social assistance (not tax based, either as cash or in kind), social insurance (e.g. health, crops), microfinance and employment support are all types of social protection modalities available. The recent (last two decades) interest and rise of social protection worldwide was in part a result of the Asian financial crisis of the late 1990s. Countries that were considered to be financial successes (e.g.

Thailand, Malaysia and Indonesia) weren't resilient enough to the economic crash and millions of households ended in poverty. Lack of social protection policies leads households to be fiscally conservative, leading to an overall slow recovery. The late 1990s accelerated interest in social and political reform for countries themselves to ensure that their most vulnerable were protected in times of shock, particularly in middle-income countries [60, 61].

In 2006, the Grameen Bank and its founder Muhammad Yunus were awarded the Nobel Peace Prize. But the Bank originated in 1976 in Bangladesh, with the objective of promoting financial independence of the poor. Grameen Bank provides small loans to under-served populations, with an emphasis on women (over 95% of loans are given to women). Now in over 43 countries, these loans are made in communities, but the responsibility of repayment of loans rests on the individual. There still exists a strong component of group solidarity because the credit to the group is discontinued if there is an individual defaulter [62, 63]. The system encourages savings and the founder has often spoken about the ability of microfinancing to enable the poor to lift themselves out of poverty and the associated long-term emotional benefits for the individual compared to receiving social assistance. Not just for poverty alleviation, this principle has also been used among people living with HIV in urban Ethiopia to ensure that PLHIV on lifelong ART can support themselves. An evaluation of WFP's PEPFAR-funded HIV operation in Ethiopia, which supports PLHIV through economic strengthening activities to prevent relapses into food insecurity and ensure sustainable long-term benefits, has provided useful operational evidence for developing and integrating social protection interventions for PLHIV.

In addition to traditional transfers (ODA or domestic), increasing number of small and large foundations, organizations and start-ups (including novel mobile apps) are raising money for specific causes and directly linking the individual donors to the beneficiaries in LMICs. Development of such ideas can be aided by crowd funding. Donations through these various platforms are impact driven and motivate individual donors by providing details about the beneficiaries and tracking the how the funds are spent. There are several examples; one philanthropic app designed by University of California, San Diego, researchers transmits tuition directly to schools in Benin connecting individual donors and recipients [64].

We will continue to see increasing social transfers and individual entitlements as countries economically develop and through direct philanthropy (increase in the supply side). But, unlike the slower shift in Western Europe towards a more individual focused society, we are seeing an accelerated pace now as countries economically develop, and individuals are simultaneously exposed to unprecedented dissemination and access to information coupled with increasing consumerism and targeted marketing (influence on the demand side).

The internet is probably the most defining technology of recent times, not only giving rise to the phenomenon of virtual communities, but also generating demand at an individual level [65]. The global trends and technology are impacting roles of traditional geographical/physical communities. Figure 28.3 summarizes the evolving dynamics for each of the community functions described in **Historical Perspectives: Communities and Health** section above. For example, improved access to information due to technology is increasing awareness and providing opportunities to individuals to educate themselves better for self-care and increase demand for more and better health services. Similarly, virtual communities (and urbanization to an extent) are creating new forums for social support not bound by physical communities and encouraging alternative social norms and rights, not necessarily driven by community expectations, but by influence of greater individual choice.

		Community function	Necessary conditions	Evolving dynamics
1	Promoting social norms & rights	Establishing cultural/social norms and rights about health	Community expectations about access to health significantly influence self-care and care-seeking behaviors	Greater individual choice (e.g., due to increasing interaction with markets and consumerism)
2	Educating for self care	Spreading knowledge about behaviors and practices to treat and prevent disease	Family and community influencers represent important source of information about health	Improved access to information about health (e.g., through technology, targeted health education campaigns), and higher expectations of health credentials
3	Generating demand for health services	Encouraging care-seeking and referring individuals to skilled care	Family and community influential represent important source of information about health	Improved access to information about health (e.g., through technology, targeted health education campaigns), and higher expectations of health credentials
4	Enabling care seeking	Reduce cost and other barriers to reaching and using services (i.e., financing, transport, childcare)	Enabling structures are community-based	Organization of enabling structures changing due to urbanization, and social transfers increasingly targeted at individual
5	Delivering health services	Filling health system gaps by providing health care services to remote or underserved populations (e.g., CHWs)	Populations are not otherwise able to access health services (e.g., geographical or financial constraints)	Roles of informal/semi-formal health services changing in unregulated, increasingly pluralistic health systems
6	Defining & monitoring quality	Defining and monitoring acceptability and quality based on social and cultural norms	Community shares common social and cultural norms	Mobility and urbanization resulting in more diverse constituency of individuals served by health system
7	Providing social support	Providing social support and encouraging healthy coping mechanisms	Friends, family and peers exist in close proximity and represent primary support network	Technology creating new forums for building supportive relationships and sharing information, particularly for individuals managing chronic diseases

Fig. 28.3 Evolving dynamics impact roles of traditional communities in health

Looking Forward: Communities Supporting Integrated Health and Nutrition

Models of Cross-Sectoral Approaches

The international community increasingly recognizes the importance of multi-sectoral approaches that focus not only on strengthening health systems, but also on addressing the social determinants of health, and at all levels of governance, from subnational to regional and global. The 17 goals and 169 targets of the SDGs elucidate the complexity and interconnectedness of the goals. Each of the other 16 goals directly or indirectly impact Goal 3, "ensuring healthy lives and promote well-being at all ages". However, all the goals of this ambitious agenda still have to be achieved from limited resources. Therefore, looking forward, a community model that makes optimal linkages with the health and other social services will be best suited to cost-effectively and holistically support the achievement of the SDGs. Figure 28.1 shows the interaction between the individual/household with the health system and the different roles of the community. A more comprehensive model incorporating other services is shown in Fig. 28.4. A model that taps sector-specific proven solutions, yet makes linkages between the various services, will best serve populations. As described in section II, social services and social protection in LMICs are dramatically increasing. Most times, the goal of such transfers is poverty alleviation, but this does present the opportunity to make inter-sectoral linkages.

There are numerous examples of community-based outreach programmes that address many of the underlying determinants of health (Fig. 28.5). Services provided range from health specific, in the case of the community health workers, to health enabling, for example community mediators and agriculture extension workers. As discussed in **Historical Perspectives: Communities and Health** section, there are an estimated 1.3 million community health workers operating around the world.

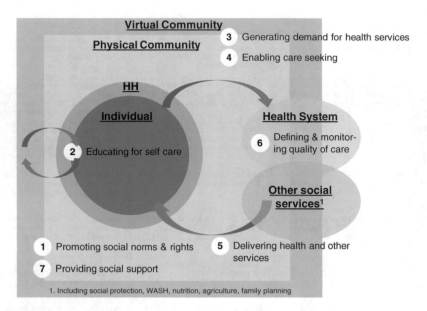

Fig. 28.4 Looking forward—a model for community-based approaches to health

Potential functions

Functions may be independent or combined

Health specific		
Basic health care	• Provide **basic health services** (prevention, disease management) • May sell basic health products	
Specialized health care	• Provide **specialized care** focused on **specific conditions** or public health needs (e.g., HIV/TB, MNCH) • May sell basic health products	
Community mediator	• Facilitate users to become aware of **rights and entitlements** and gain **better access to services**, including health care	

Health related

Other health-related services
• Deliver **agriculture extension, WASH, nutrition, education, family planning** and other services that impact health

Key considerations

Level and quality of existing health services
• Including formal health system; private, NGO, and traditional providers

Availability of resources (financial and personnel) to scale up program
• Compensation scheme
• Level of supervision and logistic support

Supply of qualified health workers
• Individuals with health-related skills
• Resources available for training

Public health needs and disease prevalence
• Including e.g., HIV/TB, maternal and child health, malaria, pneumonia, NCDs

Set enabling success factors must also be in place

Fig. 28.5 Community workers can play various functions depending on local contexts

Community development workers exist in many countries to promote social and economic development. These workers take on a diverse range of tasks and facilitative roles, including involving communities in public policy decisions, to ensuring that individuals are aware of their entitlements and assisting people in accessing these entitlements.

Agricultural extension programmes aim to deliver key information inputs to farmers and, ultimately, promote food security and drive economic growth. As of 2005, there were an estimated 500,000 extension personnel working worldwide, 95% of whom were working in public agricultural extension systems [66]. Fanzo et al. examined the integration of nutrition within extension and advisory services and workers in Africa, South Asia and the Americas [67]. In addition to providers of crop, livestock and food production/security, extension workers can also be used/considered as conduits for improved nutrition and health as they closely interact with farmers and rural communities. One opportunity is for more women (who are already engaged with farming) to be also be trained as extension workers—at present, majority of extension workers are men. Communication of good health and nutrition messaging through demonstrations, peer-to-peer engagement, trainings, and knowledge/technology transfer (e.g. bio-fortification) are different models that have attempted to integrate nutrition in the work of extension workers [67]. However, very few of these multi-sectoral approaches have been implemented at scale and the evidence on effectiveness is still being documented. The opportunity is tremendous with the global interest in "nutrition-sensitive" agriculture, but, as with all cross-sectoral work, capacity limitations and lack of incentives/motivation to add more to existing tasks impede full utilization of this potential platform [67].

Challenges and Opportunities

The road to greater policy integration will be fraught with challenges, as typical policy-making is rooted in siloed governance structures, financial flows, policy processes and power dynamics. Local governments, as well as community actors operating outside government structures, have several inherent advantages that may facilitate cross-sectoral collaboration across various stages of policy process, from problem definition and agenda setting, to policy formulation, decision-making, implementation and monitoring. Specifically, the smaller number of actors, closer proximity to programme implementation and greater functional overlap may serve to mitigate the sectoral fragmentation that pervades at the national and global levels.

The diverse cadres of health-specific and health-enabling workers have the potential to play a significant role; however, linkages between them need to be strengthened depending on the context. Some of the key considerations include existing enabling environment and available resources, capacity of the personnel and potential to address human resources gaps (Fig. 28.5). First, obviously, services and resources need to exist within a community (health and beyond health) and we are seeing that countries are increasing their own domestic resources to address the needs of their populations. Often some combination of health services exists through the following: formal public and private health systems, NGOs, traditional practitioners, CHWs, etc. Other services such as support for agriculture, WASH and nutrition may also be provided, in addition to entitlements through social protection schemes. The provision of services is often not sufficient; there can be inherent barriers to access and linkages which must be overcome, namely geographical location, lack of knowledge about available services, follow-up and affordability [68]. This is stark in South Africa, where despite the existence of several provisions for social development and health, uptake remains low. Kheth'Impilo, a community centric NGO, has been working at this community and health nexus as an effective mediator (see Box 28.2) through its patient advocate model.

For already burdened health and other social systems, communities, if effectively leveraged, can be instrumental in alleviating gaps from both the supply and demand sides. In addition to being adequately resourced in terms of services and human resource capacity, certain structural changes are imperative to empower communities to deliver good health outcomes. First, the inter-sectoral linkages that we propose (Fig. 28.5) have to be made from the planning to the implementation phase. In addition, decentralization and empowerment of local government structures is believed to not only increase the provision of services at the community level, but also increase efficiency and impact growth [69, 70]. It has been shown to increase civic awareness and engagement in local policy-making and holding government more accountable [68, 69]. Lastly, role of communities, including community health workers, needs to be formalized within larger system (health and social development).

Box 28.2 Kheth'Impilo, an NGO Linking Communities and Health Systems

Kheth'Impilo specializes in innovative solutions for health and community systems and services, particularly for marginalized communities. Their solutions include treatment, care and support for people infected and affected with HIV and TB, early childhood development, school health and trainings. One of their innovative community models is the patient advocate model designed to address the needs of poor and often illiterate people diagnosed with HIV/TB to ensure adherence to treatment.

The model consists of a network of patient facilitators and area coordinators who manage patient home visits and the associated work load. It is specifically designed to address all "systems" related to the target problem: immediate barriers in the household, community, any resource constraints and also structural issues such as ensuring sustainability through addressing unemployment, capacity/skills gaps and provision of health services [68]. In terms of health services, strict protocols are followed, including at-home HIV testing and TB screening and assessment which reduce travel to clinics, increase demand for health services and referrals, and improve clinic efficiency when patients do use clinics [68].

The patient advocate model has shown to be unique in making systemic contributions rather than providing disease-specific support. KI's community models extend existing local and national structures rather than creating parallel or new initiatives. By bolstering existing capacity, current investments are used more efficiently. The home-based testing and addressing of psycho-social barriers to treatment by following the patient extend support to the household and ultimately to the affected community. Kheth'Impilo reaches over 400,000 patients with over 3000 patient advocates. Over the last five years, it has supported over 2 million HIV tests. As a result of KI's engagement, it was found that patient mortality was reduced by 35% and loss to follow-up by 37% among patients on antiretroviral treatment who received support from patient advocates [68].

Conclusion

Despite considerable global progress against health-related Millennium Development Goals, gains made in different regions of the world have been uneven. 6.3 million deaths among children under age five, 289 thousand maternal deaths still occur each year, and 99% of these deaths occur in low- and middle-income countries (LMICs). Inadequate health systems and crippling human resource shortages pose serious bottlenecks to the achievement of health goals. Health system gaps disproportionately impact poor, marginalized populations, in both rural and urban contexts.

Compounding major health system gaps, demand-side barriers have been shown to prevent or discourage individuals from seeking care even when adequate health services exist. Religious, cultural and social norms may preclude health-promoting behaviours. Poor and vulnerable populations are less likely to enjoy access to health-related information, challenging their ability to make informed decisions about when, where and how to seek care. Costs, including treatment, transportation and opportunity cost, also represent significant obstacles to seeking care.

Both supply and demand-side gaps are impeding progress in achieving good health in societies. For decades, lay health workers and communities have stepped into fill these gaps. The global Sustainable Development Goals (SDGs) adopted in 2015 has shifted the focus from disease-specific interventions and poverty in LMICs to addressing issues of sustainability, human rights, social inclusion and justice and ensuring "no one is left behind".

Governments worldwide have rightly adopted sector-specific approaches to addressing problems with proven solutions. While interventions were aimed at communities in the past, governments are now increasing public welfare and domestic transfers to individuals. How these transfers, local programmes and public welfare platforms can be best leveraged to achieve good health and overall development pose interesting questions and debates on existing and future models of governance. Physical and virtual communities will need to be leveraged in the most optimal way.

Discussion Points

- Compare the framework of community influence (Figs. 28.1 and 28.3) in an urban setting versus rural setting.
- Explain why partnerships (SDG 17) will be key to achieving SDG 3, good health and well-being?
- As a governments increase social protection in their countries, what types of tweaks or conditions to the transfer may enable better health outcomes?
- How could the role of communities (including community health workers) be formalized within the larger health system?

References

1. Morgan LM. Community participation in health: perpetual allure, persistent challenge. Health Policy Plann. 2001;16(3):221–30.
2. Rosato M, Laverack G, Grabman LH, Tripathy P, Nair N, Mwansambo C, et al. Community participation: lessons for maternal, newborn, and child health. Lancet. 2008;372(9642):962–71.
3. Schneider H, Hlophe H, van Rensburg D. Community health workers and the response to HIV/AIDS in South Africa: tensions and prospects. Health Policy Plann. 2008;23(3):179–87.
4. MacQueen KM, McLellan E, Metzger DS, Kegeles S, Strauss RP, Scotti R, et al. What is community? An evidence-based definition for participatory public health. Am J Public Health. 2001;91(12):1929–38.
5. Chorbev I, Sotirovska M, Mihajlov D. Virtual communities for diabetes chronic disease healthcare. Int J Telemed Appl. 2011;2011:721654.
6. Demiris G. The diffusion of virtual communities in health care: concepts and challenges. Patient Educ Couns. 2006;62(2):178–88.
7. Packer CAA. Using human rights to change tradition. International Specialized Book Service Inc; 2002.
8. WHO. Health and human rights factsheet. 2015.
9. Ensor T, Cooper S. Overcoming barriers to health service access: influencing the demand side. Health Policy Plann. 2004;19(2):69–79.
10. Nualart GB. The Mahila Samakhya program: empowering education for women's equality in Indian disadvantaged communities and rural areas. Commun Pap—Media Literacy Gend Stud. 2012;1:115–32.
11. Ganle JK, Parker M, Fitzpatrick R, Otupiri E. A qualitative study of health system barriers to accessibility and utilization of maternal and newborn healthcare services in Ghana after user-fee abolition. BMC Pregnancy Childbirth. 2014;14:425.
12. Davtyan M, Brown B, Folayan MO. Addressing Ebola-related stigma: lessons learned from HIV/AIDS. Glob Health Action. 2014;7:26058.
13. Gonsalves G, Staley P. Panic, paranoia, and public health—the AIDS epidemic's lessons for Ebola. N Engl J Med. 2014;371(25):2348–9.

14. Manandhar DS, Osrin D, Shrestha BP, Mesko N, Morrison J, Tumbahangphe KM, et al. Effect of a participatory intervention with women's groups on birth outcomes in Nepal: cluster-randomised controlled trial. Lancet. 2004;364(9438):970–9.

15. Taleb F, Perkins J, Ali NA, Capello C, Ali M, Santarelli C, et al. Transforming maternal and newborn health social norms and practices to increase utilization of health services in rural Bangladesh: a qualitative review. BMC Pregnancy Childbirth. 2015;15:75.

16. Lehmann U, Sanders D. Community health workers: what do we know about them? The state of the evidence on programmes, activities, costs and impact on health outcomes of using community health workers. WHO, School of Public Health University of the Western Cape. 2007.

17. WHO. Working with individuals, families and communities to improve maternal and newborn health. 2010.

18. Gilmore B, McAuliffe E. Effectiveness of community health workers delivering preventive interventions for maternal and child health in low- and middle-income countries: a systematic review. BMC Public Health. 2013;13:847.

19. Perry HB, Zulliger R, Rogers MM. Community health workers in low-, middle-, and high-income countries: an overview of their history, recent evolution, and current effectiveness. Annu Rev Public Health. 2014;35:399–421.

20. Black RE, Victora CG, Walker SP, Bhutta ZA, Christian P, de Onis M, et al. Maternal and child undernutrition and overweight in low-income and middle-income countries. Lancet. 2013;382(9890):427–51.

21. Imdad A, Yakoob MY, Sudfeld C, Haider BA, Black RE, Bhutta ZA. Impact of vitamin A supplementation on infant and childhood mortality. BMC Public Health. 2011;11(Suppl 3):S20.

22. Monasch R, Reinisch A, Steketee RW, Korenromp EL, Alnwick D, Bergevin Y. Child coverage with mosquito nets and malaria treatment from population-based surveys in African countries: a baseline for monitoring progress in roll back malaria. Am J Trop Med Hyg. 2004;71(2 Suppl):232–8.

23. Hopkins H, Talisuna A, Whitty CJ, Staedke SG. Impact of home-based management of malaria on health outcomes in Africa: a systematic review of the evidence. Malaria J. 2007;6:134.

24. Leon N, Sanders D, Van Damme W, Besada D, Daviaud E, Oliphant NP, et al. The role of 'hidden' community volunteers in community-based health service delivery platforms: examples from sub-Saharan Africa. Glob Health Action. 2015;8:27214.

25. Lassi ZS, Das JK, Salam RA, Bhutta ZA. Evidence from community level inputs to improve quality of care for maternal and newborn health: interventions and findings. Reprod Health. 2014;11(Suppl 2):S2.

26. Perez LM, Martinez J. Community health workers: social justice and policy advocates for community health and well-being. Am J Public Health. 2008;98(1):11–4.

27. Rosenthal EL, Wiggins N, Ingram M, Mayfield-Johnson S, De Zapien JG. Community health workers then and now: an overview of national studies aimed at defining the field. J Ambul Care Manag. 2011;34(3):247–59.

28. Ingram M, Sabo S, Rothers J, Wennerstrom A, de Zapien JG. Community health workers and community advocacy: addressing health disparities. J Commun Health. 2008;33(6):417–24.

29. Farquhar SA, Michael YL, Wiggins N. Building on leadership and social capital to create change in 2 urban communities. Am J Public Health. 2005;95(4):596–601.

30. Frew E, Wolstenholme JL, Atkin W, Whynes DK. Estimating time and travel costs incurred in clinic based screening: flexible sigmoidoscopy screening for colorectal cancer. J Med Screen. 1999;6(3):119–23.

31. Peters DH, Garg A, Bloom G, Walker DG, Brieger WR, Rahman MH. Poverty and access to health care in developing countries. Ann N Y Acad Sci. 2008;1136:161–71.

32. Stein MD, Crystal S, Cunningham WE, Ananthanarayanan A, Andersen RM, Turner BJ, et al. Delays in seeking HIV care due to competing caregiver responsibilities. Am J Public Health. 2000;90(7):1138–40.

33. van Lonkhuijzen L, Stegemen M, Nyirongo R, van Roosmalen J. Use of maternity waiting home in rural Zambia. Afr J Reprod Health. 2003;7(1):32–6.

34. Decroo T, Rasschaert F, Telfer B, Remartinez D, Laga M, Ford N. Community-based antiretroviral therapy programs can overcome barriers to retention of patients and decongest health services in sub-Saharan Africa: a systematic review. Int Health. 2013;5(3):169–79.

35. Bolam A, Manandhar DS, Shrestha P, Ellis M, Costello AM. The effects of postnatal health education for mothers on infant care and family planning practices in Nepal: a randomised controlled trial. BMJ. 1998;316(7134):805–11.

36. Stanback J, Mbonye AK, Bekiita M. Contraceptive injections by community health workers in Uganda: a nonrandomized community trial. Bull World Health Organ. 2007;85(10):768–73.

37. Kwan CK, Ernst JD. HIV and tuberculosis: a deadly human syndemic. Clin Microbiol Rev. 2011;24(2):351–76.

38. Mehra D, de Pee S, Bloem MW. Nutrition, food security, social protection, and health systems strengthening for ending AIDS. In: Ivers L, editor. Food insecurity and public health. CRC Press; 2015.

39. WHO. Guideline on when to start antiretroviral therapy and on pre-exposure prophylaxis for HIV. 2015.

40. WHO. World health statistics 2015.

41. WHO. Treat, train, retain the AIDS and health workforce plan: WHO report on the consultation on AIDS and human resources for health, Geneva. 2006.

42. Gray N, Bedford J, Deconinck H, Brown, R (CMAM Forum and Anthrologica). Community engagement: the 'C' at the heart of CMAM. 2014.
43. Neupane D, Kallestrup P, McLachlan CS, Perry H. Community health workers for non-communicable diseases. Lancet Glob Health. 2014;2(10):e567.
44. Kruk ME, Paczkowski M, Mbaruku G, de Pinho H, Galea S. Women's preferences for place of delivery in rural Tanzania: a population-based discrete choice experiment. Am J Public Health. 2009;99(9):1666–72.
45. Paz-Soldan VA, Alban RE, Jones CD, Oberhelman RA. The provision of and need for social support among adult and pediatric patients with tuberculosis in Lima, Peru: a qualitative study. BMC Health Serv Res. 2013;13:290.
46. Cobb S. Presidential address-1976. Social support as a moderator of life stress. Psychosom Med. 1976;38(5):300–14.
47. Standing H, Chowdhury AM. Producing effective knowledge agents in a pluralistic environment: what future for community health workers? Soc Sci Med. 2008;66(10):2096–107.
48. Christopher JB, Le May A, Lewin S, Ross DA. Thirty years after Alma-Ata: a systematic review of the impact of community health workers delivering curative interventions against malaria, pneumonia and diarrhoea on child mortality and morbidity in sub-Saharan Africa. Hum Res Health. 2011;9:27.
49. Gilson LWG, Heggenhougen K, Owuor-Omondi L, Perera M, Ross D, Salazar L. National community health worker programs: how can they be strengthened? J Public Health Policy. 1989;10(4):518–32.
50. Walley J, Lawn JE, Tinker A, de Francisco A, Chopra M, Rudan I, et al. Primary health care: making Alma-Ata a reality. Lancet. 2008;372(9642):1001–7.
51. Mason JB, Sanders D, Musgrove P, Soekirman, Galloway R. Community health and nutrition programs. In: Jamison DT, Breman JG, Measham AR, Alleyne G, Claeson M, Evans DB, et al., editors. Disease control priorities in developing countries. 2nd ed. Washington (DC); 2006.
52. Nations U. Global trends and challenges to sustainable development post-2015. In: Nations U, editor. World Economic and Social Survey 2013: The Department of Economic and Social Affairs of the United Nations Secretariat; 2013.
53. WHO. The global burden of disease: 2004 update. 2004.
54. Children St. The urban disadvantage: state of the world's mothers 2015. Save the children. 2015.
55. Kuenne CW, Adamczyk S, Rass M, Bullinger AC, Moeslein KM. IT-based interaction platforms to foster virtual patient communities. Institut für Wirtschaftsinformatik Friedrich-Alexander Universität Erlangen-Nürnberg, 2011.
56. Finn J. An exploration of helping processes in an online self-help group focusing on issues of disability. Health Soc Work. 1999;24(3):220–31.
57. Eysenbach G, Powell J, Englesakis M, Rizo C, Stern A. Health related virtual communities and electronic support groups: systematic review of the effects of online peer to peer interactions. BMJ. 2004;328(7449):1166.
58. Vega S, Marciscano I, Holcomb M, Erps KA, Major J, Lopez AM, et al. Testing a top-down strategy for establishing a sustainable telemedicine program in a developing country: the Arizona telemedicine program-US Army-Republic of Panama Initiative. Telemed J E Health. 2013;19(10):746–53.
59. Griffiths F, Dobermann T, Cave JA, Thorogood M, Johnson S, Salamatian K, et al. The impact of online social networks on health and health systems: a scoping review and case studies. Policy Internet. 2015;7(4):473–96.
60. Bonnesen L. Cash transfers—a viable approach to development? 2012.
61. Norton A, Conway T, Foster M. Social protection concepts and approaches: implications for policy and practice in international development. Overseas Development Institute; 2011.
62. Hossain M. Credit for alleviation of rural poverty: The Grameen Bank in Bangladesh. 1988.
63. Rahman MH, Da Vanzo J. Assessing the impact of the Grameen Bank on women's status and fertility in Bangladesh. RAND research. 1993.
64. Fox T. 'Prêt-à-Payer' app to directly fund secondary schoolchildren in West Africa 2014. Available from: http://ucsdnews.ucsd.edu/pressrelease/pret_a_payer_app_to_directly_fund_secondary_schoolchildren_in_west_africa.
65. Lee H, Whitley E. Time and information technology: temporal impacts on individuals, organizations, and society. Inf Soc. 2002;18:235–40.
66. Aker JC. Dial, "A" for agriculture: a review of information and communication technologies for agricultural extension in developing countries. Agric Econ. 2011;42:631–47.
67. Fanzo J, Marshall Q, Wong J, Merchan RI, Jaber MI, Souza A, Verjee N. The integration of nutrition into extension and advisory services: a synthesis of experiences, lessons, and recommendations. Lindau, Switzerland: Global Forum for Rural Advisory Services; 2013.
68. Lucwaba K, Everts S. Siyadingana: we need each other. J Ambul Care Manag. 2015;38(3):217–8.
69. Gomez EJ. Decentralization and sub-national governance: new methodological tools and evidence for cross-regional analysis world bank thematic seminar series on decentralization and sub-national governance. Washington D C ; 2001.
70. Gomez EJ. A temporal analytical approach to decentralization: lessons from Brazil's health sector. J Health Polit Policy Law. 2008;33(1):53–91.

Chapter 29
Nutrition in Humanitarian Crises

Lynnda Kiess, Natalie Aldern, Saskia de Pee and Martin W. Bloem

Keywords Humanitarian crisis · Nutrition response · Acute malnutrition · Micronutrient deficiencies · Stunting · Vulnerability and risk · Climate change · Disasters

Learning Objectives

- Identify the key types and drivers of humanitarian crises.
- Describe the range of consequences of humanitarian crises.
- Analyze the impact of humanitarian crises on nutritional status.
- Be able to propose an appropriate nutrition response based on characteristics of a crisis.

Introduction

Never before has the world been faced with the vast number, scale and complexity of humanitarian crises than today. In 2016, the United Nations Office for the Coordination of Humanitarian Affairs (UN-OCHA) reported that the global humanitarian appeal requires US$20 billion to provide life-saving humanitarian assistance to over 87 million people across 37 countries, most of which are in conflict [1]. These anticipated needs represent a massive increase from 10 years before, in 2007, when US$4.4 billion was required to assist 26 million people [1]. And these figures do not include all the expected humanitarian needs for the El Niño weather pattern in 2016 that is affecting Southern and East Africa, Southeast Asia and Central America. In addition to more frequent crises affecting

L. Kiess (✉) · N. Aldern · S. de Pee · M.W. Bloem
Nutrition Division, World Food Programme, Rome, Italy
e-mail: lynnda.kiess@wfp.org

N. Aldern
e-mail: nataliealdern@gmail.com

S. de Pee
e-mail: Saskia.depee@wfp.org; depee.saskia@gmail.com

M.W. Bloem
e-mail: martin.bloem@wfp.org

S. de Pee · M.W. Bloem
Friedman School of Nutrition Science and Policy, Tufts University, Boston, MA, USA

M.W. Bloem
Department of International Health, Bloomberg School of Public Health,
Johns Hopkins University, Baltimore, MD, USA

© Springer Science+Business Media New York 2017
S. de Pee et al. (eds.), *Nutrition and Health in a Developing World*,
Nutrition and Health, DOI 10.1007/978-3-319-43739-2_29

larger numbers of people, a greater share of crises are complex and protracted and the people affected require prolonged support and assistance. Forced displacement due to conflict and natural disaster is also increasing, totaling 60 million people by the end of 2014 [2]. The growing humanitarian needs face further pressure, with climate change alone expected to impact crop yields, water supply, greatly intensifying droughts, floods and heat waves and also impacting on the frequency and severity of existing diseases and the introduction of new health threats [3].

Humanitarian crises (see Box 29.1 for definitions) can slow or even stop economic growth and destroy infrastructure, which can in turn hamper access to needed goods and services. A shock may disrupt access to food, damage food production and limit transportation needed for markets to function optimally. Emergencies can also impact health systems or lead to an increase in disease and disrupt household and social structures, undermining caring practices that impact on good nutrition. These disruptions are often occurring on top of already compromised systems, and each of these impacts can affect direct causes of malnutrition—increased illness, constraints on caretaking and reduced food intake or reduced dietary quality. Increases in malnutrition are hence a common consequence of humanitarian crises. There are immediate repercussions of malnutrition on morbidity and mortality, but significant impacts on child growth and development also occur, particularly in protracted crises, which can affect individuals for a lifetime and severely constrain a society's future human capacity.

Box 29.1 Definitions for Humanitarian Crises

Aggravating factors: These refer to context factors that, when present, may indicate that a deterioration in the nutrition situation is likely. These include: a general ration below mean energy requirements, crude mortality rate >1 per 10,000 per day, an epidemic of measles or whooping cough, or high prevalence of respiratory or diarrheal disease.

Assessment: A structured process of collecting and analyzing data to measure the impact of the crisis and provide an understanding of the situation and any related threats, in order to determine whether a response is required and, if so, the nature of that response. An assessment is a time-bound exercise that produces a report and recommendations to inform decision-making at a particular point in time [4].

Coping strategy: Strategies employed by individuals or households during crises to preserve productive assets which are needed to sustain a living in the future.

Disaster: A serious disruption in the functioning of a community or society involving widespread human, material, economic or environmental losses and impacts, which exceeds the ability of the affected community or society to cope using its own resources. Disaster impacts may include loss of life, injury, disease and other negative effects on human physical, mental and social well-being together with damage to property, destruction of assets, loss of services, social and economic disruption, and environmental degradation [5].

Food access: A household's ability to acquire adequate amounts of food, through any combination of home production and stocks, purchases, barter, gifts, borrowing and food aid. Food may be available but not accessible to people who do not have adequate land to cultivate or enough money to buy it.

Hazard: Natural or man-made processes or phenomena that may cause the loss of life or injury, property damage, social and economic disruption or environmental degradation.

Preparedness: Disaster preparedness minimizes the adverse effects of a hazard through effective precautionary actions, rehabilitation and recovery to ensure the timely, appropriate and effective organization and delivery of relief and assistance following a disaster.

Protracted crisis: There is no single definition of what constitutes a protracted crisis. The characterization of a protracted crisis may be based on duration, weak governance, unstable systems and/or a breakdown of local institutions. FAO and WFP, as part of the State of Food Insecurity in the World 2010 report [6], defined protracted crises as countries reporting a food crisis for eight years or more, receiving more than 10% of foreign assistance as humanitarian relief and being on the list of low-income food-deficit countries. UNHCR defines protracted displacement as situations in which refugees have been in exile for five years or more since their initial displacement and in which immediate prospects for solutions are bleak [7].

Resilience: Comes from the Latin verb resilio, literally to jump back or rebound. It was used in physics to characterize the capacity of a material to recover its initial state after a change. In international development the term means the ability of a system and its component parts to anticipate, absorb, accommodate or recover from the effects of a hazardous event in a timely and efficient manner, including through ensuring the preservation, restoration or improvement of its essential basic structures and functions [8].

Risk: The combination of the probability or frequency of occurrence of a defined hazard and the magnitude of the consequences.

Shocks: A shock is an event that can trigger decline in well-being, which can affect individuals, a community, a region or even a nation [9].

Slow-onset emergency: Disasters that take an extended period of time to produce emergency conditions which are normally accompanied by early warning signs, for example some natural disasters such as drought or economic decline [10].

Sudden-onset emergency: Disasters which occur with little or no warning, including both 'natural' disasters (e.g., earthquakes, hurricanes, floods) and man-made or 'complex' disasters (e.g., sudden conflict situations) [10].

Vulnerability: The extent to which a system, community, household or individual is susceptible to, and unable to cope with, the impact of a shock [11]. The IPCC has since changed the definition of vulnerability to the propensity or predisposition to be adversely affected [8].

Humanitarian Crises—Types, Characteristics and Consequences

Definition of Humanitarian Crisis

A humanitarian crisis or emergency has been defined as an event or series of events that represents a critical threat to the health, safety, security or well-being of a community or other large group of people, usually over a wide area [12].

Historically, humanitarian crises were viewed as short-term situations and the main objective of the humanitarian response was to save lives. The funding mechanisms for humanitarian response still reflect this 'short-term nature.' However, based on experience from the growing number of protracted crises—decades of refugee settlements in East Africa and conflict-related crises in many parts of the world that continue for years—prolonged humanitarian situations are now more and more common. In these settings, the effects of humanitarian crises become nearly 'the norm.' Equally, even when the crisis has a time-bound insult period, there may be lasting consequences of the crisis that lead to longer-term impacts on malnutrition, particularly when support to affected households is suboptimal and their recovery slow or delayed. Finally, repeated crises as seen in the Sahel droughts at the beginning of the twenty-first century (2005, 2011, 2012 and 2016) limit the ability of the poorest and most affected households to recover and erodes their resilience. Their inability to meet their daily food and nutrient requirements and to access health care and other essential social services has become nearly permanent.

There is significant rationale and momentum for greater coherence and complementarity between humanitarian, development, security and peace objectives and to link humanitarian assistance to other development-oriented interventions. In fact, the new sustainable development goals (SDGs) do not differentiate between humanitarian and development contexts. This provides an opportunity for national governments and other stakeholders to combine thinking and approaches. Addressing underlying problems of chronic poverty, inequality and vulnerability as part of humanitarian responses and similarly ensuring that emergency preparedness and recovery are considered during non-crisis periods is a critical start to building resilience, limiting conflict and strengthening governance [13]. Yet, while there are greater efforts being placed on prevention of potential crises through early warning and disaster preparedness, many crises will continue to require an immediate, large-scale humanitarian response.

Types of Crises or Shocks

Humanitarian crises can come in many different ways and forms. They can be man-made or occur as a result of natural disaster. The onset of the crisis may be sudden or slow, and the scale and duration can vary. Additionally, the carry-on impact may result in migration or affect a localized population that remains in place. These multiple characteristics and their resulting consequences are discussed in more detail in the next section. Drivers of humanitarian crises can vary from country to country and region to region, but many are common. Poverty and inequity are major drivers. Poor governance, corruption, armed conflict and political transition are also conditions that initiate or aggravate humanitarian crises. High population density and population growth and environmental degradation can also drive humanitarian crises.

Crises can be global—the financial crisis of 2008. They can be regional—El Niño in 2016. They can be local—Nepal earthquake in 2015. More and more however, there are global to local and local to global dimensions of humanitarian crises. For instance, what may start as a local crisis can rapidly become a global concern (e.g., the Syrian crisis).

It is difficult to classify humanitarian crises easily because of the great diversity in events, the variation in scale of the crisis and the variation in consequences that result due to diverse underlying drivers of the crisis in a particular location. However, typically crises are categorized as (1) man-made, (2) associated with natural hazards (commonly referred to as natural disasters) or (3) complex. Different conditions lead to natural disasters—geophysical (e.g., earthquakes, tsunamis and volcanic eruptions); hydrological (e.g., floods, avalanches); climatological (e.g., droughts); meteorological (e.g., storms, cyclones); or biological (e.g., epidemics, plagues). Natural crises can be acute or sudden onset (e.g., earthquake) or slow onset (e.g., drought). Man-made crises are disasters that are caused directly or primarily by an identifiable deliberate or negligent human action. Complex, protracted humanitarian crises are typically described as having more than one causal factor and could be a combination of man-made and natural crises. Although each protracted crisis is different, underlying causes include some combination of conflict, occupation, terrorism, natural resource pressures, climate change, inequalities, high rates of poverty and governance factors.

Consequences and Effects of Crises

The consequences and effects of humanitarian crises can be massive and complex, requiring broad responses. In the earthquake in Haiti in 2010 for instance, the United Nations and the international community provided expertise in 35 different sectors (e.g., agriculture, livelihoods, shelter, food, health) to support interventions ranging from rescue of survivors to provision of water, housing, food and restoring communication and infrastructure to cover the various different needs of people who were affected [14]. Conflict alone can undermine food security and nutrition in multiple ways:

destroying crops and livestock, disrupting markets, causing displacement, creating fear, damaging human capital and contributing to the spread of disease. Conflict also makes it difficult for governments and humanitarian actors to reach those in need. As a result, people in conflict-affected states are two times more likely to be undernourished than those living in more stable developing countries [15]. For example, there are a number of common effects and consequences of man-made, natural and complex, protracted crises.

Displacement

Displacement or movement of people as a result of a crisis can be temporary or more permanent. In the floods in Pakistan in 2010 for instance, households were temporarily relocated until flooding waters receded. Internal displacement or external migration is increasingly common with armed conflict and complex, protracted crises. Displacement has indirect consequences on many other effects of the crisis, including health, security and psychosocial impact.

Food Insecurity and Market Access

Food insecurity is a very common effect or consequence of humanitarian crises but can result from a wide range of pathways. A crisis can affect agriculture production by limiting planting, damaging fields and lowering yields. Climate change, resulting in drought or floods, can lead to these consequences, but limited access to fields—due to natural or man-made circumstances—can also influence agriculture production. Global and local prices fluctuations can also influence food production and income, as well as access to foods due to changing prices and incomes. Markets can be disrupted—either linked to goods moving to the market or related to people losing safe access to markets. There are often both immediate and long-term consequences of humanitarian crises on food security. For instance, a flood will immediately damage existing crop production. Subsequently, a lower household income could force a farmer to plant less in the subsequent season, exacerbating and extending the food security problem.

Access to Services

When service facilities are damaged, access to health care, education and other services is interrupted. These services are particularly essential for access to treatment and care for people who are being treated for chronic disease, for example diabetes, hypertension and HIV. Preventive health services such as immunization, vitamin A capsule distribution and midwifery services can also be interrupted. This can have serious longer-term public health ramifications, including a resurgence of infectious diseases such as measles in the affected areas and beyond. Children's access to education can be affected—due to physical damage to schools or an inability to access schools due to insecurity or other reasons. Access to social protection programs or agriculture extension services can similarly be interrupted.

Preparedness

The impact of a crisis depends not only on the magnitude of the crisis itself and the level of vulnerability prior to the crisis, but also on the existing capacity to plan for, predict and manage a shock. Preparedness activities seek to build capacity to provide more efficient and effective support in emergencies, as well as to mitigate the impact of an emergency before it strikes. For example, lessons learned from the 2004 Indian Ocean tsunami emphasized the need for early warning systems, which potentially could have alerted people of the approaching waves and potentially saved lives. In addition, surveillance systems could have been used for early detection of communicable disease, as well as monitoring the nutritional status of vulnerable groups [16].

Preparedness actions can include developing or improving such surveillance and warning systems, as well as investing in capacity development to enhance the ability of national actors to manage a disaster response. National disaster management plans are key preparedness tools, defining roles, responsibilities and actions to be enacted in the event of an emergency. Where rates of malnutrition are high, or the risk of deterioration of nutritional status is significant, these plans should include specific provisions for a response to protect the health and nutritional status of vulnerable groups.

Vulnerable populations often have fewer resources and less access to services, while at the same time, they live in situations that carry a high exposure to hazards (e.g., in substandard housing, in flood-prone areas, on degraded land) putting them at higher risk. Working with vulnerable groups before an emergency can support resilience through a variety of ways. For example, improving housing to better withstand weather hazards, diversifying livelihoods to raise incomes, improving nutrient intake to improve health and strengthen immune systems, and emergency trainings can support communities and individuals to better absorb and respond to shocks that may occur. See Box 29.2 for an example on the importance of preparedness in the context of El Nino.

Box 29.2 Case Study: El Niño

El Niño—a pattern of unusually warm water across the Pacific—is a phenomenon which has the power to change weather conditions around the world due to the interaction between winds and currents. The resulting changes in rainfall and temperature will have widespread impacts on food production in different regions. The 2015–2016 El Niño event has been forecast to be one of the strongest in nearly a century. The nature of the impact will differ depending on the location, but droughts driven by El Niño in Latin America, East and Southern Africa are expected to peak in late 2016 and carry the potential to decimate crop and pasture development.

Malawi is one of the countries expected to suffer poor harvests due to El Niño-driven drought. Prior to the crisis, 42.4% of children under 5 were stunted. While stunting exceeded the critical threshold, wasting prevalence stood at just 3.8%. Furthermore only 15% of children 6–23 months of age consumed a minimum acceptable diet (MAD) [17].

Given the nature of the crisis, livelihood groups which rely on rain-fed agriculture or pastures may experience significant loss to homestead production for self-consumption, as well as income. Depending on the severity of the drought and the crops most affected, the price of staple foods may increase[1] for the general population. As households with limited incomes are forced to spend more of their budgets on staple foods to cover price hikes, spending on other more micronutrient-rich foods is likely to decrease.

The use of negative coping mechanisms (e.g., selling productive assets, taking children out of school) may also increase. These actions, which are often a last resort meant to generate more income or reduce expense in the present face of a crisis, can undermine a household's ability to meet the nutrient needs of vulnerable members over the long run.

In some ways the crisis is predictable given the relatively slow-onset nature. However, the magnitude of the impact remains more difficult to predict. Early action and preparedness are needed to effectively protect the nutritional status of vulnerable groups. Given the high rates of stunting, it is particularly critical to reach pregnant and lactating women and children aged

---

[1]The Government of Malawi has a strategic grain reserve which aims to smooth these price hikes.

6–23 months. Based on MAD data, ensuring access to age-appropriate nutrient-dense foods must be a priority. When coupled with SBCC, the provision of complementary foods can help support nutrition outcomes by addressing both feeding practices (frequency) and consumption (diversity/adequacy of diet).

Impacts of a Humanitarian Crisis on Nutrition

Who Is Affected and How

Humanitarian crises will have both short-term and long-term impacts on the nutritional status of vulnerable groups such as young children, pregnant and lactating women, those with chronic illness (e.g., TB or HIV) and the elderly. Children and pregnant and lactating women have the highest nutrient requirements and have a high risk of infectious illness, the two immediate determinants of poor nutritional status. At the same time, poor nutrient intake and increased illness are two of the most common consequences of humanitarian crises, linked not just to food insecurity and increased health risks, but also to displacement and psychosocial consequences which can affect child feeding and caring practices, for instance.

While humanitarian crises can affect households across all economic classes, the poor and vulnerable suffer most in terms of bearing the brunt of consequences—increased prices, reduced food production (or extensive crop loss), inaccessibility to health or social services—and often force difficult household choices that adversely affect women, young children and elderly in particular. Vulnerable households require the greatest immediate and longer-term support to recover from the shock. Vulnerability is determined both by the potential risk and by its impact, and it may be related to age, gender, ethnicity, health status, wealth or other similar factors[2] [18].

Humanitarian crises typically strike amidst ongoing chronic problems of hunger and malnutrition in the affected countries. In addition, a crisis may exacerbate a regular seasonal hunger period or may occur during a seasonal period of higher illness (e.g., malaria or diarrhea).

The impact of a humanitarian crisis on malnutrition is determined by a number of factors that are related to the pre-crisis situation as well as the different characteristics of the crisis itself. These are described below.

Factors Affecting the Impact on Nutrition: Pre-crisis Nutrition Situation

The nutrition situation prior to the crisis will likely influence which nutrition problems become most pronounced in the immediate and longer-term aftermath of a crisis.

All forms of malnutrition, including stunting, wasting, micronutrient deficiencies (MNDs) and overweight/obesity, should be considered when gathering information to predict and understand the potential impact of a crisis on nutrition. Stunting is an indicator of vulnerability of the population, since stunted children are at higher risk of death, similar to children who are wasted [19]. This is likely linked to concurrent micronutrient deficiencies, which reduce the performance of the immune system. Even a small shock can have significant consequences on malnutrition because nutritional

---

[2]The Office for Disaster Risk Reduction, UNISDR, defines vulnerability as 'the conditions determined by physical, social, economic, and environmental factors or processes, which increase the susceptibility of a community to the impact of hazards.'

status can change very quickly. Therefore when a population with high levels of stunting and micronutrient deficiencies is exposed to a crisis, protecting nutritional status from a further deterioration is essential. Similarly, when such a population is at known risk of crises, e.g., due to a likely oncoming period of drought, improving nutritional status before the crisis starts makes good sense. This so-called prevention should focus on prevention of undernutrition, including stunting (1000-day focus, i.e., pregnant and lactating women and children under 2) and ensuring good micronutrient status (e.g., for children under 5). See Box 29.3 for an example from Nepal.

Box 29.3 Case Study: Nepal

Nutrition was already a key concern before the devastating earthquake that struck Nepal on April 25, 2015. In 2011, 41% of children under 5 were stunted, with children in rural areas more likely to be stunted (42%) than their urban counterparts (27%). In addition, 11% of children under five were wasted, and 29% were underweight. Forty-six percent of children under five were anemic and only 28% of children 6–23 months were appropriately fed, meaning they received the minimum dietary diversity and minimum meal frequency to achieve a minimum acceptable diet (MAD). Nutritional indicators for women of reproductive age were also poor, with 18% of women classified as having low BMI (<18.5 kg/m^2). Furthermore, 35% of women 15–49 years of age were anemic and only 38% of pregnant women took iron tablets for the recommended 180 days [20].

The massive 7.8 magnitude earthquake that struck Nepal in 2015 was the worst disaster to strike the country since the 1934 Nepal–Bihar Earthquake. The recent seismic event killed more than 8800 people and injured at least three times as many throughout the country. In addition to the immediate human toll, the earthquake destroyed already weak infrastructure, with 14 of 75 districts in the country reporting major damage. The crisis resulted in $10 billion in economic loss according to the Government of Nepal.

As mentioned above, the emergency came on top of already high rates of wasting, stunting and anemia among key groups. The nature of the crisis and its sudden onset impacted health systems, as well as access to basic needs such as food and water. Affected populations reported an increase in illness due to exposure to extreme hot and cold conditions due to lack of adequate housing. Furthermore, many rural communities were cut off from supply routes, negatively affecting access to markets.

Updated nutrition data (post-April 2015) were widely unavailable. However, given the pre-earthquake nutritional situation and expected impact of the earthquake, an immediate response to protect nutritional status was warranted. With the already high levels of wasting, and critical levels of stunting, the risk of rapid deterioration in nutritional status and increased wasting was extremely elevated. In addition, micronutrient deficiencies are a major contributor to morbidity and mortality and were already an issue of public health concern in Nepal before the 2015 earthquake. In affected districts with existing high levels of stunting and/or wasting, a preventative approach such as blanket supplementary feeding of specialized nutritious foods would have been appropriate.

Immediately following the earthquake, the Government of Nepal requested that the UN activate humanitarian clusters. Concerned not only by the scale of the emergency itself, but also by the risks to nutrition that the impending monsoon rains would bring, the UN Nutrition Cluster developed an integrated package of nutrition services. The package included a combination of promotion of infant and young child feeding (IYCF) practices, including for exclusive and continued breast-feeding (for mothers of children 0–5 months and children 6–23 months, respectively); distribution of a two-month supply of micronutrient powders (MNPs) for home fortification of foods for children aged 6–59 months; vitamin A supplementation for children age 6–59 months; screening children aged 6–59 months for severe acute malnutrition (SAM) using mid-upper arm circumference (MUAC), and referral of cases found; and iron and folic acid supplementation for pregnant and lactating women. This combination of education and blanket distribution of MNP together with active case finding and treatment of SAM combined prevention of micronutrient deficiencies and treatment of SAM [21].

Humanitarian crises are most commonly associated with increased numbers of children with acute malnutrition or wasting. However, where acute malnutrition rates are very low (<5%), monitoring increases in new cases or increased admissions of children to treatment facilities may not be the most sensitive indicator of the nutritional impact of a crisis (with the exception of major epidemics such as a large-scale cholera outbreak which could lead to a rapid increase in acute malnutrition). Instead, when access to food is threatened, it has been shown that households will protect their caloric intake (largely provided by cereals) and sacrifice diet diversity and diet quality [22, 23]. This can lead to a rapid onset or increase in micronutrient deficiencies. Where overweight and obesity are prevalent, management of NCDs is important but the crisis might also stimulate an increase in micronutrient deficiencies.

Factors Affecting the Impact on Nutrition: Characteristics or Effects of the Crisis

The immediate causes of undernutrition are poor dietary intake and illness. Understanding the pathway between the consequences and effects of humanitarian crises and these two immediate causes will help to explain and anticipate the potential impact on nutrition and to identify direct and complementary interventions that can prevent increases in malnutrition. Displacement, service quality and access, food insecurity and health risk are key effects that influence nutrition and are discussed below. These factors also affect how a response is designed and implemented.

Displacement

Short- or longer-term displacement can influence many factors related to nutrition. Temporary lodging areas can limit the secure, private space that is often required for breast-feeding in many cultures. In addition, displacement can affect access to cooking facilities—fuel may not be available or safely accessible, cooking equipment may be lost as a result of the crisis, or water availability may be hampered. A lack of cooking facilities often reduces the number of times households eat per day and can influence the type of foods that are prepared (e.g., easy preparation foods are preferred). This can have significant consequences for young children who need to eat a number of meals throughout the day and require a diverse diet.

Displacement can also affect access to food and markets—distances to markets may increase, frequency may decrease, and demand, competition and other behaviors of sellers may also change. This can influence the variety, price and/or regularity of food access. Displacement can lead to crowding or poor environmental conditions which could increase the risk of infections. Finally, displacement causes mental and psychological disruptions which can affect child and maternal caring practices.

Service Quality and Access

The capacity, coverage and effectiveness of the health system prior to the crisis will determine or influence whether an increased demand for services triggered by the crisis can be managed. At the same time, the crisis can often have significant impacts on the infrastructure and the human capacity of the health system, linked to security concerns and the quality of care being offered. For instance, health workers may not be able to work, they may become significantly overworked with increased caseloads, affecting quality of care, supply chains for equipment and medicines may be interrupted, or the centers themselves may be damaged. Similarly, social protection services (measures to improve and protect human capital) may be interrupted or may become overstretched.

Women, Crises and Nutrition

Women are greatly affected by humanitarian crises. They are often overrepresented in refugee and IDP communities that are formed as a result of humanitarian crises. They are primarily responsible for care of household members and often communities during crises, despite having lower social and legal status in many countries and less access to capital, goods and other means to protect themselves. They are also frequently sidelined in the planning and implementation of crisis responses in many situations. Given their role in child care and household food security, including food production, distribution and marketing, preparation, processing and storage, women's status is essential for ensuring good nutrition. Having access to security and protection services is also essential because of major risks of gender-based violence in crises. This can affect their access to markets, their ability to seek employment and their access to services provided during the emergency response.

The Nutrition Response to a Humanitarian Crisis

Increased attention has been given to nutrition as part of the humanitarian response in the past decades. In 1992, nutrition was not mentioned in any of the humanitarian appeals that were launched, in contrast to representing as much as a half billion US dollars, or more than 11%, of the total funding requests in 2012 [24].

Thresholds for a Nutrition Response

Typically, data on acute malnutrition or wasting among children under 5 years have been used to define the nutrition concerns in a humanitarian crisis—particularly to estimate relief needs, to prioritize or target geographical areas, to plan nutritional interventions and to monitor the effectiveness of nutrition assistance [25]. Global acute malnutrition (GAM) prevalence thresholds have been commonly used to guide intervention in emergencies: >15% GAM or 10–14% GAM with aggravating factors = nutritional emergency. Prevalence of wasting in children is estimated based on the 2006 WHO Child Growth Standards for weight-for-height below −2 standard deviations and/or edema (referred to as Global Acute Malnutrition) or mid-upper arm circumference (MUAC) below 125 mm [26]. MUAC is becoming more common because it is easier to collect, particularly in humanitarian crises, and is a better indicator of mortality risk [27].

While the UN WHO thresholds and tools such as the Integrated Food Security Phase Classification (IPC) still rely largely on thresholds of wasting prevalence to classify the severity of a nutritional problem in a humanitarian crisis [28], there have been practical shifts in understanding of malnutrition during crises and two major shifts are evolving.

First, there has been a shift in recognizing that it is not possible to differentiate forms or levels of malnutrition by their context, i.e., a humanitarian crisis or a non-emergency setting. Some countries have 'emergency levels' of acute malnutrition in what would be classified as non-emergency settings. And while the individual risk of mortality is highest with severe acute malnutrition or severe micronutrient deficiencies, more children die due to more moderate micronutrient deficiencies, moderate acute malnutrition and stunting because many more children are affected by these conditions. Stunting and its consequences are not only a concern for the development context, for two reasons: (1) Many crises are long-lasting and ultimately may cover a substantial part of the 1000-day period of individuals, so while called 'chronic malnutrition,' the irreversible impact of poor nutrition on health and development occurs in a relatively short period, even in crises, and (2) stunting needs to be prevented during the first 1000 days and the interventions required for that, i.e., those that ensure adequate nutrient intake, also support the immune system and lower the risk of acute malnutrition. If preventive interventions targeting this window of opportunity are not implemented during a crisis, the impact can be irreversible.

This greater understanding of the mortality risks of malnutrition and the evolving pattern of humanitarian crises worldwide have stimulated a second major shift—the importance of using data on the broader nutrition situation (wasting, stunting, micronutrient deficiencies and obesity) and data on the underlying risks (displacement, food insecurity, health situation, population density) to guide decision-making for a nutrition response.

In Fig. 29.1, the decision process for when and how to respond to acute malnutrition is presented [29]. While the first line of decision-making for this tool is still the prevalence of acute malnutrition rather than also considering stunting, micronutrient deficiencies and overweight, critical risk factors that are associated with an increased incidence of acute malnutrition are presented to guide program managers to the most optimal response plan. One of the objectives of the tool was to explicitly incorporate a range of contextual situational factors into the decision-making process, in addition to population-level data on nutritional status before and during the specific humanitarian crisis.

Increasingly there are more examples of malnutrition being considered more holistically in humanitarian responses. For instance in Indonesia during the 1998 economic crisis, the nature of the crisis was modeled to predict the impact on nutritional status (what and who would be most affected). Deterioration of diet quality was identified as the most likely nutritional consequence, and therefore, increases in micronutrient deficiencies (e.g., anemia and vitamin A deficiency) were anticipated.

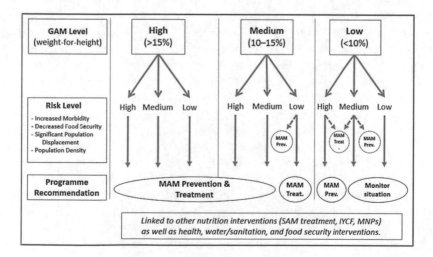

Fig. 29.1 Program recommendation for prevention of acute malnutrition and treatment of MAM. The tool may underestimate risk in slow-onset emergencies. In emergencies with severe food insecurity or epidemics where GAM is classified as low, it may be appropriate to launch blanket feeding rather than monitor the situation. From MAM Decision-Making Tool, Global Nutrition Cluster, 2014. The *dotted lines* in the diagram indicate 'additional option' (relevant in certain circumstances). Used with permission

Programs were launched early on to minimize an increase in micronutrient deficiencies [22]. In addition, response in Indonesia to the 2004 Indian Ocean tsunami considered the existing high rates of micronutrient deficiencies among women of reproductive age and young children. The tsunami was the first emergency response which included a large-scale distribution of micronutrient powders as a home fortificant to be added to semisolid or solid foods prepared for children [16]. More recently in the El Niño crisis in Central America, the existing problem of overweight/obesity is considered in the overall strategy for the food security and nutrition response [30]. The situational analysis and monitoring of the crisis impact will include measures of over- and undernutrition. The planning for food assistance rations and nutrition interventions, particularly nutrition messaging, will take into account the double burden problem in many of these countries. During the Syrian refugee crisis in Lebanon, Jordan and Iraq, significant increases in wasting have not been observed [31]. However, given the low dietary diversity and the limited availability and affordability of fortified complementary foods in these neighboring countries, there is growing awareness that other nutrition problems, including micronutrient deficiencies, child stunting, overweight and non-communicable diseases (NCDs)—all of which were prevalent in the Syrian population pre-crisis—may have increased as a result of the crisis. See Box 29.4 for an example of considering how multiple factors may be impacting nutrition in the Syrian crisis.

Box 29.4 Case Study: Syria
Even before the Syrian conflict, the country was confronted with multiple nutrition challenges. In 2009, 27.5% of children under 5 were stunted; wasting stood at 11.5% for the same age group; and 17.9% were overweight [32].

The crisis erupted in March 2011. By 2016, after more than 5 years, the protracted conflict has resulted in a massive loss of life and livelihoods. Current United Nations estimates put the number of displaced at nearly 11 million—more than half of the country's population. More than half, 4.8 million of the displaced, have fled Syria, and many now reside as refugees in neighboring countries [33].

While little assessment data are available from inside Syria, the sub-national differences in security situations are likely creating some highly localized impacts which require contextual responses. For example, transport costs for food and other goods are often influenced by armed groups which control road access and levy unofficial fines. Food that is grown in one region might be affordable locally, with high price increases in other Syrian markets to cover these transport-related costs. The varying functioning of markets is likely contributing to different food security and nutrition outcomes depending on locations.

As the conflict continues, addressing malnutrition within Syria becomes increasingly critical. Wasting rates which were poor before the crisis are likely to have deteriorated further as food and health systems are increasingly strained or nonexistent. A nutritional response within Syria considers a preventative approach on a very large scale, as well as focus on implementing malnutrition treatment services in besieged areas. A 'preventative' approach aims to prevent a predictable potential increase in malnutrition by targeting based on vulnerability (e.g., all children in a given crisis-affected area between the ages of 6–23 months), rather than targeting based on nutritional status (e.g., children 6–59 months of age are only referred to treatment for SAM when MUAC is ≤115 mm or WHZ is ≤−3).

However, the response necessary to protect the nutritional status of refugees must consider the very different contexts in which these displaced populations now live. The response is largely provided via cash based transfers, i.e., refugees are accessing foods that are available and choose based on their own preferences. Large-scale treatment is likely to become unnecessary and inappropriate if populations have access to sufficient support to meet their food and non-food needs. However, with little opportunities to generate additional income, the transfers provided to refugees must be large enough to cover all nutrient needs, and cost-effective fortified foods must be available and accessible to prevent micronutrient deficiencies among vulnerable groups. Market assessments should consider the availability of animal source foods and age-appropriate complementary foods to ensure that refugees living in camps or host communities have the means and the ability to procure and prepare foods which meet the nutrient needs of young children and that match their food preferences. Support to mothers for optimal feeding practices, including exclusive and continued breast-feeding, must be provided.

While the above considers immediate needs, long-term economic, political and social consequences of the conflict will continue to impact the underlying causes of malnutrition for many years.

Prevention and Treatment

Webb et al. have identified four objectives of nutrition action in a humanitarian crisis including reducing prevalence of acute malnutrition, reducing or preventing micronutrient deficiencies, promoting appropriate complementary care to minimize the risk of mortality among young children during illness and ensuring access to adequate, safe and nutritious foods to meet required nutrient needs [34].

There has been significant progress in improving the treatment of acute malnutrition (both severe and moderate) over the past 15 years. The development of ready-to-use foods (RUF) and a community-based approach, i.e., community management of acute malnutrition (CMAM), have made it possible to treat the majority of children in outpatient services as opposed to treatment in hospitals[3] (See Box 29.5). CMAM has led to better coverage and more effective treatment of acute malnutrition among admitted children. When SAM treatment is integrated effectively into health systems, including treatment in the community, in non-emergency contexts, it can then be scaled up during crises to prevent the mortality risk associated with malnutrition in sudden-onset crises.

Box 29.5 Revolution of Treatment of Severe Acute Malnutrition, from Clinic to Community, Enabled by Development of Ready-to-Use Therapeutic Food

Until the late 1990s, the product of choice for treatment of children with severe acute malnutrition (SAM) was therapeutic milk. The milk is to be reconstituted from powder milk several times a day by trained personnel, and children are hospitalized during their treatment, with their mother or another caretaker looking after them and feeding them the milk. The treatment could take around 3–6 weeks, which is a long time for a caretaker to be away from other family members and responsibilities. However, because of hygiene risks, possibility of errors when reconstituting the milk and unintended use, it cannot be given to caretakers for preparing and feeding at home.

In the early 1990s, a French pediatrician, Andre Briend, conceived the idea of mixing ingredients containing the nutrients required for recovering from SAM into a paste with very low water activity, which would be ready to consume and could be stored, unopened, for a long time. The low water activity prevents bacterial growth, and packaging in small servings of

---

[3]CMAM is generally described as a continuum of care with four components: (1) community outreach; (2) management of MAM (moderate acute malnutrition); (3) outpatient treatment for children with SAM (severe acute malnutrition) with a good appetite and without medical complications; and (4) inpatient treatment for children with SAM and medical complications and/or no appetite.

which one or more could be consumed per day would allow treatment of children at home, rather than as inpatients in a clinic. The ready-to-use therapeutic food (RUTF) was born, and after its equivalency to F-100 [35] or superiority to standard treatment [36] was confirmed, the formulation was finalized and the commonly used recipe includes as its ingredients peanuts, milk powder and/or whey, vegetable oil, sugar, maltodextrin and vitamin/mineral premix. The paste was packaged in foil sachets containing 500 kcal (92 g) that have a 24-month shelf-life.

WHO, WFP, SCN and UNICEF issued a joint statement endorsing RUTF for treatment of uncomplicated SAM, which means that the child has an appetite and will consume the food and is free from other medical complications that would require inpatient care, as outpatients in the community [37]. This meant that many children with SAM could now be treated at home, and the detection and follow-up for children with SAM could now be organized at community level, for example at the level of health posts rather than clinics [38]. This approach became known as community management of acute malnutrition (CMAM) and also includes treatment of moderate acute malnutrition (MAM) and prevention of acute malnutrition [39]. For detection of SAM, a color tape is used to measure the mid-upper arm circumference (MUAC), where a red result corresponds with <115 mm and indicates SAM, orange is for 115–125 mm and indicates MAM, and green is for ≥125 mm and not acutely malnourished. CMAM has markedly increased the number of children that are treated for SAM.

Meanwhile, other nutritious pastes have been developed that are similar to RUTF:

- Ready-to-use supplementary food (RUSF) for treatment of MAM—also in sachets of approximately 500 kcal, main difference is that it has less dairy and a slightly different MN content (e.g., 10% instead of 20% milk powder). Its nutrient content is based on WHO guidance issued in 2012 [40].
- Lipid-based nutrient supplement—medium quantity (LNS-MQ) for prevention of acute malnutrition, given in dosages of 250 kcal/d to children at risk of developing acute malnutrition for example in a very food-insecure lean season
- Lipid-based nutrient supplement—small quantity (LNS-SQ) used to add essential (micro) nutrients to a young child's diet to reduce the risk of undernutrition, including micronutrient deficiencies and stunting.

For MAM treatment and enhancing complementary feeding, there are also other food options available, such as fortified infant cereals (e.g., Supercereal Plus). For SAM treatment, the two main options are F100 for inpatient treatment and RUTF for outpatient treatment. Home-based care including cooking demonstrations and other care instructions for caretakers in combination with provision of vitamin/mineral supplements has also been tried, for both SAM and MAM treatment, but effects vary, depending on caretakers' access to specific foods (i.e., do they provide the required combination and amount of nutrients) and time [41, 42].

It is important to note that in addition to special nutritious foods, treatment of acute malnutrition also requires treatment and prevention of disease, and support and information for caretakers on infant and young child feeding practices, including breast-feeding, hygiene and food preparation

While these improvements in treatment of acute malnutrition are laudable, prevention of malnutrition before it occurs through a multi-sectoral approach is better. Prevention programming can reduce the number of children who become acutely malnourished, rather than only treating those who are already acutely malnourished [43, 44]. More importantly, prevention of malnutrition is an essential part of child survival interventions and required for ensuring optimal growth and development. It can protect exposed generations by ensuring appropriate nutrition during the first 1000 days (i.e., from conception until the second birthday).

Good nutrition during the first 1000 days is considered the first line of prevention against undernutrition, including wasting. When a crisis occurs, these ongoing prevention programs can be adjusted to cover a greater number of affected households/children or the package of services could be modified in response to the consequences of the crisis. In essence, any intervention to ensure optimal nutrition or to reduce the risk of undernutrition needs to address directly or indirectly the immediate causes of malnutrition—i.e., dietary intake to meet established nutrient requirements and prevention of illness, which increases nutrient needs and lowers dietary intake (reduced appetite) [45].

A wide range of programs are employed to prevent undernutrition during emergencies, including nutrition specific interventions, such as blanket supplementary feeding, and nutrition-sensitive interventions, such as improving food security and livelihoods, water and sanitation programming and improved caregiving. Good nutrition during pregnancy and lactation is also very important for reducing small-for-gestational age births and ensuring optimal growth and development during emergencies. Good nutrition among women also supports their ability to provide good care for their children.

Greater emphasis is increasingly placed on having strong system-based, multi-sectoral prevention programing in place prior to emergency onset. These systems can then be scaled up (and down) in response to crises. Equally, when prevention programming is not in place, a preventive response in an emergency can also become the basis for a longer-term prevention program post the crisis if the situation warrants.

Food Assistance and Nutrition

Food assistance is an instrument to promote food security among vulnerable households. The term food assistance is now used instead of food aid because the instruments to deliver this support have expanded beyond in-kind food transfers (e.g., actual food commodities) to include cash based transfers (e.g., cash, commodity or price vouchers). In addition to in-kind food distribution often associated with food aid, food assistance can include providing technical assistance to governments on implementing school feeding and social safety nets, and it can be linked to asset creation, work with smallholder farmers to ensure good quality produce and access to markets or developing capacity of local manufacturers of nutritious foods. Where markets are functioning, the humanitarian sector is shifting more toward cash-based transfers or open vouchers to respond better to consumer needs and preferences.

Food assistance addresses the 'food availability' and 'food access' issues of food insecurity and when operated appropriately can also contribute to the 'food stability' aspect of food security. And while the definition of food security mentions physical and economic access to nutritious food and includes 'food use,' nutrition requires more than adequate caloric intake. In most instances the intake of nutrient-dense foods (those with a high concentration of nutrients per calorie) required by young children or meeting the high requirements during pregnancy or by adolescent girls is often not specifically considered in food security programming. For cash based transfers to work effectively for nutrition, nutrient-dense foods must be available at low costs in markets or provided to households with children that cannot afford to purchase them or cannot access them. Emerging evidence shows that nutrition impacts are greatest when food security interventions (cash or in-kind) are linked to provision of specialized nutritious foods [45].

Conclusion

The number, nature, scale and complexity of humanitarian crises will continue to evolve over the next decade, particularly related to effects of climate change, poor governance and armed conflict.

There is a great need for finding better ways to execute responses to humanitarian crises, including nutrition interventions. Part of this is grounded in better programming to prevent malnutrition among the vulnerable and marginalized people prior to the onset of the crises. On equal level, there must be greater focus by world leaders on achieving international peace and justice to prevent the marked increase in protracted situations that have occurred more frequently over the past years and an investment in stability and human capacity to prevent crises and worsening of situations.

The nutrition response to humanitarian crises should reflect an understanding of the consequences of effects of the crisis as well as the nutrition situation prior to the crisis not just acute malnutrition. With the transition of malnutrition, including the increasing problem of double burden in many countries, the response should focus on the broader nutrition problem. Prevention actions should ensure optimal nutrient intake, particularly during the first 1000 days, combined with a strong multisectoral response. Protection and security of children and their caretakers is also fundamental to an effective nutrition response in humanitarian crises.

Greater investments in nutrition in non-crisis periods are needed. These programs can be expanded—similar to social protection programs (e.g., Ethiopia) during emergencies or humanitarian crises. Where these prevention programs do not currently exist, a preventive nutrition response in an emergency can be the basis for a longer-term approach.

Development of capacity in nutrition, particularly in countries affected by chronic or recurrent complex emergencies, is essential for the longer term.

Discussion Points

- Describe the different types of humanitarian crises and some of the usual consequences that arise.
- How have humanitarian crises changed over the past 10 years? What appears to be driving these changes? How might these trends change in the next 10 years?
- Figure 29.1 presents a decision-making framework for nutrition responses in humanitarian contexts. Could you mention limitations of this diagram? Describe how additional information on the nutritional situation might affect the nutrition response?
- What are the critical factors might you would consider in designing a nutrition response in a natural disaster that has a sudden onset? For a protracted complex emergency?

References

1. UNOCHA. Global humanitarian overview 2016. Geneva: UNOCHA; 2016.
2. UNHCR. Global trends report: world at war. Geneva: UNHCR; 2015.
3. Tol RJS. The economic effects of climate change. J Econ Perspect. 2009;23(2):29–51.
4. Water, Sanitation and Hygiene Cluster. WASH cluster coordination handbook: a practical guide for all those involved in the water, sanitation and hygiene cluster. Geneva; 2009.
5. International Strategy for Disaster Risk Reduction. Terminology on disaster risk reduction. UN: Geneva; 2009.
6. The State of Food Insecurity in the World. Addressing food insecurity in protracted crises. Rome: Food and Agriculture Organization; 2010.
7. Bennett C. The development agency of the future. ODI Working Paper; 2015.

8. IPCC. Summary for Policymakers. In: Managing the risks of extreme events and disasters to advance climate change adaptation [Field, C.B., V. Barros, T.F. Stocker, D. Qin, D.J. Dokken, K.L. Ebi, M.D. Mastrandrea, K. J. Mach, G.-K. Plattner, S.K. Allen, M. Tignor, and P.M. Midgley (eds.)]. A special report of working groups I and II of the intergovernmental panel on climate change. Cambridge: Cambridge University Press; 2012.
9. Coudouel A, Hentschel JS, Wodon QT. Poverty measurement and analysis, in the PRSP sourcebook. Washington DC: World Bank; 2002.
10. World Food Programme. Emergency food security assessment handbook. 2nd ed. Rome; 2009.
11. World Food Programme. Comprehensive food security & vulnerability analysis guidelines. 1st edn. Rome; 2009.
12. Humanitarian Coalition. Factsheet: what is a humanitarian emergency? Ottawa; 2016.
13. The Committee on World Food Security. Framework for action for food security and nutrition in protracted crises. Rome; 2015.
14. Government of Haiti. Haiti earthquake PDNA: assessment of damage, losses, general and sectoral needs. Port au Prince; 2010.
15. World Bank. World development report 2011: conflict, security, and development. Washington DC; 2011.
16. de Pee S, Moench-Pfanner R, Bloem MW. Indian ocean tsunami, 2004. In: Bloem MW, Semba RD, (eds.) Nutrition and health in developing countries. 2nd ed. 2008, p. 721–38.
17. Malawi MDG Endline Survey (MICS). 2014.
18. UNISDR. Terminology on disaster risk reduction. 2004.
19. Black RE, Victora CG, Walker SP, Bhutta ZA, Christian P, de Onis M, et al. Maternal and child undernutrition and overweight in low-income and middle-income countries. Lancet. 2013;328:427–51.
20. Ministry of Health and Population, New ERA and ICF International Inc. Nepal Demographic and Health Survey 2011. Kathmandu, Nepal and Calverton, Maryland: Ministry of Health and Population, New ERA, and ICF International; 2012.
21. Aguayo VM, Sharma A, Subedi GR. Delivering essential nutrition services for children after the Nepal earthquake. Lancet Global Health. 2015;3(11):e665–6.
22. Bloem MW, Darnton-Hill I. Micronutrient deficiencies—first link in a chain of nutritional and health events in economic crises. In: Primary and secondary preventive nutrition. 2001, p. 357–73.
23. World Bank. Responding to higher and more volatile world food prices. Washington DC; 2012.
24. Webb P. Malnutrition in Emergencies: the framing of nutrition concerns in the humanitarian appeals process, 1992 to 2009. Food Nutr Bull. 2009;30:379–89.
25. Young H, Borrel A, Holland D, Salama P. Public nutrition in complex emergencies. Lancet. 2004;364:1899–909.
26. WHO/WFP/UNSCN/UNICEF. Joint statement: community based management of severe acute malnutrition. Geneva; 2007.
27. Myatt M, Khara T, Collins S. A review of methods to detect cases of severely malnourished children in the community for their admission into community-based therapeutic care programs. Food Nutr Bull. 2006;27(3): S7–23.
28. World Health Organization. The management of nutrition in major emergencies. Geneva; 2000.
29. IASC Global Nutrition Cluster. Moderate acute malnutrition: a decision tool for emergencies. Geneva; 2014.
30. World Food Programme. Regional strategy for El Nino Crisis in Latin America. Rome; 2016.
31. Dolan C, McGrath M, Shoham J. ENN's perspective on the nutrition response in the Syria crisis. ENN Field Exchange 53, Geneva; 2015.
32. International Food Policy Research Institute. Global nutrition report 2015: actions and accountability to advance nutrition and sustainable development. Washington, DC; 2015.
33. OCHA Operational Reports. May 2016.
34. Webb P, Boyd E, de Pee S, Lenters L, Bloem MW, Schultink W. Nutrition in emergencies: do we know what works? Food Policy. 2014;49:33–40.
35. Diop EHI, Dossou NI, Ndour MM, Briend A, Wade S. Comparison of the efficacy of a solid ready-to-use food and a liquid, milk-based diet for the rehabilitation of severely malnourished children: a randomized trial. Am J Clin Nutr. 2003;78:302–7.
36. Ciliberto MA, Sandige H, Ndehka MDJ, Ashorn P, Briend A, Cliberto HM, Manary MJ. Comparison of home-based therapy with ready-to-use therapeutic food with standard therapy in the treatment of malnourished Malawian children: a controlled, clinical effectiveness trial. Am J Clin Nutr. 2005;81:864–70.
37. World Health Organization (WHO), World Food Programme (WFP), United Nations System Standing Committee on Nutrition (UN SCN), United Nations Children's Fund (UNICEF). Joint statement. Community-based management of severe acute malnutrition. Geneva: WHO; 2007.
38. Collins S, Dent N, Binns P, Bahwere P, Sadler K, Hallam A. Management of severe acute malnutrition in children. Lancet. 2006;368:1992–2000.
39. World Health Organization, United Nations Children's Fund. WHO child growth standards and the identification of severe acute malnutrition in infants and children; a joint statement by the World Health Organization and the United Nations Children's Fund. Geneva: WHO; 2009.

40. World Health Organization (WHO). Technical note: supplementary foods for the management of moderate acute malnutrition in infants and children 6–59 months of age. Geneva: WHO; 2012.
41. Khanum S, Ashworth A, Huttly SRA. Controlled trial of three approaches to the treatment of severe malnutrition. Lancet. 1994;344:1628–32.
42. Ashworth A, Ferguson E. Dietary counseling in the management of moderate malnourishment in children. Food Nutr Bull. 2009;30:S405–33.
43. Ruel MT, Menon P, Habicht JP, Loechl C, Bergeron G, Pelto G, Arimond M, et al. Age-based preventive targeting of food assistance and behaviour change and communication for reduction of childhood undernutrition in Haiti: a cluster randomised trial. Lancet. 2008;371:588–95.
44. Langendorf C, Roederer T, de Pee S, Brown D, Doyon S, Mamaty A, et al. Preventing acute malnutrition among young children in crises: a prospective intervention study in Niger. PLoS. 2014;11(9).
45. de Pee S, Grais R, Fenn B, et al. Prevention of acute malnutrition: distribution of special nutritious food and cash and addressing underlying causes—what to recommend when, where, for whom and how. Food Nutr Bull. 2015;36:S24–9.

Chapter 30
Ending AIDS by 2030: Partnerships and Linkages with SDG 2

Divya Mehra, Saskia de Pee and Martin W. Bloem

Keywords SDG 2 · Ending AIDS · Cascade of care · Social protection · Food security · Nutrition · Health systems strengthening · Partnerships for SDGS · HIV funding · UNAIDS strategy 2016–2021 · Key populations

Learning Objectives

- Understand the cascade of care for HIV—from transmission to retention in care.
- Gain insights into the current political, economic and programmatic environment for HIV.
- Understand the forms and roles of food and nutrition assistance in the HIV response.
- Distinguish different types of HIV-sensitive social protection options for different populations.
- Identify future HIV-related entry points through SDG 2. Compare and contrast with existing food and nutrition assistance in HIV (learning point #3).

Introduction

Tremendous success has been achieved in the fight against HIV in the last decade. By mid-2015, 15.8 million of the approximately 37 million people living with HIV were accessing treatment; AIDS-related deaths fell by 42% since its peak in 2004, and the overall new infections had fallen by 35% since 2000 and 58% among children alone [1]. Enabling policy frameworks accelerating the progress in combating the epidemic have also been successfully implemented. Recent evidence shows that treatment, particularly early treatment, is not only important for survival, but also a key strategy to prevent HIV transmission. This has made it possible to discuss 'the ending of AIDS.' In fact, the world has surpassed the AIDS target of Millennium Development Goal (MDG) 6, halting and

D. Mehra (✉) · S. de Pee · M.W. Bloem
Nutrition Division, World Food Programme, Rome, Italy
e-mail: divya.mehra@wfp.org

S. de Pee
e-mail: Saskia.depee@wfp.org; depee.saskia@gmail.com

M.W. Bloem
e-mail: martin.bloem@wfp.org

S. de Pee · M.W. Bloem
Friedman School of Nutrition Science and Policy, Tufts University, Boston, MA, USA

M.W. Bloem
Department of International Health, Bloomberg School of Public Health,
Johns Hopkins University, Baltimore, MD, USA

© Springer Science+Business Media New York 2017
S. de Pee et al. (eds.), *Nutrition and Health in a Developing World*,
Nutrition and Health, DOI 10.1007/978-3-319-43739-2_30

reversing the spread of HIV, and more countries are 'Fast-Tracking' to end the AIDS epidemic by 2030 as part of the sustainable development goals (SDGs). The HIV response has averted 30 million new HIV infections and nearly 8 million (7.8 million) AIDS-related deaths since 2000, when the MDGs were adopted [2].

Yet, access to effective HIV treatment remains one of the great challenges of our times. Approximately 22 million people living with HIV do not have access to treatment, and most of them (over 17 million) do not know that they have the virus. Furthermore, a significant number of people who are diagnosed to be HIV positive do not start treatment due to low uptake of services and in places where the 2015 WHO guidelines of test and treat have not yet been implemented; there are losses between testing and initiation of treatment. Lastly, in sub-Saharan Africa, only 65% of people living with HIV who are enrolled on ART remain on treatment as assessed after three years [3]. Issues of access, utilization of services and adherence to treatment continue through the continuum of care starting at prevention, testing, treatment initiation and long-term retention in care. Issues of retention in ART programs (also in pre-ART care) and long-term adherence to treatment and care regimens have not received adequate attention; programs that achieve high retention rates and good long-term adherence to treatment are needed and can serve as models. HIV/AIDS has claimed 36 million lives so far; it is the leading cause of death among women aged 15–49 years worldwide; sub-Saharan Africa is the most affected region, with a small population (12% of the world's population) but the highest proportion of people living with HIV (71% of all PLHIV in 2012) [4]. The 2015 WHO guidelines recommend that ART should be initiated in everyone living with HIV at any CD4 cell count based on the recent findings that treatment is an important prevention strategy as well as evidence showing that earlier use of ART results in better clinical outcomes for people living with HIV compared with delayed start of treatment. However, using those guidelines, only 40% of eligible people in low- and middle-income countries were covered by 2015 [5, 6].

Treatment is rightly the 'cornerstone of an effective response.' Adequate treatment not only allows people to live longer and healthier, but also curbs the transmission of HIV [7]. More than ever before, it is now possible to envision a world with 'zero new infections' and 'zero AIDS-related deaths' given the progress made on improved treatment. The implementation of the WHO 2010 guidelines for the prevention of mother-to-child transmission (PMTCT) can reduce the risk of transmission from 35% to less than 5% when breastfeeding, and from 25% to less than 2% in non-breastfeeding infants [8]. The rhetoric around 'the end of AIDS' is gaining significant momentum. However, to end the AIDS epidemic by 2030, a 'Fast Track' approach is necessary with clear targets for the 5 years until 2020. The 90–90–90 treatment target states that by 2020, 90% of people living with HIV know their HIV status, 90% of people who know their status will be receiving treatment and 90% of people on HIV treatment will have a suppressed viral load so their immune system remains strong and the likelihood of their infection being passed on is greatly reduced [9].

The UNAIDS Fast Track approach aims to achieve ambitious targets by 2020, including: fewer than 500,000 people newly infected with HIV, fewer than 500,000 people dying from AIDS-related illnesses and eliminating HIV-related discrimination [9]. However, in order to reach the Fast Track goals, the global community needs to look beyond health systems. Findings shared at the AIDS conference in Durban in July 2016 show the nuances and limitations of 'treatment as prevention,' if the focus is only on the medical aspect of identifying infected people and getting them on treatment. A large study in KwaZulu–Natal tested 28,000 people in a total of 22 communities every 6 months (prevalence ∼30%). In half of the communities, people who tested positive for HIV were offered medical services and ARVs close to their homes, while in the other 11 communities, HIV-positive people were only offered ARVs if they met the current government set medical criteria and went to existing clinics. The trial did not show that 'treatment as prevention' reduced infections. One of the main reasons appears to be only one-third of eligible people availed of medical services or treatment within the first three months and one-half within the first year. Furthermore, 9% of those that went to the clinic opted not to start treatment. Only 43% took up treatment, and there was no change in the incidence of new infections in the communities [10].

Just as for getting people on ARVs, and retaining them, communities can play an important role in providing leadership, particularly for key populations that have been left behind such as adolescent girls, sex workers, men who have sex with men (MSM) and injecting drug users. For example, as the epidemic among MSM rises across Asia and the Pacific (including China), community-based approaches will have to alleviate barriers to testing such as real or perceived stigma and discrimination, including from the health sector or lack of support/fear of the results [11]. Through a better understanding of 'barriers' to testing and treatment, it will be possible to reduce patient loss through the continuum of care. Global efforts are channeled toward biomedical treatment interventions, while significant work remains to be done for getting people on treatment and retaining them on care.

Current Context for HIV and Nutrition

HIV

While much remains to be done for the HIV/AIDS response, strategic shifts are occurring in the field of HIV/AIDS, global health and development in general.

First, we know that strengthening the disease-specific vertical approach for AIDS will not be enough for successfully combating the epidemic; health systems will need to be strengthened too. Under the sustainable development goals, HIV/AIDS is incorporated under the health goal, which includes a specific and ambitious target on ending the AIDS epidemic. However, there is broad agreement that HIV-sensitive targets and indicators should be included under several goals to ensure policy coherence and joint action on social, political, economic and environmental determinants of HIV, including food insecurity, poor health, poverty and inequality. The new strategy highlights that responding to HIV is a multisectoral issue with linkages to all of the sustainable development agenda. This is well outlined in the UNAIDS Strategy, where five SDGs have been selected as the key for the HIV response:

- SDG 3: Ensure healthy lives and promote well-being for all at all ages;
- SDG 5: Achieve gender equality and empower all women and girls;
- SDG 10: Reduce inequality within and among countries;
- SDG 16: Promote peaceful and inclusive societies for sustainable development, provide access to justice for all and build effective, accountable and inclusive institutions at all levels;
- SDG 17: Strengthen the means of implementation and revitalize the global partnership for sustainable development.

Furthermore, links to other SDGs have also been described [9]. In contrast to the previous UNAIDS Strategy 2011–2015 which looked at the epidemic at a global level, the updated Strategy 2016–2021 has a strong focus on varying regional, country and city contexts [9].

Second, under the 2015 WHO guidelines, all PLHIV should be on treatment and people will live longer. HIV is emerging as a chronic disease with a set of new complications and comorbidities that require sophisticated and integrated systems and expertise for disease management [12]. Deeks et al. argued for the need to rethink and develop chronic care models for HIV and link HIV treatment facilities with services for chronic diseases. This will be a substantial challenge in low resource settings where healthcare systems are already overburdened and usually mainly equipped to handle acute or disease-specific care. While it is imperative to appreciate the 'HIV as a chronic disease' paradigm, it also assumes that people are already accessing and adhering to treatment optimally, which is often not the case among the most vulnerable populations. The people most severely affected by the AIDS epidemic, including young women and adolescent girls, children, migrants and key populations, including gay men and other men who have sex with men, sex workers, people who inject drugs, transgender people and prisoners, still face barriers to accessing HIV and health services devoid of stigma and discrimination [9].

Third, despite ambitious goals and targets for ending the AIDS epidemic by 2030, HIV programming is under increasing financial strain for various reasons. AIDS is no longer the central pillar of many donor ODA strategies. Humanitarian emergencies, such as the Syrian refugee crisis, as well as the increased immigration to Europe, compete for donors' ODA funds. International financing for HIV fell from $8.6 billion in 2014 to $7.5 billion in 2015, with the USA providing two-thirds (https://blogs.worldbank.org/health). But an increasing share of HIV funding is coming from domestic sources, accounting for 57% of all HIV-related expenditure in low- and middle-income countries in 2015 (compared to 31% in 2005) [2]. Global health funding is shifting away from large-scale investment in vertical approaches that target single diseases to horizontal approaches that reinforce integration of services, maternal and child health programs, primary care and efforts to strengthen health systems overall.

Concerns have already been raised about the implications related to the rhetoric on the 'End of AIDS.' As eloquently stated in a World Bank blog, 'advocacy outran science' to create unrealistic expectations among donors, policy makers and the public alike that we have what it takes to end the epidemic [13]. In the absence of a vaccine or a cure for HIV, this epidemic will never end. Even though there is a trend toward the integration of health in an environment of declining international financing for HIV/AIDS, it is not the time to lose momentum and reverse the substantial gains made in this field. New infections have been flat lining at over 2 million annually, and several countries in Southern Africa still have a prevalence rate of over 20%.

Nutrition

While HIV/AIDS is moving toward health systems integration, food security and nutrition are gaining increasing traction globally and in national agendas. The United Nations Secretary General's Zero Hunger Challenge is aiming to achieve the vision of a Zero Hunger world by uniting around clear, measureable zero-based targets that would reject inequities and aims to eliminate childhood stunting; ensure that food is accessible to all and that food systems are sustainable. Concurrently, the Scaling up Nutrition (SUN) Movement, in 56 countries (in 2016), is galvanizing unprecedented political momentum, with national governments taking the lead to comprehensively addressing undernutrition among their populations. The 2013 Lancet Series on Maternal and Child Nutrition has emphasized the importance of also intervening during pregnancy and pre-pregnancy (adolescence and women of reproductive age) for improved nutrition outcomes among children. All of these have resulted in nutrition being front and center of the global agenda. Whereas MDG 1 combined poverty and hunger, SDG 2, *end hunger, achieve food security and improved nutrition and promote sustainable agriculture*, holistically addresses food security and nutrition.

With nutrition high on the global agenda, funding is following suit. At the Nutrition for Growth Summit in London in 2013, a commitment for US$ 4.15 billion for directly tackling undernutrition and an additional estimated $19 billion for improved nutrition outcomes through nutrition-sensitive investments by 2020 were pledged. The *Power of Nutrition*, a partnership between the Children's Investment Fund Foundation, UBS Optimus Foundation, the UK Department of International Development, UNICEF and the World Bank Group, aims to 'unlock' up to $1 billion new private and public financing for nutrition. It multiplies each new contribution four times and directs it to supporting and scaling up nutrition programming.

Opportunities Ahead

Given the present HIV/AIDS environment, there seems to be a gap between what is needed to accelerate progress in order to reach the end of AIDS by 2030 and today's global financial and political climate. As described in the UNAIDS investment framework, biomedical interventions and programs such as voluntary medical male circumcision and emphasis on treatment seem to have the strongest evidence to reduce transmission [4] and have been the priority for HIV investments. But important facts are that 22 million people in need are not on treatment; retention on treatment among PLHIV in sub-Saharan Africa after three years has been reported to be 65%; and only 39% of PLHIV know their HIV status [3]. One of the reasons for these staggering statistics is that public health resources are scarce, and as described by Magnani et al., surveillance for HIV has traditionally targeted the easily accessed populations, which in resource-limited settings includes pregnant women seeking antenatal care, those seeking medical care for sexually transmitted diseases and potentially military recruits [14]. A new strategy is required for the so far underserved populations based on context and 'knowing the epidemic.'

For such an approach, organizations and programs that raise awareness, promote and destigmatize testing will be well equipped to reach populations currently not accessed through traditional healthcare platforms. Existing initiatives, beyond those that are focused on HIV as the primary interest, should be approached with an HIV lens to assess how they can also support PLHIV or play a role in the response, either directly or indirectly. Looking ahead, there is a need to fully integrate HIV in health systems, poverty reduction, social protection and other development sectors. One example, related to food and nutrition, is that while in the past, nutrition and food assistance programs were meant to be integrated within the HIV/AIDS response, as per the UNAIDS strategy, today's environment presents a unique opportunity for approaches that focus on making the fields of nutrition and health, among others, more HIV sensitive (detailed description in the following sections). Programs with health care, education, poverty alleviation and other goals beyond HIV can play a pivotal role in targeting the underserved populations.

Another example is PMTCT: It has been acknowledged that the elimination of pediatric AIDS in the coming years is possible, but this would require an integrated and comprehensive approach. This means that the HIV/AIDS treatment and care package needs to be integrated with maternal, newborn and child health care, and family planning services would have to be scaled up substantially [15].

Comprehensively Addressing HIV/AIDS—Treatment and Beyond

The HIV/AIDS movement has experienced enormous success, and it is well positioned to be integrated with other sectors. Greater efforts are needed to ensure the integration of HIV in broad health and development efforts, including removal of parallel mechanisms.

Kim et al. [16] propose a framework to address the shortcomings in global healthcare delivery by applying a system-level analysis to care delivery value chains. Their comprehensive approach proposes to not only integrate stand-alone approaches in the shared delivery infrastructure, but also align these with the local context, including social and economic factors. They emphasize the need for 'diagonal' approaches which incorporate effective disease management with improved health systems versus horizontal or vertical approaches. Their framework includes four components: continuum of care (from prevention and screening to disease management); shared delivery infrastructure to capture synergies in required resources and address multiple health problems; understanding barriers at the community level; and leveraging the healthcare delivery system for economic and social development. They use HIV/AIDS in resource-poor settings as an example to illustrate this framework.

The 'cascade of care' and 'test and treat' concepts provide a useful framework when considering integration of HIV in other sectors [17, 18]. However, before undertaking this, current gaps and the scope of the problem need to be defined. Kranzer et al. [3] have systematically quantified the losses along the continuum of HIV care, i.e., testing, eligibility for initiating ART, pre-ART care, ART and long-term retention, recognizing that the pathway may not be a linear process since the patients may 'cycle in and out of care' as shown in Fig. 30.1.

Applying the factors proposed by Kim et al. to the continuum of care described above, we present a framework (Fig. 30.2) that defines individual-, household-, community- and health system-level considerations in all steps of the HIV cycle of care for a comprehensive response. At each step of the HIV cascade, from transmission to testing, initiation of ART and up to ongoing treatment and disease management, it is instructive to analyze individual-, household-, community- and health system-level factors in order to better prevent losses along the HIV care continuum.

Mugavero et al. [18] have presented a comparable, but distinct framework that shows the complex interplay between individual, relationship, community, health systems and policy factors as part of a 'social-ecological' perspective that impacts the process of engagement through the HIV care continuum. The authors use the framework to make a case for reforming the fragmented healthcare delivery system for HIV in the USA that is wrought with gaps and problems such as limited patient surveillance, lack of linkages between testing and medical services or support services that may be enabling for individuals to remain in care such as substance abuse treatment facilities and housing assistance, funding (e.g., insurance, government programs) and provider reimbursement. The 'case management' for PLHIV is multifaceted and multidisciplinary. If there are existing gaps in resource-rich settings, then these issues are only exacerbated in resource-limited settings.

There are significant losses at each step along the HIV continuum of care

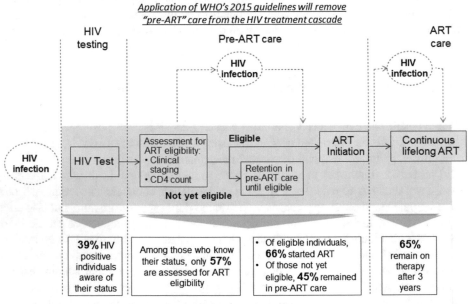

Fig. 30.1 Losses along the HIV continuum of care. From Kranzer et al. [3] (Creative Commons)

Considerations at individual, household, community and health systems levels a comprehensive HIV/AIDS response

	HIV Transmission	HIV Testing	Pre-ART C*Absence of test & treat approach*	ART Initiation & Adherence
Individual level	• Socioeconomic status • Negotiating power, position of women • Medical knowledge, attitude • Medical history, STIs • Condom use/circumcision	• Socioeconomic status • Knowledge of risk factors • Stigma • Cultural beliefs	• Socioeconomic status • Awareness / knowledge of disease progression • Monitoring of indicators • Mental wellness	• Socioeconomic status • Psychological preparedness • Substance abuse • Stigma • Cultural beliefs • Side effects
Household level	• Socioeconomic status • Support, relationships • Cultural beliefs • Education	• Socioeconomic status • Support • Attitude towards accessing health care and HIV testing	• Socioeconomic status • Food & nutrition security • Psychological support	• Socioeconomic status • Food & nutrition • Psychological support • Pressure to share • Cultural beliefs
Community level	• Social norms • Laws, policies • Support • Poverty, unemployment • Education	• Social norms towards health care • Poverty, unemployment • Laws, policies • Support	• Support groups • Community programs • Food assistance • Counseling	• Support groups • Community programs • Food assistance • Counseling
Health systems level	• Preventative facilities • Primary care clinics • PMTCT, prenatal care • Counseling • Access to healthcare • Identification of high-risk individuals • Post exposure (sexual assault)	• Avail. of healthcare • Appropriate testing, sharing results • Treatment availability • Comorbidities, STIs • PMTCT, prenatal care • Identification of others at risk	• Availability of healthcare • Therapies for delaying progression • Managing comorbidities • Patient support • On-going disease management	• Medication, including second/third line • Disease management • Psychological support • Managing comorbidities • Nutrition support

Fig. 30.2 Framework for HIV programming through the cascade of care: considerations at individual, household, community and health systems levels. From Mehra et al. [37]. Reprinted with permission from CRC Press

Our proposed framework (Fig. 30.2) draws on the considerations presented by Mugavero and colleagues, but presents a simple matrix so that each level can be parsed out throughout the care continuum to serve as a model for assessing current initiatives and identifying gaps for future programming in any given context. Although the model presents a holistic framework to address the complexities of the HIV/AIDS response, it is by no means an exhaustive list of considerations. The 4 × 4 matrix is meant to serve as a conceptual model that can be used to operationalize various aspects within a program as well serve as a point of reference to assess where there are gaps for how a particular program fits in the larger HIV/AIDS response. The framework is meant to be flexible and adjustable based on the context and 'knowing the epidemic.' For example, health system-level strengthening is more impactful for PMTCT versus the focus on individual-level issues for injecting drug users in areas of concentrated epidemics.

The framework is designed to provoke precise thinking and definitions for loosely used terminology or catchall phrases such as 'community' or 'stigma' or 'social norms.' For example 'community' may refer to the immediate geographical vicinity of where PLHIV may reside, but it could also mean virtual communities [19] or community support groups built around treatment facilities, if these happen to be away from where someone lives. Similarly, stigma could be present at the individual, community and policy levels (shown only at individual level in the framework, Fig. 30.2) impacting the testing, pre-ART care and ART adherence stages in the HIV cascade. Understanding and defining these concepts in a precise manner allows the identification of enabling (or disabling) factors that ultimately impact good HIV outcomes and support disease management. For example, understanding how communities can be effectively leveraged to support health systems and services can be very powerful for not only reducing some of the burden on the health systems, but also making linkages with 'hard-to-reach' vulnerable populations.

Lastly, this framework encourages simultaneous thinking on supply and demand side enablers and barriers. To date, supply side or biomedical treatment-focused interventions have been the emphasis. However, given that there is still much to be done, including ensuring that people know their status, eligible people start treatment, people on treatment are retained, and the most vulnerable are being reached, going forward, provision of treatment alone will not be enough; addressing the demand side and uptake factors will be equally important. The lack of focus on the demand side factors is evident in UNAIDS' investment framework, where the 'critical enablers' and 'synergies with the development sectors' have not been fully operationalized, at least in terms of guidance for programming [20]. This has led to a vicious circle: the enablers and barriers in the investment framework were not precisely defined likely due to the lack of robust evidence, and now HIV funding and programming, which is based on the investment framework that has a biomedical/treatment focus, further precludes gaining expertise and generating evidence in this area.

Application of the Matrix Framework

HIV Transmission

At the individual and household levels, several factors may be responsible for HIV transmission. Given that transmission is inextricably linked to poverty and inequality, low socioeconomic status and food insecurity could easily result in resorting to risky coping behavior such as unprotected transactional sex [21]. Women are particularly vulnerable in this situation due to systemic gender inequality, which may also hamper their negotiating power to use condoms. Education has been associated with a lower risk of acquiring HIV infection. Education also impacts an individual's knowledge of HIV/AIDS as well as attitude toward medical care, appreciation of the importance of preventative care and general well-being.

Community-level factors are equally important. These include the external political environment, local policies and laws, in addition to cultural beliefs and attitudes within a community. Cultural norms can determine local laws and, in turn, may perpetuate disabling environments which fail to address HIV. For example, stigma against MSMs or IDUs may result in punitive laws that would likely fail to curb transmission and lead to concentrated epidemics. Community-level considerations may also extend to the local attitude toward preventative behaviors, use of health systems/medical care as well as availability of risk reduction facilities within communities, e.g., availability of condoms, syringe exchange, planned parenthood, resilience building safety nets (to reduce risky coping behavior) that link with health facilities.

Health systems can play an important preventative role. PMTCT, identification of high-risk individuals and counseling would heavily rely on healthcare facilities as the 'point of contact.'

HIV Testing

Only 39% of people infected with HIV are aware of their status [3]. Therefore, it is important to understand the existing barriers for people to get tested. This can be examined both from the supply side and the demand side. On the supply side, the provision of quality health systems and facilities are at the core. But the availability of appropriate health systems (and community health workers) and facilities depend on resources within a society. Furthermore, types of available health services also depend on the level of awareness, attitudes and cultural beliefs within a community.

Only addressing the availability of health systems provides no guarantee that it would alleviate the problem of low testing. Analyzing the demand side is equally important. Individual-level factors such as socioeconomic status including food security, physical health, mental well-being, knowledge and perception of stigma based on cultural beliefs can all act as barriers to HIV testing. The most important community-level barriers may be cultural beliefs, attitude and stigma associated with HIV. This would determine the level of support that can be provided in a community such as support groups and counseling centers. In addition, the cultural beliefs can also be reflected in enabling or punitive local laws and policies.

Pre-ART Care

In the continuum of the HIV care pathway, under the 2013 WHO guidelines testing is followed by assessment of eligibility for ART for those who are diagnosed with HIV. Those eligible for ART should initiate treatment, and those not yet eligible must remain in pre-ART care. Pre-ART is the time period between when a person is tested positive for HIV until when he/she becomes eligible for ART. However, given revised guidelines in 2015 everyone living with HIV at any CD4 cell count should initiate ART. Until these guidelines are widely used globally, there may still be a period where people are in pre-ART care, which has programmatic implications. This includes three groups: (1) those who have been tested for their CD4 count know their result and are not yet eligible for ART, (2) those who have been tested for their CD4 count but do not know the result and (3) those who have not yet been tested for CD4 count but have been diagnosed with HIV. Under the new guidelines, a revised classification for this group could be defined as follows: those who have tested positive for HIV and are hence eligible for ART, but who have not yet initiated ART. This would also include the group of people (under the old guidelines) who have tested positive and are found to be eligible for treatment, but for whatever reason have not (yet) initiated treatment. This would add a fourth group to the 'pre-ART' classification. With the older guidelines, the length of the pre-ART period for the second and third groups could vary depending on the delay between testing positive for HIV infection and obtaining the CD4 count results. A later diagnosis could mean a lower CD4 count and hence a shorter pre-ART period.

Once a person has been tested for HIV, the barriers related to testing, described above, have been overcome. Where the 2015 guidelines are being implemented, testing positive would immediately result into initiating ART, regardless of CD4 count. For places where the 2015 guidelines have yet to be applied, there may be significant challenge in keeping people in pre-ART care [22], despite the fact they have already had some point of contact with the health system, and in theory could enroll and be retained in care immediately after diagnosis. Where applied, the test and treat approach will eliminate several issues related to ART care. Evidence from sub-Saharan Africa from before the 2015 guidelines shows that among those who knew their status, only 57% were assessed for ART eligibility—which means that over 40% of people were lost between the diagnosis and determining their eligibility for ART initiation and of those who were assessed and found eligible, 66% started ART, and of those not yet eligible, only 45% remained in pre-ART care [3].

Until the 2015 guidelines are universally implemented, despite the availability of health services (supply side), individual-level circumstances including discomfort related to the HIV infection and/or unwillingness, whether socioeconomic or stigma/perception related, are playing an important role in 'retention in care' losses. The pre-ART period is complicated from a programmatic perspective. The length of this period is extremely variable and dependent on many factors; starting with the availability of healthcare resources, but also strongly influenced by individual- and household-level barriers to accessing care. Significant losses are occurring in the pre-ART care period, where there is a substantial failure in linking people from diagnosis, to pre-ART care and eventually to ART. The new 2015 guidelines are a critical step in preventing losses during this step.

ART Initiation and Adherence

Initiation of ART largely depends on the success of retaining people in pre-ART care, although 'test and treat'/new WHO guidelines also provides a good model that can be effective in initiation and bypassing the issues related to pre-ART care. Once PLHIV start treatment, adherence is critical for successful outcomes. There are several demand and supply side factors that play an important role not only for starting treatment, but also for adhering to treatment regimens; these need to be appreciated more fully by healthcare providers and policy makers alike. 'Supply side'/healthcare facilities or availability and type of treatment/medication options are of prime importance and have rightly occupied a central focus in the HIV response. But this not enough, as shown by the negative outcome of the 'treatment as prevention' trial in KwaZulu-Natal, South Africa, where uptake of treatment among eligible people, even when readily available, was very low. In addition, as people are on treatment for life (spanning up to decades of treatment for young people starting treatment), adherence to treatment is equally important. Evidence shows that there are significant losses during this phase and therefore there is a need to understand 'demand side' barriers more carefully.

At the individual level, barriers can be economic, psychological and physical. Competing demands on scarce resources and poverty-related barriers such as food insecurity, homelessness and lack of means of transport all negatively impact adherence. Psychological preparedness, stigma and side effects related to medications also deter individuals from adhering to treatment. Factors at the household level may serve as additional 'demand side' barriers. These may include availability of support, interpersonal relationships, attitude toward health care, knowledge of disease, food security, sharing of medication or any form of support received through the government. The community can create an enabling environment that supports adherence. These may include provisions such as support groups, community counseling, food centers and government safety net programs for affected households and a community's knowledge, cultural beliefs and stigma. On the supply side, there are several aspects that can be strengthened beyond the provision of medication. Psychological support, counseling, management of comorbidities and side effects, emphasis on general wellness, therapeutic or supplementary nutrition support may all have an impact on supporting PLHIV to remain on treatment. The long-term costs of people on lifelong ART is an important consideration for health and national systems as PLHIV are living longer and have an increased risk of other chronic diseases [23]. Studies have shown that the risk of liver disease, cardiovascular disease and non-AIDS-related cancers are higher among PLHIV compared to the general population [24]. However, overall, ART is cost-effective as PLHIV on ART can continue to be active in the workforce [25].

Food and Nutrition in HIV Infection

Nutrition and HIV Infection

Nutrition is important at all stages of HIV infection (see also Chap. 20 on HIV and Nutrition by Paranandi and Wanke). HIV affects the immune system, which increases the risk of infections, which increases nutrient needs and at the same time increases nutrient losses and reduces nutrient intake and absorption. This deteriorating cycle can be reduced and reversed using a combination of medical treatment (biological aspect, addressing infection) and food and nutrition support (biological aspect, supporting the body and the immune system, and behavioral aspect, supporting treatment initiation, adherence and retention).

Nutrition and ART

In resource-limited settings, the HIV epidemic is often highest where malnutrition is already prevalent. Many patients first present to the clinic malnourished and with an advanced stage of disease, and malnutrition is also associated with high mortality in the early months of treatment [26–28]. The faster nutritional recovery can be achieved through ART and nutritional support, the greater the possible reduction in mortality.

As PLHIV recover and stay on lifelong treatment, adequate nutrition remains important, but the nature of nutrition challenges becomes more related to non-communicable disease (NCDs) (see Chap. 20). While many PLHIV may have been at risk of these conditions irrespective of their HIV infection, the suppressed infection as well as ongoing treatment may further increase their risk [29]. A healthy diet can contribute to managing these conditions, and regular monitoring is important. In more affluent societies, food-insecure people have a higher risk of a poor-quality diet, which increases their risk of NCDs [30].

The negative impact of HIV infection on nutritional status can be halted by ART and treatment of opportunistic infections (OIs), but for nutritional status and health to improve, people will also need to consume a balanced diet that provides the required nutrients.

An adequate nutrient intake is essential to all PLHIV before and during ART, and during early as well as later phases of treatment, in any setting. For this reason, nutrition education as well as regular assessment of nutritional status, food consumption practices and counseling tailored to individual needs is important for all PLHIV. In addition, some PLHIV may require specific food and nutrition support to treat malnutrition, i.e., rebuilding tissues (muscle mass and fat mass) and restoring bodily functions, ensure adequate nutrient intake to maintain health and nutritional status and/or support continued access and adherence to treatment and care. Where PLHIV cannot access adequately nutritious commodities, these can be provided in-kind or in the form of commodity-specific vouchers. Most care and treatment programs that include a nutrition component provide nutrition assessment and counseling, and where food support is provided, this is prioritized for malnourished PLHIV starting ART.

Enablers play an important role in increasing ART uptake and initial adherence, and as such are important for promoting universal access to treatment. Whether or not food and nutrition support have an impact on treatment success depends on many factors such as the context, clinical status of the individual, disease progression, adherence to treatment, type of food supplement and nutrient intake [31].

Applying the Matrix Framework to Food and Nutrition Assistance— Opportunities for Programming

As described in the beginning of the chapter, HIV in the coming years will likely be integrated in many sectors, and therefore, it is critical to look at food and nutrition interventions beyond just food assistance and within the broader context of structural interventions. The proposed framework (Fig. 30.2) provides a systematic way of thinking through nutrition and food assistance interventions in a holistic way; these could be HIV specific or sensitive. Figure 30.3 illustrates food and nutrition interventions at the community and health systems levels throughout the HIV continuum of care.

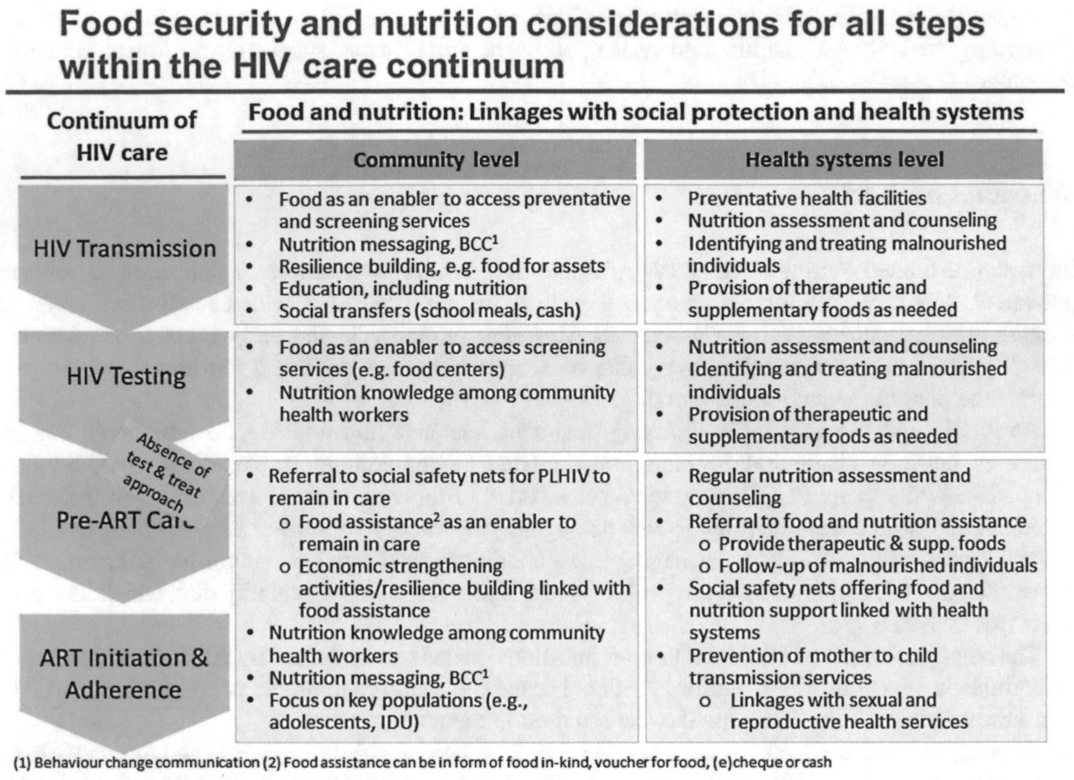

Food security and nutrition considerations for all steps within the HIV care continuum

Continuum of HIV care	Food and nutrition: Linkages with social protection and health systems	
	Community level	**Health systems level**
HIV Transmission	• Food as an enabler to access preventative and screening services • Nutrition messaging, BCC[1] • Resilience building, e.g. food for assets • Education, including nutrition • Social transfers (school meals, cash)	• Preventative health facilities • Nutrition assessment and counseling • Identifying and treating malnourished individuals • Provision of therapeutic and supplementary foods as needed
HIV Testing	• Food as an enabler to access screening services (e.g. food centers) • Nutrition knowledge among community health workers	• Nutrition assessment and counseling • Identifying and treating malnourished individuals • Provision of therapeutic and supplementary foods as needed

Absence of test & treat approach
Pre-ART Care
	• Referral to social safety nets for PLHIV to remain in care
	  o Food assistance[2] as an enabler to remain in care
	  o Economic strengthening activities/resilience building linked with food assistance
	• Nutrition knowledge among community health workers
	• Nutrition messaging, BCC[1]
	• Focus on key populations (e.g., adolescents, IDU)
		• Regular nutrition assessment and counseling
		• Referral to food and nutrition assistance
		  o Provide therapeutic & supp. foods
		  o Follow-up of malnourished individuals
		• Social safety nets offering food and nutrition support linked with health systems
		• Prevention of mother to child transmission services
		  o Linkages with sexual and reproductive health services

ART Initiation & Adherence		

(1) Behaviour change communication (2) Food assistance can be in form of food in-kind, voucher for food, (e)cheque or cash

Fig. 30.3 Food and nutrition interventions at the community and health systems levels throughout the HIV continuum of care. From Mehra et al. [37]. Reprinted with permission from CRC Press

Four main areas of focus emerge: food security and nutrition for adherence and retention in care; social protection linkages, e.g., livelihood support relevant for all stages within the HIV continuum of care; key populations; and an emphasis on linkages with sexual and reproductive health and maternal, newborn and child health.

Role of Food Security and Nutrition for Adherence

Realizing that food insecurity and poverty are important barriers to seeking a diagnosis and to starting and adhering to care and treatment, several programs provide food assistance to food-insecure PLHIV [32], which basically offset the opportunity costs of accessing treatment and compensates for the loss of income and livelihood following prolonged illness. This type of support often comes in the form of foods for the family, such as staple foods, beans or lentils, and vegetable oil, but may also come in the form of vouchers for foods or transport, or as cash. It is important to note that when PLHIV receive nutritious foods for treating malnutrition, this also supports their adherence to care and treatment.

The role of food security and nutrition as related to adherence to treatment and retention in care has been extensively reviewed by de Pee et al. [32]. Conditional food assistance among food-insecure populations was found to be an effective strategy for improving adherence. In a number of studies reviewed, food assistance was conditioned upon visits to clinic or pharmacies. As discussed by the authors, food assistance and nutrition support play a dual role for HIV: a biological intervention and/or an enabler to modify behavior that impacts adherence to treatment. While the biological

F&N impact on adherence to treatment through behavioral & biological pathways

Levels of engagement	Food and Nutrition Assistance as Enablers for Adherence to Treatment	
	Behavioural	**Biological**

Community level	• Establish social safety nets serving PLHIV (HIV sensitive / HIV specific)
	  o Food assistance[2] as an enabler to remain in care – short/medium term
	  o Economic strengthening activities linked with food assistance– longer term
	  o School feeding / Conditional Cash Based Transfer
	• Nutrition knowledge among community health workers
	• Resilience building, e.g. food for assets
	• Education, including nutrition
	• Nutrition messaging, BCC[2]
		• Linkages of the communities with the health system for longer term solutions
		  o Task shifting – Delegation of tasks to staff with lower qualifications to alleviate burden on health systems in resource limited settings (e.g. Nutrition Assessment and Counseling, NAC)
		  o Referral through community workers
		  o Nutrition support centers - community role in food distribution for beneficiaries based on clear entry and exit criteria of malnourished state
		  o Food system (e.g. shops) can handle food when health system decides eligibility

Health systems level	• Linkages with sexual and reproductive health community programs
	• Nutrition messaging, BCC[2]
	• Linkages with government social safety nets with a food assistance component for PLHIV
	  o Example: Referral to resilience building activities
	• Support to pregnant women for the prevention of mother to child transmission
		• Regular nutrition assessment
		• Referral to food and nutrition assistance
		  o Provide therapeutic and supplementary foods
		  o Follow-up of malnourished individuals
		• Nutrition counselling
		• Referral to community health workers for follow up

(1) Food assistance can be in form of food in-kind, voucher for food, (e)cheque or cash (2) Behaviour change communication

Fig. 30.4 Food and nutrition interventions impact adherence to treatment through behavioral and biological pathways: linkages between roles of communities and health systems. From Mehra et al. [37]. Reprinted with permission from CRC Press

intervention aspect is covered by health systems, the enabling environment created by food assistance takes place in the communities of PLHIV (Fig. 30.4). But the interaction and overlap between health systems and communities are imperative since treatment is for life, and health systems are significantly under-resourced and over-stretched. With regard to food support and nutrition, for instance, communities or CHWs can play a role by identifying malnourished PLHIV and conducting Nutrition Assessment and Counseling (NAC) based on criteria established by clinicians. In turn, health systems can link vulnerable PLHIV to safety nets that include a food assistance component (completing the service to NACS—for Support). An example of such a program is described below.

Focus on Social Protection—Adherence and Transmission

PLHIV are often temporarily unable to earn a living and can find themselves in a situation of economic shock that is often also associated with the healthcare costs. The impact on the most vulnerable populations is many fold worse. This situation can quickly lead to increased food insecurity, forgoing treatment, selling off assets or sending children to work instead of school. Food and nutrition assistance is therefore an essential part of a comprehensive HIV treatment and care package. But one of the concerns for food assistance programs has been the issue of sustainability as food support for PLHIV and their families can be very costly. There is increasing interest in exploring options to link PLHIV with economic strengthening activities and livelihood support once they graduate from food support, which is often linked to having recovered from malnutrition. These programs could be specifically for PLHIV or in the form of enrolling in general social protection schemes within a country.

In an initiative funded by multilateral donations and PEPFAR, WFP supports the Ethiopian Health Sector to conduct NACS for acutely malnourished PLHIV in the most underdeveloped regions of the country. During the early treatment period, food-insecure families of malnourished PLHIV receive a monthly voucher or cash allocation. Following recovery of nutritional status, clients transition from the monthly voucher or cash support to an economic strengthening program (ES), where they are trained to run a small business to boost their food security and prevent them from re-lapsing into malnutrition. During the initial period of the ES program, food-insecure PLHIV also receive a monthly food voucher or cash. In addition, food-insecure HIV-positive pregnant women as well as orphans of PLHIV receive a monthly food voucher or cash, conditioned to the adherence to PMTCT services or school attendance, respectively. Ethiopia's national HIV and AIDS authority (F/HAPCO) oversees services run by health facilities, community organizations and consumer associations. The food support component is funded by the Network of PLHIV (NEP+).

With regard to HIV transmission, it has been found that social protection (cash transfers) can play an important role in addressing 'structural drivers' associated with HIV infection risk such as poverty, food insecurity, lack of education [33]. Randomized controlled trials (RCTs) conducted in Tanzania and Malawi showed that cash transfers (conditional or unconditional) to adolescent girls were associated with lower risky behavior such as a reduction in age-disparate sex/'sugar daddy' phenomenon, lower HIV prevalence and higher proportion of negative results on tests for sexually transmitted infections [34, 35]. These RCTs were carefully implemented by researchers and their partner organizations, and the impact that was found has also been corroborated by national or government social protection entitlements. In South Africa, Cluver et al. examined the impact of the child support grant on various risky behaviors among adolescents such as prevalence of transactional sex, age-disparate sex, unprotected sex [36]. The household receipt of the child support grant was found to be associated with reduced incidence of transactional and age-disparate sex, showing that these transfers can reduce risky behavior by adolescent girls [36].

Focus on Key Populations

UNAIDS' new strategy, embedded in the SDGs framework, is a testament to the new realities of the AIDS epidemic and calls for a new phase in the response. To achieve the goals of the SDGs, the response has to ensure that people who have been thus far 'left behind' due to growing poverty and inequality, migration and humanitarian crises are all included in the response. High-risk populations, including key populations (people who inject drugs, transgender people, prisoners, gay men and other men who have sex with men and sex workers) and other vulnerable groups such as adolescent girls who are disproportionately affected by HIV/AIDS must receive special attention in the AIDS response. While HIV-sensitive social protection interventions have the capacity to impact transmission and adherence, these programs often do not reach key populations who are often marginalized, sometimes criminalized and live in contexts of increased poverty, financial instability and social exclusion.

Most of the barriers related to key populations are not rooted in the health systems, but have to be addressed at the individual, household and community levels. Enabling environments, devoid of punitive laws and discriminatory policies toward key populations is the first step. Next, all linkages between communities and health systems for effective interventions have to be made using an equality and human rights lens, with a particular focus on sexual and gender minorities.

Focus on Maternal Newborn and Child Health

Since 2000 (until 2015), over 70% of women have received ART to stop MTCT, a noteworthy achievement, given that only 36% of women received treatment in 2009 and only 1% in 2000.

In order to further reduce the number of new infections among children, linkages of preventative strategies such as family planning services with reproductive health services (antenatal care, post natal care) along with access to HIV testing, treatment and counseling and a deeper understanding of demand side barriers will be essential.

There is an opportunity to leverage MNCH programs and a role for community engagement for the integration with health systems. Looking beyond traditional service delivery, an interesting example is the Philani Child Health and Nutrition Project serving the informal settlements in the Eastern Cape, South Africa, home for close to 1 million people. The community-based non-governmental organization provides basic child health and nutrition to communities wrought with poverty, unemployment, poor housing, child malnutrition and diseases. Philani programs incorporate home-based care, antenatal programs, nutrition support and counseling and skills training (livelihood support). There are approximately 30% HIV-positive pregnant women in Philani's target communities (in 2014), and therefore, all their programs have an HIV lens when providing education, care and support.

From a perspective of community/health systems linkages, two aspects are noteworthy. First, there are opportunities in resource-limited settings to establish referral loops between communities and health facilities. Philani's 'mothers-to-be' and 'mentor mothers' programs provide support to women during and after their pregnancies to ensure good nutrition for them and their children. The community workers (chosen from the same communities and trained) are active in referring the women and children to appropriate health services as needed. In turn, the local health facilities/doctors may also refer discharged patients to the community workers for follow-up monitoring and provision of care. Second, despite the present efforts, much more can be done for PMTCT and pediatric HIV by leveraging the outreach of community workers to actively look for pregnant women and monitor children. Philani's experience shows that often they are the first point of contact for HIV-positive children and their mothers and for HIV-positive pregnant women in the communities they serve and are then able to link them to local health services for treatment. Nutrition and child health are entry points for Philani's programs.

Conclusion

While it is now possible to envision a world with 'zero new infections' and 'zero AIDS-related deaths,' based on significantly improved treatment, which also underlies the rhetoric around 'the end of AIDS,' much remains to be done. Under the revised WHO guidelines, over 22 million PLHIV who are eligible for ART do not have access yet and 17 million people do not yet know that they are infected. A large number of eligible people in need of ART do not start treatment because of low rates of testing, and losses that occur between the diagnosis of HIV and initiation of treatment. Issues of retention in ART programs and long-term adherence to treatment care regimens have often been ignored. Therefore, programs that achieve high retention rates and good long-term adherence are needed and can serve as models for other programs.

The successes achieved and lessons learned now will pave the way for future work in the field of HIV/AIDS. Emphasis on girls and women and key populations, in addition to integrating HIV care in health systems, will have to be the focus. While treatment needs to play a central role in the response, if truly getting to 'zero new infections' is the goal, demand side barriers such as poverty, food insecurity, stigma and perceptions need to be carefully understood and overcome. Opportunities of integration beyond health systems, i.e., with national social protection schemes, child grants, livelihood support and resilience building are essential in ensuring sustainability and adherence to care and treatment. The role of social protection contributing to HIV prevention needs to be further leveraged. Transfers/social assistance has the ability to reduce food insecurity along with other poverty-related drivers of risky sexual behavior, which is particularly relevant for key populations such as adolescent girls. Partnerships (the focus of SDG 17) have been the key to the successes achieved so far, and partnerships will be instrumental in continuing to address the epidemic going forward.

Discussion Points

- Explain why the linkages between communities and health systems will be essential for reaching the End of AIDS by 2030.
- Discuss the possible forms and roles of Support in addition to Nutrition Assessment and Counseling (i.e., expanding NAC to NACS).
- Discuss the scalability, affordability and sustainability of HIV-sensitive social protection.
- What demand and supply side interventions can help reduce transmission of HIV among adolescent girls?
- Apply the matrix framework (Fig. 30.1) in the context of emergencies (e.g., natural disaster, conflict, refugees camps).

Acknowledgments This chapter has been adapted from Mehra et al. [37]. Adapted with permission from CRC Press.

References

1. UNAIDS. AIDS by the numbers 2015. Joint United Nations Programme on HIV/AIDS (UNAIDS). 2015.
2. UNAIDS. How AIDS changed everything. MDG6 report. 2015.
3. Kranzer K, Govindasamy D, Ford N, Johnston V, Lawn SD. Quantifying and addressing losses along the continuum of care for people living with HIV infection in sub-Saharan Africa: a systematic review. J Int AIDS Soc. 2012;15(2):17383.
4. UNAIDS. Global Report. 2013.
5. WHO. Guideline on when to start antiretroviral therapy and on pre-exposure prophylaxis for HIV. 2015.
6. UNAIDS. UNAIDS Gapt Report. Joint United Nations Programme on HIV/AIDS (UNAIDS). 2014.
7. Karim SS, Karim QA. Antiretroviral prophylaxis: a defining moment in HIV control. Lancet. 2011;378(9809):e23–5.
8. UNAIDS. Treatment 2015. 2012.
9. UNAIDS. On the fast track to end AIDS: UNAIDS 2016–2021 strategy. 2015.
10. Cohen J. Science. Large study spotlights limits of HIV treatment as prevention. 2016 [Internet] Updated July 25 2016; cited Sep 2 2016. Available from: www.sciencemag.org/news/2016/07/large-study-spotlights-limits-hiv-treatment-prevention.
11. WHO. Promoting HIV testing among men who have sex with men in China, the 'crowdsourcing' way. 2014.
12. Deeks SG, Lewin SR, Havlir DV. The end of AIDS: HIV infection as a chronic disease. Lancet. 2013;382 (9903):1525–33.
13. Wilson D, Gorgens M. The World Bank Blog. The end of the end of AIDS. 2016 [Internet] Updated Aug 09 2016; cited Sep 2 2016. Available from: https://blogs.worldbank.org/health/end-end-aids.
14. Magnani R, Sabin K, Saidel T, Heckathorn D. Review of sampling hard-to-reach and hidden populations for HIV surveillance. Aids. 2005;19(Suppl 2):S67–72.
15. O'Hiarlaithe M, Grede, N., de Pee, S., Bloem, M.W.. Economic and social factors are some of the most common barriers preventing women from accessing maternal and newborn child health (MNCH) and prevention of mother-to-child transmission (PMTCT) services: A literature review. AIDS Behav. 2014;18:516–30.
16. Kim JY, Farmer P, Porter ME. Redefining global health-care delivery. Lancet. 2013;382(9897):1060–9.

17. Gardner EM, McLees MP, Steiner JF, Del Rio C, Burman WJ. The spectrum of engagement in HIV care and its relevance to test-and-treat strategies for prevention of HIV infection. Clin Infect Dis: an official publication of the Infectious Diseases Society of America. 2011;52(6):793–800.

18. Mugavero MJ, Norton WE, Saag MS. Health care system and policy factors influencing engagement in HIV medical care: piecing together the fragments of a fractured health care delivery system. Clin Infect Dis: an official publication of the Infectious Diseases Society of America. 2011;52(Suppl 2):S238–46.

19. Horvath KJ, Oakes JM, Rosser BR, Danilenko G, Vezina H, Amico KR, et al. Feasibility, acceptability and preliminary efficacy of an online peer-to-peer social support ART adherence intervention. AIDS Behav. 2013;17 (6):2031–44.

20. Schwartlander B, Stover J, Hallett T, Atun R, Avila C, Gouws E, et al. Towards an improved investment approach for an effective response to HIV/AIDS. Lancet. 2011;377(9782):2031–41.

21. Weiser SD, Leiter K, Bangsberg DR, Butler LM, Percy-de Korte F, Hlanze Z, et al. Food insufficiency is associated with high-risk sexual behavior among women in Botswana and Swaziland. PLoS Med. 2007;4(10):1589–97; discussion 98.

22. Rosen S, Fox MP. Retention in HIV care between testing and treatment in sub-Saharan Africa: a systematic review. PLoS Med. 2011;8(7):e1001056.

23. Magoni M, Scarcella C, Vassallo F, Lonati F, Carosi G, Castelnuovo F, et al. The evolving burden of HIV infection compared with other chronic diseases in northern Italy. HIV Med. 2011;12(3):129–37.

24. Phillips AN, Neaton J, Lundgren JD. The role of HIV in serious diseases other than AIDS. Aids. 2008;22 (18):2409–18.

25. Gonzalo T, Garcia Goni M, Munoz-Fernandez MA. Socio-economic impact of antiretroviral treatment in HIV patients. An economic review of cost savings after introduction of HAART. AIDS Rev. 2009;11(2):79–90.

26. Paton NI, Sangeetha S, Earnest A, Bellamy R. The impact of malnutrition on survival and the CD4 count response in HIV-infected patients starting antiretroviral therapy. HIV Med. 2006;7(5):323–30.

27. van der Sande MA, Schim van der Loeff MF, Aveika AA, Sabally S, Togun T, Sarge-Njie R, et al. Body mass index at time of HIV diagnosis: a strong and independent predictor of survival. J Acquir Immune Defic Syndr. 2004;37(2):1288–94.

28. Zachariah R, Fitzgerald M, Massaquoi M, Pasulani O, Arnould L, Makombe S, et al. Risk factors for high early mortality in patients on antiretroviral treatment in a rural district of Malawi. Aids. 2006;20(18):2355–60.

29. Fitch K, Grinspoon S. Nutritional and metabolic correlates of cardiovascular and bone disease in HIV-infected patients. Am J Clin Nutr. 2011;94(6):1721S–8S.

30. Drewnowski A, Darmon N. The economics of obesity: dietary energy density and energy cost. Am J Clin Nutr. 2005;82(1 Suppl):265S–73S.

31. de Pee S, Semba RD. Role of nutrition in HIV infection: review of evidence for more effective programming in resource-limited settings. Food Nutr Bull. 2010;31(4):S313–44.

32. de Pee S, Grede N, Mehra D, Bloem MW. The enabling effect of food assistance in improving adherence and/or treatment completion for antiretroviral therapy and tuberculosis treatment: a literature review. AIDS Behav. 2014;18(Suppl 5):S531–41.

33. Temim M. HIV-sensitive social protection: what does the evidence say?. Geneva: UNAIDS; 2010.

34. Baird SJ, Garfein RS, McIntosh CT, Ozler B. Effect of a cash transfer programme for schooling on prevalence of HIV and herpes simplex type 2 in Malawi: a cluster randomised trial. Lancet. 2012;379(9823):1320–9.

35. de Walque D, Dow WH, Nathan R, Abdul R, Abilahi F, Gong E, et al. Incentivising safe sex: a randomised trial of conditional cash transfers for HIV and sexually transmitted infection prevention in rural Tanzania. BMJ Open. 2012;2:e000747.

36. Cluver L, Boyes M, Orkin M, Pantelic M, Molwena T, Sherr L. Child-focused state cash transfers and adolescent risk of HIV infection in South Africa: a propensity-score-matched case-control study. Lancet Glob Health. 2013;1 (6):e362–70.

37. Mehra D, de Pee S, Bloem MW. Nutrition, food security, social protection and health systems strengthening for ending AIDS. In: Ivers L, editor. Food insecurity and public health. London: Taylor and Francis; 2014.

Part VII
Trends in Urbanization and Development, Impacts on Food Value Chains and Consumers, and Private Sector Roles

Chapter 31
How Urbanization Patterns Can Guide Strategies for Achieving Adequate Nutrition

Sunniva Bloem and Saskia de Pee

Keywords Nutrition · Urban development · Food security · Equitable growth · Obesity

Learning Objectives

- Review urban development history and its relationship with agriculture and food system development.
- Explain how recent urbanization trends differ from the past and their implications for food and nutrition security.
- Analyze how city size affects urban food systems, nutrition and poverty.
- Identify what factors besides rural food production can affect urban nutrition.

Introduction

City nutrition problems have largely been ignored by the development community since undernutrition rates have typically been higher in rural areas. Although lower, urban undernutrition rates are still high, with one in four children under the age of five being stunted [1]. Furthermore, there is a growing epidemic of obesity in cities. This epidemic has caused a large shift, including in low- and middle-income countries (LMICs), toward an increased burden of non-communicable diseases such as type II diabetes. Almost two-thirds of people living with diabetes live in cities [2]. By 2030, there will be 2.5 billion more urban inhabitants, mainly flocking to cities in Africa and Asia [3]. Both improved nutrition and sustainable cities have been included as key goals in the new sustainable development goals (SDGs). Goal 11 is to make cities inclusive, safe, resilient and sustainable, and Goal 2 is to create nutritious and sustainable food systems. However, the connection between these two goals and the rest of the SDGs has not been made clear yet. This chapter illustrates how policy

S. Bloem
The Global Alliance for Improved Nutrition (GAIN), Arthur van Schendelstraat 550,
3511 MH Utrecht, The Netherlands
e-mail: sbloem@gainhealth.org

S. de Pee (✉)
Nutrition Division, World Food Programme, Rome, Italy
e-mail: Saskia.depee@wfp.org; depee.saskia@gmail.com

3. de Pee
Friedman School of Nutrition Science and Policy, Tufts University,
Boston, MD, USA

© Springer Science+Business Media New York 2017
S. de Pee et al. (eds.), *Nutrition and Health in a Developing World*,
Nutrition and Health, DOI 10.1007/978-3-319-43739-2_31

makers and program implementers can design better nutrition strategies by analyzing past and current urbanization trends, seize the opportunity of growing cities, particularly those of medium size, and analyze dynamics between food production and access, including infrastructure, markets, global supply chains, local production and rural–urban linkages.

Achieving the Sustainable Development Goals

The individual goals of the SDGs should not be seen in isolation but instead in a comprehensive framework that acknowledges the linkages between all of them (Fig. 31.1). Improving the nutrition of all city inhabitants, especially the urban poor, is essential to achieve good health and well-being (SDG3), reduce inequalities (SDG10) and promote peace, justice and strong institutions (SDG16). Good nutrition reduces morbidity and mortality and can prevent conditions such as neural tube defects. Furthermore, if children do not get the right amount of proteins, vitamins and minerals in the first 1000 days of their life (from conception to their second birthday), they are at risk of reduced cognitive development, which affects them throughout life in terms of poorer performance at school, and lower productivity and lower incomes as adults, as well as increased risk of non-communicable diseases [4]. Improving the nutrition of the most vulnerable city dwellers, especially in the first

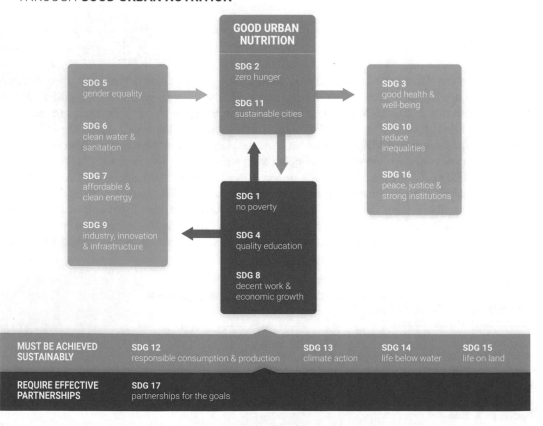

Fig. 31.1 How sustainable development goals support and benefit from good nutrition

1000 days, can have enormous impacts on reducing inequality. Urban children from the poorest quintile are twice as likely to die and three times as likely to be stunted than children from the richest quintile [5]. Providing the urban poor access to healthy foods also has the potential to reduce conflict and political unrest, as food insecurity and high inequality are the cause of many political protests. For example, the 2008 Global Food Crisis led to food riots and protests, mainly in cities, in over 43 countries around the world. These protests led to the Arab Springs in 2010, the dismissal of the Prime Minister in Haiti in 2008 and violent protests in countries such as Burkina Faso, Cameroon, Cote d'Ivoire, Guinea, Honduras, Indonesia, Kenya, Malaysia, Mozambique, Pakistan, Russia, Senegal, Thailand and Yemen [6, 7].

Ensuring everyone can access quality education (SDG4) and decent work in order to stimulate economic growth (SDG8) and eliminate poverty (SDG1) are key steps to improve urban nutrition. Unlike their rural counterparts, urban citizens are more likely to purchase the majority of the food they consume. Furthermore, the urban poor are also more likely to be employed in the informal sector in vulnerable jobs with low and unstable pay. Thus, through better education and higher and more stable income, they would be more likely to have the knowledge and means necessary to purchase healthy, nutritious, foods. Additionally, improving the nutrition of poor urban citizens early on in their life can be a great tool to improve educational levels attained by urban populations as they will be better able to learn by the time they start school. This increases their chances of finding decent work and escaping the poverty trap.

Realizing gender equality (SDG5), clean water and sanitation (SDG6), affordable and clean energy (SDG7) and improved infrastructures (SDG9) all help improve urban nutrition. However, rapid urbanization can both enable and disable progress toward these goals. We need to design cities in a way that enables the achievement of these goals in a nutrition-sensitive manner. Many women who move to cities feel more empowered than in rural areas, even when inequities still exist. We need to accelerate women's empowerment and reduce gender inequalities. Women who are in charge of their household's resources are also more likely to invest in their children's nutrition. Empowering adolescent girls can help delay early marriage, improve their nutrition and increase the likelihood for mothers to give birth to healthy babies. Rapid urbanization in low-income nations has led to many poor urban dwellers moving to slums with poor water and sanitation, little access to energy and poor infrastructures. Improving informal settlements can allow urban residents to be less at risk of diseases such as diarrhea, which reduces nutrient uptake. Furthermore, when households and businesses frequented by poor residents have access to, preferably clean, energy they are also more able to access fresh nutritious foods through refrigeration technologies. Additionally, improving transport infrastructures through roads and public transport can reduce traffic congestion and thus food waste. However, all of these factors are also affected by economic development and education which in turn are affected by nutrition.

The global goals of consuming and producing in a responsible manner (SDG12), sustainably using the oceans (SDG14), sustainably managing forests and land and halting biodiversity loss (SDG15) and mitigating climate change (SDG13) highlight that we must improve urban nutrition in a sustainable manner. Good nutrition is associated with a diverse diet, which is resource intensive. If the 5 billion people living in cities by 2030 are to access healthy, nutritious, foods such as fish, chicken, fruits and vegetables, we must make food production more efficient and green. The food system contributes 19–29% of total greenhouse gas emissions and half of that is after the food has left the farm [8]. We have to connect cities with surrounding farmlands in more efficient manners and find innovative production, distribution and storage techniques. This can reduce the impact of the entire food system on climate change and environmental degradation while still improving nutrition of the cities' poor. In order to achieve these global goals, the status quo needs to be altered. It is, therefore, that SDG17 highlights the importance of building global partnerships. The global goals are interrelated, and creating multi-stakeholder partnerships is essential to achieving them. This is clearly evident when evaluating how to improve urban nutrition.

Table 31.1 City size classifications

Type of city	Population size
Megacities	>10 million
Large	1–10 million
Medium	500,000–1 million
Small	<500,000

Urbanization Patterns

The rapid rate of urbanization in Asia and Africa is unparalleled. Cities in East Asia grew to population sizes in 10 years that it took half a century for European cities to attain [9]. The world reached a historic land mark in 2008 when the population became predominantly urban versus rural. Two-thirds of the global population will be urban by 2030, and 90% of that growth will take place in LMICs [3].

Nearly half of the urban population lives in small-sized cities, and one in eight people in the world live in the globe's megacities (see Table 31.1 for number of people of different-sized cities) [3]. There are currently a greater number of megacities located in Africa and Asia than in any other region in the world. However, the fastest growing cities in these regions (in terms of proportional increase) for the next 15 years will be large-sized cities with populations under 5 million and medium-sized cities [3].

Cities are sometimes characterized as the enemy in development. Over two-thirds of greenhouse gas emissions and global waste are created by cities despite them only inhabiting 2% of global land [10]. Rapid urbanization and limited planning and housing has led 828 million people to move to slums [11], and this figure could rise to 2 billion by 2030 if actions are not taken [12]. However, cities should also be seen as a great opportunity. They can generate enormous amounts of wealth and economic growth (70% of global domestic product) [9]. Every country in the world that is classified as high income is highly urbanized. Thus, the question policy makers should ask is not how to prevent further urbanization but instead how to make urban growth more equitable and sustainable for the cities themselves and their surrounding hinterlands?

Considering the majority of the large urban infrastructures of the swiftly emerging cities in LMICs will be built in the next two to three decades [9], it is clear policy makers must answer this question now. This can be done by analyzing urban development history of high-income countries and larger cities that have already developed in LMICs, urbanization trends, globalization, rural–urban linkages, innovative new technologies and putting both an environmental lens and a poverty alleviation lens, including health, on all initiatives. Medium-sized cities have been found to potentially generate more equitable growth than other sized cities, and they are also one of fastest growing cities. This chapter will outline why seizing the opportunity today with these medium-sized cities and ensuring they develop in a more effective manner can help create healthier and better nourished urban populations.

Nutrition Analysis of Cities

Global Nutrition Status

Whether it be overweight and obesity or undernutrition or both (termed the double burden of malnutrition), almost every nation is dealing with a nutrition problem according to The Global Nutrition Report [13]. Poorer nations are particularly at a disadvantage as they tend to be the countries that suffer from the double burden of malnutrition. Almost 2 billion adults are overweight or obese, thus bringing rates to epidemic proportions. These proportions are currently only rising and not decreasing

[13]. Furthermore, overweight and obesity are drivers of non-communicable diseases such as cardiovascular disease and type II diabetes and 66% of people with type II diabetes live in cities [2]. One in four children and adults were stunted during their childhood and 159 million children currently are stunted despite rates having decreased during the past 15 years [14]. "Hidden hunger," i.e., deficiencies of vitamins and minerals, affects almost 2 billion people, including people with undernutrition as well as people with overweight or obesity. This malnutrition does not just have implications for the health status of billions but also has severe economic costs. Medically treating obesity and associated diseases can consume up to 1/5 of healthcare budgets, while in LMICs preventing malnutrition by investing one dollar can deliver up to a 16 dollar return [13].

Global Urban Nutrition Status

The nutrition of poor city dwellers in LMICs, however, has for a long time been ignored and has predominantly been considered a rural issue [15]. This is due to a range of factors. The high level of inequality in cities and predominance of statistics calculating the average wealth and well-being of residents has led to a neglect of the plight of the urban poor in general by the development community and led to a focus on a perceived more vulnerable, poor rural base. However, many low-income urban residents can be as disadvantaged and in some cases more disadvantaged than their rural counter parts. Furthermore, gathering data that capture the diversity among the urban population is more complex compared to collecting representative data in rural areas. This has made understanding the nutrition problem in cities particularly difficult. However, new evidence has shown that despite rural rates being higher (around one in three), one in four under-fives in cities still suffer from stunting. Stunting rates in South Asian cities are as high as 39% (rural rates are 49%), and in sub-Saharan African cities, they are 30% (rural rates are 39%) [1]. Furthermore, those who are affected by stunting when they are young are more likely to become obese and suffer from non-communicable diseases as they get older. This is especially true if they gain access to processed foods that are high in fat, sugar and/or salt that are relatively cheap and easy to purchase in urban markets [16].

Due to the obesity epidemic facing both rich and poor countries, policy makers have now started to realize that urban nutrition problems require urgent attention. Cities have become places where people easily gain weight because they lack public spaces for exercise, promote more sedentary lifestyles and have food markets and retailers that often sell fried, fatty and unhealthy foods, thus making the world's urban areas obesogenic environments [17]. Data from 2010 showed that among South Asian city dwellers prevalence of obesity was 18% while it was 10% among the rural population and in sub-Saharan Africa these prevalences were 32 and 16%, respectively [18]. Global diets have changed and this change has largely been associated with urbanization. Due to easier access to markets, the industrialization of food and busy city lifestyles with long commutes, people have switched from traditional diets with more fresh foods to more convenient pre-prepared foods and more long lasting processed foods that can have high-fat, sugar and salt contents [16, 19, 20]. In addition to these foods being more convenient, LMICs have weak infrastructures for connecting rural and urban areas, which makes it more difficult to transport and store fresh foods at a low cost. Furthermore, the production of fresh foods in rural areas may be limited. Thus, poor urban consumers often find it difficult to access less processed and more, and a greater variety, of fresh foods. This dietary transition has been a driver of the obesity epidemic.

While easy access to processed foods high in sugar and/or fats fuels the obesity epidemic, food processing also offers an opportunity to add value, for example in the form of fortification, to monitor and ensure greater food safety and to extend shelf life. Greater access to animal source foods and processed, fortified, foods for older infants and young children in urban areas, including among the poor, may explain the lower prevalence of stunting in that population (32–34%) as compared to rural areas (42–36%) in Indonesia between 1999 and 2003 [21]. In Bangladesh, stunting prevalence among under-fives in urban slum areas between 1990 and 2000, however, was higher (76–62%) than among rural children (71–55%) [22]. This difference between Indonesia and Bangladesh may possibly be explained by the different level of development of the two countries in the specific time periods, which greater availability and access to animal source and processed foods in urban areas of Indonesia as compared to Bangladesh, and possibly also by different water, sanitation and hygiene situations of slum dwellers in both countries during those periods.

Consumption Trends in Cities

One distinguishing factor that separates urban food and nutrition security from rural areas is the importance of food purchasing. Despite the existence of urban agriculture, city dwellers are less able to produce their own food and spend up to 70% of their income on food in low- and middle-income countries. This makes them and their nutritional status particularly vulnerable to price and income shocks [15, 23, 24]. Low-income city dwellers of low- and middle-income countries can be more foreign trade dependent for their food purchasing and are thus more affected by global price shocks. When prices are volatile, the quality of the diet suffers because in times of high prices families often have to replace more nutritious foods with cheaper staples that provide fewer essential nutrients. For example, the prevalence of anemia among children in urban areas in Indonesia increased after the 1998 Asian economic crisis because the quality of their diets reduced [25].

In addition to the obesity epidemic, global food price shocks have played a big role in bringing attention to food and nutrition security issues of the urban poor. This is because food price shocks pose a political security risk. The 2008 global food price shocks have been highlighted as a catalyst for the protests in the Middle East in 2010 known as the Arab Spring, led to the dismissal of the Prime Minister in Haiti in 2008 and led to further food riots and protests in over 43 countries across the globe [6, 7]. Researchers have found that due to globalization and urban resident's easy access to these international markets that it is not food shortages per se but rather food access that causes food insecurity. In order to achieve inclusive urbanization, policy makers must improve access to healthy and affordable foods [26–28].

To generate the political action necessary and create more effective policies and programs, better data must be collected to reveal the complexity and severity of urban malnutrition and unearth the specific dynamics. One reason data have been particularly poor is because low-income city dwellers tend to inhabit informal settlements and are employed in the informal sector. Data from the informal economy are particularly problematic to gather because they fall outside of the realm of the "legal" formal sector. Gathering data on informal food purchasing or food security of people participating in the informal sector is even more difficult or under-prioritized [15, 29, 30].

In-depth analyses that incorporate factors such as wealth, location, gender and migrant status and their relationship with food and nutrition security of urban populations are limited. Despite the need for better data, there have been a number of studies that highlight some general trends. These findings include the fact that low-income households in cities tend to buy small quantities at a time instead of larger "bulk" purchases as their income is low and tends to fluctuate and they do not have good storage capacity. Those who do make bulk purchases tend to do it on a monthly basis and mainly buy staple foods that have a relatively long shelf life. Both informal and formal markets have started to cater for the needs of the urban poor consumers. Many small shops and street vendors can be found to buy large or normal size packages and repackage them into smaller units at a more affordable but higher than purchasing value price. Larger formal manufacturers have also now understood the purchasing power of the bottom of the pyramid due to the sheer quantity of customers and also started making smaller units of their products for retailers such as street stalls to sell to these urban consumer groups. With regard to retail, a large proportion of foods sourced by low-income urban citizens of low- and middle-income countries still tend to come from informal markets. However, this is rapidly changing as the growth of supermarkets continues to soar in these regions [31]. Another common place where city dwellers source food is from street vendors that sell ready to eat meals. They are often located in places of residence (slum areas), near transport or work sites of low-income urban workers and are considered convenient both in location and because it significantly cuts down on time to be spent on preparing food by the consumer who can be quite time constrained. Up to 2/5 of a household's food budget can be spent on food purchases away from home [30]. Time constraints affect many people whether in high-, middle- or low-income countries. For example, people in the USA, a country with one of the highest obesity rates in the world, spend on average only 30 min per day on preparing meals (including cooking and cleaning), which is the lowest among all OECD countries. Furthermore, only 51% of the population participates in cooking and cleanup [32].

Southern African Urban Food Security and Consumption Trends
One research institution that has tried to capture food consumption patterns of the urban residents of southern African cities is the African Food Security Urban Network. They have found that food insecurity for low-income urban populations can be devastatingly high (up to 80%) [28]. Urban poor households tend to purchase food from a mix of retailers including informal and formal supermarkets. However, informal retailers are frequented more often for day-to-day purchases while supermarkets are only sought out by low-income city dwellers once a month to purchase staples in bulk. Supermarkets located in areas more easily accessible by low-income segments of the urban population were also found to stock more unhealthy foods than those found in wealthy areas [57]. Thus, accessing healthy foods can be extremely hard for poor urban citizens and their dietary diversity was extremely low. Furthermore, purchasing patterns are made even more complex by the fact that formal retails have been found to source foods from informal wet markets, while informal vendors can also source foods from supermarkets. Additionally, formal supermarkets have even been found to sell food products at a lower cost than smaller informal retailers but are not frequented as often by low-income urban households because they may be located far away and inconvenient to get to [55].

Policies to improve the nutritional status of people living in citizens in LMICs must work with both the formal sector and the informal sector. However, where this balance should lie is difficult to say. The informal sector is still one of the main sources of food for urban residents especially those most vulnerable. Furthermore, it provides a substantial number of jobs for the urban poor. After decades of persistent existence and even growth it is clear this sector is unlikely to diminish and hence cannot be ignored any longer. However, supermarkets can be easier to regulate for food safety and may also sell less expensive products. Food safety is of the utmost importance because it can lead to adverse conditions such as diarrhea that can interfere with nutrient intake and utilization. Effective nutrition policies are even more difficult to formulate, considering the complex interaction between the formal and informal sector. Thus, understanding urban food systems in a city is critical to designing effective policies.

Urban Development

Urban food systems cannot be analyzed without analyzing urban development. Utilizing the vast wealth of urban development theory, the field that investigates urbanization dynamics can help shed light why urban food systems have developed the way they have and what potential solutions may be most effective. Though the density of cities and its associated general positive and negative externalities can be common across urban areas, cities are also unique and its features such as its country's national gross domestic development, the city's economic growth, geography and size can have major impacts on the food system. Analyzing these heterogeneities, particularly city size, can elucidate many of the issues facing urban food systems and suggest good entry points to improve urban food systems and nutrition.

Urban development theorists have founded two main theories that deal with city size. The first theory posits that the bigger a city is the more likely it will generate economic growth due to agglomeration economy theories and theories of economies of scale. The second is the notion that more equitable growth can be created when secondary towns are invested in versus larger cities. Recent analysis in Asia and Africa has shown that in particular medium-sized cities are large enough to exhibit both economies of scale and inclusive growth seen in secondary towns due to stronger rural–urban linkages.

Urban Development History

Cities are sometimes characterized as the enemy of or at least unrelated to agriculture; however, historically they have always developed in conjunction [33]. Cities were only able to come into existence when farmers were able to generate a surplus of food. Once people did not have to participate in the agricultural sector and only produce at subsistence level they were able to engage in non-farming activities. These people began new pursuits such as political administration, ceremonial and religious practices, craft production, marketing and trading, all of which benefit from agglomeration. Thus, people started to form towns. Initially these towns remained relatively small in size. Urban and economic growth was limited due to the Malthusian Trap where population sizes would collapse every time the food supply was not sufficient for feeding the population due to land limitations. However, the Industrial Revolution changed all of this because innovation and new technological tools allowed for agriculture to become more efficient and manufacturing activities conducted in cities more productive. Furthermore, these new breakthroughs were constantly being improved upon and the constant flow of innovation allowed cities to continue to grow, rural areas despite limited land to continue supplying enough food due to improved productivity, and people to continue benefiting from the same standard of living and even increasing it while improving their nutrition and health status.

Primate Cities

This historical trajectory of cities developing in tandem with agriculture was different, however, for low- and middle-income countries. This is because the Industrial Revolution also generated another new phenomenon: colonization and eventually globalization. New, faster and more efficient transportation allowed food supply chains to become longer than they ever had before and created a new international division of labor. Cities no longer had to be dependent on local agricultural productivity and cities in Africa and Asia under colonial regime were able to form without adequately developed national food sectors. These countries tended to exhibit primate city urbanization trends, meaning that one large city controlled most of the economic power in the country and was the central coordination point for trade. In the 1970s, cities in the global south started to become the new global manufacturing hubs because cities in the global north started deindustrializing.

This theory on the primate city phenomenon is known as Urban Primacy Theory. The theory is largely based on the work of Immanuel Wallerstein and his World Systems Approach and Dependency Theory of the 1970s [34]. Immanuel Wallerstein's World Systems Theory suggests that richer countries, termed "the core," generate their wealth by extracting natural resources including spices, food, diamonds, gold or manufactured goods such as garments from poorer countries, termed "the periphery." The periphery is characterized as having low-income workers and its economic progress is determined by its role in the World's capitalist system. Timberlake expands this theory by showing that urbanization dynamics in the periphery exhibit three main characteristics: (i) excessive urbanization; (ii) increase in tertiary and informal labor sectors; and (iii) urban primacy, i.e., having one large, dominant city [34]. The primate cities in these periphery nations are the central coordination point for extracting resources and sending them to the core. In many cases they were colonial legacies; however, globalization helped to continue this phenomenon of forming one large city versus the more dispersed urbanization pattern that was more common in high-income countries.

Secondary Towns

In the 1950s, post-colonization and after most countries had gained their independence, Import Substitution Industrialization strategies started to become the main driver of urban development. Import Substitution Industrialization strategies tend to promote urban manufacturing hubs. This is because countries utilizing this strategy want to increase economic growth by developing their local industries and try to balance their trade exports and imports. This focus on industrial and urban development ended in the 1970s when the world was hit by several oil crises and it became apparent that rural poverty had increased significantly [35].

Rapid rural population growth in Africa culminated into too few available agricultural employment opportunities and to the development of more diverse activities in small towns known as—Non-Agricultural Rural Employment (NARE) in the 1990s. These new demographic developments generated new research in the development of secondary towns [36], which was particularly focused on Africa and was significant in shedding new light on the linkages between rural and urban areas and the importance of acknowledging these linkages. These secondary cities were considered effective mechanisms to alleviate rural poverty. This is starkly different from the previous urban development theory focused on primate cities that were seen as mechanisms to generate economic wealth in the form of increasing gross domestic product. The secondary cities could be seen as a poverty alleviation tool for rural hinterlands because their smaller size and location meant they were more connected with the local food systems and were better suited to facilitate agricultural trade, services and processing activities and generate economic diversification through the development of the agricultural industrial sector in cities. In this way these cities can enhance rural productivity and income and generate an effective local urban economy [37]. Rondinelli in 1983 had already identified these characteristics of secondary towns and their potential to (i) deconcentrate urbanization, (ii) reverse polarization, (iii) alleviate some of the problems in larger cities, (iv) reduce regional inequalities, (v) stimulate rural economies and (vi) increase administrative capacity [38]. Though these insights were illustrative, they were not well understood by policy makers and never generated any effective policies in the 1990s [35].

Whether secondary towns can really be tools for reducing rural poverty is a contested topic and is context specific. Secondary towns in countries that have more centralized governments may not have enough resources to stimulate adequate economic and rural development. The public goods required might be too costly. In other circumstances, secondary towns have been shown to be unequal and offer only vulnerable informal work opportunities with low and insecure pay [37]. In other cases, secondary towns may cater more to urban than to rural populations. In Nigeria for example, secondary towns were a prominent place for urban migration from bigger cities that were considered too competitive but were therefore also too competitive for rural populations to access effectively [39]. Policy makers in the 1990s did not understand these complexities very well and thus were unable to produce coherent and adequate policies to create inclusive growth through investments in secondary towns [37].

Megacities

Though urbanization may have become somewhat more dispersed, the legacy of primate cities did not disappear and many of these cities and large secondary towns had become megacities with populations over 10 million people in the 2000s. These unprecedented enormous cities started to generate attention again. Their size and economic wealth was able to form in large part due to international trade. In this way they tended to be more a product of international dynamics than national ones [40]. Globalization allowed these cities to form far faster than the local agricultural sectors. These cities, however, also became home to enormous and vast amounts of informal settlements with poor slum conditions. This is because these cities formed at such a rapid speed with such massive numbers during decades of policies that were anti-urban (more pro-rural development) and promoted limited government intervention (structural adjustment policies). This meant that governments were unable to provide enough public goods, social protection schemes, infrastructures and housing for the influx of people, thus causing them to move to shantytowns [41].

Medium-Sized Cities

In recent years, new research has shown that medium-sized cities can potentially generate more inclusive growth. One study found that the "missing middle" cities, i.e., small-, medium- and large-sized cities, may have had slower growth than megacities during the period of 1980–2010 but they did exhibit more equitable growth. Poverty alleviation was shown to be easier in the "missing middle" cities and they were shown to be more equal [42]. Rural-to-urban migration to "missing middle" cities was also found to be a more effective tool for escaping the poverty trap than to megacities in Tanzania; half of the people who had migrated to "missing middle cities" were able to earn relatively high or middle incomes while only one out of seven people who had moved to megacities were able to escape poverty [43].

The World Bank has published several reports that show the intricacies of urban development among the "missing middle" cities [9, 44, 45]. These papers analyzed the strengths and weaknesses of small-, medium- and large-sized cities and megacities. Small-sized cities were found to lack resources to produce significant economic growth but were good platforms for processing and distribution activities for agricultural produce. Medium-sized cities are considered large enough to benefit from agglomeration theory and are more likely than their smaller counterparts to develop manufacturing industries and economic and equitable growth. Innovation and diversification can typically flourish more in large-sized cities; however, these cities, due to lack of planning, are also often burdened by poor infrastructures and congested traffic. Megacities can often generate the fastest amount of economic growth but are highly unequal. Furthermore, the location of the "missing middle" cities also played a role in their defining features. For example, smaller cities situated in clusters around larger ones might benefit from agglomeration economies but may also fall prey to more congestion [45].

There is no one-size-fits-all solution for urban development problems [46]. Size, location and context all have an impact. Furthermore, cities are not static, they change over time and so must lessons learned and policies. Analyzing these more intricate city dynamics can highlight some current general trends and indicate specific opportunities different cities might pose. For example, innovative policies may be easier to implement in medium-sized cities because their small government can implement new ideas more quickly and their limited resources require them to be more innovative. An interesting example is the city of Solo in Indonesia. Joko Widodo, currently president of Indonesia, started his career as Mayor of Solo. It is widely acknowledged that he helped facilitate a renaissance in Solo through innovative public sector reform such as engaging with street vendors to explore solutions of public space.

Chinese City Dynamics

China has one of the most intricate regulatory frameworks when it comes to rural versus urban policies. Since 1958 they have set up a system that prohibits unregulated movement between rural and urban areas. This system is known as the hukou system [58]. Depending on where you live, you are allocated a "rural or urban hukou" that allows you to be entitled to either rural or urban social services. However, this system did little to mitigate the rapid urbanization and inflow of people from rural areas that took place in the past half century. Unfortunately these rural migrants who often moved to seek better employment opportunities are more disadvantaged than their "urban hukou" carrying counterparts as many public goods were unavailable for them in the city or at least were only available at a higher cost such as education. Attaining formal employment or land rights was also much more difficult. Recognizing that the "hukou system" was not keeping pace with demographic shifts China started to reform the system in 2014. The government agreed to gradually grant 40% of the 250 million rural migrants a new "urban hukou." The majority of these new "hukous," however, were allocated to urban areas that had less than 5 million people [59]. Though the intention of this policy is to promote more balanced urbanization across the country and mitigate some congestion in the massive megacities China is home to, it fails to address why megacities have seen such a rapid influx of rural migrants. Megacities are still seen as more attractive because more resources are invested in these cities, thus creating more perceived or real opportunities [60]. Many nations have tried to ban rural-to-urban migration or blocked land expansion of cities but ended up seeing the formation of informal settlements because they did not address the core of the "problem" that is driving this migration.

The role of public and private investment in cities has a huge role to play in enticing migration and stimulating equitable or unequal growth. In China, it was found that small-sized cities and rural regions benefited from investments in medium-sized cities but were disadvantaged when investments went into megacities [61]. Furthermore, medium-sized cities were found to stimulate more sustainable growth as it stimulated the local economy better when invested wisely [62]. These findings indicate that previous investment in the primate megacities may have negatively affected rural–urban development and the environment and should be investigated to see how investments can be best used. Investing in the newly rising medium-sized cities has the potential to create positive externalities in rural areas, develop healthier urban food systems and produce more sustainable and inclusive growth.

Urban Size, Infrastructure and Food Systems

Climate change will put huge strains on the food system in the next 15 years and on the urban poor that tend to live in the most disaster prone areas that already exhibit poor housing conditions, weak infrastructures and subpar water and sanitation facilities. These strains are being exacerbated by demographic shifts of people moving from farming areas to food import dependent urban areas. Food and nutrition security will be a major tool and challenge for urban development in the next few decades [27]. Cities play a critical role in agricultural production as both the consumer and investor as a large proportion of investments come from rural household members that have migrated to urban areas and send back remittances to help support their family's small-scale farm. These small-scale farmers are very dependent on these cash remittances because they often have very limited access to credit. Furthermore, urban people can also be highly involved in the agricultural supply chain and conduct activities such as transportation, storage, processing, retailing, street vending and whole-saling. Rural–urban linkages are often strongest in small- and medium-sized cities where these cities are centers of trade and production facilities for mechanical tools and other inputs for the farming sector and are also a large consumer base [24]. These analyses of how different-sized cities interact with the food system and how they may affect their residents' nutrition status are important toward achieving both SDG2 (zero hunger and improved nutrition) and SDG11 (sustainable and inclusive cities). This chapter finds that urban nutrition and food security can be affected by the size of a city through its effect on: (1) the existing infrastructure and its relationship with urban nutrition (availability and accessibility of nutritious food, as well as availability of safe drinking water and hygiene situation of the environment) and (2) how food is sourced: international trade and local production, i.e., rural–urban connections.

An Example of Good Municipal Food and Nutrition Policy: Belo Horizonte, Brazil
Belo Horizonte is a large-sized city located in Brazil. Its city center population amassed to around 2 million in 1993 [63] and rose to 2.5 million in 2014. However, including its greater surrounding area, known as Greater Belo Horizonte, it reached to 5.7 million in 2014 making it the third largest city in Brazil [64]. In 1992 Belo Horizonte, with the introduction of a new Mayor, initiated one of the most effective municipal food and nutrition security strategies in the world led by their newly created municipal food supply agency (then called SMAB and now known as SMASAN). This new strategy put into law the right to good quality food for every citizen as a human right in 1993. Its success rests on the fact that it focused not just on calories but also good nutrition, effectively targeted and reached urban poor, and stimulated the local food economy benefiting the city and the region. Initial activities included delivering fortified flour to pregnant women, nursing mothers and young children in poor neighborhoods. This helped to significantly lower under-five child malnutrition rates in the city and allowed the government to focus on other, broader, food and nutrition security targets and activities. This included free food distributions, healthy school meals, subsidized food sales including through public restaurants, price control of food markets ensuring markets sell a range of products at a reasonable price, increasing the range and volume of agricultural production in the nearby rural areas and within the city itself, education for good nutrition practices, support for careers in the food sector, recognizing the use of land for food production and promoting urban and peri-urban agriculture [64]. Despite having 38% of households living in poverty, 18% of children under three malnourished and average child mortality rates of 35.3 deaths per 1000 live births in the early 1990s, Belo Horizonte's municipal food strategy helped to significantly increase the consumption of vegetables, decrease (between 1993 and 2005) the mortality rate of children under five by 72% and practically eliminate undernutrition and hunger [64].

Infrastructure and Its Relationship with Urban Nutrition Status

Food Waste and Cold Chains

Food waste is a serious issue in today's world. Around one-third of total food production is lost globally [27]. Most of the food that is lost tends to be perishable food, rich in vitamins and minerals, such as fruits, vegetables, seafood and other animal source foods. In the next 15 years, there will be 8.5 billion people on our planet [47], thus implying the world food demand will increase by 50% [48]. The severity of current food losses shows that both agricultural productivity and food chain efficiency will have to increase.

Where food waste is best tackled along the food chain depends on a country's income status. Richer countries should focus on the end of the supply chain as most of the food is lost in households or in retailers such as supermarkets. Some of this is driven by "best before" dates that are set at an earlier date than the products' actual shelf life and supermarkets refusing to purchase "ugly" looking but good quality fruits and vegetables. However, in low- and middle-income countries policies to reduce food waste must focus on the beginning of the supply chain to improve production, storage and transportation mechanisms. In low-income countries, most of the food is lost during production, storage and transportation. Distribution infrastructures in these countries are often poor because supply chain actors lack the technology or resources necessary to purchase better facilities such as cold chain infrastructures (refrigeration technologies across the food system). Even when cold chains exist they are often broken. Furthermore, low-income households in urban areas often lack the means to purchase personal refrigerators or do not have access to or the means to pay for the electricity that is required. Thus, these food waste issues are structural. Due to the fact that these urban food system infrastructures are so weak and generate so much food waste, food prices are inevitably higher than they could be, especially for the most nutrient dense products. This makes it even more difficult for low-income urban households to consume a healthy, nutritious diet [24]. Up to 200 million tonnes of food waste could be saved each year if poorer nations had the same cold chain technological capabilities as high-income countries [49]. It is clear that improving cold chain infrastructures in low- and middle-income countries including for the urban poor could have enormous positive impacts on urban nutrition. However, these infrastructures are energy intensive, and in order to take into account climate change and environmental risks, it is of the utmost importance that more efficient and cleaner cold chains are designed quickly. We cannot solve one problem by driving another.

It is undeniable that cold chains are one of the urban nutrition challenges. However, in what way these infrastructures can be improved upon or implemented in the first place, is also dependent on city size. According to an analysis based on the 2012 Demographic Health Survey in Indonesia, the poorest quintile of urban households are more likely to own a refrigerator when living in medium-sized cities (38%) versus small- or large-sized cities or megacities (18–24%, see Table 31.2)

Table 31.2 Poor urban household characteristics in Indonesia by city size

City size		Mega	Large	Medium	Small	Total
Household has refrigerator, %[***]	Yes (%)	18.03	24.19	37.54	22.23	
	frequency	44	105	113	996	
Sample size		244	434	301	4288	5267
Improved water source, %[***]	Yes (%)	48.57	28.80	40.59	23.89	
	frequency	119	125	123	1032	
Sample size		245	434	303	4319	5301

Data were obtained using 2012 Demographic Health Survey for Indonesia raw data and statistical software StataMP 13 [50]

[***]$p<0.01$

Poor urban household defined as belonging to the bottom two wealth quintiles of the Indonesian population

[50]. This finding highlights an opportunity for further research to be conducted to uncover why this may be the case and how to better scale up refrigerator access in cities of different sizes.

Water and Sanitation

Creating better access to improved water and sanitation facilities is a time tested nutrition-sensitive intervention to improve nutrition and is highly recommended by the Scaling Up Nutrition (SUN) Movement [51]. If people consume unhygienic water or live in areas with poor sanitation, they are at risk of contracting illnesses such as subclinical inflammation (environmental enteric dysfunction, EED) and diarrhea. These reduce a person's ability to absorb or utilize vital nutrients. One segment of the population that is at particular risk of contracting these unwanted effects from poor water and sanitation facilities are the urban poor, especially those living in slum areas. Their water and sanitation infrastructures are often so weak because they are often illegally occupying land and governments do not wish to incentivize urban migration by providing adequate sanitation and the high density of their settlements further increases risks. In addition, even in cases of formal poor urban housing, governments are reluctant to invest in sanitation as they are not "flashy" like other public works projects and working with sanitation has a stigma. Use of the world's clean water resources is already being maximized and demographic shifts will increase the pressure on these limited resources. If slum areas are not managed properly including provision of adequate infrastructures, based on the fact that currently slum areas are only expanding and can contaminate existing resources, we put our water supply at even higher risk, thus putting the urban poor in an even more vulnerable position. Furthermore, poor water and sanitation facilities also affect food safety as many informal street vendors utilize the same urban poor's infrastructures [27].

Analysis of city size dimensions of water and sanitation infrastructures in Indonesia shows that poor urban residents living in small- and large-sized cities have poorer access to improved drinking water sources than those living in medium-sized cities and megacities (see Table 31.2) [50]. Megacity poor urbanites tend to fair better in this area because public and private investments, driven by the relatively large upper and middle class, in these cities' infrastructures may also improve areas accessed by poorer urban residents. It is less clear why poor urban citizens of medium-sized cities also fair better; however, it appears to be caused by a more equitable growth that occurs in these types of cities. They are not as poor as small-sized cities that do not have the economic means to build adequate infrastructures and they are not as burdened by rapid unplanned population growth as large-sized cities that tend to have more clunky and congested infrastructures. Furthermore, large cities are often underinvested in compared to their megacity counter parts. Positive lessons learned from medium-sized cities and megacities must be utilized to scale up improved infrastructure access by the urban poor and urban food systems utilized by the urban poor in all size cities. Cities within countries, across regions and across continents should learn from each other and build partnerships and platforms that encourage the dissemination of best practices to improve urban nutrition [52].

Roads and Traffic

Roads are part of the basic building blocks of creating a food system. They are the tools that connect rural areas producing food with cities that consume a great proportion of this food. However, despite their pivotal role, roads are often forgotten in food system discussions and their impacts on nutritional status are largely unrecognized. Policies and programs in the past have focused too much on productivity and yields versus other components of the supply chain such as distribution systems. In many LMICs, distribution systems are hindered by poor road infrastructures connecting farming areas with small-sized cities. These conditions can be so horrendous that transportation times can increase up to 200%. Medium-sized cities are often in a better position than small-sized cities to produce more effective road infrastructures as they can generate enough public funds to do so and it is in the interest of many local private companies. This road infrastructure can help encourage agricultural diversification because food waste is reduced and a larger segment of the population might hence be able to afford more diverse nutritious foods. In this way farmers and urban citizens are more able to improve their diets as it has become economically feasible to produce and purchase more perishable, nutrient-rich foods.

While road infrastructures can be created and expanded more easily in megacities and surrounding areas, these cities are more likely to suffer from traffic congestion which increases distribution times and can in turn be a driver of food waste and thus limit diversification of the food supply. Additionally, diversification of production is also more difficult for local producers as the wholesale markets they sell to are often located in the centers of these megacities where traffic can be at its worst [24]. Slum dwellers are even more disadvantaged than average urban residents because it is harder for transportation vehicles to access these dense slum settlements, thus limiting their local market supply of perishable nutritious foods. Public investment in public transportation systems that reduce traffic and in roads can improve access to a more diverse diet and in that way contribute to improving the nutritional status of people living in cities, especially among the poor whose access is most constraint.

International Trade and Local Production

A higher percentage of net food importing countries are low income versus high income. The number of countries highly dependent on food imports is especially high in Africa [27]. It is clear that international trade will remain a dominant feature in the food sector in the next several decades. Furthermore, large food producers and manufacturers with head offices in the global north play a critical role in affecting access to nutritious foods for people living in cities in LMICs. They make up a significant portion of the food supply in LMICs and have the ability to not just sell unhealthy highly processed, high-sugar, high-fat and/or low-nutrient content foods but also healthier versions of basic products such as fortified staples. The food industry should be encouraged and where necessary supported, for example by tax exemptions, to develop healthy, nutritious products at an affordable price. However, these companies are not just suppliers but are also buyers in the global south as they import inputs from these areas or even set up local production facilities for the local market or for export. This investment can help develop the local food sector when producing for local markets or by transferring knowledge to other local entrepreneurs catering to this market. Policy makers should incentivize these international private actors to invest wisely to help build more nutritious urban food systems. Despite the likely continuing importance of trade, it is critical for countries to invest in local food production and strengthen rural–urban linkages because this can help stimulate more inclusive growth, increase access to nutritious foods by the urban poor and reduce the food systems effect on climate change by shortening supply chains, limiting greenhouse gas contributions and reducing waste. However, this will remain context specific as cities located in desert areas may require more intensive resources to produce locally and are therefore more costly and environmentally damaging than if they were to import foods for example.

What is defined as local production also varies. Local can mean national, regional or even urban. Urban agriculture in the form of home gardens, community and/or commercial farming plots or rooftop gardens can be a useful way to improve access to fruit and vegetable production. Staples are less likely to be grown in urban farming plots. Depending on whether peri-urban areas are considered part of cities, keeping poultry, fish and/or (small) livestock can also occur in cities. Urban horticultural activities are more easily implemented in less dense small- and medium-sized cities and ones that have less harmful industrial outputs that could contaminate soils [30]. The United Nation's Food and Agricultural Agency (FAO) estimates 800 million people participate in urban agriculture and finds that these activities can help improve nutrition and incomes of urban farmers [53].

However, the importance of urban agriculture has been fiercely attacked by many researchers and policy makers as they find that few data are available, much of the data are outdated and impact on food security is unclear [54]. For example, in southern Africa only 1% of the population obtained food from urban farms/gardens more than once a month as a source of food despite the fact that an estimated 3/5 of the urban population were found to engage in urban agriculture activities [55]. Urban agriculture should not be seen as a substitute but instead a complement of food production in rural areas as it can provide an additional source of fresh foods such as fruits and vegetables in cities.

Urban agriculture in megacities and large-sized cities is more likely in the form of high-tech initiatives known as "controlled environment agriculture," which includes hydroponics and vertical farms. Controlled environment agriculture has the potential to do less harm to the environment as it can require less water, but it is still quite costly and mainly accessible to high-income consumers. Though a lot of these innovations are being developed in high-income countries, large-sized cities in low- and middle-income countries such as Johannesburg are already experimenting with these techniques as well. Future technological advancements will hopefully lower the costs and enable scaling up.

Most people in cities still tend to purchase most of their food versus growing it themselves. The proportion of food consumed that is acquired through purchasing is more than 75%, including in small-sized cities, while in rural areas it still remains below 50% [15]. Creating better connections between rural and urban areas will be a key component of improving urban nutrition security. FAO and other international development organizations have developed a new strategy to think about urban food systems called the "city region food systems," which is a shift from their previous focus on urban farming [56]. The "city region food system" concept recognizes the centrality of urban areas in their region and their ability to coordinate and stimulate the food system in the surrounding rural hinterlands. This movement promotes the development of a positive relationship between cities and rural areas that benefits the population of both. This new concept has the potential to better translate previous academic literature on the potential of medium-sized cities, reviewed above, into more effective national and local policies. However, these policies must incorporate findings and priorities not just from stakeholders involved in food production but also from urban development actors in order to formulate and implement truly feasible and improved strategies [28]. These strategies should not just entail bringing a farmer's produce to urban markets but also develop food processing industries. Enabling local manufacturing of nutritious and safe foods can help drive economic growth and employment in urban areas, provide an additional market for farmers in rural regions and can increase access to healthier, nutritious food products for people living in both urban and rural areas.

Conclusion

In order to achieve the Sustainable Development Goals by 2030, it is clear that the world needs good nutrition for all (SDG2) and inclusive and sustainable cities (SDG11) to stimulate equitable growth and development. In the past, undernutrition was seen as a problem of the global south, but largely out grown by the global north, that no longer had to deal with undernutrition and starvation issues. Furthermore, it was seen as a challenge that predominantly faced the rural population of LMICs. Recent recognition of the scale and severity of overnutrition (overweight and obesity and associated non-communicable diseases), widespread micronutrient deficiencies and the double burden of malnutrition (under- and overnutrition occurring within the same country, households and even individuals) have shown that poor nutrition is a challenge each country must face and that should be dealt with in both urban and rural areas. The urban poor should be one of the key target groups that must not be forgotten as they are some of the most vulnerable with regard to consequences of inadequate or unbalanced nutrition. Furthermore, demographic trends show that the rapid urban growth that will occur in the next 15 years will largely take place in low- and middle-income countries. The food and nutrition sector must start building bridges to the urban development sector and vice versa in order to design and achieve effective strategies that alleviate both urban and rural malnutrition. Urban dynamics such as city size, infrastructure (including cold chains, water and sanitation, roads and transport) and global and local supply chains play significant roles in the ability of city dwellers to access nutritious foods.

Asia and Africa are home to the greatest number of megacities and to the fastest growing cities that are small and medium in size. Lessons learned from other large cities must be implemented quickly in these megacities and better platforms for sharing information among each other should be created, improved upon and utilized. Furthermore, the world cannot afford to miss the opportunity to design more efficient, sustainable and nutrition-sensitive infrastructures in these rising medium-sized cities. If policy makers manage to effectively capture this opportunity, they have the ability to stimulate inclusive growth for city dwellers and rural inhabitants alike, develop healthier and cheaper foods systems and improve the nutrition of everyone without damaging the environment.

Discussion Points

- What are and why should we care about urban nutrition problems? What has prevented policies from adequately addressing this issue in the past?
- What are the advantages and disadvantages when it comes to international trade versus local production? What are the advantages and disadvantages when it comes to formal versus informal markets?
- What types of infrastructures can enable or disable the achievement of good nutrition for people living in cities and why?
- How can urban development theory be utilized to improve food and nutrition security? What are some of the unique advantages of medium-sized cities?

Acknowledgments This chapter is partly based on Bloem S, de Pee S (2016). How urban design can contribute to improving the nutritional status of millions. Global Food Security, http://dx.doi.org/10.1016/j.gfs.2016.09.001.

References

1. Unicef. Improving child nutrition. The achievable imperative for global progress. 2013. ISBN: 978-92-806-4686-3.
2. Novo Nordisk; Steno Diabetes Center; UCL. Urban diabetes: understanding the challenges and opportunities, 2015.
3. United Nations. World urbanization prospects: the 2014 revision, highlights (ST/ESA/SER.A/352). New York. 2014. doi:10.4054/DemRes.2005.12.9.
4. Black RE, Victora CG, Walker SP, et al. Maternal and child undernutrition and overweight in low-income and middle-income countries. Lancet. 2013;382:427–51. doi:10.1016/S0140-6736(13)60937-X.
5. WHO, UNHABITAT. Urban health inequities revealed (chapter 4). In: Hidden cities unmasking and overcoming health inequities urban settings; 2010. p. 39–56,
6. United Nations. The global social crisis: report on the world social situation 2011, 2011.
7. Cohen M, Garrett JL The food price crisis and urban food (in) security, 2009.

8. Vermeulen SJ, Campbell BM, Ingram JSI. Climate change and food systems. Annu Rev Environ Resour. 2012;37:195–222. doi:10.1146/annurev-environ-020411-130608.
9. The World Bank Group. East Asia's changing urban landscape—measuring a decade of spatial growth. 2015. doi:10.1596/978-1-4648-0363-5.
10. Habitat III. The new urban agenda. 2015. https://www.habitat3.org/the-new-urban-agenda. Accessed 1 Feb 2016.
11. UN-Habitat. Prosperity of cities: state of the world's cities 2012/2013. State of the world's cities. 2012. doi:10. 1080/07293682.2013.861498.
12. Un-Habitat. The challenge of slums—global report on human settlements. London Earthscan. 2003. doi:http://dx. doi.org/10.1108/meq.2004.15.3.337.3.
13. IFPRI. Global nutrition report 2015: actions and accountability to advance nutrition and sustainable development. 2015. doi:10.2499/9780896298835.
14. Unicef, WHO, The World Bank Group. Levels and trends in child malnutrition. Midwifery. 2014:4. doi:10.1016/ S0266-6138(96)90067-4.
15. Mohiddin L, Phelps L, Walters T. Urban malnutrition: a review of food security and nutrition among the urban poor, 2012.
16. Tzioumis E, Adair LS. Childhood dual burden of under- and overnutrition in low- and middle-income countries: a critical review. Food Nutr Bull. 2014;35:230–43.
17. WHO. Report of the commission on ending childhood obesity, 2016.
18. Popkin BM, Slining MM. New dynamics in global obesity facing low- and middle-income countries. Obes Rev. 2013;14:11–20. doi:10.1111/obr.12102.
19. Satterthwaite D, McGranahan G, Tacoli C. Urbanization and its implications for food and farming. Philos Trans R Soc Lond. 2010;365:2809–20. doi:10.1098/rstb.2010.0136.
20. Dixon J, Omwega AM, Friel S, et al. The health equity dimensions of urban food systems. J Urban Heal. 2007;84:118–29. doi:10.1007/s11524-007-9176-4.
21. de Pee S, Martini E, Moench-Pfanner R et al. Nutrition and health trends in Indonesia 1999–2003, 2004.
22. Bloem MW, Moench-Pfanner R, Panagides D. Urbanization and the millennium development goals- Insights from Nutritional Surveillance data. Singapore, 2003.
23. Brinkman H-J, de Pee S, Sanogo I, et al. High food prices and the global financial crisis have reduced access to nutritious food and worsened nutritional status and health. J Nutr. 2010;140:153S–61S. doi:10.3945/jn.109.110767.
24. Cohen MJ, Garrett JL. The food price crisis and urban food (in)security. Environ Urban. 2010;22:467–82. doi:10. 1177/0956247810380375.
25. Block S, Kiess L, Webb P, et al. Macro shocks and micro outcomes: child nutrition during Indonesia's crisis. Econ Hum Biol. 2004;2:21–44.
26. McGranahan G. Urbanization and food prices, 2011.
27. Tacoli C, Thanh HX, Owusu M, et al. The role of local government in urban food security. IIED Brief, 2013.
28. Tacoli C, Vorley B. IIED briefing: reframing the debate on urbanisation, rural transformation and food security. 2015:4.
29. Ruel MT, Garrett J, Yosef S, Olivier M. Urbanization, food security and nutrition. Nutr Health Dev World. 2016.
30. Ruel MT, Garrett JL. Features of urban food and nutrition security and considerations for successful urban programming. eJADE: Electron J Agric Dev Econ. 2004;1:242–71.
31. Timmer PC. The impact of supermarkets on nutrition and nutritional knowledge: a food policy perspective. Nutr Health Dev World. 2016.
32. Society at a Glance 2011. Key Findings-United States. 2011. doi:10.1787/soc_glance-2011-en.
33. Scott AJ, Storper M. The nature of cities: the scope and limits of urban theory. Int J Urban Reg Res. 2015;39:1–15. doi:10.1111/1468-2427.12134.
34. Timberlake M. World systems theory and the study of comparative urbanisation. In: Smith MP, Feagin JR, editors. CapitalCity. Oxford: Basil Blackwell; 1987. p. 37–65.
35. Baker J, Pedersen PO. The rural-urban interface in Africa, 1992.
36. Bryceson DF, Jamal V. Farewell to farms: de-agrarianisation and employment in Africa. England: Ashgate Publishing; 1997.
37. Pederson PO. Small African towns—between rural networks and urban hierarchies. Brookfield: Avebury; 1997.
38. Rondinelli DA. Secondary cities in developing countries. Beverly Hills: SAGE; 1983.
39. Meagher K. The invasion of opportunity snatchers: the rural-urban interface in Northern Nigeria. African Stud: J Contemp; 2000.
40. Sassen S. Cities in a world economy. Los Angeles: SAGE; 2012.
41. Davis M. Planet of slums. New York: Verso; 2007.
42. Christiaensen L, Todo Y. Poverty reduction during the rural-urban transformation—the missing middle. World Dev. 2013:1–16.
43. Christiaensen L, Weerdt JD, Todo Y. Urbanization and poverty reduction: the role of rural diversification and secondary towns. Agric Econ. 2013:435–447.

44. The World Bank Group. Indonesian economic quarterly: pressures mounting, 2013.
45. The World Bank Group. Scale economies and agglomeration (chapter 4). World Development Report. 2009.
46. Henderson JV. Urbanization and the geography of development in countries. In: Joshi-Ghani A, Glaeser E (ed) Rethink cities. World Bank Publications; 2014, p. 1–30.
47. UN. UN projects world population to reach 8.5 billion by 2030, driven by growth in developing countries. In: UN news cent. 2015. http://www.un.org/sustainabledevelopment/blog/2015/07/un-projects-world-population-to-reach-8-5-billion-by-2030-driven-by-growth-in-developing-countries/.
48. United Nations. Water and food security. In: Water life. 2014. http://www.un.org/waterforlifedecade/food_security.shtml.
49. Carbon Trust. The emerging cold economy sustainable solutions for rapidly. London; 2015.
50. Bloem S. Is the goldilocks city a myth? How the degree of urbanization affects inclusive growth; The case of Indonesia. Unpubl. LSE Masters Thesis, 2014.
51. SUN Movement. Scaling up nutrition (SUN) movement strategy [2012–2015], 2012;1:7–10. doi:10.1596/978-0-8213-8077-2.
52. Rodriguez JC. The new urban: towards progressive secondary cities, 2014.
53. FAO. Urban agriculture. 2016. http://www.fao.org/urban-agriculture/en/. Accessed 3 Feb 2016.
54. Thebo AL, Drechsel P, Lambin EF. Global assessment of urban and peri-urban agriculture: irrigated and rainfed croplands. Environ Res Lett. 2014;9:9. doi:10.1088/1748-9326/9/11/114002.
55. Crush J, Frayne B. Supermarket expansion and the informal food economy in Southern African cities: implications for urban food security. J South Afr Stud. 2011;37:781–807.
56. Jennings S, Cottee J, Curtis T, Miller S. Food in an urbanised world, the role of city food systems in resilience and sustainable development, 2015.
57. Battersby J, Crush J. Africa's urban food deserts. Urban Forum. 2014;25:143–51. doi:10.1007/s12132-014-9225-5.
58. Zuo H. The earnings differential between formal and informal emloyees in urban China. Contemp Econ. 2013;7:115–24.
59. The Economist. China's cities: the great transition. Econ. 2014.
60. Henderson JV. Growth of China's medium-size cities. Brookings-whart pap urban aff. 2005:263–303.
61. Chen A, Partridge MD. When are cities engines of growth in China? spread and backwash effects across the urban hierarchy. Reg Stud. 2013;47:1313–31.
62. Cao S, Lv Y, Zheng H, Wang X. Challenges facing China's unbalanced urbanization strategy. Land Use Policy. 2014;39:412–5.
63. Brazilian Institute of Geography and Statistics (IBGE). 1993 population estimates, 1993.
64. FAO. Growing greener cities in Latin America and the Caribbean. An FAO report on urban and peri-urban agriculture in the region. Rome, Italy: FAO; 2014.

Chapter 32
Urbanization, Food Security and Nutrition

Marie T. Ruel, James Garrett, Sivan Yosef and Meghan Olivier

Keywords Urbanization · Poverty · Nutrition · Food security · Policy

Learning Objectives

- Summarize data on global trends in urban poverty, food insecurity and malnutrition
- Review the unique challenges, distinctive factors and conditions that shape poverty, food insecurity and malnutrition in urban areas
- Analyze the implications of current urbanization trends and discuss how to address the unique characteristics of urban poverty, food insecurity and malnutrition in designing programs and policies to improve the lives of urban dwellers
- Identify research gaps that need to be filled in order to better understand global urbanization trends, their consequences and their implications for programs and policies

Introduction: Global Urbanization Trends

The world has become increasingly urbanized. For the first time in history, more than half of the world's population (54%) lives in urban areas. By 2050, two-thirds (66%) will. Since 1950, the urban population has more than quintupled, increasing from 746 million to 3.9 billion in 2014. By 2050, rural–urban migration and general population growth are projected to add another 2.5 billion people

M.T. Ruel (✉) · M. Olivier
Poverty, Health and Nutrition Division, International Food Policy Research Institute,
2033K Street NW, Washington, DC 20011, USA
e-mail: m.ruel@cgiar.org

M. Olivier
e-mail: m.olivier@cgiar.org

J. Garrett
Bioversity International, Viale Tre Denari 472/a, Maccarese 00054, Italy
e-mail: j.garrett@cgiar.org

S. Yosef
International Food Policy Research Institute, 2033K Street NW, Washington, DC 20006, USA
e-mail: s.yosef@cgiar.org

© Springer Science+Business Media New York 2017
S. de Pee et al. (eds.), *Nutrition and Health in a Developing World*,
Nutrition and Health, DOI 10.1007/978-3-319-43739-2_32

to the world's urban areas [1].[1] By contrast, the world's rural population, currently at 3.4 billion, is expected to peak around 2016 and then begin to fall. Africa and Asia currently account for approximately 90% of rural dwellers, with India (857 million) and China (635 million) being home to the largest rural populations [1].

The trends and rates of urbanization vary widely by region and by national income level. In North America, Europe, and Latin America and the Caribbean, between 73 and 82% of the population currently lives in urban centers. The change in level of urbanization in these regions is expected to slow down or stagnate between now and 2050. Africa and Asia, on the other hand, have experienced a steady increase in the level of urbanization since at least 1950, and this trend is expected to continue until well beyond 2050. Currently, Africa has 40% of its population living in urban areas and Asia has 47% [1]. Between now and 2050, these two regions are expected to contribute 90% of the growth in the world's urban population [4].

These numbers set the statistical context of an urbanizing world, but with regard to food security and nutrition, they do not tell the tale. Life, in fact, is different in urban than in rural areas. This is especially true at the extremes of the rural–urban continuum. This chapter provides an overview of the unique challenges and opportunities for urban dwellers to achieve food security and optimal nutrition and discusses the implications for programs, policies and research. It starts with descriptive statistics and trends on urban poverty, food insecurity and malnutrition[2] and reviews the distinctive factors and conditions that shape food security and nutrition in urban areas, namely food systems and the determinants of food availability and access; physical activity; and the health environment, including water, sanitation and food safety. It concludes with a brief discussion of programs and policy implications, and research gaps.

Data and Trends in Urban–Rural Poverty, Food Security and Nutrition

Reliable numbers on the levels of and trends in urban poverty, food insecurity and malnutrition are scarce, especially from cross-country or global analyses. This section summarizes available information.

Poverty

From 1993 to 2002, the global rate of poverty (defined as living on <$1/day) declined from 28 to 22%, due largely to changes in rural poverty in developing countries, which dropped from 37 to 30% (compared to 13.5–13% in urban areas). During this period, urban poverty in developing countries stabilized at around 13%. However, the number of poor living in urban areas increased (from 242 million in 1993 to 291 million in 2002), while the numbers in rural areas declined (from 1031 to 890 million) over the same period.[3] Although the majority of the poor will continue to live in rural areas for decades to come, the location of poverty is clearly shifting to urban areas. The urban share of the

---

[1]The terms "urban" and "rural" are used in this chapter, *as used in the original publications*. We recognize that the distinction between urban and rural is not clear-cut and that a variety of definitions are used in the literature, some based on administrative criteria, others on different combinations of size, aspects of density or economic activity [2, 3], while many publications do not specify the definitions they use.

[2]In this paper, we use the term "malnutrition" to refer to problems of both undernutrition (deficiencies in protein, emergy and/or micronutrients) and overweight and obesity.

[3]No recent data on prevalence, numbers and trends in urban and rural poverty were found.

poor in developing countries rose from 19 to 25% from 1993 to 2002 [5].[4] In addition, statistics indicate that the poor are urbanizing faster than the population as a whole.

The location of poverty differs markedly by region. Most of the poor in Latin America already live in urban areas, whereas less than 10% do in East Asia, due largely to the numbers from China [5]. By 2020, estimates suggest that up to 85% of the poor in Latin America will live in towns and cities as will 45% of the poor in Africa and Asia [6].

Food Security

Although global data on food security disaggregated by urban and rural area are not available, some analyses provide such statistics for collections of countries. These studies indicate that urban residents do suffer from food insecurity and that food insecurity in urban areas can sometimes be more prevalent or severe there than in rural areas. A 2006 analysis of household-level data using food consumption information collected as part of household expenditure surveys[5] found that energy availability per capita (a commonly used indicator of food security) was lower in urban than in rural areas in seven of the twelve African countries studied [7]. In all but one of the countries, at least 40% of the urban population was energy deficient, with prevalence skyrocketing to nearly 90% in urban Ethiopia. Similarly, a study using nationally representative data from countries in sub-Saharan Africa, South, East and Central Asia, and Latin America found that the incidence of hunger (also defined as energy deficiency) in urban areas equaled or exceeded rural levels in 12 of 18 countries studied [8]. Urban areas in seven of these countries experienced substantially higher levels of hunger as compared to rural areas. These findings are rather surprising, given that the study also found a higher incidence of poverty in rural areas in all countries analyzed, but they serve to show that urban dwellers can also have difficulty gaining access to sufficient food, despite generally higher incomes.

It is important to note that the prevalence of food insecurity in the studies described above may have been overestimated due to two possible measurement errors: (1) the use of the same energy requirements for both urban and rural dwellers when urban dwellers tend to be less physically active and relatedly have lower total energy requirements, which would overestimate the energy deficit in urban areas; (2) failure to measure (or imprecision in measurement of) food eaten away from home. Given that eating away from home is much more common in urban than in rural areas, failure to include the composition of meals eaten outside (most surveys at that time only included amount spent on food consumed away from home, but did not have specific information on food consumed) will underestimate energy intakes in urban areas. Work is ongoing to address the latter caveat [9].

---

[4]These statistics are outdated, but our search did not identify more recent global estimates of urban and rural poverty.

[5]This study uses food consumption data from nationally representative household expenditure surveys to measure food security (defined as percentage of the population that does not consume sufficient dietary energy). The main difference between this approach and the widely used indicator of "undernourishment" developed by the Food and Agriculture Organization (FAO) is that the Smith and colleagues' approach uses actual survey data from food consumption/expenditure, whereas the FAO method is based on modeling using countries' food supply data. To define insufficient dietary energy, both methods rely on FAO/WHO/UNU 1985 "recommended energy intakes," which are age and sex specific, and different for 3 levels of physical activity: light, medium and high. (Reference: FAO/WHO/UNU 1985. Protein and energy requirements. Rome: FAO).

Nutrition

This section focuses on trends and statistics on anthropometry among women of reproductive age and preschool children, the two population groups most vulnerable to "malnutrition" and its devastating consequences for health, nutrition, cognitive development, reproduction and economic productivity throughout the life cycle [10]. We do not report on micronutrient deficiencies because we did not find any global data on urban–rural differences or trends for population micronutrient status.

Stunting and Underweight in Children

A systematic analysis of children's height and weight in 141 low- and middle-income countries (LMIC) concluded that in 2011: (1) urban children were taller and heavier than their rural counterparts in almost all countries and (2) stunting and underweight were lower in urban areas of all countries, with differences as large as 30% points [11].

When looking at trends over time in these countries, the prevalence of stunting declined from 47 to 30% between 1985 and 2011, and underweight dropped from 30 to 19%. In absolute terms, the number of stunted children fell from 239 to 163 million during this period, and the number of underweight children fell from 151 million to 105 million. The bulk of these declines occurred in rural areas, whereas the overall number of stunted and underweight children in urban areas remained largely unchanged. As a result, the *urban share* of stunted children rose from 23% in 1985 to 31% in 2011, and that of underweight children rose from 21 to 27% over this 26-year period [11].

There are marked regional differences in urban and rural levels and trends in all anthropometric indicators (Figs. 32.1 and 32.2). The largest numbers of stunted and underweight children in urban areas are currently found in Asia (South, East and Southeast Asia), although the numbers have declined markedly from 1985 to 2011. By contrast, the numbers of stunted and underweight children in urban areas of sub-Saharan Africa more than doubled over this period [11]. The heights of rural and urban children improved roughly at the same rate in most regions, except in some areas of Southern and Tropical Latin America, South Asia and Central Asia, Middle East, and North Africa, whereas the urban–rural gap decreased due to greater improvements among rural children. At the country level, the urban–rural gap in height declined in 100 countries and widened in 41 countries [11].

These findings suggest that, although the urban advantage in child nutrition remained over time in most countries and regions, there has been a gradual shift in the locus of child undernutrition from rural to urban areas, with important regional differences in the rate and nature of these changes.

Disparities in Child Nutrition Within Urban and Rural Areas

Average statistics like those presented above can mask the large disparities that exist *within* areas [12]. For example, an analysis of DHS data from 11 countries (1991–1996) showed that the odds of being stunted were between 1.3 and 3.3 times higher for children in rural as compared to urban areas, but economic differentials within urban areas ranged from 2.8 (Zambia) to 10 (Peru and the Dominican Republic) [13]. On average, urban children from the lowest socioeconomic quintile were 4 times more likely to be stunted than those from the highest quintile. Within rural areas, differentials across income classes were lower than 3.5 for all countries except Brazil (7.5). In these countries, urban children from the lowest socioeconomic quintile had rates of stunting that were either similar or worse than rural children from the same quintile. A recent analysis of DHS surveys from 47 developing countries confirms these findings and documents similar results for under-five mortality [14].

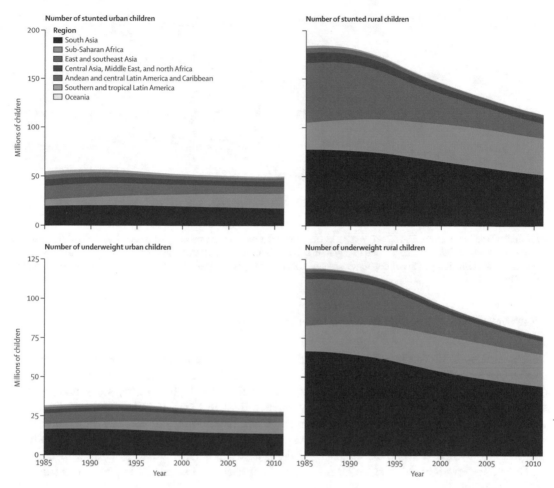

Fig. 32.1 Number of stunted and underweight children, by region and rural or urban place of residence, 1985–2011. *Source* Pacioreck et al. Children's height and weight in rural and urban populations in low-income and middle-income countries: a systematic analysis of population-representative data. The Lancet Global Health, Volume 1, Issue 5, e300–e309. Open Access

An important question that arises from these findings is why on average do urban children have better nutritional status than their rural counterparts. Several studies have examined this question over the past 20 years, analyzing different data sets and using a variety of analytical approaches. The consistent finding is that the community, household and individual determinants of child undernutrition, and the strength of their association, are largely the same in rural and urban areas. What explains the difference is the level of these determinants (e.g., maternal education, household wealth and income, and access to health services), which often favors urban dwellers [14–17]. Individual country analyses in Mozambique [18], Bangladesh and Nepal [19], and Angola, Senegal and the Central African Republic [20] confirm these findings.

These findings highlight the fact that simple averages can be misleading. They also suggest than in many countries the most vulnerable children in urban areas often live in conditions rivaling those of poor rural children. Program and policy decisions should therefore focus on the poor and most vulnerable children, wherever they live, rather than on targeting either urban or rural areas.

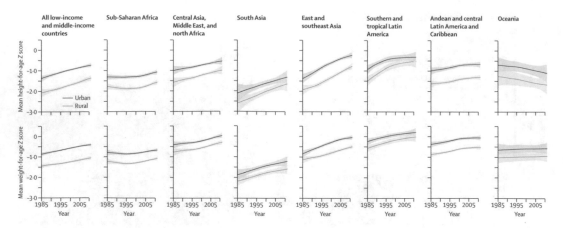

Fig. 32.2 Trends in mean HAZ and WAZ, by region and rural or urban place of residence, 1985–2011. *Source* Pacioreck et al. Children's height and weight in rural and urban populations in low-income and middle-income countries: a systematic analysis of population-representative data. The Lancet Global Health, Volume 1, Issue 5, e300–e309. Open Access

Overweight and Obesity in Children and Women

Recent estimates show that 43 million children less than 5 years of age (7%) worldwide were overweight (weight-for-height z-scores > 2) in 2011, a 54% increase from an estimated 28 million in 1990 [21]. Although the prevalence of overweight in children is highest among high-income countries (15%), as many as 32 million overweight children lived in LMIC in 2011. Regional differences show larger increases in overweight children in Africa (from 4 to 7% between 1990 and 2011) compared to Asia (from 4 to 5%), but larger numbers of affected children in Asia (17 million) compared to Africa (12 million) in 2011. Latin America remained stable over time in terms of numbers of overweight children ($\sim$ 3.8 million) and experienced a small rise in prevalence from 7 to 8%.

Urban/rural country-level comparisons using data from 80 LMIC (1998–2011) estimated that on average the prevalence of overweight children was 1.08 times higher in urban compared to rural areas (ranging from 0.44 to 1.46) [21]. Using these same data, Fig. 32.3 shows, however, that the prevalence of overweight children was *higher* in rural areas in 25 of the 80 countries analyzed (close to one-third).[6] Several of the countries where overweight was more prevalent in rural areas are classified as lower-middle-income economies by the World Bank [22]. No recent data comparing trends in child overweight in urban and rural areas were found.

Among women, the prevalence of overweight (BMI $\geq$ 25 kg/m^2) and obesity (BMI $\geq$ 30 kg/m^2) also increased since 1980, but the pace of increase, which has accelerated in the past decade, was much more dramatic than among children [23]. In 2008, it was estimated that globally, 35% of women aged $\geq$20 years (or 742.5 million) were overweight and 14% (or 297 million) were obese [24]. A recent review, which used data from 38 countries at two points in time (1991–2004 and 1998–2010), showed that mean BMI was higher among urban than rural women in most countries in both time periods, as was the prevalence of overweight [25]. The prevalence of overweight women also increased more quickly in urban areas between the two time periods in 31 of 38 countries. Similar findings were documented in previous analyses of repeated surveys (between 1989 and 2010) from 42 countries [26] and a recent analysis of 29 DHS and 4 national surveys from 1990 onward, but marked

---

[6]Data source: International Center for Equity in Health (www.equidade.org).

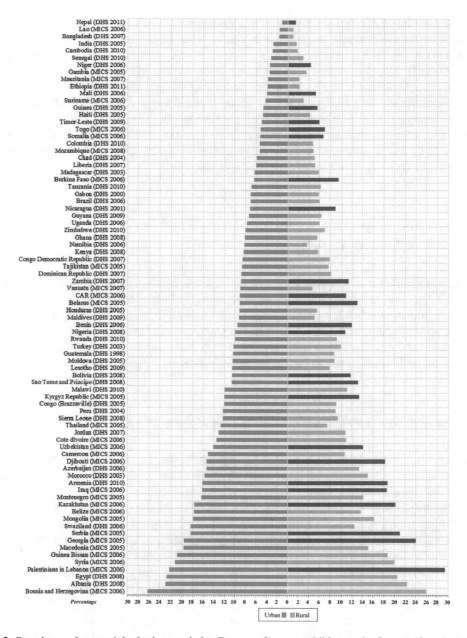

Fig. 32.3 Prevalence of overweight (body mass index Z-score > 2) among children under 5 years of age by urban and rural residence (1998–2011). *Blue* urban; *Orange* rural. *Data source* International Center for Equity in Health (www. equidade.org)

regional differences were observed. The first study showed that women in *rural* areas of Latin America, the Middle East and North Africa experienced higher increases in the prevalence of overweight than women from urban areas over the period studied, and in the second study, the rate of increase over time in the prevalence of overweight and obesity was greater in rural than in urban areas in approximately half of the countries studied [27]

One observation of changes over time is that the preponderance of obesity seems to shift from higher to lower socioeconomic levels as countries develop (rising gross national product (GNP)) [28, 29]. This crossover is particularly true for women of low socioeconomic status and happens at about $2500 GNP [29]. In Brazil, for example, a national survey in 1989 found that obesity among adults was more prevalent in the higher socioeconomic (SES) groups. Ten years later, obesity was most prevalent in the lower SES groups [30]. These findings suggest that as the nutrition transition deepens and the environment becomes increasingly obesogenic, higher socioeconomic groups who also tend to be more educated are better able to adjust—for example, they are more likely than poorer households to be health aware and to have the means to pay for healthier diets and to increase their physical activity (e.g., by enrolling in expensive gym facilities).

Challenges and Opportunities for Achieving Food Security and Optimal Nutrition in Urban Environments

This section examines the nutrition transition and related changes in urban dietary patterns and physical activity in developing countries, how these relate to changes in urban food systems and how, in turn, these processes affect food security and nutrition in urban areas. It also briefly reviews other broad categories of determinants of food security and nutrition in urban areas such as food availability (markets) and access (related to prices, incomes, urban agriculture and availability of safety nets), environmental health and access to health, water, sanitation and hygiene services, and food safety.

Food Systems, the Nutrition Transition and Urban Diets

In a process closely related to demographic and epidemiological transitions also occurring among global populations,[7] many countries have passed through or are experiencing a nutrition transition. During the nutrition transition, dietary patterns undergo significant changes, and lifestyles are characterized by lower levels of physical activity, often related to the more sedentary nature of work and motorized transportation. Diets shift from having significant proportions of complex carbohydrates, fiber and coarse grains to ones with higher amounts of saturated fats, salt, simple sugars, and processed foods. These diets usually have greater variety, with more fruits and vegetables and more animal source foods (meat, dairy, fish) [34–38]. These patterns seem to be associated to some degree with level of urbanicity, because even at similar levels of national income, those countries with higher levels of urbanization have diets with higher amounts of fats and total energy [39].[8]

In the initial stages of the nutrition transition, among the less developed countries, as diets diversify and physical activity levels go down, the problem of undernutrition starts receding (low body mass index (BMI) in adults), and problems of overweight and obesity and non-communicable diseases (NCDs), such as diabetes, heart diseases and certain cancers, emerge. In a later stage of the

---

[7]The demographic transition involves a shift from higher to lower levels of fertility and mortality. The epidemiological transition, first described by [31], involves a shift from patterns of high prevalence of infectious diseases, associated with malnutrition and poor environmental sanitation, to ones of high prevalence of chronic, non-transmissible diseases [32, 33].

[8]Consumption of total fats and oils has greatly increased in developing countries since the 1970s, even as consumption of animal fats has declined. Globally, there have been major increases in domestic production and trade in oilseeds and vegetable oil. This has been due to new technologies for oilseed production and refining processes, health concerns about consumption of animal fats and cholesterol, as well as government policies [32, 33, 39].

nutrition transition, seen in several industrialized countries, diets begin to improve and physical activity increases, as individuals (usually beginning with the wealthier and more educated segments of the population) start to make healthier food choices and purposeful changes in recreational and transport activities [37]. The pace of these different processes differs across contexts and populations, but in many countries, the rate of increase in overweight and obesity outpaces reductions in under-nutrition (e.g., child stunting, wasting, micronutrient deficiencies), thereby resulting in a "double burden" of malnutrition. This problem is characterized by the coexistence of undernutrition, including micronutrient deficiencies, and overweight and obesity and related NCD risks in the same population, communities, households and sometimes individuals [40, 41].

A number of factors drive the changes in diet and physical activity that underlie the nutrition transition. These include changes in infrastructure, technology, and culture and society, including the changing role of women, as well as economic development. These factors are briefly described below.

Urban Structure, Technology and Society

In larger cities and in more industrialized countries, urban centers have physical structures and densities that facilitate tighter distribution, transportation and information networks, allow suppliers to reach more consumers at lower cost, and encourage the quicker spread of information. Urban areas provide larger markets for food retailers and more options both for specialization among retailers and for individual retailers to market a more diverse range of foods [42]. Mass media and marketing are also more present in urban areas, influencing tastes and preferences [36]. Cities can also enjoy greater cultural diversity than many rural areas, which can increase demand for a variety of foods to meet a range of consumer tastes. As a consequence of these factors, urban residents have a greater variety of foods and food sources (e.g., supermarkets, small and convenience stores, restaurants, and street foods) available to them.

Changes in technology and society also affect the urban food environment. For example, some of the commodities distributed in urban markets require longer and more intensive agro-supply chains (from farm to fork), which introduces a range of issues related to food quality and food and water safety. Greater availability of electricity and higher incomes in urban areas mean that refrigeration is more available than in rural areas. Businesses are thus able to have wider inventories, particularly of perishables and items that need cold storage, such as dairy and meat products. Households can purchase these foods for storage at home, and so can shop on, say, a weekly, rather than daily basis [43]. Technologies have also provided for a range of processed goods, including canned and frozen items, snacks and prepared meals, as well as ultra-high temperature milk, which extends shelf-life without needing refrigeration [26].

Changing Role of Women

With more women in urban areas working in the labor force, there is increasing demand for convenience and processed foods, and for ease of purchasing [39, 44]. The physical environment as well as the workload may affect the time women spend on food-related activities such as shopping for food and preparing and enjoying meals and the time they spend on childcare [39, 45]. With both women and men working outside the home, and children going to school for extended hours, more meals are purchased and eaten outside the home (e.g., from supermarkets, restaurants, street food) and eating becomes less centered on the family [35]. With less agricultural land available, urban living is less compatible with home production and consumption than in rural areas [36].

Changing Demand for Food

The increasing demand for meat and dairy products that accompanies urbanization, compounded by rising incomes and growing populations, puts pressure on agriculture to intensify, raising demands on limited natural resources, such as land, soil and water [42]. These changes also result in increased waste, especially at the consumer end, and raise questions of how to create and support the development of healthy, sustainable food systems and appropriately address climate change. Although not given, in general, this shift means additional uses of energy in processing and transport (with increased commercialization), additional natural resource use, and need for more grains, which serve as input into animal feeds, rather than being directly consumed by humans [46].

Some of these changes relate directly to the changing urban environment, but others are connected to more general factors, such as rising national incomes and changes in the nature of market systems, rather than anything uniquely "urban." This observation highlights the continuum that exists between the "more urban" and "more rural" environments, with increasingly greater physical (e.g., roads) and virtual (e.g., communications technologies) connectivity between them. Such connectivity implies that changes that happen in one area can be transmitted to and adapted by the population in the other. We must therefore use caution when attributing aspects of food security and nutrition in cities to specifically "urban" factors rather than to more the general influences of development. Huang and Bouis [47], for example, in an analysis of data from China and Taiwan, attribute about 20% of the increases in consumption of meat, fish and dairy products to non-income or structural factors associated with living in an urban area, implying that 80% is due to these other non-geographically specific factors. Still, it is true that even some of these generic factors may be more quickly and strongly expressed in urban areas than in rural ones.

Urban Diets

As a result of the unique food environment and higher incomes in urban areas, diets tend to be different, more diverse and less affected by seasonality than rural ones. The availability of a wide range of foods and the shift away from traditional diets also meets consumer desires for greater food choices, even among the poor [34, 39]. Urban dwellers are thus more likely to meet their protein and energy requirements than rural dwellers, but they are also more likely to have imbalanced diets, often too rich in total energy, and in the proportion of energy coming from saturated fats and sugar, too high in salt, and low in fiber. Their energy-rich diets are also often poor in micronutrients, as shown in urban areas of Benin, Mali and Kenya, where the mean probability of adequacy of 11 micronutrients was low, and a large proportion of women (>80% in Burkina Faso) had inadequate intakes of B vitamins [48–50]. In more industrialized countries such as Indonesia, however, consumption of micronutrient-fortified foods such as milk and noodles was significantly higher in urban compared to rural areas, and this in turn was associated with lower odds of stunting among urban compared to rural children [51]. Globally, however, there is concern that urban dwellers are at increased risk of overweight and obesity and related risks of NCDs, while many continue to experience deficiencies in several essential micronutrients [52].

Physical Activity

An additional key risk factor for NCDs, beyond diets, is physical activity. Urban living is associated with changes in activity levels compared to life in rural areas and is believed to be associated with lower energy expenditure in aspects such as work (more sedentary jobs), domestic chores (water, electricity more readily available) and transportation (use of motorized transport), while for leisure it can go either way (e.g., urban areas may offer greater potential for outdoor physical activity, sports or gyms, but also for more sedentary leisure such as television and use of computers and video games). It is thus possible that on average changes in one domain compensate for changes in another domain and that average energy expenditure may not be that different between urban and rural areas [53]. Changes are also occurring in the rural environment, with agricultural activities becoming increasingly mechanized, employment opportunities moving away from traditional agricultural activities, and public and private motorized transport becoming more available. It is thus likely that physical activity levels are in fact declining in both urban and rural areas [53].

A global analysis of data sets from 76 countries from low-, middle- and high-income nations representing 80% of the world population in 2003 (and using the validated International Physical Activity Questionnaire) documented a worldwide population-weighted prevalence of physical inactivity[9] of 17.4%, with lower average prevalence in less developed (18.7%), compared to the most developed (27.8%) countries [54]. The study also showed higher physical inactivity among women compared to men, among elderly individuals, and among wealthier and urban countries (the authors do not specify what characteristics they used to classify countries as "urban"; they also do not disaggregate national data by urban and rural areas).

Most studies that examined the factors affecting physical activity are from industrialized countries, but they highlight the multiple factors at play, including the physical environment, perceived personal and cultural barriers, and gender and age, all of which are relevant for developing countries as well as for urban and rural areas [30, 55, 56].

Food Availability

In this section, we briefly review the role of food retailing and the food environment, including traditional and modern supply chains and foreign direct investment and globalization in influencing the availability of food in urban areas. We also touch upon the contributions of street foods and urban agriculture, although the literature on these topics is scant. We recognize the importance of the physical (built) environment as a determinant of food availability, but research so far has focused mainly on industrialized countries, and for this reason, we do not cover this topic here and refer the reader to the existing literature [57–61].

Food Retailing and the Food Environment

Traditional and Modern Supply Chains

Beginning in the 1990s, supermarkets spread quickly throughout Latin America, Central Europe and South Africa, increasing to a 50% share of food retail in the mid-2000s. By the mid-2000s, supermarkets in Southeast Asia, Central America, as well as Chile, Argentina, and Mexico had between 30

---

[9]Physical inactivity was defined as being engaged in vigorous-intensity physical activity for less than 20 min per day on at least 3 days per week, or less than 30 min per day of moderate-intensity physical activity on at least 5 days per week, or 600 MET-minutes/week combining both criteria. MET (the **metabolic equivalent of task**) is a physiological measure expressing the energy cost (or calories) of physical activities. One MET is the energy equivalent expended by an individual while seated at rest. While exercising, the MET equivalent is the energy expended compared to rest; an activity with a MET value of 5 means expending 5 times the energy than the individual would while at rest. MET minutes are derived by multiplying the number of METs for an activity by the number of minutes a person is engaged in this activity. http://www.cooperinstitute.org/2012/04/met-minutes-a-simple-common-value-to-track-exercise-progress/, accessed on February 29, 2016.

and 50% of the food market. The latest wave of supermarket expansion has been in emerging economies, mainly China, Vietnam, India and Russia. A supermarket revolution in other parts of Africa is in its nascent stages [62, 63].

These supermarket chains first established themselves in larger cities and then extended to intermediate cities and towns. Within cities, they initially established stores in higher-income areas, moving gradually to middle-income and less advantaged neighborhoods. Many of these chains are affiliated with large multinationals, such as Ahold and Carrefour. Over the past decades, as they grew, they influenced the entire supply chain. They established efficiency and cost controls, including consolidation and use of specialized and dedicated wholesale and preferred supplier systems that allowed them to compete with the more traditional wholesale and retail market and small neighborhood stores [62–65]. Some have suggested that supermarkets have also improved quality and helped to standardize products (say when buying from local producers) [66]. However, other studies suggest a weak association between supermarkets and safer food. Randolph et al. [67], for example, note that studies in East Africa and India show that a similar proportion of substandard milk samples are found in supermarket and informally marketed samples. Similarly, there is no agreement on whether supermarkets have positive nutritional impacts on consumers. While they do offer a variety of nutritious foods, including fresh produce, dairy products and animal source foods, they also present a "confusing array of new choices" [68], including abundant options in ultra-processed energy-dense/nutrient-poor obesogenic foods [69, 70].

It is important, however, to recognize that most purchases in developing countries, especially Africa and Asia, are still made through traditional shops and wet markets. These traditional systems, such as small neighborhood grocery stores, fruit and vegetable markets, meat markets, and street vendors, remain predominant, capturing 50% or more of food retailing even in these countries where modern retailing began developing earliest. As of the mid-2000s, supermarkets in sub-Saharan Africa still accounted for less than 5% of urban food expenditures and will remain a minority food supplier to urban residents for the foreseeable future [71]. This may be particularly so with regard to the urban poor. In Zambia and Kenya, for example, supermarkets still cater primarily to households in the top 20% of the income distribution [72].

There is some discussion about the appeal of traditional outlets for the future. Some studies argue that these traditional locations will stay competitive because they can charge lower prices because of lower labor, overhead and marketing costs. They also offer proximity and convenience [64, 73] and personal relationships, including extension of credit and acceptance of exchanges. Modern supermarkets, on the other hand, may have higher overhead costs for rent, labor and additional services such as processing and refrigeration, as well as higher product turnover rates due to more regulation, resulting in higher prices [74]. But larger supermarkets offer greater variety and may use a loss-leader pricing strategy to gain initial market share through packaged and processed foods and then move into high-value and more nutritious foods such as fruits, vegetables, dairy and meat [75].

In some sense, dual food systems have developed. While modern retailers have a high share of the food market in non-staples and processed products, the share in unprocessed products, such as meat and fresh produce, is lower. Reardon and colleagues [43] note that the supermarket share of the fruit and vegetable market is often roughly half that of the share for other goods (especially processed goods). In Kenya, Nicaragua and Zambia, for example, over 90% of all fruits and vegetables are purchased through traditional outlets [76]. Even in Nairobi, one of the most developed supermarket sectors, only 8% of meat purchases versus 60% of staples are made in supermarkets [77]. Fresh markets were also still the main place to buy produce in South Africa, even in the early 2000s when supermarkets already had a significant share. While 40% of marketed fruits and vegetables went through the supermarket procurement system, 7% went first to fresh markets and then to supermarkets, while 53% went through fresh markets and then to non-supermarket retailers. Latin America demonstrated a similar pattern [63, 72].

Mixed arrangements between these two systems may also exist. Domestic and international food manufacturers sell foods through traditional small neighborhood stores, while supermarkets source food from local farmers and traders. These options can take advantage of economies of scale, but may also rely on processed foods, with potential negative impacts on nutrition. An example of this is the rise of carbonated drinks in Africa, whereby manufacturers support traditional storeowners in heavily marketing their products [72].

Foreign Direct Investment and Globalization

Beyond the straightforward description of where urban dwellers buy their food, it is worthwhile to examine how the urban food environment affects food choices. Changes in lifestyles, the physical urban environment, and changes in design and operation of production, processing and marketing systems underlie such choices [57]. A number of analysts cite the growing impact of trade and globalization on consumption patterns, but the importance of imports to diets is actually rather small. In developing countries, a large majority of food, ~95%, comes from domestic sources; international trade is important at the margin of food systems [78]. The influence of multinationals and the global environment is thus felt primarily through growing foreign direct investment (FDI) rather than trade. US food companies, for example, sell five times more food through FDI sales than through exports [79]. FDI has contributed to the rise of fast food restaurants and supermarkets [80] and, in some cases, the growth of processing and marketing of global brands within the country itself. To the extent that national markets are connected to international markets, variations in international prices and global demand and supply also affect domestic food availability and pricing. Thus, even though imports may be only a small percentage of food trade, the international trade environment will still have an impact on national food offerings.

Increased advertising and increased availability and consumption of prepared food also accompany increased FDI [57, 81], potentially promoting unhealthy diets. Thow and Hawkes [82] argue that the lowering of trade barriers was critical to the expansion of processed food markets in Central America. Trade liberalization led to more food imports, particularly processed foods, and also promoted domestic meat production, thus facilitating availability and consumption of meat, dairy products, processed foods and temperate (imported) fruit in Central America. In theory, however, FDI could similarly be put to use in promotion of healthier alternatives. Supermarkets, for example, may provide an increased array of processed or prepared foods, but they also provide additional choices (and opportunities for promotion) of nutrient-rich foods such as dairy and fruits and vegetables.

Street Foods

Street foods can represent a low-cost, accessible and convenient source of food for urban residents. They can make up a significant proportion of the urban diet and are also important sources of employment, especially for women. Even when men are the vendors, they often rely on the women in the household to prepare the food [83]. After a substantial number of synthesis work and some city studies, usually dealing with food safety concerns, from the late 1980s to the early 2000s [84, 85], comprehensive research on street foods in developing countries has been limited, despite their importance.

Smaller and poorer urban families often have a higher proportion of food intake from street foods [84]. In Kenya, one study found that slum dwellers consume more street foods than those in low- and middle-income neighborhoods [50].

Street foods also provide a range of food types and can become part of the diet from a young age. In Senegal, women feed babies yoghurt, which is bought and not prepared at home, as a weaning food. Nigerian adolescents obtained between 40 and 70% of food intake of major food groups from street foods, supplying between 20 and 30% of energy [86]. And while foods are often selected because of taste and convenience, rather than nutritional value, the food energy and protein value of cooked street foods in Asia were higher than those of prepackaged processed foods [86]. This is likely due to the fact that street foods in Asia offer a variety of meals, whereas prepackaged processed foods are typically snacks rich in sugar, fat and/or salt (e.g., cookies, candies, chips). With such a significant proportion of diets coming from street foods, interventions could work to provide vendors with fresh, nutritious and less expensive locally grown ingredients, potentially boosting the role of urban agriculture and contributing to healthier urban diets.

Street foods are also an important informal sector activity and income source for the urban poor, although many middle-income residents also engage in this activity. Tinker [84] found that even in larger cities, such as Bogor, Indonesia, street food vendors can be between 15 and 20% of the labor force and create millions of dollars of revenue for the local economy. Government officials still often fail to recognize the contributions of street foods to the economy and food consumption. Many vendors face high job insecurity due to strict regulations or prohibitions on street sales as well as lack of capital to obtain proper permits. Promoting the role of street food associations in working with vendors to provide start-up capital, and providing piecemeal programs to legitimize their operations could increase food safety, provide key environmental infrastructure and ensure their livelihoods [83, 84]. A recent study in Zimbabwe, for example, found that vendors would be willing to pay for running water and electricity if the local government provided the facilities [87].

Urban Agriculture

Urban agriculture and its contribution to national production, household income, food security and diet quality are underdocumented. One recent comprehensive study [88] gathered nationally representative data from 15 developing and transition countries to examine these issues, providing one of the few reliable and recent assessments. The results show that the share of urban households that participated in agriculture (including livestock) ranged from 11% in Indonesia to nearly 70% in Vietnam and Nicaragua. In 8 of 15 countries, over 50% of urban residents practiced agriculture, and in 11 of the 15 countries, the share of urban households participating in agriculture was more than 30%. In general, rearing livestock was less common than growing crops, but not always. In urban areas of Bangladesh, Nepal, Ecuador and Nicaragua, one in three households raised livestock.

Urban agriculture accounted for 5–15% of total agricultural production in most countries and was largely geared to own-consumption rather than the market. In only four countries (Bangladesh, Madagascar, Nepal and Nicaragua) was more than one-third of production marketed; that figure varied between 15 and 26% in other seven countries. Across all households, the contribution to income was small although quite variable: The contribution to overall household income was higher than 10% in only 5 countries, of which 4 were in Africa. But among those households that practiced urban agriculture, the contribution was significant—20% or more in 7 countries.

In addition to providing income, urban agriculture can allow direct access to nutritious foods (e.g., fruit, vegetables, eggs and dairy), improving dietary diversity and guarding against seasonality shortages or shocks. Assuming that urban agriculture can, in the case of women for example, replace a non-agricultural source of employment that is more likely to be further away from home, it can also free up mothers' time, which can then be spent on food preparation and child feeding and caregiving. In the Zezza and Tasciotti [88] study, participation in urban farming was positively associated with improved dietary adequacy (using a dietary diversity score), in 10 of 15 countries.

Despite demonstrable benefits, the city environment may not favor urban agriculture. Urban agriculture is illegal in many cities, but urban residents may nevertheless use public space or vacant lots of private owners with or without their permission. Raising livestock or crops in an urban environment also encounters challenges of how to access needed inputs, such as water, and how to work safely with agrochemicals and dispose of animal or crop waste, challenges which are amplified when activities are considered illegal or undesirable and urban planners make little provision for its inclusion in the urban landscape [89, 90].

In summary, the extent and contribution of urban agriculture to national and household economy and food access varies wildly, likely reflecting space, legal, agronomic and other factors. Given that participation in urban agriculture is more concentrated among the poorest income quintiles and is negatively associated with wealth [88], it appears to serve an important role as a coping strategy and as a source of food and income that should be protected, at least in the relevant contexts.

Food Access

Urban dwellers, especially the poor, face a unique set of challenges in accessing food due to their dependence on cash, vulnerability to food price shocks, and the fragility of their employment (especially women). The impacts of these conditions on the food security and nutrition of household members will depend on such factors as whether or not the households have access to stable income sources, formal or informal safety nets, and agricultural land and other assets.

The Importance of Cash and Food Purchases

Compared to rural consumers who can often produce a considerable proportion of the food they consume, most urban consumers depend largely on food purchases. This dependence on the market is further compounded by the fact that, unlike their rural counterparts, urban residents cannot rely substantially on the exploitation of natural resources to provide for food, housing, energy or water.

Ahmed et al. [8] found the proportion of household expenditures spent on food by extremely poor urban households in 20 LMIC was more than 50% in all but two countries. The food share ranged from 48% in Guatemala to 74% in Tajikistan. And with regard to the percentage of that food that is purchased [91] showed that in the largest cities, the percentage was greater than 90% in all 5 countries analyzed, compared to a range from 29 to 59% for rural areas of Mozambique, Malawi, Nepal and Peru, and 85% in Egypt. For other, non-metropolitan urban areas, the share of total food consumption purchased ranged from 73% in Mozambique to 95% in Egypt.

Given the fact that most food is purchased in urban areas, earnings from employment (income) and food costs (mostly price but in a broad sense including ease of access and cost of time for acquiring, preparing, and eating food) play a significant role in food access. Along with the influences of marketing and, so, tastes and preferences, these economic factors influence urban consumption patterns, including food choices related to location of eating (at home or away from home) and types of food (fast food, home prepared, processed foods) [57].

Most of the economic analysis related to food consumption has focused on marketing issues, such as retail availability, and to some extent on price effects (price elasticities), but without differentiating between urban and rural consumers, and with a strong focus on industrialized countries on the issues related to marketing. Very little research has been done on the role of prices in determining overall eating patterns and health behaviors [57] or on pricing patterns across neighborhoods, urban/rural areas, food source formats or income classes, despite frequent assertions about prices of items being lower or higher in supermarkets or small stores or fast food restaurants. However, declines in relative food prices in the past decades have been significant and have likely helped to drive the changes in consumption patterns. Real-world prices for rice, sugar, soybean oil in 2000 were less than 40% of 1970 levels. Beef prices were half, and wheat prices were 60% [39]. Although prices have increased since 2004, inflation-adjusted food prices are still below levels of the food crisis of the mid-1970s [92]. Popkin et al. [80] argue that such declines are behind increased consumption of these foods, which has encouraged less healthful diets. They note, for instance, that commensurately with these price declines, individual intake of vegetable oils increased three to six times between 1985 and 2010, depending on the subpopulation studied. It is likely that consumption patterns in urban areas are a major driving force behind these numbers.

Food Price Shocks

The dependence on cash food purchases means that the urban poor are particularly vulnerable to food price shocks. Food price shocks rose to the top of the global political agenda during the food price crisis of 2007–2008, as world prices of wheat and maize tripled, compared to the levels at the beginning of 2003, and rice prices quintupled. Overall food prices rose by 64% between 2002 and mid-2008. Energy costs also climbed, which meant that not only the price of food, which has energy as a significant input cost, but also of other goods, such as transport, increased [93, 94].

While it has been commonly assumed that urban residents disproportionately suffered from these food price rises, analyses suggest that, most importantly, regardless of location it is the poor who suffer most [95]. However, even among the poor, the impact depends on a number of factors. This includes whether the household is a net food buyer; whether the household can shift from internationally traded staples, whose prices are most likely to be affected by the global price shocks, to less expensive, less traded goods such as roots and tubers; and whether the household has land, which might be used to grow crops that could actually benefit from the price rise or might otherwise be used as coping strategies [96]. The urban poor come out being disadvantaged on most of these counts: 97% of urban households are net food buyers, they spend a large proportion of their income on traded staples [96], and most do not have access to land for agriculture. Nevertheless, a simulation of a 10% rise in the price of food staples of nine LMIC indicated that the effects on urban and rural households were similar (between about a zero and 3% decline in welfare), except in Albania, Tajikistan and Vietnam, where urban households experienced a 1% point or more decline as compared to rural ones [96]. A different eight-country study found that simulated increases in food prices produced the largest increases in undernourishment (defined as dietary energy consumption falling below the minimum dietary energy requirements) among the middle-income or lowest income quintiles of both rural and urban areas [97]. Finally, a simulation analysis of four Latin American countries showed overall reductions in energy consumption resulting from the food price crisis, but no differences between urban and rural areas [98].

Urban Employment

The ability of the urban poor to obtain enough food for a healthy and active life depends primarily on their ability to earn income, yet low-paying, precarious jobs usually represent their most common employment opportunities. This exposes the urban poor to further income shocks, which will affect their ability to be food secure.

Most urban dwellers work in sectors such as petty trade, construction or manufacturing where wages are low and job tenure is insecure [99, 100]. Across developing countries, employment in the informal sector represents more than 50% of all non-agricultural employment [99]. In India, for example, 78% of the workforce is employed in the informal sector (excluding agriculture), which is mostly based in urban or semi-urban areas [101]. Non-agricultural informal employment in Latin America ranges from 42 to 75% of total employment, while averages for South and Southeast Asia hover around 70%. Women are generally more likely to be self-employed in the informal economy, and in sub-Saharan Africa, women outnumber men (51%) in the informal economy as a whole [99]. Nevertheless, formal sector jobs (government, private sector) are also important for the urban poor, particularly in some countries. Comparing data in metropolitan areas in four countries (Egypt, Ghana, Malawi and Peru), Garrett [100] found that at least as many if not a larger percentage of paid urban dwellers work in the formal, compared to the informal sector. In Egypt and Malawi, for example, more than 70% of urban jobs paid wages or salaries and only approximately 20% were self-employed.

Although informal jobs and self-employment may confer more flexibility in terms of hours worked and diversification of income, formal sector employment is likely a more stable and consistent source of income, but it tends to be less accessible for the poorest and less educated segments of the population.

Maternal Employment and Childcare

Women in urban areas are perceived to work away from home more often than those in rural areas and to be less likely to take their infant or young child along to their place of work because they often work in more formal environments (e.g., offices, factories, private homes). Whether or not this puts their children at an advantage or a disadvantage depends on the nature, stability and remuneration of the job, but equally importantly, on the type and quality of options for childcare. An analysis of data from Demographic Health Surveys (DHS) carried out in the early and mid-1990s in 11 developing countries of Africa, Asia and Latin America[10] showed that urban women were more likely to work outside the home only in Latin America (with the exception of Peru) [102]. In most of the Asian and African countries included in the sample, the percentage of women working away from home was higher in *rural* than in urban areas. However, urban mothers were less likely than rural mothers to take their child to work with them, probably because they worked in the streets or in more formal settings, like offices, factories or markets, rather than in agriculture where it might be easier to take a young child along. In Latin America, a greater percentage of urban mothers used relatives as alternative child caregivers compared to rural dwellers, but no consistent pattern was found in Asia and Africa. Hired help and institutional care were consistently higher in urban compared to rural areas in all three regions, although institutional care use was almost nonexistent in Asia and very uncommon in three of the four African countries studied, likely due to the lack of availability of these services in these countries [102].

A more comprehensive analysis comparing two urban areas Accra (Ghana) and Guatemala City (Guatemala) indicated that in both sites, women's employment and child care choices were highly influenced by the age of their youngest child [103]. Mothers with children under three years of age were less likely to be working, and if they did work, they were less likely to use formal child care as compared to mothers with older children. In Guatemala City, another important determinant of a woman's decision to work was the presence of an adult woman (a potential alternative child care-giver) in the household. In Ghana, where most urban women work in the informal sector, those who had to resume work for economic reasons when their child was still young usually took the child along to the workplace [104]. Depending on the work environment, this may or may not be positive for the child, but at a minimum it is likely to help facilitate breastfeeding, which confers important nutritional and developmental benefits to the child [105]. The number of hours a mother works each day, rather than the mother's employment status, has also been associated negatively with child

---

[10]The countries and year of survey included were for Asia: Bangladesh 1993 and Pakistan 1991; for Africa: Ghana 1993, Senegal 1992/93, Tanzania 1991/92, Zambia 1992; and for Latin America: Brazil 1996, Colombia 1995, Dominican Republic 1991, Guatemala 1995 and Peru 1992.

nutritional status in urban Dar-es-Salaam, Tanzania, but type and quality of substitute childcare was not analyzed [106].

One of the greatest threats of maternal employment to child caring is its potential negative impact on breastfeeding (a unique practice where a maternal substitute cannot be used [in most cases]). Unfortunately, there is very little research on the effects of maternal employment, and of different types and conditions of employment, on the ability of mothers to adopt optimal breastfeeding and complementary feeding practices. Earlier studies showed that maternal employment was not a main determinant of shorter breastfeeding duration or of breastmilk substitute use [107, 108]. The few studies that have looked at maternal employment and complementary feeding practices also found little evidence overall of a link between the two, or of an association between maternal employment and preventive or curative health seeking behaviors and psychosocial care, and child health and nutritional status [104, 109110111]. The key factor consistently associated with better caring practices was maternal schooling, which was not associated with employment status in the studies cited above. Again, the availability and quality of substitute child care can have tremendous effects on mitigating the potentially negative effects of maternal employment on child welfare, but this area is grossly understudied.

Additional indirect evidence that women's employment in urban areas of developing countries may not necessarily have a negative impact on child caregiving practices again comes from global urban–rural comparisons. Using DHS data from 36 countries, Smith et al. [112] found that complementary feeding practices (timing and frequency of feeding complementary foods) and health seeking behaviors were substantially better in urban compared to rural areas, even in countries where a large proportion of women were engaged in income-generating activities, often away from home. The authors attribute the urban advantage in complementary feeding and health seeking to higher maternal education, socioeconomic status and food availability, and to greater access to health services in urban compared to rural areas. Cawley and Liu [113], however, looked at this issue in the USA and found that maternal employment was associated with childhood obesity and less time spent on caregiving and food-related behaviors (e.g., women who worked spent 127 fewer minutes per day in child care and food-related behaviors, and only 15% of this difference was offset by the husband's contributions to child caregiving activities).

Overall, the scant literature on maternal employment and child nutrition and caregiving in developing countries suggests that mothers adopt a series of adaptive strategies to balance their dual role as income earner and child caregiver, such as stopping work around the perinatal period, working fewer hours or take their infant/young child to the workplace to preserve breastfeeding and ensuring adequate care. Although these adaptive strategies seem to be successful in protecting caregiving practices and children's nutritional status, they may, however, jeopardize the mothers' ability to generate income and to protect their household's livelihood and food security, especially if they are the sole income earner.

Formal and Informal Safety Nets

There is often a general perception that urban dwellers have greater access to formal safety nets. A 2014 survey analyzing data from more than 100 countries, however, shows that on average, there is less coverage of social safety nets among urban populations (21% of people covered) compared to rural populations (28%).[11] This distribution may be explained by the fact that globally, the majority of the poor still reside in rural areas, both relatively and in absolute numbers. Among other possible explanations, there could be a tendency to believe that urban populations do not need safety nets since

---

[11]World Bank, ASPIRE project: http://datatopics.worldbank.org/aspire/, accessed June 24, 2015.

more employment options are present in cities, even though jobs may be low-paying and insufficient to meet demand [114].

Compared to rural populations, it is assumed that the urban poor tend to live more transient lives: They may be rural migrants or simply move around more as circumstances change, seeking housing and jobs. The transient nature of the urban poor can present a challenge for safety net programs, as the targeted population can be difficult to locate and to maintain in the program. Nonetheless, over time some countries, such as Mexico, Colombia and Indonesia,[12] have been able to expand social protection programs originally instituted to support the poor in rural areas, to include poor households in peri-urban areas and cities. Governments are also creating policies specifically designed to support the most vulnerable urban residents, especially migrants and the unemployed, but the challenge of reaching vulnerable individuals and groups who fall outside the system remains.

Despite challenges, certain characteristics of urban areas may increase the chances of success of social assistance programs. In urban areas, information flows are generally better than in rural areas [115], making raising awareness about the program easier, and access to markets and facilities for cash transfers are also generally easier. In remote environments, traveling distances to collect transfers or to access markets can effectively diminish the value and impacts of the transfers. An accessible network of complementary services, generally more prevalent in cities compared to rural areas, can also improve the effectiveness of social assistance, especially for those programs that are conditioned on school attendance or use of health services. In Brazil, mortality from poverty-related deaths (e.g., malnutrition, diarrhea) in children under five years of age declined as the coverage of the conditional cash transfer program increased; importantly, these program effects were stronger for populations with access to a complementary healthcare service, as compared to those covered by more traditional, distant healthcare facilities [116]. NGOs and community-based organizations are often active in urban areas as well and can serve as important catalysts for improved social cooperation.

The poor may also rely on informal safety nets, which are commonly underpinned by social capital, meaning "features of social organization such as networks, norms, and social trust that facilitate coordination and cooperation for mutual benefit." [117]. These links tend to be most extensive and strong within immediate and extended family networks, because they rely heavily on social trust and reciprocity. Such links may be weaker in urban compared to rural areas, however, because of weaker identification with the community (especially when residence is temporary); higher levels of violence in urban areas, which can diminish the trust necessary for non-family collective action; and the fact that family members may live apart from one another, reducing the ability to undertake activities that do not rely on immediate reciprocity [118].

Availability and Access to Environmental and Health Services and Food Safety

The section reviews access to environmental and health services in urban areas, which are critically important for shaping food security and nutrition because they directly affect health and nutritional status.

Health services are generally more available in urban compared to rural areas of developing countries [119], but lack of access and use is often a key constraint, especially for the poorer segments

---

[12]World Bank case studies: **Indonesia**: Fernandez, Luisa (2014). "Urban Safety Net Case Study: Conditional Cash Transfer (PKH) Program in Indonesia". World Bank, Jakarta. **Colombia**. Vásquez, María Claudia (2014). "Case Study on Urban Social Protection. Conditional Cash Transfer Program in Bogotá, Colombia: "Familias en Acción". The World Bank. **Mexico**: Dávila Lárraga, Laura (2014). "Urban Social Protection in Mexico: The Human Development Opportunities Program—Oportunidades". The World Bank.

of the population. An analysis of DHS data from the 1990s from 35 countries found that overall urban dwellers were more likely than rural dwellers to use health services both for curative purposes—e.g., for childhood acute respiratory infections, fever or diarrhea—and for preventive services such as immunization [120]. A systematic review of 30 studies on inequalities in the use of maternal health care in developing countries found urban–rural differences in favor of urban dwellers for the use of skilled workers at delivery and the use of a medical setting for delivery, but less consistent results for use of antenatal care in the first trimester [121]. On the latter, one of the studies reviewed (from Jamaica) showed that urban women were *less* likely than rural women to attend antenatal care during their first trimester of pregnancy. Similarly, a recent review using data from 6 countries in sub-Saharan Africa (from late 1990s/early 2000 to 2011) documented the existence and persistence of inequalities in the use of three key maternal health services (antenatal care, facility-based delivery and modern contraception) in favor of wealthy and urban women [122]. The findings also show that countries where wealth and urban–rural inequalities decreased over time made greater strides in reducing maternal mortality than the countries where inequalities persisted.

As shown previously for other indicators, simple urban–rural comparisons mask socioeconomic disparities, which tend to be particularly large in urban areas. Within urban areas of India, for example, 83% of pregnant women in the top three wealth quartiles attended at least three prenatal healthcare visits, as opposed to only 54% in the poorest quartile, who tended to reside in slum areas [123]. Also in India, an analysis of data from the National Family Health Surveys (1992/93 and 2005/06) showed that the urban poor were at a clear disadvantage compared to the non-poor in terms of utilization of the same three maternal reproductive health services mentioned above in the African study [124].

Clearly, the greater availability of health services in urban compared to rural areas does not mean that all urban dwellers have equal access. Although healthcare access is often even more limited for many rural women, at least in India, a continuum in healthcare use has been described—from rural total, to urban poor, to urban non-poor [124].

Access to Safe Water and Good Sanitation

Many urban dwellers live in crowded, often unplanned, environments with limited access to quality water sources, poor sanitation, water drainage and waste disposal services. This makes it almost impossible to prevent contamination of water and food, maintain adequate levels of hygiene or control insect vectors of disease (such as dengue and malaria). Higher population density exacerbates the health risks of these conditions, so urban populations are particularly vulnerable [125]. Children and women, especially pregnant women, are those most affected by improper sanitation as they have a greater need for accessible, safe toilets and often take on the role of cleaning shared facilities [126]. Since improperly functioning sanitation systems are known to contaminate water sources, the issue of safe water is inextricable from that of good sanitation.

Urban child mortality has been shown to decrease as countries improve their access to safe drinking water [127]. Annually, 1.5 million children under five years of age die from illnesses related to unsafe water and poor sanitation, and in 2010 the UN General Assembly adopted a resolution that established access to safe water and sanitation as a basic human right [128]. Water- and food-borne diarrheal diseases also continue to be highly prevalent in urban areas. The prevalence of diarrhea among young children in urban areas is often high, or higher than in rural areas. A recent analysis of DHS data from 73 countries showed that children in smaller town slums were at higher risk of diarrhea than average for children living in urban or rural areas (who exhibited equal risk) [17]. Probably for this reason, improving access to sanitation in urban areas has been found to have a slightly higher impact on diarrhea in comparison with rural areas [129].

Since 1990, however, water and sanitation conditions have improved significantly. According to WHO/UNICEF [130], over 1.6 billion people gained access to improved[13] sources of drinking water between 1990 and 2012, but 750 million people still rely on unimproved sources. In 2012, in lower-income developing countries (termed less developed countries (LDCs) in the report), 84% of urban populations were using improved water sources, up from 79% in 1990. Rural populations in LDCs also gained access to improved water sources, increasing from 42 to 60% during the same period. Looking more broadly at developing regions of the world, access to improved water sources reached 95%, up from 93%, for urban populations and 80%, up from 58%, for rural populations. As of 2012, most regions had met the 2015 Millennium Development Goal (MDG) of halving the share of population without sustainable access to safe drinking water, or were on track to meet it, with the exception of sub-Saharan Africa, Oceania, and the Caucasus and Central Asia [130].

Similarly, significant progress has been made in improving sanitation. Between 1990 and 2012, almost 2 billion people worldwide gained access to improved sanitation,[14] but there are still 2.5 billion people who do not have such access and one billion people who practice open defecation [127]. Access in urban areas of LDCs increased from 38 to 48%, whereas access in rural areas continues to lag behind (having increased from a low 14 to 31% in the same period). In developing regions, access to improved sanitation increased from 64 to 73% in urban areas and from 21 to 43% in rural areas. Given population growth in urban areas, the numbers of people without sanitation in urban areas actually increased from 541 million in 1990 to 756 million in 2012, whereas in rural areas, the numbers dropped from 2.17 billion to 1.77 billion in the same period [130]. Again considering regional progress toward the global MDG, all regions except sub-Saharan Africa, Southern Asia and Oceania either were on track to meet or have met the target to halve the proportion of the population without sanitation. The number of people practicing open defecation has sharply declined by 21% during this same time period, from 1.3 billion to one billion. Open defecation in rural areas accounts for the vast majority of this occurrence; however, it is on the rise in some urban areas [130].

As noted above, although water and sanitation facilities are generally more readily available in urban compared to rural areas, there are often large differentials within urban areas in *access* to these services. In urban India, 62% of households from the three upper wealth quartiles, compared to 18.5% in the poorest quartile, had access to piped water at home [123]. Similarly, in Mombasa, Kenya, less than 20% of people living in informal settlements had access to piped and other improved sources of water compared to more than 60% among those living in formal settlements, and even within informal areas, wealthier households had much greater access to piped water [131]. Also, although water quality is generally superior in urban compared to rural areas [132], urban dwellers often have to pay for safe water. Slum areas, which are often located in unplanned areas, may be particularly affected. For example, between 1993 and 2003, slum households in Nairobi, Kenya, experienced a 33% decrease in access to piped water, while access decreased by 18 and 5% in other urban areas and in rural areas of Kenya, respectively [127]. Even when they pay for water, slum dwellers who purchased cheap bottled water have been shown to have greater risk of child morbidity, undernutrition and mortality in Indonesia, compared with those who have access to safe water or who purchased better-quality bottled water [133].

---

[13]WHO/UNICEF (2014) uses the following definition for an improved drinking water source: "…one that, by the nature of its construction, adequately protects the source from outside contamination, particularly faecal matter." Included in this grouping are (1) "piped water on premises: piped household water connection located inside the user's dwelling, plot, or yard," and (2) "other improved drinking water sources: public taps or standpipes, tube wells or boreholes, protected dug wells, protected springs, rainwater collection."

[14]WHO/UNICEF (2014) uses the following definition for an improved sanitation facility: "…one that hygienically separates human excreta from human contact." Included in this grouping are facilities that "flush/pour flush to piped sewer system, septic tank, pit latrine; ventilated improved pit (VIP) latrine; pit latrine with slab; composting toilet." Facilities that are public or shared between households are not grouped as improved.

Nevertheless, the urban and rural poor face different challenges and advantages in accessing water and sanitation. While the rural poor do not have to rely on cash income for these types of services, the urban poor do not have to travel as far to reach safe water or improved sanitation facilities [95]. However, informal urban housing areas shelter high concentrations of poor populations in need of safe water and sanitation, yet their legal status or location, that is, in areas which are flood-prone or lacking physical space for facilities, creates legal and planning challenges for improving water and sanitation services [126] and so may contribute to inequality in urban areas.

As a public good, proper sanitation has shared benefits, particularly apparent in crowded urban spaces. Collective action may be needed for residents to make their communal needs known and to manage community resources such as safe water and sanitation infrastructure. Case studies have shown that co-production, where communities and public agencies work together to address public goods problems, can be a successful model for addressing sanitation issues. Still, as noted above, the social capital required for this cooperation may be weak in informal urban settlements [125].

Food Safety

Food safety is a major concern in urban areas where supply chains are longer or otherwise originate in polluted urban areas; traceability and accountability measures are lacking or absent; and low-cost street foods are unregulated. While there is insufficient meta-analysis on food safety in urbanizing areas, research and case studies on food contamination in cities pinpoint a common set of contamination points in food value chains, such as wastewater irrigation, contaminated soils and unsanitary market conditions.

Urban/peri-urban food production may add food safety concerns to those that already exist in rural production [134]. In 2007, analysis of eleven varieties of fresh fruits from two main markets in Bangalore, India, showed contamination with unsafe amounts of heavy metals, which for cadmium exceeded by seven times the limit set by the Indian Prevention of Food Adulteration Act [135]. Studies investigating food safety in vegetables supplied to Accra and Kumasi, Ghana, and Niamey, Niger, determined that the presence of heavy metals was less of a risk for consumers than the presence of pathogens indicative of fecal contamination. The source of *Escherichia coli* present on lettuce in Niamey was believed to be from ruminant manure which was not fully composted when used to fertilize crops. Moreover, in this study, *E. coli*, streptococci and salmonella were all present in wastewater used to irrigate crops [136]. Likewise in peri-urban Mali, infant and young children's foods were found to be heavily contaminated with fecal indicator bacteria [137].

In Accra and Kumasi, studies by Amoah et al. [138] found the most significant contamination point along the lettuce supply chain was at the farm level, particularly untreated water and polluted soil, as compared to later points in the chain like the post-harvest and market levels, though these were also lacking in sanitary practices. Although some farmers used piped water to irrigate, most urban and peri-urban farmers could only irrigate from polluted water sources, in this case from drains, shallow wells near streams, or directly from the streams themselves. Samples from water sources used by farmers, with the exception of piped water, all contained levels of fecal coliform exceeding WHO standards. Even so, crops irrigated with piped water contained pathogens from application of poultry manure which was not fully composted. Due to the multiple points of contamination along the chain, this study suggests that intervention at the level of food preparation may be the most effective in mitigating risks of contaminated food.

Street food is discussed above, but it merits mention in this food safety discussion as well. The Amoah et al. surveys cited above showed that 60% of the lettuce purchased in Accra and 83% in Kumasi were bought by street vendors, where it was an ingredient in fast food meals. Although available for all income levels, this street food is most commonly purchased by males (70%) in low-income suburbs (50%); in fact, it is often the cheapest fast food in town, and for this reason, the health risks it poses are disproportionately borne by the poorest residents in these cities [138].

Studies on willingness to pay show increased consumer preference for food quality assurance, fueled by food safety concerns in urban areas. In 2009, Mergenthaler et al. found that consumers in metropolitan Vietnam were willing to pay an additional 60% of the purchase price for vegetables that did not have agrochemical residues. The authors found this willingness to pay to be higher than that reported for developed countries [139]. Food safety concerns are particularly high in China following recent food safety scares involving dangerous food additives, counterfeited products, food poisonings and sale of expired food. A survey in Beijing focusing on willingness to pay for HACCP (hazard analysis critical control point) milk products found that almost all consumers surveyed were willing to pay up to a 10% premium for HACCP products once they were educated on this quality assurance certification. A small percentage of respondents were willing to pay 30–50% premiums [140]. In 2009, sales of ultra-high temperature pasteurized milk increased by 50%. This demand was fueled by fears of adulterated milk powder which resulted in thousands of cases of sickness and infant death [141].

While higher-income populations may have available income to pay for price premiums to purchase safer food, the poor have fewer economic options and often lack electricity and/or access to refrigeration to safely store fresh or leftover food or to the use of hot water and other electric appliances to improve food safety practices [142]. Access to electricity has been shown to be a key factor in reducing child mortality in urban areas, independent of income, in an analysis of DHS data from 60 LDCs in the 1990s [143]. For rural populations, immunization coverage was the primary factor responsible for reductions in child mortality. On average, urban dwellers generally enjoy greater access to electricity than their rural counterparts; in Bangladesh, 71% of urban households have access to grid electricity, as compared to 20% of rural households. In South Africa, the urban–rural disparity is 80–50, and in Brazil, 99–77 [144].

Overall, access to safe food, control of environmental contaminants and effective quality assurance remain critical concerns for food safety in urban areas. While policy recommendations depend on the specific context at hand, it is clear that more systematic food quality assurances are needed and valued by urban inhabitants.

Implications for Policy, Programming and Research

This review highlights the dearth of information available to guide decisions about food security and nutrition policies and programs in urban areas. The slow awakening of the research community to the changing nature of urban poverty, food insecurity and malnutrition has left many research gaps to be filled. In almost every aspect of urban food security and nutrition covered here, the data and evidence are outdated, incomplete or insufficiently focused on the needs of and conditions facing the most vulnerable populations or, particularly in the case of physical activity, on the developing-country context. This includes weaknesses in terms of basic statistics about food insecurity and malnutrition, where even a clear agreed-upon indicator of food insecurity does not exist [145] and where few statistics are available about micronutrient deficiencies, which seem likely to become an even more important consideration as the focus on diet quality grows. National-, regional- or city-level data are sometimes available, but are not sufficient in number to provide global overviews or reliable rural–urban comparisons. The greatest amount of research so far seems to be around changing dietary patterns and the rise of supermarkets, although we have limited information about what the consequences of these changes are for urban versus rural consumers, or for the poorest, most food insecure and most malnourished.

In order to counter the rising challenge of the nutrition transition as well as truly achieve zero hunger and malnutrition, policymakers and programmers must better understand and take into account the challenges and opportunities found in urban areas of developing countries. They need to design policy and program instruments that can: (1) increase the availability and access of the urban poor to healthy, nutritious and safe foods and stimulate demand for high-quality diets; (2) facilitate physical activity through smart urban development that will ease access to—and affordability of— recreational facilities, encourage physical activity for daily transport and commuting and enhance safety; (3) promote and support urban agriculture where space and conditions allow; (4) support the production of safe, affordable and nutritious street foods; (5) create stable income-generating opportunities for urban dwellers, especially the poorest segments; (6) design cost-effective safety nets and other social protection programs and accurate targeting mechanisms to reach the poor to help them cope with shocks and build assets; (7) ease the trade-offs for working mothers by providing safe, affordable, accessible child care options of good quality; and (8) improve equal access of poor urban dwellers to health care, water, sanitation, waste removal and electricity.

Specifically, we urgently need updated and accurate data on the state of poverty, food insecurity and malnutrition in both urban and rural areas and among the most vulnerable populations. Disaggregation by location is needed to help policymakers and programmers make decisions regarding investments, prioritization and targeting. Figures need to provide a complete picture and so need to include data (collected over time in order to get at trends) on the multiple manifestations of malnutrition, including undernutrition, various key micronutrient deficiencies, and overweight and obesity. The figures need to be reported by gender and age groups and by income group.

We also need data and more comprehensive analyses to better understand the impacts of the rapidly changing food systems on urban livelihoods, diets and physical activity and on the nutritional status of urban dwellers. Research must help particularly to understand the conditions and unique challenges of the poor and those at most nutritional risk, who in spite of living in areas with infrastructure, basic services and fancy retail stores are often unable to access these services.

Surprisingly, little research has been done in developing countries on the urban food system and its interaction with the poor. Little comprehensive, reliable information exists about how and from where the urban poor actually access their food; what the influences on or constraints to a healthy diet are, including the effect of mass media, prices, market availability and the built environment, including electricity; and how these diets and influences vary by age and across population groups, including women, men, adolescents and those who are often outside the home for meals, such as those at school or at work.

Characteristics of the urban food system present challenges to nutrition, such as greater accessibility to highly processed foods, but also opportunities, such as having easier access to shops and so to a greater variety of foods or providing potential platforms to educate consumers and promote healthy eating choices. On a broader scale, research has been sporadic about the environmental sustainability of these urban food systems and how they interact with the local economy and local production.

Research is also needed to better understand the benefits and risks of urban and peri-urban agriculture in different contexts, and ways to support urban agriculture where it has the potential to contribute to urban livelihoods and food security, and to help poor households cope with food price fluctuations and other shocks. If appropriately supported, urban agriculture could also serve as an important vehicle for promoting production and increased consumption of nutrient-rich foods for vulnerable groups such as women and young children, and for generating income for women.

The importance of social networks and public policies and programs to the food security and nutrition of urban dwellers is also under-researched. Little is known about impacts or the costs and benefits of particular interventions on urban food security and nutrition. Research has to support efforts to design ways to identify the poor, hungry and nutritionally vulnerable; understand their needs; and provide guidance on the design and targeting of programs and expansion of services, including those of water and sanitation, that will not only be made available to them, but will also be able to access and afford.

While such services and programs are particularly important to mothers of young children, few systematic studies exist about the interaction between maternal employment and its effects on child nutrition as well as her own, the implications for older siblings who may be kept out of school to provide substitute childcare, and household welfare more generally. Research should examine more carefully how to address and ease the multiple challenges and trade-offs urban women face as they juggle between work outside the home and ensuring the food security of their household and caring for their young children. A deeper knowledge of the types of employment, informal networks and substitute childcare urban women have access to, as well a better understanding of their preferences and budgets, would help design more successful and affordable child care programs for poor urban women, and better-tailored recommendations for improving infant and young child feeding practices in urban areas, with consequent benefits for them and their families.

Conclusion

Our review confirms that the problems of urban poverty, food insecurity and malnutrition persist and are unlikely to be resolved by rapid urbanization and economic growth and development alone. Indeed, even though the prevalence of some forms of malnutrition is declining, with urban growth the numbers of urban poor and malnourished are likely to increase or at best remain constant. Undoubtedly, the location of the preponderance of the problem will shift from rural to urban areas and has already done so in Latin America. The economic disparities within urban areas, which are particularly high compared to those in rural areas, further illustrate that inclusive public sector action specifically directed at tackling urban poverty, food insecurity and malnutrition is needed, rather than simple reliance on general economic improvements. Developing countries must design comprehensive approaches to promote healthy diets and nutritious food systems and eradicate undernutrition and micronutrient deficiencies, while they also avert further rises in overweight, obesity and NCDs, and their costs in human lives and healthcare services. Governments and development partners can no longer ignore the unique features and needs of urban populations if they are to effectively address poverty, food insecurity and malnutrition globally.

Discussion Points

- What are the key research gaps that need to be filled in order to better understand the global trends in urbanization, poverty, food security and malnutrition?
- What are the most critically important features of urban life, compared to rural life, that affect poverty, food security and malnutrition in urban areas?
- What are the key factors that need to be considered when planning programs to alleviate poverty, food insecurity and malnutrition in urban areas (e.g., social safety net programs, programs to improve food security, programs to increase use of health services, or behavior change communications programs that focus on improving health and nutrition behaviors)
- What types of methods should be used to analyze the impacts of changing food systems on dietary patterns and nutrition in urban and rural areas?
- What types of policies would be most critically important to improve the economic productivity of women in urban areas while protecting their children's welfare? How should these policies be implemented and targeted?

Acknowledgments This chapter is a rewrite of "Rapid Urbanization and the Challenges of Obtaining Food and Nutrition Security," a chapter originally published in 2006 in this same book. We would like to thank Lawrence Haddad, one of the co-authors of the previous version of this chapter, and Lilia Bliznashka for her invaluable research assistance. Both are in the Poverty, Health and Nutrition Division of the International Food Policy Research Institute (IFPRI). Funding support was provided by the CGIAR Research Program on Agriculture for Nutrition and Health (A4NH), led by IFPRI.

References

1. United Nations. World Urbanization Prospects: The 2014 Revision, Highlights (ST/ESA/SER.A/352). New York: United Nations, Department of Economic and Social Affairs, Population Division; 2014.
2. Vlahov D, Galea S. Urbanization, urbanicity, and health. J Urban Health 2002;79:S1–12.
3. Razak F, Berkman L. Urban development in Sub-Saharan Africa: bearer of goods and risks. PLOS Med 2014;11 (7):1–2.
4. Potts D. The slowing of sub-Saharan Africa's urbanization: evidence and implications for urban livelihoods. Environ Urban [Internet]. 2009 [cited 2015 Jan 16];21:253–9. Available from: 10.1177/0956247809103026.
5. Ravallion M, Chen S, Sangraula P. New evidence on the urbanization of global poverty. Popul Dev Rev. 2007;33:667–701.
6. FAO. Growing greener cities. Rome, Italy: Food and Agriculture Organization (FAO); 2010.
7. Smith LC, Alderman H, Aduayom D. Food insecurity in sub-Saharan Africa. New estimates from household expenditure surveys. Research Report 146. Washington, DC: International Food Policy Research Institute; 2006.
8. Ahmed AU, Vargas-Hill R, Smith LC, Wiesmann DM, Frankenberger TR. The world's most deprived: characteristics and causes of extreme poverty and hunger. Washington, DC: International Food Policy Research Institute (IFPRI); 2007.
9. Smith LC, Dupriez O, Troubat N. Assessment of the reliability and relevance of the food data collected in national household consumption and expenditure surveys. International Household Survey Network. IHSN Working Paper, No. 008. [Internet]. 2014. Available from: http://www.ihsn.org/home/sites/default/files/resources/HCESfood%20data%20assessment%20report_DRAFT_V8_25_02_14.pdf.
10. Hoddinott J, Behrman JR, Maluccio JA, Melgar P, Quisumbing AR, Ramirez-Zea M, Stein AD, Yount KM, Martorell R. Adult consequences of growth failure in early childhood. Am J Clin Nutr. 2013;98:1170–8.
11. Paciorek CJ, Stevens G a, Finucane MM, Ezzati M. Children's height and weight in rural and urban populations in low-income and middle-income countries: a systematic analysis of population-representative data. Lancet Glob Heal [Internet]. Paciorek et al. Open Access article distributed under the terms of CC BY; 2013 [cited 2014 Dec 10];1:e300–9. Available from: http://www.ncbi.nlm.nih.gov/pubmed/25104494.
12. Katz J. Tracking nutritional changes in an urbanising world beyond 2015. Lancet Glob Heal [Internet]. Katz. Open Access article distributed under the terms of CC BY-NC-SA; 2013 [cited 2015 Jan 12];1:e245–6. Available from: http://www.ncbi.nlm.nih.gov/pubmed/25104484.
13. Menon P, Ruel MT, Morris SS. Socio-economic differentials in child stunting are consistently larger in urban than rural areas: analysis of 10 DHS data sets. Food Nutr Bull. 2000;21:282–9.
14. Van de Poel E, O'Donnell O, Van Doorslaer E. Are urban children really healthier? Evidence from 47 developing countries. Soc Sci Med [Internet]. 2007 [cited 2015 Jan 28];65:1986–2003. Available from: http://www.ncbi.nlm.nih.gov/pubmed/17698272.
15. Smith LC, Ruel MT, Ndiaye A. Why is child malnutrition lower in urban than in rural areas? Evidence from 36 developing countries. World Dev. 2005;33:1285–305.
16. Fox K, Heaton TB. Child nutritional status by rural/urban residence: a cross-national analysis. J Rural Health [Internet]. 2012 [cited 2015 Jan 28];28:380–91. Available from: http://www.ncbi.nlm.nih.gov/pubmed/23083084.
17. Fink G, Günther I, Hill K. Slum residence and child health in developing countries. Demography [Internet]. 2014 [cited 2015 Jan 28];51:1175–97. Available from: http://www.ncbi.nlm.nih.gov/pubmed/24895049.
18. Garrett JL, Ruel MT. Are determinants of rural and urban food security and nutritional status different? Some insights from Mozambique. World Dev. 1999;27:1955–75.
19. Srinivasan CS, Zanello G, Shankar B. Rural-urban disparities in child nutrition in Bangladesh and Nepal. BMC Public Health [Internet]. BMC Public Health; 2013 [cited 2015 Jan 28];13:581. Available from: http://www.pubmedcentral.nih.gov/articlerender.fcgi?artid=3729423&tool=pmcentrez&rendertype=abstract.
20. Kennedy G, Nantel G, Brouwer ID, Kok FJ. Does living in an urban environment confer advantages for childhood nutritional status? Analysis of disparities in nutritional status by wealth and residence in Angola, Central African Republic and Senegal. Public Health Nutr [Internet]. 2007 [cited 2015 Jan 28];9:187–93. Available from: http://www.journals.cambridge.org/abstract_S1368980006000371.

21. Black RE, Victora CG, Walker SP, Bhutta ZA, Christian P, de Onis M, Ezzati M, Grantham-McGregor S, Katz J, Martorell R, et al. Maternal and child undernutrition and overweight in low-income and middle-income countries. Lancet [Internet]. 2013 [cited 2013 Jun 6];382:427–51. Available from: http://linkinghub.elsevier.com/retrieve/pii/S014067361360937X.

22. World Bank. Data—Country and Lending Groups [Internet]. 2015 [cited 2015 Feb 9]. Available from: http://data.worldbank.org/about/country-and-lending-groups#Europe_and_Central_Asia.

23. Stevens GA, Singh GM, Lu Y, Danaei G, Lin JK, Finucane MM, Bahalim AN, McIntire RK, Gutierrez HR, Cowan M, et al. National, regional, and global trends in adult overweight and obesity prevalences. Popul Health Metr [Internet]. Population Health Metrics; 2012 [cited 2014 Nov 23];10:22. Available from: http://www.pubmedcentral.nih.gov/articlerender.fcgi?artid=3543235&tool=pmcentrez&rendertype=abstract.

24. WHO. Obesity: situation and trends [Internet]. website. 2015 [cited 2015 Jan 19]. Available from: http://www.who.int/gho/ncd/risk_factors/obesity_text/en/.

25. Neuman M, Kawachi I, Gortmaker S, Subramanian SV. Urban-rural differences in BMI in low- and middle-income countries: the role of socioeconomic status. Am J Clin Nutr. 2013;97:428–36.

26. Popkin BM, Adair LS, Ng SW. NOW AND THEN: the global nutrition transition: the pandemic of obesity in developing countries. Nutr Rev. 2013;70:3–21.

27. Jaacks LM, Slining MM, Popkin BM. Recent underweight and overweight trends by rural–urban residence among women in low- and middle-income countries. J Nutr. 2014;(epub ahead of print).

28. Garrett J, Ruel MT. Stunted child-overweight mother pairs: Prevalence and association with economic development and urbanization. Food Nutr Bull. 2005;26:209–21.

29. Monteiro CA, Moura EC, Conde WL, Popkin BM. Socioeconomic status and obesity in adult populations of developing countries: a review. Bull World Health Organ. 2004;82:940–6.

30. Caballero B. Emerging global epidemic of obesity: the renal perspective. Epidemic Rev. 2007;29:1–5.

31. Omran AR. The epidemiologic transition: a theory of the epidemiology of population change'. Milbank Mem Fund Q 1971;49:509–38.

32. Drewnowski A, Popkin BM. The nutrition transition: new trends in the global diet. Nutr Rev 1997;55:31–43.

33. Popkin BM, Gordon-Larsen P. The nutrition transition: worldwide obesity dynamics and their determinants. Int J Obes Relat Metab Disord 2004;28 Suppl 3:S2–9.

34. Popkin BM, Bisgrove EZ. Urbanization and nutrition in low-income countries. Food Nutr Bull. 1988;10.

35. Caballero B, Rubinstein S. Environmental factors affecting nutritional status in urban areas of developing countries. Arch Latinoam Nutr. 1997;47:3–8.

36. Mendez M a, Popkin BM. Globalization, urbanization and nutritional change in the developing world. J Agric Dev Econ. 2004;1:220–41.

37. Popkin BM, Gordon-Larsen P. The nutrition transition: worldwide obesity dynamics and their determinants. Int J Obes Relat Metab Disord. 2004;28(Suppl 3):S2–9.

38. Uauy R, Monteiro C. The challenge of improving food and nutrition in Latin America. Food Nutr Bull. 2004;25:175–82.

39. Shapouri S, Rosen S. Global diet composition: factors behind the changes and implications of the new trends. Food Secur Assess [Internet]. 2007;28–37. Available from: http://162.79.45.209/media/205655/gfa19b_1_.pdf.

40. Kolčić I. Double burden of malnutrition: a silent driver of double burden of disease in low- and middle-income countries. J Glob Health [Internet]. 2012;2:1–6. Available from: http://www.pubmedcentral.nih.gov/articlerender.fcgi?artid=3529312&tool=pmcentrez&rendertype=abstract.

41. Tzioumis E, Adair LS. Child dual burden of under- and over-nutrition in low- and middle-income countries: a critical review. Food Nutr Bull. 2014;35:230–43.

42. Stage J, Stage J, McGranahan G. Is urbanization contributing to higher food prices ? Human Settlements Working Paper Series. Urbanization and emerging populations issues—1. [Internet]. London and New York: IIED and UNFPA; 2009. Available from: http://www.iied.org/pubs/display.php?o=10573IIED.

43. Reardon T, Timmer CP, Barrett CB, Berdegué J. The rise of supermarkets in Africa, Asia, and Latin America. Am J Agric Econ. 2003;85:1140–6.

44. Schram A, Labonté R, Sanders D. Urbanization and international trade and investment policies as determinants of noncommunicable diseases in Sub-Saharan Africa. Prog Cardiovasc Dis [Internet]. Elsevier Inc.; 2013 [cited 2015 Jan 28];56:281–301. Available from: http://www.ncbi.nlm.nih.gov/pubmed/24267436.

45. Abrahams Z, Mchiza Z, Steyn NP. Diet and mortality rates in Sub-Saharan Africa: Stages in the nutrition transition. BMC Public Health [Internet]. BioMed Central Ltd; 2011;11:801. Available from: http://www.biomedcentral.com/1471-2458/11/801.

46. Godfray HCJ, Crute IR, Haddad L, Lawrence D, Muir JF, Nisbett N, Pretty J, Robinson S, Toulmin C, Whiteley R. The future of the global food system. Philos Trans R Soc Lond B Biol Sci. 2010;365:2769–77.

47. Huang J, Bouis H. Structural changes in the demand for food in Asia. Food, agriculture, and the environment. Discussion Paper 11. Washington, DC: International Food Policy Research Institute; 1996.

48. Becquey E, Martin-Prével Y. Micronutrient adequacy of women' s diet in Burkina Faso is low. J Nutr. 2010;140:2079S–85S.
49. Kennedy G, Fanou N, Brouwer ID. Dietary diversity as a measure of the micronutrient adequacy of women's diets: results from Bamako, Mali Site. Washington, DC: Food and nutrition Technical Assistance II Project, Academy for Educational Development; 2009.
50. van't Riet H, den Hartog AP, van Staveren WA. Non-home prepared foods: contribution to energy and nutrient intake of consumers living in two low-income areas in Nairobi. Public Health Nutr. 2002;5:515–22.
51. Semba RD, Moench-Pfanner R, Sun K, de Pee S, Akhter N, Rah JH, Campbell AC, Badham J, Bloem MW, Kraemer K. Consumption of micronutrient-fortified milk and noodles is associated with lower risk of stunting in preschool-aged children in Indonesia. Food Nutr Bull. 2011;32:347–53.
52. Rivera JA, Pedraza LS, Martorell R, Gil A, Bank ID. Introduction to the double burden of undernutrition and excess weight. 2014;100(suppl):1613S–6S.
53. Pratt M, Jacoby ER, Neiman A. Promoting physical activity in the senior years. Food Nutr Bull. 2004;25:183–93.
54. Dumith SC, Hallal PC, Reis RS, Kohl HW. Worldwide prevalence of physical inactivity and its association with human development index in 76 countries. Prev Med (Baltim) [Internet]. Elsevier Inc.; 2011;53:24–8. Available from: 10.1016/j.ypmed.2011.02.017.
55. Reichert FF, Barros AJD, Domingues MR, Hallal PC. The role of perceived personal barriers to engagement in leisure-time physical activity. Am J Public Health. 2007;97:515–9.
56. Duncan MJ, Spence JC, Mummery WK. Perceived environment and physical activity: a meta-analysis of selected environmental characteristics. Int J Behav Nutr Phys Act. 2005;2:1–9.
57. Popkin BM, Duffey K, Gordon-Larsen P. Environmental influences on food choice, physical activity and energy balance. Physiol Behav. 2005;86:603–13.
58. Gittelsohn J, Franceschini MCT, Rasooly IR, Ries AV, Ho LS, Pavlovich W, Santos VT, Jennings SM, Frick KD. Understanding the food environment in a low-income urban setting: implications for food store interventions. J Hunger Environ Nutr. 2008;2:33–50.
59. Moore L V., Diez Roux A V., Nettleton J a., Jacobs DR. Associations of the local food environment with diet quality—a comparison of assessments based on surveys and geographic information systems. Am J Epidemiol. 2008;167:917–24.
60. Smith DM, Cummins S, Taylor M, Dawson J, Marshall D, Sparks L, Anderson AS. Neighbourhood food environment and area deprivation: spatial accessibility to grocery stores selling fresh fruit and vegetables in urban and rural settings. Int J Epidemiol. 2010;39:277–84.
61. Bodor JN, Rose D, Farley T a, Swalm C, Scott SK. Neighbourhood fruit and vegetable availability and consumption: the role of small food stores in an urban environment. Public Health Nutr. 2008;11:413–20.
62. Reardon T. The global rise and impact of supermarkets: an international perspective. Paper prepared for "The Supermarket Revolution in Food: Good, bad or ugly for the world's farmers and retailers?" conference, Crawford Fund for International Agricultural Research, 2011.
63. Weatherspoon DD, Reardon T. The rise of supermarkets in Africa: implications for agrifood systems and the rural poor. Dev Policy Rev [Internet]. 2003;21:333–55. Available from: 10.1111/1467-7679.00214.
64. Reardon T, Berdegué JA. The Rapid Rise of Supermarkets in Latin America: Challenges and opportunities for development. Dev Policy Rev [Internet]. 2002;20:371–88. Available from: 10.1111/1467-7679.00178; 10.1111/1467-7679.00183.
65. Reardon T, Timmer P, Berdegue J. The rapid rise of supermarkets in developing countries: induced organizational, institutional, and technological change in agrifood systems. Africa (Lond) [Internet]. 2004;1:168–83. Available from: http://ideas.repec.org/a/fao/tejade/v1y2004i2p168-183.html.
66. Reardon T, Timmer P, Berdegué J. The rapid rise of supermarkets in developing countries: induced organizational, institutional, and technological change in agrifood systems. eJADE. 1AD;2:168–83.
67. Randolph T, Schelling E, Grace D, Nicholson C, Leroy J, Cole D, Demment M, Omore A, Zinsstag J, Ruel M. Role of livestock in human nutrition and health for poverty reduction in developing countries. J Anim Sci. 2007;85:2788–800.
68. Timmer P. The impact of supermarkets on nutrition and nutrition knowledge: a food policy perspective. Nutrition and Health in a Developing World 3rd Edition. In: de Pee S, Taren D, Bloem MW, editors. Nutrition and health in a developing world. 3rd ed.
69. Monteiro C, Levy R, Claro R, de Castro I, Cannon G. Increasing consumption of ultra-processed foods and likely impact on human health: evidence from Brazil. Public Health Nutr [Internet]. 2011;14:5–13. Available from: http://www.journals.cambridge.org/abstract_S1368980010003241.
70. Organization PAH. Ultra-processed food and drink products in Latin America: trends, impact on obesity, policy implications. Washington, DC: PAHO; 2015.
71. Traill W. The rapid rise of supermarkets? Dev Policy Rev. 2006;24:163–74.
72. Gómez MI, Ricketts KD. Food value chain transformations in developing countries: selected hypotheses on nutritional implications. Food Policy. 2013;42:139–50.

73. Zameer A, Mukherjee D. Food and grocery retail: patronage behavior of indian urban consumers. South Asian J Manage. 2011;18(1):119–34.
74. Goldman A, Ramaswami S, Krider R. Barriers to the advancement of modern food retail formats: theory and measurement. J Retail. 2002;281–95.
75. Minten B, Reardon T. Food prices, quality, and quality's pricing in supermarkets versus traditional markets in developing countries. Rev Agric Econ. 2008;30:480–90.
76. FAO. The state of food and agriculture (SOFA). Food Systems for Better Nutrition. [Internet]. Rome, Italy: FAO; 2013. Available from: http://www.pubmedcentral.nih.gov/articlerender.fcgi?artid=3291936&tool=pmcentrez&rendertype=abstract.
77. Ayieko M, Tschirley D, Mathenge M. Fresh fruit and vegetable consumption patterns and supply chain systems in urban Kenya: implications for policy and investment priorities. Working Paper 19. Egerton, Kenya: Tegemeo Institute of Agricultural Policy and Development; 2005.
78. Reardon T, Timmer CP. The economics of the food system revolution. Annu Rev Resour Econ. 2012;4:225–64.
79. Rayner G, Hawkes C, Lang T, Bello W. Trade liberalization and the diet transition: a public health response. Health Promot Int. 2007;21(Suppl 1):67–74.
80. Popkin BM, Adair LS, Ng SW. Global nutrition transition and the pandemic of obesity in developing countries. Nutr Rev. 2012;70:3–21.
81. Aekplakorn W, Hogan MC, Chongsuvivatwong V, Tatsanavivat P, Chariyalertsak S, Boonthum A, Tiptaradol S, Lim SS. Trends in obesity and associations with education and urban or rural residence in Thailand. Obesity. 2007;15:3113–21.
82. Thow AM, Hawkes C. The implications of trade liberalization for diet and health: a case study from Central America. Glob Health. 2009;5:5.
83. Bhowmik S. Street vendors in Asia: a review. Econ Polit Wkly. 2005.
84. Tinker I. Street foods: urban food and employment in developing countries. Oxford: Oxford University Press; 1997.
85. Simopoulos A, Bhat R, editors. Street foods. New York: Karger; 2000.
86. Bhat R, Waghray K. Bhat RV, Waghray K. Profile of street foods sold in Asian countries. World Rev Nutr Diet. 2000;86:53–99.
87. Mishra S. Street food and urban and periurban agriculture and horticulture: perspectives for a strategic coalition towards food security. Global Forum on Food Security and Nutrition Online Contribution. 2014.
88. Zezza A, Tasciotti L. Urban agriculture, poverty, and food security: empirical evidence from a sample of developing countries. Food Policy [Internet]. Elsevier Ltd; 2010 [cited 2014 Sep 3];35:265–73. Available from: http://linkinghub.elsevier.com/retrieve/pii/S0306919210000515.
89. Redwood M, editor. Agriculture in urban planning: generating livelihoods and food security. Ottawa and London: International Development Research Centre and Earthscan; 2009.
90. UNDP. Urban agriculture, food, jobs, and sustainable cities. United Nations Development Programme Publication Series for Habitat II, vol. I. New York: UNDP; 1996.
91. Garrett J, Ersado L. A rural-urban comparison of cash and consumption expenditure. (Mimeo). Washington DC: World Bank and International Food Policy Research Institute; 2003.
92. FAO. World Food Situation. FAO Food Price Index. [Internet]. Rome: Food and Agricultural Organization of the United Nations; 2015. Available from: http://www.fao.org/worldfoodsituation/foodpricesindex/en/, 27 June 2015.
93. Cohen M, Garrett J. Food price volatility and urban food insecurity. In: Seto K, Solecki W, Griffith C, editors. Handbook on urbanization and global environmental change. Tempe, Arizona: Global Institute of Sustainability.
94. Cohen MJ, Garrett JL. The food price crisis and urban food (in)security. Environ Urban [Internet]. 2010;22:467–82. Available from: <Go to ISI> ://WOS:000283511400011\nhttp://eau.sagepub.com/content/22/2/467.full.pdf.
95. Ruel MT, Garrett JL, Hawkes C, Cohen MJ. The food, fuel, and financial crises affect the urban and rural poor disproportionately: a review of the evidence. J Nutr. 2010;140:170S–6S.
96. FAO. The state of food insecurity in the world. High food prices and food security—threats and opportunities. Rome, Italy: Food and Agriculture Organization (FAO); 2008.
97. Anríquez G, Daidone S, Mane E. Rising food prices and undernourishment: a cross-country inquiry. Food Policy [Internet]. 2013 [cited 2015 Jan 28];38:190–202. Available from: http://linkinghub.elsevier.com/retrieve/pii/S0306919212000140.
98. Robles M, Torero M. Understanding the impact of high food prices in Latin America. Econ J LACEA. 2010;10(2):117–59.
99. Charmes J. The informal economy worldwide: trends and characteristics. Margin J Appl Econ Res. 2012;6:103–32.
100. Garrett J. Living life: overlooked aspects of urban employment. Food Consumption and Nutrition Division Discussion Paper 171. Washington, DC: International Food Policy Research Institute; 2004.
101. Kar S, Marjit S. Urban informal sector and poverty. Int Rev Econ Finan. 2009;18:631–42.
102. Ruel MT, Haddad LJ, Garrett JL. Some urban facts of life: implications for research and policy. World Dev. 1999;27:1917–38.

103. Quisumbing AR, Hallman K, Ruel MT. Maquiladoras and market mamas: women's work and childcare in Guatemala City and Accra [Internet]. Washington, D.C.: International Food Policy Research Institute (IFPRI); 2003. p. 48. Available from: http://www.ifpri.org/publication/maquiladoras-and-market-mamas.

104. Armar-Klemesu M, Ruel M, Maxwell D, Levin C, Morris S. Poor maternal schooling is the main constraint to good child care practices in Accra. J Nutr. 2000;130:1597–607.

105. Victora CG, Horta BL, de Mola CL, Quevedo L, Pinheiro RT, Gigante DP, Gonçalves H, Barros FC. Association between breastfeeding and intelligence, educational attainment, and income at 30 years of age: a prospective birth cohort study from Brazil. Lancet Glob Heal [Internet]. Victora et al. Open Access article distributed under the terms of CC BY; 2015;3:e199–205. Available from: http://www.thelancet.com/article/S2214109X15700021/fulltext.

106. Kulwa KBM, Kinabo JLD, Modest B. Constraints on good child-care practices and nutritional status in urban Dar-es-Salaam, Tanzania. Food Nutr Bull. 2006;27:236–44.

107. Hight-Laukaran V, Rutstein S, Peterson A, Labbok M. The use of breast milk substitutes in developing countries: the impact of women's employment. Am J Public Health. 1996;86:1235–40.

108. Winikoff B, Castle M, Hight-Laukaran V. Feeding infants in four societies. Contributions in family studies No. 14. New York: Greenwood Press; 1988.

109. Glick P, Sahn D. Maternal labour supply and child nutrition in West Africa. Oxf Bull Econ Stat. 1998;60:325–55.

110. Blau D, Guilkey D, Popkin B. Infant health and the labor supply of mothers. J Hum Resour. 1997;31:90–139.

111. Engle PL, Menon P, Garrett J, Slack A. Urbanization and caregiving: a framework for analysis and examples from Southern and Eastern Africa. Environ Urban. 1997;9:253–70.

112. Smith L, Ruel M, Ndiaye A. Why is child malnutrition lower in urban than in rural areas? Evidence from 36 developing countries. World Dev. 2005;33:1285–305.

113. Cawley J, Liu F. Maternal employment and childhood obesity: a search for mechanisms in time use data. Econ Hum Biol [Internet]. Elsevier B.V.; 2012;10:352–64. Available from: 10.1016/j.ehb.2012.04.009.

114. Gentilini U, Honorati M, Yemtsov R. How are the urban poor covered by safety nets? Preliminary evidence from survey data. Washington, DC: World Bank Group (mimeo); 2014.

115. Alderman H, Gentilini U, Gilligan DO, Hoddinott J, Karachiwalla N. Designing and implementing urban safety nets: a review of selected issues and practices (mimeo). 2014.

116. Rasella D, Aquino R, Santos C a T, Paes-Sousa R, Barreto ML. Effect of a conditional cash transfer programme on childhood mortality: a nationwide analysis of Brazilian municipalities. Lancet [Internet]. Elsevier Ltd; 2013 [cited 2015 Jan 28];382:57–64. Available from: http://www.ncbi.nlm.nih.gov/pubmed/23683599.

117. Putnam R. Bowling alone: America's declining social capital. J Democr. 1995;6:65–78.

118. Foster G. Safety Nets for children affected by HIV/AIDS in Southern Africa. In: Pharoah R, editor. A generation at risk? HIV/AIDS, vulnerable children and security in Southern Africa. 2004.

119. Godfrey R, Julien M. Urbanisation and health. Clin Med J R Coll Phys Lond. 2005;5:137–41.

120. Ruel M, Garrett J, Morris S, Maxwell D, Oshaug A, Engle P, Menon P, Slack A, Haddad L. Urban challenges to nutrition security: a review of food security, health and care in the cities. Food Consumption and Nutrition Division Discussion Paper 51. Washington DC: International Food Policy Research Institute; 1998. Ruel, M.T.

121. Say L, Raine R. A systematic review of inequalities in the use of maternal health care in developing countries. Bull World Heal Organ [Internet]. 2007;85:812–9. Available from: http://www-wds.worldbank.org/external/default/WDSContentServer/WDSP/IB/2006/02/02/000160016_20060202161329/Rendered/PDF/351170Benefit0incidence0practitioner.pdf.

122. Alam N, Hajizadeh M, Dumont A, Fournier P. Inequalities in maternal health care utilization in sub-Saharan African countries: a multiyear and multi-country analysis. PLoS ONE [Internet]. 2015;10:e0120922. Available from: http://dx.plos.org/10.1371/journal.pone.0120922.

123. Agarwal S. The state of urban health in India; comparing the poorest quartile to the rest of the urban population in selected states and cities. Environ Urban. 2011;23:13–28.

124. Kumar A, Mohanty SK. Intra-urban differentials in the utilization of reproductive healthcare in India, 1992-2006. J Urban Heal. 2011;88:311–28.

125. McGranahan G. Realizing the right to sanitation in deprived urban communities: meeting the challenges of collective action, coproduction, affordability, and housing tenure. World Dev [Internet]. Elsevier Ltd; 2015;68:242–53. Available from: http://linkinghub.elsevier.com/retrieve/pii/S0305750X14004069.

126. Satterthwaite D, Mitlin D, Bartlett S. Is it possible to reach low-income urban dwellers with good-quality sanitation? Environ Urban [Internet]. 2015;27(1):3–18. Available from: http://eau.sagepub.com/cgi/doi/10.1177/0956247815576286.

127. Fotso J-C, Ezeh AC, Madise NJ, Ciera J. Progress towards the child mortality millennium development goal in urban sub-Saharan Africa: the dynamics of population growth, immunization, and access to clean water. BMC Public Health. 2007;7:218.

128. United Nations General Assembly. General assembly adopts resolution recognizing access to clean water, sanitation as human right, by Recorded Vote of 122 in Favour, None against, 41 Abstentions [Internet]. 2010 [cited 2015 Jun 26]. Available from: http://www.un.org/press/en/2010/ga10967.doc.htm.

129. Günther I, Fink G. Water and sanitation to reduce child mortality. The impact and cost of water and sanitation infrastructure. Policy Research Working Paper 5618. Washington, D.C.: World Bank; 2011.

130. WHO/UNICEF. Progress on drinking water and sanitation. 2014 Update. Geneva (WHO) and New York (UNICEF): World Health Organization (WHO) and UNICEF; 2014.

131. WHO, UNICEF. Progress on sanitation and drinking water: 2012 update. WHO and UNICEF Joint Monitoring Programme for Water Supply and Sanitation. New York and Geneva: WHO and UNICEF; 2012.

132. Bain R, Cronk JA, Wright H, Yang T, Slaymaker J, Bartram K. Fecal contamination of drinking-water in low- and middle-income countries: a systematic review and meta-analysis. PLoS Med. 2014;11:e1001644.

133. Semba RD, de Pee S, Kraemer K, Sun K, Thorne-Lyman A, Moench-Pfanner R, Sari M, Akhter N, Bloem MW. Purchase of drinking water is associated with increased child morbidity and mortality among urban slum-dwelling families in Indonesia. Int J Hyg Environ Health [Internet]. 2009;212:387–97. Available from: http://linkinghub.elsevier.com/retrieve/pii/S1438463908000771.

134. Huang Y, Wu Y, Zhi H, Rozelle S. Small holder incomes, food safety and producing, and marketing China's fruit. Rev Agric Econ. 2008;30:469–79.

135. Mahdavian SE, Somashekar RK. Heavy metals and safety of fresh fruits in Bangalore City, India—a case study. Kathmandu Univ J Sci Eng Technol. 2008;I:17–27.

136. Diogo RVC, Buerkert A, Schlecht E. Horizontal nutrient fluxes and food safety in urban and peri-urban vegetable and millet cultivation of Niamey, Niger. Nutr Cycl Agroecosyst. 2010;87:81–102.

137. Toure O, Coulibaly S, Arby A, Maiga F, Cairncross S. Piloting an intervention to improve microbiological food safety in peri-urban Mali. Int J Hyg Environ Health. 2013;216:138–45.

138. Amoah P, Drechsel P, Abaidoo RC, Henseler M. Irrigated urban vegetable production in Ghana: microbiological contamination in farms and markets and associated consumer risk groups. J Water Health. 2007;5:455–66.

139. Mergenthaler M, Weinberger K, Qaim M. Consumer valuation of food quality and food safety attributes in Vietnam. Rev Agric Econ. 2009;31:266–83.

140. Wang Z, Mao Y, Gale F. Chinese consumer demand for food safety attributes in milk products. Food Policy. 2008;33:27–36.

141. Ortega DL, Wang HH, Olynk NJ, Wu L, Bai J, Rtega DALO, Ang HHOW, Lynk NIJO, Aping LWU, Ai JUB. Chinese consumers' demand for food safety attributes: a push for government and industry regulations. Am J Agric Econ. 2011;94:489–95.

142. Sudershan RV, Rao GMS, Rao P, Rao MVV, Polasa K. Food safety related perceptions and practices of mothers—a case study in Hyderabad, India. Food Control. 2008. 506–13.

143. Wang L. Determinants of child mortality in low-income countries : empirical findings from demographic and health surveys. 2002. 1–42.

144. Winkler H, Simoes AF, Lebre la Rovere E, Alam M, Rahman A, Mwakasonda S. Access and affordability of electricity in developing countries. World Dev. 2011;39:1037–50.

145. Leroy JL, Ruel M, Frongillo EA, Harris J, Ballard TJ. Measuring the food access dimension of food security: a critical review and mapping of indicators. Food Nutr Bull. 2015;36:167–95.

Chapter 33
The Impact of Supermarkets on Nutrition and Nutritional Knowledge: A Food Policy Perspective

C. Peter Timmer

Keywords Dietary transition · Economic growth · Food policy · Food security · Marketing system · Nutritional impacts · Role of governments · Supermarkets

Learning Objectives

- Describe the modern food supply chain.
- Explain four trends in the modern food supply chain.
- Analyze how supermarkets affect the food supply.
- Discuss how supermarkets can affect poverty and food security.

Introduction

The world of traditional food and nutritional knowledge being handed down from (mostly) mothers to daughters through household experiences is being rapidly transformed into a learning process that takes place in front of the television and in the aisles of supermarkets. How scary is that? It is, of course, possible to eat a healthy (and safe) diet from those aisles, but it is not easy. Critics such as Michael Pollan of the University of California, Berkeley, and Mark Bittman of the *New York Times* complain that the modern food industry, and its food and nutritional scientists, concentrate on getting consumers to buy highly processed foods high in salt, fat and sugar because they are very profitable. These foods are marketed aggressively, especially on children's television and via packaging in supermarkets. Most of what children know about healthy nutrition comes from these two sources. As suppliers to rich and well-educated consumers, supermarkets present serious public health challenges. As suppliers to poor and uneducated consumers, the dangers multiply. The goal of this chapter is to put these potential dangers from the rapid emergence of supermarkets in low- and middle-income countries (LMICs) into the context of the essential roles that modernizing food marketing systems play in providing food (and nutrients) to consumers. Supermarkets also offer important opportunities to improve the nutritional quality of diets.

C. P. Timmer (✉)
Economics, Harvard University, PO Box 1402, Kenwood, CA 95452, USA
e-mail: ptimmer63@gmail.com

© Springer Science+Business Media New York 2017
S. de Pee et al. (eds.), *Nutrition and Health in a Developing World*,
Nutrition and Health, DOI 10.1007/978-3-319-43739-2_33

Modern Supply Chains and the Marketing Sector

Food marketing systems need to move commodities "from the plow to the plate." The ability of particular systems to do this efficiently varies widely from country to country and even within. Some systems have "modernized" rapidly; others remain quite traditional. The pace and impact of change also varies widely within countries and regions, but in East Asia and Latin America the majority of food purchases in urban areas are now from modern retail establishments, especially supermarkets. As this chapter will emphasize, rapid changes have been taking place in the entire food marketing system (Fig. 33.1). The transformations in this system are part of a much broader set of transformations, from the structural changes that reflect the long-run dynamics of economic growth, to changed dietary patterns that accompany urbanization, higher incomes, and modern food technology. Although linked to each other, rapid changes in dietary patterns, agricultural transformation and urbanization would not be possible without modern supply chains (and integrated markets for labor, commodities and finance—topics for a separate discussion).

Markets must play three basic functions if economic growth is going to be both efficient and sustainable—(1) transforming food commodities in time, place and form (the traditional "engineering" functions of a marketing system); (2) the discovery of market prices for goods and services that determine which resources are scarce and which are abundant, and hence keep supply and demand for goods in balance; and (3) signaling to farmers and consumers, via these prices, efficient choices of what to produce and what to buy and eat. All three functions take place simultaneously (and mostly invisibly) in the food marketing system.

Modern supply chains have evolved primarily to provision supermarkets and their mainly urban consumers. Traditional supply chains and markets provisioned local consumers, both rural and urban. As populations and purchasing power move to cities, concerns for food safety and origin are increasingly reflected in the purchasing decisions of these urban and increasingly affluent consumers. The development of modern supply chains, which radically change the nature of farm-market-consumer interactions, can be an important source of income growth and job creation in both rural and urban areas. But the spread of modern supply chains can also be a challenge to food security [1–3].

Traditionally, farmers were connected to consumers by a number of marketing steps, often locally by small traders operating with minimal capital and primitive technology [4, 5]. The goal of modern

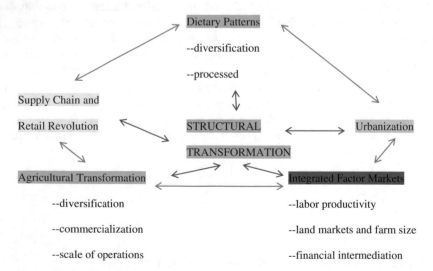

Fig. 33.1 Integrating five key components of modernizing food systems that are drivers of economic growth and structural transformation

supply chains is to reduce the number of transactions between the farmer and the consumer. A shorter supply chain can reduce costs, shorten the time between harvest and the consumer's table, and increase the efficiency of the marketing system. Tracing (and documenting) the exact flow of a commodity from the farm to retail purchases by consumers is also increasingly important to ensure food safety.

The primary functions of the marketing sector are inherently "coordination" tasks across a network of complex transactions. They require an adroit combination of public and private investments if they are to be carried out efficiently because there are substantial "public goods" dimensions to a smoothly functioning marketing system. For example, these public goods include roads and communication systems, but also the broader regulatory and legal environment, that permit low-cost transactions [6]. Historically, these investments have been made very gradually as farmers evolved from subsistence activities toward a more commercial orientation. Now that commercial activities are the norm, even in economies in which efficient marketing networks have not had time to emerge, policy makers are actively seeking new models and approaches to speed the creation of these networks. Supermarkets might already be performing this function, with little input from the public sector. This is an example where private supermarkets are supplanting the public sector in the (sub-optimal) provision of public goods, especially physical infrastructure such as cold storage facilities and food safety standards.

The marketing sector becomes increasingly important as the agricultural sector as a whole becomes *more* diversified over the course of the agricultural transformation, when compared with a representative individual farm, but significantly *less* diversified than patterns of food consumption. This increasing specialization of farms (*decreasing* diversification) is consistent with *greater* diversity at more aggregate levels because of the commercialization of agriculture.

Commercialization of agricultural systems leads to greater market orientation of farm production; progressive substitution out of non-traded inputs in favor of purchased inputs; and the gradual decline of integrated farming systems and their replacement by specialized enterprises for crop, livestock, poultry and aquaculture products. The farm-level determinants of increasing commercialization are the rising opportunity costs of family labor and increased market demand for food and other agricultural products. Family labor costs rise due to increasing off-farm employment opportunities, while positive shifts in market demand are triggered by urbanization and/or trade liberalization (Quote from Pingali and Rosegrant 1995: 171–72 [7]).

Likewise, patterns of food consumption become more diversified than patterns of domestic agricultural production because of the rising significance of international trade—that is, globalization.

The growing roles of commercialization and globalization in connecting diversity of production at the farm level with diversity of consumption at the household level spawn new problems, however. In particular, increased commercialization requires that farmers learn how to cope with a type of risk that is of little concern to subsistence farmers: the risk of fluctuating prices. At the same time, specialization in crop production increases their risk from yield fluctuations. Mechanisms for coping with risk, including contractual arrangements with supermarkets, thus play an important role in understanding the commercialization of agriculture and the government's role in it. The interplay among price fluctuations, increasing reliance on international trade, specialization of farmers in production for the market in response to price incentives and profitable new technology, and continued failure of market-based mechanisms for risk management in rural areas accounts for much of the policy interest of governments in the process of rural diversification. This policy interest in diversification is driven by widespread political concerns over lagging farmer incomes in relation to those in urban areas, but such diversification is impossible without a modern food marketing system [8].

Most countries want to speed up the gradual process of regional specialization and the development of efficient marketing systems, but they have found that government investments alone are inadequate. Well-developed, low-cost marketing systems for agricultural commodities that are accessible to all farmers with surplus output to sell require sufficient supplies of the specific commodities being marketed to justify the full investments needed to capture any economies of scale to the system. Achieving this balance is a simultaneous process, which historically has meant the gradual evolution of both the supply and demand side of the market. Supermarkets are internalizing this coordination process and speeding the rate of specialization. A private marketing system—accessible only to farmers who sell into a specific company's procurement system and supply chain—is closed to outside parties. It can expand in a coordinated way to stimulate specialized production in a region, but it will be less of a public good, and can thus be exclusionary in its benefits. The lower costs generated by specialization can confer very significant competitive advantages on regions that are both low-cost producers of a commodity and have an efficient marketing system that has adequate volume to capture the economies of scale implicit in the forward and backward linkages.[1]

The increasing dominance of modern supply chains raises concerns for both the *efficiency* and *equity* of price formation, as more and more transactions are internalized by supermarket procurement officers. Such transactions are not open and transparent, and hence concern will grow over the shift in market power toward a few, large buyers, and over the likely exclusion of disadvantaged suppliers from these arrangements. Second, however, and partially offsetting the first concern, supermarkets can also internalize consumers' desires for price stability and food safety, and hence can manage procurement contracts with price stability and safety in mind. Finally, supermarkets in LMICs will tend to be as competitive as in rich countries because much of the competition is provided by trans-national corporations themselves. Fears about monopoly control and market power seem to be ill-founded. The market for the food consumer's dollar is highly contestable, even when only a small handful of players are able to survive the cost competition.

The Rise of Supermarkets

Since the 1990s, food systems in LMICs that move food commodities from the farm to the table have been undergoing technological and institutional changes as vast and rapid as any in history. Three intersecting trends are reinforcing these changes. First, entire food systems are becoming more *private*, with a far larger role for market forces and a much smaller role for government-owned parastatals and cooperatives. Policy efforts to isolate domestic food economies from the world market have increasingly been unsuccessful in the face of market incentives for private traders. Second, food systems are becoming more *integrated*, with the same firm often dealing with farmers, traders, processors, and consumers. This integration is a stark change from food marketing sectors, especially for staple foods, that traditionally had been highly decentralized, very small scale and labor-intensive, and usually extremely competitive, although often operating at high cost because of poor infrastructure and high commercial risks. And third, food systems are becoming more *global*, with foreign direct investment (FDI) bringing state-of-the-art management and logistical techniques, as well as access to (and competition from) global markets. Globalization is more than a "buzzword" in LMICs; it is a day-to-day reality for many farmers and consumers.

The rapid spread of supermarkets is the key to understanding all three forces and how they are interacting. The rise of supermarkets and the changed role of governments in domestic food systems raise serious questions in three domains: (1) the fate of small farmers who need to diversify into higher valued products than staple grains, because "market-led diversification" now means "supermarket led"; (2) the impact on welfare of consumers (including nutritional impact, which is complicated because supermarkets can offer safer and often more nutritious foods) because consumers increasingly face a confusing array of new choices, not all of which are nutritious, when shopping in supermarkets; and finally, (3) who plans for a country's food security, the government or

---

[1]This perspective on regional specialization has been generalized and formalized in Krugman's work on economic geography. See Krugman [9].

Table 33.1 Modernizing food supply chains: Issues for food security at both the producer and consumer level

	Food grain economy (starchy staples)	Non-staple commodities (fruits and vegetables, meat/dairy/eggs/fish, processed foods)
Farm inputs/supplies	Smaller area possible Higher yields, stress tolerance Quality of food crops	More value/hectare, but what role for small farmers (what "assets" do they need to stay in?)
Farm production (management and knowledge)	Very knowledge intensive for good management practices; Access to inputs by farm size	Knowledge intensive; can there be effective extension for new technologies? Role of farm assets
Procurement/logistics and wholesalers	Less rural consumption as workers leave; More transportation and storage; Greater production instability with climate change	High transaction costs of dealing with small farmers; Issues of quality control and product traceability
Processing and value added	Milling technology How to add value; branding?	Large share of consumer food expenditure is spent in this box
Retail/consumer welfare and health dimensions	Supermarkets as suppliers of food grains? Increased price stability through private actions? Problems of access by the poor?	Modern supply chains are funneling consumer demands back up the system. The food system is less supply driven

Source Reardon [2]

supermarkets? Who should be responsible for ensuring stable supplies of staple foods, politicians or the market? Is the responsibility for improving the quality of diets strictly a matter of individual choices?

Increasingly, modern supply chains are transmitting demand signals from consumers who are shopping in supermarkets, back up the food system, level by level, to processors, farmers and input suppliers. Traditionally, each cell in the food system (Table 33.1) was connected locally by small traders operating with minimal capital and primitive technology [4, 5]. Modern supply chains are far more integrated into the farm-level procurement systems of supermarkets and are coordinated by these firms as they seek to "drive costs out of the system."

Four important trends emerge from the perspective in Table 33.1, when it is overlaid with changing food consumption patterns in a given country or region [6]. First, the vertical boxes are increasingly connected by market *and* non-market forces. One key conclusion for suppliers of agricultural input technology in the private sector is that there can be no effective demand for inputs unless farmers are able to sell surpluses into the market. This market is increasingly controlled by procurement officers for supermarket chains, and their tendency to *consolidate* suppliers may counter the effort by governments seeking to include small farmers, who are increasingly challenged as farms are split among heirs, slow economic growth offers few opportunities off the farm, and modern agricultural inputs are difficult to access because of credit needs. On the other hand, successful efforts to reduce the transactions costs of incorporating small farmers into modern supply chains may simultaneously pay dividends by making these modern inputs more accessible to farmers, and hence making small farmers more productive.

Second, there is a clear and rapid shift from the left side column of Table 33.1 to the right side—from the "starchy staple" sector to the "diversified foods" sector [10]. This shift reflects Bennett's Law—diversity of food sources in the diet increases as income increases, and the role of starchy staples decreases [11]. This dietary diversification away from starchy staples tends to improve the nutritional quality of the diet, although, in addition to more fruits, vegetables and animal-source food (dairy, eggs, fish, meat) this also means more processed foods and highly industrialized meat production, which raise nutritional, environmental, and food safety concerns. It should be noted that the tendency to produce more processed foods also opens the opportunity to improve nutritional quality through fortification and it often improves food safety.

Third, this increasingly diversified, market-driven food economy is more reflective of supply chain dynamics and consumer demand than in the past. The food marketing system is more sensitive to rapid income growth and somewhat less sensitive to population growth. Population growth is slowing quickly in most of Asia, and income growth continues at a rapid pace. In such environments, understanding how demand for individual items responds to growth in incomes will be necessary for effective planning of investments—by both the public and private sectors—all the way back the chain to input supply. Other factors that shape consumer demand for food will also be important, such as food technology, advertising, age structure, urbanization and globalization of tastes.

Fourth, as consumers increasingly use supermarkets as the source of their purchased food staples, some surprising implications arise for food security. Traditionally, staples have been purchased in small retail shops with multiple grades and varieties available. Prices fluctuated according to local supply and demand conditions and often changed daily during periods of instability. The concentration of purchasing power into a handful of supermarket chains raises the possibility that procurement officers for food staples will encourage (force) their suppliers to maintain large enough stocks so that supplies will be reliable and that prices can be kept reasonably stable. Indeed, it is easy to imagine supermarkets, especially in East and Southeast Asia, where unstable rice prices remain a threat to food security, beginning to compete for customers with a promise of "safe, reliable rice supplies, at a stable, fair price." Stable rice prices could become a private good rather than the public good they have been historically [12, 13]. When most food is purchased in supermarkets, the debate over how to provide food security—even in settings where volatile food prices can threaten it—will be transformed. We are a long way from that situation in 2015, but supermarkets are increasingly important as a supplier of basic food staples, and hence food security, in LMICs.

The Challenge to Food Security from Modern Supply Chains: A Food Policy Perspective[2]

Food policy analysis is designed to illuminate welfare trade-offs as producers, traders and consumers are buffeted by changes in technology, prices and tastes. These changes can come at the household, sectoral, national and global levels, and supermarkets in LMICs are affecting all four. A "new" food policy paradigm has emerged to help understand this impact. The original food policy paradigm focused analyses on the links between poverty and food security [14]. The new food policy paradigm stresses the "double burden" on societies facing substantial degrees of hunger and malnutrition at the same time they face rising levels of nutritional problems of affluence—obesity, heart disease, diabetes, etc. [15]. With obesity now affecting more people than hunger, this new perspective is timely.

The Food and Health Dimension

At the country level, the concern in the original food policy paradigm for keeping food prices at a level that balanced producer and consumer interests, with price stabilization around this level an important policy objective, gives way in the new food policy paradigm to equally important concerns

---

[2]Much of this section is drawn from Timmer [16].

for the budgetary consequences for governments (at national and local levels) of the health outcomes of dietary choices across entire societies.

At the household level, the traditional focus on access to foods (including intra-household access and distribution) stressed income and price variables, with a very limited role for household education and knowledge (except possibly in the derived demand for micro-nutrients). Much of the quantitative research in food policy over the past three decades has involved a search for the behavioral regularities that linked households to these market-determined variables [17, 18].

The contrast with the new concerns is sharp. Health professionals are either pessimistic about the political reality of using economic variables to influence dietary choices (one debate is over the efficiency of taxing fats and/or sugar in foods, taxing fat people, or taxing the health consequences of being fat), or are doubtful that economic incentives will actually change dietary behavior where affluence permits a wide array of choices [19]. Consequently, there is a much sharper focus on trying to change lifestyle through improved health knowledge and nutrition education. Supermarkets are becoming a part of that debate. Early evidence suggests that diets change for the worse when poorer consumers start using supermarkets, with highly processed and high-fat foods replacing less refined and more nutrient-rich foods [20, 21]. Still, there is remarkably little hard evidence on the impact of a switch from traditional markets to supermarkets on dietary patterns and nutritional well-being, especially the differential impact on children, who could benefit from improved access to dairy products and other animal protein, as well as fortified and safer foods.

The international nutrition community is engaged in a pointed debate over whether approaches to changing lifestyles through education will work. In particular, if the dietary patterns of affluence have a significant genetic component—that is, humans are "hard-wired" for an environment of food scarcity and have few internal control mechanisms over dietary intake in an environment of permanent affluence and food abundance—much more coercive efforts may be needed to change dietary behavior (and activity levels) than is implied by the education approach. On the other hand, such coercion directly contradicts consumer sovereignty and the basic principles of a democratic society. The more prominent attention in the new food policy to health problems arising from modern diets is tending to raise tensions between development economists and nutrition professionals.

Supermarkets are both the purveyors of the food abundance (and much of the "junk" food sold) and a possible vehicle for bringing about dietary change, either through improved nutrition education within stores, active promotion of healthier foods, health warnings on particular foods that cause nutritional damage, such as soft drinks with high sugar content, or even regulations on what kinds of foods are available for purchase. The rapid spread of private standards for food quality, those established by individual supermarket chains, on food safety and aspects of production technologies shows that public policy is not necessarily the fastest or most effective way to bring about changes in food marketing. These standards could easily incorporate health dimensions as well, especially if lawsuits over "fast food" contributions to obesity begin to be won by litigants. Such private standards would, in effect, have supermarkets provide a public good (although not at optimal levels). Some supermarkets in the USA are experimenting with these health themes, but even in the USA this remains a niche market. There is no evidence that supermarkets are attempting to play this role in LMICs, apart from the advertised food quality and safety standards they enforce in nearly all parts of the world where supermarkets have a significant share of food consumption.

The Poverty and Development Dimension

One of the key messages for LMICs in *Food Policy Analysis* [14] was the link between poverty and food security, at both the national and household levels. In turn, poverty was considered primarily an economic problem that could only be addressed in a sustainable fashion by linking the poor—mostly in rural areas—into the process of economic growth. A dynamic agriculture as a stimulus to forward and backward linkages within the rural economy served as the "prime mover" in this process. Through improved agricultural technology, public investments in rural infrastructure, and the end of "urban bias" that distorted incentives for farmers, policy makers could have a simple and clear approach to reducing poverty and improving food security.

With success in the rural economy, migration to urban areas would be more of a "pull" process rather than a "push," especially if favorable macroeconomic and trade policies were stimulating rapid growth in a labor-intensive manufacturing industry (and construction). In combination, these activities pulled up real wages and, when sustained, led to rapid reductions in poverty [22–24]. In many ways, this paradigm of successful structural transformation could be described as an "inclusion model" because of its focus on including the poor in the rural economy, including the rural economy in the national economy, and including the national economy in the global economy. Its greatest success was in East and Southeast Asia since the late 1960s, but the model has been under attack as the benefits of globalization seem not to be as widely shared as earlier hoped.

The failures of globalization provide another theme for the new food policy paradigm around the analytics of "exclusion." At the national level, the question is why so many countries have been "non-globalizers." The essence of the debate is whether the global economy, in the form of rich countries and transnational corporations, has excluded these countries from participating in trade and technology flows, or whether the countries themselves have been unsuccessful in the process because of domestic shortcomings in policies and governance, including corruption [25].

The debate has a local focus as well. Within an otherwise well-functioning and growing economy, many groups can be excluded from the benefits of this growth. Unskilled workers unable to graduate to higher technologies and uneducated youth unable to compete in a modern economy are a sizeable proportion of the work force in countries with poor manpower and training policies and resources. Globalization makes it more difficult for these countries to compete for trade and investment flows that would provide the first steps up the ladder of higher productivity [26].

Integrating the Food and Health Dimension with the Poverty and Development Dimension

From an economics perspective, the ultimate impact of supermarkets in LMICs will be on the level and distribution of improved welfare for consumers (producers are consumers too). What happens to small farmers, traditional traders and family-run retail shops will be factors in both the size of welfare gains and their distribution, but many other factors will also come into play. From the perspective of possible government policies to make the supermarket revolution serve farmers and consumers better, a fully informed analysis on the impact of these rapid changes in the food marketing system must incorporate all of those factors. A political process, informed (we hope) by good economic analysis, will then determine the nature of compensatory actions needed so that losers in this revolution do not end up in poverty or mobilize enough political resources to stop the technological transformation itself. The discussions about the nature and extent of these compensatory actions begin to frame a research agenda that links food policy analysis with the rapid emergence of supermarkets.

Economic progress creates winners and losers, and understanding of the process as "creative destruction" dates to Adam Smith and Joseph Schumpeter. The tensions generated during this process have continuing relevance as powerful new technologies boost productivity in rich countries and poor alike [27]. From this perspective, supermarkets are simply a vehicle for the transmission into LMICs of new technologies, potential for scale economies, and new buying patterns of consumers, and are thus the latest manifestation of a long-run process of globalization and structural transformation [24].

There are, of course, many problems with this process of economic transformation. A longstanding criticism of capitalism is that it stimulates a highly unequal process of economic growth [28]. Rich owners of financial capital and privileged workers with higher education and advanced skills are paid high returns in a market-oriented economy. What they possess is scarce, and markets reward scarcity. Individuals with only their unskilled labor to sell are plentiful. Their market wages are low and these individuals are poor. Making growth work for the poor in a market economy requires that these basic and fundamental forces be overcome, either through the sheer rapidity of economic growth or through ancillary measures to ensure that the poor connect to growth [29].

History is full of experiments on how to make an economy work for the poor, from totalitarian communism to democratic socialism, from central planning to "third way" market economies where governments provide a wide array of social services and safety nets to the population. These historical experiments have a surprising and powerful lesson: rapid economic growth that connects to the poor (now widely termed "inclusive growth") has been the *only* sustainable path out of poverty for both countries and individuals [30, 31]. The question is whether supermarkets are part of this path or part of the problem in trying to stay on it.

As an academic field, food policy analysis was "invented" to provide a framework for answering such a question. The central analytical vision of food policy, developed in the late 1970s and articulated in the early 1980s, integrated farmer, trader, and consumer decision making into the open economy, macro-framework needed for rapid economic growth [14]. Although radical at the time, the explicit goal was a sharp reduction in hunger and poverty, which would be possible if market incentives stimulated productivity and income gains in agriculture, while poor consumers were protected by stable food prices and rising real wages. The marketing sector was the key to connecting these two ends of the food system. Supermarkets were not mentioned because they were a feature of developed countries' economies and the "food policy paradigm" focused on hunger and poverty in LMICs, where supermarkets were virtually nonexistent in the early 1980s.

The analytical story, policy design, and program implementation were complicated, requiring analysts to integrate models of micro- and macro-decision making in a domestic economy open to world trade and commodity markets. At its best, the food policy paradigm sharply improved the development profession's understanding of the underlying structure and dynamics of poverty and the role of the food system in reducing it [32]. As part of this understanding, *food security* came to be seen as involving two separate analytical arenas. The first, at the "micro-household" level, required analysis of food access and entitlements. The second, at the "macro-market" level, required analysis of food price stability, market supplies, and inventory behavior. Again, in the early 1980s, supermarkets did not seem relevant to either level of analysis.

"Food policy analysis" provided policy makers a comprehensive, but intuitively tractable, vision of how to connect these two arenas—households to the macroeconomic environment—and improve food security for the consumers in their societies. As an analytical paradigm, this vision was always driven by consumer welfare. Farmers, as food producers, and middlemen in the marketing sector that transformed farm output in time, place and form, were seen as "intermediate" actors in the efficient production of consumer welfare. Thus, the food policy paradigm fit squarely within the standard framework of neoclassical economic analysis and the long-run structural transformation that underpins modern economic growth.

That paradigm has been challenged by the rapid rise of supermarkets in poor countries, and part of the challenge has been the difficulty for academic research of analyzing how supermarkets affect the food marketing system. Research that seeks to understand the impact of supermarkets on the food systems of LMICs utilizes an unconventional mix of microeconomic modeling and econometric testing with carefully structured company interviews and case studies [4, 5]. An important innovation has been the "stacked interviews" that provide statistically reliable survey data that link players and decisions along the supply chain [33].

An integrated food policy framework—incorporating both "old" and "new" issues—is needed. It can be organized around the familiar vertical structure of the food system, with farmers at the bottom, passing their produce up through the marketing system—now divided into traditional markets and

Food consumers and behavioral change

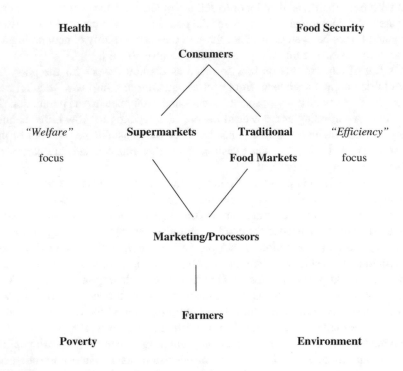

Fig. 33.2 Supermarkets and a food policy research agenda

modern retail outlets that include small-format stores such as "7-11-style" shops and supermarkets—with consumers at the top of the chain (see Fig. 33.2).

Four major policy issues confront the food system along this vertical structure: (1) health and (2) poverty concerns on the "welfare" side and (3) food security and (4) environmental concerns on the "efficiency" side. From below, the basic forces affecting small farmers are the structural transformation and the role of agriculture in that process. From above, the basic forces affecting food consumers are behavioral changes in the context of increasing affluence and choices available.

Within this framework, it is possible to identify the key linkages from supermarkets through the rest of the food system that policy makers will want to understand if they are concerned about food security. At the micro-, or household level, the issue is impact of supermarkets on poor consumers, especially the role of supermarkets in distribution of starchy staples—the main source of food security for the poor. There has been remarkably little research on this aspect of the impact of supermarkets on food security.

At the macro-level, the issue will be the impact of supermarkets on staple food supplies, price stability, and links to global grain markets. What role are supermarkets playing in these markets? Is there any way to use supermarkets (instead of parastatals, for example) to manage "macro"-food security by being the intermediary between a country's consumers and world grain markets?

A final issue asks whether supermarkets are a major factor in the health epidemic seen in affluent countries and among the affluent in poor countries. To what extent are processed foods, snack foods, sugary drinks and fatty foods, the cause of obesity, heart disease, and diabetes? Are supermarkets to blame for our rapidly rising consumption of these foods? Could they contribute to a solution?

Taken together, these questions form the core of a research agenda that is complementary to the current attention focusing on the impact of supermarkets on small farmers, and research directed at finding policy and/or program mechanisms to help them compete successfully within the global supply chain. In combination, the consumer-oriented and the producer-oriented research, linked as they are by the rapid emergence of supermarkets as the dominant players in the food marketing arena, fit comfortably within an expanded food policy paradigm.

Combining the consumer- and producer-oriented issues into the macro-dimensions of the supermarket revolution provides an opportunity to discuss the consequences of rapid supermarket development for economic growth and income distribution. These lead to policy recommendations that recognize the market power of supermarkets while also recognizing the sizeable public dimensions and mechanisms of their influence.

Economic Growth and Policy Issues

Most effects of supermarkets in LMICs are likely to play out at the firm and sector level, but macroeconomic effects will not be trivial, especially as lower food costs translate into greater real purchasing power for consumers. The impact will then be felt through differential Engel elasticities—greater stimulus to manufactured goods and modern services; gradual retardation for staple foods, traditional clothing and basic housing. Managers of supermarkets themselves are fully aware of these trends, as a stroll down any aisle will demonstrate. By passing on lower costs, or improving food quality and convenience, supermarkets can actually speed up the structural transformation and the agricultural transformation that is part of it [34].

There will also be significant efficiency effects. The mantra of supermarket procurement officers is to "drive costs out of the food marketing system." Although these "costs" are also someone's income, especially farmers and traders in the traditional agricultural marketing chain, lowering food marketing costs not only allows lower consumer costs, with the effects noted above, but they also free up productive resources that can be used in more profitable activities. This is the process by which the productivity of all economic factors of production improves, and this improvement, including in the food system, is the basic long-run source of economic growth [22].

A final growth effect may in the long run be the most important, the technology spillover effects that result from the use by supermarket managers of imported information technology and modern management techniques honed in the fierce competition of food markets in rich countries. Most of this technology arrives as part of FDI, which has been the main vehicle of rapid penetration by supermarkets into LMICs [1, 4, 5]. It is often proprietary, and supermarket owners go to great lengths to keep it internal to the company. But like most technologies, the knowledge that these tools and techniques exist is the key to rapid emulation, as local managers trained by the first wave of foreign supermarkets leave to establish their own companies and consulting firms. Thus, the spillovers from introducing modern information technologies and management techniques can occur fairly rapidly and have widespread effects across the entire economy, not just in food retailing.

Supermarkets will affect not only the efficiency of the food marketing chain, but also the distribution of benefits from the value added in the process. In general, it is very difficult to say whether these distributional changes will be positive or negative, that is, whether income distribution will improve or not.

There are two important offsetting effects. On the negative side, the evidence is clear that rapid supermarket penetration into traditional food marketing systems can quickly displace family-run, often informal retail shops, traders in traditional wet markets, and small-scale wholesalers. In most of these cases, the people displaced earn relatively low incomes and will have to make significant adjustments to find new livelihoods. The distributional effect is likely to be negative and can be substantial if these small-scale food marketing firms are numerous and widely visible. Their imminent demise can also generate significant political resistance to the spread of supermarkets, an effect already being seen throughout Asia, but with historical antecedents in the USA, Europe and Japan.

The impact of supermarket penetration on the farm sector has tended to be the most vocal issue. Experience suggests that small farmers can rapidly lose access to supermarket supply chains and thus be cut off from the growing "value added" component of retail food baskets [35]. The suggestion is that these farmers risk falling further into poverty. But this experience is not uniform. There are circumstances where small farmers have gained profitable access to modern supply chains. Keeping a significant number of small farmers in the supply chain of supermarkets in the short- to medium-run is likely to be essential for poor countries to reap widespread social benefits from the rapid domination by supermarkets. The impact on the traditional food *marketing* sector will be small relative to this impact on small farmers.

What are the potential widespread social benefits that could have positive distributional effects? The extraordinary spread and speed of supermarket penetration suggests that consumers love them, at least those consumers with adequate incomes to value the breadth of food-related quality services provided by supermarkets. It is hard to argue that low-income consumers benefit differentially, at least initially, but lower real food costs across the board (corrected for quality, safety, and convenience, all of which consumers value) clearly have an impact of greatest importance to the poor. Efforts to slow the penetration of supermarkets on behalf of small farmers and traditional agents in the food marketing chain need to keep this widespread consumer benefit in the calculus. At the same time, significantly more evidence is needed on whether food-poor consumers have access to these benefits [20, 21].

There are few policy implications that are specific to managing the supermarket revolution. This chapter argues that the rapid emergence of supermarkets—and their associated supply chains that include both multi-national and local firms—is a particularly visible element of a long-term and on-going process of technological change and structural transformation that has raised living standards wherever it has succeeded. To be sure, this process requires active attention on the part of policy makers so that the underlying infrastructure and policies that stimulate this change—and the safety nets to cushion its impact on the poor and those who lose out—are in place. Many of these government efforts will be part of a more general approach to good social and economic policies that maintain equitable distribution of rapid economic growth.

Beyond that, policy makers need to be careful not to "choose winners" or "reward losers." The process of economic development is dynamic and unpredictable, full of "creative destruction" and exciting innovations [27]. There will be winners and losers in the process, but only innovation and technical change can raise living standards in the long run.

That said, the supermarket revolution does affect food security in several important ways. First, supermarkets (and the associated changes in food supply chains) may change a number of important characteristics of the food system, even as food policy *objectives* remain little changed. These objectives are the rapid alleviation of hunger and poverty in a sustainable environment that improves health and life expectancy.

For example, the drivers of change may now be multinational corporations rather than domestic marketing boards; the policy levers may be nutritional education, emphasis on activity levels in schools to prevent childhood obesity, even more coercive taxes and regulations; and agricultural choices may be more influenced by quality standards and relationships with procurement officers than price policies and extension agents. These changes require that policy analysts in the fields of agriculture, food and nutrition also have a broader perspective—and a broader set of skills—than before.

There are also likely to be some common themes for the "new" food and nutrition policy analyst—the food system is more consumer-driven than before, the marketing system is even more important as the efficient vehicle for transmitting consumer desires back to farmer opportunities, but there are fewer players in the new marketing system. However, the old problems—building human capital through education, improving the institutional environment for risk management, and stimulating technical change while managing its consequences—remain front and center on the agenda. The supermarket revolution both complicates these problems—models of atomistic competition are even less relevant than before—while it offers important new opportunities for societies to meet their food and nutrition policy objectives.

Conclusion

The food system changes considerably when societies develop from being predominantly agrarian to being more industrialized and urbanized. The distance between food producers and consumers increases and consumers demand more convenient, diverse, healthy and safe foods. Supermarkets play a major role in linking actors along the food chain to consumers, not only by ensuring supplies become available in-time and in good condition for purchasing, especially by urban consumers, but also by driving what becomes available, how and providing information to consumers, including through marketing. The rapid emergence of supermarkets in low- and middle-income countries hence plays an essential role in providing food (and nutrients) to consumers, but there are also negative effects, including increased availability and marketing of high-fat, high-sugar and salty foods, in supermarkets and beyond. In essence, the modernization of the food system, which is to a large extent led by supermarkets and their interaction with actors along the supply chain, shortens the distance between food producers and consumers but in a way that reduces the number of players and the influence of public sector entities. On the positive side, supermarkets and modern supply chains offer significantly enhanced food safety, the opportunity to fortify basic food staples with essential vitamins and minerals, and the potential to stabilize food prices, thus contributing to food security. On the negative side, supermarkets and modern supply chains offer an enticing array of "junk foods" that are likely contributors to the obesity epidemic and rapid spread of non-communicable diseases. Government policies can shape both the positive and negative dimensions at the margin, but most of the dynamics of supermarket growth are stimulated by technological changes and consumer demands that are beyond the control of governments.

Discussion Points

- What is the link between supermarkets and farmers? How can the growth of supermarkets support and hinder the farmers and other traditional members of the food supply chain?
- Should small farmers see themselves more as producers or consumers? What are the implications for how they perceive themselves?
- How can the modern food supply chain be used to improve and hinder healthy dietary patterns? What are the global market forces that would influence these patterns?
- How are public and private sectors working or not working together regarding the modern food supply and this impact on development, food security and safety?

Acknowledgments This chapter, significantly revised from the first edition, had its origins in a paper presented at the Sixth National Workshop on Food and Nutrition, Indonesian Academy of Sciences (LIPI), Jakarta, Indonesia, May 17–19, 2004. In over a decade since then, the "supermarket revolution" has continued to accelerate. Recent reviews are in Reardon and Timmer, 2012 and 2014 [3, 5].

References

1. Reardon T, Timmer CP, Barrett CB, Berdegue JA. The rise of supermarkets in Africa, Asia, and Latin America. Am J Agric Econ. 2003;85(5):1140–6.
2. Reardon T. Linking food market transformation to improved food security in Asia. Presentation at the ASEAN Food Security Conference, Singapore. Organized by Nathan Associates, Arlington, VA with support from USAID; 17 June 2010.
3. Reardon T, Timmer CP. Five inter-linked transformations in the Asian agrifood economy: food security implications. Global Food Secur. 2014;. doi:10.1016/j.gfs.2014.02.001.
4. Reardon T, Timmer CP. Transformation of markets for agricultural output in developing countries since 1950: How has thinking changed? In: Evenson RE, Pingali P, editors. Chapter 55 Handbook of agricultural economics, vol. 3: Agricultural development: farmers, farm production, and farm markets. Amsterdam: Elsevier Press; 2007. p. 2807–55.
5. Reardon T, Timmer CP. The economics of the food system revolution. Ann Rev Resour Econ. 2012;4:14.1–40.
6. Timmer CP. Food security and scarcity: why ending hunger is so hard. Philadelphia, PA: University of Pennsylvania Press; 2014.
7. Pingali PL, Rosegrant MW. Agricultural commercialization and diversification: processes and policies. Food Policy. 1995;20(3):171–85.
8. Timmer CP. Farmers and markets: the political economy of new paradigms. Am J Agric Econ. 1997;79(2):621–27.
9. Krugman P. Geography and trade. New York: Norton; 1993.
10. Chaudhri R, Timmer CP. The impact of changing affluence on diets and demand patterns for agricultural commodities. Staff Working Paper no. 785. Washington, D.C.: World Bank; 1985.
11. Bennett MK. The world's food. New York: Harper; 1954.
12. Timmer CP. Food price policy: the rationale for government intervention. Food Policy. 1989;14(1):17–27.
13. Timmer CP. Reflections on food crises past. Food Policy. 2010;35(1):1–11.
14. Timmer CP, Falcon WP, Pearson SR. Food policy analysis. Baltimore, MD: Johns Hopkins University Press for the World Bank; 1983.
15. Maxwell S, Slater R. editors. Food policy old and new. Dev Policy Rev. 2003;21:5–6.
16. Timmer CP. Do supermarkets change the food policy agenda? World Dev. 2009;37(11):1812–19. (Special Issue on agrifood industry transformation and small farmers in developing countries, Reardon T, Barrett CB, Berdegué JA, Swinnen JFM, editors).
17. Timmer CP. Is there 'curvature' in the slutsky matrix? Rev Econ Stat. 1981;62(3):395–402.
18. Bhargava A. Food, economics and health. Oxford: Oxford University Press; 2008.
19. Ludwig DS, Friedman MI. Always hungry? Here's why. New York Times: Sunday Review; 18 May 2014. p. 1.
20. Asfaw A. Supermarket purchases and the dietary patterns of households in Guatemala. IFPRI Discussion Paper 696. Washington, DC; 2007.
21. Michelson HC. Small farmers, NGOs, and a Walmart world: welfare effects of supermarkets operating in Nicaragua. Am J Agric Econ. 2013;95(3):628–49.
22. Timmer CP. Agriculture and economic growth. In: Gardner B, Rausser G, editors. Handbook of agricultural economics, vol. II. Amsterdam: North-Holland; 2002. p. 1487–546.
23. Timmer CP. Agriculture and pro-poor growth: an Asian perspective. Working Paper No. 63, Washington, DC: Center for Global Development; 2005.
24. Timmer CP. A world without agriculture: the structural transformation in historical perspective. Henry Wendt distinguished lecture. Washington, DC: American Enterprise Institute; 2009.
25. Resnick D, Birner R. Does good governance contribute to pro-poor growth? A review of the evidence from cross-country studies. DSGD Discussion Paper No. 30. Washington, D.C.: International Food Policy Research Institute; Feb 2006.
26. Goldberg PK, Pavcnik N. Distributional effects of globalization in developing countries. J Econ Lit. 2007;XLV (1):39–82.
27. McCraw T. Prophet of innovation: Joseph Schumpeter and creative destruction. Boston: Harvard Business School Press; 2007.
28. Piketty T. Capital in the twenty-first century (trans. by Arthur Goldhammer). Cambridge, MA: The Belknap Press of Harvard University Press; 2014.
29. Easterly W. Inequality does retard economic growth. Center for Global Development Working Paper. Washington, DC; 2003.
30. Besley T, Cord L, editors. Operationalizing pro-poor growth: synthesis and country experiences. London: Palgrave MacMillan; 2006.
31. Ferreira FHG, Ravallion M. Global poverty and inequality: a review of the evidence. Policy Research Working Paper Series 4623, The World Bank; 2008.

32. Eicher CK, Staatz JM, editors. International agricultural development. 3rd ed. Baltimore: Johns Hopkins University Press; 1998.
33. Reardon T, Chen K, Minten B, Adriano Lourdes. The quiet revolution in staple food value chains: enter the dragon, the elephant and the tiger. Mandaluyong City, Philippines: Asian Development Bank; 2012.
34. Timmer C Peter. The agricultural transformation. In: Chenery H, Srinivasan TN, editors. Handbook of development economics, vol. 1. Amsterdam: North-Holland; 1988. p. 275–331.
35. Reardon T, Barrett CB, Berdegue JA, Swinnen JFM. Agrifood industry transformation and small farmers in developing countries: introduction to a special issue. World Dev. 2009;37(11):1717–27.

Chapter 34
Value Chain Focus on Food and Nutrition Security

Jessica C. Fanzo, Shauna Downs, Quinn E. Marshall, Saskia de Pee
and Martin W. Bloem

Keywords Food value chains · Nutrition · Value chains · Agriculture · Food processing · Private sector

Learning Objectives

- Define the concepts of food value chains.
- Describe the actors in food value chains and the different typologies of food value chains in the developing world.
- Elucidate why food systems and diets have evolved in the context of value chains.
- Analyze how nutrition-focused value chains can address nutrition and improve diets.
- Develop a nutrition-focused food value chain framework.

J.C. Fanzo (✉)
Berman Institute of Bioethics and School of Advanced International Studies,
Johns Hopkins University, 1717 Massachusetts Ave., #730, Washington, DC 20036, USA
e-mail: jfanzo1@jhu.edu

S. Downs
Berman Institute of Bioethics, Johns Hopkins University, 1809 Ashland Avenue,
Baltimore, MD 21205, USA
e-mail: sdowns5@jhu.edu

Q.E. Marshall · S. de Pee · M.W. Bloem
Nutrition Division, World Food Programme, Rome, Italy
e-mail: quinn.marshall@wfp.org

S. de Pee
e-mail: Saskia.depee@wfp.org; depee.saskia@gmail.com

M.W. Bloem
e-mail: martin.bloem@wfp.org

M.W. Bloem
Department of International Health, Bloomberg School of Public Health,
Johns Hopkins University, Baltimore, MD, USA

S. de Pee · M.W. Bloem
Friedman School of Nutrition Science and Policy, Tufts University, Boston, MA, USA

© Springer Science+Business Media New York 2017
S. de Pee et al. (eds.), *Nutrition and Health in a Developing World*,
Nutrition and Health, DOI 10.1007/978-3-319-43739-2_34

Introduction to Value Chains

What Are Value Chains?

The value chain describes the full range of activities that the specific actors involved undertake to bring a product from its design and conception to its end use by the consumer. This includes activities such as design, production, marketing and distribution. The activities that comprise a value chain can be contained within a single actor or divided among different actors. Value chain activities can produce goods or services and can be contained within a single geographical location or spread over wider areas [1].

Value chains have focused mainly on a supply chain in which value is added to the product as it moves through the chain. Most commonly, value chains are thought of as a series of activities and actors along the supply chain, and what and where value is added in the chain for and by these activities and actors. The point of the value chain is to create and build value at every step as a product moves through the chain. Depending on the commodity, there are a series of activities and actors involved with what and where value is added in the chain, for and by these activities and actors.

Michael Porter first described value chains in the 1980s as a way to identify how and where value can be increased in an internal business chain. Porter defines the value chain as made of primary activities and support activities (Fig. 34.1). Primary activities involve inbound logistics (getting the material in for adding value by processing it), operations (which are all the processes within the manufacturing), outbound (which involves distribution to the points of sale), marketing and sales (which sell it, brand it and promote it) and service (which maintains the functionality of the product, post-sales).

The support functions, which feed into all the primary functions, are the infrastructure, human resources, technology and procurement. These support activities, often undervalued, can change the value of products by the quality of those services. Both the primary and support activities allow a "company" or "business" to charge a margin, which partly comes from the value addition of the primary and support functions and partly from the advantage that the company gains due to communication of the value addition to the consumer (through advertisement and branding, trust, etc.).

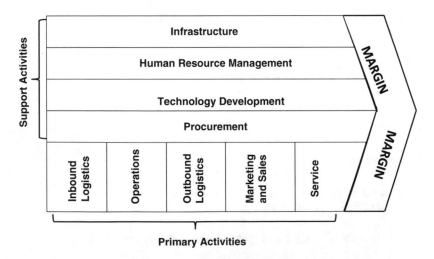

Fig. 34.1 Basic model of Porter's value chain. From Porter and Millar [2]. Reprinted with permission

The major goal is that the margin should be the amount a consumer is willing to pay above the sum of the costs of all the said activities in the value chain [2].

What Are Food Value Chains?

Food value chains (FVC) are the full range of activities that are required to bring a food product from conception, through the different phases of production, to delivery to final consumers and disposal after use [3]. Production is actually growing, raising or making of the product. Processing is refining, altering and potentially creating value of the product. Manufacturing is the process in which the product is produced at a larger scale. FVCs should be distinguished from food supply chains. Food supply chains are a generic term for the sum of the many food production, manufacturing and marketing links from farm to table. Those links include equipment dealers, seed suppliers, food processors, distributors and even government regulators. The term "food value chain" is a permutation of the food supply chain concept in that quality of the end product is prioritized. Therefore, every actor in the chain is invested in making sure the chain produces a valuable food product for the consumer.

What Is Value?

Value chains have always played an important role in the food system, particularly from an economic perspective. Taking a value chain approach necessitates understanding a market system in its totality: the firms that operate within an industry—from input suppliers to end market buyers; the support markets that provide technical, business and financial services to the industry; and the business environment in which the industry operates.

The end markets into which a product or service is sold—whether local, regional or international—provide the opportunities and set the parameters for economic growth. Generally, there are multiple actual and potential end markets, each with different demand characteristics and returns.

The terms "value" and "values" are used in different ways when referring to food value chains:

1. "Value-added" is used to characterize food production and processing that involves the conversion of raw products through processes that give the resulting product an "incremental value" in the market place. An "incremental value" is realized from either higher price or expanded market.
2. "Value-added" is also used to characterize food products that have incremental value in the marketplace by differentiating them from similar products based on food production and processing attributes such as geographical location; environmental stewardship; food safety; or functionality.
3. The words "value" and "values" are also used to characterize the nature of certain business relationships among interacting food business enterprises, rather than any attribute of the product itself.

Food Value Chain Actors and Typologies

Actors Across the Food Value Chain

FVCs involve many actors: farmers, processors, wholesalers, distributors, retailers and consumers (Fig. 34.2). These actors influence the way in which food is produced, processed, distributed,

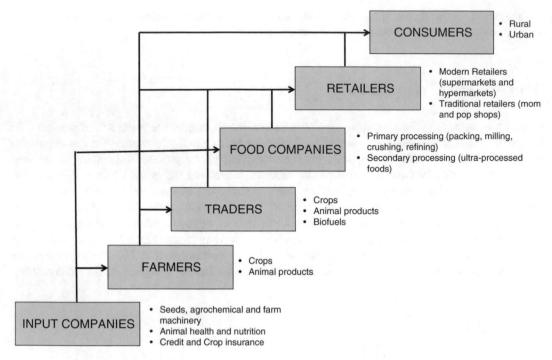

Fig. 34.2 Range of actors in the food value chain. *Source* Adapted from KPMG 2013 [5]

marketed and consumed and whether or not nutritious foods are available, affordable and acceptable. In addition to these actors, policy actors (not depicted in the figure) can also shape FVCs. For example, agriculture policies affect what is grown, raised, processed and sold, which subsequently influences the food environment in which consumers make decisions about what to eat [4]. Thus, the decisions made by one group of actors have implications for the other actors along the value chain. Moreover, these actions need to be responsive to consumer demand and preferences. The FVC is often discussed from the producer's perspective—the *supply* side. Little emphasis is placed on how informed consumers can play a role in influencing the value chains, and how changes in the *demand* for specific foods can influence the processes and outputs of value chains. In order to increase consumption of nutritious foods, both the supply and demand sides of the value chain need to be considered. The private sector—from large multinational companies to small, local agri-business enterprises—is central to linking one end of the chain to the other.

The Role of the Private Sector

In 2011, Porter published an article in the Harvard Business Review entitled "Creating Shared Value: Redefining Capitalism and the Role of the Corporation in Society" [6]. The article posits that companies can create shared value by creating economic value in a way that concomitantly creates value for society by addressing its needs and challenges [6]. Given that the private sector actors are integral to FVCs, there is an opportunity for creating shared value in terms of nutrition.

The role of the private sector in both the primary and secondary activities of the FVC is key. The food and beverage industry spans the entire value chain approach—from food production, to processing, storing to delivering to the consumer. "With rising consumer incomes, urbanization and the need for preservation and convenience, the food industry will play an expanding role in processing agricultural outputs into food products. The logistics and distribution capabilities of food companies offer an unparalleled worldwide reach into urban and, increasingly, rural markets" [7]. The industry's role is in the driver seat to maximize nutritional outcomes throughout the entire value chain. Supermarkets can improve the food marketing chain as well as distribute the value-added benefits of foods. "Entire food systems are becoming more private, with a far larger role for market forces and a much smaller role of government-owned parastatals and cooperatives" [8].

Types of Food Value Chains

Developing country FVCs have experienced a rapid transformation in recent years. Only a few decades ago, most food was grown for household food consumption among smallholder farmers living in rural areas. Food was also purchased at small, localized markets [9]. That has changed. Now, most food purchased by consumers has travelled longer distances and has touched several different actors across a FVC. This has been influenced by changes in food consumption patterns prompted by rapid urbanization, income growth and expansion of modern retailers, processors and distributors [9]. Furthermore, more and more households are moving out of rural areas into urban centers, where they utilize modern supermarkets and are diversifying their diets, sometimes both positively and negatively. The demand for higher-valued, nutrient-rich products such as meats, dairy, fruits and vegetables is increasing. In addition, the markets for packaged, processed and ready-to-eat foods are expanding, including breakfast cereals, confectionaries, ready-to-eat meals and carbonated soft drinks, among others [3]. Rural populations also depend on FVCs for their food purchases because most of them, including the poor, are net-food buyers and are employed in the food sector [9].

Gomez and Ricketts [9] developed a typology that assigns FVCs that focus on providing nutritious foods to consumers into four broad categories to reflect the aforementioned transformations. The simplified version of the four typologies is shown in Table 34.1 and includes traditional, modern, modern-to-traditional and traditional-to-modern FVCs.

Consumers purchasing food through traditional value chains most often purchase food directly from smallholder farmers and traders in local or regional wet markets or from traditional retailers such as "mom and pop" shops, street vendors or roadside stands [10–12]. Traditional FVCs are mainly informal and are common in small rural markets located relatively close to production regions but may also travel longer distances to reach urban consumers, primarily in lower-income neighborhoods [13]. Traditional markets may help increase access to affordable nutritious foods such as fruits and vegetables, with the potential to lead to improvements in micronutrient intakes, particularly of B vitamins and vitamin C; however, given the lack of post-harvest and distribution infrastructure there may be limited year-round availability of diverse foods that can enhance diet quality [9].

Table 34.1 Typology of food value chains for nutrition

Type	Description
Traditional	Traditional traders buy primarily from smallholder farmers and sell to consumers and traditional retailers in wet (mostly local) markets
Modern	Domestic and multinational food manufacturers procure primarily from commercial farms and sell through modern supermarket outlets
Modern-to-traditional	Domestic and multinational food manufacturers sell through the network of traditional traders and retailers (e.g., mom and pop shops)
Traditional-to-modern	Supermarkets and food manufacturers source food from smallholder farmers and traders

Modern FVCs are largely driven by the expansion of modern retailers in developing countries, primarily in urban areas [9]. They involve both domestic and multinational food manufacturers and wholesalers, in addition to commercial agribusinesses and farms [14, 15]. These value chains are often more streamlined and have greater economies of scale than traditional value chains and are able to offer a year-round, wide assortment of fresh and processed and packaged food products; however, they are unlikely to reach all consumers (i.e., lower-income consumers) [9]. Although the traditional FVCs often still dominate low- and middle-income countries, growth in modern value chains has been high [16]. Modern value chains can impact nutrition outcomes both positively and negatively by providing year-round availability of a wide variety of foods, mainly for high- and middle-income households living in urban areas and by contributing to overnutrition by enhancing the availability of inexpensive, processed and packaged foods that are often high in sugar, salt and unhealthy fat [9].

Modern-to-traditional value chains often involve distribution of primarily processed and packaged foods produced by food manufacturers and sold through traditional retailers [9]. Modern-to-traditional FVCs allow for year-round distribution of processed and packaged foods, targeting lower-income consumers in urban areas as well as remote markets in rural areas [9]. Increasing access to processed and packaged foods through modern-to-traditional FVCs has the potential to decrease undernourishment in rural areas while at the same time potentially increasing overnutrition in urban areas [9]. Nevertheless, these FVCs provide an opportunity for implementing processed and packaged food fortification initiatives targeting micronutrient deficiencies.

Traditional-to-modern FVCs consist of smallholder farmers and traders selling primarily high-value crop and livestock products to supermarkets and food manufacturers [9]. Smallholder farmers and traders' participation in these FVCs may increase incomes leading to reductions in undernutrition particularly through indirect ways such as increased opportunities for off-farm employment in commercial farms and post-harvest businesses [9]. However, smallholders often face difficulties in terms of achieving the product quality and uniformity standards the modern retailers and manufacturers require [17, 18]. The World Food Programme's (WFP) Purchase for Progress (P4P) initiative is trying to address these barriers among smallholders in several countries as part of its procurement of staple crops for food aid. Box 34.1 provides an overview of the P4P initiative.

Box 34.1 An overview of World Food Programme's P4P Initiative

The WFP, the largest humanitarian agency worldwide, is a major staple food buyer. WFP buys these staple foods locally whenever their price, quality and quantity criteria can be met. The P4P initiative aims to increase local procurement and achieve higher development gains with WFP's procurement footprint by buying food in a smallholder-friendly way. Farmers often face challenges gaining access to formal markets, and the P4P tries to address these barriers by focusing on the following three main pillars:

1. Demand: Test innovative ways of buying staple foods and promote marketing opportunities for smallholder farmers
2. Supply: Support farmers to achieve better yields, reduce their post-harvest losses and improve the quality of their crops
3. Learning and Sharing: Gather and share lessons on effective approaches to connect smallholder farmers to markets in a sustainable way.

P4P has been found to lead to positive changes in the lives and livelihoods of participating smallholder farmers by providing them with crucial resources and encouraging them to work together as part of farming organizations.

Global Context of Food Systems and the Evolution of Nutrition

Diet Shifts and Value Chains

There is a rapid transition occurring in dietary and activity patterns globally, paralleled by major demographic and socioeconomic changes. Dietary changes include an increase in the consumption of animal-based products, vegetable oils, sugar, sugar-sweetened beverages (SSB) and ultra-processed, fast and street foods. Much of this shift is due to growing urbanization, increased availability of fast food outlets and marketing and promotion of processed food products [19]. These changes, together with a decrease in activity levels—driven largely by increases in sedentary job opportunities, increased use of motorized transportation and decreased active transportation (i.e., walking and cycling) likely due to insufficient infrastructure (e.g., sidewalks), and lack of leisure time—have resulted in rising levels of obesity in many countries (including low- and middle-income) [20–25].

Low- and middle-income countries are now facing multiple burdens of malnutrition [21, 26]—a high prevalence of undernutrition (and often associated infectious diseases) as well as a considerable rise in overweight and obesity (and the associated non-communicable diseases (NCDs) such as cardiovascular and coronary heart disease, diabetes and various cancers) [21, 23, 27]. While urbanization, sedentary lifestyles and the lack of infrastructure and security of poor neighborhoods and slums contribute to these trends in transitioning economies, rises in overweight and obesity are now found in both urban and rural communities and there are only marginal differences between the ratio of overweight and obesity levels in urban and rural populations [28]. Countries with marked levels of low birth weight and stunting arc sensitive to the consequences of changing diets and activity patterns [29]. The trends in obesity are crippling some of the poorest countries, which are still reeling from undernutrition and infectious diseases [28, 30].

Alongside increases in the prevalence of overweight and obesity in low- and middle-income countries, there have also been marked changes to the food supply. Multinational food companies manufacturing ultra-processed foods have begun focusing on low- and middle-income countries as a source of growth as profit gains begin to stagnate in high-income countries [31]. This has led to an increase in the availability, affordability and acceptability of these foods in many countries and has transformed the food environment [31, 32]. Many of these products are targeted to the poor by using smaller package sizes, with a low unit price, and ensuring that the products are available in both traditional and modern retailers.

Changes in the types of food we eat, and shifts in our diet will drive a new "demand" of how food is grown, processed and consumed [19]. While populations are growing, overall wealth among that growing population is also increasing, particularly in places like India, China and Brazil. With this increase in wealth comes an increased demand for higher quality, nutrient-rich products such as meat, dairy products, and oils as well as ultra-processed food consumption. Americans account for just 4.5% of the world's population, but eat approximately 15% of the meat produced globally [33]. On average, the USA consumes 124 kg meat/capita/year compared to the global average of 38 kg/capita/year [34]. The countries that consume the least amount of meat are in Africa and South Asia, where the highest burden of undernutrition lies, with consumption in some countries as low as 8.5 kg/person/year in Ethiopia and 3 kg/person/year in Bangladesh [35]. While there may be a need to grow more crops in a sustainable way, there is also a need to ensure that food is available and accessible in a more equitable way, that food that is grown, provided and sold is both safe and of better nutritional quality, and consumers demand more nutritious foods [36]. These changes will come with ethical and environmental costs to society in some way.

In middle- and high-income countries, attention and publicity are increasing to promote better quality diets (in terms of nutrition but also sustainability). However, it is clear that the cost of such diets is currently high [19] and even the costs of basic diets in much of the world remains higher than daily wages [37]. In South Africa, a middle-income country, a nutritious and healthy diet costs 69% more than a typical South African diet [19]. Even in high-income countries, some cannot meet the dietary guidelines, particularly fresh fruit and vegetable recommendations, and energy-dense foods high in fat, sugar and salt are often less expensive and provide more energy per dollar spent than nutrient-rich foods [19, 38].

Changes in value chains and their influence on the obesogenic environment have undoubtedly contributed to these shifts in dietary patterns. In today's environment, energy-dense but otherwise nutrient-poor foods are increasingly accessible and affordable [19]. The obesogenic environment is one of the major explanations for the increasing prevalence in obesity [39]. Disadvantaged, vulnerable and poor families often find themselves in environments that are obesogenic. They have less access to healthy foods, have jobs that don't allow time to prepare and consume healthy meals, and live in environments that do not promote physical activity.

Although value chains are currently geared, in many ways, toward the production of foods that contribute to the obesogenic environment, there is a potential to reorient them to improve the availability, affordability and acceptability of nutritious foods. Although, FVCs for nutrition have most often been thought of in terms of increasing access to micronutrients (e.g., biofortified staple crops), they can also be used to promote (or discourage) consumption of foods within the context of obesity and NCDs and have an important role in addressing the double burden of malnutrition.

Value Chains for Nutrition

Why Food Value Chains Can Contribute to Nutrition

FVC approaches are already used in international development with the objective of enhancing the livelihoods of food producers, but they rarely consider diet quality and nutrition [3]. In low- and middle-income countries, the FVC approach has mainly been thought of through economic, cash crop terms. Yet more can be done within the value chain model, including ensuring that better partnerships with unique sets of players can add value by bringing more nutrition to the value chain. By including nutrition as an outcome of value chains, demand and supply "ends" of the chain can be linked, (with the producer and consumer often being the same person), with a focus on ensuring that the nutritional needs of the population are met.

FVCs touch all four aspects of food and nutrition security: production, access, acceptability and quality of foods. In the recent Lancet series on child and maternal nutrition, value chains were highlighted as a potential way to leverage agriculture to improve nutrition, particularly with regards to traditional value chains for micronutrient-rich foods [40]. Many poor households predominantly consume staple-based diets and lack access to fruits and vegetables, animal-source or wild foods of high nutrient content [3, 41]. In order for the agricultural sector to play a more effective role in terms of improving access, acceptability and quality of diets and more nutrient-rich foods that are lacking in diets of poor households, there needs to be a greater focus on what happens to foods being produced all the way to their consumption [3]. Economic constraints, insufficient supply and demand of affordable nutritious foods, lack of nutrition sensitiveness along the agricultural value chain, and limited appropriate information on nutrition for consumers to change behavior are critical factors that limit poor population's access to nutritious foods. Food and nutrient losses along the value chain, which may be caused by ineffective or inefficient harvesting, storage, processing and handling, are other factors that affect the availability, cost and hence affordability of nutrient-rich foods.

Value for Nutrition

Adopting value chain approaches can be an effective way to identify the causes of inadequate food availability, affordability and acceptability and to implement effective solutions and create long-term, sustainable benefits for nutrition [3]. Perhaps much of this adoption can occur through the agriculture sector. However, it should be noted that commonly, value chain approaches (particularly those approaches rooted in agriculture) focus on the processes and actors involved from the producer's perspective (i.e., the supply side). Very little attention is paid to the role of consumers and how they can influence the value chain through increased demand for nutritious foods. Figure 34.3 depicts some of the ways in which nutrition interventions can leverage agriculture-focused value chain activities to address the double burden of malnutrition at both the market and household level (i.e., consumer).

The ultimate goal of supply-side initiatives is to improve food availability at household level and to increase household income (i.e., food access). However, evidence has shown that improvements in food supply and household income alone are not sufficient to improve nutritional status. Thus, to reflect a nutrition "lens" on the smallholder value chain, the demand side of the equation—the smallholder farmer as consumer of nutritious foods—must also be considered.

The demand side relates to household decisions regarding purchase of food, allocation of resources to different household members and knowledge of safe and nutritious food preparation and child-feeding practices. Demand-side interventions focus on awareness, behavioral change, knowledge transfer and empowerment in order to increase demand for nutritious foods and improve dietary intake. Resources controlled by women, as well as nutrition education, are critical across the entire chain. Because the smallholder value chain focuses on both demand- and supply-side issues, the value chain is articulated not as a linear process but as a circle, which acknowledges that the smallholder farmer is both the target producer and a consumer of the nutritious foods produced. In this context, "value" is defined not only in terms of economic impact (e.g., income earned) but also as a social impact through improved nutritional status and better health.

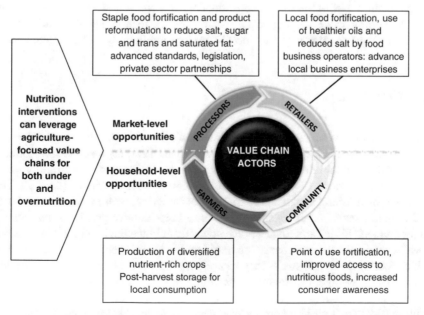

Fig. 34.3 Examples of how nutrition interventions can leverage agriculture-focused value chains. *Source* Adapted from USAID Feed the Future, Rwanda [42]

The links between what is produced on the farm, the consumer who buys that food and the income received by the producer does not stop at production [3]. Food is stored, distributed, processed, retailed, prepared and consumed in a range of ways that affect the access, acceptability and nutritional quality of foods for the consumer. Value chains are thus fundamental to consumption, dietary and nutrition perspectives and not only in terms of the supply of foods. Little emphasis has been given to how consumers can play a role in influencing value chains and how changes in the demand for specific foods can influence the processes and outputs of value chains. Demand for healthier products can be increased when consumers value these higher quality products, which is linked to food preferences. Food preferences are influenced by exposure to eating behaviors of parents, caregivers, peers and role models, to the availability of foods inside and outside the home, to cultural and social norms as well as to new information and marketing [43]. By targeting food preferences through social marketing, modeling of healthy eating behaviors and other mechanisms, demand for more nutritious foods can be increased.

In addition to the role of consumer demand in influencing value chains, there has also been little attention given to how actors, particularly women along the value chain can be better informed on enhancing the nutritional value of local foods. Food and nutrition systems need to be rethought by creating new business paradigms that engage smallholder farmers from a livelihoods perspective but also from a health and nutrition perspective.

Nutrition Value Chain Actors

Figure 34.4 presents the sequence of processes and the main actors involved in a basic value chain with a lens on nutrition, which takes food from the farm to the consumer [44, 45]. It also depicts the two main pathways in which value chains can improve nutrition outcomes: (1) by improving consumption of the nutritious foods produced by smallholders and (2) by generating income which enables consumers to purchase healthier foods. There are various incentives (and disincentives) that can help stimulate activity among value chain actors to produce and consume more nutritious foods, including organizational incentives (e.g., consolidating to increase competitive advantage), financial incentives (e.g., adding value, cutting costs, seeking profit), technological incentives (e.g., technological innovations) and regulatory/policy incentives (e.g., regulations, policies, legal decisions) [44].

Entry and Exit Points

Typically, poor households subsist on monotonous staple-based diets; they lack access to nutritious foods, such as fruits, vegetables, animal-source foods (fish, meat, eggs and dairy products), fortified foods or wild foods of high nutrient content. Lack of diversity in the diet is strongly associated with inadequate intake (and risks of deficiencies) of essential micronutrients [46–48]. The resulting deficiencies have far-reaching health and nutrition consequences, both in the short and the long term.

One of the main uses of value chain analysis is to help identify points in the chain that can be "leveraged for change" [44]. Targeting leverage points can reduce the likelihood that nutrients are lost or exit the value chain as well as enhance the nutritional value of specific nutrient-rich foods. Exiting points, such as food and nutrient losses that occur along the value chain, are caused by ineffective or inefficient harvesting, storage, processing or handling, reducing availability and raising the price of nutrient-rich foods. The poor are at highest risk of exposure to unsafe food, and since malnourished and micronutrient-deficient children are most susceptible to the health risks associated with unsafe

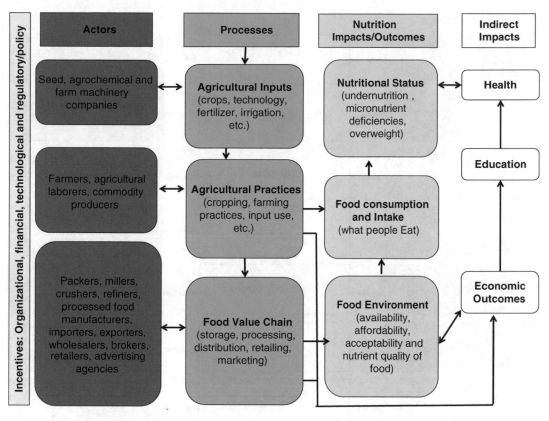

Fig. 34.4 Food value chains for nutrition. *Source* Adapted from Hawkes 2009 [44], Hawkes et al. [45]

food or water, they have the most to gain from improvements in the nutritional value and safety of foods [3].

It is also important to understand potential entry points: to enhance (or prevent losses) in the nutritional value of foods during processing or to fortify (or restore the nutrient content of) foods formulated for special groups (such as complementary foods for young children or nutrient-rich foods for pregnant women or people living with HIV). Entry points to educate and raise awareness among the different actors in the value chain are also important in terms of stimulating demand for the target products. Economic constraints, lack of knowledge and information, and related lack of demand for nutritious foods are critical factors that limit poor populations' access to such foods. Figure 34.5 shows ways in which more nutrition can enter or exit FVCs.

As FVCs have become more popular in terms of improving nutrition in development, tools to help extension workers, non-governmental organizations and researchers to apply value chain analysis in the field have been developed. These tools help guide value chain analysis and identify potential leverage points in the chain. By mapping the FVC, it is possible to identify areas where nutrients are lost or exit the value chain and to identify potential solutions to try to mitigate these loses. IDS and GAIN recently developed a "Nutritious Agriculture by Design" tool[1] that aims to help program planners put a nutrition focus on agricultural programs and the Value Chains Knowledge Clearing House[2] provides tools for farmers, practitioners and researchers to help guide value chain analysis.

---

[1]http://nutritiousagriculture-tool1.gainhealth.org/.

[2]http://tools4valuechains.org/.

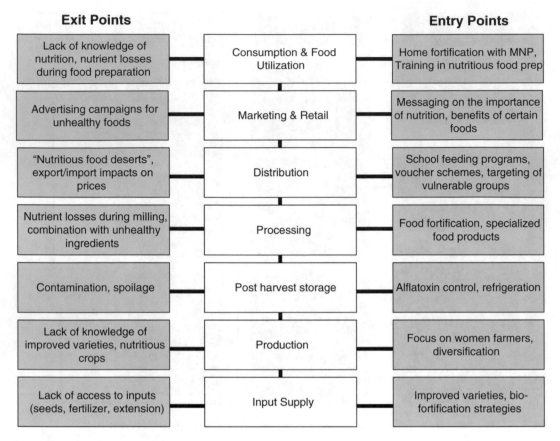

Fig. 34.5 Exit and entry points along the value chain for nutrition

Nutrition-Focused Food Value Chains

Figure 34.6 adapts Porter's value chain to a more nutrition-focused chain. The primary activities encompass the FVC from inputs into agricultural production to food retailing, marketing and labeling. The secondary activities relate to the supportive factors that increase the likelihood of adding nutrition value along the FVC. Throughout the nutrition-focused FVC, there are opportunities for creating shared value in terms of both economic and nutritional goals.

Primary Activities

Inbound Logistics

Inbound logistics encompass inputs into production and agricultural production itself. The actors involved in these processes include seed, irrigation and farming equipment companies as well as plant breeders, farmers and laborers, among others. Adding nutrition value at this stage of the FVC can be achieved by producing nutrient-rich crops and by maximizing yields of those crops. For example, HarvestPlus has developed specific crop and nutrient combinations (e.g., rice biofortified with zinc in Bangladesh and India, maize biofortified with provitamin A in Nigeria and Zambia) to deliver specific

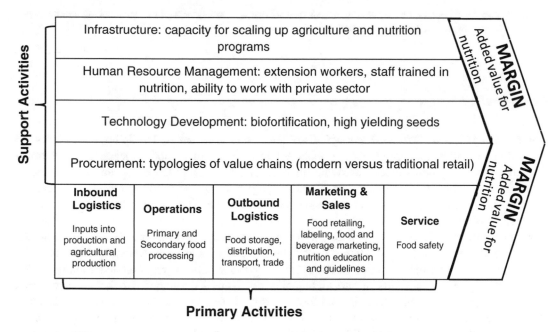

Fig. 34.6   Nutrition-focused food value chain framework. Adapted from Porter and Miller [2]

micronutrients to populations at risk of micronutrient deficiency in Africa and Asia [49]. Golden rice—rice that has been genetically modified to be high in beta-carotene in order to reduce vitamin A deficiency—provides another example of adding value in terms of nutrition before food leaves the farmgate. Importantly, a key factor in increasing the uptake of vitamin A rich orange sweet potato in Uganda and Mozambique was that the crop was high yielding, drought tolerant and virus resistant, and consumers who received education on the nutritional value of the food and were encouraged to try it reported to enjoy the taste of the food, which increased farmers' willingness to produce this nutrient-rich variety [50, 51].

Operations

Operations include both primary and secondary food processing and the actors (mainly the food industry) involved in these processes. Adding nutrition value at this point in the value chain can be achieved both by fortifying processed foods with micronutrients and by ensuring healthier inputs are used in processed foods (e.g., using less salt, limiting trans fat, etc.). The private sector has a key role to play at this point in the FVC.

New partnerships working across the value chain are emerging such as the new partnership between PepsiCo and World Food Programme on the development of locally sourced chickpea-based ready-to-use foods for treating malnutrition in Ethiopia. Danone has partnered with Grameen Bank to develop a social business model that delivers nutrients to those who may be at risk for micronutrient deficiencies in Bangladesh through their dairy production, along with nutrient-rich biscuits and snacks. However, we need more of these types of models, and more partnerships to inject nutrition into the many agri-food value chains across the developing world.

There is an urgent need for major donors from the private sector, foundations, and the development community to invest in a twenty-first century approach to nutrition science.

—Yach et al. [52].

Outbound Logistics

Outbound logistics include food storage, distribution, transport and trade. Outbound logistics can occur directly after food production (inbound logistics) or after food processing (operations), depending on the product type. Improving nutrition at this stage of the FVC can be achieved by increasing access to nutrient-rich foods. Ensuring proper storage of foods to reduce wastage, distributing food more efficiently and ensuring that there are roads and adequate infrastructure in place to transport food can help increase access to nutritious foods. For example, a dairy farming development assistance project in Zambia—which aimed to reduce household food insecurity among vulnerable groups through increased incomes generated from the sale of milk and other dairy-related products—improved storage and transportation through technologies for milk aggregation and cooling [3, 53]. This led to improved availability of safe, high-quality, cooled milk through milk collection centers and increased farmer profits, diet diversity and food security [3, 53]. In Singapore, the Healthy Hawkers Programme led to an increase in the availability and affordability of healthier oils for use by street vendors after the Health Promotion Board worked with oil manufacturers to produce a blended oil with 25% less saturated fat than the oil typically used (palm oil) by vendors. In order to bring down the cost of the blended oil, the Health Promotion Board worked with manufacturers to share logistic services, including storage and delivery resources, which led to the oil being comparable in price to palm oil [4].

Marketing and Sales

This is a very important step in the FVC to improve acceptability as well as the availability and affordability of nutritious foods. Food retailers play a key role in terms of increasing access to foods that have a higher content of essential nutrients, such as vitamins and minerals, without having a higher energy density compared to similar foods. In urban populations, supermarkets are critically important and are playing a role in coordinating markets and price determination [54]. In rural populations, local markets, smallholder farms and small "mom and pop" shops are important in terms of accessing nutritious foods such as fruits and vegetables and health products.

Food and beverage marketing—both by food industry and governments—can improve consumer acceptability of foods; however, the types of foods "marketed" by these two types of actors are often quite different. Governments and NGOs can influence consumers' perceptions of the nutrition value of foods by implementing regulation, mass media campaigns, adopting nutrition guidelines and nutrition education. For example, when the USA adopted mandatory labeling of trans fat, it raised consumer awareness [55], which then led to an increase in consumer demand for trans fat-free foods [58]. This in turn resulted in the food industry reformulating many of their products [56]. In Mozambique, a HarvestPlus Reaching End Users project increased the production, availability and consumption of orange-fleshed sweet potato among rural households [57]. More than 50% of consumers who purchased sweet potato in 10 markets indicated that they bought it because of its associated nutritional and health benefits, which they had learned about from the educational messages (radio ads, programs, promotion events, market signs and murals) implemented as part of the project [3, 57]. Building demand for nutritious foods is a key component of value chains for nutrition, particularly when their appearance or taste differs from the foods that consumers are accustomed to eating (e.g., golden rice) [58].

Secondary Activities

The secondary activities consist of infrastructure, human resource management, technology development and procurement. In terms of adding nutrition value in the value chain, these activities aim to support the primary activities in the chain and increase the uptake of activities that are likely to improve the availability, affordability and acceptability of nutritious foods. For example, ensuring that there is sufficient infrastructure in place increases the likelihood of being able to successfully scale up nutrition-sensitive agricultural programs and initiatives. For example, the Scaling Up Nutrition (SUN) movement focuses on increasing in-country capacity to implement interventions aimed at improving nutrition outcomes, while the SUN Business Network supports SUN countries to develop plans for collaborating with business on these approaches. As part of the movement, SUN countries mobilize resources to enable prioritization of nutrition interventions. Given that many of the initiatives aimed at creating nutrition value along the FVC involve various sectors and disciplines, ensuring that staff are trained in the importance of nutrition as well as being able to work with the private sector is important. Many of the initiatives involving biofortification are joint ventures among governments, NGOs and the private sector. In addition to improving infrastructure and human resource management, ensuring technology development, and its uptake, by actors in the FVC as well as streamlining the value chain by improving procurement can help increase access to nutritious foods. For example, reducing post-harvest losses is an important point for intervention along value chains, particularly in low- and middle-income countries where a substantial proportion of food is lost before leaving the farm gate [59].

Conclusion

Value chains are not a new concept and many working in agriculture and business have been utilizing not only the concept, but have put value chains into practical use. Yet, very little has been done to ensure nutrition is included and linked into the chain. This is likely a reflection of the cross-disciplinary nature of FVCs. The analysis of FVC requires an understanding of nutrition, agriculture, food technology, economics, marketing, etc. However, the training received by nutritionists in these other areas is often insufficient. Because of this, there are still many unanswered questions that require research, more operational understanding and collaborative investigation. Nevertheless, FVCs for nutrition have a role to play in terms of identifying innovative ways to improve the availability, affordability and acceptability of nutritious foods both in the context of under- and overnutrition, and there is currently a push for conducting FVC analyses in an integrated manner with various stakeholders. This will require buy-in from various actors in the value chain and will need to target both supply and demand-side dynamics. There is likely a role for policy in terms of supporting actions along the FVC that can contribute to healthier consumption patterns; however, there is also a role for the private sector. Applying a business-lens to nutrition may help to identify opportunities for integrating nutrition into FVCs with the goal of increasing the availability, affordability and acceptability of nutritious foods for the population.

Discussion Points

- What are the opportunities and barriers to increase the consumer demand for and consumption of nutrient-rich foods among the poor? Does nutrition knowledge and awareness of consumers play a role in influencing the value chain? Where do they get their information from and what sources/value chain actors do they trust?

- What role does industry play in ensuring access to nutritious foods? What role should commercial farmers/producers/processors/distributors play in value chains that are more nutrition focused? What role do women play as they play dual roles as producers and consumers?
- How can food be enriched, processed, preserved to increase their nutritive potential along the value chain? How can nutrient losses be avoided along the value chain? How expensive are these alterations to foods? Are consumers willing to pay for more nutritious foods?
- How can value chains be better used to produce specialized nutritious foods for children under two, pregnant mothers and special needs populations such as People Living with HIV?
- Where do supermarkets play a role for poor and vulnerable populations?
- How can nutrition be balanced (economies of scale/trade-offs) with economic gains, intensification of agricultural production systems and more complicated value chain systems (i.e., USA)?

References

1. Global Value Chains Initiative. 2014. Available here: http://www.cggc.duke.edu/projects/gvc.php.
2. Porter ME, Millar VE. How information gives you competitive advantage. Harvard Bus Rev. 1985;63(4):149–60.
3. Hawkes C, Ruel MT. Value chains for nutrition (2020 conference paper 4). Washington, DC: International Food Policy Research Institute; 2011.
4. Hawkes C, Thow AM, Downs S, Ling AL, Ghosh-Jerath S, Snowdon W, Jewell J. Identifying effective food systems solutions for nutrition and noncommunicable diseases: creating policy coherence in the fats supply chain. SCN News. (40):39–47.
5. KPMG International. The agricultural and food value chain: entering a new era of cooperation. London, UK; 2013.
6. Porter ME, Kramer MR. Creating shared value. Harvard Bus Rev. 2011;89(1/2):62–77.
7. Yach D, Acharya T. Strengthening food security in a developing world. In: USAID frontiers in development. Washington DC; 2010.
8. Timmer P. The transformation of food supply chains. In: Pritchard B, Ortiz R, Shekar M, editors. Routledge handbook of food and nutrition security. Routledge: New York.
9. Gómez MI, Ricketts KD. Food value chain transformations in developing countries: selected hypotheses on nutritional implications. Food Policy. 2013;42:139–50.
10. Reardon T, Henson S, Gulati A, Hawkes C, Blouin C, Drager N, Dubé L. Links between supermarkets and food prices, diet diversity and food safety in developing countries. Trade Food Diet Health Perspect Policy Options. 2010;111–130.
11. Reddy G, Murthy M, Meena P. Value chains and retailing of fresh vegetables and fruits, Andhra Pradesh. Agric Econ Res Rev. 2010;23:435–60.
12. Gorton M, Sauer J, Supatpongkul P. Wet markets, supermarkets and the "big middle" for food retailing in developing countries: evidence from Thailand. World Dev. 2011;39(9):1624–37.
13. Ruben R, van Tilbur A, Trienekens J, van Boekel M. Linking market integration, supply chain governance, quality, and value added in tropical food chains. In: Ruben R, van Boekel M, van Tilbur A, Trienekens J, editors. Tropical food chains: governance regimes for quality management. Wageningen: Wageningen Academic Publishers; 2007. P. 13–46.
14. Reardon T, Timmer CP. Transformation of markets for agricultural output in developing countries since 1950: how has thinking changed? Handbook Agric Econ. 2007;3:2807–55.
15. Reardon T, Gulati A. The supermarket revolution in developing countries: Policies for "competitiveness with inclusiveness" (No. 2); 2008.
16. Euromonitor International. Examining the impact of the growth of modern grocery retailers on the wider retail landscape. 2012.
17. Reardon T. The rapid rise of supermarkets and the use of private standards in their food product procurement systems in developing countries. Agro-food Chains Netw Dev. 2006.
18. Reardon T, Swinnen JF. Agrifood sector liberalisation and the rise of supermarkets in former state-controlled economies: a comparative overview. Dev Policy Rev. 2004;22(5):515–23.
19. Keats S, Wiggins S. Future diets: implications for agriculture and food prices. Report, London: Overseas Development Institute. http://www.odi.org/sites/odi.org.uk/files/odi-assets/publications-opinion-files/8776.pdf.
20. Lenfant C. Can we prevent cardiovascular diseases in low-and middle-income countries? Bull World Health Organ. 2001;79(10):980–2.

21. Popkin BM, Du S. Dynamics of the nutrition transition toward the animal foods sector in china and its implications: a worried perspective. J Nutr. 2003;133(11):3898S–906S.
22. Marshall SJ. Developing countries face double burden of disease. Bull World Health Organ. 2004;82(7):556–56.
23. WHO (World Health Organization. "Obesity and overweight." Fact sheet No. 311, May 2013. Geneva: WHO; 2013.
24. Laverty AA, Palladino R, Lee JT, Millett C. Associations between active travel and weight, blood pressure and diabetes in six middle income countries: a cross-sectional study in older adults. Int J Behav Nutr Phys Activity. 2015;12(1):65.
25. Kohl HW, Craig CL, Lambert EV, Inoue S, Alkandari JR, Leetongin G, Kahlmeier S & Lancet Physical Activity Series Working Group. The pandemic of physical inactivity: global action for public health. The Lancet. 2012;380 (9838):294–305.
26. Yach D. Food industry: friend or foe? Obes Rev. 2014;15(1):2–5.
27. Lim SS, Vos T, Flaxman AD, Danaei G, Shibuya K, Adair-Rohani H, Aryee M. A comparative risk assessment of burden of disease and injury attributable to 67 risk factors and risk factor clusters in 21 regions, 1990–2010: a systematic analysis for the global burden of disease study 2010. Lancet. 2013;380(9859):2224–60.
28. Popkin BM, Adair LS, Ng SW. Global nutrition transition and the pandemic of obesity in developing countries. Nutr Rev. 2012;70(1):3–21.
29. Adair L, Fall C, Osmond A, Stein R, Martorell R, Ramirez-Zea M, Sachdev HS, et al. Associations of linear growth and relative weight gain during early life with adult health and human capital in countries of low and middle income: findings from five birth cohort studies. Lancet. 2013;382:525–34.
30. Walker P, Rhubart-Berg P, McKenzie S, Kelling K, Lawrence RS. Public health implications of meat production and consumption. Public Health Nutr. 2005;8(04):348–56.
31. Stuckler D, McKee M, Ebrahim S, Basu S. Manufacturing epidemics: the role of global producers in increased consumption of unhealthy commodities including processed foods, alcohol, and tobacco. PLoS Med. 2012;9(6): e1001235.
32. Igumbor EU, Sanders D, Puoane TR, Tsolekile L, Schwarz C, Purdy C, Hawkes C. "Big food", the consumer food environment, health, and the policy response in South Africa. PLoS Med. 2012;9(7):e1001253.
33. Stokstad E. Could less meat mean more food? Science. 2010;327(5967):810–1.
34. Wilkinson P, Smith KR, Davies M, Adair H, Armstrong BG, Barrett M, Chalabi Z. Public health benefits of strategies to reduce greenhouse-gas emissions: household energy. Lancet. 2009;374(9705):1917–29.
35. FAO (Food and Agriculture Organization). "FAOStat." Rome: FAO; 2014.
36. FAO (Food and Agriculture Organization) 2013. "The State of Food and Agriculture." Rome: FAO; 2013. http://www.fao.org/publications/sofa/2013/en/.
37. Brinkman HJ, de Pee S, Sanogo I, Subran L, Bloem MW. High food prices and the global financial crisis have reduced access to nutritious food and worsened nutritional status and health. J Nutr. 2010;140(1):153S–61S.
38. Aggarwal A, Monsivais P, Drewnowski A. Nutrient intakes linked to better health. PLoS ONE. 2012;7(5):e37533. doi:10.1371/journal.pone.003753.
39. WHO (World Health Organization. WHO Technical Report Series; 916. Geneva: WHO; 2003.
40. Ruel MT, Alderman H. Nutrition-sensitive interventions and programmes: how can they help to accelerate progress in improving maternal and child nutrition? Lancet. 2013;382(9891):536–51.
41. Dewey KG, Adu-Afarwuah S. Systematic review of the efficacy and effectiveness of complementary feeding interventions in developing countries. Matern Child Nutr. 2008;4(s1):24–85.
42. USAID Feed the Future. 2014. http://www.bdsknowledge.org/dyn/bds/docs/804/RwandaFTFStrategicReview.pdf.
43. Hawkes C, Smith TG, Jewell J, Wardle J, Hammond RA, Friel S, Kain J. Smart food policies for obesity prevention. The Lancet. 2015.
44. Hawkes C. Identifying innovative interventions to promote healthy eating using consumption-oriented food supply chain analysis. J Hunger Environ Nutr. 2009;4(3–4):336–56.
45. Hawkes C, Turner R, Waage R. Current and planned research on agriculture for improved nutrition: a mapping and a gap analysis. London: DFID; 2012.
46. Ruel MT. Operationalizing dietary diversity: a review of measurement issues and research priorities. J Nutr. 2003;133(11):3911S–26S.
47. Leakey RR. Potential for novel food products from agroforestry trees: a review. Food Chem. 1999;66(1):1–14.
48. Arimond M, Ruel MT. Dietary diversity is associated with child nutritional status: evidence from 11 demographic and health surveys. J Nutr. 2004;134(10):2579–85.
49. HarvestPlus. Biofortification Progress Briefs. 2014. Available at: http://www.harvestplus.org/content/new-progress-briefs-biofortification-released.
50. Harvest Plus. 2010. http://www.harvestplus.org/content/orange-sweet-potato-faces-bright-future-africa-0.
51. Tomlins K, Ndunguru G, Stambul K, Joshua N, Ngendello T, Rwiza E, Amour R, Ramadhani B, Kapande A, Westby A. Sensory evaluation and consumer acceptability of pale-fleshed and orange-fleshed sweetpotato by school children and mothers with preschool children. J Sci Food Agric. 2007;87(13):2436–46.

52. Yach D, Khan M, Bradley D, Hargrove R, Kehoe S, Mensah G. The role and challenges of the food industry in addressing chronic disease. Globalization Health. 2010;6:10.
53. Swanson R. Final Evaluation of Dairy Development FFP DAP for Vulnerable Populations in Zambia. 2009. Available at: http://www.fsnnetwork.org/sites/default/files/final_evalution_of_zambia_title_ii.pdf.
54. Timmer P. The impact of supermarkets on farmers, consumers and food security in developing countries. In: Semba R, Bloem B, editors. Nutrition and health in developing countries 2nd edition. Totowa NJ: Humana Press; 2008. P. 739–752.
55. Eckel RH, Kris-Etherton P, Lichtenstein AH, Wylie-Rosett J, Groom A, Stitzel KF, Yin-Piazza S. Americans' awareness, knowledge, and behaviors regarding fats: 2006–2007. J Am Diet Assoc. 2009;109(2):288–96.
56. Mozaffarian D, Jacobson MF, Greenstein JS. Food reformulations to reduce trans fatty acids. N Engl J Med. 2010;362(21):2037–9.
57. HarvestPlus. Disseminating orange-fleshed sweet potato Findings from a HarvestPlus Project in Mozambique and Uganda; 2012. Available at: http://www.harvestplus.org/sites/default/files/HarvestPlus_OFSP_Brief_English_2012_v2_small.pdf.
58. USAID. Microlinks. 2014. Available at: https://www.microlinks.org/good-practice-center/value-chain-wiki/applying-value-chain-approach-food-utilization.
59. Parfitt J, Barthel M, Macnaughton S. Food waste within food supply chains: quantification and potential for change to 2050. Philos Trans R Soc B Biol Sci. 2010;365(1554):3065–81.

Chapter 35
Role of Foundations and Initiatives by the Private Sector for Improving Health and Nutrition

Kalpana Beesabathuni, Kesso Gabrielle van Zutphen and Klaus Kraemer

Keywords Foundations · Initiatives · Private sector · Health · Nutrition · Shared value · Advocacy · Open innovation · Public–private partnerships · Corporate social responsibility · Conflicts of interest · Social impact bonds · Development impact bonds

Learning Objectives

- To understand the types of private sector donors who provide financial and in-kind resources and technical know-how to development activities.
- To learn and be able to distinguish various approaches of private sector-supported nutrition and health programs.
- To identify innovations in private sector-supported nutritional interventions.

Introduction

In the last decades, a wide range of non-state actors ranging from non-governmental organizations (NGOs) to multi-national firms have become key players in development, the private sector being one of them. Contributions from the private sector to development in low- and middle-income countries (LMICs) are receiving increasing attention, and the private sector is increasingly being recognized as a fundamental contributor to health and nutrition more specifically, by moving beyond its core function as a driver of economic growth through corporate social investment in the form of private foundations and initiatives [1, 2]. The "private sector" is a broad term encompassing a range of diverse actors, and its definitions vary. Its stakeholders include the for-profit private sector and private foundations [3]. While the former operates on a for-profit basis, private foundations are commonly defined as "a non-governmental, non-profit organization having a principal fund of its own, managed by its own trustees and board of directors, and established to maintain or aid social, educational,

K. Beesabathuni
9th Floor, Infinity Tower A, DLF Phase 2, Gurgaon 122002, Haryana, India
e-mail: kalpana.beesabathuni@sightandlife.org

K.G. van Zutphen
46 rue de Carouge, Geneva 1205, Switzerland
e-mail: kesso.vanzutphen@gmail.com

K. Kraemer (✉)
PO Box 2116, Basel 4002, Switzerland
e-mail: klaus.kraemer@sightandlife.org

© Springer Science+Business Media New York 2017
S. de Pee et al. (eds.), *Nutrition and Health in a Developing World*,
Nutrition and Health, DOI 10.1007/978-3-319-43739-2_35

charitable, religious, or other activities serving the common welfare" [4 (p. 11)]. They are generally entirely funded by their parent corporations. Additionally, there is a growing presence of high-level family foundations that are now providing funds directed at development. These families either have their own high net worth or bring together funders from multiple sources. This chapter will essentially focus on private foundations and initiatives that are funded by a corporate entity.

While foundations have largely remained absent from global governance literature while other non-state actors such as firms and international NGOs have been the subject of ever-increasing research, the phenomenon of philanthropic private foundations as a key player in the health realm is not new [5]. Foundations such as Rockefeller Foundation and Ford Foundation were early players and leaders in the field of health, with Rockefeller Foundation being established over a century ago for instance [5]. As this chapter will illustrate, the health sector continues to be a core focus for private foundations [5]. Today's largest private global health foundation is the Bill & Melinda Gates Foundation with an endowment of US$41.3 billion as of June 30, 2015 [6]. The total amount paid out by the foundation for all grants in 2014 was US$3.86 billion, of which $1.11 billion was for global health and $1.92 billion for global development which comprises nutrition. In fact, 3% of the foundation's global development budget is dedicated to nutrition programs [6, 7]. In 2007, the amount spent by the Gates Foundation on global health was almost as much as WHO's annual budget (approximately $1.65 billion) and was substantially more than the total grant spending of the Rockefeller Foundation across all programmatic areas in the same year ($0.17 billion) [8]. Although the influence of the Gates Foundation is of a different order, the Ford Foundation, W.K. Kellogg Foundation, Robert Wood Johnson Foundation and Rockefeller Foundation are known as today's largest private global health foundations [9]. Nearly 2500 corporate foundations incorporated in the USA have total assets of US$25 billion. These foundations paid out US$5.4 billion in grants in the year 2013 [10].

There is a wide range of incentives for the for-profit private sector's philanthropic engagement in LMIC to improve health and nutrition; three common reasons refer to (1) risk mitigation, (2) exploring business opportunities and (3) increasing staff satisfaction. With regard to risk mitigation, a company can choose to address risk for example in response to civil society or consumer pressure to protect its brand from bad publicity or simply because it can positively influence how customers perceive the brand and increase customer loyalty [3]. Likewise, private foundations and initiatives can choose to respond to social factors that can impact the workforce of a company, including their families and broader communities and thus the client base of the company [3]. Secondly, to address health and nutrition challenges is increasingly presented as a business opportunity for companies, coinciding with the incentive of making profit and an increased focus on innovations that respond to new demands and societal needs and which ensure sustainability. Furthermore, the 2010 United Nations (UN) Millennium Development Goal (MDG) Summit Joint Statement underlines that the leading companies of the future will be "those that do business in a way that addresses the major development challenges" [11 (p. 20)]. Thirdly, staff satisfaction in the form of contributing to something good which employees can feel proud of, is an equally important incentive for the private sector to engage in development activities. It can motivate employees and make them feel more engaged with their company, especially if it offers them the chance to participate actively in such efforts [3, 12].

In recent decades, an increasing number of corporate foundations have started to provide funding to LMIC. The nature of Corporate Social Responsibility (CSR) has changed over the years from providing one-time grants to communities around the parent companies' operational geographies, to building a portfolio of strategic programs with a mission of longer-term social development. Moreover, while it is typically perceived that corporate foundations only serve as a humanitarian arm, our experience and research indicates that foundations have also played a critical role as social intrapreneurs[1] in advancing much needed science, technology and delivery models in LMIC with a focus on vulnerable groups and that several of them function as intrapreneurs with a social mission. In fact, as will be seen throughout this chapter, private initiatives and foundations can have a positive impact on health and nutrition outcomes through a variety of processes and roles including and not limited to: the provision of goods and financial and in-kind resources, the advance of advocacy tools, driving innovation and novel approaches, and their role in public–private partnerships (PPPs) [3].

According to the 2015 Global Nutrition Report, there is little evidence of private sector contributions to improving nutrition [7]. Due to lack of peer-reviewed literature on the role of private sector for improving nutrition, this chapter draws on documented case studies. The foundations and initiatives that were chosen as case studies and examples for this chapter were selected from the 2015 list of Fortune Global 500—an annual list of the 500 largest companies in the world as compiled by FORTUNE magazine, companies listed in the Access to Nutrition Index (ATNI) and Scaling Up Nutrition (SUN) Business Network. Priority was given to the ones whose vision and mission focused on food- and nutrition-related activities in LMIC and the ones who majorly fund global health- and/or nutrition-related activities. With regard to the section on PPPs, part of the content stems from a qualitative research study that was conducted in India on the identification of major barriers for PPPs in public health nutrition.

The chapter first explores how corporate foundations and initiatives can improve health and nutrition through the provision of goods and financial and in-kind resources, followed by how the health and nutrition advocacy tools they develop not only improve nutrition-specific outcomes but also set the scene for further engagement at national and global level. Third, the chapter looks at how private initiatives and foundations' drive for innovation and novel approaches have already shown improvements for health and nutrition and are expected to continue to yield promising results in the future. Fourth, the proliferation of PPPs specifically for health, described as a "collaborative partnership where […] each partnership brings together at least three parties, among them a corporation (and/or industry association) and an intergovernmental organization to achieve a health creating goal on the basis of a mutually agreed division of labor" will be highlighted with a particular focus on how foundations in PPPs are increasingly contributing to advances in health outcomes and how transparency and credibility have played a key role in enabling this process [14]. Further, corporate foundations with their unique position as the interface between public and private sectors due to their experience in development programs could also act as a third party in PPPs. Last but not least, the chapter will close by giving an insight into the various ways through which the private sector and private foundations and initiatives in particular can have negative consequences for nutrition, thereby stressing the importance of accountability mechanisms to mitigate conflicts of interest and to incentivize the private sector to improve nutrition and health outcomes.

Provision of Goods and Financial and In-Kind Resources

Over the years, foundations have transformed from being purely vehicles for providing philanthropic services to entities that can influence companies to align with the ecosystem of LMIC and improve consumers' access to essential public health goods and services. By matching the challenges in public health to the strengths of the private sector, these foundations can create a shared value by creating

---

[1]An intrapreneur is an "entrepreneur within a large firm, who uses entrepreneurial skills without incurring the risks associated with those activities. Intrapreneurs are usually employees within a company who are assigned a special idea or project, and are instructed to develop the project like an entrepreneur would. Intrapreneurs usually have the resources and capabilities of the firm at their disposal. The intrapreneur's main job is to turn that special idea or project into a profitable venture for the company" [13].

economic value for a corporate while also generating value for society by addressing its needs [15]. In fact, leading companies are starting to find ways to create shared value around access to public health goods and services by improving the health of vulnerable populations while also creating short- and long-term value for the business, thereby recognizing both private and public sector needs [15]. The following paragraph illustrates how shared value offers corporations the opportunity to utilize their skills, resources and management capability to lead social progress through two activities: first the provision of commercial goods, and second its contribution to needed financial and in-kind resources [15].

Britannia Industries Limited was first established in 1892 in Kolkata as a small bakery that produced biscuits. Britannia is now one of India's biggest brands and food-products corporations selling products in over 5 categories (dairy, cakes, biscuits, breads and rusk) to more than half of the Indian population through 3.5 million retail outlets, and about 50% of Britannia's product portfolio is fortified with micronutrients [16]. Through its health and nutrition initiatives, Britannia aims to improve people's nutritional status: It provides food-based solutions such as the fortification of popular products, and it makes these more accessible and available and advocates for people's "right to nutrition." Britannia first started manufacturing iron-fortified biscuits for the school-feeding programs of the United Nations World Food Programme (WFP), and it then fortified all its commercial baked products with vitamins, iodine and iron, and also removed trans fats. Biscuits are extremely popular in India with 90% of urban and rural households consuming them. They thus appear to be an ideal vehicle for the delivery of essential micronutrients for people who may have an inadequate micronutrient intake [17]. A school-feeding fortification program supported by the Global Alliance for Improved Nutrition (GAIN), Britannia, and the Naandi Foundation came to the conclusion that the best way to address anemia among children was to fortify Britannia Tiger biscuits with iron as these were extremely popular among school children. Britannia managed to produce an iron-fortified Tiger biscuit to be sold at the identical price as the existing non-fortified product [18]. In a 2009 pilot study, Britannia found that together with treatment for hookworms, the consumption of their fortified Tiger biscuits improved iron status by 25% among more than 300 anemic children within a 90-day period [19].

Another example refers to the Unilever Foundation, which through its partnerships with five leading global organizations, namely Oxfam, Population Services International (PSI), Save the Children, United Nations Children's Fund (UNICEF) and United Nations World Food Programme (WFP), has contributed to scalable social change and extended the delivery of lifesaving solutions through the manufacture of soap, such as the Lifebuoy brand and Pureit (household water purification systems) [20]. In order to reach its aim of doubling the size of its business while reducing its environmental footprint and increasing its social impact simultaneously, Unilever recognizes that it must work in partnership with other stakeholders who share the same goal and leverage each other's skills, expertise and resources [21, 22]. One such example refers to the collaboration between Unilever Foundation and PSI, a global health organization, who both work together to avert preventable deaths (e.g., diarrheal diseases and acute respiratory infections) of which 2 million children under 5 die each year, by teaching the importance of hand-washing with soap and increasing access to safe drinking water and sanitation [23]. With PSI's more than 40 years of on-the-ground experience and Unilever's Lifebuoy soap products and communication materials, this joint initiative is an ideal match to encourage children to get into the habit of washing their hands with soap at critical times of the day in a consistent and correct manner. In 2013, Lifebuoy's 'Help A Child Reach 5' campaign that teaches lifesaving hand-washing habits was launched in a village in the Indian state of Madhya Pradesh called Thesgora that has one of the highest rates of diarrhea in India. After one year, an independent evaluation was done by AC Nielsen among 1485 households with children aged below 12 years. According to the evaluators, the overall diarrhea incidence in Thesgora dropped from 36 to 5% [24]. Partnerships with NGOs, microfinance institutions, cooperatives and women self-help groups thus helped in improving awareness, and increasing access by making them available at affordable price points or loans as well as at local purchase points.

Likewise, the Ajinomoto Group, a Japanese food and chemical corporation which was founded with the aim of helping people to "Eat well, Live well" by contributing to significant advances in health and food, is working in different parts of the world to improve nutrition as part of its CSR activities [25]. The Ghana Nutrition Improvement Project launched in 2009 is a social business that is designed to bring solutions to serious social problems in LMIC, such as malnutrition, through sustainable business activities. It does so with three goals in mind: the development of a new market, innovation—the project involves the manufacture and sale of the KOKO Plus, a complementary food supplement, which should be added to traditional porridge to mitigate the nutritional deficiency of the meal for a child, and setting up multi-sector partnerships with local government, academia, aid agencies, international organizations and businesses [25, 26].

Shifting the focus to foundations and initiatives' role as contributors of financial resources, Ajinomoto set up the Ajinomoto International Cooperation Network for Nutrition and Health (AIN) program in 1999 and has a support program in the form of a grant program, which aims at improving food-, nutrition- and health-related outcomes in local communities in LMIC [27]. Through workshops, the program trains volunteers and other human resources to undertake health- and nutrition-friendly activities that are compatible with local food customs and cultures [27].

Another example refers to the Power of Nutrition, an independent fund that aims to mobilize one billion dollars to address undernutrition. The fund was launched in April 2015, and the first $200 million will be provided by carefully selected partners including the Children's Investment Fund Foundation (CIFF), UBS Optimus Foundation, the UK's Department for International Development (DFID), UNICEF and the World Bank Group (WBG). In fact, contributions include $55 m from CIFF, up to £32 m ($47 m) from the DFID, and up to Swiss Francs 25 m ($26 m) from the UBS Optimus Foundation. The fund accepts donations and grants from a mix of private and public investors and has developed an innovative matching offer that guarantees that every dollar in private funding is multiplied up to six times with new financing secured from other funders. The fund also mobilizes resources toward governments from LMIC who seek financial support for their national nutrition programs [28, 29].

With regard to in-kind contributions, Britannia Nutrition Foundation (BNF) founded in 2009 to fight against malnutrition among underprivileged children works toward reducing child malnutrition among India's most vulnerable and underprivileged populations by raising awareness about malnutrition [16]. BNF also delivers awareness-building initiatives that aim to address the lack of knowledge on malnutrition. During the annual national nutrition week, BNF organizes a symposium, which serves as a tool for creating a space and platform for action. A variety of stakeholders from different fields attend the event such as economists, speakers who work in social development, nutrition and medicine, as well as key opinion leaders [30].

Public Health Advocacy

Public health advocacy can be defined as the activity of overcoming substantial structural barriers to public health objectives [31]. It is not primarily oriented at changing the knowledge, attitudes or behaviors of individuals, but rather the legislative, fiscal, physical and social environments in which individual knowledge, attitude and behavior change can take place [31]. One of the main challenges in public health nutrition is the lack of political will and commitment. Advocacy tools that clearly communicate the issue, using evidence-based content and stories and infographics that translate the urgency of addressing the problem, as well as tools which communicate programmatic and policy solutions can help convince decision makers and key stakeholders about the need to take action. Numerous private initiatives and foundations are increasingly engaging, coordinating and strengthening efforts at local, national and international level, to raise awareness about health and adequate

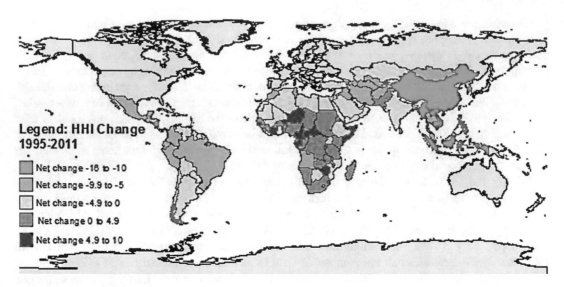

Fig. 35.1 Global map presenting net change in Hidden Hunger Index (HHI) scores, 1995–2011. This figure illustrates the magnitude of change in HHI between 1995 and 2011. It shows that the top performers were largely from East and South Asia, and most of the worst performers were African countries [32]

nutrition among the public and policy makers. As the following section will demonstrate, one way this has been done is through the development of advocacy tools.

One example specifically related to nutrition refers to the Hidden Hunger Index (HHI). The HHI was developed in consultation with academics and decision makers from a range of global institutions, including UN agencies, academia, US government agencies and international NGOs and is an example of how to translate scientific findings to a visual graphic that calls for policy makers to take action [32]. *Sight and Life* foundation (a nutrition think tank primarily supported by DSM) developed maps and indices of global hidden hunger, which reveal the burden of micronutrient deficiencies and how they contribute to the disease burden (see Fig. 35.1). The HHI is a useful tool for the SUN countries to set priorities and monitor progress [32]. The existing global political will to put nutrition on the health agenda and the acknowledgement of seeing nutrition as a fundamental determinant to the achievement of the MDGs and their successors, the Sustainable Development Goals (SDGs), has been manifested by the increasing support for the SUN Movement. More importantly, SUN's main stakeholders, that are national governments themselves, require tools that will allow them to make evidence-based budget and policy decisions [32]. The HHI provides valuable information for policy makers to help them prioritize interventions, as well as beneficial information for public health programmers as a basis for action, and the monitoring and evaluation of programs. In fact, by revealing where the burden of micronutrient deficiencies are and their contribution to disease, the index enables the development of appropriate interventions, such as multiple micronutrient supplementation for pregnant women, home fortification with micronutrient powders for preschool-age children, and food fortification for the general population, which can effectively target those populations most affected by micronutrient deficiencies, and therefore acts as powerful advocacy tool to reduce the burden of hidden hunger [32].

The SUN movement launched in 2010 works through four different country-level networks (Civil Society, Donor, UN System and Business), in a collective effort to see a world without hunger and malnutrition. In order to do so, these networks support their respective national governments by participating in multi-stakeholder platforms and they ensure alignment and coherence between their national strategies and activities [33]. The SUN Business Network, convened by WFP and GAIN, is comprised of large national companies and multi-nationals who are committed to support governments' efforts to scale up nutrition. It aims to mobilize and intensify efforts from the business community in support of the SUN Movement [34]. To do this, the network has produced a number of resources that include: a Guide to Business Engagement aimed at country stakeholders to help inform the development of local strategies to engage business in local nutrition plans; a toolkit of best practice for nutrition in the workforce which builds the case for investing in nutrition workplace programs through nutrition policies including maternity protection and breastfeeding support for instance; a toolkit for implementing policies and interventions to support lactation in the workplace [35]. In celebration of the World's Breastfeeding Week in 2015 which focused on women and work, the UN Foundation organized a webinar with the private sector and the global development community, focused on supporting innovations that enable working women to breastfeed. The company Philips was inspired by the significant potential breastfeeding has to save children's lives and, as a result, made a commitment to Every Woman Every Child in 2014 that pledged, among other elements, to research and support breastfeeding practices for women in Africa [36]. As a follow-up of the webinar, 29 SUN Business Network members have committed to putting good nutrition at the center of business practice. By June 2016, these businesses will support breastfeeding mothers and improve policies for maternal health [36]. Moreover, the SUN Business Network provides advice to SUN country policymakers and it supports governments' efforts to scale up nutrition through its global advocacy activities, through high-level outreach events during the World Economic Forum (WEF), the UN General Assembly and the SUN Global Gathering, and played a coordinating role for business in the Second International Conference on Nutrition (ICN2) [34]. As a result of this platform, SUN countries are increasingly developing plans to engage business in national plans. In 2015, the SUN Business Network assisted eleven countries to set up national business networks whose aim is to identify the areas where stakeholders and businesses can support current national nutrition strategies in being more open to the role that the private sector and other stakeholders can play as a crucial partner to scale up nutrition. Furthermore, 29 countries have asked for further support from the SUN Business Network and the Movement to engage better with business to scale up nutrition. Globally, there are 164 companies committing to scaling up nutrition, of which 44 are multi-national companies with global commitments which will be tracked through the Global Nutrition Report and 122 are companies that have pledged to develop commitments at national level [37, 38]. By being the only global platform for businesses commitments to scaling up nutrition and which tracks business commitments annually, the SUN Business Network has served as a powerful advocacy platform that enables and promotes further collaboration between business and other actors to scale up nutrition at all levels. The network also serves as a platform for businesses to express their commitment in taking part in this process.

Often there is a deficit of qualified personnel, suitable infrastructure or effective planning and management skills in LMIC. The following examples demonstrate how private foundations address this gap. The Nestlé Foundation for the Study of Problems of Nutrition in the World was founded in 1966 by a donation from the Nestlé company on the occasion of its 100th anniversary. The foundation is financially and operationally independent of the company since its inception. It is self-constituting and is managed by a council consisting of at least 5 internationally well-established scientists. The foundation initiates and supports research capabilities in human nutrition with public health relevance in LMIC [39]. One of the foundation's main objectives is the transfer of scientific and technological knowledge to target countries. In fact, at least 75% of the budget of the foundation's sponsored research projects in collaboration with scientists at universities and research institutes in high-income countries must be earmarked for use within LMIC. Additionally, financial support is provided for higher education and for research projects by faculty in the early stage of their careers and who are yet to prove their capabilities [40].

Another example refers to the Sir Dorabji Tata Trust (SDTT), which supports a variety of causes, individuals and institutions in a wide array of areas. Its partnership with the Madsen's Institute for Tribal and Rural Advancement (MITRA) is a strategic alliance for malaria control and community health in south Orissa (India) for building institutional capacity. This partnership has led to establishment of a malaria resource center that provides technical assistance to NGOs in south Orissa (India) for them to carry out community-based malaria control programs using the Mal-Mal approach [41, 42]. This approach rests on the discovery that reduction of malaria prevalence can lead to improvements in nutritional status at the community and individual level. In fact, data show that the 16 districts of Orissa listed as having high malaria prevalence are also known for their high burden of malnutrition, suggesting that there could potentially be correlation and causal pathway whereby chronic or recurrent malaria is a cause for malnutrition and that anything done to prevent and treat malaria may also positively impact nutrition status. The screening and treatment of malaria could hence decrease both malaria and malnutrition at the same time [42]. Mal-Mal camps for children were offered in MITRA's project villages in the peak transmission months, where children with malaria were detected with malaria parasitaemia and treated with effective treatment embedded within a regular growth-monitoring program. An annual round of Mal-Mal camps has been conducted by MITRA in 50 villages since 2010. Based on a review of 74 nutritionally at-risk children who received the MITRA protocol in 2009, data from the regular MITRA growth-monitoring program during the first year of the Mal-Mal approach showed that throughout the year, the number of children losing weight halved while those gaining weight significantly increased [42]. This is a good example that reveals that in some cases, processes need to be docile and flexible to enhance and create an enabling environment that will make space for the desired public health outcomes. Corporate foundations, such as the Tata Trust in this case, can play a key role in facilitating this process by supporting program activities and financial management through its employees and seed funding, which in turn enables and facilitates the establishment and setup of facilities (such as the malaria resource center) which can provide critical inputs to strategic thinking and developing new approaches such as the Mal-Mal approach. Most importantly, the success of such approaches can be leveraged and/or scaled up and used as the scientific evidence needed to promote policies, methods and new perspectives on how to improve nutrition outcomes [42].

Driving Innovation and Novel Approaches

Private foundations and initiatives are drivers of innovation, which can respond to and address the health and nutrition challenges faced by vulnerable populations in LMIC in a variety of ways. Foundations' financial and operational independence makes them agile which is required to promote and advance innovation, allowing them to take risks that governments and traditional donors may be reluctant to take, as well as to invest in long-term results-based projects [2]. Foundations also often refer to innovation to explain their work and their method to providing support and assistance. The Rockefeller Foundation has even celebrated its centenary with the slogan "Innovation for the next 100 years" [2]. Interestingly, foundations and initiatives' innovative approaches may have an impactful and significant effect on health and nutrition if the new ideas and approaches they develop are being taken over and scaled up by traditional donors or national governments once proven worthwhile, and also individuals, households and communities, including through the use of commercial channels. The role of foundations as innovators may imply support for the translation of current and new knowledge and ideas into new fields, the identification of new issues and challenges, or evaluating new approaches for addressing specific issues, for example via support for pilot projects as the following section will show [2]. With the help of a few examples, this section will explore several innovative pathways through which foundations and initiatives can have a positive impact on health and nutrition outcomes in LMIC, namely the discovery and development of novel approaches, innovation catalysts, open innovation activities and upcoming novel approaches.

Several foundations focus on innovation and include it as a criterion for selecting programs or projects for funding. One such example is Syngenta Foundation's Kilimo Salama program, which introduced insurance against drought, excess rain and field crop diseases such as blight or aflatoxin, and other potential risks for 187,000 smallholder farmers in Kenya and Rwanda between 2009 and 2013 [43]. The outcome of this program was that it made the farmers more confident in investing in better-quality inputs and to access agricultural loans. In fact, results showed that insured farmers invested 20% more in their farms and earned 16% more income than their uninsured neighbors [43]. *Sight and Life* has equally been active in promoting and delivering innovative thinking and solutions. In the Kenyan refugee camp Kakuma, the WFP and *Sight and Life* in collaboration with Johns Hopkins School of Public Health researched the potential barriers to micronutrient powder (MNP) use. The findings of this study were published in the report entitled "A Qualitative Study Examining Low Micronutrient Powder Uptake at Kakuma Refugee Camp," which identified different ways to improve the multiple micronutrient powders' (MNPs) distribution program [44]. A recommendation was made "to improve upon the existing [...] box and sachet material." Indeed, while the existing MixMe™ sachets are well designed to protect the MNP from degradation under difficult environmental conditions, as well as humidity, light and temperature thanks to its layers of PET, composite aluminum and polyethylene foil; the same protective packaging attributes are not environmentally friendly as the sachets cannot be recycled, repurposed, burned, biodegraded or composted [45]. To this end, and as part of the global movement to implement environmentally sensitive activities, *Sight and Life* addressed this issue by launching an open innovation challenge in 2012, which welcomed more sustainable packaging concepts for MNPs, while fulfilling cost-per-unit requirements and maintaining product stability under harsh conditions. The three winners' ideas proved to be innovative and efficacious concepts [45]. As a follow-up, a "double sack" economical packaging for MNPs is currently undergoing stability assessment.

As governments and local bodies do not always have the resources to test out innovative solutions, private foundations can serve as helpful innovation catalysts through the greater freedom they have in taking risks and in considering long-term programs [46]. The Novartis' foundation symposium in 2014 was on the theme of "sustainable healthcare interventions: from blueprint to lasting impact" which resulted in a rich exchange of experiences and ideas on developing innovative healthcare solutions, and further commitment for the foundation's role as a catalyst to try out innovative healthcare solutions and then convince governments to expand them [47]. The Novartis Foundation pioneers the blueprint of the solution, validates it and gets it going. For instance, the foundation piloted and is accelerating the novel use of mobile phones to improve access to primary healthcare through training and healthcare consultations in remote communities in Ghana by overcoming geographical barriers through information and communication technologies. This project also set up a teleconsultation center to provide structured decision-making assistance to health workers in rural areas and adapted this to the existing mobile health platform, which utilizes text messages to provide vital health information of patients from a mobile phone to a database [47]. Despite the positive impact that telehealth systems may have on patients' health, they also present risks to the security and privacy of patients' health information. The main privacy risk is that of a lack of control over the collection, use and sharing of data [48]. For instance, home telehealth devices may collect and transmit information on activities in the household that a patient does not wish to reveal, such as substance abuse. Smartphone apps may also share data on location to third parties. Security risks involve unauthorized access to data during collection, transmission or storage. Despite the efforts that are being made to create as safe as possible apps and devices, many still contain significant flaws giving malware and hackers opportunities to threaten the security of telehealth systems. Systems' security must significantly improve to prevent mal-intending individuals from accessing and misusing information, and regulations need to be put in place to provide secure and strong risk and privacy protections for patients and users [48].

Pharmaceutical companies, for instance, are increasingly sharing financing, intellectual property and expertise, a phenomenon known as "open innovation." In fact, "in contrast to classic closed innovation, whereby an enterprise generates, develops, and brings to market its own ideas, in the new open innovation model, an enterprise utilizes in-house ideas as well as those of its network partners and seeks ways to bring products and services to market by deploying multiple pathways" [49 (p. 2)]. Although the era of open innovation has begun for many firms, we still lack a clear understanding of the mechanisms, inside and outside of the organization, i.e., when and how to fully profit from the concept [50]. Similarly, to encourage innovation in targeting neglected diseases in LMIC and in order to foster new ways of thinking and approaches on how research is done, GlaxoSmithKline (GSK) has launched an open innovation strategy with the aim of promoting change beyond GSK by sharing resources, know-how, intellectual property and expertise with the global scientific and research community. GSK's specialist Research & Development (R&D) facility at Tres Cantos in Madrid offers laboratory space to external scientists and academics that are also targeting diseases that LMIC suffer from. The Tres Cantos Open Lab Foundation was established by GSK to support new external scientists coming into the laboratory, and all projects supported by the foundation must add to research that helps discover and develop new medicines for diseases in LMIC. Although the facility currently solely focuses on diseases in LMIC, GSK has started to adapt open innovation models to apply to other areas of medical challenge such as rare diseases [51].

With regard to upcoming novel approaches, one emerging area in public health to explore and that has been successful in other areas such as education and recidivism is the concept of a social development bond or a social investment bond (SIB) for innovative financing of health and nutrition programs. According to the Center for American Progress, a SIB or "Pay for Success" contract connects private investment with nonprofit service providers and governments to produce improved social outcomes that generate government savings. Reliable performance measures are required to evaluate whether the program is effective [52]. A bond-issuing organization enters into a contract with the government to provide social services. It then issues the bonds to private investors who will receive principal repayment and a return on their investment from performance-based payments if the benchmarks are achieved. The investors provide the working capital to this SIB issuing organization, which in turn funds the NGO service providers [50]. The government only makes payment to the bond-issuing organization if and when social or environmental performance targets have been met. If the interventions fail, investors lose some or all of their investment. One of the key challenges of SIBs is to identify interventions with sufficiently high net benefits that would ensure that investors earn their desired rates of return. The Rockefeller Foundation has been an early leader of the ecosystem of SIBs since 2009, when the foundation made a grant to Social Finance UK who launched the first-ever SIB aimed at lowering recidivism rates at Peterborough Prison. The Ministry of Justice and the Big Lottery Fund ensured the private investors received their required financial return [53]. Other first social impact bonds showed encouraging results, and three programs that focused on education and teenagers were deemed a success. Not only did the children's literacy skills and school attendance improve, but investors were also able to make return on their investments. SIBs are also being tested in the USA and other high-income countries as a more cost-efficient method to solve social problems [52]. Over the last three years, the Rockefeller Foundation has helped to set up the SIB ecosystem in the USA by providing support in a variety of ways such as planning grants to service providers and intermediaries; funding research focusing on social applications, political trajectories, the investor landscape; and supporting governors' and mayors' offices to increase their capacities to execute bonds [53].

A version of SIBs, called "Development Impact Bonds" (DIBs), aims to help tackle complex social issues in LMICs. Perhaps one of the best known is the Global Alliance for Vaccines and Immunization (GAVI). Through its partner body, the International Finance Facility for Immunization, GAVI has raised more than $5 billion from private investors, including Vodafone, JP Morgan, la

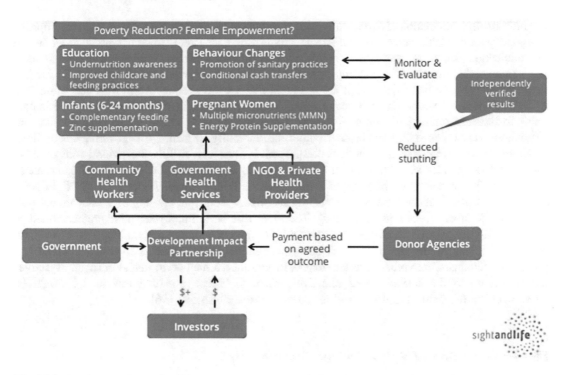

Fig. 35.2 Development impact bond for stunting prevention. This figure portrays the different methods a DIB structure can use to address the current issues in the nutrition environment, whereby the Development Impact Partnership (DIP) holds investments and contracts with investors, outcome funders, service providers and donor agencies. An array of relationships are enhanced among the DIP, the donor agencies and partner governments, and payments for a range of effective interventions to prevent stunting are channeled through the DIP. According to the attained outcomes, the donors pay investors including a return through the DIP. Adapted from [55]

Caixa Foundation [54]. Several country donors including the USA, as well as the Gates Foundation, have committed over $6.3 billion to repay these private investors if programs prove successful [54].

Early in 2014, the Center for Global Development convened a workshop with experts in nutrition and innovative financing to explore DIBs in nutrition [55]. This expert team further described how DIB is one possible approach to solve three key challenges in addressing malnutrition (see Fig. 35.2). Firstly, although donors have committed at the 2013 Nutrition for Growth summit to spend more than 4 billion USD through 2020, there is still a significant shortage of more than 5 billion USD that is required to scale up access to ten nutrition interventions in 34 focus countries [55]. A DIB can thus leverage the support of new investors to contribute to this funding gap. Secondly, where there is evidence on effective interventions, there is a looming chasm between the science on the one hand and the knowledge on how to get products and services where they are most needed on the other hand [55]. Because private investors, who have fewer terms and processes, with quicker decision making, finance a DIB, there is more flexibility to adapt dynamically to the changing context in the field than there would be under traditional government contracts. Thirdly, the multi-sectoral nature of nutrition requires the coordination of many actors that are fragmented and may also be competitive. A DIB provides a platform for coordination for public, private and nonprofit stakeholders with clear roles for each of them and a precise focus on agreeable outcomes. Finally, since success is linked to investor financial returns, tracking and monitoring of data becomes vital and could help the nutrition community build a stronger evidence base for a variety of interventions [55].

Traditionally, foundations have been active in activities along the value chain that can improve access to public health goods for vulnerable groups such as R&D, low-cost production, health communication, social marketing and advocacy, and distribution channels. Foundations are most likely to be early adopters of social impact bonds or DIBs as it provides a collaborative mechanism for public–private partnerships, which are scarce in the nutrition sector. Moreover, according to a study conducted by Social Finance, many foundations are attracted by the ability of social impact bonds to increase funding for the social sector with a focus on outcomes rather than outputs and surprisingly, as a lever to improve broader public accountability by leading the governments to direct resources to most effective interventions [53]. Further, this area fulfills the natural role of most foundations as an "idea shop" that take the risk of proving a concept before government can scale it. Although DIBs for development have yet to be tested, the UBS Optimus Foundation, CIFF, Educate Girls and Instiglio launched the first Development Impact Bond pilot to improve educational outcomes in Rajasthan (India) in June 2014. The DIB will be a three-year pilot project aimed at addressing high dropout rates and poor education [56]. The UBS Optimus Foundation explained that, in addition to improving the lives of children, the foundation's interest is to test the model and potentially demonstrate to other investors that DIBs could be a method to invest in social objectives and contribute to the scaling up of effective programs. It is hoped that this model would be extrapolated to the field of nutrition and health once proven effective [56].

The Proliferation of Public Private Partnerships

The latter half of the 1990s witnessed a growing number of initiatives involving collaboration between the public and corporate sectors with the aim of overcoming public and market "failures" of international public health, using global public–private partnerships (PPPs) to revolutionize development and global health [1]. More recently, these partnerships have expanded to the nutrition sector, with an increasing number of PPPs that aim to address the double burden of malnutrition. Although PPPs in nutrition are still being perfected, PPPs can play a critical role in tackling malnutrition, increasing the chance of survival and the possibility of healthier and more productive communities and nations. This section will look at some of the successes of private foundations and initiatives in this field.

Some of the areas in which the public sector readily welcomes partnerships with the private sector are areas in public health infrastructure, logistics and education. The Abbott Fund and the Government of Tanzania formed one such successful PPP for over 10 years to strengthen the country's healthcare system [57]. Key improvements included modernizing Muhimbili National Hospital, building new laboratories at 23 regional-level hospitals and supporting more than 20,000 healthcare worker trainings in HIV care and treatment. An independent evaluation conducted by the government found that approximately one in three people receiving HIV treatment were cared for at one of more than 90 sites that were established as a result of this partnership [57].

Sight and Life's association with WFP started prior to the PPP between WFP and DSM in early 2006, when it supported WFP's Indian Ocean Tsunami relief operations. At the invitation of *Sight and Life*, WFP came to Switzerland to discuss with DSM their activities in feeding the hungry of the world. This topic generated enormous interest [58]. WFP and DSM have partnered since 2007 with the aim to develop sustainable and cost-effective, nutritious food solutions for the hungry poor. The partnership was strengthened and extended in 2013 for another three years during which it enabled WFP to double the number of people reached with improved nutrition, from 15 to 25–30 million annually by 2015 [59]. In December 2015, this partnership was renewed for three more years [60]. As one of WFP's Global efforts and seek to reach twice as many people who benefit from improved nutrition, DSM combines scientific and technical expertise in the area of high-nutrient products and financial seed support to help improve the nutritional value of the WFP food distributions to the most vulnerable [60]. Importantly, the partnership has leveraged the company's decades of technical expertise to improve the quality of WFP food supplies through tailor-made and innovative food fortification interventions, which WFP continues to purchase from a range of suppliers through competitive tendering [59]. *Sight and Life* plays a unique role in providing scientific scrutiny to the partnership and allows the partnership to advocate its impact and accelerate the nutrition agenda forward [59].

Another illustration yet different in its approach relates to the Global Alliance for Vaccines and Immunization's (GAVI) newest PPP, namely the GAVI Matching Fund, which is supported by the Bill & Melinda Gates Foundation and by the British Government through DFID. By 2015, every donation to GAVI through the Matching Fund by the private sector partner, its customers, employees and business partners is matched either by the Bill & Melinda Gates Foundation or by the British Government (in the case of UK companies' donations). Together, the Bill & Melinda Gates Foundation and DFID have pledged approximately $130 million to match these donations. Through the GAVI Matching Fund, GAVI raised US$210 million for the 2011–2015 period [61]. The Fund has been extended into the 2016–2020 period with a US$75 million funding from the Bill & Melinda Gates Foundation, 10 million Euros from the Dutch Government and a further US$76 million from the Government of Japan in May 2016 [61, 62]. This will enable GAVI to deliver additional life-saving vaccines to LMIC. The totality of funds goes to GAVI for immunization programs in the poorest countries [63].

Recently, India has witnessed an increase in the number of PPPs in several sectors predominantly in infrastructure. There are no PPPs in nutrition, and the public sector investment is very low despite an alarming malnutrition situation and dismal state of state-spending on nutrition. In fact, less than 1.5% of state development expenditure and less than 2.5% of the total revenue expenditure of the states is incurred on nutrition [64]. In a recent qualitative research study conducted in India to explore and identify barriers to private investment in the nutrition space (see Fig. 35.3), one of the major barriers identified for the absence of PPPs in public health nutrition is the lack of transparency and trust among the stakeholders, notably between the private and public sectors [64]. This mistrust was generated because many civil society and government actors have experienced private sector behavior that has undermined public policy and public health agendas. Private sector foundations that are better connected to the area of public health than other divisions within corporations can play a critical role in understanding the needs of the public sector and can act as a facilitator between the sectors. Foundations are able to build a common vocabulary with the public sector and thus have the opportunity to build trust toward a PPP.

Project Laser Beam, the five-year multi-million dollar PPP to find new solutions to persisting problems in the area of undernutrition, was launched in 2009 by the WFP, Unilever, GAIN, Mondelez International Foundation and DSM. Over the five-year partnership, the project implemented 18 interventions, with approximately 1.74 million new beneficiaries (i.e., new to nutrition support) in Bangladesh and Indonesia. The project also uncovered crucial lessons that can help accelerate progress in tackling undernutrition using a cross-sectoral approach, one essential learning being that "implementing a decentralized consensus-driven operating model" that is "managed by a neutral external third party" is crucial to operate efficiently as described below [65]. This neutral external third party was Accenture Development Partnerships: A business unit within Accenture that provides technology and business services to the international development sector, on a nonprofit basis. WFP was the only partner who initially managed and coordinated the partnership and also implemented nutrition interventions. This put additional workload and burden on a single partner. As a result of this imbalance, a decentralized operating model was developed to manage Project Laser Beam. A secretariat was hosted by Accenture Development Partnerships (the external third party), who provided global program and partnership management for the project. The team supported new partner engagements, designed and supported the implementation governance structure, supported

The Existing landscape			
There are existing models of successful public private partnerships in nutrition in India.	◔	◑	○
These successful models have had impact at a local level.	◔	◑	○
It is very important in the present context to have public private partnerships specific to nutrition in India	◑	◕	◔
Transparency is key to building a successful PPP in nutrition	●	●	●
Shared goals, partner equity and accountability are the other major attributes of building a successful partnership in the nutrition	●	●	◕
Barriers to and benefits of Private Sector involvement			
Lack of trust among stakeholders is the primary barrier to building a successful PPP in nutrition in India	◕	◕	◑
Conflict of interest, lack of standards and regulations for private sector engagement are the other barriers	◔	◕	◕
Services in the nutrition are more welcome than making products for a successful PPP	●	●	●
Improving coverage of beneficiaries, logistics and manpower deployment are the major areas in which private sector can contribute to a PPP in nutrition in India	◕	●	◑
Way Forward : Central and State Governments openness to Private Sector			
There will be considerable changes in policy making by the central government to encourage more PPPs in nutrition	◕	○	◔
Maharashtra is the most promising state in terms of its policies to welcome PPPs in Nutrition	◑	●	◕
Madhya Pradesh and Bihar governments have high potential in engaging with private sector for public health nutrition	◔	◕	◑
Potential Private Sector Involvement in different verticals in Nutrition			
Governance and co ordination	○	○	○
Science and Strategy	◔	◔	◑
Operationalizing programs	○	○	○
Monitoring and Evaluation	●	◕	◑
Media and Nutrition Education	◕	●	●
Legend: _Strongly Disagree_ ○ ——→ ● _Strongly Agree_			

Fig. 35.3 Key findings on barriers to PPP in nutrition. This figure depicts the key findings resulting from a study aimed at identifying barriers to PPPs in nutrition in India. Stakeholders from the private and public sector (government), and civil society (non-governmental organizations and institutions that manifest interests and will of citizens) involved in the nutrition sector were interviewed, and results revealed that the major barriers are related to trust between the public and private sector and the lack of government guidelines to engage the private sector. Monitoring and evaluation scored high because of private sector's prevalent practice of using technology for analytics in supply chain, gaining consumer insights and for communicating with consumers [64]

GAIN in developing the monitoring and evaluation frameworks, coordinated activities undertaken by the secretariat, facilitated as a neutral body, partnership engagements at global and national levels, and developed the approach for the Project Laser Beam country operating models and the secretariat. By focusing on each partner's core competency, Accenture Development Partnerships enabled them to use their strengths and manage their designated interventions. In fact, the burden of a single partner having to coordinate the partnership was relieved, and transparency across the partnership was improved [66].

Similarly, the ATNI, that provides a framework to monitor the world's 25 largest food and beverage manufacturers on their nutrition-related commitments, recommends companies to increase their efforts to address malnutrition beyond philanthropy. ATNI suggests that companies that are expanding their footprint in lower-income countries, in consultation with local stakeholders and in alignment with national efforts, leverage the experience, skills and scale of their core business functions to implement PPPs so as to make their products more accessible and culturally appropriate for lower-income consumers at risk of or suffering from malnutrition [67].

Standards for Private Sector Involvement

As seen throughout the chapter, there are numerous ways through which private initiatives and foundations can positively contribute to health and nutrition outcomes. And as new ways of collaborations (e.g., PPPs) are being welcomed and show their effectiveness when they are framed in a context of trust and transparency, the debate around whether or not and to what extent the private sector should be involved in areas that have intrinsically been under the jurisdiction of the public sector remains very relevant. In fact, ultimately, businesses' primary concern is to create value for their shareholders and investors and likewise, it is evident that those who donate money have a set of priorities that are of interest to them in making such donations [15]. When this imperative is not aligned with advancing public health, conflicts of interest come to surface. Therefore, the range of activities pursued by businesses can have both positive and negative outcomes for nutrition and health [7].

One common example refers to Medecins Sans Frontieres (Doctors Without Borders, MSF) which, although strategically engaged with the Gates Foundation, is one of the few major global health actors not accepting Gates funding. MSF believes that its financial independence from the foundation enables it to voice criticism or concerns on specific issues over which the foundation has enormous influence [68]. The 10-year multi-billion dollar "Global Vaccines Action Plan" adopted in May 2012, largely funded by the Gates Foundation, was heavily criticized by MSF who found it too focused on new vaccines, thereby neglecting the fundamental need to improve basic public health and immunization programs in LMIC. MSF hoped to draw attention to this issue ahead of the 2012 World Health Assembly [7]. Moreover, a study published in 2011 investigating the scope of potential conflicts of interests that exist among several private foundations that are major funders of global health, had observed that the Bill and Melinda Gates Foundation had substantial holdings in the Coca-Cola Corporation, and had also participated in grants that encouraged communities in LMIC to become business affiliates of Coca-Cola [15]. Such findings underline the importance of having regulated environments when engaging with private sector foundations and initiatives especially when we know that sugary drinks such as those produced by Coca-Cola are strongly associated with obesity and diabetes in LMIC [15].

Such issues have helped the world to think about the need for global guidelines and precautions that would mitigate if not prevent these competing interests from having negative repercussions on global health. It is essential to improve private foundations and initiatives' transparency and accountability for nutrition and health outcomes. Nevertheless, ensuring accountability in nutrition and health can be a challenging task for numerous reasons, one of them being that in order for commitments and actions to be monitored within these cross-sectoral domains, leaders from different sectors (e.g., education, agriculture and health) need to work in a coordinated and coherent way at all levels [69]. Another obstacle for driving accountability is the lack of trust across key stakeholder groups in donor organizations, government, civil society and business.

With regard to nutrition, the nutrition community has developed various tools, frameworks and organizational approaches to advance accountability and transparency. Some of these mechanisms are currently being used by private foundations and initiatives in particular. They are for example used by the SUN Movement, the ATNI described earlier in this chapter, the Hunger and Nutrition Commitment Index (HANCI) which compares and ranks LMICs whose undernutrition and hunger status is alarming or severe, and the 2015 Global Nutrition Report which laid out the issues of lack of transparency, trust and quality commitments between key stakeholders, and added a section dedicated to the private sector, proposing a set of recommendations to advance accountability and trust across the nutrition landscape. Approaches and tools such as the SBN, ATNI and HANCI serve as essential building blocks for further learning and improvement in the first years of the SDGs [69]. Shifting the focus to the global level and private foundations and initiatives more specifically, in 1999, more than 20 years after the adoption of the original Sullivan Principles, United Nations Secretary General Kofi Annan unveiled the new "Global Sullivan Principles" according to which some companies have developed their own corporate social responsible guidelines, while other NGOs work toward the development of international standards such as the International Organization for Standardization (ISO) of which ISO 26000 specifically relates to social responsibility and is designed to provide guidance on how business and organizations can operate in an ethical and transparent way that contributes to the welfare and health of a society [70]. There is also the Council on Foundations, a national (US-based) nonprofit association of more than 1700 grant-making foundations and corporations. As the leading advocate for philanthropy, the council strives to increase the effectiveness, stewardship and accountability of this sector while providing its members with the services and support they need to reach the common objectives [71]. A few strategies have been identified as a way to mitigate the potential conflict of interests in private foundations to negatively impact global health decision making. A first method is referred to as "divestment" whereby private foundations are strongly discouraged to invest in companies that stand to profit from the tax-exempt foundation's agenda or in companies that produce products that have well-established correlations with public health outcomes such as sweet foods, sugary drinks and tobacco [15]. More transparency suggests that private foundations and initiatives should adopt full disclosure, or transparency, and ensure that all individuals on foundation boards recuse themselves from decisions related to their affiliate companies. And last but not least, it is crucial to align community needs with aid. Despite having made many declarations to do so, private foundations tend to work in "silos" and prioritize a set of issues that their founder or governing director decides is a priority. Foundation program portfolios and investment should be in line with the priorities and needs of the intended beneficiaries of its support [15].

Conclusion

It was the aim of this chapter to give an overview of how private foundations and initiatives can significantly and positively contribute to long-term investments in health and nutrition outcomes in LMIC by leveraging companies' knowledge and resource networks. As was shown throughout this chapter, this impact can manifest itself through the provision of goods and financial and in-kind contributions by foundations and initiatives toward various projects and programs, through the advance in advocacy tools, through a variety of innovations such as the development of novel approaches, open innovations and catalytic roles, and finally through the proliferation of PPPs, which have the potential for mobilizing resources, tapping into the development and delivery capacity of the private sector and scaling up nutrition interventions quickly and efficiently along many other benefits.

Worthwhile to mention is that collaboration is essential to the success and sustainability of a foundation's efforts—engaging with diverse partners in the private, public and nonprofit sectors is essential to foster innovation at a global, national and local level. Nevertheless, as was mentioned in the previous section, in order for corporate foundations' role to be further strengthened and improved in the public health ecosystem in the future, conflicts of interest must be mitigated and addressed [15]. Transparency and accountability are key elements that encourage this process, and efforts must be made across all sectors to acknowledge the interests of all stakeholder groups, namely civil society, government, donor organizations and the private sector [69]. Foundations can also work toward more trust and accountability by adopting reporting mechanisms where the social impact of investment (and not solely coverage of beneficiaries) is measured. Independent audits can also regularly measure the scope and management of conflicts of interest with private foundations, and a widely shared and monitored public health code of ethics could provide guidance to mitigate conflicts of interest [9]. Other measures include setting up organizational structures that are independent from their parent company, building inclusive partnerships with government, not-for-profit organizations and companies operating in LMIC with common goals and values, and striving for transparency by divestment and alignment of foundation investments with community needs. It is hoped that foundations and initiatives will continue to strive for sustainability and develop new and adaptable models, which can be scaled up effectively to speed up progress where it is most needed.

Discussion Points

- How are private sector products linked to development?
- Describe how global standards for philanthropy strengthen additional support from the private sector.
- How would you approach a development project that would be soliciting funds from a corporation? Can you describe a product or program that a corporation would be interested in supporting its development and why?
- Analyze the role that private foundations have had with leveraging national and international support for a nutrition program.

Acknowledgments The authors would like to thank Rahul Dutta for his collaboration and qualitative research on public private partnerships in public health nutrition in India. We also appreciate Svenia Sayer-Ruehmann's creative support for the figures in this chapter.

References

1. International Trade Forum. New developments in philanthropy: how private foundations are changing international development. http://www.tradeforum.org/New-Developments-in-Philanthropy-How-Private-Foundations-are-Changing-International-Development/. Accessed 2 Apr 2015.
2. Lundsgaarde E, Funk E, Kopyra A, Richter J, Steinfeldt H. Private foundations and development cooperation—insights from Tanzania. Bonn: DIE; 2012. http://www.die-gdi.de/uploads/media/Studies_69.pdf. Accessed 3 Apr 2015.
3. Davies P. The role of the private sector in the context of aid effectiveness. OECD; 2011.
4. Andrews FE. Philanthropic foundations. 1st ed. New York: Russel Sage Foundation; 1956.
5. Moran M. Private foundations and development partnerships. London: Routledge; 2014.
6. Gates Foundation. Annual report 2014 [Internet]. Bill & Melinda Gates Foundation, 2015 [cited 18 Oct 2015]. Available from: http://www.gatesfoundation.org/Who-We-Are/Resources-and-Media/Annual-Reports/Annual-Report-2014.

7. International Food Policy Research Institute. Global nutrition report 2015: actions and accountability to advance nutrition and sustainable development. Washington, DC: International Food Policy Research Institute; 2015.

8. McCoy D, Kembhavi G, Patel J, Luintel A. The Bill & Melinda Gates Foundation's grant-making programme for global health. Lancet. 2009;373(9675):1645–53.

9. Stuckler D, Basu S, McKee M. Global health philanthropy and institutional relationships: how should conflicts of interest be addressed? PLoS Med. 2011;8(4):e1001020.

10. Aggregate Fiscal Data of Corporate Foundations in the US, 2013. [cited 4 Jan 2016]. Available from: http://data.foundationcenter.org/#/foundations/corporate/nationwide/total/list/2013.

11. WBCSD. Delivering results: moving towards scale. WBCSD; 2010.

12. WHO. Private enterprise for public health opportunities for business to improve women's and children's health. A short guide for companies. Geneva: The Partnership for Maternal and Newborn Child Health, WHO; 2012. http://www.who.int/pmnch/topics/part_publications/private_enterprise_for_public_health_guide.pdf. Accessed 2 Apr 2015.

13. Investopedia. Intrapreneur. http://www.investopedia.com/terms/i/intrapreneur.asp. Accessed 6 Apr 2015.

14. Buse K, Walt G. Global public–private partnerships: part I—a new development in health? Bull World Health Organ. 2000;78(4).

15. Porter ME, Kramer MR. Creating shared value. Harvard Bus Rev. 2011;89(1/2):62–77. https://hbr.org/2011/01/the-big-idea-creating-shared-value. Accessed 2 Apr 2015.

16. Britannia.co.in. Company Overview|Britannia Industries Limited—Official Website [Internet]. 2015 [cited 7 Oct 2015]. Available from: http://britannia.co.in/about-us/overview.

17. Hystra. Marketing nutrition for the base of the pyramid. Introducing successful practices for improved access to nutritious complementary foods: key lessons from case studies [Internet]. Paris: Hystra; 2014. Available from: http://www.gainhealth.org/wp-content/uploads/2015/02/Marketing-Nutrition-for-Base-of-Pyramid-report.pdf.

18. GAIN. Shaping markets to combat undernutrition [Internet]. Geneva: GAIN; 2011. Available from: http://www.gainhealth.org/wp-content/uploads/2014/04/54.-Shaping-Markets-to-Combat-Undernutrition.pdf.

19. Britannia. Britannia fortifies biscuits to improve public health. http://sharedvalue.org/examples/tiger-micronutrient-fortified-biscuits. Accessed 3 Apr 2015.

20. Unilever. Engaging with stakeholders [Internet]. Unilever global company website. 2015 [cited 7 Oct 2015]. Available from: https://www.unilever.com/sustainable-living/the-sustainable-living-plan/our-approach-to-reporting/engaging-with-stakeholders/.

21. Unilever. Global partnerships [Internet]. Unilever global company website. 2015 [cited 7 Oct 2015]. Available from: https://www.unilever.com/sustainable-living/transformational-change/global-partnerships/.

22. Unilever. Health and hygiene [Internet]. Unilever global company website. 2015 [cited 7 Oct 2015]. Available from: https://www.unilever.com/sustainable-living/the-sustainable-living-plan/improving-health-and-well-being/health-and-hygiene/.

23. Unilever. PSI: saving lives through hand washing with soap and clean drinking water [Internet]. Unilever global company website. 2015 [cited 7 Oct 2015]. Available from: https://www.unilever.com/sustainable-living/transformational-change/global-partnerships/psi-saving-lives-through-handwashing-with-soap-and-clean-drinking-water/.

24. Unilever. Unilever Lifebuoy campaign achieves dramatic results. http://www.unilever.com/mediacentre/pressreleases/2014/unileverlifebuoycam. Accessed 3 Apr 2015.

25. Ajinomoto. About Us|Ajinomoto Group [Internet]. Ajinomoto.com. 2015 [cited 7 Oct 2015]. Available from: http://www.ajinomoto.com/en/aboutus/?scid=av_ot_pc_comehead_aboutus.

26. Ohara A. Case study: Ajinomoto Co.: better nutrition, brighter future in Ghana. Business call to action, 2013? Accessed 4 Apr 2015.

27. Ajinomoto. The Ajinomoto International Cooperation Network for Nutrition and Health (AIN) program. https://www.ajinomoto.com/en/activity/csr/ain/ainkoubo.html. Accessed 4 Apr 2015.

28. World Bank. New fund targets billion dollars for children's nutrition [Internet]. 2015 [cited 12 Oct 2015]. Available from: http://www.worldbank.org/en/news/press-release/2015/04/16/new-fund-targets-billion-dollars.

29. The Power of Nutrition. Guaranteeing that investments are matched 4-6x [Internet]. The power of nutrition. 2015 [cited 12 Oct 2015]. Available from: http://www.powerofnutrition.org/how-we-work/.

30. Dasra. Inclusive India Awards. Dasra; 2012. Accessed 4 Apr 2015.

31. Chapman S, Lupton D. The flight for public health. London: British Medical Journal Publishing; 1994.

32. Ruel-Bergeron J, Stevens G, Sugimoto J, Roos F, Ezzati M, Black R, et al. Global update and trends of hidden hunger, 1995–2011: the hidden hunger index. PLoS One. 2015;10(12).

33. SUN Business Network. About|Sun Business Network [Internet]. Sunbusinessnetwork.org. 2015 [cited 19 Oct 2015]. Available from: http://sunbusinessnetwork.org/about/.

34. Scaling Up Nutrition. Business Network [Internet]. Scaling up nutrition. 2014 [cited 19 Oct 2015]. Available from: http://scalingupnutrition.org/the-sun-network/business-network.

35. SUN Business Network. Resources|Sun Business Network [Internet]. Sunbusinessnetwork.org. 2015 [cited 19 Oct 2015]. Available from: http://sunbusinessnetwork.org/resources/.

36. SUN Business Network. Breastfeeding women and work: how can business make it work? Sun Business Network [Internet]. Sunbusinessnetwork.org. 2015 [cited 19 Oct 2015]. Available from: http://sunbusinessnetwork.org/news-items/breastfeeding-women-and-work-how-can-business-make-it-work/.

37. SUN Business Network. SUN Business Network Company Commitments|Sun Business Network [Internet]. Sunbusinessnetwork.org. 2015 [cited 19 Oct 2015]. Available from: http://scalingupnutrition.org/the-sun-network/business-network.

38. SUN Business Network. SUN Business Network Company Commitments|Sun Business Network [Internet]. Sunbusinessnetwork.org. 2015 [cited 19 Oct 2015]. Available from: http://sunbusinessnetwork.org/sun-resources/sbn-company-list/.

39. Nestle Foundation. About the Foundation. http://www.nestlefoundation.org/e/about.html. Accessed 3 Apr 2015.

40. Nestle Foundation. Guidelines for grant applications to the Nestle Foundation [Internet]. 1st ed. Lausanne: Nestle Foundation; 2015 [cited 7 Oct 2015]. Available from:http://www.nestlefoundation.org/e/docs/Guidelines_for_Grant_application_FINAL_20081006.pdf   http://www.cof.org/sites/default/files/documents/files/CorporateGuide.pdf.

41. Chacko P. Health and a lot more—the Mitra programmes being supported by the Sir Dorabji Tata Trust and the Allied Trusts are a rare bright spot in a blighted region rife with inequities and disparities [Internet]. Tata. 2011 [cited 7 Oct 2015]. Available from: http://www.tata.com/ourcommitment/articlesinside/3DeulgYpo1E=/TLYVr3YPkMU.

42. Oommen J. Mal-Mal approach to malnutrition. http://infochangeindia.org/agenda/malnutrition/mal-mal-approach-to-malnutrition.html. Accessed 6 Apr 2015.

43. Syngenta Foundation for Sustainable Agriculture. "Kilimo Salama" becomes ACRE. http://www.syngentafoundation.org/index.cfm?pageID=562. Accessed 4 Apr 2015.

44. Kodish S, Gittelsohn JA. Qualitative study examining low micronutrient powder (MNP) uptake at Kakuma refugee camp, vol 42. Johns Hopkins Department of International Health, Bloomberg School of Public Health; 2011.

45. Perry MA. Partnership for more sustainable packaging inspires innovation challenge. Sight Life. 2013;27(2).

46. OECD. Philanthropic Foundations and Development Co-operation. Dev Assist Committee J. 2003;4(3). http://www.oecd.org/development/stats/22272860.pdf. Accessed 3 Apr 2015.

47. Novartis Foundation. Moving from innovation to lasting impact. http://www.novartisfoundation.org/news/more/922/moving-from-innovation-to-lasting-impact. Accessed 3 Apr 2015.

48. Hale T, Kvedar J. Privacy and security concerns in telehealth. AMA J Ethics. 2014;16(12):981–5.

49. Dandonoli P. Open innovation as a new paradigm for global collaborations in health. Globalization Health. 2013;9(41). http://www.globalizationandhealth.com/content/9/1/41. Accessed 3 Apr 2015.

50. Enkel E, Gassmann O, Chesbrough H. Open R&D and open innovation: exploring the phenomenon. R&D Manage. 2009;39(4):311–6.

51. GSK. Open innovation. http://www.gsk.com/en-gb/research/sharing-our-research/open-innovation/. Accessed 4 Apr 2015.

52. Liebman JB. Social impact bonds. A promising new financing model to accelerate social innovation and improve government performance. Washington, DC: Center for American Progress; 2011. https://cdn.americanprogress.org/wp-content/uploads/issues/2011/02/pdf/social_impact_bonds.pdf. Accessed 3 Apr 2015.

53. Hughes J, Scherer J. Foundations for social impact bonds how and why philanthropy is catalyzing the development of a new market [Internet]. Boston: Social Finance; 2014. Available from: http://www.socialfinanceus.org/sites/socialfinanceus.org/files/Foundation%20for%20Social%20Impact%20Bonds,%202014.pdf.

54. Bowden A. Innovating with development impact bonds [Internet]. Conscious Company Magazine; 2015 [cited 7 Oct 2015]. Available from: http://www.consciouscompanymagazine.com/blogs/press/18338685-innovating-with-development-impact-bonds.

55. Center for Global Development. Exploring development impact bonds in nutrition: workshop 24 Feb 2014 briefing note (2/18/14). CGD; 2014.

56. Perakis R. First development impact bond is launched [Internet]. Center for Global Development; 2014 [cited 7 Oct 2015]. Available from: http://www.cgdev.org/blog/first-development-impact-bond-launched.

57. Abbott Fund. Public-Private partnership for health care in Tanzania. http://www.abbottfund.org/project/17/83/Mentoring-for-Health-Care-in-Tanzania? Accessed 4 Apr 2015.

58. Sight and Life. Sight and Life annual report 2006: expanding strengths from 20 years of Sight and Life. Basel: Sight and Life; 2006.

59. Bahl K, Jayaram S, Brown B. DSM-WFP: a partnership to advance the global nutrition agenda. Washington, DC: Results for Development Institute; 2014.

60. DSM. A brighter future for people most at risk [Internet]. DSM; 2016 [cited 5 Jan 2016]. Available from: http://www.dsm.com/corporate/sustainability/nutrition-challenge/partnerships/world-food-programme.html.

61. Gavi Alliance. The GAVI Matching Fund [Internet]. GAVI Alliance; 2016 [cited 14 June 2016]. Available from: http://www.gavi.org/funding/matching-fund/.
62. Gavi Alliance. Gavi welcomes contribution of US$76 million from Government of Japan [Internet]. GAVI Alliance; 2016 [cited 14 June 2016]. Available from: http://www.gavi.org/library/news/statements/2016/gavi-welcomes-contribution-of-usd-76-million-from-government-of-japan/.
63. GAVI Alliance. The GAVI Matching Fund. A public-private partnership to save children's lives. GAVI Alliance; 2013.
64. Dutta R. Public private partnerships in nutrition—perspectives from India. Presented at the Micronutrient Forum. Addis Ababa; 2014.
65. WFP, Unilever, Mondelez International, DSM, GAIN. Project laser beam: lesson from a five-year, global public-private partnership addressing child undernutrition. Final conclusion. Project laser beam. 2014.
66. Accenture. Project laser beam—partnership to reduce child under nutrition—accenture [Internet]. Accenture.com. 2015 [cited 12 Oct 2015]. Available from: https://www.accenture.com/us-en/success-project-laser-beam-reduce-child-under-nutrition.aspx.
67. Access to Nutrition Index. 2013. http://www.accesstonutrition.org/. Accessed 9 Apr 2015.
68. Doctors Without Borders. Do you take money from the Gates Foundation? [Internet]. MSF USA; 2014 [cited 7 Oct 2015]. Available from: http://www.doctorswithoutborders.org/news-stories/newsletter/do-you-take-money-gates-foundation.
69. Sight and Life. Goodbye MDGs Hello SDGs [Internet]. Sight Life Magazine; 2015 [cited 5 Jan 2016]; 29(2):42–8. Available from: http://www.sightandlife.org/fileadmin/data/Magazine/2015/29_2_2015/Sight_and_Life_Magazine_29_2_2015.pdf.
70. International Organization for Standardization. ISO 26000—social responsibility—ISO [Internet]. Iso.org. 2015 [cited 6 Oct 2015]. Available from: http://www.iso.org/iso/home/standards/iso26000.htm.
71. Council on Foundations. Increasing impact, enhancing value: a practitioner's guide to leading corporate philanthropy [Internet]. Arlington: Council on Foundations; 2012. Available from: http://www.cof.org/sites/default/files/documents/files/CorporateGuide.pdf.

Part VIII
Ethics—Critical to Making Progress in Public Health

Chapter 36
Ethics in Public Health Research

Tanya Doherty and Mickey Chopra

Keywords International research collaborations · Research ethics · Informed consent · Confidentiality · Standards of care

Learning Objectives

- To understand the basic ethical principles relevant to research involving human participants and to apply them to real-world ethical dilemmas in health research.
- To be informed about international guidance documents on research ethics.
- To stimulate thinking and discussion of ethical issues by (future) researchers particularly those involved with international collaborative studies through use of case studies.
- For students and researchers to become more familiar with a range of real-world dilemmas and debates in international health research, especially in low- and middle-income countries.

Introduction

Scientific research has produced substantial social benefits. It has also posed some troubling ethical questions. During the last century, there have been a number of notorious cases in which participants have been harmed as a consequence of unethical clinical research. Public attention was drawn to these issues by reported abuses of human subjects in biomedical experiments, especially during the Second World War. During the Nuremberg War Crime Trials, the Nuremberg code [1] was drafted as a set of standards for judging physicians and scientists who had conducted biomedical experiments on concentration camp prisoners. The central feature of the Nuremberg Code was the protection of the integrity of the person participating in research. The Nuremberg Code was endorsed by the World Medical Association (WMA) which published the Declaration of Helsinki [2] in 1964. The

T. Doherty (✉)
Health Systems Research Unit, South African Medical Research Council, Francie van Zijl Drive,
Parow, Cape Town, South Africa
e-mail: Tanya.doherty@mrc.ac.za

M. Chopra
World Bank, Washington, DC, USA
e-mail: mchopra@worldbank.org

© Springer Science+Business Media New York 2017
S. de Pee et al. (eds.), *Nutrition and Health in a Developing World*,
Nutrition and Health, DOI 10.1007/978-3-319-43739-2_36

Declaration, which has been amended nine times, sets out the principles to be observed in research on human participants and has become the cornerstone of research related to health care. The principles in the Declaration of Helsinki have been incorporated into many of the forms of guidance that have subsequently been drawn up to govern the conduct of research related to health care.

The objective of ethical guidance is to provide an ethical framework: A set of principles that allows us to evaluate the actions and policies of individuals and bodies such as international organizations, academic institutions and government agencies. These principles seek to identify the considerations that should apply to individuals and agencies when making decisions or adopting policies. They constitute a framework for articulating the duties, obligations, claims and expectations of those involved in research related to health care.

During the last few decades, there has been a significant increase in the number of international collaborative health research studies involving high-income country (HIC) sponsors and scientists and low and middle-income country (LMIC) institutions and subjects. The inherent inequality of the relationship between these two groups of actors has drawn attention to the ethics of research sponsored (or conducted) by groups in HIC but carried out in LMIC. A major question that has arisen concerns whether it is appropriate to apply the same set of ethical standards and procedures that are used for studies in HIC, to studies conducted in LMIC settings, where the cultural and social context may be different.

In light of the increase in collaborative research, some institutions have developed ethical guidelines that are aimed specifically at international collaborative research. The Council for International Organisations of Medical Sciences (CIOMS), in collaboration with WHO, recognized the special circumstances which arise when applying the Declaration of Helsinki to research undertaken in LMIC settings and proposed guidelines to address them in 1982 [3]. These guidelines sought to direct the conduct of research involving human participants in a way that would recognize the social, economic, legal, regulatory and administrative arrangements that exist in LMICs. In the USA, the ethical issues which arise when clinical research sponsored by the USA is undertaken in LMIC settings were given detailed consideration in the US National Bioethics Advisory Commissions (NBAC) report entitled: Ethical and policy issues in international research: clinical trials in developing countries [4]. The NBAC report emphasizes the ethical and logistical problems that arise where research related to health care in LMIC settings is externally sponsored. It is clear that the development of an adequate system of ethical review and oversight is a necessary condition of a defensible practice of international collaborative research in the decades ahead.

The aim of this chapter is to generate awareness and openness of discussion that may engage researchers from HICs and LMICs in an effort to increase understanding and promote guidelines that acknowledge both similarities and differences. The topics covered represent a wide range of ethical issues in public health research.

Basic Ethical Principles

The expression "basic ethical principles" refers to those general judgments that serve as a basic justification for the many particular ethical prescriptions and evaluations of human actions. Three basic principles are particularly relevant to the ethics of research involving human participants: the principles of respect of persons, beneficence and justice.

Respect for Persons

Respect for persons incorporates at least two ethical convictions: first, that individuals should be treated as autonomous agents, and second, that persons with diminished autonomy are entitled to protection.

An autonomous person is an individual capable of deliberation about personal goals and of acting under the direction of such deliberation. To respect autonomy is to take other people's interests into account, to support a sense of self-respect and self-worth and to encourage individuals to develop and express their capacities. To show lack of respect for an autonomous agent is to use individuals as a means either to our own ends or to the welfare of others, to increase risk of illness or death or to misinform.

However, not every human being is capable of self-determination. The capacity for self-determination matures during an individual's life, and some individuals lose this capacity wholly or in part because of illness, mental disability or circumstances that severely restrict liberty. Respect for the immature and the incapacitated may require protecting them as they mature or while they are incapacitated.

Some persons are in need of extensive protection, even to the point of excluding them from activities which may harm them; other persons require little protection beyond making sure they undertake activities freely and with awareness of possible adverse consequence. The extent of protection afforded should depend upon the risk of harm and the likelihood of benefit. The judgment that an individual lacks autonomy should be periodically re-evaluated and will vary in different situations.

In most cases of research involving human participants, respect for persons demands that individuals enter into research voluntarily and with adequate information. In some situations, however, application of the principle is not obvious. The involvement of prisoners as subjects of research provides an important example. On the one hand, it would seem that the principle of respect for persons requires that prisoners not be deprived of the opportunity to volunteer for research. On the other hand, under prison conditions they may be subtly coerced or unduly influenced to engage in research activities for which they would not otherwise volunteer. Respect for persons would then dictate that prisoners be protected. Whether to allow prisoners to "volunteer" or to "protect" them presents a dilemma. Respecting persons is often a matter of balancing competing claims urged by the principle of respect itself.

Beneficence

Persons are treated in an ethical manner not only by respecting their decisions and protecting them from harm, but also by making efforts to secure their well-being. The term "beneficence" is often understood to cover acts of kindness or charity that go beyond strict obligation. In this context, beneficence is understood in a stronger sense, as an obligation. Two general rules have been formulated as complementary expressions of beneficent actions in this sense: (1) do not harm and (2) maximize possible benefits and minimize possible harms. The problem posed by these imperatives is to decide when it is justifiable to seek certain benefits despite the risks involved and when the benefits should be foregone because of the risks.

The obligations of beneficence affect both individual investigators and society at large, because they extend both to particular research projects and to the entire enterprise of research. In the case of particular projects, investigators and members of their institutions are obliged to give forethought to the maximization of benefits and the reduction in risk that might occur from the research investigation. In the case of scientific research in general, members of the larger society are obliged to recognize the longer-term benefits and risks that may result from the improvement in knowledge and from the development of novel medical, psychotherapeutic and social procedures.

Justice

Who ought to receive the benefits of research and bear its burdens? This is a question of justice, in the sense of "fairness in distribution" or "what is deserved." An injustice occurs when some benefit to which a person is entitled is denied without good reason or when some burden is imposed unduly.

During the nineteenth and early twentieth centuries, the burdens of serving as research participants fell largely upon poor ward patients, while the benefits of improved medical care flowed primarily to private patients. Subsequently, the exploitation of unwilling prisoners as research subjects in Nazi concentration camps was condemned as a particularly blatant injustice. In the USA, in the 1940s, the Tuskegee syphilis study [5] used disadvantaged, rural black men to study the untreated course of a disease that was by no means confined to that population. These subjects were deprived of demonstrably effective treatment in order not to interrupt the study, long after such treatment became generally available.

Against this historical background, it can be seen how conceptions of justice are relevant to research involving human participants. For example, the selection of research participants needs to be scrutinized in order to determine whether some classes (e.g., welfare patients, particular racial and ethnic minorities, or persons confined to institutions) are being systematically selected simply because of their easy availability, their compromised position or their manipulability, rather than for reasons directly related to the problem being studied. Finally, whenever research leads to the development of therapeutic devices and procedures, justice demands both that these not provide advantages only to those who can afford them and that such research should not unduly involve persons from groups unlikely to be among the beneficiaries of subsequent applications of the research.

Application of Ethical Principles

The basic ethical principles described above should not be thought of as rules to be applied mechanistically. By their nature, they call for interpretation and exercise of judgment. Most importantly, they need to be applied within research settings. This leads to the consideration of the following requirements: informed consent, confidentiality, standards of care and responsibility to the study community.

These requirements, however, also need to take into consideration the special circumstances of research undertaken in LMIC settings and sponsored by HICs. Research ethics committees or institutional review boards to oversee public health research have been established in most LMICs over the past few decades, but these may be less well established, less supported financially and have different requirements than those in HICs [6, 7]. This leads to a danger that the conduct of research may fail to adequately protect participants from LMICs.

The basic bioethical principles may have different meanings in different settings, and foreign investigators and funders need to be sensitive to these different perspectives. Given the urgency of research on conditions such as HIV/AIDS, careful examination of both the interpretation of existing principles and the evolution of new guidelines is critical. This poses a challenge to researchers and ethicists from both donor and recipient organizations. The remainder of the chapter will focus on the ethical requirements for research with a focus on the challenges and key areas of uncertainty.

Informed Consent

Respect for persons has been described as a basic ethical principle. In research, this duty requires that we do not act against a person's wishes. His or her consent to participate in research must thus be obtained. When externally sponsored research is undertaken in LMICs, a range of issues arise in seeking consent to take part in research. With regard to informing potential participants, concepts that are common in research such as use of placebos or the idea of randomization may be unfamiliar to participants in the setting in which the research is being conducted. With regard to the voluntary nature of consent, it may be common in a particular context for a spouse or senior member of the family to make decisions regarding health care (and by extension, to research) for the whole family or household. In addition, access to better health care and other benefits that might be made available through participation in research may act as powerful inducements hampering the true voluntary nature of a participant's consent.

Informed consent implies that the researcher and participant have entered into a voluntary agreement without any element of coercion and that the participant is fully knowledgeable of the implications of participation. Consent, however, is only effective if a meaningful exchange of information takes place. If the obtaining of consent is largely ceremonial, or if the researcher merely pays lip service to the concept, then the autonomy of subjects is disregarded and the process does not offer adequate protection. Given that participation is the key to informed consent, it is necessary to ensure a proper climate for the communication process.

Communicating information about a choice and its implications can be difficult and time-consuming, but it allows valid, informed decisions. Widespread illiteracy is not a barrier to comprehension, especially since informed consent is more an interactive process than one that depends on reading. When appropriate, oral or pictorial depiction of concepts such as randomization could be used to improve understanding.

Ideally, each potential research subject should comprehend the nature of the investigation before providing valid informed consent. This information should be communicated and interpreted at an appropriate level of understanding so that it does not become overwhelming and senseless. The pre-recruitment counseling for research conducted on patients seeking medical care should include information explicitly emphasizing that non-participation in the research project will in no way compromise the care provided at the institution.

We should not rely solely on individual informed consent to educate people about studies, especially community trials. Baseline knowledge in the community should be enhanced by more open discussions of the topic in places like community meetings, because the more people understand the subject, the less anxious they are when given individual information as part of their invitation to participate. Moreover, the importance of community structures within many African societies should be acknowledged and a process of dual consent may give more legitimacy to a study than individual consent alone.

The following case study provides examples of how a process of community information can be combined with innovative methods of individual consent. The case is based on an article by Preziosi et al. [8].

Case Study 1

In the process of this study that aimed to evaluate a new pertussis vaccine in a rural community in Senegal, the researchers wanted to assess the incorporation of clear procedures for obtaining individual informed consent from parents. In this part of Senegal, consent for all previous research with human subjects had been obtained from community leaders on behalf of all eligible members of the community. Individuals could subsequently decline to participate.

At the start of the study, meetings were held by the field staff and physicians in each village to provide information and obtain consensus. All residents were invited. Presentations were given simultaneously in Sereer and French. Each presentation included a review of the activity of the research organization in the study area, information about vaccination and a description of the study. To illustrate the principle of randomization and the possibility that one of the vaccines might fail, the presenters used a familiar agricultural example: the evaluation of fertilizers or seed varieties on randomized plots, a procedure familiar to farmers in the area. After these meetings, the researchers began to inform the mothers further and to give them a distinct opportunity to refuse to participate. During one vaccination session, a pilot evaluation of the feasibility of obtaining individual oral informed consent was conducted. Subsequently, a physician fluent in Sereer routinely presented the information at each monthly vaccination session and recorded the mother's answers as witnessed by the vaccination nurse. From that point until the last vaccination in the study, the mother of each child eligible for inclusion in the vaccine study was asked whether she had been informed about it and if so how. If she had not, the study was explained to her and she could then decide whether or not to participate. Throughout the study, whole-cell DTP-poliovirus vaccine (which was the standard of care at the time) was available for the infants of mothers who declined to be included in the study or to have subsequent doses administered. The interventions were evaluated at the end of the study to determine the feasibility and validity of seeking individual informed consent.

Results of this evaluation showed that mothers were generally in agreement with vaccination and to the participation of their children in the study. Certain questions raised indicated their difficulty in understanding the concept of a double-blind study: They wanted to choose one of the vaccines for their children or at least to know which vaccine was given in order to be able to make their own judgments about both vaccines. In general, the results of this study indicate that the parents understood the study sufficiently to make informed choices. During the meetings, comments by community residents emphasized their understanding of the principles of the vaccine study after these principles were illustrated with better-known examples drawn from agriculture. The increased acceptance of vaccination overall suggested a positive effect of the information sessions held by the researchers.

The consent process described in the case provided each mother with an opportunity to make an individual choice for her child within the context of community consensus, which is consistent with the social organization of the community. To rely solely on communal consent for research is not widely accepted in ethical guidelines [3], and the use (or abuse) of cultural relativism to obviate the need for eliciting informed consent from individuals has been severely criticized [9]. In this situation, given the nature of the intervention (vaccination), individual informed consent was appropriate as a means to ensure autonomy and prevent exploitation of this society. The NBAC report [4] (recommendation 3.6) provides some guidelines as to the role of others in the consent process. It states: "*Where culture or custom requires that permission of a community representative be granted before researchers may approach potential research participants, researchers should be sensitive to such local requirements. However, in no case may permission from a community representative or council replace the requirement of a competent individual's voluntary informed consent.*"

In a cluster randomized trial of a participatory women's group intervention in Nepal [10], the researchers held a series of meetings with members of the District Development Committee, the Chief District Officer and local stakeholders to explain the aims and design (community randomization) of the trial. This was followed by meetings with the chairpersons of the 24 village development committees (unit of randomization) involved in the study who gave signed consent on behalf of their communities. Enrollment into the study was done by a team of field interviewers who visited homes within the selected villages, explained the study to eligible women and asked for individual consent to participate.

In the two examples given above, obtaining individual informed consent with community consensus was appropriate and served many benefits beyond the autonomy that it gave to the participants.

Confidentiality

Researchers are required to ensure that the information that they gather from participants is protected to prevent undue harm or negative consequences from participation in the research. This relates to the basic ethical principle of beneficence. This is particularly important where research is being carried out with vulnerable or identifiable population groups such as individuals with HIV/AIDS. Breaking of confidentiality is a risk to subjects which can cause people to become social outcasts, stigmatized and various other adverse social consequences. These risks are different depending on the subject under study and feelings surrounding this in the particular culture or society.

Maintaining the confidentiality of information obtained from health research poses unique challenges to researchers especially where they may uncover practices during the conduct of field work that may be substandard or even place patients at risk. The following case raises issues regarding the maintenance of confidentiality in a research study involving a vulnerable participant group.

Case Study 2

Background

To determine the level of vertical HIV transmission, a local non-governmental research group in Uganda designs a study that uses a prospective cohort study design to follow HIV-positive women from late pregnancy until their infants reach one year. The study will cover ten villages in an area where government prevention of mother-to-child HIV transmission (PMTCT) services are provided through the district hospital, some rural hospitals and a few primary healthcare centers.

Recruitment Methods

The study team proposes to set up a recruitment system which will use two main sources to find HIV-positive pregnant women: (1) community-based health workers and women's groups and (2) health workers who are providing PMTCT services.

All health providers who provide PMTCT services and who agree to be part of the recruitment process will be given an instruction sheet explaining the purpose and methods of the study. They will discuss the study with women who test HIV positive during antenatal VCT and obtain their consent to be interviewed at home by the research team. Health providers will give the researchers the names of those who agree to participate but will not provide a list of those who refuse to be interviewed. Information sources within the community will be asked to serve as intermediaries to schedule an interview between the researchers and the consenting women.

As some of the women may have changed their mind about being interviewed after their original consent, a second layer of protection from unwanted attention is afforded to the women by adopting the following measures: (1) during the interview, attention will be focused on the pregnancy and the health of the infant rather than issues related to HIV and (2) artificial privacy will be created during the interview by using a "team" of interviewers where one person conducts the actual interview, while the other members of the team engage family members in dummy interviews. Women will be free to discontinue the interview at any time without prejudice.

Deliberations of the Ethical Review Committee

The study is presented to the ethical review committee of the international funder following its approval by the local ethical review board. All but one member of the ethical review committee, an anthropologist who has worked extensively in Uganda, approve the study. She is concerned that there is some chance that the confidentiality of the women may be compromised and wants assurances that the records that identify the research subjects will be kept confidential. The study group responds that all records will be kept under lock and key in the main offices of the NGO, which is nowhere near the study site.

In the case described above, the researchers used a variety of individuals to recruit participants into the study including healthcare workers and community workers. This may have threatened the confidentiality of the participants as it is not clear whether the community workers were aware of the aims of the research or the HIV status of the women. The Declaration of Helsinki [2] addresses the issue of confidentiality in the following recommendation: *"The right of research subjects to safe-guard their integrity must always be respected. Every precaution should be taken to respect the privacy of the subject, the confidentiality of the patient's information and to minimize the impact of the study on the subject's physical and mental integrity and on the personality of the subject."*

There are many dilemmas that confront researchers in their attempts to uphold confidentiality. Public health research in particular often involves observational data collection within facilities. If during data collection a researcher uncovers a situation in a clinic where bad practice places patients at risks, he/she faces a dilemma. The researcher knows what they are seeing is wrong yet they have an ethical obligation to protect the confidentiality of the healthcare workers and the health center. Researchers often face role confusion between observing/reporting and implementing/taking action. In participatory/social science research, this role can be particularly unclear as researchers work closely with participants in a collaborative relationship. The main obligation of the researcher is to maintain the confidentiality of the participants/study sites, yet to what extent should this be upheld? Are there times when it would be appropriate to disclose information and how is that decision made? In all cases, the need to protect confidentiality needs to be balanced against the risk to individual patients.

Disclosing the names of health centers that have been involved in research, especially where poor practices/care has been observed, may have serious implications for the health workers who staff these centers. Their jobs may be threatened, and they may face criticism from the management. Yet, without knowing which the "problem" health centers are, would it be possible for the management to make the necessary changes to improve the quality of care? This is a complex dilemma, but one that researchers will increasingly be faced with as health systems research grows and the realities of service provision are brought to light.

Standards of Care

What standard of care to provide to participants in research has become an increasingly debated topic as more research is being conducted in LMICs. Should participants receive the best current treatment available anywhere in the world, or treatment based on an alternative standard of care which takes local circumstances into account? Where the best current treatment is inexpensive and simple to deliver, the answer is clear [11]. However, for many diseases and conditions, such a standard of care is routinely available to only a small proportion of the world's population and may be difficult to provide in LMICs.

This raises the question: What would be an ethically sound comparison group against which to compare a new treatment/intervention? If an established treatment exists for a condition, is there ever any justification to test a new treatment against a control group that receives no treatment? The following case highlights this dilemma.

Case Study 3

Since the early 1990s, several randomized controlled trials have evaluated the efficacy of perinatal ARV prophylaxis regimens for the PMTCT. The first of these, the PACTG 076 trial conducted in the USA and France, evaluated the efficacy of antenatal and intrapartum zidovudine to the mother and 6 weeks of postnatal zidovudine to infants versus placebo. All mothers fed their infants formula milk. At 18 months, transmission was 7.6% in the zidovudine group and 22.6% in the placebo group. This was the first randomized controlled trial to prove the efficacy of an intervention to reduce the incidence of HIV infection in infants.

When the results of the PACTG 076 trial became available, a number of randomized placebo-controlled trials of ARVs to reduce MTCT were already underway in Africa and Thailand. In September 1997, a paper by Lurie and Wolfe [12] and an editorial by Angell [13] in the New England Journal of Medicine criticized placebo-controlled trials of short-course zidovudine given to HIV-infected pregnant women to prevent mother-to-child HIV transmission. The trials were designed to determine whether relatively affordable and more feasible shorter courses of zidovudine given to pregnant women in LMICs would reduce the risk of mother-to-child transmission. They were conducted in countries where conventional local antenatal care did not include antiretroviral treatment. The trial designs had been approved by ethics committees in the countries in which the trials were conducted. Research in which the control group would be provided with a placebo would be deemed unethical in HICs where antiretroviral treatment is available and the long-course zidovudine as assessed in PACTG 076 would be considered the standard of care.

The critics of the trials of a short course of treatment argued that it was unethical to give the control group a placebo when it had already been demonstrated that the longer courses reduced transmission of the virus. The CDC, NIH, UNAIDS and a wide range of individuals rejected this view for several reasons [14–17]. Firstly, the 076 regimen was a complex, expensive, three-phase regimen that would be difficult to implement in resource-poor settings; secondly, the 076 trial was undertaken in a non-breastfeeding population which is very different to the situation in African contexts where the majority of women breastfeed and other risk factors such as micronutrient deficiencies and sexually transmitted infections are more frequently present.

When deciding on an appropriate standard of care for a control group in a randomized trial, the context in which the research is to be conducted needs to be carefully evaluated. A suitable standard of care can only be defined in consultation with individuals working in the country and must be justified to local research ethics committees.

The NBAC report [4] refers to the provision of treatment for control groups. "*Researchers and sponsors should design clinical trials that provide members of any control group with an established effective treatment, whether or not such treatment is available in the host country. Any study that would not provide the control group with an established, effective treatment should include a justification for using an alternative design. Ethics review committees must assess the justification provided, including the risks to participants, and the overall ethical acceptability of the research design.*"

The issue of standards of care also arises with regard to preventive interventions, such as participants in a vaccine trial, and this has been hotly debated very recently in relation to Ebola vaccine trials. The unprecedented Ebola epidemic that occurred in West Africa in 2014–15 spurred the development of Ebola vaccine candidates, and difficult questions emerged about how to design clinical trials and who should be the first to get the vaccine. Many scientists said that with Ebola, it would not be ethical to use the standard procedure for testing a vaccine's efficacy: a randomized placebo-controlled trial, in which some trial subjects would be assigned to a control group that does not receive the actual vaccine [18]. Since animal experiments had suggested that Ebola vaccines could well offer protection, keeping them from health workers facing a disease as deadly as Ebola was considered by some to be unethical.

Some scientists proposed an alternative trial design known as stepped wedge, which takes advantage of the common reality that a large-scale study cannot give everyone the vaccine on the exact same date. Stepped-wedge trials compare the rates of infection in people already vaccinated with those who have yet to receive the vaccine. In this design, all participants will receive the vaccine by the end of the study. The pharmaceutical company argued against this approach as it would take longer to complete a stepped-wedge trial than a standard RCT and the analysis would be more complex. They proposed using an "active control," a proven vaccine (for instance, against hepatitis B) that would at least protect participants against another virus. The ultimate decision taken was to proceed to an RCT with an active control once the phase I trials were complete as this design provided the fastest and most acceptable route to determine whether the vaccine was safe and effective.

These are complex questions that researchers have to face. The important principle to keep in mind when considering these issues is not to exploit those who are vulnerable. This can be achieved by providing the universal standard of care where possible, choosing an alternative trial design, or at least providing the same level of care that is available in the national public health system, and attempting to improve standards of care both during and after the research process, in particular through a comprehensive dissemination plan including recommendations based on the research findings, targeted at policy makers.

Responsibility to the Study Community After Completion of Research

Not all research will have results that can be translated directly into practice. However, research related to health care is usually designed to obtain results that will lead to an improvement in the prevention, diagnosis or treatment of a disease. One issue that arises when considering whether it is acceptable to undertake research in a LMIC setting is whether the intervention being studied is likely to be affordable in that country if shown to be effective. Researchers also need to consider whether it is appropriate to conduct research if the benefits of that research will not be made available to the community in which the research was undertaken.

The case below addresses the issue of researchers' responsibilities to study communities. Central questions to keep in mind while reading the case are: What benefits should be provided to the research participants, and by whom, after their participation in the trial has ended, and what, if anything, should be made available to others in the host community or country?

Case Study 4

Background Information

Vaccination against *Plasmodium falciparum* is the intervention with the greatest potential to reduce malaria-associated severe morbidity and mortality in areas with the most intense transmission. Infants and young children at risk of *P. falciparum* in Africa and non-immune travelers to areas endemic for *P. falciparum* and *Plasmodium vivax* represent the extremes of target groups in whom malaria vaccines would be useful.

So far, only one vaccine, a multistage synthetic peptide, has shown any evidence of protection. Phase I studies of this candidate vaccine in the USA have been encouraging: Immunization of human subjects shows evidence of a strong immune response. No safety studies have been performed in children under 6 months. Furthermore, no synthetic peptide vaccine has previously been given to this age group.

In order to progress in the critical path of vaccine development and testing toward the implementation of a new vaccine in malaria control programs, a multinational pharmaceutical company is in the process of designing a randomized double-blind placebo-controlled efficacy trial of the vaccine when given alongside the EPI scheme.

A country in East Africa where malaria is endemic has expressed interest in participating in the vaccine research effort, and their scientists and the pharmaceutical company investigators are collaborating on a study protocol to see whether the vaccine is effective in reducing deaths due to malaria in the under-5 population.

Site Selection and Recruitment

This study will be conducted in a town in the south of the country where there is intense year-round malaria transmission. The incidence of clinical malaria rises steeply after the first month of life, and the incidence in infants attending local health facilities for malaria and severe anemia, a common manifestation of malaria, is 0.7 and 0.6 episodes per child year, respectively. In this town, a district hospital provides curative health services and an active mother and child clinic (MCH) delivers routine childhood immunizations and offers a monthly weighing clinic. Malaria control efforts are based on prompt diagnosis and chloroquine treatment, although 60% of parasite strains in the area are resistant to chloroquine.

The researchers will recruit participants at the MCH clinic. Researchers will explain the trial to mothers, when they bring their children for their first immunization. After receiving written informed consent from the mother, a child will receive a first dose of SPf66 or placebo (aluminum hydroxide), when they present for the first EPI immunization at around one month of age. Second and third doses will be given at 2 and 7 months of age, respectively.

Parents will be advised to attend the clinic if their child experiences any health problems (such as fever or diarrhea). Children who develop malaria (as determined by both clinical findings and microscopy) will be treated in the district hospital according to national guidelines (chloroquine therapy). The study will look at cases of malaria as the main study endpoint.

A few months prior to the proposed start of the trial, the pharmaceutical company investigators visit the host country in order to meet with representatives from the Department of Health to finalize the research protocol. The representatives from the Department of Health request that if the vaccine is effective, all children in this country should benefit from the results of the study by receiving free doses of the vaccine for five years following the completion of the trial.

The researchers find this to be an extreme request. They explain that they have a limited budget for their research and they cannot afford to pay for the cost of vaccination coverage of the whole population of 45 million. They emphasize that they are currently conducting trials for other treatments aimed at the LMIC market, and it would be unfair to provide free treatment to one country and not to another.

The issue of benefits to study subjects on completion of a trial has become a complex debate among international researchers. Some have argued that interventions proven to be beneficial to participants during a study should be made available to them at the completion of the study [19]. Continued access to experimental medications is one way in which subjects may benefit from research participation. However, participation in research does not necessarily entitle subjects to continue receiving treatment, nor does it obligate investigators to provide continued treatment; to do so would be to blur the line between research and clinical care. Importantly, researchers should develop explicit dissemination strategies to inform participants and host communities of the results of the research results. Having participated in the research and assumed risks, the participants and host community have a right to know what was found and its implications for public health policy and practice.

If the vaccine company in the above case was unable to provide broad population benefits by making the vaccine available to the Ministry of Health free of charge on completion of the trial, are there other benefits they could provide such as upgrading of the district hospital to deal more effectively with malaria cases, or assisting with other control measures such as provision of bed nets?

The NBAC report [4] refers to the issue of post-trial benefits and recommends (4.1) that: "*Researchers and sponsors in clinical trials should make reasonable, good faith efforts before the initiation of a trial to secure, at its conclusion, continued access for all participants to needed experimental interventions that have been proven effective for the participants. Although the details of the arrangements will depend on a number of factors (including but not limited to the results of a trial), research protocols should typically describe the duration, extent, and financing of such continued access. When no arrangements have been negotiated, the researcher should justify to the ethics review committee why this is the case.*" The Declaration of Helsinki [2] offers a similar guideline. It states that: "*At the conclusion of a study, every patient entered into the study should be assured of access to the best proven prophylactic, diagnostic and therapeutic methods identified by the study.*"

It can be seen from the above guidelines that the ethical obligation to provide the intervention to others in the community who might benefit from it is considerably less strong, but a plan to do so would help reduce the risk of exploitation. The NBAC report [4] makes the following recommendation regarding post-trial benefits (recommendation 4.2): "*Research proposals submitted to ethics review committees should include an explanation of how new interventions that are proven to be effective from the research will become available to some or all of the host country population beyond the research participants themselves. Where applicable, the investigator should describe any pre-research negotiations among sponsors, host country officials, and other appropriate parties aimed at making such interventions available. In cases in which investigators do not believe that successful interventions will become available to the host country population, they should explain to the relevant ethics review committee(s) why the research is nonetheless responsive to the health needs of the country and presents a reasonable risk/benefit ratio.*"

Determining who should be responsible for providing post-research benefits to research participants and host communities or countries is an especially difficult problem.

Researchers or sponsors of research include a diverse set of individuals and entities, with different resources, roles and responsibilities in the research process. These differences will influence the nature of the obligations that each party should shoulder. A researcher's basic and generally accepted responsibility on completion of a study is one of advocacy by ensuring that the issue of access to effective interventions and other post-trial benefits is considered at each stage of the research process, especially the planning and design stages. This means discussing with relevant parties the potential for making effective interventions available and serving as an advocate, assuming that the trial results are positive.

The fundamental goal of public health research is to improve the health and quality of care provided to individuals and communities. Researchers should therefore discuss and develop plans prior to the undertaking of studies regarding the long-term benefit to participants and the wider community. Raising the quality of health care available to those in LMICs, given current inequities, cannot be achieved in the short term. However, through the conduct of research that is responsive to the needs of LMICs together with attempts to make these interventions affordable and accessible, we could move closer to this goal.

Ethical Review Processes

An effective system for the review of the ethics of research is a crucial safeguard for participants in research. The accepted method of ensuring that unethical research is prevented is through the establishment of a system in which research ethics committees undertake independent review of scientific protocols. It is important for ethics committees to be independent of government and sponsors of research. Furthermore, international collaborative research should be subject to review in both the country hosting the study and at the international collaborating partners' institution. The reality, however, is that ethics committees are often absent, under-resourced or ineffective in many LMICs.

There are three levels of assessment that should be considered for all research proposals:

- Relevance to priorities in health care within the country where the research is proposed to be conducted.
- Scientific validity.
- Ethical acceptability.

Although ethics committees are not constituted to take policy decisions on, for example, whether the findings of a research project could be implemented in the country, they should determine whether the implications of the research have been considered including the possibility of introducing to the wider community, treatment shown to be effective. In addition, they should request justification for research that does not include provisions for the development of expertise in research within the country where it is undertaken.

There is also a role for ethics committees to assess the scientific rigor of research. Ethical review mechanisms should ensure that the scientific design of the research realizes social value for the primary participants of the research and that the scientific design is appropriate for achieving the research objectives and is feasible within the social, political and cultural context. Research that is not appropriately designed will fail to provide answers to questions posed by the research and thus have limited or no benefit to participants or the wider community.

An ethics committee's primary task is to assess the ethical acceptability of research proposals with particular attention paid to the following: the predictable risks involved for participants, the anticipated benefits to participants, the provisions within the design relating to the care and protection of participants, the procedures for recruitment and selection, the processes for obtaining informed consent and provision for refusing consent and or withdrawing it during research and provisions for protecting the security and confidentiality of participant data.

The mere presence of an ethics committee is not enough to ensure that research will be adequately reviewed. Committees may be ineffective for a variety of reasons including a lack of financial and human resources, a lack of training in and experience with reviewing the ethics of research. Furthermore, if a committee has limited independence and no clear framework of guidance to work within, there is a danger that they take ad hoc rather than principled decisions.

For research ethics committees to function effectively, committee members must receive adequate training. As ethics committees often have a high turnover of staff, regular training programs are needed. A number of programs are being established to develop expertise in the field of medical ethics from organizations such as the National Institutes of Health (NIH) in the USA, the World Health Organization and the Wellcome Trust. International organizations need to continue to expand their programs for establishing, training and monitoring the development of research ethics committees.

Careful reflection by HIC scientists about the ethics of conducting research in developing countries is essential, but it must go hand in hand with true collaborative partnerships and the establishment of systems of review by researchers in the host countries. To encourage the development of ethical theory and practice in public health research in LMICs, local experts, medical and non-medical, must become more actively involved in screening research proposals and in studying examples where ethical dilemmas and conflicts are highlighted in order to draw on important lessons and to improve research practice.

Conclusions

Researchers, sponsors and others who are involved in research related to health care are often faced with diverse and sometimes conflicting guidance. It is important to consider all ethical questions in the context of an ethical framework that can provide a guide to use when determining how to apply guidelines. A major priority is the development of national ethical guidance and the strengthening of the process of ethical review of research, which will provide a further layer of protection to participants in research.

Discussion Points

- What are the common challenges in conducting international collaborative research and what mechanisms could be put in place to mitigate these?
- What role do ethical review processes play in international collaborative research studies? What are the functions of the local and international ethical review structures?
- What considerations should be taken into account when seeking informed consent for research undertaken in LMICs?
- What considerations should be taken into account when deciding on the standard of care to offer participants in a control group?
- What the responsibilities of a researcher and research sponsor on completion of a study?

References

1. The Nuremberg Code: Trials of War Criminals Before the Nuremberg Military Tribunals Under Control Council Law No. 10. Washington: US government printing office; 1949. p. 181–2.
2. World Medical Association. Declaration of Helsinki: ethical principles for medical research involving human subjects. Adopted 18th WMA General Assembly, Helsinki, Finland, June 1964. Amended 52nd WMA general assembly, Edinburgh, Scotland. France: Ferney-Voltaire; Oct 2000.
3. Council for International Organizations of Medical Sciences. International guidelines for ethical review of epidemiological studies. CIOMS; 1991.
4. National Bioethics Advisory Commission. Ethical and policy issues in international research: clinical trials in developing countries. NBAC; 2001.
5. Brandt AM. Racism and research: the case of the Tuskegee syphilis study: Hastings center report 8, no. 6; 1978.
6. Emanuel EJ, Wendler D, Killen J, Grady C. What makes clinical research in developing countries ethical? The benchmarks of ethical research. J Infect Dis. 2004;189(5):930–7.
7. Hyder AA, Wali SA, Khan AN, Teoh NB, Kass NE, Dawson L. Ethical review of health research: a perspective from developing country researchers. J Med Ethics. 2004;30(1):68–72.
8. Preziosi MP, Yam A, Ndiaye M, Simaga A, Simondon F, Wassilak SG. Practical experiences in obtaining informed consent for a vaccine trial in rural Africa. N Engl J Med. 1997;336(5):370–3.
9. Lurie P, Bishaw M, Chesney MA, Cooke M, Fernandes ME, Hearst N, et al. Ethical, behavioral, and social aspects of HIV vaccine trials in developing countries. JAMA. 1994;271(4):295–301.

10. Manandhar DS, Osrin D, Shrestha BP, Mesko N, Morrison J, Tumbahangphe KM, et al. Effect of a participatory intervention with women's groups on birth outcomes in Nepal: cluster-randomised controlled trial. Lancet. 2004;364(9438):970–9.

11. Nuffield Council on Bioethics. The ethics of research related to healthcare in developing countries. London: Nuffield Council on Bioethics; 2002.

12. Lurie P, Wolfe SM. Unethical trials of interventions to reduce perinatal transmission of the human immunodeficiency virus in developing countries. N Engl J Med. 1997;337(12):853–6.

13. Angell M. The ethics of clinical research in the Third World. N Engl J Med. 1997;337(12):847–9.

14. DeCock K, Shaffer N, Wiktor S, Simonds RS, Rogers M. Ethics of HIV trials. Lancet. 1997;350:1546–7.

15. Merson MH. Ethics of placebo-controlled trials of zidovudine to prevent perinatal transmission of HIV in the Third World. N Engl J Med. 1998;338:836.

16. Perinatal HIV Intervention Research in Developing Countries Workshop Participants. Science, ethics, and the future of research into maternal-infant transmission of HIV-1. Lancet 1999;353:832–835.

17. Varmus H, Satcher D. Ethical complexities of conducting research in developing countries. N Engl J Med. 1997;337:1003–5.

18. Cohen J, Kupferschmidt K. Ebola vaccine trials raise ethical issues. Science. 2014;346(6207):289–90.

19. National Bioethics Advisory Commission. When research is concluded—access to the benefits of research by participants, communities, and countries. In: Ethical and policy issues in international research: clinical trials in developing countries. Washington DC: US Government Printing Office; 2001.

Index

A

Accenture Development Partnerships, 783–785
Acceptable Range of Macronutrient Distribution (ARMD), definition, 587
Access to Nutrition Index (ATNI), 773
Acquired immune deficiency syndrome (AIDS), 414, 419–420
    advanced AIDS, 450
    End of AIDS, 668
    HIV wasting, 451
    United Nations Programme on (UNAIDS), 415
        combination prevention, 426
    WHO plan, Three by Five, 415
Acrodermatitis enteropathica, 273, 274
Activity-based costing ingredients (ABC-I) approach, 619
Adequate intake (AI), 161, 330, 587
    calculation for, 96
Adolescent Girls' Anaemia Control Programme, 569
Adolescents, 124, 126, 129–130, 559
    adolescent growth and nutritional status in relation to pregnancy, 565–567
    child marriage and adolescent pregnancy, 561
    delivery platforms, 571
        community- and health-based delivery platforms, 572
        school-based platforms, 571–572
        social safety nets or social protection programs, 572–573
    determinants of growth of, 564–565
    global data on adolescent nutrition, 562–563
    growth and development of, 564
    intervention strategies and delivery platforms, 567–568
    micronutrient deficiencies and anemia in low- and middle-income countries, 567
    nutrition-sensitive interventions, 570
        anthelmintic treatment, 570
        optimizing interval between pregnancies, 571
        postponing age at marriage and first pregnancy, 570–571
    nutrition-specific interventions, 568
        dietary intake, improving, 569–570
        iron and folic acid status, 568–569
    pregnant adolescents, nutrition of, 570
    unique lives and needs of, 560–561
    and youth, 560
Adult-onset diabetes, 150, 152, 154
Adult weight classifications, 97
African countries, nutrition capacity in, 73–74
African Nutrition Leadership Programme (ANLP), 80
Aga Khan Development Network (AKDN), 80
Agenda for Sustainable Development (2030), 367
Agriculture, urban, 718–719
Agriculture development programs, 604
Air displacement plethysmography (ADP) technology, 96
Ajinomoto Group, 775
Alma-Ata declaration, 625
Alpha(1)-acid glycoprotein (AGP), 105, 269
1 α-hydroxylation, 300
Alpha-linolenic acid (ALA), 322, 325, 330
American with Disabilities Act (ADA), 525
Amylase, 166–167
Anemia, 172, 176, 243, 569
    in adolescents, in low- and middle-income countries, 567
    assessment of, 241, 242
    control of, 252–256
    detection, by clinical examination, 243
    and HIV infection, 428
    in pregnancy, 477
    prevalence, 244
    small for gestational age and, 508
    and TB, 443
    as vitamin A deficiency disorder, 210–211
Anorexia nervosa, 470, 472
Anthelmintic treatment, in adolescents, 570
Anthropometric measures, 96, 124, 125, 126, 131
    for adults and aging, 96–98
    for birth outcomes and pregnancy, 98–99
    for children, 99–101
Anti-tuberculosis therapy (ATT), 438
Antioxidants, 475
Antiretroviral drugs (ARVs), 341, 371, 415, 416, 425
Antiretroviral therapy (ART), 341, 415, 423–424, 457, 459–460, 674, 675
Arachidonic acid (AA), 322, 326

© Springer Science+Business Media New York 2017
S. de Pee et al. (eds.), *Nutrition and Health in a Developing World*,
Nutrition and Health, DOI 10.1007/978-3-319-43739-2

Asian countries, nutrition capacity in, 74–75
Asthma, 198, 324
Attention deficit disorder (ADD), 542
Attention deficit/hyperactivity disorder (ADHD), 526,
    542
    feeding/nutritional problems, 542–543
    growth deviants, 543
Atwater, Wilbur Olin, 10
Autism, 526, 529. *See also* Autism spectrum disorders
    (ASDs)
Autism spectrum disorders (ASDs), 543
    feeding/nutritional problems, 543–544
    growth deviants, 544
    symptoms, 533
Average for gestational age (AGA) infants, 98
Avon Longitudinal Study of Parents and Children
    (ALSPAC), 541

B
Baby-Friendly Hospital Initiative (BFHI), 374, 375
Baby-friendly hospitals (BFHs), 374–375
Bacillus Calmette–Guerin (BCG) vaccine, 396, 397, 402,
    403, 405, 406
    historical perspective, 387
Balanced energy and protein (BEP) supplementation, 569
Balanced protein–energy (BPE) supplementation, 493,
    495
The Barker Hypothesis, 512
Bedaquiline, 404
Behavior change communications (BCC) strategy, 73,
    605, 614
Beneficence, ethical principles, 795
Benefit:cost analysis, 34
Benefit:cost ratios, nutrition interventions, 34, 41
Bennett's law, 741
Benoiston de Châteauneuf, Louis François, 7
Beriberi, 11–12, 14
β-apocarotenals, 182
Beta-carotene, 182, 541
    food sources, 187
Bifidobacteria, 350
Bilharzia. *See* Schistosomiasis
Biofortification, 171, 216–217, 280
Biomarkers, 105–107
    and dietary intake, 107
    and environmental factors, 105
    and obesity, 106
    proteomics, 106
    and time, 106
Bitot's spots, 208, 209, 211
Blegvad, Olaf, 16
Blinding, 50
Bloch, Carl, 16
Body mass index (BMI), 96–97, 99–100, 562, 563, 710
    in HIV, 461, 462
    measure of overweight and obesity, 144–145
    risk for TB and, 438, 439
Bovine TB, 392

Breast cancer, 479–480
    obesity, 479
    vitamin D supplementation and, 480
Breast milk substitute, 362, 372
Breastfeeding, 11, 35, 205, 208, 337, 338, 361, 459, 777.
    See also Human milk
    and 2030 Agenda for Sustainable Development, 367
    benefits
        for child, 339–340
        for mother, 340
    community and global issues affecting, 370–371
    definitions and recommendations, 361–362
    essential fatty acids in, 327
    and HIV transmission, 341, 429
    infant feeding after 12 months, 365
    and infant health, 363–364
    initiation, 365–366
    Kangaroo method, 366–367
    and maternal health, 364–365
    nutrient content of breast milk, 362–363
    promotion and support, 340–341
    protection, promotion and support, 371
        policies and guidelines, 372–374
        promotion programs, 374–376
    socioecological model and social determinants, 371
    suboptimal, 35, 37
    trends, 367
        global and regional trends, 367–370
    vitamin D deficiency, 299, 302, 304
Bretonneau, Pierre Fidèle, 9
Britannia Industries Limited, 774
Britannia Nutrition Foundation (BNF), 775
British Public Health Act (1848), 8
Buffalo milk, 339, 341

C
C-reactive protein (CRP), 105, 269
Cachexia
    in HIV, 454
    tuberculosis and, 440–441
Calcium, 538
    deficiency signs and symptoms, 103
    pregnancy and, 476
Calmette, Léon Charles Albert, 405
Candida albicans, 366
Capacity development, 67
    achieving international goals
        and targets, 68–69
    advocacy and leadership, 79–80
    approaches to develop
        individual capacity, 77
        institutional capacity, 81–82
        systemic capacity, 82
    assessing nutrition capacity, 70
        in African countries, 73–74
        in Asian countries, 74–75
        capacity for addressing obesity and
            non-communicable diseases, 75

global health workforce and capacity to deliver nutrition services, 70–72
multi-country nutrition initiatives, 72–73
building on what we know, 76
burden of malnutrition, 67–68
complex nexus of contributing factors, 68
curriculum and credentials for development needs, 78–79
defining, 69
innovative approaches to education and training, 80–81
levels of, 69
monitoring and evaluating, 82–84
new knowledge and skills to address post-2015 challenges, 77
new ways of working with other disciplines, 77–78
Caritat, Marie Jean Antoine Nicolas, 4
Carotenoids, 107, 182, 188
Casein proteins, 342, 349
Catechol-O-methyltransferase (COMT) gene, 533, 534
CD4 count, 424–425, 429, 455
CD4 receptor, 418
CD4+ T cells, 395, 400, 418
Centers for Disease Control and Prevention (CDC), 414
Cephalopelvic disproportion (CPD), 474
Cerebral palsy (CP), 525, 544
feeding/nutritional problems, 545
growth deviants or nutritional deficits, 545–546
Cervical cancer, 480
Chadwick, Edwin, 7, 7–8
Chapin, Charles, 10
Child growth
assessment, 119
importance of zinc for, 274
Child health, 127, 506, 508, 631
Child Health Days, 214
Child Health Epidemiology Reference Group (CHERG), 506
Child marriage and adolescent pregnancy, 561
Child mortality, 506, 548, 714
reduction of, vitamin A and, 16–18
Child nutrition
disparities in, urban and rural areas, 708–709
services, 73
zinc supplementation, 275
Children
anthropometric measures for, 99–101
HIV infection in, 429–430
preventive zinc supplementation in, 275–276
tuberculosis in, 443–444
Chinese city dynamics, 695
Cholera, 8, 9
Chromium, 104
deficiency signs and symptoms, 103
recommendations for
older men, 588
older women, 589
Chronic diseases, 516

in aging, 585
and diet and nutrition in LMICs, 585–586
non-transmissible disease epidemiology in low-income country, 585
relationship of chronic disease to diet and nutrition in LMICs, 585–586
Cities, nutrition analysis of, 688
consumption trends in cities, 690–691
global nutrition status, 688–689
global urban nutrition status, 689–690
City region food system, 700
Climate variability and agriculture, relationship between, 68
Cod liver oil, 16–17, 438
Cognitive function
economics of malnutrition and cognitive impairment, 34
iodine role in brain development, 290
Colostrum, 338, 362
Combination prevention, 425–426
Communities, 625
historical perspectives, 626, 627
access barriers, overcoming, 630
defining and monitoring quality of care, 632
health services, delivering, 630–632
home care and care seeking, educating for, 629–630
social norms and rights, promoting, 627–628
social support, providing, 632–634
shifting dynamics, 634
focus shifting from communities to individuals, 637–638
physical communities, changing dynamics of, 635–636
sustainable development goals (SDGs), 634–635
virtual communities, 636–637
supporting integrated health and nutrition, 639
cross-sectoral approaches, models of, 639–642
Community- and health-based delivery platforms, for adolescents, 572
Community-based management of acute malnutrition (CMAM), 631–632, 659
Community-driven quality, 632
Community health workers (CHWs), 629–630
history of, 633–634
Competency-based training and education, 78
Complementary feeding, 173, 206, 362
Conditional cash transfer (CCT) programs, 572–573
Condorcet, Marquis de, 4
Confidentiality, ethics in public health research, 799–800
Contagion, origins of concept, 8–9
Contagionist theory, 8
Convention on the Rights of Persons with Disabilities (CRPD), 548
Convention on the Rights of the Child (CRC), 547
Convergence model, 387
Copper deficiency, 278

signs and symptoms, 103
Copy number variants (CNVs), 532
Corporate social responsibility (CSR), 772
Cost–benefit analysis, 35–36
Cost-effectiveness, 34, 36, 606
Cost-effectiveness analysis, nutrition interventions,
    41–43
Council for International Organisations of Medical
    Sciences (CIOMS), 794
Counterfactual, 612
Cow's milk, 341–342
    and linear growth, 344–345
    malnutrition, 348–349
    pregnant and lactating women, 348
    SAM and MAM
        in prevention and treatment of, 345–347
        use of cow's milk ingredients in foods for, 351
    school milk programs for prevention of
        undernutrition, 348
Cretinism, 290
Cross-sectoral approaches, models of, 639–642
Curriculum and credentials for development needs,
    78–79
CYP27B1 mRNA, 300
Cytochromes, function, 236

D

Dairy ingredients, recommended use of, 351
    cost-effectiveness of milk content, 352–353
Dairy products, 312
D'Alembert, Jean le Rond, 4
Declaration of Helsinki, 794, 800, 804
7-Dehydrocholesterol, 299
Delamanid, 404
Demographic dividend, 560
Demographic Health Surveys (DHS) surveys, 145
Demographic transition, 585
Development Impact Bonds (DIBs), 780–781
Developmental disabilities (DDs), 523
    attention deficit/hyperactivity disorder (ADHD), 542
        feeding/nutritional problems, 542–543
        growth deviants, 543
    autism spectrum disorders (ASDs), 543
        feeding/nutritional problems, 543–544
        growth deviants, 544
    cerebral palsy (CP), 544
        feeding/nutritional problems, 545
        growth deviants or nutritional deficits, 545–546
    definition, 524–526
    Down syndrome (DS) or trisomy 21, 546
        growth deviants, 546
    epidemiology
        cultural perceptions, 530–531
        discrepancies, 530
        etiology, 531
        in low-income and middle-income countries,
            526–530
    etiology, 531

environmental exposures, 532
from epigenetics/epigenomics, 534–535
gene-environment interactions (GxE), evidence
    for, 533
genetics and genomics, 531–532
potential to prevent developmental disabilities,
    535–536
nutritional implications for, 536
    folic acid, 540–541
    iodine, 541
    iron, 540
    macronutrients, undernutrition in terms of,
        536–537
    micronutrients, undernutrition with respect to,
        538–539
    vitamin A deficiency, 541–542
outcomes, 548
    education, inclusion, or exclusion, 550–552
    employment, 552–553
    morbidities and mortalities, 548–550
    sociopolitical, policies, and conventions adopted by
        countries' regulations, 547–548
    spina bifida, 546
    growth deviants, 547
Deworming and enhanced vitamin A (DEVTA), 195
DIAAS (digestible indispensable amino acid score), 342
Diarrhea, 23t
    prevention and treatment, 629
    relative risk of suboptimum breastfeeding, 339
    zinc deficiency and, 268
Diderot, Denis, 4
Dietary diversification, 212–213, 279–280, 568
Dietary intake, measuring, 95–96
    biomarkers and, 107
    long-term trends, 18–19
Dietary reference intakes (DRI), 160, 189
    adequate intake level (AI), 161
    estimated average requirement (EAR), 160–161
    groups and circumstances with higher nutrient needs,
        162–163
    recommended dietary allowance (RDA), 160
    recommended nutrient intake (RNI), 160
    upper intake level (UL), 161–162
Digestible Indispensable Amino Acid Score (DIAAS),
    165
1,25-Dihydroxyvitamin D (1,25-(OH)2D), 300
Direct nutrition interventions, 490–495
    preterm birth (PTB), 491, 493
    small for gestational age and birth size, 493–494
    still birth and perinatal mortality, 495
Directly Observed Therapy Short-Course (DOTS),
    401–402
Disability-adjusted life years (DALYs), 35, 41–42
Divalent metal transporter (DMT1), 238
Docosahexaenoic acid (DHA), 322, 325, 326–327
    in breast milk, 339
    supplementation during pregnancy, 328
Down syndrome (DS), 546

growth deviants, 546
Dried skimmed milk (DSM), 349, 351, 353
Drug-resistant virus, 425
Dual-energy X-ray absorptiometry (DEXA) scan, 96

E
Ebola virus disease (EVD), 628
Economics
  malnutrition
    cognitive impairment, 34
    productivity losses, 36
  nutrition interventions
    benefit:cost ratios, 34, 41
    cost-effectiveness analysis, 41–43
    overview of costs, 37
    recommendations, 42
Education and training, innovative approaches to, 80–81
Effectiveness trials, 50, 608
Efficacy trials, 50
Eicosapentanoic (EPA) acid, 322
Eijkman, Christian, 12, 14
Elders in low–middle-income countries, 579
  biology of aging, 581
  burden of chronic diseases in aging, 585
    non-transmissible disease epidemiology in low-income country, 585
    relationship of chronic disease to diet and nutrition, 585–586
  deficiency and undernutrition states in low-income country elderly, 592–594
  demography of aging of populations, 583–584
  dietary intakes assessment in older subjects, 590–591
  evolutionary paradoxes, 580–581
  excess and overnutrition states, 594–595
  good nutritional status, addressing, 595
  nutrient intake recommendations
    for older men, 588
    for older women, 589
  nutritional requirements, nutrient intake recommendations and guidelines for healthful eating, 586–590
  patterns of dietary consumption in later life, 591–592
  senescence of tissue and organ function with aging, 581
    function of alimentary and digestive tract in aging, 582–583
  successful aging
    normative aging, 583
    frail aging, 583
ELISA techniques, 241
Ellison, Joseph, 16
ENACT course, 80
Encyclopédie, 4
Energy and protein, 120, 488
  pregnancy, 474
Energy availability, 472
Energy density, 166–167
  increasing, 167–168

eNutrition Academy, 80
Enzymes, sources of, 165
Epidemiological transition, 585, 586
Epilepsy, 529
Essential fatty acids, 165, 321
  effect of n-6 and n-3 fatty acids in pregnancy, lactation, and infancy, 325–326
  immunomodulation, 323
  long-chain polyunsaturated fatty acids in human milk, 326–328
  metabolism, 322–323
  n-3 and n-6 PUFA dietary intakes and disease, associations between, 324
    asthma, 324
    noncommunicable diseases, 324
  polyunsaturated fatty acids, 323
    n-3 and n-6 PUFA, 324, 325–326
  requirements, 329
  and specific needs in developing countries, 329–330
Essential nutrients, 51, 55
  and active compounds, 165
Estimated Average Requirement (EAR), 96, 160–161, 176, 265, 586
Estimated Energy Requirement (EER), 587
Ethambutol, 404
Ethics, in public health research
  basic ethical principles
    beneficence, 795
    justice, 794, 796
    respect for persons, 795, 796–797
  confidentiality, 799–800
  informed consent, 796–798
  responsibilities after completion of research, 802–804
  review of research proposals, 804, 805–806
  standards of care, 800–802
Evaluation research, using results from, 622
Evidence-based medicine (EBM), 48–51, 53–54
  drawbacks, 53
Evidence for nutrition-specific interventions and programs, 53–60
  assessing impact of programs for improving nutrition, 59
  choosing a control group for, 54–55
  evidence-based medicine paradigm, 53–54
  magnitude of nutrient intervention, 56
  outcome focused interventions, collecting and interpreting 'right' evidence, 56
  stunting, 59–60
Exercise. *See* Female athlete triad
Extensively drug-resistant TB (XDR-TB), 386
External validity of RCTs, 50, 57
Extrapulmonary TB (EPTB), 392, 397, 400, 403

F
F-75, 346–347
F(-)100 (therapeutic milk), 163, 164, 346–347
Factors affecting impact on nutrition
  characteristics/effects of crisis, 633

displacement, 655
  service quality and access, 655–656
  women, crises and nutrition, 656
pre-crisis nutrition situation, 653–655
FAO/WHO Codex Alimentarius Commission, 174
Farr, William, 6
Fat, in milk, 343–344
Female athlete triad, 472
Ferritin, 237, 241, 256
Fetal growth restriction (FGR), 131–132, 503
First pregnancy, postponing age at marriage and,
    570–571
Fisher, Ronald A., 6
Fluoride deficiency signs and symptoms, 103
Folic acid, 540–541
  costs of interventions, 37
  deficiency, 35
  improving, in adolescents, 568–569
  supplementation, 568
Food access, 719
  cash and food purchases, importance of, 719
    food price shocks, 720
  formal and informal safety nets, 722–723
  urban employment, 720
    maternal employment and childcare, 721–722
Food and Agriculture Organization (FAO), historical
    perspective, 22
Food and available energy, 94–95
Food availability, 715
  foreign direct investment and globalization, 717
  street foods, 717–718
  traditional and modern supply chains, 715–717
  urban agriculture, 718–719
Food balance sheets, 94
Food-based dietary guidelines (FBDG), 164, 166
Food fortification, 255–256, 312, 477, 758, 776
  biofortification, 171, 217
  with iron and folic acid, 568
  with vitamin A, 193, 215, 313
  with vitamin D, 299, 312, 313
  with zinc, 278–279
Food insecurity, 92
  HIV and, 453
  and tuberculosis, 439–440
  and undernutrition, 428
Food policy analysis, 745
Food production, history of growth, 18
Food safety, 726–727
Food security, 707
  in HIV, 453
Food systems, nutrition transition and urban diets, 712
  changing demand for food, 714
  changing role of women, 713
  physical activity, 714–715
  urban diets, 714
  urban structure, technology and society, 713
Food value chain, 755
  actors across, 755–756

nutrition-focused, 764
  private sector, role of, 756–757
  types of, 757–758
Food waste and cold chains, 697–698
Ford Foundation, 772
Foreign direct investment (FDI), 740, 747
  and globalization, 717
Forensic medicine, 21
Fortification, 171
  biofortification, 171
  considerations for, 172–173
  home-fortification/point-of-use fortification, 172
  industrial fortification of foods for general population,
      171–172
  iron, 255–256
  setting nutrient level for, 174
  standards, specifications and quality control for,
      174–175
  vitamin A, 215, 216
Fortification Rapid Assessment Tool (FRAT), 215
Fortified blended food (FBF), 163
Frail aging, 583
Frank, Johann Peter, 5
Free erythrocyte protoporphyrin (FEP), 241

G
Gene-environment interactions (GxE), evidence for, 533
  from epigenetics/epigenomics, 534–535
Genovesi, Antonio, 7
Geographical communities, defined, 626
Gestational diabetes (GD), 508
GlaxoSmithKline (GSK), 780
Glisson, Francis, 299
Global acute malnutrition (GAM) prevalence thresholds,
    656
Global Alliance for Improved Nutrition (GAIN), 774
Global Alliance for Vaccines and Immunization (GAVI),
    780, 783
Global Food Security Index, 94
Global Fund for AIDS, Tuberculosis (TB) and Malaria
    (GFATM), 415, 416–417
Global health workforce and capacity to deliver nutrition
    services, 70–72
Global Hunger Index, 97
Global Vaccines Action Plan, 785
Glutathione (GSH), 349
Goat's milk, 339, 342
Godwin, William, 4
Goiter
  iodine deficiency, 289, 290, 294
  rate in iodine assessment, 291
Goldberger, Joseph, 15
Gonadotropin-releasing hormone (GnRH), 471
Graduate education, historical perspective, 21
Grameen Bank, 638
Graunt, John, 6
Grijns, Gerrit, 12
Growth retardation, 510, 516

health and social consequences, 134–135
interventions, 135–136
measures and indicators
fetal growth, 121–123
high weight-for-height, 125
international reference population, 125, 126
interpretation, 124–125, 130–131
low height-for-age, 124–125
low weight-for-height, 125
overweight, 125
mental development effects, 120
prevalence in developing countries
geographic distribution, 131–134
intrauterine growth restriction, 123
stunting, 124–125
underweight, 125, 134
socioeconomic status correlation, 120
vitamin A deficiency, 209–210
Guérin, Camille, 405
Gynecologic morbidity, 479

H
Halley, Edmund, 6
Harrison's sulcus, 307
HarvestPlus, 764, 766
Hazard Analysis and Critical Control Points (HACCP), 62
Health Organization of the League of Nations, 22
Health system, defined, 417
Healthy growth and development, promoting, 135–136
Height-for-age z-scores (HAZ), 99
Helen Keller International (HKI), 81, 609, 610, 616
Helicobacter pylori infection, 583
HemoCue system, 243
Hemoglobin, 105, 508, 538
function, 236
iron deficiency testing, 243, 244
Hemosiderin, 237
Henle, Jacob, 10
Hepatitis B virus (HBV) and HIV infection, 427–428
Hepatitis C virus (HCV) and HIV infection, 428
Hepcidin, 239, 240, 257
Hidden Hunger Index (HHI), 776
High birth weight (HBW) infants, 98
High-density lipoprotein (HDL), 458
High energy biscuits (HEB), 164
High energy foods with low or high nutrient density, 168
Highly active antiretroviral therapy, 415
HIV, 413, 628
access to care and treatment, 416–417
health systems strengthening, 417
anti-HIV antibodies, 419
biology of, 418
and breastfeeding, 341
clinical history of, 418
acquired immune deficiency syndrome (AIDS), 419–420
acute HIV infection, 418–419

clinical latency/chronic asymptomatic HIV infection, 419
early HIV infection, 418–419
early symptomatic infection, 419
continuum of care, 421
antiretroviral therapy (ART), 423–424
comprehensive HIV care, 421–422
HIV counseling and testing, 422–423
linking to care, 423
viral suppression, CD4 count monitoring and resistance testing, 424–425
enteropathy, 452
global epidemiology of, 420
history, 414–415
HIV-1, 417
HIV-2, 417
HIV wasting, 451
malnutrition and, 348–349
nutrition and, 667–668, 674–675
overlapping epidemics, 427
anemia, 428
food insecurity and undernutrition, 428
hepatitis B virus (HBV), 427–428
hepatitis C virus (HCV), 428
schistosomiasis, 429
TB/HIV coinfection, 427
prevention, 425, 426–427, 631
treatment as, 425
testing, 672–673
transmission, 418, 672
tuberculosis risks, 388
women and children, 429–430
HIV/AIDS movement, 669–672
HIV and HIV/TB co-infection, 449
background, 449–450
cachexia in, 454
food security in, 453
impact of fully suppressed HIV viral load on nutrition/metabolism, 458
macronutrients
deficiencies in, 461
interventions in, 455–456, 462
and malnutrition, 460–463
micronutrients
deficiencies in, 454, 461–462
interventions in, 456–457, 462–463
mortality and weight loss and, 451
nutrition
and ART in, 457
nutrition programs and, 457–458
nutritional assessment in, 455
nutritional status in, 461
outcomes in, 461
protein energy malnutrition in, 453–454
resting energy expenditure/metabolic abnormalities in, 454
vulnerable populations, 458
children, 458–460

during pregnancy, 460
weight loss in, 451–452
Home-fortification, 172, 568
Home-fortification technical advisory group (HF-TAG),
169
Home-processing methods, 167
Homestead food production (HFP) program, 609, 610,
616
Hopkins, Frederick Gowland, 13, 14
Household- or institutional-level fortification, 568
Household food insecurity access scale (HHFIAS), 95
Household penetration of adequately iodized salt (HHIS),
291
Human milk, 337. *See also* Breastfeeding
benefits
for child, 339–340
for mother, 340
breastfeeding promotion and support, 340–341
composition, 338–339, 341
fat, 343–344
lactose, 342–343
minerals, 343
protein, 342
HIV and, 341
lactose, 350–351
recommended use of dairy ingredients, 351
cost-effectiveness of milk content, 352–353
specific effects of whey in undernutrition, 349–350
Humanitarian crises, 647
consequences and effects of crises, 650
access to services, 651
displacement, 651
food insecurity and market access, 651
definition of, 648–650
factors affecting impact on nutrition.*See* Factors
affecting impact on nutrition
nutrition response to, 656
food assistance and nutrition, 661
prevention and treatment, 659–661
thresholds for, 656–659
preparedness, 651–652
types of crises/shocks, 650
who and how, 653
Hydrocarbon carotenoids, 182
Hydrogen peroxidases, 236
25-Hydroxyvitamin D3 (25(OH)D3), 299
Hygiene, 3, 20, 21
Hypertensive disorders, 508
Hyperthyroidism, 290–291
Hypocalcaemia, 307
Hypothyroidism, 290
Hypotonia, 307

I
Immune function and morbidity, importance of zinc for,
274
Impact evaluation, 61–63
Implementation science, 34
Inadequate nutrient intake, correcting, 170
fortification, 171–175

increasing contribution from nutrient-rich,
unprocessed, foods, 170–171
supplementation, 175
Individual capacity development, 77
Industrial fortification of foods, 171–172
Infant feeding after 12 months, 365
Infant mortality history of social reform, 11
Infectious diseases, 3, 10, 20
morbidity, 207
Informal education, 79
Informed consent, ethics in public health research,
796–798
Institut Pasteur, 21
Institutional capacity, developing, 81–82
Insulin-like growth factor 1 (IGF-1), 345
Integrated Child Development Services (ICDS), 569
Integrated Food Security Phase Classification (IPC), 656
Intelligence and cognition in children born SGA,
514–515
Interferon-gamma (IFN-γ), 403
Interferon-gamma release assays (IGRAs), 402–403
INTERGROWTH-21st Project, 123, 505
International Baby Food Action Network (IBFAN), 367
International Classification of Functioning Disability and
Health (ICF), 525
International Classification of Functioning Disability and
Health for Children and Youth (ICF-CY), 526
International Food Policy Research Institute (IFPRI), 609
International Network of Food Data Systems
(INFOODS), 591
International trade and local production, 699–700
International Vitamin A Consultative Group (IVACG),
168
Interphotoreceptor retinoid binding protein (IRBP), 184
Intervening to improve nutrition, 52
Intrauterine growth restriction/retardation (IUGR), 98,
123, 503, 509, 538
epidemiology, 123
measures, 123
Iodine, 165, 538
absorption and transport, 288
costs of interventions, 37
deficiency, 35. *See also* Iodine deficiency
deficiency signs and symptoms, 103
excess, 294
food sources, 288
functions. *See* Iodine functions and brain
development
intake requirements, 291–293
iodized oil
injection, 294
oral, 289, 290, 294
iodized salt, 288, 291, 292, 293
potassium iodide administration, 294
pregnancy and, 478
prophylaxis and treatment, 293–294
requirements and prevalence, 291–293
thyroid hormones, 287
Iodine deficiency
assessment, 35

goiter rate, 291
  thyroid-stimulating hormone level, 291
  urine concentrations, 288
and clinical manifestations
  cretinism, 290
  goiter, 289, 290, 294
effects
  in adults, 290–291
  in childhood, 290
  on pregnancy and infancy, 289–290
history of study, 287, 288
pathophysiology
  goitrogens, 288
  intake, 289
public health significance, 292
Iodine deficiency disorder (IDD), 287, 289, 541
Iodine functions and brain development, 288, 292–293
  growth and development, 287, 289
  metabolism, 288
Iron
  absorption, 238–239
  biological functions, 235–240
  costs of interventions, 37
  deficiency. *See* Iron deficiency
  deficiency signs and symptoms, 103
  functional, 237
  functions
    cytochromes, 236
    enzymes, 236
    hemoglobin, 236
    myoglobin, 236
  homeostasis, regulation of, 239–240
  metabolism and regulation of, 236–240
  overload, 256–257
  pregnancy and, 476–477
  storage, 237–238
  supplementation, 568
  transport, 237
  turnover and loss, 238
Iron and folic acid (IFA), 491, 493, 494, 495, 497, 568–569
Iron deficiency, 35, 540
  clinical examination, 243
  control
    fortification, 255–256
    helminth infection, 251–252
    nutrition education and promotion, 255
    supplementation, 252–255
  definition, 235, 241
  delayed cord clamping, 256
  diagnosis of anemia, 243
  functional consequences
    birth outcomes, 249–250
    child behavior and development, 250
    heavy metal absorption, 251
    infection, 251–252
    mortality, 249–250
    work performance and productivity, 250–251

hemoglobin field testing, 243
  overview of tests, 241
  pathogenesis
    intake, 244, 247–248
    iron loss, 238
    iron requirement increase, 237, 247
  prevalence, 244, 245–246
  prospects for study, 258
  risk factors, 244, 247
Iron deficiency anemia, 242
  assessment, 241–244
  definition, 241
  functional consequences
    child behavior and development, 250
    heavy metal absorption, 251
    infection, 251–252
    work performance and productivity, 250–251
  intervention strategies for prevention and treatment of, 252
  maternal mortality, 249
  prevalence, 244, 245–246, 248–249
Iron regulator proteins (IRPs), 239–240
Isoniazid preventive therapy (IPT), 401, 404

J
Joint United Nations Programme on AIDS (UNAIDS), 415, 667
Joints, 101, 297, 582
  fixed contractures of, 545
  swollen joints, 325
  and PTB, 392
Justice, ethical principles, 794, 796

K
Kaiser–Permanente (K-P) diet, 543
Kangaroo method, 366–367
Kaposi sarcoma, 414
Keratomalacia, 209
Kheth'Impilo, 642
Kilimo Salama program, 779
Koch, Robert, 10, 387
Kwashiorkor, 15, 102

L
Lactase, 350–351
Lactating women, 348
Lactose, 342–343, 350–351
Lancet estimates, 40
Lancet Series on Maternal and Child Nutrition, 603
Large for gestational age (LGA) infant, 98
Last menstrual period (LMP), 504–505
Latent TB infection (LTBI), 391, 397, 398
Latent tuberculosis infection (LTBI), 438
Life years saved (LYS), 35
Linear growth
  assessment, 132
  cow's milk and, 344–345
  growth stimulating factors in milk, 165

Linoleic acid (LA), 322
Lipid-based nutrient supplements (LNS), 167, 491
Lister Institute, 21
Liver X receptor (LXR), 323
Long-chain polyunsaturated fatty acids in human milk, 326–328
Low birth weight (LBW), 98
    epidemiology, 123
    iron deficiency, 237
    and small-for-gestational age, 108–109
Low birth weight (LBW) rate, 122
Low dietary calcium intakes, 302–304
Low-income and middle income countries (LMICs), 146
    elders in. *See* Elders in low–middle-income countries
    obesity trends in, 147–151, 153–154
    prevalence of
        developmental disabilities in, 526–530
        obesity in, 146–147
Lunin, Nicholai Ivanovich, 13, 14

M
Macronutrients
    deficiencies, and HIV and HIV/TB co-infection, 461
    interventions
        in HIV and HIV/TB co-infection, 455–456, 462
        and TB, 441–442
    and risk of tuberculosis, 440
Madsen's Institute for Tribal and Rural Advancement (MITRA), 777
Magendie, François, 10
Magnesium
    deficiency signs and symptoms, 103
    pregnancy and, 478
Mainstreaming Nutrition Initiative, 73
Malaria control, 629, 631
Malnutrition, 91, 125, 127, 131, 136, 348–349, 450
    burden of, 67–68
    causes of, 57
    community, household and individual measures, 92
    deficiency signs and symptoms, 103
    double-burden of, 92
    economics, productivity losses, 36
    global measures, 107
        low birth weight and small-for-gestational age, 108–109
        micronutrient deficiencies, 110
        overweight/obesity, 110
        spectrum of malnutrition across regions, 111
        undernourishment, 108
        undernutrition, 109
    HIV and HIV/TB co-infection and, 460–463
    and outcomes of tuberculosis, 439
    prevention and treatment, 629
    and risk of tuberculosis, 439
    specific indicators of nutritional status, 94
        anthropometric measurements, 96–101
        biomarkers, 105–107
        clinical signs of malnutrition, 101–104
        diet, 95–96
        food and available energy, 94–95

functional outcomes, 107
    treatment of, 631–632
Malthus, Thomas Robert, 5
Manicus, August Henrick, 8–9
Mantoux tuberculin skin test, 402
Marriage, postponing age at, 570–571
Marten, Benjamin, 387
Maternal, newborn and child health (MNCH) outcomes, 487
Maternal death, 474
Maternal employment and childcare, 721–722
Maternal health, 506, 508
    breastfeeding and, 364–365
Maternal morbidity, 474
Maternal mortality, 249, 473, 475, 476, 477–478
Maternal newborn and child health, 679
Maternal nutrition
    assessment of, 488–490
    and birth outcomes, 487
    before conception, 495–496
    evidence from programs, 497–498
    nutrition interventions during pregnancy. *See* Maternal nutrition interventions during pregnancy
    role of intergenerational effects, 497
Maternal nutrition interventions during pregnancy, 490
    direct nutrition interventions, 490–495
        preterm birth (PTB), 491, 493
        small for gestational age and birth size, 493–494
        still birth and perinatal mortality, 495
    nutrition-related factors during pregnancy, 495
Maternal–infant bonding, 364
Maternity waiting homes (MWHs), 630
Matrix framework application to food and nutrition assistance, 675
    key populations, focus on, 678
    maternal newborn and child health, focus on, 679
    role of food security and nutrition for adherence, 676–677
    social protection, focus on, 677–678
McKeown, Thomas, 20
McNamara, Robert, 22
Mean dietary energy requirements (MDER), 94
Measles
    case fatality rates over time, 22
    history of study, 8–9
Medecins Sans Frontieres (MSF), 785
Medical Police, 5, 21
Mediterranean diet, 482
Mellanby, Edward, 16, 17
Men who had sex with men (MSM), 414, 667
Menstrual cycle, 471
    anorexia nervosa, 472
    female athlete triad, 472
    overnutrition and obesity, 473
Metabolomics, 107
5,10-Methylenetetrahydrofolate reductase (*MTHFR*) gene, 533
Metropolis Water Act of 1852, 9
mHealth (mobile-health) revolution, 81
Miasma, history of concept, 8–9

Microbiology, historical perspective, 10
Microcytic anemia, 251
Micronutrient deficiencies, 92, 110, 539
    and anemia in adolescents in low- and middle-income
        countries, 567
    in HIV, 454
    in HIV and HIV/TB co-infection, 461–462
Micronutrient interventions
    in HIV and HIV/TB co-infection, 456–457, 462–463
    in TB, 442–443
Micronutrient powders (MNPs), 47, 254, 779
Micronutrients, 34, 35, 36, 254–255
    and risk of tuberculosis, 440
Mid-upper arm circumference (MUAC), 99–101, 125,
    352, 353, 656
Midday meal program, 173
Milk protein, 342, 347
Minerals, 165
    in milk, 343
Moderate acute malnutrition (MAM), 162, 353
    cow's milk in prevention and treatment of, 345–347
Modern-to-traditional value chains, 758
Morbidity
    gynecologic, 479
    maternal, 474
    obstetric, 473–474
    reproductive, 473
    small for gestational age and, 512
        long term, 512–513
        short term, 512
Mortality, 3
    child, 506, 548, 714
    HIV, 451
    maternal, 249, 473, 475, 476, 477–478
    perinatal, 495
    from severe malnutrition, 458
    small for gestational age and, 510
    trends in developed countries, 20–21, 23
Mother-to-child transmission (MTCT) of HIV, 371
Multicentre Growth Reference Study (MGRS), 26, 126
Multi-country nutrition initiatives, 72–73
Multidrug-resistant tuberculosis (MDR-TB), 386,
    404–405
Multiple micronutrient powder (MNP), 607
Multiple micronutrients (MMN), 478, 491, 494, 499
Multiple (stunting), 35
    costs of interventions, 37
Murat, Joachim, 7
Muscle accretion, 353
    whey protein and, 350
Mycobacterium africanum, 396
Mycobacterium canettii, 396
Mycobacterium caprae, 396
Mycobacterium microti (voles), 396
Mycobacterium orygis, 396
Mycobacterium pinnipedii (seals), 396
Mycobacterium tuberculosis (MTB), 387, 437, 442
    transmission of, 392–394

Mycobacterium tuberculosis complex (MTBC), 396
Myoglobin, function, 236
Myopathy, 307

N
N-3 and N-6 fatty acids, 321–323
    effect in pregnancy, lactation, and infancy, 325–326
N-3 and N-6 PUFA dietary intakes and disease,
    associations between, 324
    asthma, 324
    noncommunicable diseases, 324
Naandi Foundation, 774
NADH dehydrogenase, 236
National Bioethics Advisory Commission (NBAC), 794,
    798, 804
National Institutes of Health (NIH), historical
    perspective, 21, 22
National Weekly Iron and Folic Acid Supplementation
    Programme, 569
Neonatal care, 629
Nestlé Foundation, 777
Neural tube defect (NTD), 495, 540, 568
Neurobehavioral development, importance of zinc for,
    275
Newman, George, 11, 19
Night blindness, 208
Non-Agricultural Rural Employment (NARE), 693
Non-communicable diseases (NCDs), 68, 75, 324, 471,
    585, 632, 675
Non-transmissible disease epidemiology in low-income
    country, 585
Normative aging, 583
Nuremberg code, ethics, 793
Nutrient deficiencies, determining, 168–170
Nutrient density, 167
    increasing, 167–168
Nutrient needs, 159
    ascertaining impact of measures to correct dietary
        deficiencies, 175–176
    determining (risk of) nutrient deficiencies, at
        population level, 168–170
    dietary reference intakes (DRI), 160
        adequate intake (AI) level, 161
        estimated average requirement (EAR), 160–161
        groups and circumstances with higher nutrient
            needs, 162–163
        recommended dietary allowance (RDA), 160
        recommended nutrient intake (RNI), 160
        upper intake level (UL), 161–162
    energy density, 166–167
        increasing, 167–168
    high energy foods with low or high nutrient density,
        168
    inadequate nutrient intake, correcting, 170
        fortification, 171–175
        increasing contribution from nutrient-rich,
            unprocessed, foods, 170–171
        supplementation, 175

Nutrient needs (*cont.*)
    meeting nutrient requirements from diet, 163
      selecting foods that can meet nutrient
        requirements, 164–166
      single foods that meet all nutrient intake
        recommendations, 164
    nutrient density, 167
      increasing, 167–168
Nutrition Assessment and Counseling (NAC), 677
Nutrition evidence in context, 47
    evidence-based medicine (EBM), 48–51, 53–54
    evidence for nutrition-specific interventions and
      programs, 53–60
    impact evaluation, 61–63
    trends and context, importance of, 60–61
Nutrition programs and HIV, 457–458
Nutrition-related factors during
    pregnancy, 495
Nutrition science, 51–52
Nutrition surveillance, 59
Nutrition transition, 144
Nutrition value chain actors, 762
Nutritional assessment in HIV, 455
Nutritional deficiencies, 15
Nutritional effect of zinc fortification, 278
Nutritional immunology, 15–16
Nutritional problems in utero and during early life, 471
Nutritional science, historical perspective, 10–11
"Nutritious Agriculture by Design" tool, 763

O
Obesity, 106
    in children and women, 710–712
    overnutrition and, 473
    overweight and. *See* Overweight and obesity
    pubertal onset, 471
Obstetric morbidity, 473–474
OneHealth, 39
Open innovation, 780
Opportunistic infections (OI), 449, 675
Oral rehydration solution (ORS), 361
Orr, John Boyd, 19
Osteomalacia, rickets, 298
Ovarian cancer, 480–481
    micronutrients, 481
    obesity, 480–481
Overnutrition, 91, 92
    diagnosing, 594–595
    and obesity, 473, 479
Overweight and obesity, 92, 110, 124, 143
    in children and women, 710–712
    comparative approach, 145–146
    epidemiologic transition, 143
    implications for public health, 150
      genetic component, 154
      interactions of obesity and activity, 152–154
      physical activity, 152
    lower and middle income countries (LMICs), 146
      obesity trends in, 147–151, 153–154
      prevalence in, 146–147
    measures, 144–145
    research and policy implications, 155
    survey design and sample, 145
Ovulation and menstruation. *See* Menstrual cycle
Oxytocin, external administration of, 364

P
Panum, Peter Ludwig, 8–9
Pasteur Institute, historical perspective, 21
Pasteur, Louis, 10
PDCAAS method (protein digestibility corrected amino
    acid score), 342
Pediatric TB, 400–401
Peer-reviewed research studies, 49
Pellagra, 15
PEPFAR (President's Emergency Plan for AIDS Relief),
    415, 416–417
Peptide YY, 440
Performance-based incentives, 81
Perinatal mortality, still birth and, 495
Peroxisome proliferators-activated receptor (PPAR), 323
Pervasive developmental disorders (PDDs), 529
Pharmaceutical companies, 780
Physical activity, 454, 714–715
    overweight and obesity, 152
Phytate:zinc molar ratio, 267
Plasma and serum zinc concentration, 268–269
Plausibility, 608
Pneumocystis carinii pneumonia (PCP), 414
Point-of-use fortification, 172, 568
Polyunsaturated fatty acids (PUFA), 323, 327, 491
    in milk, 343
Population growth, mortality decline, 20
Porter, Michael, 754, 756
    value chain, 754
Potassium iodate, 293
Poverty, 706–707
    and development dimension, 743–744
    integrating food and health dimension with, 744–747
Poverty and hunger index, 94
Pre-ART care, 673
Preconception, 496
Preeclampsia, 474, 508
Pregnancy, 473
    adolescent growth and nutritional status in relation to,
      565–567
    calcium, 476
    energy and protein, 474
    and HIV, 460
    iodine, 478
    iron and vitamin B, 476–477
    magnesium, 478
    multiple micronutrients, 478
    nutrition interventions during. *See* Pregnancy,
      nutrition interventions during
    optimizing interval between pregnancies, 571

overnutrition and obesity, 479
postponing age at marriage and first pregnancy,
    570–571
and TB, 444
vitamin A, 475
vitamin D, 475–476
vitamins C and E, 475
weight gain during, 99
zinc, 274–275, 477–478
Pregnancy, nutrition interventions during, 490
    direct nutrition interventions, 490–495
        preterm birth (PTB), 491, 493
        small for gestational age and birth size, 493–494
        still birth and perinatal mortality, 495
    nutrition-related factors during pregnancy, 495
Pregnant adolescents, nutrition of, 570
Pregnant and lactating women, 348
Prelacteal feeding practices, 366
Premenstrual syndrome (PMS), 473
Premenstrual tension (PMT). See Premenstrual syndrome
    (PMS)
Preterm birth (PTB), 491, 493
Preterm milk, 363
Prevention of mother-to-child transmission of HIV
    (PMTCT) programs, 429, 459, 666
Preventive health and nutrition programs, 59
Preventive medicine, historical perspective, 6, 7
Private sector, 771
    driving innovation and novel approaches, 778–782
    proliferation of public private partnerships, 782–785
    provision of goods and financial and in-kind
        resources, 773–775
    public health advocacy, 775–778
    standards for private sector involvement, 785–786
Probability, 6
Program effectiveness trials, 608
Program managers, 77, 78
Program theory framework and program impact
    pathways analysis, 608
    designing, 609
    using, 610
Programs, nutrition-sensitive, 603
    comprehensive evaluation framework, 610
        challenge of finding valid counterfactual, 612
        choosing indicators, 615
        ensuring appropriate sample size, 615
        importance of time, duration, and timing, 614–615
        selecting evaluation design, 612–613
    cost of program, 619
        differences in priorities, expectations, and
            incentives, 620
        differences in time constraints and time frames,
            620–621
        evaluation and program implementation toward
            common goal, 619
        independence of evaluators, 621–622

defined, 603
designing process evaluation, 616
drawing sample, 618
evaluation research, using results from, 622
key challenges in evaluating, 604
    assessing benefits beyond targeted beneficiaries,
        606–607
    complexity, 605
    differing points among program implementers and
        evaluators, 606
    efficacy trials, 607–608
    long impact pathways and time frames, 605
    program effectiveness trials, 608
    trade-offs between implementation constraints and
        evaluation rigor, 605–606
probability, 608, 613
program theory framework and program impact
    pathways, 608
    designing, 609
    using, 610
selecting data collection methods and tools, 617–618
sharing and feeding results to program implementers,
    618–619
summarizing results from process evaluation, 618
timing and time frames, importance of, 616–617
understanding pathways to impact, 615–616
Progressive Era regulations, 22
Propensity score matching (PSM), 613
Prostate cancer, 325, 481–482
Protein, 165
    in breast milk, 342
Protein Digestibility Corrected Amino Acid Score
    (PDCAAS), 165
Protein energy malnutrition (PEM), 102
    in HIV, 453–454
    risk for TB, 440
Protein malnutrition, 15
Proteomics, 106
Provider-initiated counseling and testing (PICT), 422
Pubertal onset, 470
    nutritional problems in utero and during early life,
        471
    obesity, 471
    vitamin D deficiency, 471
Puberty, defined, 564
Public health, historical perspective, 257
    graduate education, 21
    idea of progress, 4–5
    international organizations, 21–23
    statistics, 6–7, 8
Public health advocacy, 775–778
Public–private partnerships (PPPs), 773
    proliferation of, 782–785
Pulmonary TB (PTB), 392, 396, 398–404
Purified protein derivative (PPD), 402
Pyrazinamide, 404

Q

Quaker Service Team, 100
Quality-adjusted life years (QALYs) saved, 35
Quetelet, Adolphe, 6

R

Ready-to-use foods (RUF), 659
Ready-to-use supplementary foods (RUSF), 278, 352
Ready-to-use therapeutic food (RUTF), 163, 168, 278, 346–347, 352, 631
Recommended Dietary Allowance (RDA), 160, 586
Recommended Nutrient Intake (RNI), 56, 160, 174, 188, 586
    RNI/RDA, 160
Reproductive and maternal health, 631
Reproductive health, 469
    menstrual cycle, 471
        anorexia nervosa, 472
        female athlete triad, 472
        overnutrition and obesity, 473
    pregnancy, 473
        calcium, 476
        energy and protein, 474
        iodine, 478
        iron and vitamin B, 476–477
        magnesium, 478
        multiple micronutrients, 478
        overnutrition and obesity, 479
        vitamin A, 475
        vitamin D, 475–476
        vitamins C and E, 475
        zinc, 477–478
    premenstrual syndrome (PMS), 473
    pubertal onset, 470
        nutritional problems in utero and during early life, 471
        obesity, 471
        vitamin D deficiency, 471
    reproductive organ cancers, 479
        breast cancer, 479–480
        cervical cancer, 480
        ovarian cancer, 480–481
        prostate cancer, 481–482
        uterus cancer, 481
    reproductive well-being, 470
    sexually transmitted infections (STIs), 479
Reproductive morbidity, 473
Resistin, 440
Resonance Raman spectroscopy (RRS), 107
Respect for persons, ethical principles, 795, 796–797
Respiratory transmission, 392
Resting energy expenditure/metabolic abnormalities in HIV, 454
Retinoic acid response element (RARE), 185
Retinoids, 182
Retinol activity equivalent (RAE), 186

Retinol-binding protein (RBP), function, 184, 189
Retinol in urine, 207
Rickets
    bony deformities associated with, 307, 308
    causes, 297, 298
    clinical features, 307
    definition, 298
    diagnosis, 308–309
    epidemiology
        geographic distribution, 302–304
        vitamin D synthesis, 299–304
    historical background, 298–299
    osteomalacia, 298
    pathogenesis, 303
    pathophysiology, 307
    prevention, 310–312
    prospects for study, 312–313
    public health importance, 305–307
    treatment, 310
Rifampicin, 404
Risk–benefit analyses, 52
Roads and traffic, 698–699
Robert Wood Johnson Foundation, 772
Rockefeller Foundation, 21, 772, 780
Rowe, John, 583

S

SABLA, 570
Safe water and good sanitation, access to, 724–726
Safety nets, formal and informal, 722–723
Sanitary movement, historical perspective, 7–8
Sanitation, water and, 698
Saturated fatty acids (SFAs), 343
Scaling Up Nutrition (SUN) Business Network, 773, 776–777
Scaling Up Nutrition (SUN) Movement, 73, 81, 668, 698, 767
Schistosomiasis, 429
School-based platforms, for adolescents, 571–572
School milk programs for prevention of undernutrition, 348
Sedgwick, William, 10
Selenium deficiency signs and symptoms, 103
Selenium toxicity, 106
Service Availability and Readiness Assessment (SARA), 70
Severe acute malnutrition (SAM), 34, 162, 353
    community management of, 41
    cow's milk in prevention and treatment of, 345–347
Sexually transmitted disease (STD), 479
Sexually transmitted infections (STIs), 479
Shattuck, Lemuel, 8
Sheep milk, 339, 341, 342
Shock, Nathan, 581
Sickle cell anemia, 565
Sir Dorabji Tata Trust (SDTT), 777

Small for gestational age (SGA), 98, 108, 122–123, 503
 assessing, 504–506
 and birth size, 493–494
 and development, 513
  child development, 513–515
  long-term performance, 516
 epidemiology and determinants, 506
  fetal factors, 510
  maternal factors. *See* Small for gestational age (SGA) maternal factors
  placental factors, 509
 and morbidity, 512
  long term, 512–513
  short term, 512
 and mortality, 510
 symmetric and asymmetric, 510
Small for gestational age (SGA) maternal factors
 anemia, 508
 gestational diabetes (GD), 508
 preeclampsia, 508
 toxins, 509
 undernutrition, 508–509
Small intestine, absorption of zinc from, 268
Small-quantity LNS (LNS-SQ), 172, 174
Snow, John, 9
Social behavior change communication (SBCC), 59
Social investment bond (SIB), 780
Social medicine, 5
Social protection, 677–678
Social safety nets/social protection programs, for adolescents, 572–573
Society for Nutrition Education and Behavior (SNEB), 78
Socioeconomic status (SES), 91, 366, 564
 as barrier to HIV testing, 673
 breastfeeding promotion, 372
 indicators of, 390
 nutrient interventions, 177
 stunting correlation, 120, 124
 unprotected transactional sex, 672
 vitamin A deficiency, 201, 203
Sodium–iodide symporter (NIS), 288
Southern African urban food security and consumption trends, 691
Spina bifida, 546
 growth deviants, 547
Standard deviation, 6
Standards of care, ethics in public health research, 800–802
State Medicine, 21
Statistics, historical perspective in public health, 6–7, 8
Stein-Leventhal syndrome, 470
Still birth and perinatal mortality, 495
Stockholm Birth Cohort, 516
Street foods, 717–718
Streptomycin, 387

Stunted and plump, 92
Stunting, 33, 56, 59–60, 120, 125, 269–270, 497, 708
Sub-Saharan Africa, HIV in, 420
Suboptimal breastfeeding, 35, 37
 costs of interventions, 37
Successful aging, 583
Succinate dehydrogenase, 236
Sudden infant death syndrome (SIDS), 134
Super Cereal Plus, 62
Supermarkets, on nutrition and nutritional knowledge, 737, 757
 challenge to food security from modern supply chains, 742
 economic growth and policy issues, 747–749
 food and health dimension, 742–743
 modern supply chains and marketing sector, 738–740
 poverty and development dimension, 743–744
  integrating food and health dimension with, 744–747
 rise of supermarkets, 740–742
Sustainable Development Goals (SDGs), 69, 84, 107, 634–635, 643, 649, 665, 666, 685, 686–687, 776
 applying matrix framework to food and nutrition assistance, 675
  food security and nutrition for adherence, role of, 676–677
  key populations, focus on, 678
  maternal newborn and child health, focus on, 679
  social protection, focus on, 677–678
 HIV
  and AIDS movement, 669–672
  current context for, 667–668
  matrix framework, application of, 672
   ART initiation and adherence, 674
   HIV testing, 672–673
   HIV transmission, 672
   pre-ART care, 673
  nutrition
   and ART, 675
   current context for, 668
   and HIV infection, 674–675
  opportunities ahead, 669
Symmetric and asymmetric SGA, 510–511
Syngenta Foundation's Kilimo Salama program, 779
Systematic review, 49, 53
Systemic capacity, developing, 82
Systemic iron homeostasis, 240

T
Takaki, Kanehiro, 12, 13
Targeted fortification, 568
TB/HIV coinfection, 427, 463
 burden countries, 405
 macronutrients
  deficiencies in, 461
  interventions in, 462

TB/HIV coinfection (*cont.*)
  and malnutrition, 460–461
  micronutrients
    deficiencies in, 461–462
    interventions in, 462–463
  nutritional status in, 461
  outcomes in, 461
TBXpert Project, 403
Testing before use/consumption, 52
Thames, contamination of, 9
Thames Water, 9
Therapeutic zinc supplementation, 277
Thrifty phenotype, 512
Thyroid hormones, 287, 288, 289, 290–291
Thyrotropin (TSH), 289
Tolerable Upper Intake Level, 587
Toll-like receptors (TLRs), 305, 323
Total daily energy expenditure (TDEE), 454
Trade-offs between implementation constraints and
  evaluation rigor, 605–606
Traditional birth attendants (TBAs), 629
Traditional-to-modern FVCs, 758
Traffic, roads and, 698–699
7-Transdomain chemokine receptor, 418
Transthyretin, function, 184
Trends and context, importance of, 60–61
Tres Cantos Open Lab Foundation, 780
Trisomy 21, 546
  growth deviants, 546
Tuberculin skin test (TST), 402–403
Tuberculosis (TB), 385, 631
  control strategy, 401–402
  convergence model, 387
  diagnosis, 402–403
  epidemiology, 388
    geographic distribution, 388
    global drug resistance, 389
    global tuberculosis, 388
    Mycobacterium tuberculosis, transmission of,
      392–394
    risk factors, 390, 394–395
    risk groups, HIV infection, 388
  factors contributing to global tuberculosis burden, 386
  global incidence of, 389
  global threat, 385–386
  historical perspective, 386–388
    Bacilli Calmette-Guérin vaccine, 387
    cod liver oil therapy, 438
    treatment, 387, 438
  in HIV-positive individuals, 399
  malnutrition and, 348–349
  pathogen, 396–397
  pathogenesis and clinical manifestations, 397
  pediatric TB, 400–401
  prevention, through vaccination, 405–406
  seasonal dependence of, 396
  symptoms and stages of, 399
  therapy, 404–405
  vulnerable populations, 389

  children, 390
  diabetes, 392
  disparities in other settings, 391
  high-risk populations, 391–392
  indigenous peoples, 390
  race and ethnicity, 389–390
  role of migration, 391
  urban and rural disparities, 390
Tuberculosis (TB) infection, 437
  and cachexia, 440–441
  food insecurity and, 439–440
  history, 438
  macronutrients
    interventions and, 441–442
    and risk of, 440
  malnutrition
    and outcomes of, 439
    and risk of, 439
  micronutrients
    interventions in, 442–443
    and risk of, 440
  treatment, 443
  vulnerable populations, 443
    children, nutrition and TB, 443–444
    pregnancy, nutrition and TB, 444

U
Ultraviolet (UV) light, 393
  B radiation, 299
Under-five mortality rate (U5MR), 169
Undernourishment, 92, 108
Undernutrition, 33, 92, 109, 163
  and benefit–cost of interventions, 41–43
  costs of, 34–38
    interventions to reduce, 38–41
  maternal, 488
  school milk programs for prevention of, 348
  small for gestational age and, 508–509
  specific effects of whey in, 349–350
  SUN estimates, 39
Underweight in children, 708
United Nations AIDS (UNAIDS) Fast Track approach,
  666
United Nations Children's Fund, 81
United Nations International Children's Emergency Fund
  (UNICEF), historical perspective, 22
United Nations Multiple Micronutrient Preparation
  (UNIMMAP), 444
United Nations Office for the Coordination of
  Humanitarian Affairs (UN-OCHA), 647
United Nations REACH program, 73
United States Public Health Service, 22
United States Special Supplemental Nutrition Program
  for Women Infants and Children, 375–376
Universal fortification, 568
Upper intake level (UL), 161–162
Urbanization, food security and nutrition, 635, 637, 705
  disparities in child nutrition within urban and rural
    areas, 708–709

food access, 719
  cash and food purchases, importance of, 719
  food price shocks, 720
  formal and informal safety nets, 722–723
  maternal employment and childcare, 721–722
  to safe water and good sanitation, 724–726
  urban employment, 720
food availability, 715
  food retailing and food environment, 715
  foreign direct investment and globalization, 717
  street foods, 717–718
  traditional and modern supply chains, 715–717
  urban agriculture, 718–719
food safety, 726–727
food security, 707
food systems, nutrition transition and urban diets, 712
  changing demand for food, 714
  changing role of women, 713
  physical activity, 714–715
  urban diets, 714
  urban structure, technology and society, 713
global urbanization trends, 705–706
implications for policy, programming and research, 727–729
overweight and obesity in children and women, 710–712
poverty, 706–707
stunting and underweight in children, 708
Urbanization patterns, 685, 688
  cities, nutrition analysis of, 688
    consumption trends in cities, 690–691
    global nutrition status, 688–689
    global urban nutrition status, 689–690
  infrastructure and its relationship with urban nutrition status, 697
    food waste and cold chains, 697–698
    roads and traffic, 698–699
    water and sanitation, 698
  international trade and local production, 699–700
  sustainable development goals, achieving, 686–687
  urban development, 691
    history, 692
    medium-sized cities, 694–695
    megacities, 694
    primate cities, 692–693
    secondary towns, 693–694
  urban size, infrastructure and food systems, 696
Urinary iodine concentrations (UICs), 291
Uterus cancer, 481
  obesity, 481

V

Vaccines, 405–406, 785, 802
  Bacilli Calmette-Guérin vaccine, 387
Value chain, 754–755, 760
  contribution of food value chains to nutrition, 760
  entry and exit points, 762–763

food value chain
  actors across, 755–756
  private sector, role of, 756–757
  types of, 757–758
global context of food systems and evolution of nutrition, 759
  diet shifts and value chains, 759–760
nutrition-focused food value chains, 764
nutrition value chain actors, 762
primary activities, 764
  inbound logistics, 764–765
  marketing and sales, 766
  operations, 765
  outbound logistics, 766
secondary activities, 767
Value Chains Knowledge Clearing House, 763
Value for nutrition, 761–762
Very low birth weight (VLBW) infants, 98
Villermé, Louis René, 7
Virtual communities, 626
Vision, vitamin A role, 184, 185
Vitamin A, 614
  absorption and transport, 183–184
  in breast milk, 363
  costs of interventions, 37
  deficiency. *See* Vitamin A deficiency
  deficiency signs and symptoms, 103
  food sources, 186–188
  functions
    gene regulation, 184–185
    overview, 182
    visual cycle, 184, 185
  history of study, 10, 11, 13, 14, 197–200
  intake recommendations, 186–188
  metabolism, 184
  newborn dosing, 195–196
  pregnancy and, 475
  structure and nomenclature, 182–183
  supplementation, historical perspective, 15–18
Vitamin A deficiency, 35, 181, 541–542
  anemia, 209–210
  breastfeeding studies, 205, 206
  child morbidity and mortality impact, 193–195
  complementary feeding, 206–207
  growth retardation, 209–210
  infant morbidity and mortality impact, 195–196
  infectious disease morbidity, 207, 209
  maternal morbidity and mortality impact, 197
    risk for TB, 440
  prevalence
    geographic distribution, 192
    neonates, 191–192
    overview, 181–182
    preschool children, 190–191
    school-aged children, 192
    women, 192–193
  prevention

dietary diversification, 212–213
  fortification, 215, 216
  overview, 212
  supplementation, 213–214
risk factors
  age, 202–203
  gender, 203
  location, 202
  periodicity in risk, 203–204
  socioeconomic status, 203
xerophthalmia, 208
  conjunctival xerosis with Bitot's spots, 208, 209
  corneal xerosis, ulceration, and necrosis, 208–209
  night blindness, 208
  treatment, 211–212
Vitamin A deficiency disorders (VADD), 188–189, 190
Vitamin B complex
  deficiency signs and symptoms, 103–104
  pregnancy and, 476–477
Vitamin B1, 363, 444
  deficiency signs and symptoms, 103
  EAR for, 161
  function and maternal deficiency, 539
Vitamin B2, 103, 444
  deficiency signs and symptoms, 103
  function and maternal deficiency, 539
Vitamin B3, 278, 444, 456
  deficiency signs and symptoms, 103
Vitamin B6, 103, 110, 279, 363, 444
  deficiency signs and symptoms, 103
  function and maternal deficiency, 539
Vitamin B9, 104, 594
  deficiency signs and symptoms, 104, 105
Vitamin B12, 444, 476, 595
  in breast milk, 363
  deficiency signs and symptoms, 104, 105
  function and maternal deficiency, 539
Vitamin C
  deficiency signs and symptoms, 104, 457
  pregnancy and, 475
Vitamin D, 493
  in breast milk, 363
  deficiency, 592
    breast-feeding, 299, 302, 304
    genetic predisposition, 312–313
    geographic distribution, 302–304
    and puberty, 471
    risk for TB, 440
  deficiency signs and symptoms, 103
  non-skeletal actions of, 311
  pregnancy and, 475–476
  synthesis and metabolism, 299–304
Vitamin D binding protein (DBP), 299
Vitamin E
  deficiency, risk for TB, 440
  pregnancy and, 475
Vitamin K deficiency signs and symptoms, 103

Vitamins, 165. *See also individual vitamins*
  functions, 539
  history of study, 11–14
Vocational training of nutrition workforce, 79
Voluntary counseling and testing (VCT), 422
Von Liebig, Justus, 10
Von Voit, Carl, 10

W
Wald, George, 201
Wallerstein, Immanuel, 693
Wasting, 109, 125, 134
  HIV wasting, 451
Water and sanitation, 698
Weight-for-age z-scores (WAZ), 99
Weight-for-height/length z-scores (WHZ), 99
Weight gain during pregnancy, 99
Weight loss, 364
  etiology, 451–452
  and HIV, 451
Whey protein, 349–350
Whistler, Daniel, 299
Williams, Cicely, 15
W.K. Kellogg Foundation, 772
Workforce requirements in nutrition sector, estimating,
  71
  demand-based approach, 72
  service-target approach, 72
  worker-to-population ratio, 72
World Bank, historical perspective, 22
World Breastfeeding Trends Initiative (WBTi), 72, 367
World Food Programme, 81
World Health Assembly (WHA), 368
World Health Organisation (WHO), 22
WPC80, 352

X
Xerophthalmia, 185, 208
  conjunctival xerosis with Bitot's spots, 208, 209
  corneal xerosis, ulceration, and necrosis, 208–209
  night blindness, 208
  treatment, 211–212
Xpert MTB/RIF assays, 402, 403

Y
Yunus, Muhammad, 638

Z
Z-score, growth data interpretation, 127
Zidovudine (AZT), 415
Zinc
  costs of interventions, 37
  deficiency, 35, 103. *See also* Zinc deficiency
  pregnancy and, 477–478
Zinc deficiency, 265
  assessment of, 268
    dietary intake, 269

plasma and serum concentration, 268–269
stunting, 269–270
causes of, 266
    absorption from small intestine, 268
    inadequate dietary intake, 267
    physiological requirements, conditions increasing,
        267
estimates of requirements, 265–266
importance of, 273
    for child growth, 274
    for immune function and morbidity, 274

for neurobehavioral development, 275
for pregnancy outcome, 274–275
intervention strategies, 275
    biofortification, 280
    dietary diversification and modification, 279–280
    food fortification with, 278–279
    preventive supplementation in children, 275–276
    preventive supplementation in pregnant women,
        276–277
    therapeutic supplementation, 277
prevalence of, 270–273